Harrison's

POCKET MEDICAL DICTIONARY

For Medical and Allied Healthcare Professionals

Harrison's

POCKET MEDICAL DICTIONARY

For Medical and Allied Healthcare Professionals

CBSPD
Dedicated to Education

CBS Publishers & Distributors Pvt Ltd

• New Delhi • Bengaluru • Chennai • Kochi • Kolkata • Lucknow • Mumbai
• Hyderabad • Jharkhand • Nagpur • Patna • Pune • Uttarakhand

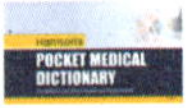

ISBN: 978-93-94525-69-6

First Edition: 2025

Published by **Satish Kumar Jain** and produced by **Varun Jain** for

CBS Publishers and Distributors Pvt Ltd
4819/XI Prahlad Street, 24 Ansari Road, Daryaganj, New Delhi 110 002, India.
Ph: +91-11-23289259, 23266861, 23266867 Website: www.cbspd.com
Fax: 011-23243014
e-mail: delhi@cbspd.com; cbspubs@airtelmail.in.

Corporate Office: 204 FIE, Industrial Area, Patparganj, Delhi 110 092
Ph: +91-11-4934 4934 Fax: 4934 4935
e-mail: feedback@cbspd.com; bhupesharora@cbspd.com

Branches

- **Bengaluru:** Seema House 2975, 17th Cross, K.R. Road, Banasankari 2nd Stage, Bengaluru-560 070, Karnataka
  Ph: +91-80-26771678/79 Fax: +91-80-26771680 e-mail: bangalore@cbspd.com
- **Chennai:** 7, Subbaraya Street, Shenoy Nagar, Chennai-600 030, Tamil Nadu
  Ph: +91-44-26680620, 26681266 Fax: +91-44-42032115 e-mail: chennai@cbspd.com
- **Kochi:** 68/1534, 35, 36-Power House Road, Opp. KSEB, Cochin-682018, Kochi, Kerala
  Ph: +91-484-4059061-65 Fax: +91-484-4059065 e-mail: kochi@cbspd.com
- **Kolkata:** Hind Ceramics Compound, 1st Floor, 147, Nilganj Road, Belghoria, Kolkata-700056, West Bengal
  Ph: +033-2563-3055/56 e-mail: kolkata@cbspd.com
- **Lucknow:** Basement, Khushnuma Complex, 7-Meerabai Marg (Behind Jawahar Bhawan), Lucknow-226001, Uttar Pradesh
  Ph: +0522-4000032 e-mail: tiwari.lucknow@cbspd.com
- **Mumbai:** PWD Shed, Gala No. 25/26, Ramchandra Bhatt Marg, Next to J.J. Hospital Gate No. 2, Opp. Union Bank of India, Noor Baug, Mumbai-400009, Maharashtra
  Ph: +91-22-66661880/89 Fax: +91-22-24902342 e-mail: mumbai@cbspd.com

Representatives

- **Hyderabad** +91-9885175004
- **Nagpur** +91-9421945513
- **Pune** +91-9623451994
- **Jharkhand** +91-9811541605
- **Patna** +91-9334159340
- **Uttarakhand** +91-9716462459

Printed at : Goyal Offset Works Pvt. Ltd. Haryana

Special Contribution

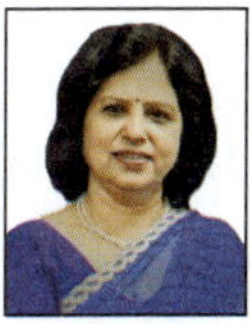

Anju Dhir BSc (Med), MSc (Micro), PhD (Biotech)

Ex-Lecturer (Microbiol)
Shivalik Institute of Nursing
Shimla, Himachal Pradesh
Product Manager and Medical
Developmental Editor
CBS Publishers & Distributors Pvt Ltd.

Preface

Congratulations on choosing Harrison's Pocket Medical Dictionary, a unique, progressive way of teaching and learning of medical terminology. The approach you will find in this book makes use of the latest and most authoritative information regarding learning and retaining medical terminology. This is a book that promotes acquisition of medical terms. The book is written with a focused attention on the most commonly encountered medical terminology and language by a student as well as a professional. The book will certainly advance the career-specific subsets of the medical language. The best way to actively learn medical language is through experiencing it such as in clinical scenarios.

The vocabulary in this book is based on the context of real-world healthcare. The medical terminology is centered around patient care, including the assessment of health, diagnosis, treatment, disease, illness, and injury. The health and allied health professional learners can walk around with this handy Harrison's Pocket Medical Dictionary while they care for patients.

Medical terminology includes technical, specific, standardized, and precise words, terms, and phrases that are used in medical educational and professional world. The use of career-specific language leads to effective and meaningful communication among care providers and their colleagues.

Acknowledgments

We extend our deepest gratitude to all those who contributed to the creation and success of **Harrison's Pocket Medical Dictionary**. The culmination of their dedication, expertise, and collaborative spirit has been instrumental in bringing this comprehensive resource to reality. We acknowledge the collaborative efforts of healthcare experts, educators, and linguistic professionals who have contributed to the development of this comprehensive resource.

We would like to thank **Mr Satish Kumar Jain** (Chairman) and **Mr Varun Jain** (Managing Director), M/s CBS Publishers and Distributors Pvt Ltd for providing us the platform in bringing out the book. We have no words to describe the role, efforts, inputs and initiatives undertaken by **Mr Bhupesh Aarora**, Sr. Vice President – Publishing and Marketing (Health Sciences Division) for helping and motivating us.

We would like to thank Dr Anju Dhir (Sr. Product Manger & Medical Developmental Editor), for making efforts to compile the terms and give an updated look to this book.

We would like to thank Ms Nitasha Arora (Publishing Head and Content Strategist – Medical and Nursing), Ms Daljeet Kaur (Assistant Publishing Manager), Mr Shivendu Bhushan Pandey (Sr. Manager and Team Lead), Mr Ashutosh Pathak (Sr. Proofreader cum Team Coordinator) for their valuable guidance and supervision throughout this endeavor.

Besides, we extend our heartfelt appreciation to the dedicated editorial team of CBS comprising Ms Surbhi Gupta (Editorial Team Lead), Mr Pankaj Singh, Ms Supriya Jha and Ms Ritu Maurya whose unwavering commitment to precision, thorough research, and thoughtful refinement have been integral to the creation of this Medical Dictionary.

Our special thanks are due to Ms Pooja Sharma, Mr Chaman Lal, Mr Prakash Gaur, Mr Phool Kumar, Mr Girish Pandey, Mr Chander Mani, Mr Ravinder Kumar, Ms Babita Verma and Ms Khushi for typesetting and designing the layout; Ms Tanya, Mr Rahul Negi, Mr Manoj Kumar Chaudhary, Mr Vikram Chaudhary and Mr Arun Kumar for drawing catchy figures for this dictionary. We are also thankful to the proofreaders Mr Sachin Kumar Yadav, Mr Shubham Tripathi and Mr Vijay Prajapati who have contributed to this book by proof checking.

Last but not least, we extend gratitude to our valued readers, for choosing **Harrison's Pocket Medical Dictionary** as their companion in the exploration of medical vocabulary. Your trust in our publication is a testament to our shared commitment to advancing knowledge and fostering a deeper understanding of medical, nursing and allied health sciences.

Thank you team, your collective efforts have made it a valuable resource for students, professionals, and enthusiasts alike.

Guide to Abbreviations

Abbreviation	Expansion
adj	Adjective
dent	Dental
ECG	Electrocardiogram
F	French
H	Hindi
L	Latin
mol	Molecular Biology
pl	Plural
psy	Psychiatry
radio	Radiology

Contents

TABLES

Annexures

ANNEXURE 1

AIIMS/ICMR COVID-19 National Task Force/Joint Monitoring Group Clinical Guidance for Management of Adult COVID-19 Patients

Adult patient diagnosed with COVID-19

Mild disease

Upper respiratory tract symptoms and/or fever without shortness of breath or hypoxia

Home Isolation and Care (Refer to relevant guideline)

Must do
- Physical distancing, indoor mask use, strict hand hygiene
- Symptomatic management (hydration, antipyretics, antitussive)
- Stay in contact with treating physician
- Monitor temperature and oxygen saturation (by applying a SpO_2 probe to fingers)

Seek immediate medical attention if:
- Difficulty in breathing or SpO_2 <93%
- High grade fever/severe cough, particularly if lasting for >5 days
- A low threshold to be kept for those with any of the high-risk features*

May do

Therapies based on low certainty of evidence especially for those with high-risk of progression*
- Inhalational Budesonide (given *via* Metered dose inhaler/dry powder inhaler) at a dose of 800 mcg BD for 5 days) to be given if symptoms (fever and/or cough) are persistent beyond 5 days of disease onset

***High-risk for severe disease or mortality**
- Age >60 years
- Cardiovascular disease, hypertension, and CAD
- Diabetes mellitus and other immunocompromised states (such as HIV)
- Active tuberculosis
- Chronic lung/kidney/liver disease
- Cerebrovascular disease
- Obesity

If cough persists for >2–3 weeks, investigate for tuberculosis and other conditions

Moderate disease

Any one of:
1. Respiratory rate ≥24/min, breathlessness
2. SpO_2: 90% to ≤93% on room air

Admit in ward

Oxygen support:
- Target SpO_2: 92–96% (88–92% in patients with COPD)
- Preferred devices for oxygenation: Nonrebreathing face mask
- Awake proning encouraged in all patients requiring supplemental oxygen therapy (sequential position changes every 2 hours)

Anti-inflammatory or immunomodulatory therapy:
- Inj. Methylprednisolone 0.5–1 mg/kg in 2 divided doses (or an equivalent dose of dexamethasone) is usually for a duration of 5–10 days
- Steroids can have risk of secondary infection such as invasive mucormycosis when used too early, at higher dose or for longer than required

Anticoagulation:
- Conventional dose prophylactic unfractionated heparin or low molecular weight heparin (weight based, e.g., enoxaparin 0.5 mg/kg/day SC). There should be no contraindication or high risk of bleeding

Monitoring:
- **Clinical monitoring:** Breathing rate, hemodynamic instability, change in oxygen requirement
- **Serial CXR:** HRCT chest to be done only if there is worsening
- **Lab monitoring:** CRP, D-dimer, blood sugar 48–72 hourly; CBC, KFT, LFT 24–48 hourly

Severe disease

Any one of:
1. Respiratory rate >30/min, breathlessness
2. SpO_2 <90% on room air

Admit in HDU/ICU

Respiratory support:
- Consider use of NIV (Helmet or face mask interface depending on availability) in patients with increasing oxygen requirement, if work of breathing is low
- Consider use of HFNC in patients with increasing oxygen requirement
- Intubation should be prioritized in patients with high work of breathing/if NIV is not tolerated
- Use institutional protocol for ventilatory management when required

Anti-inflammatory or immunomodulatory therapy:
- Inj. Methylprednisolone 1–2 mg/kg IV in 2 divided doses (or an equivalent dose of dexamethasone) usually for a duration 5–10 days
- Steroids can have risk of secondary infection such as invasive mucormycosis when used too early, at higher dose or for longer than required

Supportive measures:
- Maintain euvolemia (if available, use dynamic measures for assessing fluid responsiveness)
- If sepsis/septic shock: Manage as per existing protocol and local antibiogram

Monitoring:
- **Clinical monitoring:** Work of breathing, Hemodynamic instability, Change in oxygen requirement
- **Serial CXR:** HRCT chest to be done only if there is worsening
- **Lab monitoring:** CRP, D-dimer,blood sugar 48–72 hourly; CBC, KFT, LFT 24–48 hourly

After clinical improvement, discharge as per revised discharge criteria

ANNEXURE 2

Fever of Unknown Origin

FUO is defined as:

- Fever >38.3°C (101°F) on at least two occasions.
- Illness duration ≥3 weeks.
- No known immunocompromised state.
- Diagnosis is uncertain after thorough history taking, physical examination and obligatory investigations, including blood culture (n = 3), urine culture, CXR, abdominal ultrasound and tuberculin skin test.

Etiology	**Infectious causes (15–25%)** • Abscess—usually in abdomen or pelvis due to risk factors, like cirrhosis, steroid or immunosuppressive medications, recent surgery, diabetes • Osteomyelitis • Bacterial endocarditis—culture negative in 2–5%, especially in *Coxiella burnetii, Tropheryma whipplei, Brucella, Mycoplasma, Chlamydia, Histoplasma, Legionella, Bartonella,* HACEK organisms which required either special media or longer than usual incubation • Prostatitis, dental abscesses, sinusitis, and cholangitis are sources of occult fever • TB, HIV/AIDS, CMV, EBV, malaria, typhoid fever, dengue fever, hepatitis A, Lyme disease, syphilis, psittacosis (bird exposure) and rat-bite fever **Neoplastic causes (<20%)** • Lymphomas (especially non-Hodgkin's lymphoma, most common cause) • Solid tumors: RCC most common, also breast, liver, colon, pancreas or liver metastases • Malignant histiocytosis **Collagen vascular diseases (15–25% of cases)** • SLE • RA • Rheumatic fever • Vasculitis, especially temporal (giant cell) arteritis • Juvenile rheumatoid arthritis (JRA), Still's disease **Miscellaneous causes (15–20% of cases)** • Drug fever: Commonly antibiotics, antihistamines, antiarrhythmics, methyldopa, phenytoin, dilatin and NSAIDs • Sarcoidosis • Inherited Familial Mediterranean fever • Factitious • Pulmonary embolism

Contd...

Investigations	**Initial investigations** • **Bloodwork:** CBC with differential and smear, electrolytes, BUN, Creatinine, calcium profile, LFTs, ESR, CRP, muscle enzymes, RF, ANA, serum protein electrophoresis, Fe, transferrin, TIBC, B_{12} • **Cultures:** Blood (× 2 sets), urine, sputum, stool C&S, other fluids as appropriate VDRL, heterophile Ab (mononucleosis), CMV antigenemia tests, HIV serology, PPD and CXR. *If no diagnostic clues from the above, proceed with further investigations including:* • CT chest, abdomen and pelvis with contrast • Colonoscopy *If no diagnostic clue from the above, proceed with further investigations including:* • 67-Gallium scan • 111 Indium PMN scan • FDG PET scan
Management	• Treatment is directed at the specific cause found from the above investigations. • If no diagnosis with the above, consider empiric therapy versus watchful waiting. • Prognosis for most patients with FUO persisting without a diagnosis is very good without intervention. • **Empirical therapies may include:** Anti-TB therapy, broad spectrum antibiotics, colchicine, NSAIDS, steroids.

Conceptual Diagnostic Algorithm for FUO

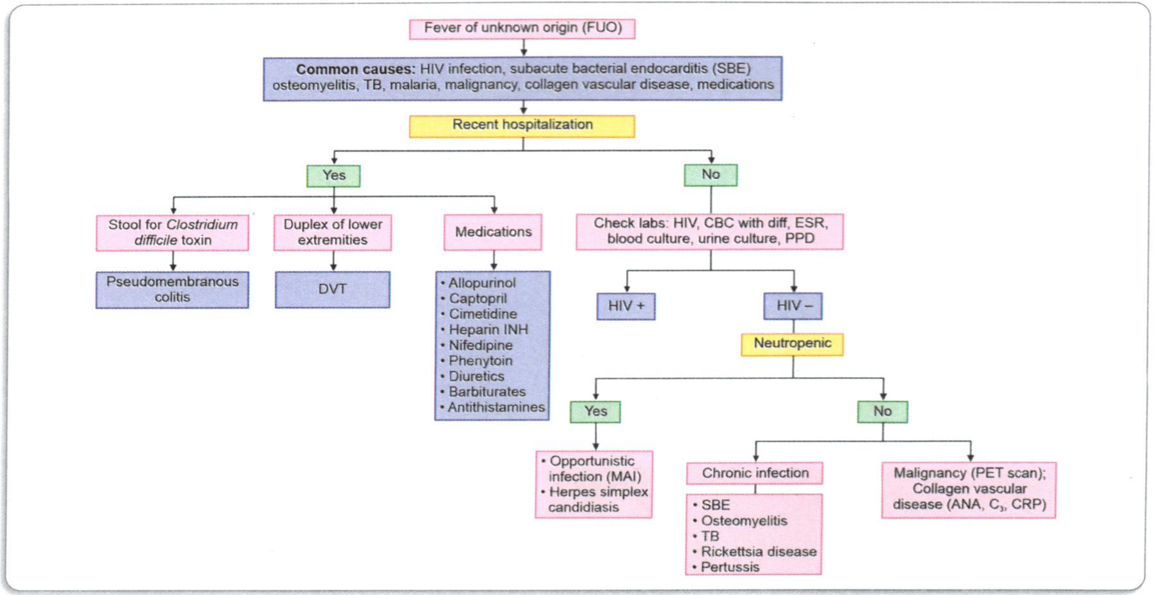

ANNEXURE 3

Adult Basic Life Support Algorithm for Healthcare Provider

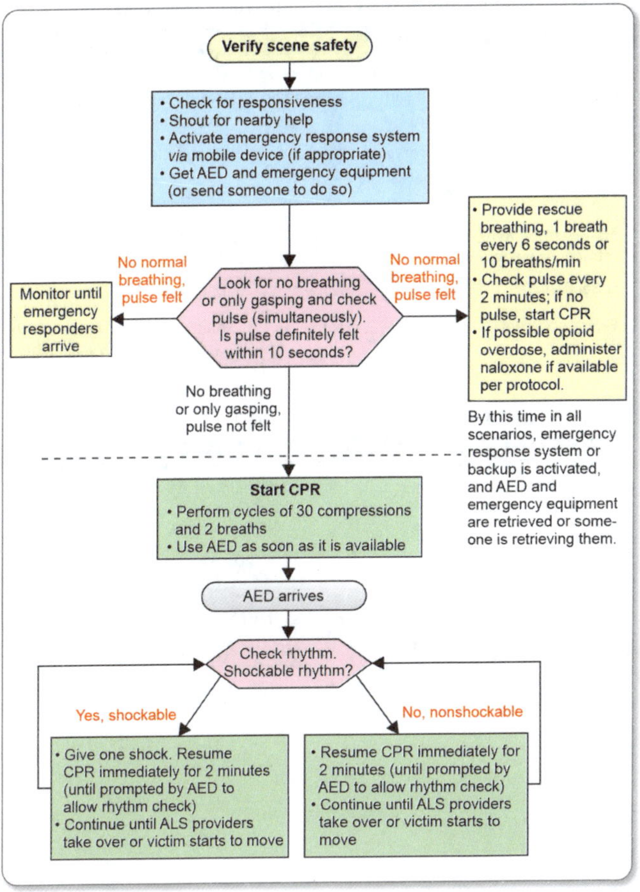

ANNEXURE 4

Mechanical Ventilation

Silverman-Anderson scoring of respiratory distress in preterm babies

Parameter	Score 0	Score 1	Score 2
Upper chest retraction (observe if upper chest is synchronized with abdomen during inspiration)	Synchronized movement	Upper chest lags during inspiration	See-saw movement of upper chest
Lower chest retraction (observe for retractions in the rib spaces below mid-axillary line)	None	Just visible	Marked
Xiphoid retraction (observe for retractions below xiphoid)	None	Just visible	Marked
Nasal flaring	None	Minimal	Marked
Expiratory grunt	None	Audible with stethoscope	Audible with unaided ear

Downes' scoring of respiratory distress in newborn (both term and preterm babies)

Parameters	Score 0	Score 1	Score 2
Respiratory rate	<60/min	60–80/min	>80/min
Cyanosis	Nil	In room air	In >40% FiO_2
Air entry	Normal	Mild decrease	Marked decrease
Grunt	None	Audible with stethoscope	Audible with unaided ear
Retraction	Nil	Mild	Moderate

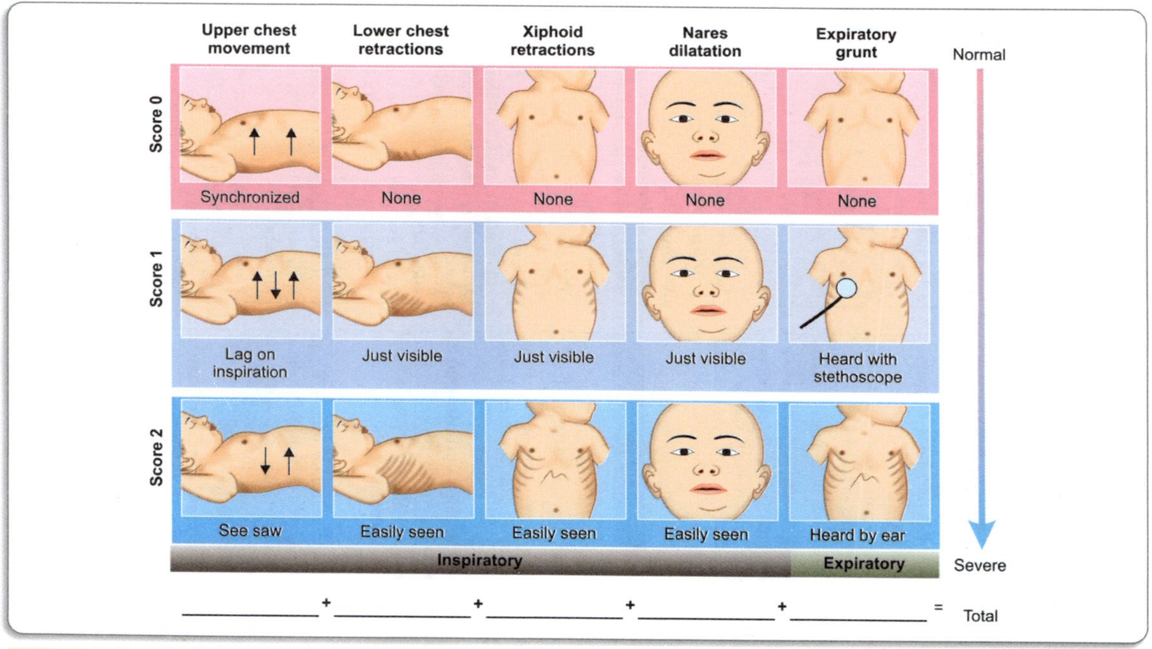

Silverman-Anderson scoring

ANNEXURE 5

List of Prohibited Drugs

Manufacture and Sale through Gazette Notifications Under Section 26A of Drugs & Cosmetics Act, 1940 by The Ministry of Health and Family Welfare, Government of India

Banned Drugs

Analgin: All formulations containing Analgin for human use.

Fixed dose combination of **Flupenthixol + Malitrecen** for human use

Pioglitazone and all formulations containing **Pioglitazone** for human use

Dextropropoxyphene and formulations containing Dextropropoxyphene for human use

Amidopyrine

Fixed dose combinations of vitamins with anti-inflammatory agents and tranquilizers

Fixed dose combinations of Iron with **Strychnine**, **Arsenic** and **Yohimbine**

Fixed dose combinations of **Yohimbine** and **Strychnine** with **Testosterone** and vitamins

Fixed dose combinations of **Atropine** in **Analgesics** and **Antipyretics**

Fixed dose combinations of **Strychnine** and **Caffeine** in tonics

Nialamide

Fixed dose combinations of crude **Ergot** preparations except those containing **Ergotamine**, **Caffeine**, analgesics, antihistamines for the treatment of migraine, headaches

Fixed dose combinations of vitamins with anti TB drugs except combination of **Isoniazid** with **Pyridoxine Hydrochloride** (vitamin B_6)

Fixed dose combinations of **Penicillin** with **Sulfonamides**

Contd...

Fixed dose combinations of **Chloramphenicol** with any other drug for internal use

Fixed dose combinations of **Corticosteroids** with any other drug for internal use

Fixed dose combination of **Histamine** H_2 receptor antagonists with antacids except for those combinations approved by Drugs Controller, India

All Pharmaceutical preparations containing **Chloroform** exceeding 0.5% w/w or v/v whichever is appropriate

Fixed dose combination containing more than one antihistamine

Fixed dose combination of **Salbutamol** or any other drug having primarily bronchodilatory activity with centrally acting antitussive and/or antihistamine

Fixed dose combination of **Metoclopramide** with systemically absorbed drugs except fixed dose combination of metoclopramide with **aspirin/paracetamol**

Preparations claiming to combat cough associated with asthma containing centrally acting antitussive and/or an antihistamine

Fixed dose combination containing **Pectin** and/or **Kaolin** with any drug which is systemically absorbed from GI tract except for combinations of Pectin and/or Kaolin with drugs not systemically absorbed

Dover's Powder IP and Dover's Powder Tablets IP

Contd...

Antidiarrheal formulations containing **Phthalylsulfathiazole** or **Sulfaguanidine** or **Succinyl Sulfathiazole**

Liquid oral antidiarrheals or any other dosage form for pediatric use containing **Diphenoxylate Loperamide** or **Atropine** or **Belladona** including their salts or esters or metabolites **Hyoscyamine** or their extracts or their alkaloids

Fixed dose combination of antidiarrheals with electrolytes

Patent and proprietary oral rehydration salts other than those confirming to the following parameters:
Patent and proprietary oral rehydration salts on reconstitution to one liter shall contain:
Sodium: 50–90 millimoles.
Total osmolarity: 240–290 millimoles.
Dextrose: Sodium molar ratio—Not less than 1:1 and not more than 3:1

Patent and proprietary oral rehydration salts shall not contain mono or polysaccharides or saccharine sweetening agent

Fixed dose combination of **Diazepam** and **Diphenhydramine Hydrochloride**

Phenylpropanolamine and its formulation for human use

Nimesulide formulations for human use in children below 12 years of age

Fixed dose combination of a drug, standards of which are prescribed in the Second Schedule to the said Act with an Ayurvedic, Siddha or Unani drug.

Fixed dose combination of **Analgin** with any other drug

Fixed dose combination of **Oxyphenbutazone** or **Phenylbutazone** with any other drug

Tegaserod and its formulations for human use

Fixed dose combinations of **Sodium Bromide/Chloral Hydrate** with other drugs

Contd...

Fixed dose combination of **Sedatives/hypnotics/anxiolytics** with analgesics-antipyretics

Fixed dose combination of **Estrogen** and **Progestin** (other than oral contraceptive) containing per tablet estrogen content of >50 mcg (equivalent to **Ethinyl Estradiol**) and **progestin** content of >3 mg (equivalent to **Norethisterone Acetate**) and all fixed dose combination injectable preparations containing synthetic **Estrogen** and **Progesterone**. (Subs. By Noti. No. 743 (E) dt 10-08-1989).

Combination of anabolic **Steroids** with other drugs

Phenacetin

Demeclocycline liquid oral preparations

Oxytetracycline liquid oral preparations

Methapyrilene, its salts

Penicillin skin/eye ointment

Tetracycline liquid oral preparations

Methaqualone

Practolol

Fixed dose combinations of antihistaminic with antidiarrheals

Fixed dose combinations of vitamins with analgesics

Fixed dose combinations of any other **Tetracycline** with vitamin C.

Fixed dose combinations of **Hydroxyquinoline** group of drugs with any other drug except for preparations meant for external use

The patent and proprietary medicines of fixed dose combinations of essential oils with alcohol having percentage higher than 20% proof except preparations given in the Indian Pharmacopoeia

Fixed dose combination of **Ethambutol** with INH other than the following: INH Ethambutol 200 mg, 600 mg, 300 mg, 800 mg

Contd...

Fixed dose combination of any anthelmintic with cathartic/purgative except for **piperazine/santonin**

Fixed dose combination of laxatives and/or antispasmodic drugs in enzyme preparations

Fixed dose combination of centrally acting, antitussive with antihistamine, having high atropine like activity in expectorants

Liquid oral tonic preparations containing **glycerophosphates** and/or other phosphates and/or central nervous system stimulant and such preparations containing alcohol >20% proof

Chloralhydrate as a drug

Antidiarrheal formulations containing **Kaolin** or **Pectin** or **Attapulgite** or **Activated Charcoal**

Antidiarrheal formulations containing **Neomycin** or **Streptomycin** or **Dihydrostreptomycin** including their respective salts or esters

Liquid oral antidiarrheals or any other dosage form for pediatric use containing halogenated **hydroxyquinolines**

Patent and proprietary cereal-based oral rehydration salts on reconstitution to one liter shall contain:
Sodium: 50–90 millimoles.
Total osmolarity: Not >290 milliosmoles.

Precooked rice—equivalent to not <50 g and not >80 g as total replacement of **Dextrose**.
Patent and proprietary oral with rehydration salts (ORS) specifications and labeled with the indication for "Adult Choleretic Diarrhea only"

Fenfluramine and **Dexfenfluramine**
Rimonabant Rosiglitazone

Sibutramine and its formulations for human use, and **R-Sibutramine** and its formulations for human use

Contd...

(*)Human Placental Extract and its formulations for human use.

Cisapride and its formulations for human use

Mepacrine Hydrochloride (Quinacrine and its salts) in any dosage form for use for female sterilization or contraception

Fixed dose combination of **dextropropoxyphene** with any other drug other than antispasmodic and/or nonsteriodal antiinflammatory drugs (NSAIDs)

Gatifloxacin formulations for systemic use in humans by any route including oral and injectable

List of Drugs Prohibited for Import

Nialamide

Practolol

Methapyrilene and its salts

Mepacrine Hydrochloride (**Quinacrine** and its Salts) in any dosage form for use for female sterilization or contraception

Rimonabant

Chloral Hydrate as a drug

Phenacetin

Methaqualone

Fenfluramine and **Dexfenfluramine**

Other Pharmaceutical Items Prohibited from Manufacturing, Sale and Distribution

Cosmetics Licensed as toothpaste/tooth powder containing tobacco

Fixed dose combination of vitamin B_1, vitamin B_6 and vitamin B_{12} for human use

Contd...

**Prohibition revoked vide Gazette Notification GSR No. 418(E) dated May 30, 2011.*

Fixed dose combination of **Pancreatin** or **Pancrelipase** containing amylase, protease and lipase with any other enzyme
Fixed dose combination of **Phenobarbitone** with any antiasthmatic drugs
Fixed dose combination of **Phenobarbitone** with **Ergotamine** and/or **Belladona**
Fixed dose combination of **Nalidixic acid** with any antiamoebic including **Metronidazole**
Fixed dose combination of **Cyproheptadine** with **Lysine** or **Peptone**
Valdecoxib and and its formulation
Letrozole for induction of ovulation in anovulatory infertility
Parenteral preparations fixed dose combination of **streptomycin** with **Penicillin**

Contd...

Fixed dose combination of hemoglobin in any form (natural or synthetic)
Fixed dose combination of **Nitrofurantoin** and **trimethoprim**
Fixed dose combination of **Phenobarbitone** with **Hyoscine** and/or **Hyoscyamine**
Fixed dose combination of **Haloperidol** with any anticholinergic agent including **Propantheline Bromide**
Fixed dose combination of **Loperamide Hydrochloride** with **Furazolidone**
Astemizole **Terfinadine** **Fenformin** **Rofecoxib**
Diclofenac and its formulations for animal use

Source: *https://drugs.delhi.gov.in/drugs/banned-drugs*

ANNEXURE 6

Medical Abbreviations

Abbreviation	Meaning
a.c.	before meals
add.	add let there be added
ad lib.	Latin, "at one's pleasure"; as much as one desires; freely
agit.	agitate (stir or shake)
alt. d., alt. dieb.	every other day; on alternate days
alt. h., alt. hor.	every other hour; at alternate hours
a.m.	morning, before noon
BDS, b.d.s.	twice daily
b.i.d., b.d.	twice daily
bis ind.	twice a day
bucc.	buccal (inside cheek)
cap., caps.	capsule
c.m.	tomorrow morning
c.n.	tomorrow night
DAW	dispense as written (i.e., no generic substitution)
dil.	dilute
emuls.	emulsion
garg.	gargle
gtt(s)	drop(s)
h, hr, hor.	hour
hor. alt.	every other hour (every second hour; at alternate hours)
hor. decub.	at bedtime
ID	intradermal
IJ, inj.	injection
IM	intramuscular

Contd...

Abbreviation	Meaning
IN	intranasal
inf.	infusion (extraction)/ intravenous infusion
IP	intraperitoneal
IT	intrathecal
IV	intravenous
lat. dol.	to the painful side
lin	liniment
liq.	solution
lot.	lotion
mane	in the morning
mcg	microgram
mist.	mixture
mod. prescript.	in the manner directed
nebul	a spray (such as for insufflation)
noct.	at night
non rep.	no repeats (no refills)
NS	normal saline (0.9%)
1/2NS	half-normal saline (0.45%)
o.m.	every morning
o.n.	every night
p.	continue
per	by or through
p.c.	after meals
p.o.	by mouth or orally
p.r., PR	rectally
p.r.n., PRN	as needed
p.v., PV	vaginally
q.1 h, q.1°	every 1 hour (can replace '1' with other numbers)

Contd...

Abbreviation	Meaning
q.a.d.	every other day
q.a.m.	every morning (every day before noon)
q.d./q.1.d.	every day
q.d.a.m.	once daily in the morning
q.d.p.m.	once daily in the evening
q.d.s.	4 times a day
q.p.m.	every evening (every day after noon)
q.h.	every hour
q.h.s.	every night at bedtime
q.i.d.	4 times a day
rep., rept.	repeats
SC	subcutaneous

Contd...

Abbreviation	Meaning
SL, s.l.	sublingually, under the tongue
s.o.s., si op. sit	if there is a need
stat	immediately
supp.	suppository
susp.	suspension
syr.	syrup
tab.	tablet
t.d.s., TDS	3 times a day
t.i.d., t.d.	3 times a day
t.i.w.	3 times a week
top.	topical
TPN	total parenteral nutrition
vag.	vaginally
w/o	without

ANNEXURE 7

Normal Values

Vital Signs and Body Mass Index

Blood Pressure: Systolic/Diastolic (mm Hg)	
At physician's office (average 5 measurements)	$<140/90$
Ambulatory BP monitor	$<135/85$
With diabetes	$<130/80$
Heart Rate (HR) or Pulse (Beats/min)	
Bradycardia	<60
Normal	60–80
Tachycardia	>100
Respiration Rate (RR) (Breaths/min)	
Bradypnea	<12
Normal (eupnea)	12–18
Tachypnea	>18
Body Temperature (°C)	
Fever	>37.5
Normal	36.5–37.5 (approximate)
Hypothermia	<35.0
Body Mass Index (BMI) (kg/m^2)	
Underweight	<18.5
Normal	18.5–24.9
Overweight	25.0–29.9
Obesity class I	30.0–34.9
Obesity class II	35.0–39.9
Obesity class III (extreme, morbid)	≥ 40.0

Common Blood Tests with Normal Range	
Tests	**Range**
Albumin	3.5–5.0 g/dL
Alkaline phosphatase (ALP serum)	35–100 U/L
Ammonia – NH_3	20–70 µg/dL
Amylase (serum)	<160 U/L
Aspartate aminotransferase (AST)	0–35 U/L
Bicarbonate (HCO_3) (Serum)	24–30 mEq/L
Bilirubin serum total	1.5 mg/dL
Bilirubin, conjugated (Direct)	<0.4 mg/dL

Contd...

Common Blood Tests with Normal Range	
Tests	**Range**
Blood Urea Nitrogen (BUN)	7–22 mg/dL
Calcium serum total	8.7–10.3 mg/dL
Ionized	4.2–5.2 mg/dL
Carbon dioxide pressure, arterial ($PaCO_2$)	35–45 mm Hg
Chloride serum	98–106 mEq/L
Cholesterol, total desirable	<200 mg/dL
Borderline high	201–240
High	>241
Cholesterol, LDL	
High risk patients (Framingham risk score)	<77.3 mg/dL or >50% reduction
Intermediate risk patient if LDL ≥3.5	<77.3 mg/dL or 50% reduction
Low risk patient if LDL	≥5.0 >50% reduction from baseline
Cholesterol, HDL	
Low	<40 mg/dL
Creatine Kinase serum (CK also CPK)	5–130 U/L
Copper	70–155 μg/dL
Creatinine, serum	
Male	0.8–1.4 mg/dL
Female	0.56–1.0 mg/dL
Creatinine clearance (Adult)	75–125 mL/min
Ferritin	10–250 ng/mL
Folic Acid (Folate)	3–16 ng/mL
Gamma Glutamyl Transferase (GGT)	
Female	5–36 U/L
Male	8–61 U/L
Glucose, fasting	59–105 mg/dL
Normal	<120 mg/dL
Glucose, postprandial	
Normal	<120 mg/dL
Glycosylated Hemoglobin – HbA1c	
Normal	4–6%
Iron	60–178 μg/dL
Iron-Binding Capacity, Total – TIBC	251–460 μg/dL
Lactic Acid (Lactate plasma venous)	9–16 mg/dL
Lactate Dehydrogenase serum (LDH)	95–195 IU/L
Magnesium serum	1.82–2.31 mg/dL
Osmolality serum	280–300 mOsm/kg
Oxygen partial pressure, arterial – PaO_2	85–105 mm Hg

Contd...

Common Blood Tests with Normal Range	
pH - arterial	7.35–7.45 pH
Phosphorus, inorganic	2.5–4.5 mg/dL
Potassium	3.5–5.0 mEq/L
Protein, total	
Plasma	6.0–8.0 g/dL
Urine	<150 mg/24 hrs
Triglyceride	<195 mg/dL
Uric Acid	3.0–7.0 mg/dL
Blood Urea Nitrogen (BUN)	7–22.4 mg/dL
Hematocrit	
Female	37–46%
Male	42–52%
Hemoglobin	
Female	12.3–15.7 g/dL
Male	14.0–17.4 g/dL
Erythrocyte Sedimentation Rate	
(ESR Westergren)	5–36 U/L
Female	<10 mm/hr
Male	<6 mm/hr
Bleeding Time (IVY)	<9 minutes
Clotting Time	5–15 minutes
Fibrinogen	175–400 mg/dL
Prothrombin Time (PT)	10–13 seconds
Partial Thromboplastin Time (PTT)	28–38 seconds
Thrombin Time	14–16 seconds

Note: *Values and units of measurement listed in these tables are derived from several resources. Substantial variation exists in the ranges quoted as 'normal' and may vary depending on the assay used by different laboratories. Therefore, these tables should be considered directional only. Some values vary by gender, age, time of day and condition.*

ANNEXURE 8

Incubation Period of Various Communicable Diseases

Sl. no.	Communicable diseases	Causes	Incubation period
	Respiratory infections		
1.	Measles	Rubeola	10 days from exposure to onset of fever, and 14 days to appearance of rash (average is 7 days)
2.	Smallpox	Variola	Range 7–19 days
3.	Viral Rhinitis (Common cold)	Different viruses	12 hours–5 days (average 48 hours)
4.	Severe Acute Respiratory Syndrome (SARS)	SARS-associated corona virus	3–10 days, usually 4–6 days
5.	Chicken pox	Varicella-zoster virus	14–16 days
6.	Shingles (varicella zoster virus, second outbreak of chicken pox	Varicella-zoster virus	2–3 weeks and is usually 14–16 days
7.	Rubella (German measles)	RNA virus of the Togaviridae virus family	2–3 weeks
8.	Mumps	Myxovirus parotiditis	2–3 weeks
9.	Influenza	Influenza virus (A, B, C, D)	18–72 hours
10.	Pandemic Influenza A (H1N1 - Swine flu)	Influenza virus (A)	2–3 days
11.	Diphtheria	*Cornybacterium diphtheriae*	2–6 days
12.	Pneumonia	*Streptococcus pneumoniae*	12 hours or as long as 3 days after exposure to the flu virus
13.	Pertusis (whooping cough)	*B. pertussis*	7–14 days
14.	Meningococcal meningitis	*N. meningitidis*	3–4 days

Contd...

Sl. no.	Communicable diseases	Causes	Incubation period
15.	Respiratory tract infection	Rhinoviruses and group A streptococci	1–5 days
16.	Influenza and parain-fluenza	Influenza virus and parainfluenza virus	1–4 days
17.	Respiratory syncytial disease	Respiratory syncytial virus (RSV)	1 week
18.	EBV disease	Epstein-Barr virus (EBV)	4–6 weeks
19.	Tuberculosis	*Mycobacterium tuberculosis*	3–6 weeks
	Intestinal infections		
20.	Acute diarrhea, often with fever and cramps	Salmonella	Usually 6–48 hours
21.	Cholera	*Vibrio cholerae*	Few hours to 5 days
22.	Hepatitis	Hepatitis A virus	14–50 days, average 4 weeks
23.	Hepatitis	Hepatitis B virus	50–180 days, usually 2–3 months
24.	Hepatitis	Hepatitis C virus	2 weeks–6 months
25.	Hepatitis	Hepatitis E virus	3–8 weeks
26.	Hepatitis	Hepatitis D virus	Usually between 2–8 weeks In case of co-infection with hepatitis B: about 45–160 days
27.	Hepatitis	Hepatitis G virus	
28.	Poliomyelitis	Poliovirus	7–14 days
29.	Typhoid fever (Entric fever)	*Salmonella typhi*	10–14 days
	Food poisoning		
30.	Salmonella food poisoning	*Salmonella typhimurium*	12–24 hours
31.	Staphylococcal food poisoning	*Staphylococcus aureus*	1–8 hours
32.	Botulism	*Clostridium botulinum*	18–36 hours
33.	*Clostridium perfrin-gens* food poisoning	*Clostridium perfringens*	6–24 hours

Contd...

Sl. no.	Communicable diseases	Causes	Incubation period
34.	Cereus food poisoning	*Bacillus cereus*	1–6 hours
35.	Amoebiasis	*Entamoeba histolytica*	2–4 weeks
36.	Ascariasis	*Ascaris lumbricoides*	18 days to several weeks
37.	Hook worm infection	*Ancylostoma duodenale*	5 weeks–9 months
38.	Whip worm infection	*Trichuris trichiura*	60–90 days
	Arthropod-borne infection		
39.	Dengue	*Aedes aegypti*	8–10 days
40.	Malaria	*Plasmodium vivax, P falciparum, P malariae, P ovale, Plasmodium knowlesi*	12 days for falciparum 14 days for vivax 17 days for ovale
41.	Lymphatic filariasis	Culex, anopheles, and aedes mosquito	8–16 months
42.	Zika virus disease	Zika virus	Few days–1 week
	Zoonoses		
43.	Rabies	Rabies virus	1–3 months
44.	Monkey pox	Monkey pox virus	Usually 7–14 days but can range from 5 to 21 days
45.	Nipah virus	Paramyxoviridae	4–14 days
46.	Japanese encephalitis	Group B arbo virus	5–15 days
47.	Yellow fever	Flavi virus fibricus	3–6 days
48.	KFD	Group B flavi viruses	Between 3 and 8 days
49.	Chikungunya	Group A virus-aedes mosquitoes	4–7 days
50.	Brucellosis	4 species infect man-*B melitensis, B abortus, B suis, B canis*	1–3 weeks
51.	Leptosiprosis	Spirocheates	10 days
52.	Plague	Y. pestis	Bubonic plague: 2–7 days Septicaemic plague: 2–7 days Pneumonic plague: 1–3 days
53.	Human salmonellosis	Salmonella	6–72 hours
54.	Rickettsial zoonoses	Rickettsiae	5–10 days

Contd...

Sl. no.	Communicable diseases	Causes	Incubation period
55.	Scrub typhus	*Rickettsia tsutsugamushi*	10–12 days
56.	Murine typhus	*Rickettsia typhi*	1–2 weeks
57.	Indian tick typhus	*Rickettsia conorii*	3–7 days
58.	Q fever	*Coxiella burnetii*	2–3 weeks
59.	Taeniasis	*T. saginata, T. solium, Taenia asiatica*	8–14 weeks
60.	Hydatid disease	*Echinococcus granulosus* *Echinococcus multilocularis*	Months to years
61.	Leishmaniasis	Leishmania	1–4 months
		Surface infections	
62.	Trachoma	*Chlamydia trachomatis*	5–12 days
63.	Scabies	*Sarcoptes scabiei* (itch mite)	6 weeks before onset of itching. Re-exposure— symptoms develop in 1–4 days
64.	Methicillin resistant *Staphylococcus aureus* infection	Methicillin resistant *Staphylococcus aureus* (MRSA)	1–10 days
65.	Tetanus	*Clostridium tetani*	6–10 days
66.	Leprosy (Hansen's disease)	*Mycobacterium leprae*	3–5 years
67.	Conjunctivitis (pink eyes)	*Mycobacterium leprae*	24–72 hours
		Sexually-transmitted diseases	
68.	Syphilis	*Treponema pallidum*	10–90 days, usually 3 weeks
69.	AIDS	Human immunodeficiency virus	<1–15 + years

Color Plates

Skeletal System

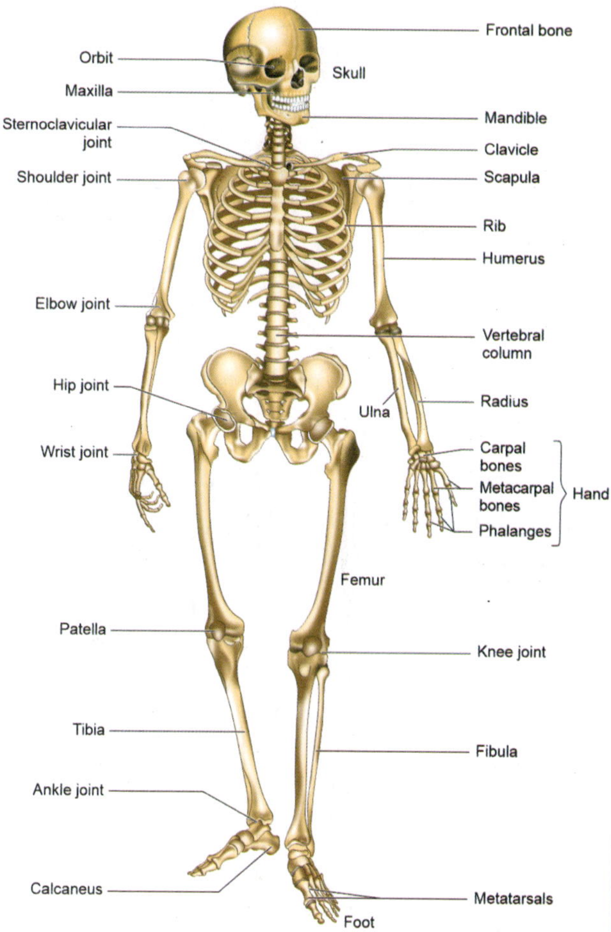

Arterial System

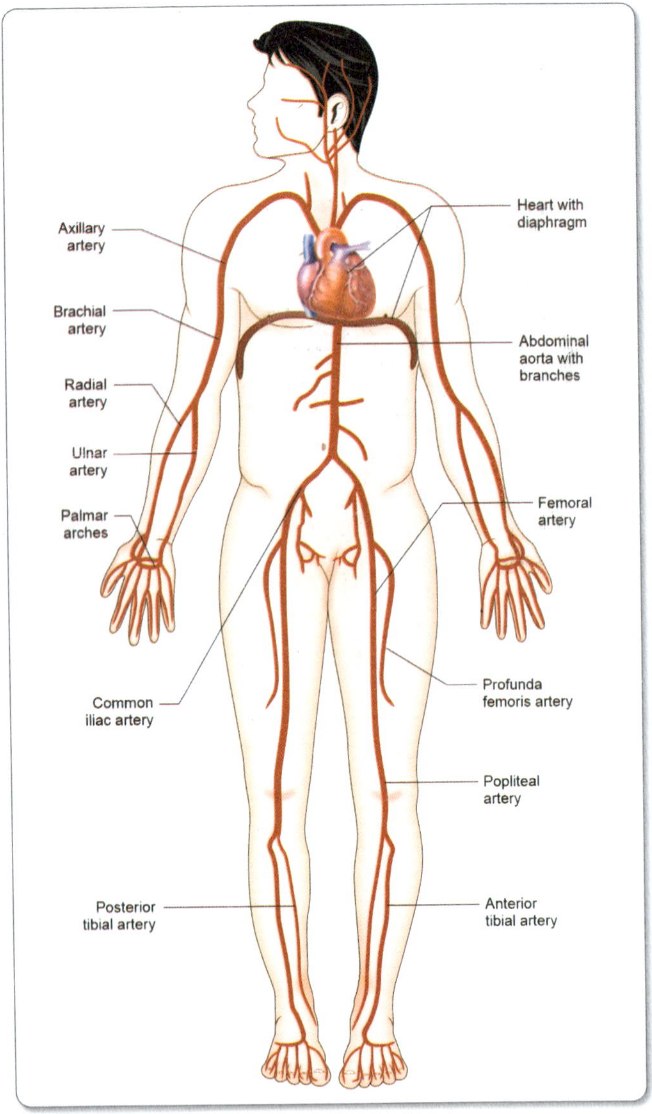

Venous System

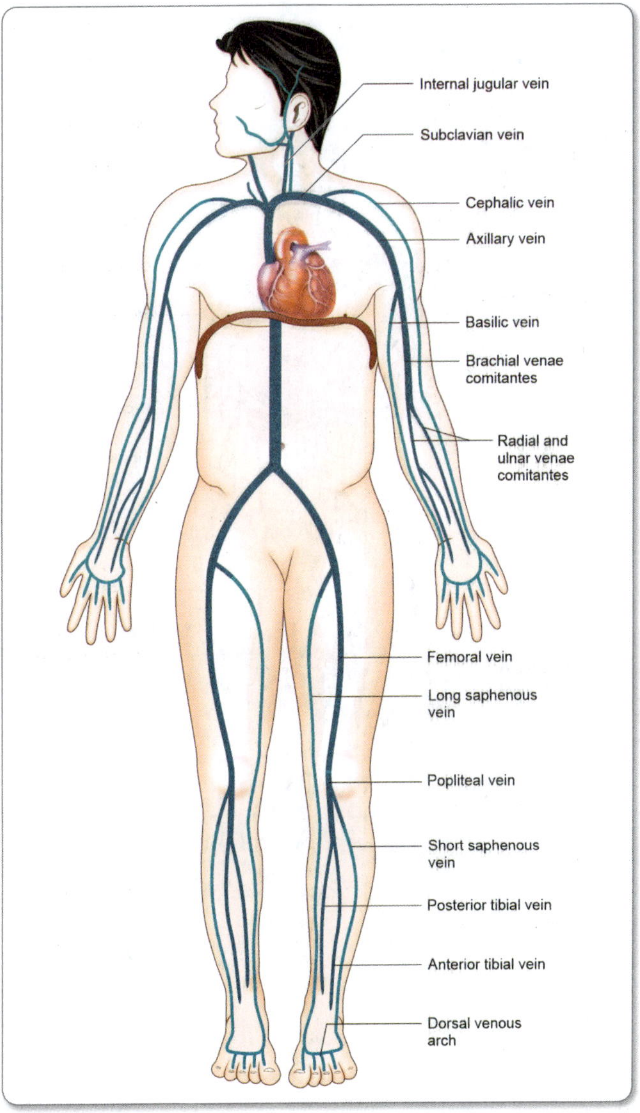

Muscular System

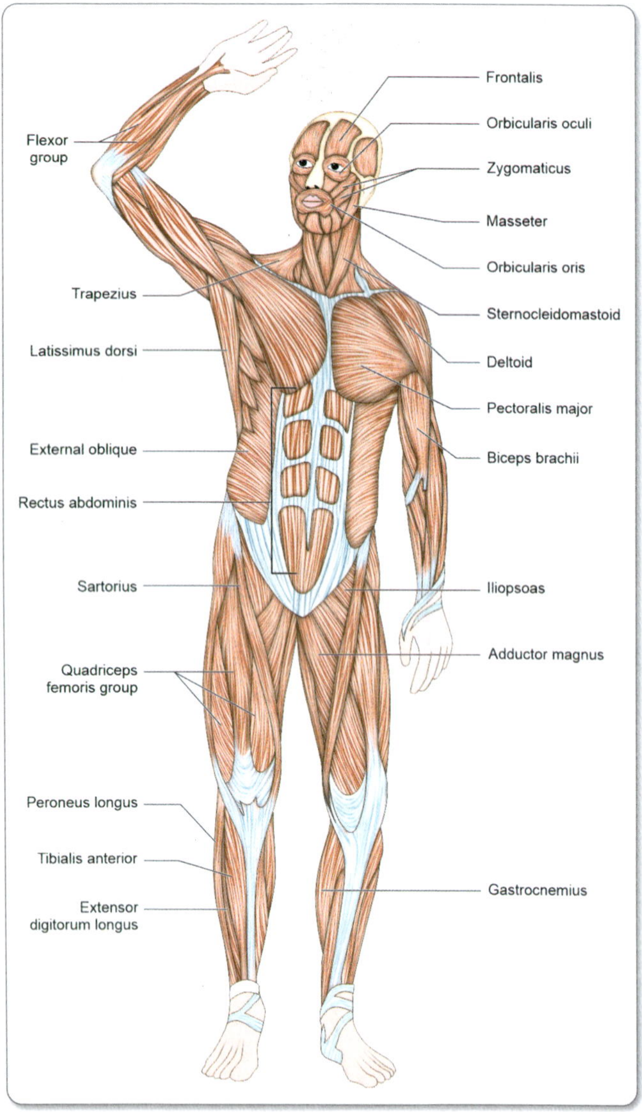

Respiratory System

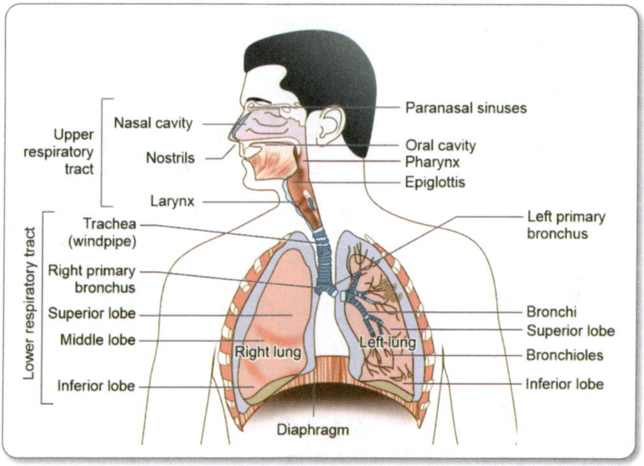

Renal System

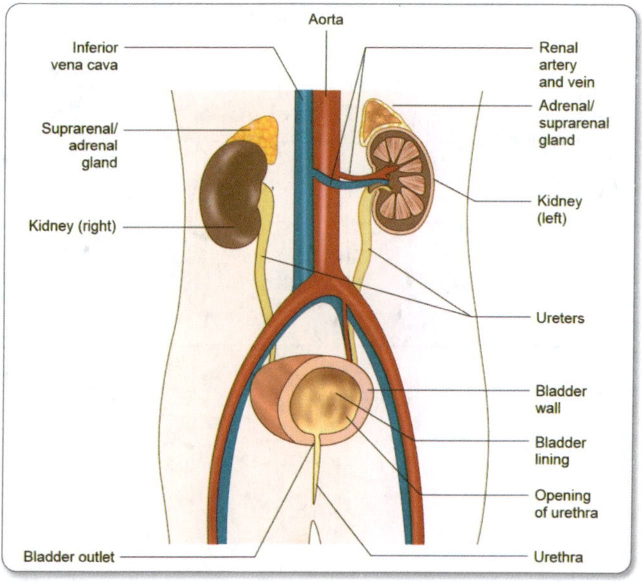

Endocrine System

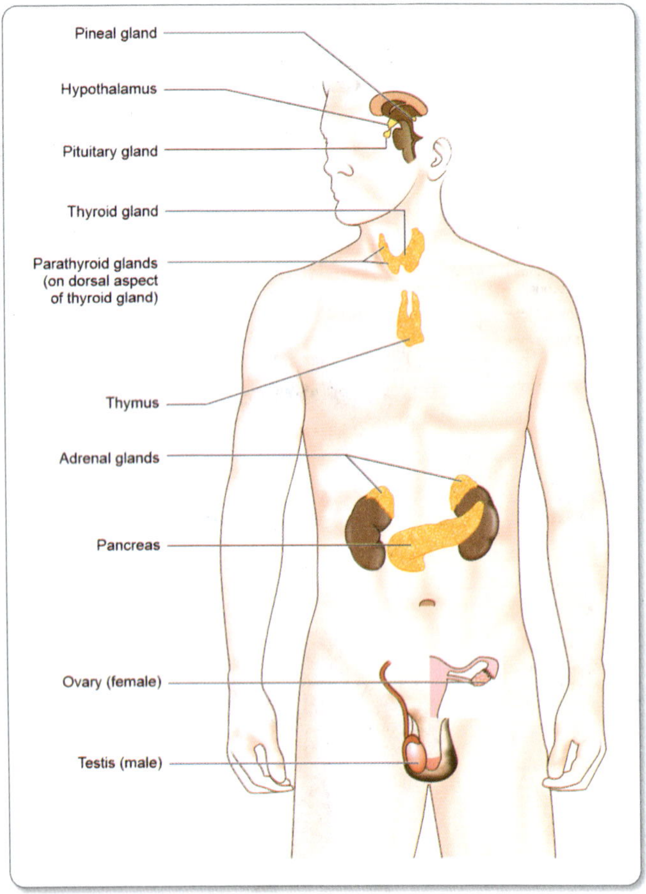

A

A Anterior, area, aqua, ampere, accommodation, arterial blood gas.

A Symbol for Angstrom unit, alveolar gas, adenosine.

Ab Antibody, Abdomen.

Abarticulation (*ab-ahr-tik"u-la-shen*) The act of dislocating a joint.

Abasia (*a-ba'se-a*) Inability to walk due to impaired coordination.

Abdomen (*ab-do'men*) Belly; the portion of the trunk between the pelvis and thorax.

Abdomen angina Intermittent severe ischemia resulting in colicky abdominal pain within half an hour after taking food and lasting for an hour or two.

Abdomen apoplexy Acute hemoperitoneum.

Acute abdomen Sudden onset of severe pain in the abdomen requiring surgical intervention.

Pendulous abdomen Markedly relaxed anterior wall of the abdomen hanging over the lower part.

Scaphoid abdomen Hollowed anterior wall of abdomen, making abdomen boat shaped.

Surgical abdomen Acute abdomen.

Abdominocentesis (*ab-dom'i-no-sen-te'sis*) Abdominal paracentesis, puncture of the abdomen with a trocar to remove fluid from the abdominal cavity through the cannula.

Abdominohysterectomy (*ab-dom"i-no-his'ter-ek'to-me*) Removal of the uterus through abdominal incision; removal of the uterus *via* an incision made in the abdominal wall rather than *via* the vagina.

Abdominoperineal Pertaining to the abdomen and perineal region.

Abdominoplasty (*ab'domino-pla'sti*) A type of cosmetic surgery in which excess fat and skin are removed from the abdominal area; tummy tuck.

Abdominoscopy (*ab-dom'i-nos'ko-pe*) Examination of the abdominal cavity and its contents by the use of an endoscope; peritoneoscopy.

Abdominothoracic (*ab-dom'i-no-tho-ra'sik*) Pertaining to the abdomen and thorax.

Abdominovaginal (*ab-dom"i-no-vaj'i-nel*) Relating to the abdomen and to the vagina.

Abdominovesical (*ab-dom"i-no-ves'i-kal*) Relating to the abdomen and the urinary bladder.

Abducens (*ab-du'sens*) Drawing away from the midline of the body.

Abducens nerve The sixth cranial nerve supplying lateral rectus muscle.

Abduct (*ab-dukt*) To draw away from the median plane of the body.

Abduction (*ab-duk'shun*) Lateral movement away from the median plane of the body or the axial line of an extremity.

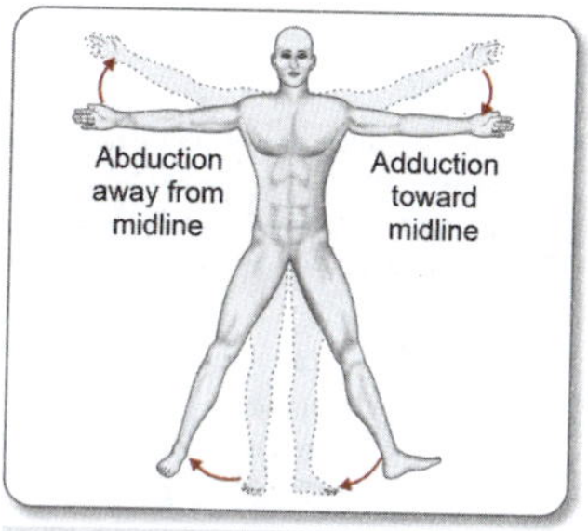

Abduction and adduction

Abductor (*ab-duk'tor*) A muscle that on contraction draws the part away from the median plane of the body or the axial line of an extremity.

Aberrancy (*ab-er'an-se*) The quality or state of being aberrant.

Aberrant (*ab-er'ant*) Deviating from the normal; wandering off; certain ducts, vessels or nerves taking an unusual course.

Abiotrophy (*ab-e-ot'ro-fe*) Premature degeneration of tissues and cells.

Ablation (*ab-la'shun*) Removal or destruction of a part.

Ablepharia A congenital absence of eyelids (partial or complete).

Ablepsia (*a-blep'se-a*) Blindness.

Abortifacient (*a-bor-ti-fa'shent*) Any drug or measure used to induce abortion.

Abortion (*a-bor'shun*) Termination of pregnancy before the fetus is capable of maintaining an independent existence. The fetus is not viable until the seventh calendar month.

Complete abortion An abortion in which all products of conception are expelled.

Criminal abortion Induction of abortion without any clear medical indications.

Habitual abortion Three or more consecutive spontaneous abortions.

Imminent abortion Impending abortion characterized by bleeding and pain, with effaced and patulous cervix.

Incomplete abortion An abortion in which some portion of the placenta or of the embryo has been retained in the uterus.

Induced abortion Termination of pregnancy before the fetus is viable.

Inevitable abortion An abortion in which the ovum has been detached and felt in the cervix or there is escape of amniotic fluid and the process of abortion cannot be arrested.

Missed abortion Death of fetus before completion of 20 weeks of gestation and retention of the products of conception for a variable time.

Saline abortion Termination of pregnancy during the second trimester by replacing 200 mL amniotic fluid with 200 mL of 20% saline solution stimulating uterine contractions.

Septic abortion Abortion in which there is an infection of uterine contents.

Spontaneous abortion Abortion without any apparent cause.

Therapeutic abortion Performance of abortion when the continuance of pregnancy would involve risk to the life or to the physical and mental health of pregnant woman or when the fetus has a known condition incompatible with life.

Threatened abortion Hemorrhage during early pregnancy unaccompanied by pain or dilatation of the cervix.

Tubal abortion Detachment of the ovum from its base and expulsion through the abdominal ostium.

Abortus (*ab'or-tus*) Number of pregnancy losses before 20 weeks regardless of cause.

ABO system Consist of A and B antigens on red blood cells and their corresponding antibodies in the sea of people who do not express these antigens.

Abrasion (*a-bra'zhun*) Scraping away of skin or mucosa.

Abreaction (*ab're-ak-shun*) Recollection of repressed memories and the release of and from the emotions that are associated with experiences buried in the unconscious.

Abruptio (ablatio) abrutio (*a-brup'she-o*) Tearing away.

Abruptio placentae Premature detachment of a normally situated placenta after 20th week of gestation.

Abscess (*ab-ses*) A localized collection of pus in any part of the body as a result of infection by pyogenic organisms.

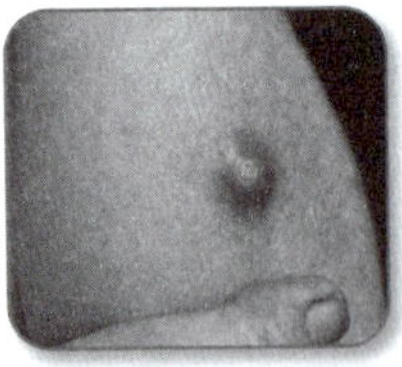

Abscess

Alveolar abscess Abscess in dentoalveolar process.

Amoebic abscess Liquefactive necrosis of liver or organs containing amoebae.

Appendicular abscess An intraperitoneal abscess resulting from extension of infection in appendicitis, especially with perforation of the appendix.

Brodie's abscess Deep seated bony swelling from chronic osteomyelitis situated near a joint named after Sir Benjamin-Brodie, London surgeon.

Cold abscess An abscess without usual signs of inflammation.

Collar-stud abscess A cystic swelling in the neck that has connection with tuberculous lymphadenitis. The diseased node(s) beneath the cervical fascia being connected by a small opening in the fascia to a more superficially placed 'cold' abscess. Similar abscess may be seen in localized cellulitis of the fingers or hand.

Cryptic abscess Abscess in crypts of Lieberkuhn of large intestinal mucosa as in ulcerative colitis.

Dental abscess Abscess with fetor, local tenderness and some degree of trismus.

Diffuse abscess A collection of pus not circumscribed by a well-defined capsule.

Ischiorectal abscess A redness and swelling between the anal verge and the ischiorectal tuberosity.

Lung abscess A localized collection of pus in the parenchyma of the lung as a result of tissue necrosis and suppuration from a pyogenic infection.

Perforating abscess An abscess that breaks down tissue barriers to enter adjacent areas.

Peritonsillar abscess Extension of tonsillar infection beyond the capsule with abscess formation; quinsy.

Popliteal abscess Abscess in popliteal space which is often deep seated, giving slight fullness of the space. The patient inclines to keep the knee joint somewhat flexed and full extension causes pain.

Potts' abscess Tuberculous abscess of the spine.

Psoas abscess An abscess, usually tuberculous, originating in tuberculous spondylitis and extending through iliopsoas muscle to the inguinal region.

Pyemic abscess Abscess resulting from pyemia, septicemia or bacteremia.

Ring abscess An acute purulent corneal inflammation wherein a central necrotic area is surrounded by an annular girdle of leucocytic infiltration.

Satellite abscess An abscess having relation to a parent abscess.

Stellate abscess Star-shaped necrotic area surrounded by epitheloid cells in the enlarged glands in lymphogranuloma venereum.

Stitch abscess An abscess around a stitch or suture.

Tropical abscess Amoebic abscess.

Tuberculous abscess An abscess caused by tubercle bacilli.

Wandering abscess An abscess occurring at a distance from the primary focus of a disease, and pus burrows along fascial planes.

Abscission (*ab-si'shun*) Removal by excision.

Absorption (*ab-sorp'shun*) Taking up of liquids by solids or of gases by solids or liquids; removal of antibody from serum by addition of an antigen or removal of an antigen by addition of an antibody.

Abulia (*a-bu'li-a*) Loss or impaired ability to perform voluntary actions or to make decisions.

Acalculia (*a-kal-ku'li-a*) A form of aphasia with an inability to do mathematical calculations.

Acantha (*a-kan'tha*) Spine or spinous process.

Acanthion (*a-kan'-the-on*) The tip of the anterior nasal spine.

Acanthosis (*ak'an-tho'sis*) Increased thickness of the prickle cell layer of the skin.

Acanthosis nigricans Hyperpigmented, hyperkeratotic growth on the skin flexures as a skin manifestation of internal malignancy.

Acapnia (hypocapnia) (*a-kar'de-a*) Absence of carbon dioxide in the blood.

Acardia Congenital absence of the heart.

Acariasis (*ak'a-ria-sis*) Any disease caused by an infestation with a burrowing mite, *Sarcoptes scabei*.

Acaricide (*a-kar'i-sid*) An agent that destroys acarids.

Acarid (*ak'a-rid*) Any member of the subgroup of the arthropod class Arachnida that includes the mites and ticks.

Acarina (*ak'a-ri'na*) Ectoparasites such as mites or ticks, which act as vectors of diseases.

Acarus (tyroglyphus) (*ak'ar-us*) A genus of mites.

Acatalasia (*a"kat-a-la'ze-a*) A metabolic disorder characterized by a total or near total loss of catalase activity in erythrocytes; a rare inherited disorder marked by the absence of enzyme, catalase. It makes the gingival and oral tissues to be susceptible to bacterial infection leading to gangrene and destruction of alveolar bone.

Acceptor (*ak-sep'tor*) A compound that will take up a chemical group from another compound.

Accessory nerve (spinal accessory nerve) Eleventh cranial nerve.

Accommodation (*a-kom'o-da'shun*) Adaptation or adjustment.

Accommodation reflex Constriction of the ciliary muscles causing contraction of the pupil and convergence of eyes in accommodation to a near vision.

Accouchement (*a-kush-mawn*) The act of giving birth to a baby.

Acentric (*a-sen'trik*) Not central; a chromosome without a centromere.

Acephalus (*a-sef'a-lus*) A headless fetus.

Acervulus cerebri A collection of granules of calcium containing material that is sometimes found within the pineal gland as its calcification proceeds (normally after 17 years).

Acetabulum (cotyloid cavity) (*as'e-tab'u-lum*) A cup-shaped depression on the lateral surface of the innominate bone (hip bone) that provides the socket into which the head of the femur rotates.

Acetaminophen (paracetamol) (*a-set'a-min'o-fen*) A synthetic preparation having antipyretic and analgesic properties.

Acetazolamide (*as'et-a-zol'a-mid*) A drug that inhibits the enzyme carbonic anhydrase, used as a diuretic and to reduce raised intraocular tension.

Acetoacetic acid A ketone body formed in excess and appearing in urine in starvation or diabetic ketoacidosis.

Acetohexamide (*as'e-to-heks'a-mid*) An oral hypoglycemic agent that stimulates pancreatic insulin secretion; useful in the treatment of type 2 diabetes.

Acetone (*as'e-ton*) Dimethyl ketone having a sweet fruity odor. It is produced when fats are not properly oxidized as in diabetes and after prolonged fasting.

Acetone body Ketone body.

Acetonuria (*as'e-to-nu're-a*) Presence of acetone bodies in the urine.

Acetylcholine (ACh) (*as'e-til-ko'len*) A choline ester that acts as a neurotransmitter at neuromuscular junction in the parasympathetic nervous system and sympathetic paraganglionic fibers (cholinergic fibers). It is inactivated by the enzyme cholinesterase.

Acetylcysteine (*as'e-til-sis'te-in*) A mucolytic agent.

Acetylsalicylic acid (*a-se'til-sal'i-sil'ik*) Aspirin.

Achalasia (Cardiospasm) (*ak'a-la'ze-a*) Failure to relax.

Achalasia of the cardia Failure of the cardia (lower esophageal) sphincter to relax restricting the passage of food to the stomach.

Achilles (*a-kil'ez*) The strong tendon connecting gastrocnemius and soleus muscles to the heel named after Achilles, hero of Iliad whose vulnerable spot was his heel.

Achlorhydria (*a'klor-hi'dre-a*) Absence of free hydrochloric acid in the stomach.

Acholia (*a-ko'le-a*) A condition in which little or no bile is secreted or the flow of bile into the digestive tract is obstructed.

Acholuria (*a-ko-lu're-a*) Absence of bile pigments in the urine.

Achondroplasia (*a-kon'dro-pla'se-a*) A genetic disorder characterized by short stature and disproportionately short limbs but normal trunk.

Achromatic (*ak'ro-mat'ik*) Colorless; not containing chromatin; difficult to stain; nondispersion of light into constituent components.

Achromtopsia (*a-kro"ma-top'se-a*) A rare, bilateral inherited retinal degeneration affecting all three types of cone photoreceptor cells that results in reduced visual acuity, photophobia, hemeralopia, and severe loss of color discrimination.

Achylia (*a-ki'le-a*) Absence of chyle.

Achylia gastrica Absence or decrease in secretion of gastric juice.

Achylia pancreatica Absence or decrease in pancreatic secretion.

Acid-base balance The pH of the extracellular fluid is maintained at about 7.4 despite production of up to 100 mmoL of hydrogen ions each day by an average adult. Homeostasis is maintained by short-term mechanisms in the form of buffers involving bicarbonate and phosphate system and hemoglobin and long term compensation involving the kidney and normal lung function.

Acidemia (*as-i-de'me-a*) An increase in the hydrogen ion concentration or a fall in pH below normal.

Acid-etch technique Using an acidic substance to prepare the tooth's enamel for the application of dental adhesive.

Acid-fast Not decolorized easily by acid-alcohol after staining as acid-fast bacteria, classic example being *Mycobacterium tuberculosis.*

Acidophil (*a-sid'o-fil*) Acidophilic; an acid-staining cell of the anterior pituitary; a bacteria growing well in an acid medium.

Acidophilic (*a-sid'o-fil'ik*) Having affinity to acid; pertaining to a cell capable of being stained by acid dyes.

Acidosis (*as'i-do'sis*) A state of increased acid content of the blood.

Acinus (*as'i-nus*) The smallest division of a gland; the basic respiratory unit of pulmonary tissue taking part in gas exchange. It is the portion of the lung distal to and supplied by a single terminal bronchiole. It includes several generations of respiratory bronchioles, alveolar ducts and alveolar sacs. Alveoli project from them. Liver acinus is the smallest functional unit of lever.

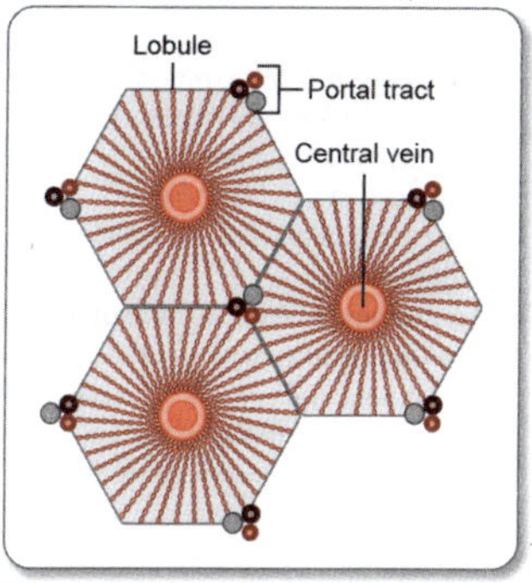

Liver acinus

Aclasis (*a-kla'sis*) A state of continuity between normal and abnormal tissue.

Acne (*ak'ne*) An inflammatory follicular, popular and pustular eruption involving the sebaceous apparatus.

Acne conglobata A chronic disease characterized by the presence of comedones, papules, nodules, cysts and scarring on chest, shoulders, back and nape of the neck, found in men during late puberty.

Acne excoriate Acne associated with extensive excoriations, seen in young females.

Acne neonatorum Acne on the nose and cheek in newborns around 3 months, mostly males.

Acne vulgaris Common during adolescence, characterized by comedones, papules, pustules, nodules and cysts on face. There is increase in size of sebaceous glands and increased secretion of sebum with inflammatory changes.

Drug Acne Acneiform lesions from drugs such as corticosteroids, phenytoin.

Occupational Acne Exposure to oils and tars among workers producing acne at site of contact with the skin.

Tropical Acne Variant of acne with large painful cysts, nodules and pustules leading to scarring and seen on the back, nape of neck, buttocks, thighs and arms.

Aconite (*ak'o-nit*) A powerful alkaloid from the root of Aconitum.

Acoustic (*a-kus'tik*) Pertaining to sound or to sense of hearing.

Acoustic meatus The opening of the auditory canal.

Acoustic nerve Vestibulocochlear nerve.

Acoustic reflexometry A procedure to measure the level of sound transmitted and reflected from the middle ear.

Acoustic reflex threshold A test for measurement of the intensity of a sound at which stapedius muscle contracts.

Acoustic trauma Injury to hearing by loud noise.

Acoustic nerve Vestibulocochlear nerve.

Acquired (*a-kwird*) Developed as a result of factors acting from outside.

Acquired Immune Deficiency Syndrome Acquired immunodeficiency syndrome (AIDS) An infection with the human immunodeficiency virus (HIV-1 and HIV-2) resulting in the development of AIDS. The infection is transmitted by sexual infects CD4 + helper lymphocytes resulting in a decrease in their numbers and there is failure of most aspects of immune function, particularly cell mediated immunity. There is defect and reduced response by B lymphocytes, monocytes and macrophages. It presents with fatigue, fever, malaise weight loss, diarrhea, lymphadenopathy, opportunistic infections and Kaposi sarcoma. The condition is diagnosed by demonstration of the presence of antibodies to HIV in serum (ELISA test) and confirmed by immunoblot (western blot) test which also detects the presence of anti HIV antibodies.

Acrania Absence of fetal skull, which results in brain tissue being exposed to amniotic fluid.

Acriflavine A topical antiseptic.

Acro Combining word for extremity; top.

Acrocentric (*ak'ro-sen'trik*) Location of a centromere at one end of a chromosome.

Acrocyanosis (*ak'ro-si-a-no'sis*) Cyanosis of the hands and feet due to spasm of the arterioles.

Acrodermatitis (*ak'ro-der-ma-ti'tis*) Dermatitis of the extremities.

Acrodynia (*ak'ro-din'e-a*) A toxic neuropathy following exposure to mercury in infants and young children characterized by pain and swelling, and pink coloration of the fingers and toes, listlessness, irritability, profuse sweating and failure to thrive.

Acromegaly (*ak'ro-meg'a-le*) A condition caused by the growth hormone (GH), secretion from a pituitary tumor in adult. GH acts by stimulation of secretion of insulin-like growth factor 1 and its binding proteins from liver. It is characterized by large hands and feet, growth of lower jaw, and skull, skin thickening, increased sweating, enlargement of lips, nose and tongue and visceromegaly.

Acromion (*a-kro'me-on*) The lateral projection of the spine of the scapula that articulates with the clavicle and forms the highest point of the shoulder.

Acroparesthesia (*ak'ro-par'es-the'ze-a*) Tingling and numbness in the extremities.

Acrosclerosis (*ak'ro-skl'er'o-sis*) A combination of Raynaud's disease and scleroderma affecting distal parts of the extremities, and of the neck and face.

Acrosome (*ak'ro-som*) A cap like-lysosomal structure on the head of a spermatozoa that contains enzymes to digest the membrane of the ovum.

ACTH (Adrenocorticotropic hormone, adrenocorticotropin, corticotropin) Anterior pituitary that stimulates the adrenal cortex to produce adrenalcortical hormones.

Actin (*ak'tin*) A muscle protein found in the myofibrils. Along with myosin, it causes contraction and relaxation of muscle. It occurs in globular (G-action) and fibrous (F-actin) forms.

Actinobacillus (*ak'ti-no-bas'i-lus*) Small gram-negative coccobacillus of genus schizomycetes capable of infecting domestic animals, rarely man.

Actinomyces (*ak'tin-o-mi'sez*) A genus of bacteria containing gram-positive filaments belonging to the genus of schizomycetes. They cause various diseases in humans and animals.

Actinomyces antibioticus A species of Actinomyces from which the antibiotic actinomycin is produced.

Actinomyces bovis A species of actinomyces responsible for actinomycosis in cattle.

Actinomyces israelii A species of Actinomyces that causes human actinomycosis. It is gram-positive, anaerobic branching, filamentous bacterium that exists as a normal flora in the oral cavity.

Actinomycin (*ak'tin-o-mi'sin*) A highly toxic antibiotic produced from *A. antibioticus* effective.

Actinomycosis (*ak'tin-o-mi-ko'sis*) A chronic suppurative and granulomatous infection by Actinomycosis israelii. It involves face and neck commonly. The organisms invade lungs, pleura, ileocecal and pelvic regions. The abscesses discharge pus containing sulfur granules. It is treated with penicillin.

Actinotherapy (*-ther'a-pe*) Phototherapy.

Action Potential Potential antagonistica ability to oppose or result of the action, as in a drug or muscle.

Active Transport The process of movement of molecules against a concentration or electrochemical gradient.

Actomyosin (*ak'to-mi'o-sin*) A protein complex of actin and myosin in the muscle fibers.

Acupuncture (*ak'u-punk'chur*) A Chinese procedure in which specific areas of the body along the peripheral nerves are pierced with fine needles to relieve pain, to produce surgical anesthesia and to promote treatment.

Acute (*a-kut*) Rapid onset with severe symptoms and sharp course.

Acute confusional state A global impairment in mental function with varying degrees of impaired level of consciousness and memory defect especially for recent events leading to disorientation in time and place.

Acute congestive glaucoma A condition noted in middle aged persons, commonly women having hypermetropia with small eyeballs and presents with severe headache, neuralgic pains and vomiting. The eyes are red and lids edematous. The anterior chamber is shallow and pupils dilated and vertically oval. The eyeball is stony hard.

Acute disseminated encephalitis An acute complication of viral infection or vaccination affecting entire brain and spinal cord or focally affecting a nerve or cord root.

Acute mountain sickness A symptom complex of less than a week duration associated with rapid ascent to greater than 2500–4500 meters, characterized by marked frontal throbbing headache, nausea, vomiting and insomnia. There may be retinal hemorrhage and sometimes life-threatening high altitude pulmonary edema or cerebral edema. The person has to be descended immediately and treated with dexamethasone.

Acute necrotizing ulcerative gingivitis A condition characterized by progressive necrosis of oral tissues seen in individuals with poor oral hygiene.

Acute phase protein A group of proteins which show characteristic change in response to inflammation and tissue injury.

Acute radiation injury syndrome A disorder noted in nuclear reactor accidents which may be asymptomatic with chromosomal aberrations, asymptomatic with mild decrease of leucocytes and platelets, or nausea, anorexia and vomiting, or bone marrow depression.

Acute renal failure A sudden failure of the kidney to maintain normal biochemical homeostasis in the body. It is characterized by a failure to excrete waste products of metabolism leading to an increase in the levels of blood urea, and serum creatinine. The condition may be prerenal, renal or postrenal.

Acute respiratory distress syndrome A severe, life-threatening catastrophe occurring suddenly in patients without any evidence of previous lung diseases following a variety of unrelated pulmonary injuries. Adam's apple (laryngeal prominence). The condition is characterized by marked dyspnea, progressive hypoxemia, reduced pulmonary compliance, marked impairment in oxygen transportation despite ventilatory assistance and roentgenographic evidence of bilateral pulmonary infiltrates.

Acute respiratory failure An inability to keep the arterial blood gases at normal level while breathing ambient air at sea level and the individual exhibits partial pressure of oxygen below 60 mm Hg with or without an elevation of carbon dioxide tension above 49 mm Hg in the arterial blood. Acute respiratory failure may develop from inadequate gas exchange (type I) and/or inadequate eventilation (type II). The former is associated with hypoxemia, seen in diseases affecting the peripheral gas exchanging parts of the lungs, and the latter with hypoxemia and hypercarbia, seen in obstructive pulmonary diseases, neuromuscular diseases and disorders of chest bellows.

Acute abdomen Sudden onset of severe pain in the abdomen requiring surgical intervention.

Acyclovir (*a-si'klo-vir*) An antiviral agent used in the treatment of herpes simplex infections of genitals and herpes infections of the skin.

Acute rheumatism Synonyms to rheumatic fever, occurs as a result of inadequate treatment of streptococcal sore throat.

Adamantinoma (*ad'a-man'ti-no'ma*) Ameloblastoma, a benign tumor of the jaw especially mandible arising from enamel forming cells.

Adam's apple (laryngeal prominence) Laryngeal prominence formed by the two laminae of the thyroid cartilage.

Adams-stokes syndrome Also called Stokes-Adams syndrome; an abrupt, transient loss of consciousness due to sudden but pronounced decrease in cardiac output.

Adaptation (*ad'ap-ta'shun*) Adjustment of an organism to its environment; ability of the eyes to adjust to variations in the intensity of light; property of certain receptors becoming less responsive or cease to show any response to constant intensity of stimulation; proper fitting of dentures or restorative material to the teeth; adjustment of the microorganism to a new environment.

Color adaptation The adaptation of the vision in dark of in reduced illumination.

Genetic adaptation The progeny of a mutant organism better adapted to a new environment, especially seen in drug resistant organisms.

Light adaptation Adjustment of the eye to vision in bright light.

Phenotypic adaptation Alteration in the properties mutation or to a change in the environment.

Photopic adaptation light adaptation.

Retinal adaptation Adjustment of the eye to dark adaptation.

Addiction (*a-dik'shun*) Psychological or physical dependence on a substance (alcohol, drug) or practice (eating, gambling) which is beyond voluntary control.

Addison's disease A disease resulting from deficiency in the secretion of either glucocorticoids or mineralocorticoids initially and later of any class of adrenocortical hormones. It may present with an acute adrenal crisis (circulatory shock with severe hypotension, hyponatremia and hyperkalemia) or chronic features (weight loss, malaise, weakness, anorexia, nausea, pigmentation and decrease in body hair). The condition is treated by glucocorticoid replacement therapy and mineralocorticoid; named after Thomas Addison who described the disease when he was a medical student in Edinburgh.

Adduct (*a-dukt*) To draw toward the median line or the main axis of the body or limb; an inclusion product.

Adductor (*a-duk'tor*) A muscle that draws a part toward the midline.

Aden-(adeno) Combining word for gland.

Adenine (*ad'e-nin*) A major purine found in RNA and DNA.

Adenitis (*ad'e-ni'tis*) Inflammation of a lymph node or a gland.

Adenocarcinoma (*ad'e-no-kar'si-no'ma*) A malignant condition of the epithelial cells in glandular tissue or glandular pattern.

Adenohypophysis (*ad"-no-hi-pofi-sis*) The anterior part of the pituitary gland, secretes many hormones, including ACTH, prolactin, and somatotropin.

Adenoidectomy The surgical removal of the adenosis; one of the common to surgical procedures done on kids along with the removal of tonsils.

Adenoid (pharyngeal tonsils) (*ad'e-noid*) Hypertrophied lymphoid tissue situated at the roof of the nasopharynx, present at birth and gradually undergoes atrophy; nasopharyngeal tonsil.

Adenoma (*ad'e-no'ma*) A benign epithelial tumor in which the tumor cells form glands or gland-like structures in the stroma.

Acidophilic adenoma A tumor of eosinophilic chromophil cells of the anterior pituitary associated with gigantism and acromegaly.

Adenoma sebaceum Benign growth from the epithelium of sebaceous glands.

Basal cell adenoma A benign, encapsulated slow growing painless salivary gland tumor especially in the parotid gland.

Basophilic adenoma A tumor of basophilic cells of the anterior pituitary associated with Cushing's syndrome.

Bronchial adenoma A tumor arising either in the main or lobar bronchus from the duct epithelium of bronchial mucous glands and includes three histologically distinct types of tumors: Carcinoid, cylindroma and mucoepidermoid tumors. The tumor may obstruct bronchial passage or grow out as a dumb-bell tumor or bleed.

Chromophil adenoma A pituitary basophilic or an eosinophilic adenoma.

Chromophobe adenoma A tumor of chromophobe cells of the anterior pituitary.

Hurthle cell adenoma A tumor of thyroid gland containing eosinophil-staining cells.

Islet adenoma A tumor of pancreas that may contain beta cells and lead to hypoglycemia.

Villous adenoma Large polyp arising from mucosa of large intestine.

Adenomyosis (*ad'e-no-mi'o-sis*) A benign ingrowth of the endometrium into the uterine muscles.

Adenosine (*a-din'o-sen*) Purine nucleotide consisting of adenine and ribose and is a component of RNA; a cardiac depressant.

Adenosine deaminase (ADA) (*a-den'o-sen de-am'i-nas*) A protein that is produced by cells throughout the body and is associated with the activation of lymphocytes, a type of white blood cell that plays a role in the immune response to infections.

Adenosine diphosphate ADP is an organic compound in metabolism, is essential to the flow of energy in living cells.

Adenosine triphosphate Also known as 5'-adenylic acid, consist of a phosphate grows, the sugar ribose and adenine; it is a nucleotide.

Adenosis N. (Pl. Adenoses) (*ad'e-no'sis*) Proliferation of the acini of the glands.

Adenovirus (*ad'e-no-vi'rus*) Any virus belonging to the family of adenoviridae. Adeno-pharyngo-conjunctival (APC) virus is an example.

Adhesion (*ad-he'shun*) A property of uniting two surfaces of parts as in wound healing; a fibrous band holding parts together; substance adhering to each other.

Adiadochokinesis The inability to perform rapid alternating movement of muscles.

Adie's syndrome (holmes-adie syndrome) A neurological disorder characterized by atomically dilated pupil. In most patients the pupil is larger than the normal. The autonomic nervous system is affected.

Adipocere (*ad'i-po-ser"*) The adipose tissue of dead bodies.

Adipose (*ad'i-pos*) Body fat.

Adiposis (liposis) (*ad'i-po'sis*) Excessive accumulation of fat in the body.

Aditus (*ad'i-tus*) An entrance to a cavity or channel.

Adjuvant (*adj'u-vant*) A nonspecific immune enhancer; the agent added to a drug affects the action of active ingredient in a predictable manner.

Freund's complete adjuvant A water in oil emulsion with inclusion of killed mycobacteria to further enhance antigenicity.

Freund's incomplete adjuvant A water in oil emulsion in which the antigen solution is emulsified in mineral oil.

Adjuvant therapy Additional cancer treatment given after the primary treatment to lower the risk of reoccurrence of cancer.

Adnexa (*ad-nek'sa*) Things connected, appendages.

Adrenal gland (suprarenal glands) A triangular secretory organ on the superior surface of the kidneys. Each consists of an outer cortex and inner medulla, each having different functions. The cortex in response to ACTH of anterior pituitary secretes cortisol and androgens.

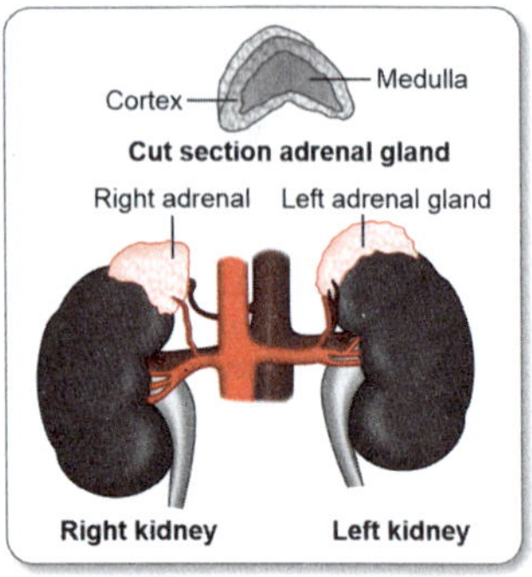

Adrenal gland

Adrenaline (*a-dren'a-lin*) A stress hormone produced within the adrenal gland that quickens the heart beat, strengthens the force of the heart's contraction, and opens up the bronchioles in the lungs, among other effects; an endogenous adrenal hormone and a synthetic vasoconstrictor.

Adrenergic (*ad'ren-er'jik*) Acting through the agency of adrenaline or noradrenaline.

Adrenergic bronchodilator A drug that acts on the sympathetic receptors to relax bronchial smooth muscle.

Adrenergic drug A sympathomimetic agent.

Adrenergic fibers Autonomic nerve fibers that release the neurotransmitter noradrenaline and in some regions, dopamine.

Adrenergic nerve A nerve controlling the release of noradrenaline at its synapses.

Adrenergic receptor A site in a sympathetic effector cell that reacts to adrenergic stimulation. They are alpha- adrenergic responding to sympathomi-metic stimuli and beta-adrenergic inhibiting the sympathomimetic activity.

Adrenocorticotropic hormone (adrenocorticotropin) (ACTH) Anterior pituitary that stimulates the adrenal cortex to produce adrenocortical hormones.

Adrenogenital syndrome Congenital adrenal hyperplasia characterized by virilization in female and precocious puberty in male children. There is a congenital deficiency of enzymes leading to a metabolic block in hormone synthesis.

Adrenolytic (*-lit'ik*) Inhibiting the activity of adrenergic nerves or interfering with the response of adrenaline.

Advancement (*ad-vans'ment*) A surgical procedure in which a tendon or a skin flap is detached from its attachment and sutured to a point further forward.

Adventitia (tunics adventitia) (*ad'ven-tish'e-a*) Outermost connective tissue coat of a blood vessel.

Adventitious (*ad'ven-tish'is*) Acquired; not natural; coming from without.

Adventitious breath sounds Sounds audible in disease but not present in normal persons. They may arise in the lungs (wheeze, crackles) or in the pleura (pleural rub).

Aedes (*a-e'dez*) A genus of mosquitoes, some of them are vectors of diseases.

Aedes aegypti A vector of dengue fever and yellow fever.

Aer- (Aero-) Combining form for the word air, gas.

Aerobe (*ar'ob*) Microorganism that can live and grow in presence of free oxygen. adj. **aerobic**.

Fecultative aerobes Microorganisms that can live in presence or absence of oxygen.

Obligate aerobes Microorganisms that require oxygen for growth.

Aerobic Using oxygen; surviving in presence of oxygen.

Aerobic exercise Intense exercise facilitating re-synthesis of high energy compounds in presence of oxygen.

Aerodontalgia (*ar'o-don-tal'je-a*) Pain in the teeth due to an alteration of atmospheric pressure.

Aeroneurosis A functional nervous disorder of flight personnel that is caused by emotional stress and is characterized by symptoms such as restlessness, abdominal pain and diarrhea.

Aerophagia (*ar'o-fa'je-a*) Excessive and repetitive air swallowing.

Aerosol (*ar'o-sol*) A suspension of fine liquid or solid particles in air which gets dispersed over a wide surface on inhalation into the lungs. β-adrenergic bronchodilators, anticholinergic bronchodilators and corticosteroids can be administered in the form of an aerosol.

Afebrile (*a-feb'ril*) Without fever.

Affect (*afekt*) The experience of emotion expressed by the patient. It is variable over time in response to changing emotional states and is observed by other.

Appropriate affect Existence of harmony between the emotional tone and the accompanying idea, thought or speech.

Inappropriate affect Disharmony between emotional tone with the idea, thought or speech accompanying it.

Afferent (*af'er-ent*) Directed from periphery toward center such as nerves or signals.

Afibrinogenemia (*a-fibrin-o-je-neme-a*) Absence or deficiency of fibrinogen in the blood, leading to its incoagulability.

Aflatoxin (*af'la-tok'sin*) Toxic products of fungi, particularly *Aspergillus flavus* and Aflatoxin parasiticus which contaminate groundnuts, cereals or pulses stored in damp environment.

Afterbirth (*af'ter-birth*) The placenta and membranes that are expelled from the uterus after childbirth.

Aftercare Care of a patient after a stay in hospital or if a person on release from prison.

Afterimage (*af'ter-im"aj*) An illusory percept that lingers at the precise retinotopic location of a stimulus after the stimulus has disappeared.

Afterpains (*af'ter-panz*) Cramplike pain noted after childbirth due to contractions of the uterus.

Agammaglobulinemia (*a-gam-a-glob'u-li-ne'me-a*) Absence of or markedly diminished levels of gamma globulin in the blood, due to an abnormal B lymphocyte function.

Agar (*ag'ar*) Polysaccharide forming stable gel, used in solid culture media in bacteriology.

Agenesis (*a-jen'e-sis*) Absence of an organ, failure to form or imperfect development of an organ.

Agglutination (clumping) (*a-glu'ti-na'shun*) Adhesion together of small particles to form visible clumps by antibodies.

Agglutinin (*a-glu'ti-nin*) An antibody found in the blood that attaches to an antigen found on red blood causing them to clump together; a substance capable of agglutinating organic particles.

Anti-Rh agglutinin An agglutinin produced in plasma by Rh-negative mothers carrying an Rh-positive fetus or following transfusion of Rh-positive blood into an Rh-negative person.

Cold agglutinin A red blood cell agglutinin that acts only at low temperatures.

Agglutinogen (*a-glu'tin'o-jen*) Any substance that stimulates the production of agglutinin.

Aglossia (*a-glos'e-a*) Congenital absence of the whole tongue.

Agnathia (*ag-na'the-a*) The complete or virtual absence of the mandible.

Agnosia (*ag'no-sia*) Inability to recognize familiar faces, locations or objects.

Agonal (*ag'o-nal*) Relating to great pain, especially the agony of death.

Agonist (Prime Mover) (*ag'o-nist*) A muscle in a state of contraction; a drug capable of combining with receptors and stimulating physiologic activity.

Agoraphobia (*ag'o-ra-fob'e-a*) Fear of open spaces.

Agranulocytosis (*a-gran'u-lo-si-to'sis*) A symptom complex of severe depression of neutrophils often associated with infection. It is characterized by severe prostration, fever, necrotic lesions in the mouth and throat and almost complete absence of neutrophils in peripheral blood.

Agraphia (Dysgraphia) (*a-grafe-a*) Loss of power of writing in spite of normal muscles of writing.

Agromania An abnormal desire to live alone, especially in an isolated area.

Ague (*a'gu*) Malaria; a chill.

AID Artificial insemination by donor.

AIDS Acquired Immune Deficiency Syndrt A Syndrome

AIH Autoimmune hepatitis.

Ainhum (*i'num*) Linear groove at the base of the fifth toe with swelling of distal part as if tied by a ligature and severe pain. The groove invades circumferentially to cause auto amputation, noted in bare footed males, in Africa.

Air embolism A serious condition, when one or more air bubbles enter a vein or artery and block it.

Air Sickness A type of incompatibility disorder causing cold sweats, nausea and vomiting during the flight.

Akathisia (*ak'a-thi'sea*) Inability to sit still with motor restlessness.

Akinesia (*a'ki-ne'se-a*) Absence or poverty of movements; adj. **akinetic**.

Ala Alanine.

Ala (*a'la*) A winglike structure; pl. **alae.**

Ala nasi The broad and lateral flaring wall of each nostril.

Alactasia (*alak-ta'ze-a*) Inability to absorb lactose due to an abnormality of brush-border of small intestine leading to an osmotic diarrhea.

Alanine (*al'a-nen*) One of the amino acids found widely in proteins.

Alastrim Variola minor, which is virologically distinct from variola major; less virulent form of smallpox.

Albers-schonberg disease (*al'bars-skon' barg*) A hereditary condition characterized by increased bone density secondary to defective resorption named after Albers-Schonberg, German radiologist.

Albinism (*al'bi-nizm*) Congenital absence of pigment in the skin, hair and eyes due to tyrosine abnormality in production of melanin.

Oculocutaneous albinism A condition without melanin, inherited as an autosomal recessive trait, characterized by white skin, deficient pigment in the hair, iris and retina, poor vision, photophobia, and rotary nystagmus.

Albino (*al-bi'no*) An individual with albinism.

Albumin (*al-bu'min*) A simple protein distributed widely in tissues and fluids of plants and animals.

Blood albumin A serum albumin.

Egg albumin Albumin of egg whites.

Human albumin Sterile preparation of serum albumin obtained by fractionating blood plasma proteins from healthy blood donors.

Serum albumin The principal protein found in the blood plasma.

Albuminuria (Proteinuria) (*al'bu-mi-nu're-a*) Sign that protein is leaking through the kidney, most often through the glomeruli, or a sign of significant kidney disease.

Albumose Any of various products of enzymatic protein hydrolysis.

Albuterol (*al-bu'tar-ol*) A selective sympathomimetic bronchodilator, inhaled to relax bronchial muscles and ease breathing during an asthma attack.

Alcaptonuria Black urine disease; a very rare inherited disorder that prevents the body fully metabolizing tyrosine and Phenylalanine.

Alcohol (*alko-hol*) Derived from Arabic word al-koh'l. One of a series of organic chemical compounds containing hydroxyl (-OH) functional group.

Absolute alcohol A solution containing 99% alcohol.

Benzyl alcohol Colorless liquid used as a bacteriostatic and as a local anesthetic.

Cetyl alcohol Solid alcohol used as an emulsifying agent.

Dehydrated alcohol A volatile liquid used as a solvent and injected into nerves and ganglia for relieving pain.

Denatured alcohol Ethyl alcohol rendered unfit for consumption.

Ethyl alcohol Ethanol, ordinary grain alcohol.

Isopropyl alcohol A volatile liquid used as a solvent and disinfectant.

Methyl alcohol Methanol, liquid obtained by distillation of wood.

Wood alcohol Methanol.

Alcoholics Anonymous A self-help program for fighting addiction to alcohol.

Alcoholism (*-izm*) A disorder characterized by alcohol abuse, dependence or addiction.

Aldomet (Methyldopa), reduces both supine and standing blood pressure.

Aldosterone (*al-dos'ter-on*) A mineralocorticoid hormone secreted by adrenal cortex. Its major action is in the regulation of electrolyte and water balance by promoting the retention of sodium and excretion of potassium in the distal convoluted renal tubules.

Aldosteronism (*al-dos'te-ro-nizm*) Hyperaldosteronism, a disorder caused by excessive secretion of aldosterone.

Primary aldosteronism Conn's syndrome.

Secondary aldosteronism Extra adrenal stimulation of aldosterone secretion as in nephrotic syndrome, cardiac failure, cirrhosis and hypoproteinemia.

Aleppo boil Delhi boiler desert boil is cutaneous leishmaniasis

Aleukemic (*a'lu-ke'mik*) A rare condition in which malignant white cells invade the skin before they appear in the peripheral blood or bone marrow.

Alexia (*a-lek'se-a*) Loss of ability to understand the meaning of written or printed words or sentences.

Alexin (cefalexin); an antibiotic used to treat bacterial infections indifferent parts of body; it acts by preventing bacterial cell wall formation.

Alexithymia Inability or difficulty to describe one's emotions or moods.

ALG Anti-lymphocyte globulin.

Algesimeter (*al'je-sim'e-ter*) An instrument for measuring the degree of sensitivity to a painful stimulus.

-Algid (*al'jid*) Chilly; cold.

Alimentary system Digestive system from mouth to anus consisting of esophagus, stomach, small and large intestines and rectum.

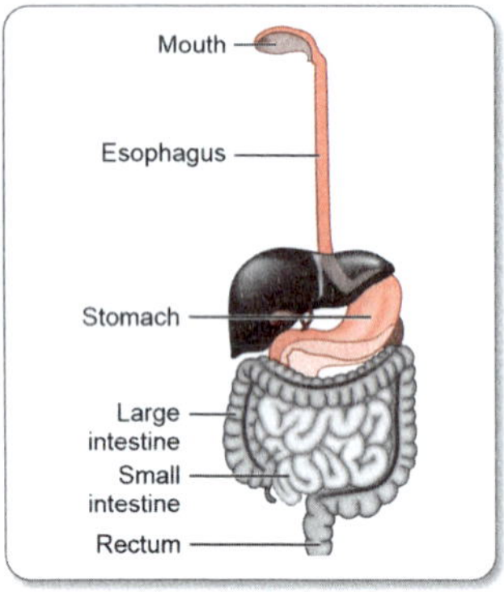

Alimentary system

Alizarin (alizarin carmine) (*a-liz'a-rin*) A hydroxyl anthraquinone compound isolated from the plant Rubia cordifolia.

Alkalemia (*al-ka-le'me-a*) A fall in H^+ ion concentration of the blood or a rise in pH.

Alkalinuria (*al'ka-li-nu're-a*) The passage of alkaline urine.

Alkaloid (*al'ka-loid*) Heterocyclic nitrogen-containing plant product having pharmacologic activity and the examples are atropine, nicotine, caffeine, cocaine, strychnine, morphine and quinine.

Vinca alkaloids Alkaloids produced by *Vinca rosea*; vincristine and vinblastine are used in treatment of malignancy.

Alkalosis (*al'ka-lo'sis*) An increase in base or decrease in acid.

Metabolic alkalosis An increase in plasma bicarbonate concentration. There is marked loss of acid other than H_2CO_3 from the stomach and kidney and a fall in plasma chloride.

Respiratory alkalosis A condition where CO_2 in the arterial blood is below normal range. There is hyperventilation and pH is raised.

Alkaptonuria (Alcaptonuria) (*al-kap"-to-nu're-a*) A rare genetic metabolic disorder characterized by the accumulation of homogentisic acid in the body.

Allantois (*a-lan'to-is*) A vestigial fetal membrane developing from the sac.

Allele (allelomorph) (*a'lel*) One of two or more variations of a gene located at a particular site of chromosome.

Allergen (*al'er-jen*) An antigenic substance capable of producing hypersensitivity (immediate and late) reaction.

Allergy (*al'er-je*) An immunologic response in a susceptible person to exposure to an allergen. The exposure to antigen in atopic individuals stimulates peripheral lymphoid tissues to synthesize IgE antibodies. They possess two Fab and Fc pieces. They get fixed by Fc piece to the mast cells. The cytoplasmic matrix of the mast cells is filled with granules. Any further exposure to the same antigen leads to the union of antigen with the antigen receptors on Fab portion of two molecules of IgE antibody. There is degranulation of the cells following entry of calcium and release of mediators of anaphylaxis; an acquired hypersensitivity to certain drugs and biologic products.

Allesthesia (*al'es-the'ze-a*) Experiencing sensation remote from the a place where stimulus is applied; stimulus in one limb being referred to opposite limb.

Allogeneic (*al'o-je-ne'ik*) Pertaining to different gene constitutions within the same species.

Allograft (*al'o-graft*) Homograft; a graft such as organ, tissues or cells donated from genetically distinct individual of the same species.

Alloimmune (*al'o-i-mun*) Specifically immune to an allogenic antigen.

Alloisoleucine An amino acid that exists as two enantiomers. It occurs in healthy serum only in trace amounts, except for individuals suffering from maple syrup urine disease.

Allopathy (*al'op'a-the*) A system of treating diseases by producing a pathologic reaction that is antagonistic to the disease being treated.

Alloplasia (*al'o-plas'ze-a*) The development of tissues at a site where such tissue does not occur.

Allopurinol (*al'o-pur'i-nol*) A drug capable of inhibiting xanthine oxidase and bringing down the serum and urinary level of uric acid. Used in the treatment of gout.

Allorhythmia (*al'o-rith'me-a*) Irregularity of the heart recurring regularly.

Allostasis (*alo-sta-sis*) Ability to achieve stability of body systems through change.

Alloxan (*a-lok'san*) An oxidation product of uric acid capable of destroying islets of Langerhans in experimental animals and producing diabetes.

Allylestrenol (altyloestrenol) A steroid used to prevent premature labor in pregnant women.

Alopecia (baldness) (*al'o-pa'she-a*) Absence or loss of hair from skin areas where it is normally found; a disease that happens when the immune system attacks hair follicles and causes hair loss.

Alopecia aerate Circumscribed loss of hair on the scalp and beard.

Alopecia capitis totalis Total loss of hair on the scalp.

Alopecia medicamentosa Diffuse hair loss of the scalp due to administration of cytotoxic agents.

Alopecia totalis Total loss of hair of the scalp.

Alopecia universalis Total loss of hair from all parts of the body.

Cicatricial alopecia Loss of hair associated with scarring.

Male pattern alopecia Hair loss in males, which begins in the frontal region and progresses to leave behind a horse shoe area of hair remains in the back and temples due to the influence of androgenic hormone.

Aloxiprin A drug used for the treatment of inflammation and pain associated with musculoskeletal issues and joint pain.

Alpha-fetoprotein (AFP) (*alfa-fe'to-pro'ten*) (AFP) A plasma protein formed in fetal liver, yolk sac, and gastrointestinal tract and by hepatocellular carcinoma.

Alprazolam (*al-pra'zo-lam*) A benzodiazepine, works by increasing the action of a chemical messenger (GABA) which suppresses the abnormal and excessive activity of the nerve cells in the brain.

Alprenolol A nonselective beta-blocker used in the treatment of edema, hypotension, ventricular tachycardias and atrial fibrillation.

ALS Advanced life support, an emergency care that may include airway management, defibrillator and use of drugs and medication; antilymphocytic serum; amyotrophic lateral sclerosis.

Altitude sickness (mountain sickness) Physical distress from difficulty adjusting to lower oxygen pressure at high altitude.

Aluminum hydroxide An antacid used to treat heartburn, upset stomach, acid indigestion or sour stomach.

Alveolitis (*al-ve'o-li'tis*) Inflammation of alveoli; inflammation of a tooth socket.

Cryptogenic fibrosing alveolitis A fibrosing lesion from the beginning.

Extrinsic allergic alveolitis A hypersensitivity reaction occurring at the peripheral gas exchanging parts of the lungs in response to repeated inhalation of antigens contained in finely particulate organic dusts of wide variety and other agents by a susceptible individual. External agents like spores of thermophilic actinomycetes and other fungi, moulding stored vegetable matters (hay, bagasse) and animal protein (avian, bovine, porcine or insect material) act as antigens.

Fibrosing alveolitis An inflammatory process of the lung with predominant involvement of alveolar walls. It is characterized by inflammatory cellular thickening of the alveolar walls with marked tendency to fibrosis (mural) or the presence of a large number of large mononuclear cells (desquamative).

Alveolus (*al-ve'o-lus*) Pl. **alveoli**; a small cavity; a sac-like dilatation.

Alveolus dentalis Tooth socket.

Pulmonary alveolus Terminal blind ending structures of the respiratory bronchioles where gas exchange takes place.

Alveus (*al've-us*) A channel or groove.

Alzheimer's Disease (*alts'hi-merz*) A condition with atrophy of brain particularly the cerebral cortex and hippocampus, characterized by gradual impairment of memory and dementia, named after Alois Alzheimer, German neurologist.

Amanita (*am'a-ni'ta*) A genus of fungi, many members of which are poisonous.

Amantadine (*a-man'ta-den*) An antiviral agent used in prophylaxis against influenza A virus and in the treatment of Parkinsonism.

Amaurosis (*am'aw-ro'sis*) Blindness occurring without any apparent cause. adj. **amaurotic**.

Amaurosis fugax A temporary loss of vision from a transient ischemia due to carotid artery insufficiency.

Ambivalence (*am-biv'a-lens*) Coexistence of two opposing impulses toward the same thing in the same person at the same time.

Amblyomma (*am'ble-om'a*) A genus of hard-bodied ticks.

Amblyopia (*am'ble-o'pe-a*) Reduction or dimness of vision without any detectable organic lesion.

Amblyoscope (Orthoptoscope, Synoptophore) (*am'ble-o-skop*) An instrument to measure binocular vision and for stimulation of vision in the amblyopic eye.

Amoeba (*a-me'ba*) A pseudopod forming protozoa of the class sarcodina found in water. It constantly changes its shape by sending out finger-like processes of protoplasm for mobility and to obtain food. Some species of the genus amoeba such as entamoeba, iodamoeba and acanthamoeba are parasites of man.

Amoebiasis (*am"e-bi'a-sis*) A disease caused by *Entamoeba histolytica*, a pathogenic intestinal ameba. It spreads between humans by its cysts. It gives rise to amebic dysentery or extraintestinal amebiasis such as amebic liver abscess. The amebic cysts gain entry into the body by fecal oral route. The vegetative trophozoites emerge from the cysts in the colon, and invade the mucous membrane and produce flask-shaped ulcers. Amebae reach the liver through portal venous system and cause destruction of parenchyma of the liver to produce an amebic abscess. The liquid contents are chocolate brown in color.

Amebocyte (*a-me'bo-sit"*) A cell having amoeboid form or movements.

Ameboma (*am"e-bo'me*) A rare complication of amebic colitis presenting as a mass of granulation tissue with peripheral fibrosis and a core of inflammation related to amebic chronic infection.

Amelia (*a-me'le-a*) Congenital absence of a limb or limbs.

Ameloblast (*a-mel'o-blast*) A cylindrical epithelial cell found in the innermost layer of the enamel.

Ameloblastoma (*a-mel'o-blas'to'ma*) A benign but locally invasive tumor of enamel organ. Multicystic ameloblastoma of the left mandible.

Amelogenesis (*amė-lo-jen'i-sis*) The formation of dental enamel.

Amnioscope (*am-ne-o-skop*) An endoscope to visualize the fetus and amniotic fluid.

Amenorrhea (*a-menö-reä*) Absence or abnormal cessation of the menstruation.

Lactation amenorrhea Absence of menstruation incidental to lactation.

Physiologic amenorrhea Absence of menstruation during pregnancy.

Primary amenorrhea Failure of menstruation to occur at puberty.

Secondary amenorrhea Cessation of menstruation in a woman who was menstruating earlier.

Amentia (*a-menshe-a*) Mental retardation; mental disorder characterized by confusion, disorientation and sometimes stupor.

Amethocaine An ester local anesthetic used to anesthetize eye, ear, nose and throat before starting surgery or procedure.

Ametropia (*am'i-tro'pe-a*) A refractory error with failure of parallel rays to get focused on retina.

Amiloride A type of diuretic that helps prevent losing too much potassium, and used in hypertension and heart failure.

Aminacrine A flourescent anti-infective dye used as a topical antiseptic and experimentally as a mutagen, an intracellular pH indicator and a small molecule MALDI matrix.

Amino acid Organic compounds containing both amino (NH_2) and a carboxyl (COOH) group. Amino acids are essential building blocks for proteins and polypeptides.

Branched-chain amino acid Essential amino acids leucine, isoleucine and valine. They bypass liver and are available for the cells from the circulation.

Dispensable amino acid Amino acids that can be synthesized in the body by transamination if there is sufficient supply of amino group.

Essential amino acid Amino acids that cannot be synthesized by the organism and are to be supplied in the diet. They are histidine, isoleucine, leucine, lysine, methionine, cysteine, phenylalanine, tyrosine, threonine, tryptophan and valine. Arginine is also needed in infants.

Indispensable amino acid Amino acids required in the diet.

Nonessential amino acid Amino acid that may be synthesized by the organism.

Aminoglutethimide (*a-me"no-gloo-teth'i-mid*) A substance that inhibits cholesterol metabolism, thus of production of adrenocortical hormone.

Aminoglycosides (*a-me"no-gli'ko-sid*) Any of a group of antibiotics derived from *Streptomyces* or produced synthetically. Streptomycin, gentamicin, tobramycin, netilmycin, amikacin and neomycin possess similiar structure and adverse effects.

Aminopeptidase Catalyses the cleavage of amino acids from the aminoterminus of protein and peptidase substrates.

Aminophylline (*am'i-nof'i-lin*) A mixture of theophylline and ethylenediamine used as a bronchodilator.

Amitosis (*am'i-tosis*) A direct cell division by simple cleavage of the nucleus.

Amitriptyline (*am'i-trip'ti-len*) A tricyclic antidepressant.

Amnesia (*am-ne'ze-a*) Partial or total inability to recall past experiences. It may be organic or emotional in origin.

Anterograde amnesia Amnesia in reference to the events following injury or disease.

Dissociative amnesia Patchy and inconsistent memory loss and is a characteristic feature of a loss of personal identity.

Retrograde amnesia Amnesia in reference to the events that occurred before the injury or disease.

Transient amnesia Loss of memory for a period of time due to a toxic confusional state, psychological fugue state or postictal period after a seizure.

Transient global amnesia An abrupt discrete and reversible loss of short-term memory function.

Amnihook A 12 inches long, curved hook at the top. It resembles a crochet hook. Used to break the amniotic sac, to allow the fluid to escape.

Amniocentesis (*am'ne-o-sen-te'sis*) Aspiration of fluid from the amniotic sac by transabdominal or transcervical approach guided by ultrasound scanning. It is a prenatal diagnostic procedure performed to study genetic and biochemical disorders, and to determine fetal maturity.

Amnion (*am'ne-on*) The innermost of the membranes that envelop the embryo in uterus and filled with amniotic fluid.

Amnioscope (*am-ne-o-skop*) An endoscope to visualize the fetus and amniotic fluid.

Amniotic cavity The fluid-filled cavity of the amnion.

Amniotic fluid (Liquor amnii) The albuminous, transparent fluid in the amnion protects the fetus from injury, helps in maintenance of an even temperature and prevents development of any adhesions between the amnion and the fetus.

Amniotomy (*am'ne-ot'o-me*) Artificial rupture of the fetal membranes to induce labor.

Amobarbital (Amylobarbitone) (*am'o-bar'bi-tal*) An intermediate acting sedative.

Amodiaquine hydrochloride (*am'o-di-a-kwin*) An antimalarial and anti-inflammatory agent.

Amok (*amuck*) *psy* A dissociative episode characterized by a period of brooding followed by an outburst of violent, aggressive or homicidal behavior directed at people and objects.

Amoxicillin (*a-mok'si-sil'in*) An analog of ampicillin with a similar antibacterial spectrum. It is reliably absorbed from the gastroinstestinal tract.

AMP Adenosine monophosphate.

Ampere (*am'per*) A unit of electric current produced by one volt acting through a resistance of one ohm, named after Andre Ampere.

Amphetamine (*am-fet'a-men*) A sympathomimetic amine having CNS stimulating effects.

Amphiarthrosis (*am-fe-ar-thro-sis*) An articulation permitting little motion as the opposing surfaces of bone are connected by fibrocartilage, such as articulation of the bodies of the vertebrae.

Amphoric Breath Sounds A variant of bronchial breathing having a hollow reverberatory quality, audible over an open pneumothorax and over a thin walled cavity communicating with a bronchus.

Amphotericin B (*am'fo-ter'i-sin*) An antibiotic preparation used in the treatment of systemic fungal infections. It is administered by intravenous infusion in increasing daily doses.

Ampicillin (*amp'i-sil'in*) A semisynthetic penicillin having a bactericidal action against both gram-positive and some gram-negative organisms. It is susceptible to degradation by beta-lactamases.

Ampule (ampoule) (*am'pul*) A small sealed glass container that preserves its contents sterile, such as medication for parenteral administration.

Ampulla (*am-pula*) A flask-like dilatation of a tubular structure. pl. **ampullae.**

Ampulla of ductus deferens Dilatation of vas deferens when, it approaches its fellow prior to it is joined by the duct of seminal vesicle.

Ampulla of thorns One of the small terminal expansion of an interlobar arteries in the splenic pulp.

Ampulla of uterine tube The wide portion of fallopian tube near the fimbriated end.

Hepatopancreatic ampulla The dilatation formed by unction of the common bile duct and main pancreatic duct proximal to their opening into the duodenum; ampulla of Vater.

Membranous ampulla The dilatations at one end of each of the three semicircular ducts (anterior, posterior and lateral) where they connect with the utricle.

Osseous ampulla The dilatation of one end of each of the three bony semicircular canals (anterior, posterior and lateral), each contains a membranous ampulla.

Rectal ampulla Dilated portion of the rectum just above the anal canal.

Amputation (*am'pu-ta'shun*) The surgical removal of limb/or part of a limb or an outgrowth.

Above knee (AK) A division of femur in the supracondylar region at midthigh.

Below knee (BK) A division of tibia and fibula distal to tibial tuberosity.

Chopart's amputation Amputation of the foot through midtarsal joint.

Congenital amputation Amputation of fetal parts as a developmental defect.

Double-flap amputation Amputation in which a flap is cut from the soft parts on either side of the limb.

Dupuytren's amputation Amputation of arm or shoulder joint.

Flap amputation An amputation in which flaps of muscle and skin are made to cover the end of the bone.

Guillotine amputation Amputation performed by a circular incision through the skin, and the muscles and bone are kept and left open for dressing.

Primary amputation Amputation performed before inflammation sets in.

Secondary amputation Performed during suppuration.

Spontaneous amputation Amputation as a result of disease process rather than external trauma as in leprosy or diabetes mellitus.

Syme's amputation Of the foot at the ankle joint with removal of the malleoli.

Traumatic amputation Resulting from accident.

Amsacrine (*am'sa-kren*) Belongs to the class of compounds known as acridines.

Amygdala (amygdaloid nucleus) *a-mig'da-la*) An almond shaped structure; corpus amygdalo deum; tonsilla cerebelli; lymphatic tonsils.

Amylase (*am'i-las*) An enzyme that catalyzes the hydrolysis of starch into smaller molecules.

Amyl nitrite A vasodilator, used in angina by inhalation.

Amyloid (*am'i-loid*) Any of a group of chemically diverse proteins that appear microscopically homogeneous, that get deposited in the walls of blood vessels especially in association with reticuloendothelial tissue.

AA Amyloid Secondary amyloid derived from serum protein.

AL Amyloid Amyloid made up of light chain immunoglobulin.

Amyloidosis (*am'i-loi-do'sis*) A disease associated with amyloid deposition.

Primary amyloidosis Monoclonal overproduction of a normal immunoglobulin light chain; often presents with nephrotic syndrome, renal impairment, restrictive cardiomyopathy, malabsorption, macroglossia, and peripheral neuropathy.

Reactive amyloidosis Deposition of normal protein, amyloid A component. It is produced in the liver in response to long-standing inflammation. It is associated with nephrotic syndrome, progressive renal impairment and hepatosplenomegaly.

Amylopectin (*am'i-lo-pek'tin*) Insoluble branched chain starch, found in cereals.

Amylose (*am'i-los*) An unbranched long polysaccharide, or sugar, chain.

Amyotonia congenita (Floppy Baby Syndrome) Congenital disease of children exhibiting general hypotonia of the muscles.

Amyotrophy (*a'mi-ot'ra-fe*) Atrophy of muscle.

Diabetic amyotrophy Severe and progressive weakness and wasting of the proximal muscles of lower limbs accompanied by pain.

An Prefix, without, or -less.

Anabolic *(a-na-bä-lik)* Marked by or promoting metabolic activity concerned with the biosynthesis of complex molecules

Anabolism *(a-nab'o-lizm)* A metabolic activity in which the simple substances are converted into complex compounds by the cells.

Anacidity *(an'a-sid'i-te)* Lack of normal acidity.

Anacrotism *(a-nak'ro-tizm)* An abnormal type of pulse exhibiting a prominent notch on its ascending limb.

Anaerobe *(an'e-rob)* Microorganism that grows optionally without oxygen.

Facultative anaerobes Microorganisms that can grow under either anaerobic or aerobic condition.

Obligate anaerobes Microorganisms that can grow only in complete absence of oxygen.

Anaerobic *(an'er-o-bic)* Energy production body's production of energy when needed amounts of oxygen are not readily available.

Anal *(a'n-1)* Relating to the anus.

Anal canal The terminal portion of the large intestine that opens out in anus. It remains closed except during defecation or passage of flatus.

Anal fissure Traumatic and ischaemic damage to anal mucosa resulting in a mucosal tear in the midline posteriorly. There is severe pain on defecation, bleeding, mucus discharge and pruritus.

Anal fistula Fistula-in-ano, an indurated track with external opening and internal orifice in the anal canal.

Anal reflex An immediate contraction of the anal sphincter on scratching the skin around the anus.

Anal tag Swollen skin at the distal end of an anal fissure. It is often accompanied by pain on defecation and fresh bleeding.

Analeptic *(an'a-lep'tik)* Restorative; a central nervous stimulant.

Analgesia *(an'al-je'ze-a)* Absence of pain sensibility.

Analgesic *(an'al-je'sik)* Substance relieving pain; insensitive to pain.

Analgesic nephropathy Tubulointerstitial inflammation associated with papillary necrosis caused by ingestion of analgesics such as acetaminophen, aspirin and phenacetin and manifest in hematuria, renal colic and pyelonephritis.

Analog *(an'a-log)* A drug whose effect mimics that of another, having a dissimilar chemical structure; a part or organ possessing similar function as another, but of different origin.

Analogous *(a-nal'o-gus)* Resembling in appearance or function.

Analysand *(s-nal'i-sand)* One who is undergoing psychoanalysis.

Analysis *(a-nal'i-sis)* Separating complex material into constituent parts and identifying them; determination of concentration of one arterial constituent in a mixture.

Blood gas analysis The determination of oxygen and carbon dioxide concentrations and pH, using O_2, CO_2 and pH electrodes. HCO_3 is determined by a nomogram.

Anamnesis *(an'am-ne'sis)* History taking from a patient; faculty of memory.

Anaphase *(an'a-faz)* Stage of mitosis or meiosis with division of centromere in which daughter chromosomes move toward the poles of the cell.

Anaphylactoid reaction An anaphylaxis-like reaction occurring as a non-immune reaction.

Anaphylaxis *(-fi-lak'sis)* A hypersensitivity reaction that occurs upon exposure to an antigen to which the body has previously formed an IgE antibody.

Anaplasia *(-pla'z-e-a)* A loss of differentiation of cells and their orientation to one another as in tumor tissue.

Anasarca *(an'a-sar-ka)* Edema involving the whole body; dropsy.

Anastomosis *(a-nas'to-mo'sis)* A communication between two vessels by collaterals; an opening between two organs or spaces, which can be natural or resulting from injury, surgery or disease. Example: Roux-en-Y Gastric anastomosis between stomach and small bowel.

Anatomical deadspace The air remaining in the conducting system, from nose to the beginning of respiratory bronchioles, does not participate in the gas exchange and that part of the ventilation is considered wasted. However, it helps in saturation of the inspired air with moisture brings it to the level of body temperature, and enables the removal of particulate matter.

Anatomy (*a-nat'a-me*) The structure of an organism; the branch of science dealing with morphology or structure of organisms.

Applied anatomy Application of anatomical knowledge in diagnosis and treatment.

Comparative anatomy Comparison of homologous structures of different animals.

Descriptive anatomy Description of individual parts of the body.

Developmental anatomy Embryology.

Gross anatomy Study of structures by naked eye.

Microscopic anatomy Histology.

Pathologic anatomy Anatomy studied in relation to function.

Radiological anatomy Study of body through X-ray imaging.

Surface anatomy Study of the configuration of the surface of the body in its relation to deeper structures.

Surgical anatomy Applied anatomy in relation to surgical diagnosis and treatment.

Topographic anatomy The study of parts in their relation to surrounding parts.

Anatropia (*an'atro'pe-a*) An upward deviation of visual axis of one eye when other eye is fixing.

Anconeus (*ang-ko'ne-us*) Short extensor of elbow. *see* Table of muscles.

Ancylostoma (ankyloatoma) (*an"-si-los'to-ma*) A parasitic nematode worm and commonly known as the old world hookworm.

Ancylostomiasis (*an-si-los-to-mi'a-sis*) *see* Ankylostomiasis.

Androgen (*an'dro-jen*) Masculinizing hormone.

Androsterone Metabolite of testosterone.

Anencephaly (*an'en-sef'a-le*) The congenital absence of a major portion of the brain, skull and scalp.

Anergy (*an'er-je*) A condition in which T cells have decreased or absence of lymphokine secretion when the T cell receptor is engaged by an antigen.

Anesthesia (an"es-the'ze-a) Loss of sensation with or without loss of consciousness.

Basal anesthesia Parenteral administration of sedatives as premedication to produce a state of depressed consciousness; short of general anesthesia.

Block conduction anesthesia Injection of local anesthetic agent in close proximity of a nerve supplying the area (nerve block) or encircling the operative field (field block) to inhibit nerve transmission.

Caudal anesthesia Regional anesthesia produced by injection of a local anesthetic agent into the epidural space *via* sacrococcygeal notch.

Closed circuit anesthesia Inhalation anesthesia in which there is continuous rebreathing of an anesthetic in a closed system with removal of CO_2.

Dissociated anesthesia Loss of sensation of pain and temperature with preservation of touch sensation as in syringomyelia.

Endotracheal anesthesia Anesthesia produced by introduction of gaseous mixture through a tube inserted into the trachea.

Epidural anesthesia Regional anesthesia produced by injection of a local anesthetic between the vertebral spines and beneath ligamentum flavum into the extradural space.

General anesthesia A state of unconsciousness and loss of ability to perceive pain produced by administration of anesthetic agents by intravenous or inhalation route.

Girdle anesthesia Anesthesia distributed in the form of a band around the abdomen.

Glove-and-stocking anesthesia Loss of sensation in the area that would be covered by a glove and stocking as in peripheral neuropathy.

Infiltration anesthesia Local anesthesia produced by injection of anesthetic directly into the tissues.

Inhalation anesthesia General anesthesia produced by inhalation of vapor or gaseous anesthetic agents such as ether, nitrous oxide and methoxyflurane.

Insufflation anesthesia Maintenance of inhalation anesthesia by blowing a mixture of gases or vapors into the airway.

Local anesthesia Regional anesthesia produced by direct infiltration of an anesthetic into the operative field.

Open anesthesia Application usually by dropping of volatile anesthetic agent onto gauge held over the nose and mouth and there is no significant rebreathing.

Primary anesthesia The first stage of anesthesia before loss of consciousness.

Pudendal anesthesia A type of local anesthesia produced by blocking the pudendal nerve on either side near the ischial spine.

Rectal anesthesia General anesthesia produced by instillation into the rectum of liquid inhalation anesthetics.

Refrigeration anesthesia Local anesthesia induced by lowering temperature of a part of body to near freezing either by spraying it with ethyl chloride or by immersion in ice.

Regional anesthesia Nerve or field block by anesthetic agent to produce a circumscribed area of anesthesia.

Retrobulbar anesthesia Injection of a local anesthetic behind the eyeball.

Saddle block anesthesia A type of spinal anesthesia limited to buttocks, perineum and inner surfaces of thigh produced by injection of anesthetic agent into fourth lumbar space.

Segmental anesthesia Anesthsia limited to an area supplied by one or more spinal nerve roots, due to neurologic lesion.

Spinal anesthesia Loss of sensation produced by disease of spinal cord; anesthetic into the subarachnoid space of the spinal canal.

Splanchnic anesthesia Anesthesia produced by injection into splanchnic ganglia.

Tactile anesthesia Loss of sense of touch.

Thermal anesthesia Loss of heat sense.

Topical anesthesia Local anesthesia induced by direct application of local anesthetic solutions, ointments or jellies.

Traumatic anesthesia Loss of sensation from nerve injury.

Twilight anesthesia A state of light anesthesia.

Anesthesiologist (*an'es-the'ze-ol'o-jit*) A medical specialist trained in anesthesiology.

Anesthetic (*an"es-thet'ik*) Any agent that produces a local or general loss of sensation, including pain.

Anesthetist (*a-nes'the-tist*) A doctor or nurse who gives an anesthetic to a patient.

Aneuploidy (*an'u-ploi'de*) A congenital or acquired alteration in the number of chromosomes that deviates from multiple of a haploid of chromosomes.

Aneurysm (*an'u-rizm*) Localized rounded distension of a vessel in continuity of its lumen.

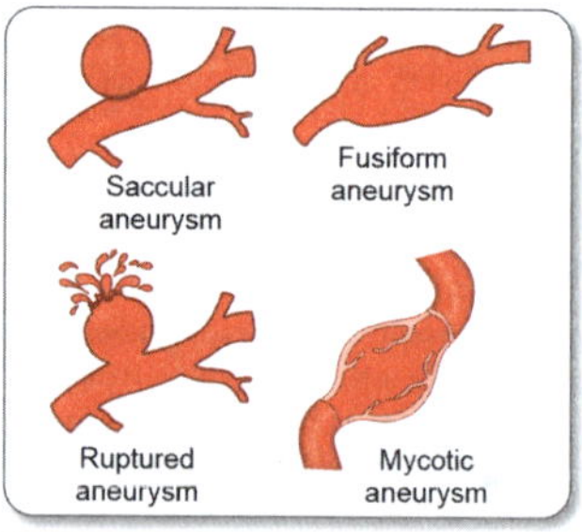

Aneurysm

Abdominal aortic aneurysm Localized dilatation of the wall of abdominal aorta.

Aortic aneurysm An abnormal dilatation of the aortic wall due to atheroma, Marfan's syndrome, or aortitis.

Arteriovenous aneurysm A dilated arteriovenous shunt.

Berry (saccular) aneurysm Aneurysmal bulging from the bifurcation of cerebral arteries particularly in the region of circle of Willis, and they develop from defects in the media of the arterial wall.

Cirsoid aneurysm A dilatation of a group of vessels due to congenital malformations.

Dissecting aneurysm Splitting of an arterial wall with entry of blood through an intimal tear.

Fusiform aneurysm A rare, sausage like expansions of the entire blood vessels on all sides.

Mycotic aneurysm Aneurysm due to impaction of a septic embolus.

Popliteal aneurysm A cystic swelling of the popliteal space exhibiting an expansile impulse.

Rasmussen's aneurysm Dilated artery traversing a pulmonarytuberculous cavity causing massive hemoptysis.

Ventricular aneurysm Persistent occlusion of the infarct-related artery causes thinning and stretching of the infarcted segment of the ventricle.

Angi- (angio) Combining word for vessel.

Angiitis (vasculitis) (*an'je-i'tis*) Inflammation of a vessel, refers to a blood or lymph vessel; vasculitis.

Angina (*an-ji-na*) A severe constricting pain referring to angina pectoris; sore throat.

Abdominal angina Intermittent cramping abdominal pain, frequently occurring after food, caused by inadequacy of mesenteric circulation.

Angina pectoris Discomfort due to transient myocardial ischemia and occurs when there is an imbalance between myocardial oxygen supply and demand. Coronary atheroma is the most common cause.

Crescendo angina Unstable angina showing rapidly worsening angina at rest or prolonged and severe chest pain without ECG or enzyme abnormalities.

Ludwig's angina Cellulitis under deep cervical fascia.

Noctural angina Angina developing either soon after patient lies down due to an increase in venous return that increases myocardial oxygen demand beyond the capacity of supply or several hours later due to an increase in myocardial oxygen demand or vasospasm.

Postprandial angina Angina developing during or soon after meals due to an increased oxygen demand in splanchnic vascular bed.

Prinzmetal angina A variant of angina pectoris in which pain occurs during rest, severe and of longer duration associated with ECG abnormalities with elevation of ST segment.

Stable angina Characterized by central chest pain that is precipitated by exertion and promptly relieved by rest. The pain may radiate to the neck, and often accompanied by discomfort in the arms, wrists and sometimes hand.

Unstable angina Acute coronary insufficiency in which the symptoms are intermediate in severity between stable angina pectoris and myocardial infarction.

Variant angina A form of angina attributed to a local magnesium deficiency.

Vincent's angina An ulcerative infection of tonsils and pharynx.

Walk-through angina Angina occurring during exercise, but disappearing with continued exercise.

Angina pectoris Discomfort due to transient myocardial ischemia and occurs when there is an imbalance between myocardial oxygen supply and demand. Coronary atheroma is the most common cause.

Angiocardiography (*an'je-o-kar'de-og'ra-fe*) Radiographic imaging of the heart and blood vessels following injection of radio-opaque solution.

Angiodysplasia (*an'je-o-dis-pla'zhea*) Development of vascular malformations in the proximal colon and it is associated with aortic valve disease. There is acute and profuse bleeding that stops spontaneously.

Angiogenesis (*an'je-o-jen'i-sis*) Development of blood vessels in the embryo.

Angiography (*anje-og'ra-fe*) A radiologic procedure used to visualize the interior of blood vessels following injection of a contrast medium.

Coronary angiography Performed to detect stenoses and guide revascularization procedures in patients with coronary artery disease.

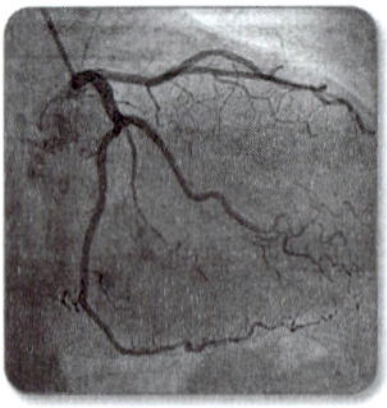

CT angiography of coronary artery

Digital subtraction angiography (DSA) A technique whereby images obtained before contrast injection are digitized and subtracted from postcontrast images.

Pulmonary angiography To diagnose pulmonary emboli, contrast medium is passed down a catheter inserted *via* the femoral vein into the main pulmonary artery renal a performed to investigate renal artery stenosis, following injection of contrast material into the aorta.

Angioid (*an'je-oid*) Resembling blood vessel.

Angiokeratoma (*an'je-o-ker'a-to'ma*) Telangiectatic wart.

Angiology (*an'je-ol'o-je*) The study of vessels of the blood, as related to blood vessels and lymphatics.

Angioma (arteriovenous malformation) (*an'je-o'ma*) Vascular tumor of blood vessels.

Cavernous angioma Cavernous hemangioma.

Telangiectatic angioma Angioma with dilated vessels.

Angioneurotic edema (angioedema) (*an'je-o-e-de'ma*) Development of urticaria and edematous areas of skin, mucous membrane or viscera. It is caused by dilatation and increased permeability of the capillaries.

Angioplasty (*an'je-o-plas'te*) A procedure used to open blocked coronary arteries caused by coronary artery disease. Example: Balloon angioplasty.

Angiospasm (*an'je-o-spazm*) Vasospasm; spasmodic contractions of a blood vessel with increase in blood pressure.

Angiotensin (*an'je-o-ten'sin*) Decapeptide with vasoconstrictive activity produced by enzymatic action of renin upon angiotensinogen.

Angiotensin I A decapeptide produced by the action of renin on angiotensinogen, a mild vasopressor and promotes release of aldosterone.

Angiotensin II An octapeptide produced from angiotensin I by angiotensin converting enzyme, a powerful vasopressor and promotes release of aldosterone a II receptor antagonists drugs act by blocking the action of angiotensin II on heart, peripheral vasculature and kidney.

Angle (*ang'gl*) A figure or space formed by the junction of two lines or planes.

Angle of Treitz Sharp curve at the duodenojejunal junction.

Cardiophrenic angle The medial inferior corner of thoracic cavity bordered by the heart and diaphragm.

Carrying angle The angle made at the elbow by extending the long axis of the forearm and the upper arm.

Cerebellopontine angle The angle formed by the junction of the cerebellum and the pons.

Costal angle The meeting point of lower border of the false ribs with the axis of sterum.

Costovertebral angle The angle formed on either side of vertebral column between the last rib and lumbar vertebrae.

Iridocorneal angle The acute angle between iris and cornea at the periphery of the anterior chamber of the eye.

Mandibular angle The angle formed by the lower margin of the body and the posterior margin of the ramus of the mandible.

Sternal angle Junction of the manubrium with the body of the sternum and it corresponds with the attachment of the second costal cartilage on either side of the sternum; Louis angle.

Visual angle Angle formed by lines drawn from the nodal point of the eye to the edges of the object viewed.

Angstrom (*ang'strom*) A unit of length used for atomic dimensions and light wave, named after Angstrom, Swedish physicist.

Anhidrosis (anidrosis) (*an'hi-dros'is*) Failure to sweat.

Anhidrotic (*an'hi-drot'ik*) An agent which suppresses sweating; reduction or absence of sweat glands.

Anhydrase (*an'hidr'ase*) An enzyme that catalyzes the removal of water from a compound.

Anhydremia (*an'hi-dre'me-a*) Deficiency of water in the blood.

Anileridine A synthetic opioid and strong analgesic medication. It is a narcotic pain reliever used to treat moderate to severe pain.

Anima (*an'i-ma*) The soul.

Animus (*an'i-mas*) A feeling of hate or anger toward someone or something.

Aniridia (*an'i-rid'e-a*) Congenital absence of iris.

Aniseikonia (*an'i-si-ko'ne-a*) Inequality of retinal images of both eyes.

Anisocytosis (*-si-to'sis*) Inequality in the size of red cells, which is prominently seen in megaloblastic anemia.

Anisomelia (*an-i-so-me'li-a*) Inequality of two paired limbs.

Anisometropia (*an-i'so-ma-tro'pe-a*) Inequality in the refractive power of both eyes.

Ankle (*ang'k'l*) Tarsus; the region of joint between leg and foot.

Ankylosing spondylitis Chronic inflammatory arthritis with a predilection for sacroiliac joints and spine. There is progressive stiffening and fusion of axial skeleton.

Ankylosis (*ang'ki-lo'sis*) Immobilization of joint by fibrous or bony union.

Artificial ankylosis Arthrodesis bony a union of bony surfaces resulting in complete immobility.

Extracapsular ankylosis Stiffness of a joint due to rigidity of the surrounding tissues.

False ankylosis Fibrous ankylosis.

Fibrous ankylosis Decreased mobility of the joint due to proliferation of the surrounding fibrous tissues.

Intracapsular ankylosis Stiffness of the joint due to adhesions between the articular surfaces of the joint.

Ankylostoma (*an'kil-os'to-ma*) A genus of nematodes of the family Ankylostomatidae, whose members are intestinal parasites of them *Ankylostoma duodenale Necator americanus* belonging to the suborder Strongylata causes ankylostomiasis.

Annulus (*an'u-lus*) Pl. **annuli**. A small ring or an encircling structure.

Annulus fibrosus Major outer part of intervertebral disk made of cartilage; ring of attachment of cardiac valve.

Anodontia (*an'o-don'she-a*) Congenital absence of some or all of the teeth.

Anodyne (*an'o-din*) Relieving pain; a medicine that relieves pain.

Anomaloscope An instrument used to test color blindness. It quantifies and characterizes color blindness.

Anomalous pulmonary venous drainage A rare congenital defect. Also known as Total Anomalous Pulmonary Venous Return (TAPVR). The four pulmonary veins drain abnormally to the right atrium through an abnormal connection.

Anomaly (*a-nom'a-le*) Deviation from normal especially as a result of congenital or hereditary defects.

Anomia (*a-nom'e-a*) Inability to produce correct word.

Anonychia (*an'o-nik'e-a*) Congenital absence of nail.

Anopheles (*a-nof'e-lez*) A genus of mosquitoes belonging to anophilinae subfamily, many of which are vectors of malaria.

Anoplasty (*a'no-plas'te*) Reconstructive surgery of the anus.

Anorchism (*an-or'kizm*) Absence of testes.

Anorchidism (*an-or'ki-diz"m*) The unilateral or bilateral partial or complete absence of testicular tissue, with or without rudimentary epididymal and spermatic cord remnants, in the presence of internal Wolffian duct development and normal external genitalia.

Anorexia (*an'o-rek'se-a*) A nervosa a psychoneurotic condition which develops during adolescence and affects predominantly girls who want to maintain a slim figure. It is characterized by weight loss, avoidance of high-calorie diet, distortion of body image and amenorrhea.

Anorexia nervosa A nervosa a psychoneurotic condition which develops during adolescence and affects predominantly girls who want to maintain a slim figure. It is characterized by weight loss, avoidance of high-calorie diet, distortion of body image and amenorrhea.

Anosmia (*an-oz'me-a*) Loss of sense of smell.

Anovular (Anovulatory) (*an-ov'u-ler*) Without ovulation.

Anoxemia (*an'ok-se'me-a*) A state of insufficient oxygen in the blood. It develops from one or more mechanisms such as alveolar hypoventilation, ventilation perfusion imbalance, right-to-left shunt and diffusion abnormalities.

Anoxia (*a-nok'se-a*) A deficiency of oxygen in a body tissue.

Anemic anoxia Due to decrease in hemoglobin in the blood.

Anoxic anoxia Due to reduced oxygen pressure in high altitudes.

Histotoxic anoxia An inability of tissue cells to utilize oxygen.

Stagnant anoxia Ischemic hypoxia.

Ansa (*an'sa*) Pl. **ansae**. Any structure in the form of a loop or an arc.

Ansiform In the form of a loop or an arc.

Ant- (Anti-) Combining word for counteractive, against.

Antabuse (Disulfiram) used in the treatment of alcohol use disorders by producing unpleasant side effects and sensitivity to alcohol.

Antacid (*an'ta-sid*) Substance neutralizing acid in the stomach and duodenum and are combinations of calcium, aluminium and magnesium salts.

Antagonist (*an-tag'o-nist*) Something opposing the action of another, such as muscle (antagonist muscle) or drug. α-Adrenergic antagonist α-blocker, β-adrenergic antagonist β-blocker (antagonist muscle).

Antazoline Antihistamine agent used for the symptomatic treatment of nasal congestion and allergic conjunctivitis.

Ante- Combining word for before.

Anteflexion (*an-te-flek'shun*) A bending forward of an organ, especially of the body of the uterus.

Antemortem (*an'temor'tem*) Before death.

Antenatal (*an'te-natal*) Before birth.

Antepartum (*an'te-par'tum*) Before delivery.

Antepartum hemorrhage Bleeding from or into the genital tract occurring from 24 to weeks of pregnancy and prior to delivery.

Anterior (*an-ter'e-or*) Before in relation to time or space; ventral; front surface of the body.

Anterior chamber In front of aqueous cavity of the eye, between the cornea and iris.

Anterior horn cell Motor neuron cell in the anterior horn of the gray matter of the spinal cord, whose axon innervates skeletal muscle.

Anteversion (*an'te-ver'zhun*) Turning or tilting forward.

Anthelix (antihelix) (*ant'he-liks*) An elevated ridge of cartilage anterior to the posterior part of the auricle helix.

Anthelmintic (*ant'hel-min'tik*) An agent that destroys or expels intestinal worms.

Anthracosis (*an'thra-ko'sis*) A blackening of lungs by carbon dust in city dwellers.

Anthracycline (*an'thra-si'klen*) Antineoplastic antibiotics that include daunomycin and doxorubicin.

Anthralin (*an'thra-lin*) A man-made version of a natural substance found in Goa powder, which is from the araroba tree.

Anthrax (*an'thrax*) An occupational disease of farmers, butchers and dealers in hides, hair, wool and bonemeal, and a disorder of domestic animals infected by inhalation or ingestion of spores of *Bacillus anthracis*. Initially there is an itchy papule on the skin which becomes a vesicle containing serosanguinous fluid. It dries to form a thick black eschar. It can give rise to pharyngitis, laryngitis or bronchopneumonia.

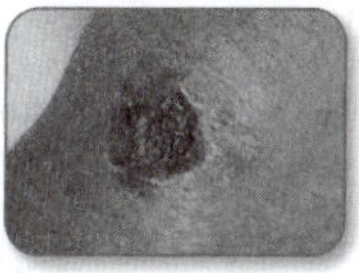

Anthrax lesion

Anthrop- (Anthropo-) Combining word for man.

Anthropometry (*an'thro-pom'e-tre*) Measurements of human body and parts, such as skull, bone, height and weight.

Anthropozoonosis Disease that is transmissible from an animal to a human or vice versa under natural conditions.

Antibiotic (*an'te-bi-ot'ik*) A chemical substance derived from mold or bacteria that kills or inhibits the growth of microorganisms.

Aminoglycoside antibiotic Bactericidal agents that have been administered parenterally for systemic treatment.

Antibiotic resistance Ability of microorganisms to resist the effects of antibiotics.

Antibiotic sensitivity test Response of the culture of bacteria to the antibiotic.

Beta-lactam antibiotic Penicillins and cephalosporins containing a four-membered β-lactam ring. They are bactericidal killing bacteria by interfering with their cell wall synthesis.

Broad spectrum antibiotic Effective against a wide range of bacteria.

Macrolide antibiotic Used to treat infections caused by gram-positive organisms. Erythromycin, clarithromycin, azithromycin and spiramycin are examples.

Tetracycline antibiotic Bacteriostatic agent inhibiting the growth of gram-positive and gram-negative bacteria.

Antibody (*an'ti-bod-e*) (Ab) Immunoglobulin with ability to react with specific antigen and are classified as agglutinin, bacteriolysin, hemolysin, opsonin or precipitin on the mode of their action. Antibodies are synthesized by B-lymphocytes that have been stimulated by the antigen bound to a cell surface receptor.

Anticardiolipin antibody Anti- phosphatid antibodies.

Antimitochondrial antibody Antibodies directed against mitochondrial antigens.

Antineutrophil cytoplasmic antibody (ANCA) Antibodies to proteinase 3 resulting in granular staining of neutrophil cytoplasm, found in vasculitis, Wegener's granulomatosis and rapidly progressive idiopathic glomerulonephritis.

Antinuclear antibody (ANA) Autoantibodies directed against nuclear components such as DNA, RNA and histones.

Antiphospholipid antibody A group of heterogeneous autoantibodies that are primarily directed against a complex antigen of which β_2-glycoprotein-1 is an essential component, found in SLE, primary antiphospholipid syndrome and recurrent cerebral ischemia.

Blocking antibody IgG reacting with an antigen, preventing it from reacting with IgE and prevent hypersensitivity reaction.

Complement-fixing antibody Activation of complement by IgM and IgG in the classic pathway and by IgA by alternate pathway, heterophite an antibody directed against heterophite antigens.

Immune antibody Induced by immunization.

Incomplete antibody An antibody that binds to bacteria or erythrocytes, but does not result in agglutination; an univalent antibody fragment, such as Fab fragment.

Monoclonal antibody A highly specific antibody formed by fusing a myeloma cell to a cell producing an antibody against a desired antigen.

Natural antibody Antibodies that react with antigens to which the individual had no exposure.

Neutralizing antibody Antibody on mixing with homologous infectious agent reduces the infectious titer.

Protective antibody Antibody responsible for immunity to an infectious agent as seen in passive immunity.

Anticholinergic (*an'ti-ko'lin-er'jik*) Antagonist to the action of parasympathetic or other cholinergic nerve fibers.

Anticholinesterase (*an'ti-ko'lin-es'ter-as*) Inhibitor of breakdown of acetylcholine by inhibiting the enzyme acetylcholinesterase.

Anticoagulant (*an'te-ko-ag'u-lant*) Prevent clotting of blood; any substance which prevents blood coagulation.

Anticonvulsant (*an'te-kon-vul'sant*) Agent preventing or arresting convulsions.

Antidepressant (*an'ti-de-pres'ant*) Drugs used in the treatment of depressive illness and they include tricyclic compounds lamitriptyline, imipramine, 5HT reuptake inhibitors (fluoxetine) monoamine oxidize inhibitors (phenelrine) and nor adrenergic and 5HT reuptake inhibitors (venlafaxine).

Antidiuretic hormone (ADH) Acts to maintain blood pressure, blood volume and tissue water content by controlling the amount of water and salts in the body.

Antidote (*an'ti-dot*) An agent that neutralizes a toxin or poison.

Chemical antidote A substance that unites with a poison to term a harmless chemical compound.

Mechanical antidote A substance that prevents the absorption of a poison.

Physiologic antidote Substance counteracting the effects of poison by production of opposing physiologic effects.

Universal antidote A substance that is effective against many poisons, such as activated charcoal.

Antidromic (*an"te-drom'ik*) Conducting impulses in a direction opposite to the normal.

Antiemetic (*an'te-e-met'ik*) Preventing or relieving nausea and vomiting; an agent that prevents or relieves nausea and vomiting.

Antigen (*an'ti-jen*) (Ag) Substance that is able to produce specific detectable immune reaction. adj. **antigenic**.

Australia antigen Hepatitis B surface antigen.

Blood group antigen Antigen found on the surface of erythrocytes that determine a blood grouping reaction with specific antiserum.

Capsular antigen Antigen found in the capsule of certain microorganisms.

Carcinoembryonic antigen (CEA) A glycoprotein of embryonic endodermal origin found in certain carcinomas.

Complete antigen Antigen capable of stimulating the formation of antibody with which it reacts.

Flagellar antigen The heat labile antigen associated with bacterial flagella.

Hepatitis-associated antigen (HAA) Surface antigen of hepatitis B virus; Australia antigen.

Hepatitis B core antigen (HBc Ag) Antigen found in the core of hepatitis B virus (Dane particle).

Hepatitis B e antigen (HBe Ag) An antigen of DNA core of hepatitis B virus.

Hepatitis B surface antigen (HBs Ag) A surface coat antigen of the hepatitis B virus.

Heterophile antigen An antigen common to more than one species.

Histocompatibility antigen Genetically determined isoantigens found on the surface of nucleated cells of most tissues.

Human lymphocyte antigen (HLA) Histocompatibility antigens on the surface of nucleated cells determined by a region on chromosome 6 having several genetic loci (A, B, C, DP, DQ, DR, MB, MT, and Te) that have a strong influence on human allotransplantation.

Incomplete antigen Haptene.

O antigen Somatic antigen of nonmotile bacteria.

Oncofetal antigen Carcinoembryonic antigen.

Organ-specific antigen Tissue specific antigen with a specificity to a particular organ.

Partial antigen Haptene.

Prostate specific antigen (PSA) An endopeptidase secreted by the epithelial cells of prostate.

Sensitized antigen A complex formed when antigen combines with specific antibody.

Somatic antigen Antigen in the body of a bacteria.

Species-specific antigen Antigenic components in the tissues and fluids that distinguish the species.

Tissue-specific antigen Organ specific antigens.

Tumor-specific antigen An antigen produced by certain tumors.

Viral antigen Antigen that is intimately associated with virus.

Antihemophilic factor (Factor VIII) Blood clotting protein.

Antihistamine (*an'te-his'ta-min*) Drug that blocks the effects of histamine.

Anti-Inflammatory (*an'te-in-flam'a-tor'e*) Drugs to reduce inflammation without directly antagonizing the causative agent.

Antiketogenic hormones The hormones which inhibit the formation of ketone bodies in the human body. Insulin prevents the formation of ketone bodies.

Antilymphocyte serum (ALS) Serum containing antibodies directed against lymphocytes that promote some degree of immunosuppression, used to reduce the occurrence of rejection of transplanted organs.

Antimetabolite (*an'ti-me-tab'o-lit*) A substance that competes with or antagonizes a particular metabolite.

Antimitotic A type of drug that blocks cell growth by stopping mitosis.

Antimutagen The agents that interfere with the mutagenicity of a substance.

Antimycotic (*an'ti-mi-kot'ik*) Antagonistic to fungi.

Antioxidant (*an'te-ok'si-dant*) Agents that protect against cell damage caused by oxygen free radicals.

Antiperistalsis (*an"te-per'i-stal'sis*) Reversed peristalsis.

Antipruritic (*an"te-proo-rit'ik*) Preventing or relieving itching.

Antipyretic (*an"te-pi-ret'ik*) Reducing fever; antifebrile; preventing or alleviating fever.

Antisepsis (*an"ti-sep'sis*) The destruction or inhibition of microorganisms on living tissues, thereby limiting or preventing the harmful results of infection.

Antiseptic (*an"ti-sep'tik*) An agent capable of preventing infection by inhibiting growth of infectious agents.

Antiserum (*an'ti-se-rum*) Serum containing one or more specific antibodies.

Antispasmodic (*an"te-spaz-mod'ik*) Preventing or relieving spasm.

Antitoxin (*an"te-tok'sin*) Antibody formed in response to poisonous substances of biologic origin such as diphtheria, gas gangrene, botulism or tetanus.

Antitragus (*an"te-tra-gus*) A projection of the auricle posterior to the tragus.

Antitussive (*an"te-tus'iv*) Drugs that suppress or relieve coughing.

Antivenin (antivenene) (*an"te-ven'in*) An antitoxin specific for an animal or insect venom.

Antrectomy The resection or surgery of the main stomach referred to as antrum, to treat gastric diseases causing the damage.

Antroscope (*an'tro-skop*) An instrument for visualization of maxillary antrum.

Antrostomy (*an'tros'to-me*) Creation of a permanent opening for drainage from maxillary sinus into inferior meatus.

Antrum (*an'trum*) Any nearly closed cavity having bony walls; pyloric end of the stomach.

Antrum of Highmore Maxillary sinus.

Antrum of stomach An upward sloping segment beyond angular notch on lesser curvature, and the mucosa does not secrete acid.

Mastoid antrum A cavity in the petrous portion of the temporal bone, communicating posteriorly with the mastoid cells and anteriorly with the middle ear.

Puncture of antrum Puncture of maxillary sinus by inserting a trochar near the floor of the nose through the sinus wall to drain fluid.

Anus (*a'nus*) The opening of the rectum through which fecal material is excreted. It is the lower opening of the alimentary tract found in the fold between the buttocks.

Artificial anus An opening into the bowel formed by colostomy.

Imperforate anus Anal atresia.

Anvil (*an'vil*) Incus, the second of the three small bones found in the middle ear.

Anxiety (*ang-zi'te*) Feeling of apprehension from the anticipation of danger, which may be internal or external.

Anxiety neurosis A predominant causeless fear and uncertainty free floating a pervasive unfocussed fear not attached to any idea.

Aorta (*a-or'ta*) The main trunk of the systemic arterial system. It arises from the base of the left ventricle and passes upward as the ascending aorta, then takes a turn backward and left as the arch of the aorta, and passes down as descending aorta. It has thoracic and abdominal portions and terminates at the left side of the body of the fourth vertebra by dividing into right and left common iliac arteries.

Abdominal aorta Gives branches to the abdominal organs and pelvic organs.

Ascending aorta Gives right and left coronary arteries to supply the myocardium.

Thoracic aorta Gives branches such as bronchial, esophageal, pericardial and nine pairs of intercostal arteries.

Aortic arch The part of aorta between the ascending and descending aorta. Gives three branches as innominate artery, left common carotid artery and left subclavian artery.

Aortic regurgitation Aortic insufficiency.

Aortic stenosis Narrowing of the aortic valve. It may be congenital, rheumatic or due to calcification of the aortic valve. The condition develops slowly and leads to hypertrophy of the left ventricle. There is fixed outflow obstruction and is associated with an ejection systolic murmur.

Aortic valve The semilunar valve between the left ventricle and the ascending aorta and it closes at the end of systole.

Aortitis (*a'or-ti'tis*) Inflammation of the aorta.

Aorto aortitis Condition affecting the aortic arch or thoracoabdominal aorta and its branches or both and exhibit features of cough, breathlessness, hemoptysis and pain.

Aortography (*a-or-tog'ra-fe*) Radiographic visualization of aorta and its branches after injection of a contrast medium.

APC Antigen-presenting cell; gene adenomatous polyposis coli gene.

Aperient (*a-per'e-ent*) Mild purgative.

Apex (*a'peks*) Pl. **apices**. The pointed extremity of a conical or pyramidal structure.

Apex beat Apical impulse.

Apex of lung Apical segment of the lung rising 2–3 cm above the clavicle.

Apex of heart Lowermost and outermost part of the heart formed by the left ventricle.

Apex Beat Apical impulse.

APGAR Score A simple test to evaluate neonate's postpartum status and potential for survival in the neonatal period by giving 0–2 marks to each of five parameters: Appearance, pulse, grimacereflex, activity or muscle tone and respiratory effort. Higher score is better. It is acronym of Virginia Apgar, US anesthetist.

Aphakia (*a-fa'ke-a*) Absence of lens of eye.

Aphasia (dysphasia) (*a-fa'zhea*) Total loss of the spoken speech due to dysfunction of the central mechanism in the brain.

Amnestic aphasia Inability to remember words.

Auditory aphasia Inability to understand spoken words in presence of normal hearing.

Broca's aphasia Expressive aphasia with impaired speech production with lesion in posterior end of left inferior frontal gyrus.

Conduction aphasia A lesion in the association tracts between motor and speech centers result in skipping or repeating words on substitution of one word to another.

Expressive aphasia Motor aphasia or Broca's aphasia.

Fluent aphasia Inability to understand the spoken word, but able to produce an incoherent speech.

Global aphasia A combination of a grossly nonfluent aphasia and fluent aphasia.

Jargon aphasia Aphasia in which nonsense words are repeated.

Motor aphasia Broca's aphasia.

Nominal aphasia Difficulty in finding correct name for an object.

Sensory aphasia Loss of ability to comprehend the meaning of written or spoken words.

Syntactical aphasia Inability to arrange words in proper sequence.

Wernicke's aphasia Sensory aphasia due to an injury to Wernicke's area in the temporal lobe of dominant hemisphere.

Aphonia (*a-fo'ne-a*) Loss of voice.

Aphtha (*af'thah*) Pl. **aphthae**. Small ulcers on the mucous membrane of the mouth.

Apical abscess Most common form of dental abscess, caused by infection of the root canal of the tooth.

Apical ballooning syndrome An acute, reversible cardiac dysfunction that is noted in postmenopausal females.

Apicectomy (*a'pi-sek'to-me*) Excision of air cells in the apex of the petrous part of the temporal bone.

Aplasia (*a-pl'zhea*) Lack of development of an organ or tissue; improper or defective regeneration.

Apnea (*ap'ne'-a*) Temporary cessation of breathing.

Sleep apnea Absence of airflow at the nose and mouth for at least 10 seconds during sleep and they are repetitive. It may be central due to cessation of respiratory efforts of the chest due to failure of rhythm genesis or obstructive due to obstruction to extrathoracic airway at the level of oropharynx or mixed.

Apneusis (*ap-noo'sis*) A sustained inspiratory effort leading to an abnormal respiration.

Apocrine (*ap'o-krin*) Coiled tubular glands, such as sweat glands.

Apomorphine (*ap'o-mor'fen*) A morphine derivative that acts as an emetic and expectorant.

Aponeurosis (*ap'o-noo-ro'sis*) An expanded fibrous sheet that attaches muscle to a bone or other tissue.

Apophysis (*a-pof'i-sis*) Pl. **apophyses**. A projection from a bone; bony outgrowth without an independent center of ossification.

Apophysitis (*a-pofi-zi'tis*) Inflammation of an apophysis.

Apoplexy (*ap'o-plex'se*) Sudden stroke; an effusion of blood into a tissue or organ.

Apoptosis (*a-pop-to'sis*) An intrinsic program of cell death. It is characterized by chromatin condensation and DNA degradation.

Apothecary (*a-poth'e-kar'e*) A druggist or pharmacist.

Appendectomy (*ap'en-dek'to-me*) Surgical removal of vermiform appendix.

Appendicitis (*a-pen'di-si'tis*) An inflammation of the mucous membrane or lymph follicles of the vermiform appendix. It may be obstructive (colicky abdominal pain later shifting to the right iliac fossa, nausea, vomiting, fever) or nonobstructive (continuous dull aching pain in the abdomen, aggravated by movement).

Appendicostomy (*a-pen'di-kos'to-me*) Surgical opening into the intestine through the tip of appendix.

Appendicular (*ap"en-dik'u-lar*) Relating to an appendage and especially a limb.

Appendix (vermiform appendix) (*a-pen'diks*) Pl. **appendices**. Various appendages to organs; when unqualified refers to vermiform appendix.

Appendix epiploica A number of small sacs of the peritoneum distended with fat projecting from serous coat of the large intestine along taeniae coli.

Vermiform appendix A short blind ended, worm-like intestinal diverticulum extending from the blind end of the cecum.

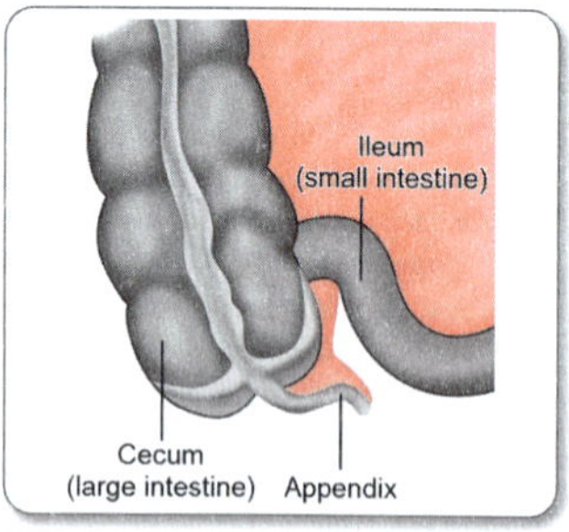

Vermiform appendix

Applanation (*apla-na'shun*) Abnormal flattening of the corneal surface.

Apperception (*ap'er-sep'shun*) Comprehension modified by one's own emotions; process of understanding through linkage with previous experience.

Appestat (*ap'i-stat*) Brain center concerned in controlling appetite.

Apposition (*ap'o-zish'un*) Positioning of things in proximity; the condition of being placed together; the relationship of fracture fragments to one another.

Apraxia (Dyspraxia) (*a-prak'se-a*) An inability to execute purposeful movements without impairment of muscle power, sensation or coordination.

Aproctia Congenital absence of the anus or its opening.

Aprosexia (*ap'ro-seksia*) Inability to concentrate.

Aprotinin (*ap'ro-tin'in*) A hemostatic agent that inhibits the fibrinolytic enzyme plasmin.

Apyrexia (*a'pi-rek-se'a*) Absence of fever.

Aqueduct (*ak'we-dukt*) A conduit or canal.

Aqueous humor Transparent fluid found in the aqueous chambers of the eye and it is produced by the ciliary processes.

Arachidonic acid (*a-rak'i-don'ik*) A 20-carbon polyunsaturated fatty acid with 4 double boosts, found in the phospholipid component of cell membranes, precursor of prostaglandins and leukotrienes.

Arachnidism An injury caused by venom from spider's bite.

Arachnodactyly (*a-rak'no-dak'ti-le*) Abnormally long and slender toes.

Arachnoid (Arachnid Mater) (*a-rak'noid*) Resembling a cob-web; arachnoid membrane.

Arachnoid mater A delicate fibrous membrane interposed between the duramater and the pia mater, which cover the brain (an encephali) and spinal cord (a spinalis). It is closely applied to dura, but there is a subarachnoid space between arachnoid and pia mater.

Arachnoiditis (*a-rak'noi-di'tis*) Inflammation of arachnoid membrane.

Arbor (*ar'bor*) A tree-like; arthropod-borne.

Arborvirus (*ar'bor-virus*) RNA viruses which multiply in both vertebrate host and insect vector; arthropod-borne viruses.

ARC AIDS related complex.

Arc-eye Conjunctivitis and keratitis from exposure to welding arc.

Arch (arche, archi, archo) Any anatomical structure having a curved outline.

Aortic arch The curved part between the ascending aorta and descending aorta; a series of arterial channels encircling the embryonic pharynx of potentially six pairs 1 and 2 disappear; pair 3 takes part in the formation of carotids, 4th becomes the arch of the aorta, 5th disappears and 6th forms the proximal part of the pulmonary arteries, and until birth, the ductus arteriosus.

Plantar arch The arterial arch formed by the external plantar artery naming across the bases of metatarsal bones and the deep branch of dorsalis pedis artery.

Pulmonary arch The fifth aortic arch on left side becoming pulmonary artery.

Supraorbital arch Bony arch formed by the upper margin of the orbit.

Zygomatic arch Arch formed by temporal process of the zygomatic bone and zygomatic process of the temporal bone.

Archenteron (*ark-en'ter-on*) Gastrocele; primitive digestive cavity of embryo.

Arcus (*ar'kus*) An arch.

Arcus alveolaris mandibulae The arch formed by the alveolar process of the mandible or maxilla.

Arcus dentalis Dental arch.

Arcus juvenilis An opaque grayish ring at the periphery of the cornea in young individuals.

Arcus plantaris Plantar arch.

Arcus senilis An opaque, grayish ring at the periphery of the cornea within the sclerocorneal junction frequently occurring in elderly persons.

Areola (*a-re'o-la*) Any small area; a circular area of diffuse pigmentation, as around the nipple of the breast or around a wheal or the part of iris around the pupil.

Areolar tissue A type of connective tissue that is present throughout the human body.

Argasidae (*ahr-gas'i-de*) A family of arthropods, the soft ticks.

Argentaffin cells (*ar-jen'ta-fin*) Refers to cells that reacts with silver and get stained brown or black.

Aregentaffin reaction A staining that involves reduction of ammoniacal silver to metallic iron, used to identify APUD system.

Argentaffinoma (Carcinoid) (*ar'jen-taf'i-no-ma*) Carcinoid tumor.

Arginine (*ar'ji-nen*) An amino acid found in proteins. It participates, in urea cycle to produce urea, and in the synthesis of creatine.

Argyll Robertson pupil Unequal, irregular, miotic pupils having presence of accommodation reflex but absence of light and ciliospinal reflexes, noted in neurosyphilis named after Douglas Mo-ray Cooper Lamb Argyll Robertson, Scottish physician.

Argyria (*ar-ji're-a*) Silver poisoning with slate-gray discoloration of skin and deeper tissues.

Ariboflavinosis (*a-ri'bo-fla'vi-no'sis*) A condition caused by deficiency of riboflavin in the diet presenting with cheilitis, angular stomatitis and magenta tongue.

Arnold-Chiari malformation Structural defect in posterior foss, hindbrain. It is a condition in which brain tissue extends into the spinal canal, present at birth.

Arousal (*a-rou'zal*) The act of stimulating someone sexually.

Arrhenoblastoma (*a-re'no-blas-to'ma*) A rare tumor of ovary that secretes male sex hormone to cause virilization.

Arrhythmia (*a-rith'me-a*) Loss or an irregularity of rhythm.

Cardiac arrhythmia A disturbance in the electrical activity of the heart. It may be paroxysmal or continuous. It may cause bradycardia or tachycardia. Arrhythmia may be supraventricular (sinus, atrial or junctional) or ventricular.

Reperfusion arrhythmia Arrhythmia occurring in the damaged heart following thrombolysis or angioplasty due to reperfusion.

Respiratory arrhythmia Disturbance in normal quiet rhythm of inspiration and expiration becoming abnormal as in Cheyne-Stokes breathing, and Riot's breathing.

Sinus arrhythmia Phasic alteration of the heart rate during respiration. There is an increase in sinus rate during inspiration and decrease during expiration.

Arsenic (*ar'se-nik*) A highly poisonous, steel-gray metal, symbol As atomic no. 33. Acute poisoning results in shock and death. Chronic poisoning is associated with skin pigmentation, hyperkeratosis of palms and soles, transverse lines on the finger nails and peripheral neuropathy.

Arter-arteri-, arterio Combing word for artery.

Arteriectomy/Arteriotomy A surgical excision of an artery or part of an artery. May be performed for diagnostic purpose or to reconstruct a blocked artery.

Arteriogram (*ar'te-re-o-gram*) A radiogram an artery taken after injection of radio-opaque substance into an artery.

Arteriography (*ar-ter'e-og'ra-fe*) Radiographic visualization of artery.

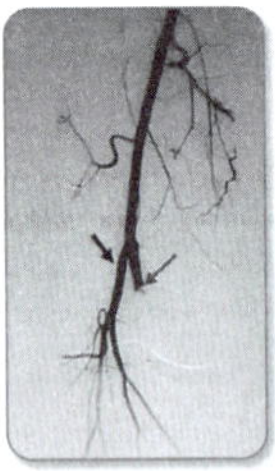

Arteriography of popliteal artery

Arteriole (*ar-ter'e-ol*) A minute branch of an artery with muscular wall; a terminal artery continuous with the capillary network.

Arteriolitis Inflammation of the arterioles, which may complicate severe hypertension.

Arterioplasty (*ar-ter'e-o-plas'te*) Surgical reconstruction of the wall of an artery.

Arteriosclerosis (*ar-ter'e-o-skle-ro'sis*) Arterial hardening.

Arteriovenous anastomosis A direct connection between arterioles and venules, by passing the capillary network, through muscular microvessels that are 20–130 pm wide.

Arteriovenous aneurysm A dilated arteriovenous shunt.

Arteriovenous malformation An abnormal connection between arteries and veins, usually in the brain or spine.

Artery (*ar'ter-e*) Pl. **arteries**. A vessel carrying blood away from the heart. There are two divisions: pulmonary and systemic. Pulmonary and umbilical arteries convey deoxygenated blood. Systemic arteries carry oxygenated blood to the different parts of the body.

Arthr (Arthro) Combining word for joint; articulation.

Arthralgia (*ar-thral'jea*) Pain in the joint.

Arthrectomy Surgical excision of a joint.

Arthritis (*ar-thri'tis*) Pl. **arthritides**, adj. **arthritic**. Inflammation of a joint.

Acute septic arthritis Bacterial infection of the joint presenting with hot, painful, tender, swollen joint.

Degenerative arthritis Osteoarthritis.

Gouty arthritis An inflammatory arthritis from crystals of monosodium urate monohydrate derived from hyperuricemic body fluids.

Gonococcal arthritis Arthritis usually of knee joint produced by gonococcal infection.

Infective arthritis Septic arthritis and arthritis associated with specific infections such as gonorrhea, brucellosis, tuberculosis, leprosy, and syphilis.

Juvenile idiopathic arthritis Inflammatory arthritis of children.

Juvenile rheumatoid arthritis Arthritis with an age of onset less than 16 years that may present as oligoarthritis, polyarthritis with systemic manifestations such as hepatosplenomegaly and lymphadenopathy.

Lyme arthritis Large joint arthritis from *Borrelia burgdorferi*.

Palindromic arthritis Transient recurrent arthritis of large joints, of undetermined etiology.

Psoriatic arthritis A seronegative inflammatory arthritis found in patients with psoriasis.

Reactive arthritis Arthritis following an enteric infection Reiter's disease is characterized by reactive arthritis.

Rheumatoid arthritis Chronic inflammatory polyarthritis. There is symmetrical, deforming polyarthritis affecting small and large synovial joints, with associated systemic disturbances. There is presence of circulating antiglobulin antibodies (rheumatoid factor). The course of the disease is prolonged with exacerbations and remissions.

Syphilitic arthritis Painful peri articular swelling or painless effusion (congenital syphilis) joint involvement (acquired syphilis).

Tuberculous arthritis Joint involvement in tuberculosis.

Arthrodesis (*ar"thro-de'sis*) Refers to orthopedic surgery in which two or more bones in a joint are fused to become one larger bone.

Arthrodial joint (gliding joint) A gliding joint, or a synovial joint that allows only gliding movement in the plane of the articular surfaces.

Arthrodysplasia (*ar'thro-dis-pla'ze-a*) A hereditary disorder characterized by deformity of various joints.

Arthrography (*ar-throg'ra-fe*) Radiography of a joint; radiography of a synovial joint after injection of a contrast medium.

Arthrogryposis (*ar'thro-gri-po-sis*) A fixation of joint by contractures and fusion.

Arthropathy (*ar-throp'a-the*) Any joint disease.

Arthroplasty (*ar'thro-plas'te*) Creation of an artificial joint; plastic repair of a joint to restore its integrity and function.

Arthropyosis (*ar'thro-pi-o'sis*) Formation of pus in a joint cavity.

Arthroscope (*ar'thro-skop*) An endoscopy for examining the interior of a joint.

Arthrostomy (*ar-thros'to-me*) Surgical creation of a temporary opening into a joint cavity to facilitate drainage.

Articulation (*ar'tik"yu-la'shun*) The place of union between two or more bones as in joint. It may be immovable (synarthrosis), slightly movable (amphiarthrosis) or freely movable (diarthrosis); pronunciation of words and sentences.

Articulator An instrument designed to perform mechanical reproduction of jaw movement using cast stone models of dentition.

Artifact (artefact) (*ar'ti-fakt*) A substance or signal that interferes with or obscures the interpretation of a study; any abnormality in histology and radiography produced by the technique used; anything produced artificially.

Artificial Not natural.

Artificial insemination Depositing of sperm of the partner or of a donor—in the female reproductive tract in an attempt to impregnate.

Artificial reproduction Artificial insemination, ovum donation, *in vitro* fertilization, surrogate motherhood, and cryopreserved embryo transplantation.

Artificial sphincter An inflatable cuff implanted around the upper urethra to squeeze the urethra shut and provide urinary control.

Artificial tears A solution containing 0.5% carboxymethyl cellulose or 5% polyvinyl alcohol for treatment of xerophthalmia.

Artificial respiration Breathing induced by some manipulative technique when natural respiration has ceased or is faltering. It is used on a patient with a beating heart or as part of the CPR to achieve the internal respiration.

Asbestosis (*as-bes-to'sis*) A diffuse interstitial fibrosis of lung parenchyma caused by exposure to asbestos. The fibrosis is diffuse with airspace enlargement or honeycombing.

Ascariasis (*as'kar-ri'a-sis*) Round worm infestation. The nematode *Ascaris lumbricoides* is a pale yellow worm of 20 cm and gains entry by eating food contaminated with immature ova. They hatch in the duodenum and larva migrate through the lungs ultimately reach small intestine and mature. The presentation may be abdominal discomfort, passage of worms in stools or vomiting of worms, intestinal obstruction, blockage of bile or pancreatic duct and obstruction of appendix.

Ascaris (*as'ka-ris*) A genus of round worm that is parasitic in small intestine of humans.

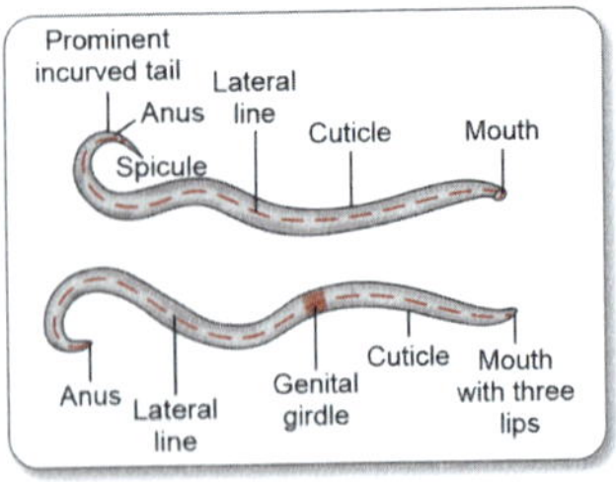

Ascaris

Ascites (hydroperitoneum) (*a-si'tez*) Accumulation of free fluid in the peritoneal cavity. It causes abdominal distension with fullness of flanks. Its presence is demonstrable by shifting dullness on percussion and a fluid thrill when the amount of fluid is large. Cirrhosis of liver, nephrotic syndrome, congestive heart failure, hypoproteinemia, tuberculosis, malignancy form the common causes for ascites. Ascites is a physical sign.

Ascorbic acid (*a-skor'bik*) Vitamin C; antiscorbutic vitamin preventing scurvy.

Asepsis (*a-sep'sis*) A condition without any living pathogenic microorganisms.

Asherman syndrome Cessation of menstruation and/or infertility caused by intrauterine adhesions, named after Israeli Gynecologist Joseph Asherman.

Asparaginase (*as-par'a-jin-as*) An enzyme catalyzing the hydrolysis of asparagine to aspartic acid and ammonia; an enzyme from *Escherichia coli* used in the treatment of acute leukemia.

Asparagine (*as-par'a-jen*) A nonessential amino acid occurring in proteins.

Aspartic acid (aspartate) (*a-spar'tik*) Aminosuccinic acid, amino acid found in the protein.

Asperger's syndrome *psy* Children who have autistic behavior without problems with language.

Aspergillosis (*as'per-jil'o-sis*) A disorder initiated by inhalation of the spores liberated by the fungi of Aspergillus, mainly *Aspergillus fumigatus* the clinical manifestations depend on the immunological reactivity of the individual and present as hypersensitivity reaction of aspergillus (allergic bronchopulmonary asper gillosis, bronchocentric granulomatosis, and mucoid impaction of bronchus, extrinsic allergic alveolitis, and asthma) saprophytic colonization (aspergilloma) or tissue invasive aspergillosis.

Aspergillus (*as'per-jil'us*) A mould-like fungus with a worldwide distribution in the soil and decaying vegetation. The spores of size of two to three microns in diameter are arranged like a holy water sprinkler at the end of a filament. The spores get separated readily and present in air in large numbers especially during winter months and can be readily inhaled. *Aspergillus fumigatus* is the common example. Other species are *A. niger, A. terreus* and *A. nidulans.*

Aspermia (*a-sper'me-a*) Lack of expulsion of semen following ejaculation.

Asphyxia (*as-fik'se-a*) Condition produced by lack of oxygen in air and it results in hypoxemia and hypercapnia.

Aspiration (*as'pi-ra'shun*) The act of inhaling; removal of fluid or gas by suction from body cavity.

Aspiration pneumonia Inhalation of acidic gastric contents in comatose patients, leading to acute inflammation of lung parenchyma.

Vacuum aspiration Removal of uterine contents by application of vacuum.

Aspirin (acetylsalicylic acid) (*as'pi-rin*) Acetylsalicylic acid, widely used analgesic and antipyretic. It inhibits platelet aggregation, used prophylactically in small doses in coronary artery disease, transient ischemic disease and thromboembolic condition of the brain.

Assay Analysis of the chemical composition or strength of substance.

Assimilation (*a-sim'i-la'shun*) Conversion of nutrient substances into living tissue; *psy* absorption of new experience.

Association area Association cortex.

Astasia (*as-ta'zhea*) Inability to stand due to muscular incoordination.

Aster (*a'ster*) The star-shaped arrangement of microtubules that is characteristic of a mitotic or meiotic spindle own tissue.

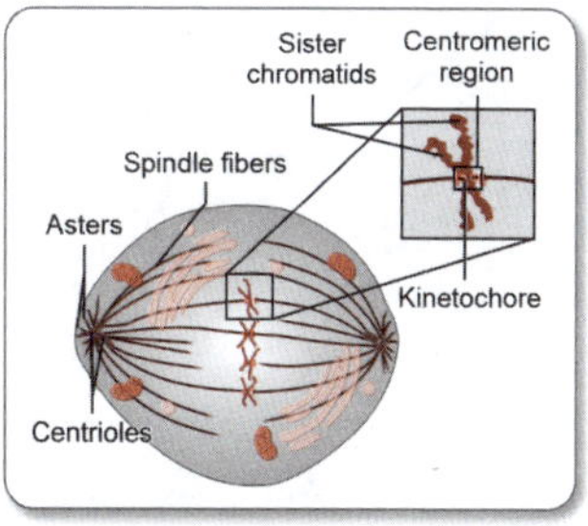

Asters pattern in mitotic cell division

Asthenia (*as-the'ne-a*) Loss of strength; disability.

Asthenopia (*as'thi-no'pe-a*) Weakness of eyes accompanied by pain, headache and dimness of vision.

Asthma (*az'mah*) Bronchial asthma a complex and heterogeneous syndrome characterized by episodic intrathoracic airways obstruction, airways hyperresponsiveness and airways inflammation resulting in occurrence of dyspnea and wheezing which varies widely over time either spontaneously or in response to treatment.

Aspirin-sensitive asthma Asthma following aspirin or NSAIDs. It develops without any previous history of asthma or atopy.

Exercise induced asthma Initiation or exacerbation of bronchospasm by exercise. Dyspnea may be a relatively occult manifestation of hypersensitive airways.

Extrinsic atopic asthma Exposure to antigen in atopic individuals stimulates peripheral lymphoid tissues to synthesize IgE, and initiate asthma.

Extrinsic nonatopic asthma Constant exposure to a large amount of antigen may stimulate appearance of antibodies, which combine with allergens to form immune complexes and initiate asthma.

Intrinsic asthma Asthma in middle aged in whom an extrinsic allergen cannot be identified nocturnal a asthma associated with deep, nocturnal worsening.

Occupational asthma Asthma due to inhalation of airborne dusts, vapors and fumes encountered in work place.

Astigmatism (*a-stigma-tizm*) A lens having different curvatures in different meridians; a condition of unequal curvatures in the refractive surfaces of eye and prevent the focusing of ray, at a single point in retina.

Astragalus (*as-trag'a-les*) A preparation or extract of this root; talus *see* Table of bones.

Astringent (*a-strin'joint*) A medicine which draws togethers, constricts, binds.

Astrocyte (astroglial cell) (*as'tro-sit*) Spider cell, forms the structural framework for the neurons. Their foot processes are closely associated with blood vessels to form the blood-brain barrier.

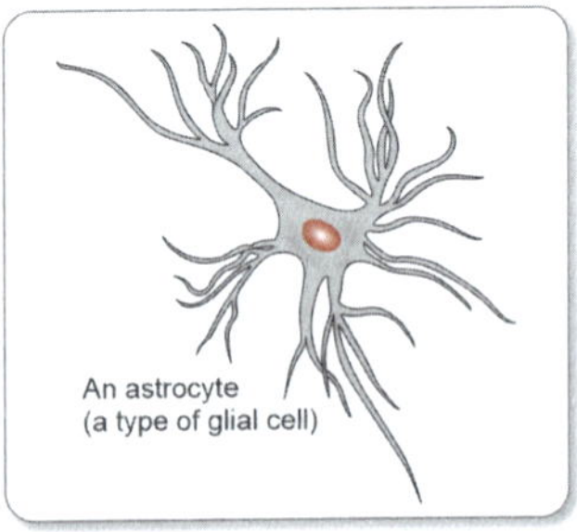

Astrocyte

Astrocytoma (*as'tro-si-to'ma*) A diffuse and infiltrating tumor which may be solid or partly cystic occurs at any age. In children it occurs in the cerebellum.

Malignant astrocytoma Glioblastoma multiforme, which undergoes degenerative changes, and occurs in cerebrum of adults. It contains all types of glial cells.

Asymptomatic Without signs or symptoms of disease.

Asynclitism (*a-sin'kli'tizm*) Oblique presentations of the fetal head during labor; maturation of the nucleus and cytoplasm of blood cells at different times.

Asyndesis (*a-sin'de-sis*) A disorder of language wherein the related elements of a sentence can not be brought together.

Asynergy (*a-sin'er-je*) Lack of coordination between different parts or organs.

Asystole (*a-sis'to-le*) Cardiac arrest, absence of heart beat.

Ataraxia A state of serene calmness.

Atavism (*a'ta-vi-zm*) Recurrence of a trait found in a remote ancestor but not in near generations.

Ataxia (*a-tak'se-a*) Imperfect control over voluntary actions.

Ataxia-telangiectasia An autosomal recessive condition characterized by sinopulmonary infections, choreoathetosis, slurring speech and muscle atrophy and oculocutaneous telangiectasia.

Cerebellar ataxia Ataxia due to cerebellar disease, with ataxic gait.

Friedreich's ataxia Friedreich's ataxia is an inherited progressive nervous system disorder causing loss of balance.

Frontal ataxia Inability to walk normally due to frontal lobe lesions, walks with slow, short shuffling steps, dragging feet on the ground.

Kinetic ataxia A motor ataxia.

Motor ataxia Incoordination occurs only during movement.

Sensory ataxia Loss of proprioception, ataxia is apparent in the affected limb on closure of eyes.

Static ataxia Limb outstretched horizontally sways up and down.

Atel- (*atelo*) Combining word for incomplete, imperfectly developed.

Atelectasis (*at'e-lek'ta-sis*) Collapse, referring to lung; failure of expansion of lung in neonate.

Ateliosis Failure to achieve perfection.

Atenolol (*a-ten'o-lol*) A β-blocker medicine, used to treat high blood pressure and irregular heartbeats.

Atheroma (*ath'er-o'ma*) Atherosclerosis, a patchy focal disease of the arterial wall. Coronary arteries are at high-risk.

Atherosclerosis (*ath'er-o"-skle-ro'sis*) A condition caused by intramural deposition of LDL, secondary to exposure of smooth muscle to lipid, resulting in platelet induced smooth muscle proliferation, formation of fibrotic plaques and calcification.

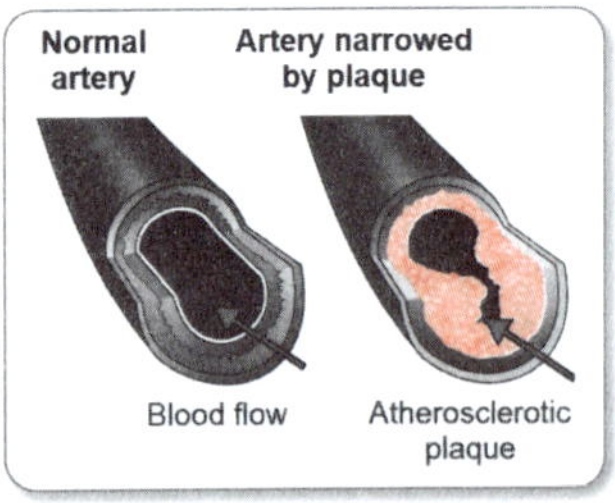

Atherosclerosis

Athetosis (*ath'i-to'sis*) Slower writhing movements of the limbs.

Athlete's foot Dermatomycosis of the toe webs and soles of the feet of athletes resulting in maceration, erosion and pruritus. *Trichophyton rubrum* is the common causative agent.

Athyreosis (*a-th're-o'sis*) Hypothyroidism.

Atlas (*at'las*) The first cervical vertebra; *see* Table of bones.

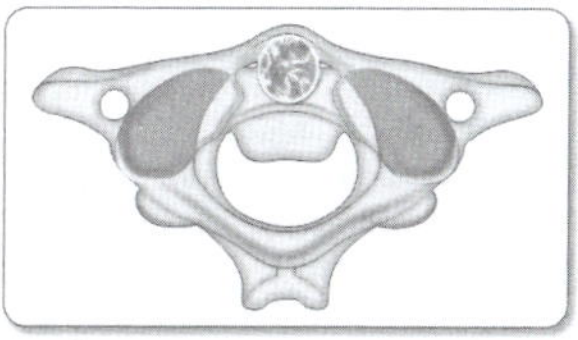

Atlas bone

Atony (*at'o-ne*) Lack of tone or strength.

Atopy (*at'o-pe*) A genetic predisposition to develop an immediate hypersensitivity against substances of day-to-day exposure from the environment and there is an increased production of IgE. Common examples of diseases of atopy are bronchial asthma, allergic rhinitis, and atopic dermatitis.

ATP Adenosine Triphosphate

Atresia (*a-tre-zhea*) Congenital absence of a normal opening or normally patent lumen.

Atrioventricular bundle (av bundle, bundle of His) A branch of nerve cells that extends from AV node. It receives the electrical signal from the AV node and carries it to the Purkinje fibers.

Atrioventricular node Electrically connects the heart's atria and ventricles to coordinate beating on the top of the heart.

Atrium (*a'tre-um*) Pl. **atria**. A chamber, or cavity to which several chambers are connected; upper smaller chamber of the heart on either side which receives blood from vena cavae (right) and from pulmonary veins (left) and convey it to the ventricles of the same side; tympanic cavity that lies deep to the tympanic membrane; a part of gas exchanging portion of the lung, the alveolar duct from which alveolar sacs open.

Atrophy (*at'ro-fe*) Wasting wherein there is diminution in the size of a cell, tissue, organ or part.

Atropine (*at'ro-pen*) An anticholinergic alkaloid obtained from *Atropa belladonna* used as a smooth muscle relaxant. It is antisecretory, mydriatic and anticholinergic.

Attachment disorder A behavioral disorder that affects the ability to form and maintain relationships.

Attenuation (*a-ten'u-a'shun*) Diminution of an effect; reduction of virulence.

Attrition The act of weakening or exhausting by constant harassment abuse of attack.

Audi (audio) Combining word for hearing.

Audiogram A graph showing the results of pure-tone hearing test.

Audiometer (*aw'de-ome-ter*) An instrument to test the power of hearing.

Auditory (*aw'de-ta'ri*) Acuity and clarity at which a particular sound can be heard.

Auditory nerve Runs from cochlea to the brain stem. It is 8th cranial nerve and transmits sounds and equilibrium information from inner ear to the brain.

Auerbach's plexus (myenteric plexus) (*ow'er-baks*) Autonomic plexus found between the layers of gut muscle from midesophagus downward that exhibits a motor control of peristalsis, named after Leopold Auerbach, German anatomist.

Aura (*aw'rah*) A subjective (illusionary or hallucinatory) or objective (mator) event making the onset of epileptic attack or migraine.

Aural (*aw'r'l*) Pertaining to or perceived by ear; pertaining to aura.

Auricle (*aw'ri-k'l*) Part of the external ear not contained within the head; the pinna, or flap of the ear.

Auriscope (*aw'ri-skop*) Otoscope.

Auscultation (*aws'kul-ta'shun*) Listening for sounds made by different structures of the body directly (by applying ear) or indirectly (through stethoscope).

Auscultatory gap Interval of absolute or relative silence occasionally found on listening over an artery during deflation of the blood pressure cuff. It begins at a variable point below the systolic pressure and continues from 10mm–50 mm.

Australia antigen Hepatitis B virus antigen first isolated from an Australian aborgine. It is found in hepatocyte cytoplasm.

Aut- (auto-) Combining word for self.

Autism (*aw'tizm*) A condition wherein the subjective, self-centerd trends of thought dominate the person.

Autoagglutination (*aw'to-a-gloo'ti-na'shun*) Clumping of an individual's cells by his own serum, as in auto-hem-agglutination.

Autoantibody (*aw'to-an'ti-bod'e*) An antibody produced in response to and reacting against an endogenous body constituent.

Autochthonous (*aw-tok'tha-nas*) Pertaining to autochthons; indigenous.

Autoclave (*aw'to-klav*) An apparatus for effective sterilization by steam under pressure.

Autocrine (*aw'to-krin*) A secretion of a cell which binds to the receptors and influence the function of cell type that produced it.

Autogenous vaccine A vaccine prepared from cultures of microorganisms obtained from an individual and then used to immunize that same individual against further spread and progress of some microorganisms.

Autograft (*aw'to-graft*) A graft of tissue obtained from another site in or on the body of an individual receiving it, autologous graft.

Autoimmune disease Conditions in which immune system mistakenly damages healthy cells in a body.

Autoimmunity (*aw"to-i-mun'i-te*) Reaction of an organism's immune system to self-antigens and there is production of autoantibody. It is closely linked to connective tissue disease.

Autoinoculation (*aw"to-in-ok'u-la'shun*) Inoculation with microorganisms from one's own body.

Autointoxication A state of being poisoned by toxic substances produced within the body.

Autologous (*aw-tol'a-gus*) Related to self.

Autologous blood Transfusion collection and reinfusion of the patient's own blood.

Autologous blood donation Donation of a person's own blood before scheduled surgery to make the blood available in case a transfusion is necessary during or after surgery.

Autologous bone marrow transfusion A treatment modality for leukemia patients, a cytopreserved bone marrow taken from the patient during remission is reinfused during relapse.

Autologous transplant A patient receiving a transplant of his or her own tissue.

Autolysis (*aw-tol'i-sis*) Destruction of cells as a result of the action of autolysin; enzymatic digestion of cells.

Automatism (*aw-tom'a-tizm*) Automatic performance of acts representative of unconscious symbolic activity.

Autonomic nervous system The part of nervous system that controls involuntary body functions. It has two divisions as sympathetic or thoracolumbar division and the parasympathetic or craniosacral division a triad dilated pupils, moist palms and tachycardia, noted in schizophrenics.

Autoploidy Having sets of chromosomes that originated within the same species only.

Autopsy (necropsy, postmortem) (*aw'top-se*) The postmortem examination of a body; necropsy.

Autoradiograpy (radioautopphy) (*aw"to-ra"de-og'ra-fe*) A technique using X-ray film to visualize molecules or fragments of molecules that have been radioactively labeled.

Autoscopy A visual experience where the subject sees an image of self in external space, viewed from within his/her own physical body.

Autosome (*aw'to-som*) Nonsex chromosome.

Autotransfusion (*aw"to-trans-fu'zhun*) Transfusion back into the body of blood removed.

Autotrophic (lithotrophic) (*aw"to-tro'fik*) Relating to a living thing that can make its own food from simple chemical substances such as carbon dioxide.

Autovaccination Vaccination of an individual by material from the individual's own body or with a vaccine prepared from such material.

Autovaccine (autogenous vacine) (*aw'to-vak'sen*) A vaccine prepared from cultures of organisms isolated from the patient's own tissues or secretions.

Auxesis (*awk-se'sis*) Increase of cell size without cell division.

Auxiliary liver transplantation A technique in which all or part of the graft is placed in the abdomen and the native liver being left in situ.

Auxotrophic (*awk"so-tro'fik*) The inability of an organism to synthesize a particular organic compound required for its growth by itself.

AV block Atrioventricular block. Any delay in conduction or failure of an electrical impulse to reach the ventricular conduction system.

First-degree AV block A delay in conduction with prolonged PR interval and all the P waves are conducted to the ventricle.

Second-degree AV block There are dropped beats as some impulses from atria fail to reach ventricle.

Third-degree AV block No atrial beats are conducted to the ventricle.

Avascular (*a-vas'ku-ler*) Not vascular; without blood.

Avascularization (*a-vas"ku-ler-i-za'shun*) Loss of vascularity, as by scarring.

Aversion therapy A form of psychological treatment in which the patient is exposed to a stimulus while simultaneously being subjected to some form of discomfort.

Avitaminosis A condition resulting from a deficiency of a particular vitamin.

Avoidant (*a-void'ant*) Tending to avoid intimacy or interaction with others especially as a means of coping with anxiety or stress.

Avulsion **(Evulsion)** (*a-vul'shun*) A tearing away of a part of structure.

Axilla (*ak-sil'a*) Pl. **axillae**. The armpit.

Axis (*ak'sis*) Pl. **axes**. The line passing through the center of a body or about which a structure revolves; central line of the body; second cervical vertebra; an artery that divides immediately upon its origin.

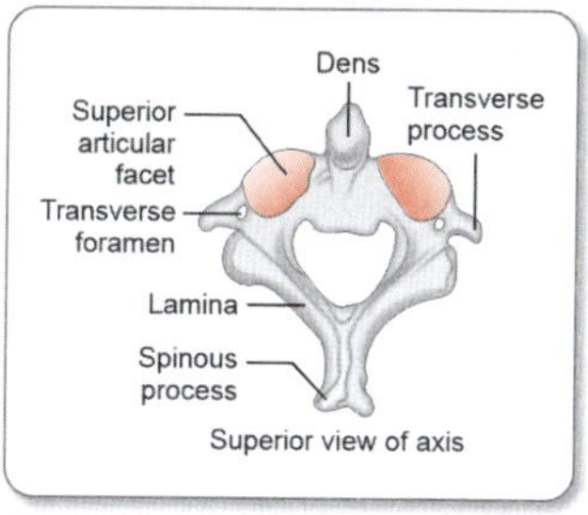

Axis bone (C2 vertebra)

Axitinib A third-generation selective inhibitor of VEGF receptors 1–3 and is indicated for the treatment of patients with advanced renal cancer.

Axolemma (*ak'so-lem'a*) The surface membrane of an axon.

Axon (*ak'son*) The axis of the body; long outgoing process of nerve cell by which impulses travel away from a neuron; vertebral column.

Axoplasm (*ak'so-plasm*) The cytoplasm of an axon.

Azapetine Belongs to the class of benzapines. It is a potent arterial vasodilator in the treatment of peripheral vascular diseases.

Azathioprine (*az'ah-thi'o-pren*) A cytotoxic and immunosuppressive agent used in the treatment of leukemia, auto immune diseases and organ transplantation.

Azelastine (*a-zel'-e-sten*) A second-generation antihistamine approved for treatment of allergic rhinitis.

Azithromycin (*az-ith"ro-mi'sin*) A macrolide antibiotic active against certain gram-negative organisms, including *H. influenzae*. Its serum half life is prolonged allowing once —daily administration.

Azo-(azoto) (*az'ot*) Nitrogen.

Azoospermia (aspermia) (*a-zo'o-sper'me-a*) Absence of spermatozoa in the semen; failure of spermatogenesis azotemia high blood urea.

Azotemia (*az"o-te'me-e*) Elevation, or buildup of, nitrogenous products (BUN-usually ranging 7 – 21 mg/dL), creatinine in the blood, and other secondary waste products within the body.

Azoturia (*az'o-tu're-a*) An increased excretion of nitrogen compound and urea in the urine.

Azurophil (*azh-u'ro-fil*) Red blood cells containing granules that stain readily with an azure dye.

Azurophilia (*azh'u-ro-fil'e-a*) A condition in which blood contains cells having azurophilic granules.

Azygos vein A blood vessel that carries blood from the back walls of the chest and abdomen to the heart.

B

Babinski reflex (*ba-bin-ske*) Dorsiflexion of the big toe at the metacarpophalangeal joint on stimulation of the sole of the foot due to the contraction of the extensor hallucis longus. It is accompanied by the extension and spread of the other toes like a fan indicating a lesion of the pyramidal tract, described by Joseph Babinski, French neurologist.

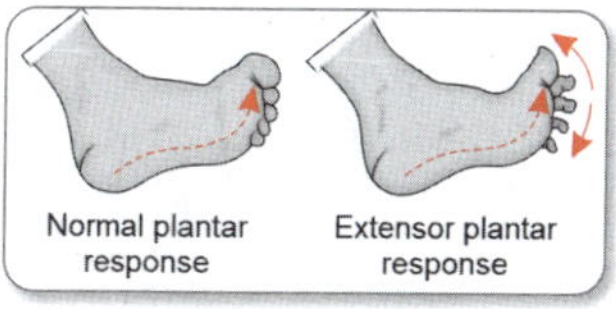

Babinski reflex

Bacille Calmette-Guerin Attenuated strain of *Mycobacterium bovis* used in the preparation of BCG vaccine named after Albert Calmette and Camille Guerin, French bacteriologists.

Bacillemia (*bas-i-leme-a*) The presence of bacilli in the circulating blood.

Bacilluria (*bas-i-lu're-a*) The presence of bacilli in the urine.

Bacillus (*ba-sil'us*) Rod-shaped bacterium belonging to the family of Bacillaceae. It is aerobic, and **gram-positive**; pl. **bacilli.**

Acid-fast bacillus A group of bacteria showing characteristics of acid fastness.

Bacillus anthracis A bacillus pathogenic to man causing anthrax.

Bacillus cereus An aerobic spore-forming bacillus that may cause opportunistic infection in an immunocompromised host.

Bacillus melaninogenicus A gram-negative nonspore forming organism responsible for lung abscess and Vincent's angina.

Bacillus subtilis A laboratory contaminant, generally nonpathogenic.

Ducrey's bacillus Also known as *Haemophilus ducreyi* responsible for soft chancre or chancroid infection.

Friedlander's bacillus Also known as *Klebsiella pneumoniae* causing necrotizing pneumonia.

Hansen's bacillus Also known as *Mycobacterium leprae*, causative agent of leprosy.

Koch-weeks bacillus Also known as *Haemophilus aegyptius*, causative agent of infectious conjunctivitis.

Tubercle bacillus Also known as *Mycobacterium tuberculosis*, causative agent of tuberculosis.

Typhoid bacillus Also known as *Salmonella typhi*, causative agent of typhoid fever.

Bacitracin (*bas-i-tra'sin*) An antibiotic produced by *Bacillus subtilis* and it is applied locally in infections from hemolytic streptococci and staphylococci.

Backbone (spinal column, spine, vertebral column) The vertebral column.

Baclofen (*bak'lo-fen"*) A gamma-aminobutyric acid (GABA) agonist used as a skeletal muscle relaxant.

Bacteremia (*bak-ter-e'me-a*) The presence of bacteria in the blood, whether associated with active disease or not.

Bacteria (*bak-te're-a*) Any microorganism of the class schizomycetes.

Bactericidal (*bak-ter-i-si'dal*) Destructive to or destroying bacteria.

Bacteriological index (*bak-tere-o-logi'cal in'deks*) Smears obtained from 4 skin lesions, from both earlobes and nose, which are stained for presence of acid-fast bacilli. It is estimated as 0 (no bacilli in any field) 1+ (few bacilli in few fields), 2+ (few bacilli in all 100 fields), and 3+ (many bacilli found in all fields). For the scores of 7, sites are added and divided by 7. If the score is <2, the case is paucibacillary leprosy; and if score is 2 or more, it is multibacillary leprosy.

Bacteriology (*bak-te're-o'lo-ge*) The branch of science concerned with the study of bacteria.

Bacteriolysin (*bak-te're-ol'i-sin*) An antibacterial antibody, causing lysis of bacteria.

Bacteriophage (phage) (*bak-te're-o'fag*) A virus with specific affinity for bacteria. Bacteriophages are widely distributed in nature.

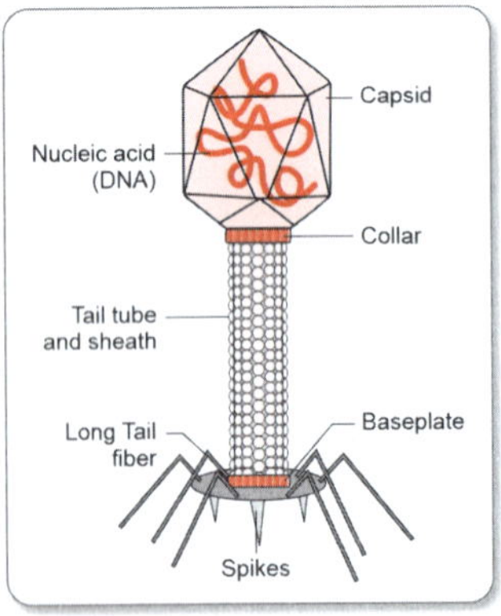

Bacteriophage

Bacteriostatic (*bak-te-re-o-stat'ik*) An agent inhibiting the growth or multiplication of bacteria.

Bacterium (*bak-te're-um*) Pl. **bacteria**; nonspore forming single-celled organism that multiplies by simple cell division. It may be spherical, rod-shaped or spiraliform. The spherical cocci and other bacilli are nonmotile and spiral forms are motile.

Bacteroides (*bak-ter-oyd'ez*) Anaerobic filamentous nonsporulating gram-negative bacteria found as normal flora in the oral cavity and colon, and as secondary invader in the necrotic tissue.

Bacteroides fragilis Is an important example of the genus.

Bacterium (*bak-te're-um*) Pl. **bacteria**; nonspore forming single-celled organism that multiplies by simple cell division. It may be spherical, rod-shaped or spiraliform. The spherical cocci and other bacilli are nonmotile and spiral forms are motile.

Bagassosis (*bag-a-so'sis*) Occupational respiratory disorder caused by inhalation of sugarcane dust containing *Thermoactinomyces sacchari*, a fungus. It is characterized by fever, dyspnea and malaise.

Baghdad sore Oriental sore due to *Leishmania tropica*.

Balanitis (*bal-a-ni'tis*) Inflammation of the glans penis or glans clitoridis, associated with a purulent discharge. Example, Amoebic balanitis.

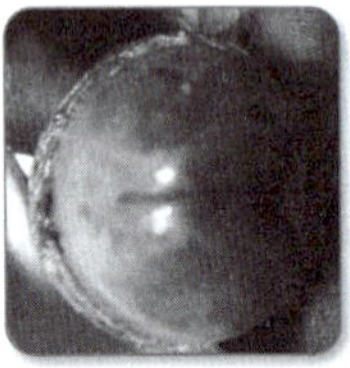

Amoebic balanitis

Balanoposthitis (*bal'a-no-pos-thi'tis*) Inflammation of the glans penis and overlying prepuce.

Balantidiasis (*bal'an-ti-di'a-sis*) Infection of large intestine by protozoan parasites of the genus *Balantidium*. It presents with abdominal pain, diarrhea, vomiting and loss of weight and is treated with tetracyclines or metronidazole.

Balantidium (bal-an-tid'e-um) A ciliated protozoan parasite found in the large intestine. *B. coli*, a species of *Balantidium*, is the largest protozoan parasite causing balantidiasis.

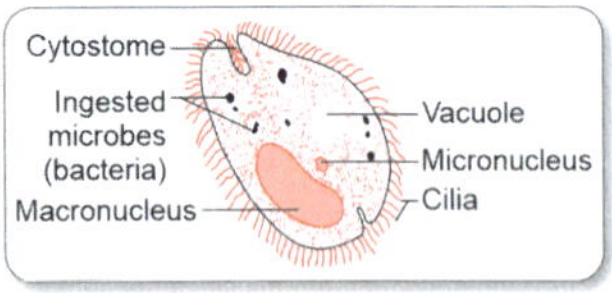

Balantidium coli

Baldness (*bawld'ness*) Lack of or loss of hair on head.

Balloon angioplasty A technique to reopen arteries narrowed by atheromatous plaques by inserting and inflating a balloon catheter inside the blood vessels.

Balloon catheter A catheter with a balloon near its tip used to open a narrowed artery or intestine or to drain an obstructed organ such as urinary bladder.

Ball and socket joint A synovial joint in which one rounded bone head moves within the concavity of another bone, such as in hip and shoulder joints.

Ballistocardiograph (*ba-lis'to-kar'de-o-gra-f*) An instrument used to take ballistocardiogram.

Ballotment (*bal'ot-mon'ent*) A palpatory method to toss an organ and feel, especially a floating organ such as kidney, or fetus.

Balneotherapy A type of hydrotherapy such as a warm bath in the evening.

Bamethan A vasodilator drug belonging to haloalkanes group.

Bandage (*ban'dej*) A roll of gauze used to wrap any part of the body as a dressing.

Adhesive bandage A small flexible sheet of material consists of a medical dressing of plain absorb cut gauze held in place by a fabric tape coated with adhesive.

Bandage lens Contact lens used as corneal dressing.

Figure-of-eight-bandage A type of medical bandage typically used to secure dressings or splints, in which the successive turns cross each other as in the figure eight.

Four-tailed bandage A bandage consisting of a strip of cloth split in two on both ends.

Many-tailed bandage A bandage or binder with split ends used for the trunk and limbs; a piece of roller to which slips are stitched in an overlapping pattern.

Roller bandage A tightly rolled, circular bandage of varying widths and materials, often prepared commercially.

Scultetus bandage A strip of material such as gauze used to protect, immobilize, compress, or support a wound or injured body part.

Spica bandage A bandage, applied in successive V-shaped crossings and is used to immobilize a limb especially at a joint.

Spiral reverse bandage A spiral bandage where the bandage is folded back on itself by 180° after each turn.

Velpeau bandage A bandage used to support and immobilize the arm when the clavicle is fractured.

Bandl's ring A constriction located at the junction of the thinned lower uterine segment and thick retracted upper uterine segment which is associated with obstructed labor.

Banti's disease (*ban'tez*) Congestive splenomegaly with cirrhosis, described by Italian pathologist, Guido Banti.

Barber's itch An infection of hair follicles in the face by staphylococci, presenting with papules and pustules; folliculitis barbae; a dermatomycosis caused by a fungus— Trichophyton, *tinea barbae.*

Barbiturate (*bar-bit'u-rat*) A salt of barbituric acid that is depressant of the central nervous system. It is used as a sedative or hypnotic, named after Saint Barbara.

Bariatrics (*bar'e-a'triks*) Scientific study of obesity and its related disorders.

Baritosis Pneumoconiosis due to inhalation of barium dust.

Barium enema Use of barium sulfate as an enema to enable X-ray and fluoroscopic examination of the colon.

Barium sulfate A radiopaque barium compound used in roentgenography of the gastrointestinal tract.

Barium X-ray examination Any of a group of imaging procedures that are used to diagnose diseases of gastrointestinal tract using barium sulfate as a contrast medium.

Baroreceptor (baroceptor) (*bar'o-re-sep'ter*) A sensory nerve ending in the wall of the auricle of the heart, aortic arch, carotid sinus and vena cava sensitive to stretching of the wall from an increased pressure within.

Barotitis (*bar'o-ti'tis*) Acute vertigo due to otitis media or the passage of water into the middle ear at depths of 5–20 m; inflammation of the middle ear due to sudden changes in barometric pressure as may occur while flying or diving.

Barotrauma (*bar'o-traw'ma*) Injury to the eustachian tube and the tympanic membrane due to an imbalance between ambient pressure and intratympanic pressures.

Barr body Sex chromatin mass found in the nuclei of the somatic cells of normal females, described by Murray Barr, a Canadian anatomist. It represents an inactivated X-chromosome.

Barrett's esophagus Occurrence of columnar epithelium lining of a segment of esophagus occasionally accompanied by peptic ulceration. The patient has an increased risk of development of adenocarcinoma, named after Norman Barrett, British surgeon.

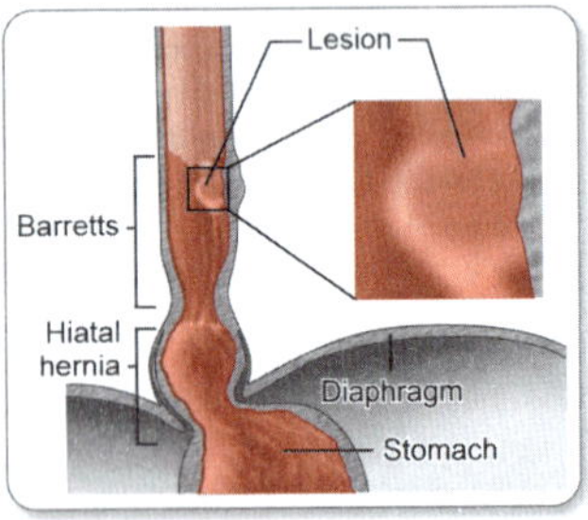

Barrett's esophagus

Bartholinitis (*bar'to-lin-i'tis*) Inflammation of Bartholin's glands.

Bartholin's glands (greater vestibular glands) A pair of pea-sized vulvovaginal glands that secrete a fluid that lubricates the vagina during sexual arousal. These glands are felt on palpating the posterior part of the labia majora between the finger and thumbs.

Bartonellosis (*bar'to-nel-o'sis*) A disease caused by *Bartonella* and transmitted by the bite of sandfly. It presents with fever, hemolytic anemia and multiple eruptions on the skin and mucous membranes and responds to antibiotics such as chloramphenicol.

Basal cell carcinoma A skin cancer that develops on areas of skin exposed to sun, such as face.

Basal ganglia Part of extrapyramidal system containing corpus striatum (caudate and lentiform nuclei), amygdaloid nuclei and the putamen.

Basal metabolism The amount of energy required when the person is at rest to maintain vital body functions.

Basement membrane A structure involved in cell growth, adhesion and differentiation, consists of a multimolecular layer composed of collagen glycoprotein, fibronectin and proteoglycans and is subjacent to epithelium and endothelium.

Base pairing Two bases which form a 'rung of the DNA ladder'. A DNA nucleotide is made of a molecule of sugar, a molecule of phosphoric acid and a molecule of base. The bases are the 'letters' that spell out the genetic code. In base pairing, adenine always pairs with thymine, and guanine with cytosine; two nucleotides (always a pyrimidine with a purine) that are paired and held together by a hydrogen bond.

Basilar artery The single posterior arterial trunk formed by union of two vertebral arteries at the base of the skull.

Basilar membrane Cellular structure giving a base for spiral organ of Corti.

Basion (*ba'se-on*) Midpoint of the anterior border of the foramen magnum.

Basophil (*ba'so-fil*) A granular leukocyte that stains with basic dyes that may have a role in some allergic reaction, and constitutes 0.5% to 1% of leukocytes; a type of cell found in the anterior lobe of the pituitary that produces corticotropin.

Basophilia (*ba-so-fil'e-a*) An abnormal increase in the number of basophils in the blood or in an organ.

Bathyesthesia (*bath'e-es-the'ze-a*) Deep sensibility.

Battered child syndrome Unexplained or inappropriately explained physical trauma and other manifestations of severe repeated physical abuse of children, usually by parents.

Battered woman syndrome Repeated episodes of physical assault of a woman by husband or partner.

Bazin's disease (*ba-zin'*) Erythema induratum described by a French dermatologist, Antoine Bazin.

BCG *Bacille Calmette-Guerin.*

BCG vaccine A freeze-dried vaccine of a live, attenuated strain of *Mycobacterium bovis* used in children for immunization against tuberculosis.

Beclomethasone (*bek"lo-meth'a-son*) An inhaled corticosteroid used as maintenance treatment in the prophylaxis of asthma attacks.

Becquerel (*bek"a-rel*) The SI unit of measurement of radioactivity.

Bedbug (*bed'bug*) A blood-sucking arthropod and it elicits pruritus; small, flat, parasitic insects from the genus *Cimex* that feed solely on the blood of people and animals while they sleep.

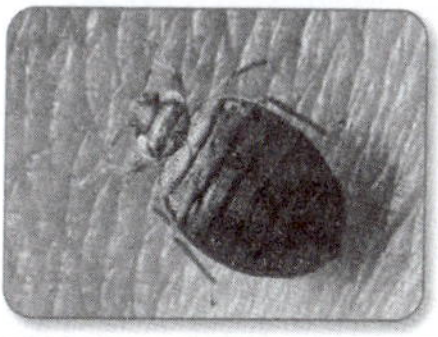

Bedbug

Bed occupancy A 24-hour patient occupancy in a hospital inpatient service.

Bedsore (decubitus ulcer, pressure sore) Decubitus ulcer, pressure sore; ischemic necrosis and ulceration of tissue especially over a bony prominence.

Bedwetting Enuresis.

Behaviorism (*be'havi-ur'izm*) A system of psychology in which all behavior, normal and abnormal, is seen as a set of conditioned reflexes separate from individual's will.

Behcet's disease (*be'sets*) Diffuse vasculitis causing orogenital lesions and uveitis in young males, described by a Turkish dermatologist, Hulusi Behcet.

Behavior modification Behavioral therapy designed to change the learned behavior of an individual.

Behavior therapy Treatment of psychoneurosis by attempts to modify behavior; psychotherapy that helps a person to change the way he or she responds to certain circumstances.

Bejel (endemic syphilis) (*bej'l*) A nonvenereal form of syphilis affecting children, caused by a strain of *Treponema pallidum.*

Beck triad (*bek*) A symptom complex of cardiac tamponade consisting of high venous pressure, low arterial pressure and a small quiet heart, described by Claude Beck, US physician.

Bel (*bal*) A unit of measurement of the intensity of sound and is expressed as a logarithm of the ratio of two sounds of acoustic intensity and is expressed in decibels.

Belle indifference A conversion disorder in which patient shows lack of concern towards their symptoms.

Beclomethasone (*bek"lo-meth'a-son*) An inhaled corticosteroid used as maintenance treatment in the prophylaxis of asthma attacks.

Bell's palsy Lower motor neuron facial paralysis which is associated with immobility of one half of the face.

Belly (*bel'e*) The abdomen or abdominal cavity; the fleshy central part of a muscle.

Belly button Umbilicus.

Belly tap Abdominal tap.

Benazepril (*ben-a'ze-pril*) An ACE inhibitor administered orally in the form of its hydrochloride for the treatment of hypertension.

Bence Jones protein Thermosensitive urinary protein in multiple myeloma, described by an English physician, Henry Bence Jones. A precipitate form when urine is heated to 50° – 60°C and it disappears on further heating. It reappears on cooling.

Bendroflumethiazide (*ben'dro-flu'meti'a-zid*) A thiazide diuretic.

Bends (*bendz*) Pain in the limbs and abdomen noted following rapid reduction of air pressure. It is caused by bubbles of nitrogen in blood and tissues.

Benedict test A test to demonstrate presence of sugar in the urine, described by American chemist, Stanley Benedict. 5 mL of fresh Benedict's copper sulphate-based reagent is taken in a test tube and boiled. 8 drops of urine added to it by a dropper. Then it is heated to vigorous boiling and allowed to cool. The presence of reducing substance is revealed by the appearance of a precipitate varying from light green turbidity to a red precipitate. If the reduction is due to glucose, the amount is assessed as 0.5, 1.0, 1.5 and 2% when it shows light green turbidity, green, yellow and red precipitate, respectively.

Benedikt syndrome A syndrome of ipsilateral hemiplegia with oculomotor palsy and contralateral tremors due to involvement of the third nerve and red nucleus, described by Moritz Benedikt, an Austrian physician.

Benign (*be-nin*) Nonmalignant, mild.

Benign lymphadenopathy Any nonmalignant regional or generalized enlargement of lymph nodes.

Benign prostatic hypertrophy A nonmalignant enlargement of the prostate due to excessive growth of prostate tissue, presents in elderly males as nocturia, difficulty in initiating urination and diminished force of urinary stream.

Benign tumor A growth that does not spread to other parts of the body. However, it can grow to a large size.

Bennett fracture A fracture through the base of the first metacarpal bone and into the carpometacarpal joint, named after Edward Bennett, Irish surgeon.

Benzaldehyde (*ben-zal'de-hid*) A colorless liquid aldehyde with the odor of bitter almonds, used in the manufacture of dyes and perfumes.

Benzalkonium chloride (*ben"zal-ko'ne -em*) A white or yellowish white mixture of chloride salts obtained as a bitter aromatic powder or gelatinous pieces that is used as an antiseptic and germicide.

Benzathine penicillin Long-acting penicillin.

Benzocaine (*ben'zo-kan*) A local anesthetic derived from aminobenzoic acid.

Benzodiazepine (*ben'zo-di-az'e-pen*) A psychotropic drug possessing hypnotic and sedative action.

Benzoic acid (*ben'zoyc*) A white crystalline material used in keratolytic ointments and in food preservation.

Benzphetamine (*benz-fet'a-men*) A sympathomimetic amine with pharmacologic activity similar to the prototype drugs of this class used in obesity, the amphetamines.

3,4-benzpyrene A carcinogenic polycyclic hydrocarbon.

Benzthiazide A thiazide diuretic used in the treatment of high blood pressure and edema.

Benztropine (*benz'tro-pen*) An anticholinergic drug used to treat Parkinson's disease (PD) and extrapyramidal symptoms, except tardive dyskinesia.

Benzyl benzoate A colorless liquid used as a topical scabicide.

Berger's disease Idiopathic, focal glomerulonephritis with mesangial deposits of IgA.

Beri-beri (*ber'e-ber'e*) A disease caused by a deficiency of thiamine in diet, derived from a Sinhalese word. There is failure of metabolism of glucose aerobically and there is accumulation of pyruvic and lactic acid.

Berylliosis (*ber'il-le-o'sis*) Beryllium poisoning. Acute inhalation causes a generalized acute inflammatory reaction in the respiratory tract and alveoli. Chronic disease, following inhalation in a low dose over a long time causes progressively increasing dyspnea and fatigue.

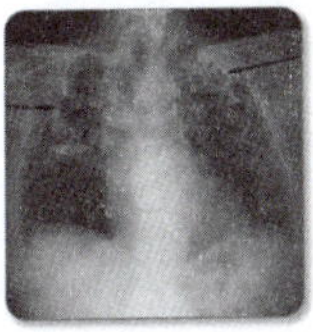

Berylliosis

Beta blocker Beta adrenergic blocking agents that lower blood pressure.

Betamethasone (*be'ta-meth'a-son*) A synthetic glucocorticoid used as a topical anti-inflammatory agent.

Bethanechol (*be-than'a-kol*) A direct-acting parasympathomimetic agent that is FDA approved for the treatment of post-operative urinary retention, postpartum urinary retention, and overflow incontinence caused by neurogenic atony of the bladder.

Bethesda system A system for reporting cervical or vaginal cytologic findings and diagnoses, named after Bethesda, Maryland, USA, headquarters of National Institute of Health.

Bevacizumab (*beva-siz'u-mab*) A monoclonal antivascular endothelial growth factor antibody used in combination with antineoplastic agents for the treatment of many types of cancer.

Bezoar (*be'zor*) A ball of entangled material formed in the stomach and intestine, such as a hair ball (trichobezoar), ball of hair and vegetable fiber (trichophytobezoar) or food ball (phytobezoar).

Bi- Bismuth.

Biceps (*bi'seps*) A muscle having two heads.

Biceps brachii Muscle of the upper arm with two heads. It flexes the arm and forearm and supinates hand.

Biceps femoris One of the hamstring muscles lying posterolaterally in the thigh. It flexes knee and rotates it outward.

Biceps groove A groove between the greater and lesser tubercles of the humerus for the passage of biceps tendon.

Biceps reflex Contraction of biceps muscles on percussing its tendon.

Biconcave (*bi'kan'kav*) Concave on each side.

Biconvex (*bi'kon'veks*) Convex on each side.

Bicornuate (*bi-kor'nu-at*) Having two horns, especially of uterus with body partly divided into two.

Bicuspid (*bi-cus'pid*) Having two cusps.

Bicuspid tooth A premolar tooth having two cusps on the grinding surface and a flattened root. There are two premolars on either side of jaw between the canines and molars.

Bicuspid valve Mitral valve between the left atrium and left ventricle of the heart.

Bifocal (*bi-fo'kal*) Lens having two parts with different focusing powers.

Bifurcation (*bi-fur-ka'shun*) The site at which a single structure separates into two branches.

Bigeminal pulse Two coming in couples where second beat is weaker. It is due to premature contraction and is followed by a pause. It is noted in partial heart block and digitalis toxicity.

Bigeminy (*bi-jem'i-ne*) Occurring in pairs. adj. **bigeminal**.

Atrial bigeminy An arrhythmia consisting of repetitive sequence of one atrial premature complex followed by a narrow sinus impulse.

Ventricular bigeminy An arrhythmia consisting of repeated sequence of one ventricular premature complex followed by a normal beat.

Bilateral (*bi-lat'er-al*) Having two sides; appearing on two sides.

Bile (*bil*) Gall, secretion of the liver consisting bile salts, bilirubin, cholesterol, phospholipid and electrolytes, which aid in the emulsification of fats.

Bile acids Acids such as cholic, glycocholic and taurocholic acids which occur as salts in bile. They help in digestion of fats.

Bile duct Intercellular passages that convey bile from the liver to the hepatic duct which joins the duct from gallbladder (cystic duct) to form common bile duct that opens into the duodenum.

Bile pigments Highly colored substances such as bilirubin and biliverdin found in bile that are derived from hemoglobin. They impart brown color to the stools.

Bile salts Alkali salts of bile such as sodium glycocholate and sodium taurocholate.

Bilharzia (*bil-har'ze-a*) Blood fluke, *Schistosoma*, described by Theodor Bilharz, a German physician.

Biliary (*bil'e-ar-e*) Relating to the bile, or bile duct or gallbladder.

Biliary atresia A birth defect in which the bile ducts fail to develop or underdeveloped.

Biliary calculus Gallstone.

Biliary cirrhosis A form of cirrhosis of the liver resulting from destruction of intrahepatic bile ducts (primary) or secondary to prolonged obstruction.

Biliary colic Severe pain in upper right abdomen caused by passing of gallstones by gallbladder's attempt to expel gallstones.

Biliary sludge Bile in a gel form that contains numerous crystals of calcium bilirubinate granules, cholesterol crystals and glycoproteins and essential precursor to the formation of gallstones.

Biliary tract The organs and ducts in which the bile is formed, concentrated and carried from the liver to the duodenum.

Biliary colic Severe pain in upper right abdomen caused by passing of gallstones by gallbladder's attempt to expel gallstones.

Bilious (*bil'yus*) Relating to bile; a disorder affecting the bile.

Bilirubin (*bil-i-roo'bin*) An orange-yellow bile pigment formed as a degradation product of hemoglobin.

Bilirubinemia (*bil'i-roo-bin-e'me-a*) The presence of bilirubin in excess amounts in the blood .

Biliuria (choiuria) (*bil'i-u're-a*) The presence of bile acids or bile salts in the urine.

Biliverdin (*bil-i-ver'din*) A green pigment produced by catabolism or hemoglobin which later gets reduced to bilirubin.

Bimanual (*bi-man'u-al*) Performed by both hands.

Binaural (*bin-aw'ral*) Pertaining to both ears.

Binder (*bind'er*) A broad bandage; an inert substance that holds a mixture of solid particles together.

Binocular (*bin-ok'u-lar*) Pertaining to both eyes.

Bioassay (*bi'o-as'a*) Determination of the effectiveness of a specific sample of a drug on a live animal or an isolated organ preparation.

Bioavailability (*bi'o-a-val'a-bil'i-te*) The degree to which a drug is available to act on the target organ. It is affected by the route of administration, rate of metabolism, lipid solubility and binding proteins.

Biochemistry The science dealing with living organisms and of chemical changes occurring in them.

Biofeedback (*bi"o-fed'bak*) A learning technique wherein a desired response is learnt on the basis of the information received from the eyes or ears on the status of an autonomic body function.

Bioflavonoid (*bi"o-flavo-noid*) A vitamin that maintains the resistance of cell and capillary walls to permeation.

Biological response modifier Molecules that modulate the immune response.

Biology (*bi-ol'o-je*) The science of life and living things.

Molecular biology Branch of biology dealing with analysis of the structure and development of biological systems.

Bionics (*bi-on'iks*) bioelectronics.

Bioprosthesis (*bi'o-pros-the'sis*) A prosthesis (as a porcine heart valve) consisting of an animal part or containing animal tissue.

Biopsy (*bi-op-se*) Removal of a piece of tissue from the body and examining it a microscopically after staining, for purpose of diagnosis.

Aspiration biopsy Removal of tissue by a needle and syringe.

Brush biopsy Removal of a tissue by brushing.

Needle biopsy Removal of tissues by a needle attached to a syringe.

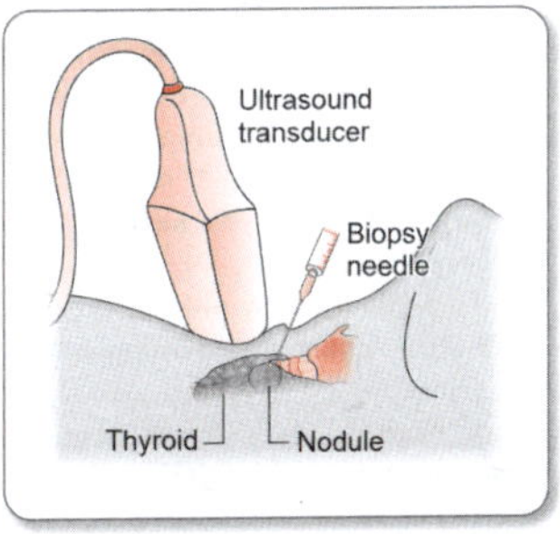

Needle biopsy

Percutaneous transthoracic needle aspiration biopsy Using a fluoroscopically guided aspiration needle to obtain a sample of a tissue from a pulmonary lesion.

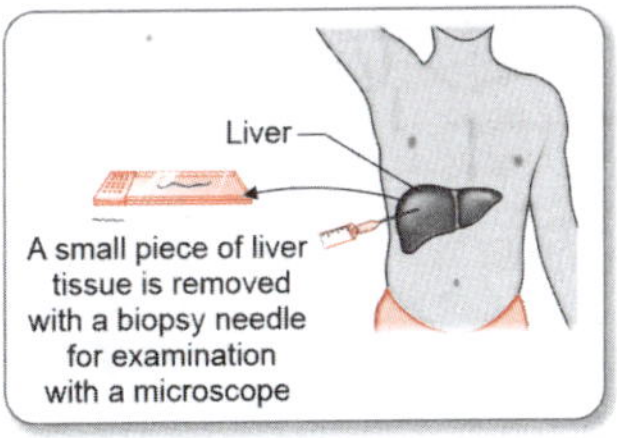

Percutaneous needle biopsy

Punch biopsy Removal of a small bit of tissue by a hollow punch.

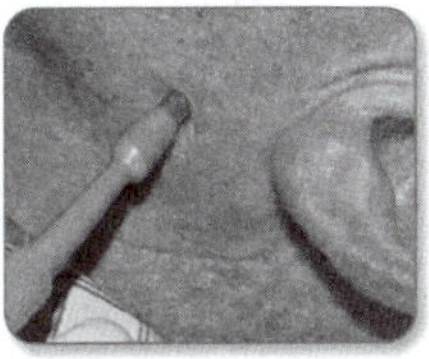

Punch biopsy

Sternal biopsy Biopsy of bone marrow of the sternum either by puncture or trephine.

Biostatistics (*bi'o-sta-'tis'tiks*) Vital statistics; application of statistical methods to analyze biologic data.

Biot's breathing (*be-oz*) An irregular respiration that can become slow or rapid, shallow or deep with irregular pauses, found in meningitis, named after Camille Biot, French physician.

Biotechnology Use of molecular biology and other advanced multidisciplinary sciences to produce products and processes.

Biotin (*bi'o-tin*) A member of B complex involved in carboxylase reactions and is essential for the metabolism of fat and carbohydrates. Liver, kidney, milk, egg yolk and yeast are rich in biotin. Biotin deficiency causes scaly dermatitis, muscle pain and anorexia.

Biperiden (*bi-per'i-den*) A white crystalline muscle relaxant $C_{21}H_{29}NO$ used especially to reduce the symptoms (as tremors, akinesia, and muscle rigidity) associated with Parkinson's disease.

Bipolar (*bi-po'lar*) Having two poles.

Bipolar affective disorder A disorder wherein the patient exhibits both maniac and depressive episodes.

Bipolar cells Primitive cells found in the bone marrow that are yet to terminally differentiate and are capable of giving rise to erythroid and megakaryotic daughter cells.

Bipolar traits Personality traits that represent extreme opposites of expression.

Birefringence (*bi're-frin'jens*) The splitting of a ray of light into two.

Birquet syndrome A somatization disorder running a chronic and fluctuating course with pain, vomiting, nausea, headache, dizziness, menstrual irregularities and sexual dysfunction seen in women.

Birth (*burth*) The act of being born; passage of a child from uterus.

Birth canal The canal through which fetus passes in birth and it comprises the cervix, vagina and vulva.

Birth certificate A legal record of the birth of a child.

Birth control pill Oral contraceptive containing synthetic estrogen and progesterone or synthetic progesterone alone.

Birth defect A congenital anomaly.

Birth injury An injury sustained by the neonate during the birth process.

Birth mark Nevus, mole.

Birth rate The number of live births per 1,000 estimated mid-year population in a given year.

Birth weight Weight recorded within the first hour of life, and is considered the single most important determinant of its chances of survival, healthy growth and development. It should be at least 2.5 kg.

High birth weight Birth weight over 4 kg.

Low birth weight Birth weight less than 2.5 kg. Such babies are those born prematurely and those with fetal growth retardation.

Multiple birth The birth of two or more offspring produced in the same gestation period.

Birth control Birth control Prevention of conception or implantation of fertilized ovum or termination of pregnancy.

Premature birth Birth of a premature baby.

Birth mark Nevus, mole.

Birth rate The number of live births per 1,000 estimated mid-year population in a given year.

Bisacodyl (*bis-ak'o-dil*) A cathartic having direct effect on the colon.

Bisexual (*bi-seks'u-al*) Having gonads of both sexes, in one person; hermaphrodite; a person who is sexually attracted to others of either sex.

Bistoury (*bis'too-re*) A long narrow straight or curved surgical knife.

Bite guard A plastic dental appliance that fits over the biting surface of the upper or lower teeth.

Bite lock (*bit'lok*) A dental device to retain bite rims. Also known as a ramp or turbo, prevent damage to metal braces by restricting the upper and lower teeth from touching.

Bitewing (*bit'wing*) A dental X-ray film designed to show the crowns of the upper and lower teeth simultaneously.

Bivalent (*bi-va'lent*) Associated in pairs.

Black death Plague.

Black eye Beefy red eye from extravasated blood which extends beyond the orbital margins. There may be hemorrhage in the conjunctiva.

Blackfan-Diamond syndrome Inherited disorder with erythroid hypoplasia and anemia.

Black head A black tipped semisolid sebum that obstructs the opening of a hair follicle.

Black water fever Production of dark brown-black urine due to intravascular hemolysis seen in falciparum malaria.

Bladder (*blad'der*) A hollow muscular organ commonly referred to urinary bladder.

Atonic bladder Loss of bladder control with loss of bladder sensation. There is overflow incontinence with dribbling. It develops in spinal cord lesion above S_2 in acute stage.

Automatic bladder Sudden complete reflex evacuation of bladder. There is absence of bladder distension and its capacity is small. It develops in spinal cord lesion above S_2 in chronic stage.

Autonomous bladder Overflow incontinence with absence of bladder sensation. There is loss of bladder control noted in spinal cord or cauda equina $S_{2,3,4}$ lesions.

Bladder cancer Most common site of urinary tract for malignancy. It is a transitional cell carcinoma which spreads locally by direct invasion. Painless hematuria is the presenting symptom.

Bladder irrigation The washing out of the bladder by water or medicated solution.

Bladder stone Large round stone in the bladder.

Neurogenic bladder Any dysfunction of the urinary bladder due to lesions of CNS or nerve supply to bladder.

Pear-shaped bladder Extensive compression of the urinary bladder from an excess tissue in the pelvis giving a pear-shape to the bladder following intravenous pyelogram.

Urinary bladder Musculomembranous distensible reservoir situated in the pelvic cavity. It receives urine from kidneys through ureters and stores it for some time and then discharges out through urethra.

Bladder training A behavioral modification program used to treat stress incontinence.

Bladder worm Cysticercus, the young tapeworm of Genus Taenia. It has smell, sac-like vesicle resembling a bladder.

Blalock-Taussig shunt An anastomosis of a subclavian artery to the pulmonary artery on the same side in cyanotic heart disease characterized by reduced pulmonary flow such as tetralogy of Fallots and pulmonary atresia, named after Alfred Blalock, US surgeon and Halen Taussig, US pediatrician.

Blastema (*blas-te'ma*) A heterogeneous cell mass that through migration and proliferation transiently forms at the injury site and undergoes morphogenesis to form the missing organ.

Blastocele (*blas'to-sel*) The fluid-filled cavity of the mass of cells produced by cleavage of a fertilized ovum.

Blastocyst (*blas'to-sist*) An early stage of embryo wherein there is a two-layer sphere of cells surrounding a fluid-filled cavity.

Blastomere (*blas'to-mer*) One of the cells that are produced during cleavage of a zygote and that form the morula.

Blastomycosis (*blas'to-mi-ko'sis*) Systemic infection caused by blastomyces. It may present like a pneumonitis or as a long-term illness affecting the lungs, skin and bones.

Blastopore (*blas'to-por*) A mouth-like opening of the archenteron on the surface of the embryo during the invagination of the archenteron.

Blastula (*blas'tu-la*) An early stage of development through which a zygote develops into an embryo. It is a fluid-filled sphere formed by a single layer of cells. It is the form in which embryo gets implanted in the wall of the uterus.

Bleeding (*bled'-ing*) Flow of blood from an injured vessel; hemorrhage.

Blennophthalmia Inflammation of the mucous membrane of the eye; conjunctivitis.

Blennorrhagia (biemiorrhea) (blen'o-ra'je-a) Excess discharge of mucus.

Blennorrhea (blen'o-re'a) Discharge from the urethra or vagina due to gonorrhea.

Bleomycin An antitumor drug.

Blepharitis (blef'ar-i'tis) Inflammation of the hair follicles and glands along the border of the eyelids. The eyelids become red, tender and sore with sticky exudate.

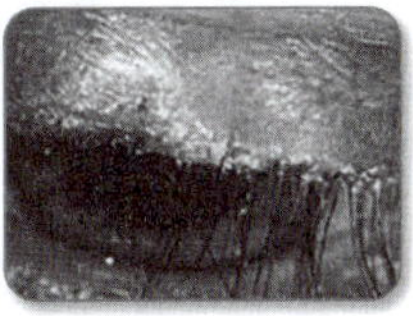

Seborrheic blepharitis

Blepharon Greek word for eyelid.

Blepharophimosis (blefa-ro-fi-mo'sis) A congenital anomaly in which the eyelids are underdeveloped such that they cannot open as far as usual and permanently cover part of the eyes.

Blepharoplasty (tarsoplasty) (*blef'a-ro-plas"te*) A surgical rejuvenating procedure that may be performed on the upper and/or lower eyelids; surgical removal of wrinkled skin on the eyelid.

Blepharospasm (*blef'a-ro-spa-sm*) Spasm of the orbicularis oculi causing closure of the eyelids.

Blindness Inability to see from injuries to the eye, corneal opacity, cataract, glaucoma and muscular degeneration.

Blind spot Optic disk devoid of rods and cones.

Blister (*blis'ter*) An elevation of the epidermis containing fluid.

Block (*blok*) Obstruction; a method of regional anesthesia to stop passage of sensory impulses; to obstruct any passage or opening.

Block dissection Removal of local lymphatic drainage area with tumor as a single block of tissue.

Caudal block Extradural injection of anesthetic agent.

Epidural block Single injection in lumbar spaces.

Spinal block Subarachnoid block causing rapid anesthesia.

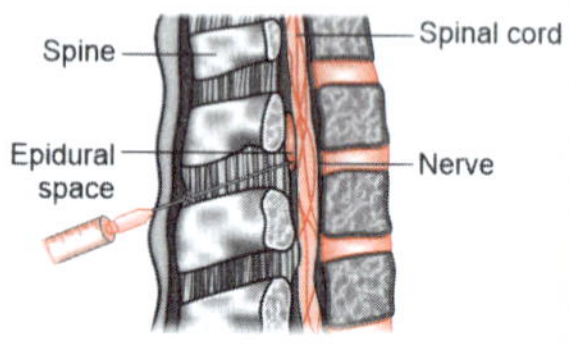

Production of epidural block with injection – needle stopping before dura

Blocking *psy* Abrupt interruption in learn of thinking before a thought or idea is finished, after a brief pause, person indicates no recall of what was being said or was going to be said.

Blocking antibody Antibody (IgG) that combines with antigen preventing access of other antibodies.

Blood (*blud*) The liquid pumped by the heart through the circulatory system consisting of arteries, veins and capillaries. It consists of a clear yellow fluid (plasma) and formed elements (red blood cells, white blood cells and platelets). The major functions of the blood is to transport oxygen and nutrient substances to the cells and remove from the cells carbon dioxide and other waste products for elimination.

Arterial blood Oxygenated blood found in the pulmonary veins, the left chambers of the heart and the systemic arteries.

Blood agar A culture medium consisting of blood and nutrient agar used for cultivation of microorganisms.

Blood-borne pathogens Pathogenic microorganisms found in the blood that can cause disease in humans.

Blood capillaries Hair-like vessels that convey blood from the arterioles to the venules.

Blood circulation The circuit of blood in the body through which blood circulates.

Blood clot The end result of blood clotting consisting of a semisolid mass of erythrocytes, leukocytes and platelets that are enmeshed in an insoluble fibrin network.

Blood dyscrasia A condition wherein the constituents of blood are abnormal in structure and function.

Blood fluke Flatworm of genus *Schistocerca*.

Blood gas Gas dissolved in liquid part of the blood. It includes oxygen, carbon dioxide and nitrogen.

Blood gas analysis Determination of the concentration and pressure of oxygen and carbon dioxide and bicarbonate levels in the arterial blood.

Blood gas tension partial pressure of a gas in the blood.

Blood level The concentration of a drug or other substance in the plasma, serum or whole blood.

Blood osmolality The osmatic pressure of blood. The normal values in serum are 280 to 295 mOsm/L.

Blood pH The hydrogen ion concentration of the blood and the normal values are 7.38 to 7.44.

Blood smear A drop of blood spread on a slide for examination.

Blood transfusion The replacement of blood or one of its components.

Blood urea nitrogen (*BUN*) the level of nitrogen in the blood in the form of urea.

Blood vessel Any one of the network of muscular tubes that carry blood such as arteries, arterioles, veins, venules and capillaries.

Cord blood Blood in the umbilical vessels at the time of delivery of the infant.

Occult blood Blood found in minute quantity that is detectable only by chemical tests.

Venous blood Blood that has given up its oxygen to the cells and is carrying carbon dioxide.

Whole blood Blood from which none of the elements has been removed.

Blood bank An unit concerned with collecting, processing and storing blood for transfusion.

Blood-brain barrier The phenomenon by which several substances found in the blood including drugs fail to reach neurons and cerebrospinal fluid.

Blood cell (blood corpuscle) Any of the formed elements of blood.

Blood clotting The conversion of blood from a free flowing liquid to a semi-solid gel.

Blood coagulation An important process that prevents excessive bleeding when a blood vessel is injured.

Blood corpuscle A blood cell, either red or white blood cell.

Blood count Determination of the number of red and white blood cells per cubic millimeter of blood.

Blood donor A person donating blood.

Blood group The classification of blood based on the presence or absence of genetically determined antigens located on the surface of the erythrocyte. There are a number of human blood group systems, each system is determined by a series of two or more genes that are closely linked on a single autosomal chromosome. ABO blood group discovered by Karl Landsteiner is of great significance in blood transfusion. The population is divided into four blood groups as A, B, AB and O. The Rhesus (Rh) system is of value in obstetrics.

Blood plasma Liquid portion of blood.

Blood poisoning A life-threatening complication of an infection, sepsis.

Blood pressure The pressure exerted by the flow of blood as it is pumped by the heart through the main arteries.

Basal blood pressure Blood pressure obtained after making the patient to rest for about an hour in bed or after a sedative to allay anxiety.

Blood pressure estimation Gives an indication of the overall cardiovascular status as it depends upon cardiac output and peripheral resistance caused by the values of blood pressure obtained when the patient is examined in a clinic without any prior preparation.

Blood transfusion The replacement of blood or one of its components.

Blood vessel Any one of the network of muscular tubes that carry blood such as arteries, arterioles, veins, venules and capillaries.

Bloom syndrome Immunodeficiency disease with reduction in immunoglobulin levels.

Blotting (*blot'ing*) A technique for transferring DNA (Southern blotting), RNA (Northern blotting), or proteins (Western blotting) from an agarose or polyacrylamide gel to a nylon membrane.

Blount's disease Breaking and fragmentation of the medial tibial epiphysis, named after Water Blount, US orthopedic surgeon; tibia vara.

Blue baby A neonate with cyanosis or any etiology.

BMI Body mass index.

Boas's sign In cholecystitis, there may be an area of hyperesthesia posteriorly. The tenderness extends from about 2.5 cm lateral to the spines of the vertebrae to the posterior axillary line, and vertically from the level of the 11th thoracic to the 1st lumbar spine.

Boari flap Tubularization of a flap of bladder to extent from the bladder to extend from the bladder to the ureteral orifice; useful in management of lower ureteric strictures and can be performed as either open or laparoscopic operation.

Boceprevir (*bo-sep're-vir*) A hepatitis C virus NS3/4A protease inhibitor used in combination with other medications to treat chronic hepatitis C genotype 1 infection.

Body (*bod'ē*) The whole physical structure of an individual with all organs; a cadaver or a corpse; the largest or main part of any organ.

Body contour surgery Surgical procedures performed to improve body shape by removing fat and skin.

Body dysmorphic syndrome *psy* A psychiatric disorder characterized by preoccupation with an imagined physical defect.

Body fluid A fluid contained in the three compartments of the body such as plasma, interstitial fluid between the cells and intracellular fluid within the cells.

Body mechanics Study of muscular actions and functions of muscles in maintaining the posture of the body.

Body plethysmograph A device permitting rapid estimation of the volume of air in the thorax.

Donovan's Body Intracellular bacillus (*Calymmatobacterium donovani*) see in histiocyte in the genital skin of patients affected with granuloma inguinale.

Howell-Jolly body A cytopathological finding of basophilic nuclear remnants (cluster of DNA) in circulating erythrocytes.

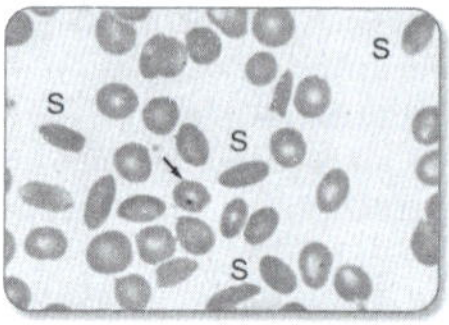

Howell-Jolly body

Boerhaave syndrome (*boor'ha-ve*) Spontaneous rupture of the esophagus leading to mediastinitis and pleural effusion. Usually associated with violent retching and vomiting, named after Hermann Boerhaave, Danish physician.

Boil (*boil*) Furuncle, infection of a hair follicle by staphylococci. It is characterized by redness, swelling, heat and tenderness.

Bolus (*bo'lus*) A rounded mass of food material; material injected intravenously and rapidly at one time for a quick response; a rounded soft mass of pharmaceutical preparation ready to swallow.

Bombay phenotype The O_h phenotype, a variant of the ABO antigens on red cells. These red cells do not agglutinate with antisera containing anti-A, anti-B or anti-'H' type antibody. These red cells lack the H antigen and H substance. The condition was described in Mumbai.

Bonding Development of an emotional attachment between parents and newborn; *dent* application of synthetic material on teeth.

Bone (*bon*) The dense, hard tissue forming the skeleton; any distinct piece of the skeleton of the body (*see* **Table**).

Bone age Radiologic study of estimation of biologic age based on the stage of development of ossification centers of the wrist bones and long bones of extremities.

Bone cancer A skeletal malignancy occurring primarily as a sarcoma or as metastasis from cancer elsewhere in the body.

Bone cell Osteocyte, a nucleated cell with spidery processes in the septate lacuna of bone.

Bone cyst A cystic structure replacing the bone.

Bone density The concentration of protein and mineral salts in bone; their concentration is lowered in osteoporosis.

Bone densitometry The measurement of bone mass or density.

Bone graft A surgical procedure in which a piece of bone is removed from one part of the body to repair the bone damaged in another part.

Bone marrow transplant Transplantation of bone marrow from healthy donors to stimulate production of blood cells.

Bone spur An abnormal bony excrescence often found in heel; an overgrowth of bone; osteophyte.

Bone marrow (marrow) Soft tissue found within bone cavities and it is the site of blood cell production.

Bony labyrinth Bony, rigid, outer wall of the inner ear in the temporal bone; having 3 parts—vestibule, semicircular canals and cochlea.

Borax (*bor'aks*) A white powder used, for example, in the making of glass and as a cleaning chemical.

Borborygmus *(bor'bo-rig'mus)* Rumbling noise or gurgling sound produced by the movement of fluid and gas through the intestines. pl. **borborygmi**.

Borderline (*bor'dar-lin*) Any condition that cannot be placed in one of usually two categories.

Borderline hypertension That range of systolic and diastolic blood pressures which are not benefited by therapy.

Borderline leprosy Dimorphous leprosy borderline lesions between two extremes of leprosy such as tuberculoid and lepromatous leprosy.

Borderline personality A personality disturbance in which one lies between a neurotic, capable of coping with his environment and apsychotic who has lost contact with reality and there is persistent instability in emotions, relationships and behavior.

Borderline tumor A growth with low malignant potential.

Bordetella (*bor'de-te'la*) Gram-negative coccobacillus, named after a French bacteriologist, Jules Bordet.

Bordetella pertussis Causative agent of whooping cough.

Boric acid (*bor'ik*) A weakly acid crystalline compound derived from borax, used as a mild antiseptic and in the manufacture of heat-resistant glass and enamels.

Table: Bones

Name	Region	Character	Articulations
Atlas	Neck	Ring-shaped first cervical vertebra under skull, having no body	Occipital bone above and axis vertebra below
Axis	Neck	Second cervical vertebra with used body of atlas as odontoid process	With atlas above and 3rd cervical vertebra below
Calcaneus	Foot (heel)	Largest of the tarsal bones, irregular in shape	With talus and cuboid bone
Capitate	Wrist	Central carpal bone with rounded head	With metacarpals distally and other carpal bones proximally

Contd...

Name	Region	Character	Articulations
Carpals	Wrist	Eight in number, small irregular bones scaphoid, lunate, triquetral, pisiform trapezoid, capitate, trapezium and hamate arranged in two rows of 4 each	With radius proximally and metacarpals distally
Clavicle	Front of shoulder	Horizontally placed long bone, with concavo-convex curve, in the upper part of a thorax	With sternum, scapula and first rib
Coccyx	Tip of the vertebral column at lower end	Triangular in shape, formed by fusion of last 4 vertebrae	With sacrum
Concha inferior	Lateral wall of nasal cavity	Thin curved piece of bone attached on the lateral wall of nasal cavity	With ethmoid, lacrimal and palatine processes of maxilla
Cuboid	Foot	Irregular cubical bone placed laterally	With calcaneus, cuneiform and 4th and 5th metatarsal bones
Cuneiform	Foot	Three in number, medial, intermediate and lateral, wedge-shaped bones	With bases of 1st to 4th metatarsal bones and other tarsal bones
Ethmoid	Skull	Single bone below frontal bone extending into nasal cavity contributing to nasal septum and forming superior and middle nasal conchae	With sphenoid, frontal, vomer, maxilla, lacrimal and nasal bones
Fabella	Knee	A small rounded sesamoid bone, present in the lateral head of gastrocnemius near its origin	With femur, reduces friction of tendon with bone
Femur	Thigh	Longest bone of the skeleton	Forms hip joint with *os-innominatum* and knee joint with tibia and patella distally
Fibula	Leg	Thin long bone placed laterally in leg	With tibia at both ends and also with talus distally

Contd...

Name	Region	Character	Articulations
Frontal	Skull	Single bone on the anterior part of skull, having frontal air sinus in it	With parietal, sphenoid, maxilla, ethmoid, zygomatic, lacrimal and nasal bones
Hamate	Wrist	Carpal bone, hammer-shaped, placed medially in distal row of carpal bones	With bases of 4th and 5th metacarpal bones and other carpal bones
Hip bone	Pelvis	Irregular bone formed by fusion of 3 bones ischium, ilium and pubis. Bones of two sides together with sacrum form bony pelvis	Hip joint, with head of femur, sacroiliac joint with sacrum and symphysis pubis with pubic bone of other side
Humerus	Arm	Long bone with head, greater and lesser trochanter at upper end and trochlea and capitulum at lower end	Forms shoulder joint with glenoid cavity of scapula and elbow joint with radius and ulna distally
Hyoid	Front of neck	U-shaped small bone to which muscles of the tongue and ribbon muscles of neck are attached	Suspended by ligament and muscles having no articulation with any bone
Ilium	Pelvis	Flat bony part of hip bone having crest and spines	With sacrum behind contributes to upper part of acetabulum which articulates with head of the femur
Incus	Small bone in the middle ear cavity	Anvil-shaped	With malleus and stapes
Ischium	Pelvis	Part of hip bone below and behind acetabulum	Contributes to lower part of acetabulum which articulates with head of the femur
Lacrimal	Skull	Thin small flat bone contributes to medial wall of orbit near its margin	With ethmoid, frontal and maxilla
Lunate	Wrist	Half moon-shaped carpal bone in the proximal row of carpals	With radius and triquetral to form wrist joint and with other carpal bones forms intercarpal joints

Contd...

Name	Region	Character	Articulations
Malleus	Small bone in the middle ear cavity	Hammer-shaped, placed laterally in contact with tympanic membrane	With incus
Mandible	Lower jaw	Horse shoe-shaped, having body, ramus and condyloid-coronoid processes. Body has sockets for teeth	With temporal bone forming temporomandibular joint, also with 16 teeth in adult
Maxilla	Upper jaw	Irregular paired bone below orbit and on lateral side of nasal cavity having maxillary air sinus in it, carries upper teeth	With ethmoid, frontal, vomer, lacrimal, nasal, palatine, zygomatic, maxilla of opposite side and inferior concha
Metacarpal	Hand	Five short-long bones, heads of which form knuckles	Distally articulates with bases of proximal phalanges, proximally articulates with distal row of carpal bones
Metatarsal	Foot	Five short-long bones of foot with concavity on plantar surface	Distally articulates with bases of proximal phalanges, proximally articulates with tarsal bones
Nasal	Skull	Small paired bone, together forming bridge of the nose	With frontal, ethmoid and maxilla
Navicular	Foot	Boat-shaped tarsal bone with a tuberosity on medial side	With talus proximally and 3 cuneiform bones distally
Occipital	Skull	Single bone at the back of skull, and at the base of skull having large foramen magnum.	With sphenoid, both parietals and temporal bones
Palatine	Skull	Paired bone forming posterior part of hard palate	With ethmoid, sphenoid, vomer, maxilla and palatine of opposite side
Patella	Knee	Largest sesamoid bone, irregularly rectangular, placed in the tendon of quadriceps femoris, forms knee cap	With femur

Contd...

Name	Region	Character	Articulations
Phalanges	Fingers and toes	Short-long bones, 3 in each fingers and toes, 2 in thumb and big toe arranged as proximal, middle and distal	With heads of metacarpal and metatarsal, with other phalanges proximal and distal to them
Pisiform	Wrist	Smallest sesamoid bone placed medially in proximal row of carpal bone	With triquetral bone
Pubic	Pelvis	Lower anterior part of hip bone, having body and 2 rami enclosing obturator foramen	With pubic bone of opposite side forming symphysis pubis bone
Radius	Forearm	Long bone placed laterally in forearm	Proximally with ulna and humerus distally with ulna and carpal bones-scaphoid and lunate
Ribs	Chest wall	Twelve pairs of thin ribbon-shaped bones (tinning posterolateral wall of chest)	Posteriorly all ribs articulate with corresponding vertebrae, anteriorly upper 7 ribs with sternum through costal cartilages, lower 3 ribs with costal cartilages of rib above and last 2 ribs are floating
Sacrum	Lower back	Wedge-shaped triangular bone formed by fusion of 5 vertebrae below lumbar vertebrae	With 5th lumbar vertebra above, coccyx below and ilium on the two sides
Scaphoid	Wrist	Boat-shaped carpal bone placed laterally in proximal row of carpal bones	With radius proximally and with other carpal bones
Sesamoid	In the tendons of muscles of extremities	Small, rounded or flat bones developing in the long tendons near the joints	
Sphenoid	Base of skull	Single, irregular bone having body and wing-shaped extensions forming part of lateral wall of orbit	With frontal, occipital, ethmoid, vomer, palatine, parietal, temporal and zygomatic bones

Contd...

Name	Region	Character	Articulations
Stapes	Middle ear	Smallest bone, stirrup-shaped, placed medially in middle ear cavity	With incus laterally, covers oval window of vestibule of internal ear medially.
Sternum	Chest	Flat bone placed in midline of anterior wall of chest, comprising 3 parts—manubrium, body and xiphoid process	With clavicle and upper 7 pairs of ribs on each side
Talus	Ankle	Large tarsal bone having no muscular attachment	With tibia, fibula, calcaneus and navicular
Tarsal bones	Ankle-foot	Irregular bones of foot, arranged in rows—talus, calcaneus, navicular, cuboid and 8 cuneiforms	Forms ankle joint with tibia-fibula, intertarsal joints with each other and tarsometatarsal joints with bases of metatarsal bones
Temporal	Lateral side of skull	Paired irregular bone having mastoid, squamous, petrous, tympanic and zygomatic parts, contains middle and internal ear	With occipital, sphenoid, mandible, parietal and zygomatic bones
Tibia	Leg	Larger long bone in leg placed medially	With femur and fibula proximally and talus and fibula distally
Trapezium	Wrist	Carpal bone of the distal row placed laterally	With trapezoid and scaphoid and with bases of 1st and 2nd metacarpals
Trapezoid	Wrist	Carpal bone of distal row, trapezoid shape	With capitate, scaphoid, trapezium and bases of 2nd metacarpal bone
Triquetral	Wrist	Small 3 facet triangular carpal bone of proximal row of carpal bones	With hamate, lunate, pisiform and articular disk of wrist joint
Ulna	Forearm	Long bone placed medially in forearm	Proximally with radius forming superior radioulnar joint and with humerus forming elbow joint distally with radius and articular disk

Contd...

Name	Region	Character	Articulations
Vertebrae	Vertebral column	Irregular bones having body, neural arches, transverse processes, spine and vertebral canal. 7 cervical, 12 thoracic, 5 lumbar, 5 sacral fused to form sacrum and lower 3–5 coccygeal fused as coccyx	1st cervical with occipital, 5th lumbar with sacrum, all vertebrae with adjacent vertebrae above and below. Thoracic also articulates with ribs
Vomer	Skull	Thin sheet-like bone forming posteroinferior part of nasal septum	With sphenoid and ethmoid
Zygomatic	Skull	Irregular bone forming bony prominence of cheek and lower margin of orbit	with frontal, sphenoid, maxilla and temporal bone

Bornholm disease (devil's grip, epidemic myalgia, epidemic pleurodynia) (*born'hom*) Pleurodynia with involvement of intercostal muscles first noted in Danish island, Bornholm.

Borrelia (*bor-rel'e-a*) A spirochete causing relapsing fever, described by a French bacteriologist, Amedee Borrel; ***B. burgdorferi*** causative agent of Lyme disease; ***B. duttonii*** causative agent of tick-borne relapsing fever; ***B. recurrentis*** causative agent of louse-borne relapsing fever; ***B. vincenti*** causative agent of cancrum oris.

Botulism (*boch'u-lizm*) Food poisoning due to botulin produced by the growth of *Clostridium botulinum* in improperly preserved or canned foods. The manifestations consist chiefly of vomiting and paresis of skeletal, ocular, pharyngeal and respiratory muscles.

Infant botulism A potentially life-threatening disease caused by a bacterium called *Clostridium botulinum*.

Wound botulism A rare condition and occurs when the *Clostridium* spores get into an open wound and are able to reproduce in an anaerobic environment.

Bouchard' nodes Swelling of the middle joint of the finger.

Bougie (*boo'zhe*) A slender flexible cylindrical instrument introduced to dilate the constricted region such as urethra, or esophagus.

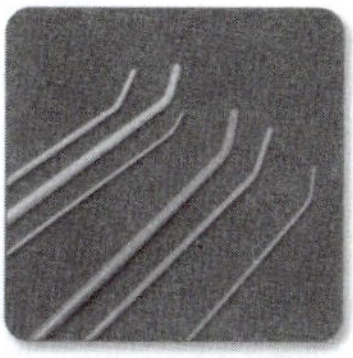

Bougies

Bowel (*bo'wel*) The intestine.

Bowel movement Evacuation of feces.

Bowel sounds The normal sounds associated with movement of intestinal contents.

Bowen disease (*bau'nz*) A persistent progressive but potentially malignant intraepidermal carcinoma.

Bowleg (*bo'leg*) Genu vara.

Bowman capsule (*bo'manz*) Glomerular capsule described by an English physician, Sir William Bowman.

Brace (*Bras*) Mechanical support for damaged bones and ligaments.

Carpal tunnel brace A brace that looks like a fingerless glove. It stabilizes your wrist in a straight and sometimes slightly bent-back position.

Collar brace An instrument used to support the neck and spine and limit head movement after an injury.

Brachial (*bra'ke-al*) Pertaining to the arm.

Brachial artery The principal artery of upper arm.

Brachialis (*bra'ke-al'is*) A muscle of the arm lying beneath biceps brachii.

Brachial plexus A network of lower four cervical and the first thoracic spinal nerves that control the muscles of the upper limb.

Brachiocephalic artery (innominate artery) Artery that branches off the aorta in upper chest; it is first branch of aorta and resembles the handle of a cane.

Brachiocephalic vein (innominate vein) Paired vein and helps return oxygen-poor blood from head, neck and arms back to the heart. It begins at the meeting point of subclavian vein and internal jugular vein.

Brachium (*bra-ke-um*) The arm or anatomical structure resembling an arm.

Brachy A combining word for short.

Brachycephaly (*brak'e-se-fal-i*) Short head.

Brachytherapy (*brak"e-ther'e-pe*) Heat treatment with ionizing radiations; Treatment with ionizing radiation whose source is near or on the surface of the body at a close distance.

Brady A combining form of word meaning slow.

Bradycardia (*brad'e-kar'de-a*) Slow heartbeat exhibiting slow pulse rate, less than 60/min. Noted in myxedema, obstructive jaundice, raised intracranial tension, digoxin toxicity, and complete heart block.

Relative bradycardia Normal relation of increase in pulse rate of 10 beats for each half degree centigrade rise of temperature is not maintained and pulse rate is relatively slow compared to the temperature. It is seen in typhoid, meningitis, dengue fever, cerebral abscess and in viral infections.

Bradycardia-tachycardia syndrome Heart rate alternating between abnormally slow and abnormally rapid rhythm.

Bradykinesia (*brad'e-kin-ne'se-a*) Marked slowness of movement.

Bradykinin (*brad'e-ki'nin*) A plasma kinin.

Braille (*bral*) A system of reading and writing that enables the blind to see by using the sense of touch, named after Louis Braille, blind French education.

Brain (*bran*) Highest controlling center of nervous system. It is a large soft mass of nerve tissue contained within the cranium. It consists of cerebrum, cerebellum, midbrain, pons and medulla. It is composed of neurons and neuroglia. Gray matter is composed of neuron cells and is concentrated in the cerebral cortex and nuclei and basal ganglia. White matter is composed of neuron processes which form tracts connecting parts of the brain with each other and with the spinal cord.

Brain abscess A pocket of infection in a part of the brain.

Brain damage Degeneration or death of nerve cells in the brain.

Brain edema Swelling of the brain due to an increase in its water content.

Brain fever Meningitis.

Brain scan The use of radioisotopes injected into circulation to detect abnormalities in the brain.

Brain shift Displacement of parts of brain by expanding lesion.

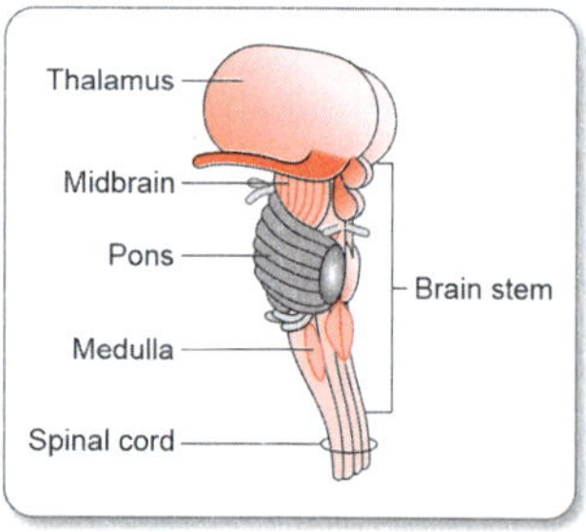

Brain stem

Brainwashing Intense psychological indoctrination.

Brain death The irreversible cessation of all brain functions while heart continues beating. There is lack of response to stimuli, lack of all reflexes, absent respirations and an isoelectric electroencephalogram.

Brain stem The stem-like part of midbrain comprising pons and medulla oblongata that connects cerebral hemispheres with the spinal cord.

Brain tumor Any intracranial space occupying lesion such as neoplasm, cyst, or abscess.

Branchial cyst A cyst that arises at the site of one of the embryonic pharyngeal pouches due to a developmental anomaly.

Braxton Hicks contractions Painless uterine contractions without cervical dilatation in latter half of pregnancy, named after Braxton Hicks, UK obstetrician.

Brandt Andrews method A technique for expelling the placenta from the uterus.

Breakbone fever Dengue fever.

Breast (*brest*) Anterior aspect of the chest; mammary gland.

Breast augmentation Enlarging breasts for cosmetic purposes.

Breast crawl Human babies when kept in skin-to-skin contact between their mother's breasts can initiate breast feeding on their own.

Breast examination A process in which the breasts and their accessory structures are observed and palpated to find out any change or abnormality that could indicate malignant condition.

Breastfeeding The act of providing milk to a new born or infant from mother's breasts.

Breast implant An inert sac filled with silicone covered by polyurethane foam used to augment cosmetically the female contour; a soft pouch, filled with saline or silicone that is surgically implanted beneath the skin and muscle of the chest wall to form a reconstructed breast after mastectomy.

Breast milk Contains 88% water, 3.5% fat, lactose, protein 1.0–1.5%, sterile, provides IgA and is more easily digestible.

Breast mouse Fibroadenoma of the breast, an extremely mobile swelling of rubbery hard consistency.

Breast pump A device for withdrawing milk from the breast.

Breast reconstruction Any surgical method used to create a new breast after mastectomy.

Breast reduction A surgical procedure performed in order to decrease the size of breast.

Breast self-examination A monthly routine in which a woman follows several steps to detect any changes or lumps in her breast; BSE.

Breast shadows Artifacts on chest radiography of women caused by breast tissue.

Breastbone The long flat bone that forms the center front of the chest wall; it is attached to the collar bone and the first seven ribs.

Breast cancer A malignant neoplasm of breast tissue in women between the age of 30 and 50 may present as a small painless lump, thick or dimpled skin or nipple retraction, nipple discharge, ulceration and enlarged axillary lymph nodes, metastases through the lymphatics to axillary lymph nodes and to bone, lung, liver and brain. The extent of disease determines therapy. Surgery may be radical or simple mastectomy. Radiation or chemotherapy are adjuvant therapy.

Breathing (*brething*) The act of respiration; inhalation and exhalation.

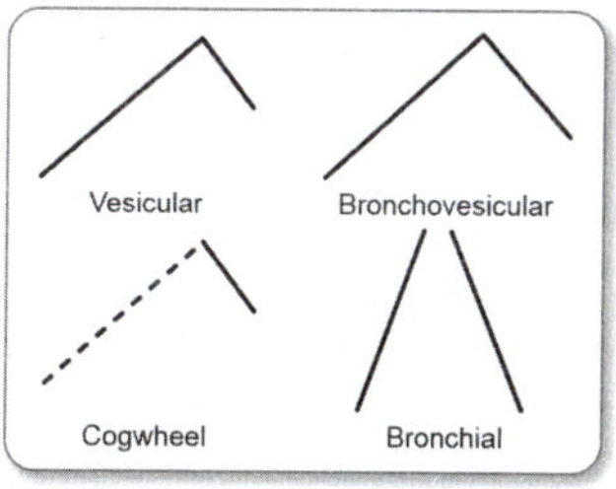

Breathing

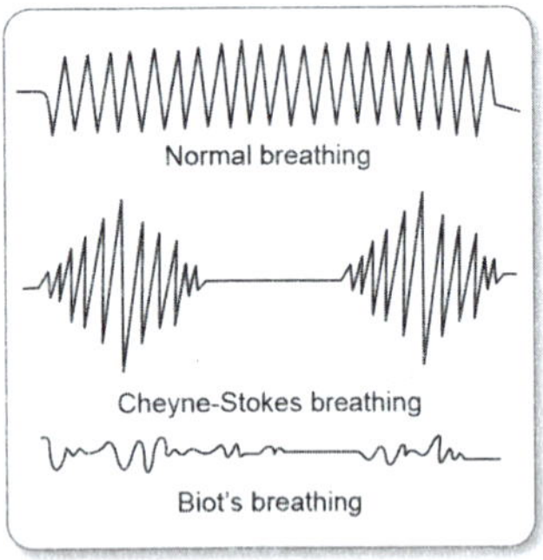

Breathing rhythm

Abdominal breathing Seen in men. There is downward excursion of the diaphragm with inspiration and free movement of the abdominal wall. It is more evident in paralysis of intercostal muscles, ankylosing spondylitis, pleurisy and fibrosis of the lung.

Biots breathing An irregular respiration which may become slow or rapid, shallow or deep with irregular pauses, seen in meningitis, named after Camille Biot, French physician.

Bronchial breathing Sounds heard when the normal dampening effect of the air-containing alveoli is lost. The expiratory phase is longer as long as, or longer than inspiration. There is a pause between inspiration and expiration. The quality of the sound may be hollow or tubular. The breathing may be high pitched or low pitched.

Bronchovesicular breathing An intermediate type of breathing exhibiting features of both vesicular and bronchial breathing.

Cavernous breathing Low pitched bronchial breathing heard over cavities.

Cheyne-Stokes breathing (*chan'stoks*) A periodic form of respiration wherein the successive respirations gradually become deeper and deeper and then diminish until there is temporary cessation of the respiration. It is noted in raised intracranial tension, narcotic poisoning of the respiratory centers, severe pneumonia, cardiac and renal failure, also when patient is asleep or comatose, named after John Cheyne, Scottish physician and William Stokes, Irish physician.

Cogwheel breathing Breathing instead of being steady, appear jerky and inspiratory phase appears broken in nervous individual and in conditions of pleural adhesions.

Costal breathing Participation of intercostal muscles in the respiration, seen in women. It is encountered in paralysis of the diaphragm, peritonitis, ascites and diaphragmatic paralysis; thoracic respiration.

Kussmaul's breathing Increased rate and depth of breathing in diabetic ketoacidosis and renal failure.

Puerile breathing In children, the breath sounds are harsher than in adults.

Pursed lip breathing Slow exhalation promoting emptying of the lungs and retarding collapse of conducting airways.

Tubular breathing A high pitched bronchial breathing heard over an area of consolidation.

Vesicular breathing Heard over the chest as a breezy rustling sound, inspiratory phase is fairly intense, longer and of low pitch. The expiratory phase is shorter with its length being equal to a third of the length of inspiration. The inspiration is harsher than expiration and its intensity is greater than that of expiration. There is no gap between inspiration and expiration. These sounds are heard on the greater part of the normal lung, except over trachea and the region where major bronchi are situated near the surface of the chest wall.

Breath sounds The sounds heard through a stethoscope placed over the lungs during breathing.

Breech (*brech*) Buttocks.

Breech presentation Position of the fetus presenting with buttocks.

Bregma (*breg'ma*) The junction of the coronal and sagittal sutures on the skull; anterior fontanelle.

Brenner's tumor (*bren'erz*) A benign fibroepithelioma of the ovary named after Fritz Brenner, German pathologist.

Bridge (*brij*) A narrow band of tissue; a dental appliance that replaces a missing tooth and it is attached to adjacent teeth for support; a structure that connects two distant points, including parts of an organ.

Bright disease Acute glomerulonephritis, described by an English physician, Richard Bright.

Briquet's syndrome Somatization disorder is a chronic psychiatric condition in which patients experience physical symptoms that have no apparent physiological cause.

Broca's area (*bro'kas*) Speech center in the brain, described by a French anatomist, Pierre Broca.

Brodie's abscess A deep-seated bony swelling situated near a joint in chronic osteomyelitis, named after Sir Benjamin Brodie, English surgeon.

Brodmann's areas (*brod'manz*) Division of cerebral cortex into 47 different areas that are associated with specific neurologic functions, named after Korbinian Brodmann, German anatomist.

Bromhexine Mucolytic agent.

Bromide (*bro'mid*) A binary compound of bromine with another element or a radical including some (such as potassium bromide) used as sedatives.

Bromism (*bro'mizm*) Poisoning by bromine or a bromine compound.

Bromodiphenhydramine (*bro"mo-di" fen-hi'dra-men*) An ethanolamine antihistamine with antimicrobial property. Bromodiphenhydramine is used in the control of cutaneous allergies.

Brompheniramine (*brom"fen-ir'a-men*) Antihistamine used to treat hypersensitivity reactions (as rhinitis).

Bronchial (*brong'ke-al*) Pertaining to bronchi or bronchioles.

Bronchial adenoma A benign tumor of the lung situated near the hilum. It arises either in the main or lobar bronchus from the duct epithelium of bronchial mucous glands. It appears as a polypoid mass causing dry irritant cough and hemoptysis.

Bronchial tree The branching, tree-like structure of airways in the lungs.

Bronchial washing Irrigation of the bronchi and bronchioles to collect cells for cytologic study and to cleanse the region.

Bronchiectasis (*brong'ke-ek'ta-sis*) Abnormal and permanent distortion and dilatation of the subsegmental airways. There is distinction of the components of bronchial wall. The condition develops insidiously and the manifestations depend on the degree of dilatation, infective episodes and secretion. There is profuse purulent expectoration and it has a postural relationship.

Dry bronchiectasis Bronchiectasis without infection presents with hemoptysis.

Bronchiloquy (*brong-kil'o-kwe*) A modification of the voice sounds, by which they are intensified and heightened in pitch.

Bronchiole (*brong'ke-ol*) Pl. **bronchioles**; finer division of a bronchus. They are membranous and branch more frequently at a few millimeter distance. Smooth muscle forms its wall. There are no mucous glands.

Respiratory bronchiole Last division of bronchial tree. It contains both bronchiolar epithelium and alveoli in their walls. It ends by dividing into two or more air sacs.

Terminal bronchiole The airway immediately proximal to the respiratory bronchiole. This last purely conducting structure supplies an acinus.

Bronchiolitis (*brong'ke-o-li'tis*) Inflammation of the bronchioles.

Bronchiolitis obliterans organizing pneumonia (BOOP) An infiltrative lung disease with a subacute clinical course where the granulation tissue plugs within the lumens of small airways.

Bronchitis (*brong-ki'tis*) Inflammation of the bronchi.

Acute bronchitis Bronchitis having a short clinical course with cough, expectoration and fever. Often caused by the spread of upper respiratory viral infections to the bronchi.

Chronic bronchitis Chronic or recurrent excess mucus secretion into the bronchial tree without a demonstrable cause either local or general occurring on most of the days during at least three months of the year for at least two successive years. It is caused by protracted bronchial irritation by cigarette smoke and airborne particulate and gaseous pollutants. There is bronchial mucous gland hyperplasia with chronic productive cough.

Bronchoconstrictor A substance that causes the airways to narrow.

Bronchodilator (*brong'ko-dil-a-ter*) A drug that widens the constricted bronchial passages by relaxing the smooth muscles, beta-adrenergic receptor agonists, methylxanthine and anticholinergic are examples.

Bronchography (*brong-kog'ra-fe*) Roentgenography of the bronchial tree after instilling, a radiopaque medium into a bronchus.

Bronchophony (*brong-kof'o-ne*) Voice sounds heard through the stethoscope on a large bronchus and it can be heard in other regions of the chest in consolidation of the lung.

Bronchopneumonia (*brong'ko-nu-mo'ne-a*) A combination of bronchiolitis and pneumonia.

Bronchoscope (*brong'ko-skop*) An instrument to visualize the interior of the airways, to aspirate secretions, to remove foreign body and to perform brush or biopsy.

Bronchospasm (*brong'ko-spazm*) Spasmodic contraction of the bronchial smooth muscle of the airways causing the airways to narrow.

Bronchospirometry (*brong'ko-spi-rom'e-tre*) Determination of the ventilatory function tests by a spirometer.

Bronchus (*brong'kus*) Air passage arising from the trachea which divides into lobar bronchi and in turn into segmental and subsegmental bronchi; pl. **bronchi**.

Intermediate bronchus Descending right main bronchus after giving upper lobe bronchus.

Large bronchus Proximal five generations of bronchial division, contain abundant cartilage forming a complete ring in their walls and contain a large number of mucous glands.

Segmental bronchus Bronchi leading to the segments of the lobes of the lung.

Small bronchus Next 10 generations of bronchial division after large bronchi, contain sparse amount of cartilage in their walls and collapse easily. Number of mucous glands are less.

Bronze baby syndrome (*brong*) A condition in which the skin, serum and urine develop a dark, grayish-brown discoloration following phototherapy in infants with cholestasis.

Brown-Sequard's syndrome (*brown'sa-karz*) Hemisection of spinal cord causing ipsilateral spastic paralysis with loss of vibration and position sense and contralateral loss of pain and temperature, named after Charles Brown-Sequard, French physiologist.

Brucella (*bro-sel'a*) Nonmotile gram-negative genus of microorganisms belonging to the family of Brucellaceae, described by David Bruce, British army surgeon.

Brucellosis (malta fever, mediterranean fever, undulant fever) (*broo'sel-o'sis*) An infection caused by *Brucella abortus* which is usually spread to humans by ingestion of raw milk from infected cattle and cause both a bloodstream infection and an intracellular infection. It presents with fever, sweating, weakness, headache, anorexia, pain in the limbs and back and splenomegaly. Tetracycline, streptomycin and rifampicin are useful in the treatment.

Brudzinski's sign (*brood-zin'skez*) Passive flexion of the neck causing flexion of limbs in meningitis, named after Jozef Brudzinski, Polish physician.

Brugada syndrome (*bru'ga-da*) An inherited arrhythmogenic disease with polymorphic ventricular tachycardia characterized by typical electrocardiographic pattern of ST-segment elevation >2 mm in precordial leads V1 through V3, incomplete bundle branch block in the right precordial leads and an increased risk of sudden cardiac death as a result of ventricular fibrillation.

Brugia (*broo'je-a*) A genus of filarial worms.

Brugia malayi Nematode of filariasis that infects man and other animals, and microfilariae not confined to night.

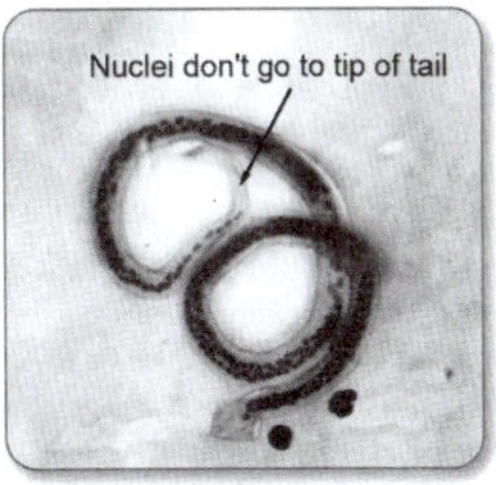

Brugia malayi—microfilaria

Bruise (contusion) (*brooz*) A superficial injury.

Bruit (*broot*) An abnormal sound or a murmur heard on auscultation.

Arterial bruit Systolic bruit audible over normal arteries with increased blood flow as in thyrotoxicosis or over the site where the lumen is narrowed as in renal artery stenosis or carotid stenosis.

Systolic bruit Arterial bruit.

Brunner's glands (*brun'erz*) Submucosal glands in the first part of duodenum secreting alkaline fluid on stimulus of acid in the lumen, named after Johann Brunner, Swiss anatomist.

Brush border (*brush*) Layer of absorbing surfaces of small intestine and first convoluted tubules of the kidney, consists of tightly packed microvilli.

Bruxism (*bruk'sizm*) Rhythmic or spasmodic grinding of the teeth especially during sleep.

Bryant's triangle When the patient lies in the dorsal position, a plumb line is drawn toward the floor from the anterior superior iliac spine (base- line), and another line to the tip of greater trochanter from the anterior superior iliac spine. Then a line is drawn by shortest route from the tip of greater trochanter to the baseline (horizontal line). A difference in the horizontal line on both sides is useful to note shortening in femoral head or neck, named after Sir Thomas Bryant, British surgeon.

Bubo (*boo'bo*) An enlarged and inflamed lymph node in the axilla or groin.

Tropical bubo Inflamed lymph nodes along the iliac vessels in LGV.

Bubonic plague Common type of plague characterized by painful, swollen lymph nodes (buboes) in the axilla, groin or neck.

Buccal (*buk'al*) Pertaining to the cheek.

Buccal administration Drugs administered by tablet held in the mouth.

Buccal smear Scraping of epithelium of oral mucosa for sex chromatin.

Buccal glands Minor salivary glands located on the inner side of the cheeks.

Buccinator (*buk'sina'ter*) The main muscle of the cheek.

Buclizine (*bu'kli-zen*) An antihistamine and antiemetic drug for the treatment of allergy symptoms and prevention of nausea and vomiting.

Budd-Chiari syndrome (*bud'ke-ar'e*) Obstruction to the venous outflow of the liver owing to occlusion of the hepatic vein described by Austrian pathologists, George Budd and Hans Chiari.

Buerger disease (*bur'gerz*) Thromboangitis obliterans, named after Leo Buerger, US urologist. It is a combination of thrombosis, inflammation and obliteration of small and medium-sized arteries. The disease begins in distal small arteries and spreads upward. Lower limbs are commonly affected and it occurs in young smokers.

Buffer (*buf'er*) A substance maintaining original hydrogen-ion concentration of its solution upon adding an acid or base.

Bulb (*bulb*) A rounded mass.

Bulbar (*bul'ber*) Pertaining to medulla oblongata.

Bulbar palsy Motor neuron disease affecting medulla and lower four cranial nerves.

Bulbourethral glands A pea sized gland in the male located behind and to the side of the urethra that discharges seminal fluid into the urethra.

Bulimia (*bu-lim'e-a*) Episodes of uncontrolled excessive hunger.

Bulla (*bul'ah*) A large vesicle; sharply demarcated avascular area in the lung with a wall thickness less than 1 mm and an internal diameter more than 1 cm; a large blister; a large projecting structure.

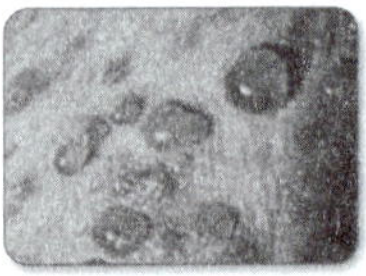

Bullae

Bundle (*bun-del*) A collection of fibers.

Bundle branch block A type of heart block in which interruption to the flow of electrical impulses through the right or left bundle of His delays activation of the appropriate ventricle that widens QRS complex and makes alteration in QRS morphology. Right bundle branch block is a common normal variant but left bundle branch block signifies an underlying heart disease; the wire-like branch that carries these impulses and splits into left and right bundles.

Bundle of His A band of atypical cardiac muscle fibers arising from AV node extending along the AV groove to the top of interventricular septum where it divides into right and left bundle branches, named after Wilhelm His, German physician.

Bunion (*bun'yun*) Abnormal prominence of the inner aspect of the first metatarsal head.

Buphthalmos (hydrophthalmos) (*buf-thol'mos*) Enlargement of whole eye, seen in infantile glaucoma; oxy eye.

Bupivacaine (*bu-piv'a-kan*) A widely used local anesthetic agent, often administered by spinal injection prior to total hip arthroplasty.

Bur (burr) (*bur*) A rough, prickly case around the seeds of certain plants, as the chestnut or burdock.

Burkitt's lymphoma Massive jaw lesions and extranodal abdominal involvement, caused by Epstein-Barr virus. It is characterized by sheets of monotonous small round cells punctuated by a 'starry sky' pattern.

Burn (*burn*) Tissue injury caused by heat, electricity, chemicals, radiation or gases. The effect depends on the type, duration, and intensity of the agent and the part of the body involved. The effect may be local or local and systemic. Superficial burns cause damage to the outer layers of the epidermis (first degree). The damage in second-degree burns extends through the epidermis into the dermis. However, it does not interfere with regeneration of the epidermis. Full thickness of the skin including the tissue beneath, it is affected in third-degree burn. There is destruction of epidermis, dermis and underlying tissues.

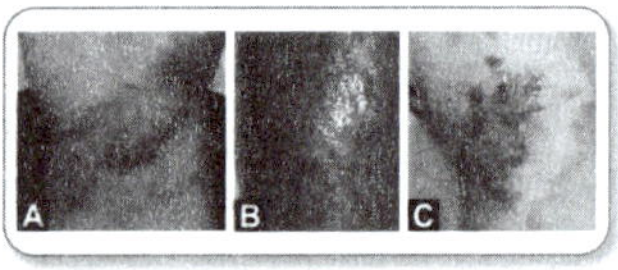

*Burns: **A.** First degree; **B.** Second degree; **C.** Third degree*

Burr (*burr*) A devise that rotates at high-speed, used to cut tooth or bone.

Burr cells Erythrocytes with scalloped margins may appear in renal failure.

Burr hole A hole made to relieve pressure inside the skull or to gain access to brain.

Bursa (*bur'sa*) A sac filled with a viscid fluid located at the sites of friction and prevents friction between tissues around a moving joint; pl. **bursae**.

Anserine bursa Bursa related to the insertion of the tendons of the gracilis, sartorius and semitendinosus muscles, likened to a goose's foot.

Patellar bursa Formed by several bursae located in the region of the patella; includes the suprapatellar infrapatellar, and prepatellar bursae.

Psoas bursa Bursa in the groin beneath inguinal ligament.

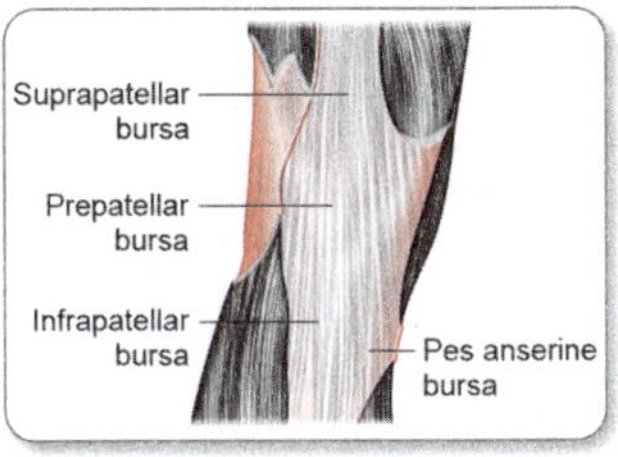

Patellar bursa

Semi-membranous bursa Swelling in the medial side of the popliteal space.

Bursitis (*ber-si'tis*) Inflammation of a bursa.

Achilles bursitis Painful swelling nearer to *os calcis*.

Infrapatellar bursitis Clergyman's knee. Tenderness and swelling below the patella at the insertion of quadriceps tendon.

Ischiogluteal bursitis Swelling and tenderness over ischiogluteal bursa, and is detected when the hip is flexed.

Metatarsal bursitis Pain and swelling situated more anteriorly over the metatarsal heads.

Olecranon bursitis A localized swelling over the olecranon.

Prepatellar bursitis Housemaid's knee; localized pain and swelling in the anteroinferior part of the patella.

Subachilles bursitis Painful swelling bulging out on either side of the Achilles tendon.

Buspirone (*bu-spi'ron*) An anxiolytic agent used for short-term treatment of generalized anxiety and second-line treatment of depression.

Busulfan (*bu-sul'fan*) Alkylating cytotoxic agent, used in chronic myeloid leukemia.

Butabarbital (butabarbitone) (*bu-ta-bar'bi-tal*) A barbiturate used short-term to treat insomnia, or as a sedative before surgery.

Butacaine A para aminobenzoic acid containing local anesthetic. It has more rapid onset of action and a more prolonged onset of action than cocaine.

Butterfly fragment A wedge-shaped fragment of a long bone which is split off the main fragments encountered in a comminuted fracture.

Butterfly bandage A small piece of adhesive tape with broad wing-shaped ends to hold the edges of a superficial wound together.

Butterfly rash A photosensitive facial rash seen in SLE. It consists of an erythematous blush or scaly reddish patches on the malar region extending over nasal bridge.

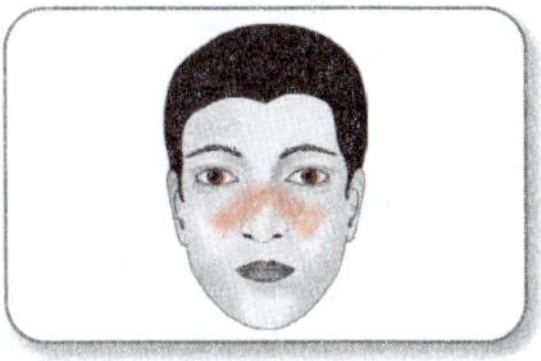

Butterfly rash

Byssinosis (*bis'i-no'sis*) An occupational lung disease in textile workers exposed to dust of cotton, flax, hemp or jute.

C

Cabergoline (*ka-bur'go-len*) A dopamine receptor agonist that is used to treat hyperprolactinemic conditions of various causes.

Cachet (*ka-sha't*) The state of being respected or admired.

Cachexia (*ka-keks'e-a*) Severe wasting and weakness.

Cacosmia (*ka-koz'me-a*) An unpleasant smell.

Cadmium (*kad'me-am*) Metallic element used in many alloys and plating, inhalation of the fumes may lead to fever, albuminuria and fibrosis of the lung.

Caffeine (*kaf'en*) An alkaloid present in coffee, amcolate, tea and cola drinks. It stimulates central nervous system, gastric secretion and raises free fatty acids in plasma. It acts by increasing the activity of beta-2 adrenoreceptors.

Caisson disease A clinical complex caused by rapid body decompression with intravascular boiling of 'nitrogen' noted in Scuba divers, workers in high pressure environment and high-altitude pilots. It is characterized by headache, nausea, vomiting, vertigo, tinnitus, dyspnea, convulsions and shock; decompression sickness.

Calamine (*kal'a-min*) A pink powder containing zinc oxide used externally in various skin conditions as a soothening agent. It is protective and astringent.

Calcaneus (heel bone) (*kal-ka-ne-us*) The heel bone that articulates with cuboid bone and with the talus.

Calcaneoapophysitis (*kal-ka'ne-o-a-pof'e-zi-tis*) Pain and inflammation of the posterior portion of the calcaneus at the place of insertion of the Achilles tendon.

Calcaneodynia (*kal-ka-ne-o-din'e-a*) Pain in the heel when standing or walking.

Calcaneotibial (*kal-ka'ne-o-tib'e-al*) Pertaining to the calcaneus and tibia.

Calcar (*kal'kar*) A spur-like process.

Calcicosis (*kal'si-ko'sis*) Pneumoconiosis produced by inhalation of dust from limestone.

Calciferol (*kal-sif'er-ol*) Vitamin D2; a synthetic preparation used in the treatment of vitamin D deficiency and hypocalcemic tetany.

Calcification (*kal'si-fi-ka'shun*) Deposition of calcium salts in body tissues and making them hard.

Arterial calcification Deposition of calcium in the arterial walls.

Dystrophic calcification Process of deposition of calcium and other minerals in the cellular debris.

Eggshell calcification Presence of shell-like calcification in the periphery of the lymph nodes, seen in hilar lymph nodes in silicosis.

Metastatic calcification Calcification of soft tissue with transference of calcium from bone.

Monckeberg's calcification Deposition of calcium in the media of arteries.

Rice grain calcification Multiple, small, ovoid calcifications resembling grains of rice in the soft tissues, may be seen in cysticercosis.

Calcinosis (*kal'si-no'sis*) A condition characterized by abnormal deposition of calcium salts in tissues.

Calcinosis circumscripta Subcutaneous calcification.

Tumoral calcinosis Soft tissue calcification that usually involves the particular tissues.

Calcitonin (*kal'si-to'nin*) A thyroid hormone necessary to maintain a dense, strong bone matrix and to regulate the level of calcium in the blood.

C-gene related peptide CGRP, a regulatory peptide of CNS and lung.

Calcium (*kal'se-um*) Lime, Ca. A metallic element atomic number 20, atomic weight

20, a major component of limestone. Calcium phosphate forms 75% of body ash and 85% of mineral matter in bones. Calcium gives firmness and rigidity to bones and teeth, and is necessary for blood coagulation, enzyme activation and acid-base balance. It is necessary for lactation, neuromuscular functions, and membrane permeability. Milk and milk products, and fish are good dietary sources of calcium.

Calcium carbonate Tasteless, odorless powder of precipitated chalk used as antacid and as an antidote to corrosive acid poisoning.

Calcium chloride Solution of calcium salt, used to raise calcium level of the blood. It is administered intravenously in conditions like hypocalcemic tetany.

Calcium cyclamate An artificial sweetening agent.

Calcium gluconate Odorless and tasteless calcium powder.

Calcium glycerophosphate Calcium salt of glycerophosphoric acid as a dietary supplement and in drug formulations.

Calcium hydroxide White powder used as an astringent, and cavity liner.

Calcium lactate A white odorless and tasteless powder.

Calcium oxalate Crystalline calcium.

Calcium oxide A corrosive mineral.

Calcium phosphate A white amorphous powder used as an antacid in gastric hyperacidity.

Calcium saccharin An artificial sweetener.

Calcium antagonist (Calcium channel blockers) medicines used to lower blood pressure. These stop calcium from entering the cells of the heart and arteries.

Calculosis (*kalku-lo'sis*) The formation of or the condition of having a calculus or calculi.

Calculus (*kal'ku-lus*) Pl. **calculi**. Any abnormal concretion, commonly refferred to a stone found within the body. It is composed of mineral salts and may occur in urinary and biliary systems and as a hard deposit on the teeth.

Biliary calculus Gallstone, cholelith. Composed of cholesterol. Bilirubin or calcium may be deposited in such stones.

Dental calculus Calcium deposits on teeth.

Hemic calculus A stone formed from coagulated blood.

Pancreatic calculus A stone in the pancreas, formed of calcium carbonate.

Renal calculus A renal stone found in the kidney that may block urinary flow.

Salivary calculus A calculus in the salivary duct especially that of the submandibular gland noted while eating.

Urinary calculus A stone in any part of the urinary system.

Vesical calculus A stone in the bladder.

Calibrator (*kal'i-bra'tor*) An instrument for measuring the inside diameter of tubes or orifices.

Caliper (caliper) (*kal'i-per*) An instrument to measure the diameters of arm or pelvis; weight bearing splints that permit walking.

Callosity (callus) (*ka-los'i-te*) A circumscribed thickened and hypertrophied horny layer of the skin. It occurs on the flexor surfaces of hands and feet and is caused by friction or pressure.

Callus (*kal'us*) Callosity; the osseous material woven across and around the ends of a fractured bone that is ultimately replaced by true bone in the healing process; keratotic thickening of skin.

Calor (*ka'lor*) heat.

Calorie (*kal'o-re*) A unit of energy content of foods or the amount of energy expended by an organism.

Large calorie KcL. The amount of heat required to change the temperature of 1 kg of water from 14.5° to 15.5°.

Small calorie cal. The amount of heat required to change the temperature of 1 gram of water.

Calorimeter (*kal'o-rim'e-ter*) An instrument to determine the amount of heat exchanged in a chemical reaction or by the animal body in specific conditions.

Calot's triangle (*kal-oz*) A triangle formed by the cystic artery superiorly, the cystic duct inferiorly and the hepatic duct medially, a dangerous area in cholecystectomy named after Jean-Francois Calot, French surgeon.

Calvaria (*kal'va're-a*) The dome-like superior portion of the cranium composed of the superior portions of the frontal, parietal and occipital bones, and covered by the scalp.

Calyx (*ka'lix*) Pl. **calyces**. Any cup-like organ or cavity; a cup-like extension of the renal pelvis that encloses the papilla of a renal pyramid.

Camphor (*kam'for*) An antipruritic agent.

Campimetry (*kamp-ime'-tre*) Perimetry an ophthalmological test that allows us to measure the visual field.

Campodactylia (*kampo-dak-til'e-a*) Flexion deformity of the fingers or toes.

Campylobacter (*kam'pi-lo-bak'ter*) A gram-negative, motile, spirally curved, rod-shaped bacteria of the family Spirillaceae, reclassified as helicobacter.

Canal (*ka-nal*) A narrow tubular passage or channel.

Adductor canal A triangular space between the adductor longus and vastus medialis muscles. It extends from the apex of the femoral triangle to the popliteal space. It transmits femoral vessels and the saphenous nerve.

Alimentary canal The digestive tract from the mouth to the anus.

Alveolar canal One of the several canals in the maxilla that transmits the posterior superior alveolar blood vessels and nerves to the upper teeth.

Anal canal The terminal portion of the rectum opening at the anus.

Birth canal The passage way consisting of the cervix, vagina and vulva through which the fetus passes during delivery.

Bony semicircular canal One of the several canals located in the bony labyrinth of the internal ear. It encloses the semicircular ducts that open into the vestibule. They are enclosed within the petrous portion of temporal bone.

Canal of Lambert One of several bronchioalveolar communications in the lung.

Carotid canal A canal in the petrous portion of the temporal bone that transmits the internal carotid artery to the cranial cavity.

Central canal A small canal in the middle of the spinal cord.

Cervical canal A canal in the cervix of the uterus extending from the internal os to the external os.

Condylar canal A canal in the occipital bone for passage of emissary vein from transverse sinus and it opens anterier to the occipital condyle.

Craniopharyngeal canal A canal in the fetal sphenoid bone that contains the stalk of Rathke's pouch.

Ethmoidal canal One of the two grooves lying between the ethmoid and frontal bones. The anterior ethmoidal canal transmits the anterior ethmoidal vessels and nasociliary nerve and posterior ethmoidal vessels and nasociliary nerve are transmitted through posterior ethmoidal canal.

External auditory canal External auditory meatus transmitting the sound waves.

Facial canal Canal in the internal acoustic meatus of temporal bone transmitting the facial nerve.

Gastric canal A longitudinal groove on the lesser curvature of the stomach.

Haversian canal One of the many minute canals found in compact bone each surrounded by lamellae of bone. Contains blood vessels, lymphatics, nerves and sometimes marrow, constitutes haversian system; a canal in the mandible that carries a neurovascular bundle to the teeth.

Hyaloid canal A canal in the vitreous body of the eye which serves as a lymph channel in fetus.

Hypoglossal canal A canal in the occipital bone transmitting hypoglossal nerve and a branch of the posterior meningeal artery.

Incisive canal A short canal in the maxillary bone transmitting nasopalatine nerve and the branches of great palatine arteries to the nasal fossa.

Infraorbital canal A canal in maxilla lying in the floor of the orbit transmitting the infraorbital nerve and artery.

Internal auditory canal A canal in the petrous portion of the temporal bone that transmits the acoustic and facial nerves and the acoustic artery.

Intestinal canal The alimentary canal from pyloric opening to the anus.

Lacrimal canal Lacrimal duct.

Mandibular canal A canal in the mandible that transmits the inferior alveolar blood vessels and nerve to the teeth.

Maxillary canal Alveolar canal.

Nasolacrimal canal Canal lying between the lacrimal bone and inferior nasal conchae containing the nasolacrimal duct.

Nutrient canal Opening on the surface of compact bone through which blood vessels reach medullary cavity of long bones.

Obturator canal An opening in the obturator membrane of the hip bone that transmits the obturator vessels and nerve.

Pharyngeal canal Canal between the sphenoid and palatine bones that transmits branches of the sphenopalatine vessels.

Portal canal Area between adjoining liver lobules consisting of connective tissue and interlobular branches of the hepatic artery, portal vein and bile duct.

Pterygoid canal A canal of the sphenoid bone transmitting the pterygoid vessels and nerve.

Pterygopalatine canal A canal between the maxillary and palatine bones that transmits the descending palatine nerve and artery.

Pudendal canal A canal on the pelvic surface of the obturator internus muscle that transmits pudendal vessels, named after Alcock Pudenda.

Root canal Passage in the root of a tooth through which nerve and blood vessels pass.

Sacral canal A cavity within the sacrum.

Semicircular canal One of several canals located in the bony labyrinth of the internal ear. It encloses superior, posterior and lateral semicircular ducts that open into the vestibule. They are found within the petrous portion of the temporal bone.

Spinal canal Vertebral canal.

Spiral canal of cochlea Bony labyrinth of the inner ear containing a spiral tube of 30 mm long that makes a two and three quarters turn about a central bony axis. It contains the scala tympani, scala vestibuli and cochlear duct.

Uterine canal The cavity of uterus.

Vaginal canal The cavity of the vagina.

Vertebral canal The cavity formed by the foramina of the vertebral column that contains the spinal cord and its meninges.

Volkmann's canal Small canal found in bone through which blood vessels pass from periosteum.

Canaliculus (*kan'a-lik'u-lus*) Pl. **canaliculi.** A small channel or canal.

Cancellous (*kan-cel'us*) A bony plate composed of cancellous bone.

Cancer (*kan'ser*) Any of a group of diseases caused by unrestricted multiplication of cells in an organ or tissue that can spread throughout the body.

Cancer grading Degree of cancer cell differentiation.

Cancer screening A program to detect cancer in its asymptomatic stage.

Cancer staging Extent of dissemination of cancer. T (tumor), N (regional extension to nodes), M (metastases) classification is used in staging of cancer according to size, and spread.

Cancrum (canker) (*kang' krum*) A rapidly spreading ulcer.

Cancrum oris Gangrene-like lesions in the mouth in malnourished children caused by *Borrelia vincenti*.

Candela (*kan-del'a*) The basic SI unit of luminous intensity.

Candida (*kan'di-da*) A genus of yeasts that develops a pseudomycelium and reproduces by budding. They form part of normal flora of the mouth formerly called monilia.

Candida albicans A small oral budding fungus, causative agent of candidiasis.

Candidiasis (*kan'di-di'a-sis*) Thrush; any organ of the body can be invaded by candida, but vaginal and oral thrush are the common forms.

Cutaneous candidiasis Occurs in intertriginous areas.

Chronic mucocutaneous candidiasis Occurs in children with T cell defect characterized by hyperkeratotic plaque-like lesions on the skin and endocrinopathies.

Oropharyngeal candidiasis White plaques of fungus on the pharynx and palate. Rare in healthy, complicates treatment with broad-spectrum antibiotics, oral and inhaled corticosteroids and is found when immunity is defective. It may spread to the esophagus and lung.

Vaginal candidiasis Dysuria, white, thick, 'cheesy' odorless discharge and irritation with inflammation of vulva and cervix.

Canine (*ka'nin*) Pertaining to a dog.

Canine tooth Any of the four teeth found between incisors and molars in upper and lower jaw.

Canities (*kan-ish'e-ez*) Whiteness of hair.

Canker A small, shallow sore inside the mouth or at the base of gums.

Cannabis (*kan'a-bis*) Marijuana.

Cannula (*kan'u-la*) A tube or sheath enclosing a trocar; a thin, flexible tube inserted into the body to withdraw or introduce fluids.

Canthus (*kan'thus*) Pl. **canthi**. The angle at either end of the slit between the eyelids.

CAOS Computer-assisted orthopedic surgery.

Cap (*kap*) A covering.

Knee cap Patella.

CAPD Continuous ambulatory peritoneal dialysis.

Capgras syndrome Delusional belief that a friend, family member, etc has been replaced by a twin imposter.

Capillary (*kap'i-lar'e*) Pl. **capillaries**. Any of the tiny blood vessels that connect the ends of the arterioles with the beginnings of the venules.

Capillary permeability The ability of a substance to diffuse through capillary walls into tissue spaces.

Capnograph (*kap'no-graf*) A monitoring device that measures the concentration of carbon dioxide in exhaled air and displays a numerical readout and waveform tracing.

Capnography Continuous recording of the carbon dioxide level in exhaled air in mechanically ventilated patients.

Capitate (*kap'i-tat*) Head-shaped.

Capitate bone The largest of the carpal bones, situated at the base of the palm of hand articulating with the third metacarpal.

Capitellum (*kap'i-tel'um*) The round eminence at the lower end of the humerus articulating with the radius.

Capitulum (*ka-pit'u-lum*) Pl. **capitula**. A small rounded articular end of a bone.

Capping (*kap'ing*) Placing a protective substance over the exposed pulp of a teeth; placing an artificial crown on a tooth for cosmetic purpose; induction of a person into nursing profession.

Capreomycin A weak antituberculosis drug administered parenterally in drug resistant cases of tuberculosis. It has cross resistance with kanamycin and viomycin.

Capsule A sheath; a special container made of gelatin, to dispense a single dose of a drug.

Glomerular capsule The glomerular capsule of the kidneys, named after William Bowman, a surgeon and anatomist.

Joint capsule The sleeve-like membrane that encloses the bony ends in a diarthrodial joint. It consists of an outer fibrous layer and an inner synovial layer and contains synovial fluid.

Lens capsule A transparent, structureless membrane that surrounds and encloses the lens of the eye.

Capsulitis (*kap'su-li'tis*) Inflammation of a capsule.

Capsulotomy (*kap'su-lot'o-me*) Cutting of a capsule of the lens or a joint.

Captopril An antihypertensive agent that blocks the conversion of angiotensin I to angiotensin II.

Caput succedaneum Edematous swelling of the fetal scalp that crosses the suture lines.

Carbachol (*kar'ba-kol*) A direct acting miotic agent administered ophthalmically to decrease intraocular pressure after cataract surgery, and to induce miosis during surgery.

Carbamazepine (*kar-ba-maz'e-pen*) A drug used in the treatment of trigeminal neuralgia and temporal lobe epilepsy.

Carbenicillin (*kar'ben-i-sil'in*) A semi-synthetic penicillin.

Carbenoxolone A synthetic derivative of glycyrrhizinic acid. It acts by protecting the mucosal barrier from acid-pepsin attack and increasing mucosal mucin production.

Carbimazole (*kar'bima-zol*) An imidazole derivative, antithyroid used in the treatment of thyrotoxicosis.

Carbinoxamine (*kar'bin-ok'sa-men*) An antihistamine used to relieve symptoms of allergy, hay fever, and the common cold.

Carbohydrate (*kar'bo-hi'drat*) One of a group of chemical substances, including glucose, glycogen, starches, dextrines and celluloses, that contain only carbon, oxygen and hydrogen. It is the main source of energy.

Carbol fuchsin (*kar'bol-fuk'sin*) A mixture of an aqueous solution of phenol and an alcoholic solution of fuchsin used as a stain in microscopy especially in staining bacteria.

Carbolic acid (*kar-bolik*) Alternative name for phenol, especially when it is used as an antiseptic or disinfectant.

Carbon dioxide CO_2, the final metabolic product of carbon as a colorless and odorless gas compound present in food. It is eliminated through the lungs mostly and a small amount in the urine and sweat.

Carbon dioxide solid therapy Snow used for therapeutic refrigeration.

Carbon monoxide CO, a poisonous gas resulting from the inefficient and incomplete combustion of coal. It is colorless, odorless and tasteless making it difficult to detect by senses.

Carbon monoxide poisoning Causes impairment of consciousness, hypertonia and hyper reflexia, coma, focal neurologic damage, myocardial ischemia, and cardiac arrhythmias, treated with 100% oxygen with mechanical ventilation.

Carbon tetrachloride CCl_4, a clear colorless liquid having an etheral odor. It is toxic causing acute atrophy of the liver and kidney.

Carboplatin (*kar'bo-plat"in*) A platinum containing cytotoxic agent used in treatment of ovarian cancer.

Carboxyhemoglobin (*kar-bok'si-he'mo-glo'bin*) A compound formed by union of carbon monoxide and hemoglobin.

Carboxylase (*kar-bok'si-las*) An enzyme that catalyzes the removal of carboxyl group from amino acids.

Carbuncle (*kar'bung'kl*) Large multilocular boil of the skin and deeper tissues. It terminates in a slough and suppuration. It is associated with systemic manifestations.

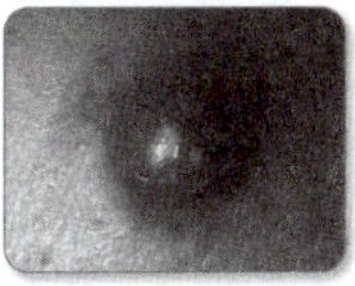

Carbuncle

Carcinoembryonic antigen (CEA) A glycoprotein of fetal endoderm, may be found elevated, may indicate recurrence of certain type of cancers.

Carcinogen (*kar-sin'o-jen*) Any substance or agent that produces cancer or increases the risk of development of cancer.

Carcinogenesis (*kar-sin'o-jen'e-sis*) The production of cancer.

Carcinoid (*kar'si-noid*) A tumor arising from argentaffin cells found in the intestine, associated with secretion of serotonin.

Carcinoid syndrome A symptom complex caused by carcinoids arising from the enterochromaffin system, most common in the ileum whose metastases to the liver release vasoactive substances such as serotonin, bradykinin, histamine, and prostaglandin. It presents with cutaneous flushing, diarrhea, small bowel obstruction, bronchospasm, endocardial fibrosis involving the right sided cardiac valves and right ventricular wall leading to heart failure.

Carcinoma (*kar'si-no'ma*) A malignant tumor arising from cells in the surface layer or lining membrane of an organ. They tend to infiltrate and metastasize to distant organs or parts of the body.

Alveolar cell carcinoma A variety of lung cancer.

Basal cell carcinoma Skin malignancy that rarely metastasizes.

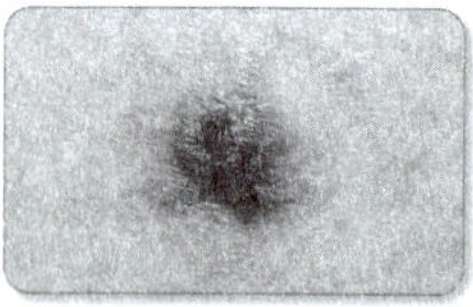

Basal cell carcinoma

Bronchogenic carcinoma A malignant tumor originating in the bronchus. The examples are squamous cell carcinoma, adenocarcinoma, small cell carcinoma and large cell carcinoma.

Carcinoma in situ Malignant cell changes noted in the epithelial tissue that do not extend beyond the basement membrane.

Carcinoma en cuirasse A markedly indurated carcinoma involving a broad expanse of skin and subcutaneous breast tissue that is covered by papules and nodules progressing into morphea-like plaques.

Epidermoid carcinoma A tumor on surface, such as the skin or bronchus.

Giant cell carcinoma A tumor characterized by presence of unusually large cells.

Medullary carcinoma A soft tumor composed of cells with little fibrous tissue.

Mucinous carcinoma Malignant tumor in which the glandular tissue secretes mucin.

Oat cell carcinoma A variety of poorly differentiated small cell carcinoma that contains small oat-shaped cells.

Scirrhous carcinoma Hard carcinoma.

Squamous cell carcinoma An epidermoid carcinoma developing from squamous cells.

Carcinosarcoma (*kar'si-no-sar-ko'ma*) A malignant tumor containing elements of both carcinoma and sarcoma. These highly aggressive tumors are carcinomas and the cells display sarcoma-like spindling.

Carcinomatosis (*kar'si-no'ma-to'sis*) A preterminal condition characterized by widespread dissemination of carcinoma in the body.

Cardia (*kar'de-a*) Junction of upper part of the stomach and esophagus; heart.

Cardiac (*kar'de-ak*) Pertaining to the heart; pertaining to the cardia.

Cardiac ablation A technique for correcting abnormal heart rhythms by destroying the tissue within the heart responsible for setting the faulty pace.

Cardiac aneurysm Stretching of fibrotic area due to earlier myocardial infarction.

Cardiac arrhythmia An abnormality of cardiac rhythm. It may be in the form of bradycardia or tachycardia.

Cardiac asthma Dyspnea and wheeze from bronchial endothelial edema in left ventricular failure.

Cardiac cachexia Loss of lean body mass that occurs in some patients with moderate to severe heart failure.

Cardiac catheterization Percutaneous intravascular insertion of a catheter into any chamber of the heart to monitor its function and to inject a contrast medium for imaging.

Cardiac cirrhosis Hepatocellular atrophy, centrilobular necrosis and extensive fibrosis caused by repeated and/ or prolonged congestive heart failure.

Cardiac compensation The ability of the heart to compensate for impaired function of the valves through the reserve power.

Cardiac enzymes A group of three enzymes CPK (its isoenzyme CK-M8), AST and LDH which rise and fall in the same order over a period of weeks following myocardial infarction.

Cardiac failure A condition resulting from the inability of the heart to pump sufficient amount of blood to meet the demands of the tissues. It may be high output failure when the demands are excessive as in thyrotoxicosis and anemia or low output failure when the heart itself is defective, following myocardial infarction.

Cardiac glycoside A drug used in the treatment of rhythm disorders or heart failure.

Cardiac hormones *see* Atrial natriuretic peptides.

Cardiac hypertrophy Enlargement of the heart.

Cardiac index Cardiac output in L/ min body surface area in sq. meters.

Cardiac insufficiency Inadequate cardiac output due to failure of the heart to function properly as in valvular abnormalities.

Cardiac massage Rhythmic strong pressure on the lower end of sternum in cardiac arrest.

Cardiac output The amount of blood discharged from the left or right ventricles per minute.

Cardiac plexus The nerve plexus at the base of the heart with the branches of the vagus nerves and sympathetic trunks. It provides nerve supply to the heart.

Cardiac reserve The capacity of the heart to increase its output to meet the body requirement.

Cardiac siphon The intracavernous and supraclinoid segments of the internal carotid artery.

Cardiac transplantation Transplantation of the heart in younger patients with severe intractable heart failure whose life expectancy is <6 months.

Cardiac troponin T A muscle protein whose presence can be detected in the blood following myocardial infarction. It is a rapid test to indicate myocardial damage at a very early stage.

Cardiac arrest Sudden stoppage of pumping action of the heart requiring institution of basic life support followed by advanced life support measures; sudden death due to cardiac causes.

Cardiac cycle The period from the commencement of one heart beat to the beginning of next beat includes systole, the contraction of atria and ventricles to move blood forward and diastole, the period during which the cavities are refilled with blood.

Cardiac muscle Myocardium; involuntary, striated muscle.

Cardiac reflex An involuntary response of alteration in heart rate following stimulation of sensory nerve endings in the wall of the carotid sinus which slows the heart rate, and stimulation of vagus fibers by increased venous return resulting in increased heart rate.

Cardinal veins Also known as the ducts of cuvier are veins that drain into the sinus venosus during embryonic development.

Cardiology (*kar-de-ol'o-je*) The study of pathophysiology, diagnosis and treatment of heart diseases.

Cardiomyopathy (*kar'de-o-mi-op'a-the*) Any disease that affects the heart muscle.

Alcoholic cardiomyopathy Development of cardiomyopathy in the alcoholics who consume large quantities of alcoholic beverages.

Dilated cardiomyopathy An impaired ventricular contraction leading to progressive left sided, and later right sided heart failure. Arrhythmia, thromboembolism and sudden death are common.

Hypertrophic cardiomyopathy A familial disorder characterized by inappropriate and elaborate ventricular hypertrophy with malalignment of the myocardial fibers. The hypertrophy may be generalized or confined to interventricular septum or apex.

Obliterative/Restrictive cardiomyopathy Impaired ventricular filling as the ventricles are 'stiff'. The atrial pressure rises and there is atrial hypertrophy, dilatation and later atrial fibrillation.

Puerperal cardiomyopathy Deterioration of cardiac status with successive pregnancies and development of cardiomyopathy during later stages of pregnancy or during puerperium.

Cardiomyotomy Surgical treatment for achalasia cardia wherein the muscles surrounding the cardioesophageal junction are cut.

Cardioplegia (*kar'de-o-ple'je-a*) Temporary arrest of cardiac function by hypothermia, medication or electrical stimuli to reduce the need of oxygen by heart muscle during surgery requiring cardiopulmonary bypass.

Cardiopulmonary bypass Provision of an extracorporeal device like a heart-lung machine to pump blood while a surgical procedure being carried on the heart.

Cardiospasm (*kar'de-o-spasm*) Disordered motor function of the distal end of the esophagus and failure of the esophageal orifice of the stomach to relax.

Cardiotocography (*kar'de-o-to-kog'ra-fe*) A continuous electronic record of the baby's heart rate obtained *via* an ultrasound transducer placed on the mother's abdomen.

Cardiotomy syndrome (postcardiotomy syndrome) Inability to wear from cardiopulmonary bypass or need for mechanical support following cardiac surgery.

Cardiovascular system (circulatory system) The network of structures consisting of the heart and blood vessels, that pumps blood and transports it throughout the body.

Cardioversion (countershock) (*kar'de-o-ver'zhun*) Synchronized electric shock applied to terminate cardiac arrhythmias defibrillation.

Carfilzomib An anti-cancer medication acting as a selective proteasome inhibitor.

Caries (*kar'i-ez*) Gradual decay and disintegration of a tooth or bone.

Caries spine *see* Pott's spine.

Dental caries *see* Dental caries.

Carina (*ka-ri'na*) A structure with a projecting central ridge.

Carina tracheae A ridge at the lower end of the trachea at its bifurcation as major bronchi.

Carisoprodol (*kar'i-so-pro'dol*) A centrally acting muscle relaxant used to relieve the discomfort associated with various musculoskeletal conditions.

Carminative (*kar-min'ativ*) A pleasant tasting agent preventing gas formation in the gastrointestinal tract.

Carmustine An anti-neoplastic nitrosurea compound; also called BCNU.

Carneous mole A fleshy mass in the uterus consisting of pieces of placenta and products of conception that have not been expelled after miscarriage.

Caroli's syndrome Autosomal recessive disorder presenting Caroli's disease in association with congenital hepatic fibrosis.

Carotenemia (xanthemia) (*kar'o-te-ne'me-a*) Presence of carotene in the blood leading to yellowish discoloration of the skin, and not of conjunctiva.

Carotenoid (*ka-rot'e-noyd*) Resembling carotene; pigment varying from light yellow to red color found in plants and animals. The examples are beta carotene in carrots, lycopene in tomatoes and lutein in spinach and are antioxidants.

Carotid artery Pertains to the right and left common carotid arteries that supply to the head and neck.

Carotid body A collection of cells at the bifurcation of the common carotid artery that respond to the changes in oxygen concentration in the blood and to changes in blood pressure.

Carotid sinus Slight dilatation at carotid bifurcation.

Carotidynia (*kar-ot'i-dine-a*) Spontaneous episodes of dull ache originating in the middle of the neck on one side and radiating to ipsilateral face, ear, jaw, tooth or down the neck. It is accompanied by tenderness on palpation over the carotid artery and induration of the overlying tissues.

Carpal (*kar-pal*) Pertaining to the wrist.

Carpal bone One of the eight bones that make up the wrist.

Carpal boss A bony growth on the dorsal surface of the third metacarpocarpal joint.

Carpal tunnel A canal in the wrist where the carpal bones form a concavity bridged by flexor retinaculum through which the flexor tendons and the median nerve pass.

Carpal tunnel syndrome Occurrence of tingling, pain and numbness in the region of the median nerve distribution of the hand. It is caused by compression of the median nerve as it passes between the bones and ligament at the front of the wrist.

Carphology (floccillation) (*kar-fol'o-je*) The action of grasping at imaginary objects or plucking at one's bed linen, a characteristic of people affected by delirium.

Carpopedal spasm Spasm of hands and feet as in tetany.

Carpus (*kar'pus*) The joint between the arm and hand made up of eight bones of the wrist.

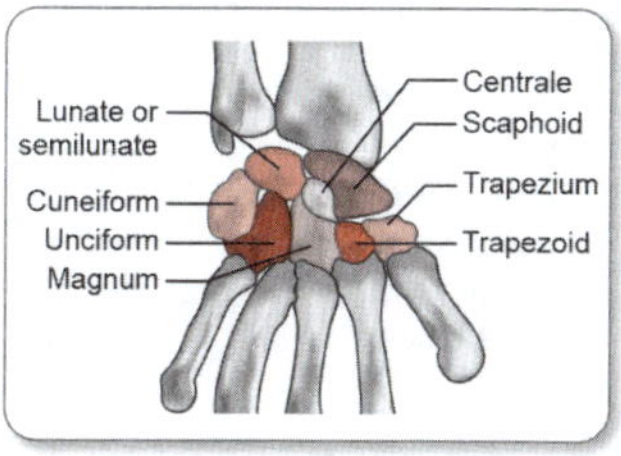

Carpus

Carrier (*kare'-ar*) An individual who harbors a specific microorganism without exhibiting any clinical features of the disease and is potentially capable of spreading the organisms to others; an insect passively carrying an infectious agent; a substance that when combined with another transport substance can pass through the cell membrane; a heterozygote carrying a recessive gene together with its normal allele; an apparatus or instrument used for transportation of some material such as an amalgam.

Convalescent carrier A person harboring an infective agent during recovery from the disease caused by the organism.

Genetic carrier One whose chromosomes contain a pathologic mutant gene that may be transmitted to child.

Healthy carrier A person harboring an infectious agent without suffering from the disease.

Incubatory carrier A person who harbors and spreads an infective agent during the incubation period of a disease.

Cartilage (*kar'ti-lij*) A specialized type of dense connective tissue consisting of cells embedded in a firm and compact matrix or ground substance. It can withstand considerable pressure or tension. It forms part of the skeleton and is seen in the costal cartilages of the ribs, in the nasal septum, in the external ear, larynx, trachea, bronchi, between the vertebral bodies and covering of the articular surfaces of bones.

Articular cartilage The thin layer of smooth, elastic cartilage on the joint surfaces of a bone as in a synovial joint.

Costal cartilage A cartilage that connects the ends of a true rib with the sternum or the end of rib with costal cartilage above.

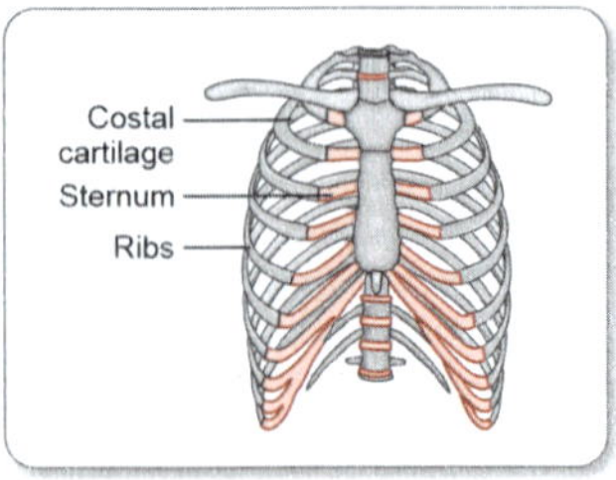

Rib cage: Showing costal cartilage

Cricoid cartilage Signet ring-shaped lowermost cartilage of the larynx.

Cuneiform cartilage One of the small pieces of cartilage lying in the aryepiglottic fold of the larynx.

Fibrous cartilage Fibrocartilage.

Hyaline cartilage A bluish white, flexible, glossy, transparent cartilage.

Semilunar cartilage Medial or lateral crescentic cartilage of the knee joint between the femur and tibia.

Thyroid cartilage A shield-shaped large cartilage of the larynx found in front of the middle of the neck known as Adam's apple.

Yellow cartilage A network of yellow elastic fibers that hold cartilage cells.

Caruncle (*kar'ung-kal*) A small fleshy eminence, often abnormal.

Lacrimal caruncle A small reddish elevation on the conjunctiva near the inner canthus, at the medial angle of the eye.

Sublingual caruncle A protuberance on either side of the frenum of the tongue containing the openings of the ducts from submandibular and sublingual salivary glands.

Urethral caruncle A highly vascular, small papillary growth that may sometimes develop in the urinary meatus in female.

Carvedilol (*kar'va-dilol*) A β-adrenergic blocking agent (β-blocker) used to treat heart failure, hypertension, and left ventricular dysfunction after a heart attack.

Case Occurrence of disease; a patient; an enclosing structure.

Caseation (*ka'se-a'shun*) The process of conversion of a necrotic tissue into a granular amorphous cheesy mass associated with a tuberculous lesion also seen in histoplasmosis; the precipitation of casein during coagulation of milk.

Casein (*ka'-se-in*) The principal milk protein that supplies all the amino acids necessary for growth and development.

Cassette (*ka-set*) A flat, light proof box with an intensifying screen for holding X-ray film; a case for film or magnetic tape; a segment of eukaryotic DNA that can be substitued by another sequence by transposition.

Cast A positive copy of teeth and jaw over which denture bases are made; making an accurate metallic reproduction of a wax pattern of a dental appliance, tooth; material moulded to the shape of the part in which it has accumulated; a rigid casing applied to a part of the body to immobilise a fracture or dislocation.

Epithelial cast An aggregation of renal epithelium filled with granules or fat droplets seen in acute nephritis.

Granular cast Substance following degeneration of a hyaline cast.

Hyaline cast A urinary cast that is pale, transparent and having homogeneous rounded ends.

Red blood cell cast A urinary cast composed mainly of red blood cells.

Urinary cast A cast found in the urine, formed from precipitation of proteins in the renal tubules.

White blood cell cast A leukocyte cast found in urine in pyogenic infections of the kidney.

Castor oil Oil from the plant *Ricinus communis* used internally as a laxative and externally as an emollient.

Castration (*kas-tra'shun*) Excision of one or both testicles or ovaries.

CAT Computerized axial tomography.

Cat bite fever An infection by *Pasteurella multocida* acquired by cat bite, is characterized by an abscess at the site of inoculation and focal arthralgia.

Catabolism (*ka-tab'o-lizm*) A process of metabolism wherein the complex chemicals are broken down into simpler forms usually with the release of energy, and byproducts such as water and carbon dioxide.

Catalase (*kat'a-las*) Enzyme catalyzing decomposition of hydrogen peroxide to water and oxygen.

Catalepsy (*kat'a-lep'se*) An abnormal trance-like state in which the muscles of the face, body, and limbs remain in a rigid position.

Catalyst (*kat'a-list*) A substance that hastens the rate of a chemical reaction without getting altered in the reaction. These are effective in small amounts and are not used up in the reaction.

Cataphoria (*kat'a-for'e-a*) A tendency of the visual axes or both eyes to deviate below the horizontal plane in absence of stimulus. adj. **catophoric**.

Cataplexy (*kat'a-plek"se*) Sudden loss of muscle power following a strong emotional stimulus.

Cataract (*kat'a-rakt*) Opacity of the lens of the eye, its capsule or both.

Capsular cataract Cataract occurring in the capsule.

Hypermature cataract Overripe cataract.

Immature cataract An early cataract which is not fully matured to require treatment.

Mature cataract Opaque lens with dense changes in anterior cortex of the lens preventing visualization of the posterior portion of the lens and posterior portion of eye.

Nuclear cataract A cataract in which the nucleus of the lens is opacified.

Overripe cataract Stage following mature cataract where the lens is solidified and shrunken.

Radiation cataract A cataract caused by exposure to radiation.

Ripe cataract Mature cataract.

Senile cataract A cataract developing in an elderly person.

Catarrh (*ka-tar*) Inflammation of the mucous membrane of the oronasopharyngeal mucosa.

Catastrophic illness Prolonged illness usually considered to be life threatening.

Catatonia (*kat-a-to'ne-a*) Motor anomalies in non-organic disorders, wherein there is increased tone and fixed postures.

Catecholamine (*kat'e-kol'a-men*) One of the biologically active amines, epinephrine (adrenaline), norepinephrine (noradrenaline) and dopamine, which have important effect on nervous system.

Catgut (*kat'gut*) Sheep intestine twisted for use as an absorbable ligature.

Catharsis (*ka-thar'sis*) Purgative action of the bowel; emotion release.

Cathartic (*ka-thar'tik*) A purgative producing bowel movements.

Cathartic colon A colon affected by long-term abuse of cathartics and laxatives characterized by intractable diarrhea, hypokalemia, protein-losing enteropathy, cachexia and potentially increased constipation.

Cathepsin (*ka-thep'sin*) Soluble lysosomal or secreted proteases that can be classified based on their active site functional residue.

Catheter (*kath'e-ter*) A hollow, flexible tube passed through the body for evacuating fluids or injecting them into body cavities or vessels. It is made up of rubber, plastic, metal or elastic web.

Arterial catheter A catheter inserted into an artery to inject medication or radioactive contrast material, to remove blood or to measure pressure.

Balloon catheter A double-lumened catheter surrounded by a balloon.

Cardiac catheter A long catheter passed through the lumen of a blood vessel into the chambers of the heart.

Central venous catheter A catheter inserted into the superior vena cava to permit intermittent or continuous monitoring of central venous pressure.

Condom catheter A specially designed condom that includes a catheter bag.

Double channel catheter A catheter providing for inflow and outflow.

Eustachian catheter A catheter passed into the eustachian tube through the nasal passage.

Female catheter A catheter of 12.7 cm long used to pass into a woman's bladder.

Foley catheter A urinary tract catheter with a balloon at one end. After insertion of the catheter, the balloon is filled with sterile water to prevent it leaving the bladder, named after Frederic Foley, US urologist.

Indwelling catheter Any catheter allowed to remain inside a vein, artery or body cavity.

Intravenous catheter A catheter inserted into a vein to administer fluids or medications.

Male catheter A catheter of 30.5 to 33 cm length used to pass into a man's bladder.

Pacing catheter A catheter inserted into a vein or pulmonary artery that contains wires or leads for providing electrical stimuli from an external cardiac pacemaker.

Self-retaining catheter A bladder catheter designed to remain in place.

Swan-Ganz catheter A thin, flexible flow-directed catheter using a balloon to carry it through the heart to pulmonary artery and is positioned in a small arterial branch. Pulmonary wedge pressure is measured in front of inflated and wedged balloon.

Catheterization (*kath'e-ter-i-za'shun*) Insertion of a catheter into the body to drain, or inject fluids or to perform certain procedures such as widening of narrowed arteries.

Cat-scratch disease Illness caused by the scratches or bite of cats, there is occurrence of a papule, and regional lymphadenopathy. It0 is thought to be caused by a bacterium and is a self-limiting illness.

Cauda (*kaw'da*) A tail or tail-like structure.

Cauda equina The terminal portion of the spinal cord and the roots of the spinal nerves below L_1 nerve.

Caudal (*kaw'dal*) Pertaining to any tail-like structure; inferior in position.

Caul (*kawl*) A portion of the amnion, or bag of waters, which is sometimes found around the head of a child after birth.

Causal agent Any entity that produces effect or is responsible for events or results.

Causalgia (*kaw-sal'je-a*) Severe and rare burning pain and trophic skin changes from injury to peripheral nerve fibers.

Caustic (*kaw'stik*) Corrosive agent particularly alkali that destroys the living tissue.

Cauterize (*kaw'ter-iz*) To burn with a hot iron, electric current, fire, or a caustic, especially for curative purposes.

Cauterization (*kaw'ter-i-za'shun*) Application of a caustic chemical, an electric current, a hot iron or freezing to the tissues in order to destroy them, to stop them from bleeding or to promote their healing.

Cavernitis (*kaver-ni'tis*) An inflammation of the corpus cavernosum is relatively rare and must be differentiated from a tumor, abscess, thrombosis or embolism of the penile vessels.

Cavernosography Radiography of penis following injection of a contrast material into the corpus cavernosa.

Cavernosometry (*kaver-no-som'e-tre*) The measurement of pressure within the corpora cavernosa of the penis during infusion.

Cavernous breathing Low pitch bronchial breath sound heard over superficial large cavity with patent bronchus, abscess and bronchiectatic cavity with patent bronchi.

Cavernous sinus On either side of pituitary traversed by internal carotid artery and 3rd to 6th cranial nerves.

Cavity (*kav'i-ti*) A hollow space.

Abdominal cavity The ventral cavity in the abdomen containing all abdominal organs.

Alveolar cavity Tiny air sacs at the end of the bronchioles.

Amniotic cavity The fluid-filled cavity around the developing embryo.

Articular cavity The synovial cavity of a joint.

Dental cavity A hole in the tooth caused by caries.

Oral cavity The cavity of the mouth.

Pelvic cavity The cavity of the pelvis. It consists of major pelvic cavity lying between the iliac fossa above iliopectineal line and minor pelvic cavity lying below the ileopectineal line or the inlet of the pelvis.

Pericardial cavity The potential space between the visceral pericardium and parietal pericardium.

Peritoneal cavity The potential space between the parietal peritoneum lining the inner aspect of abdominal wall and the visceral peritoneum covering the visceral organs.

Pleural cavity The potential space between the parietal pleura lining the inner surface of the thoracic cavity and the visceral pleura covering the lungs.

Pulmonary cavity Irregular air-filled structures with a wall thickness greater than 1 mm.

Serous cavity The space between the two layers of serous membranes such as pleura, pericardium or peritoneum.

Spinal cavity The cavity containing the spinal cord.

Thoracic cavity The space enclosed within the walls of thorax above the diaphragm.

Tympanic cavity Middle ear cavity.

Uterine cavity The cavity of the body of the uterus.

Cavity varnish A solution of natural or synthetic resin in an organic solvent like acetone, ether, or chloroform.

CBW (chemical and biological warfare) The use of chemicals, bacteria, viruses, toxins, or poisons to injure or kill soldiers or civilians.

C cell tumor Calcitonin secreting tumor of thyroid.

CD Cluster of differentiation, name of surface antigens of human leukocytes characterized by monoclonal antibodies enabling leukocytes and other hemopoietic cells to be categorized by the expression on the cell surface.

CD 4/CD 8 Ratio of circulating T lymphocytes with 'helper cell' determinants (CD4 antigen) on the cell surface to T lymphocytes with 'suppressor cell' determinants (CD8 antigen).

CD4 receptor Receptors on T4 lymphocytes to which the human immunodeficiency virus binds producing an infection.

Cecostomy (*se-kos'to-me*) A surgical procedure in which an opening is created in the cecum to relieve cecal distension produced by intestinal pseudo-obstructions or, rarely, distal obstruction or by profound paralytic ileus.

Cecum (*se'kum*) A blind pouch forming the first part of the large intestine, located below the entrance of ileum at the ileocecal valve. Vermiform appendix is at its lower end.

Cefaclor (*sefa-klor*) A second generation cephalosporin used to treat a wide variety of infections in the body.

Cefadroxil (*sefa-droks'il*) A cephalosporin antibiotic used in the treatment of various bacterial infections, such as urinary tract infections, skin and skin structure infections, and tonsillitis.

Cefixime (*se-fik'sem*) An antibiotic, is a third-generation cephalosporin like ceftriaxone and cefotaxime.

Celiac (*se'le-ak*) Related to a serious autoimmune disease that occurs in genetically predisposed people where the ingestion of gluten leads to damage in the small intestine.

Celiac disease A illness caused by an immune reaction to eating gluten.

Celioscopy (*se"le-osko-pe*) Examination of the abdominal cavity by surgical insertion of an endoscope through the abdominal wall.

Cell Basic structural unit of all animals/body containing a mass of protoplasm containing a nucleus or nuclear material; a small enclosed cavity like an air cell.

Acantholytic cell An epithelial cell that has separated from another epithelial cell and consequently has become round.

Alpha cell A cell present in the anterior lobe of the pituitary and pancreas. In the latter, it is concerned with the secretion of glucagon.

Ameloblast cell Cell concerned with production of enamel of tooth crown.

Argentaffin cell A cell in the epithelium of the stomach, intestines and appendix that secretes serotonin.

Beta cell A cell found in the islets of Langerhans concerned with secretion of insulin; a cell found in anterior lobe of pituitary.

Betz cell Giant pyramidal cells in the motor area of the cerebral cortex whose axons form the corticospinal tract, named after Vladimir Betz, Russian anatomist.

Bipolar cell A neuron having two processes, an axon and a dendrite, found in the retina of the eye and in the cochlear and vestibular ganglia of the acoustic nerve.

Burr cell An erythrocyte having spicutes over its surface.

Caterpillar cell Large multinucleated giant cell with lengthwise chromatin clumping in nucleus seen in heart in acute rheumatic fever.

Cementoblast cell One of the cells concerned with secretion of parathyroid hormone; one of the secretory cells found in gastric glands and secrete pepsin; a chromophobe cell of pituitary.

Chromaffin cell A cell found in adrenal medulla where granules stain brown with potassium dichromate.

Clue cell An epithelial cell of the vagina coated with coccobacillary organisms.

Cone cell A light receptor cell in the retina.

Delta cell Somatostatin secreting cell found in islets of Langerhans.

Endothelial cell One of the flat cells that line the blood and lymph vessels.

Ependymal cell One of the cells of the developing neural tube that gives rise to the ependyma.

Faggot cell Malignant promyelocyte containing numerous Auer rods seen in acute myelogenous leukemia.

Foam cell A cell that contains vacuoles and lipid substance.

Ganglion cell A neuronal cell found in ganglion.

Goblet cell An epithelial cell with a large globule of mucin giving it an appearance of goblet.

Golgi cell A multipolar nerve cell in the cerebral cortex and posterior horns of the spinal cord.

Gustatory cell An epithelial cell in a taste bud.

Hair cell An epithelial cell having fine non-motile cilia found in the maculae and the organ of Corti of the membranous labyrinth of the inner ear. They act as receptors for the senses of position and hearing.

Hairy cell Leukocytes possessing multiple cytoplasmic projections on the cell surface, found in hairy cell leukemia.

HeLa cell A cell from a strain continuously cultured from a patient's carcinoma of the cervix. The name has come from the first two letters of the patient's first and last names, Henrietta Lacks.

Helper T cell A type of T lymphocytes required for the production of antibodies against certain antigens.
Hyperchromatic cell Densely staining cell which contains more than the normal number of chromosomes.
Interstitial cell One of the many cells found in the connective tissue of the ovary and the seminiferous tubules of the testis concerned with hormonal secretion.
Islet cell A cell of the islets of Langerhans of the pancreas.
Juvenile cell The early developmental cell of a white blood cell.
Juxtaglomerular cell A modified smooth muscle cell found in the wall of the afferent arteriole leading to a glomerulus of the kidney. It secretes renin when there is a fall in blood pressure and activates the renin-angiotensin mechanism.
Killer T cell A type of T lymphocytes that directly kill organisms.
Kupffer cell Specialized cells localized in liver involved in he breakdown of red blood cells.
LE cell A polymorphonuclear leukocyte containing an amorphous round body.
Labile cell A cell which is continuously replicating, found in tissues which undergo high turnover such as gastrointestinal tract.
Leydig cell The testosterone-secreting cell of the testis.
Littoral cell A macrophage found in the sinuses of lymphatic tissue.
Lutein cell A cell of the corpus luteum of the ovary, containing fatty yellowish granules.
Mastoid cell One of the air spaces in the mastoid process of temporal bone.
Memory cell A cell derived from B or T lymphocytes that has the ability to recognize a foreign antigen to which the body has been previously sensitized. They stimulate plasma cells to produce antibodies.
Microglia cell A neuroglial cell found in the brain and spinal cord capable of phagocytosis.
Myeloma cell A cell found in the bone marrow of patients with multiple myeloma.
Myoepithelial cell A spindle-shaped contractile epithelial cell found in the salivary, sweat and mammary glands.
Natural killer cell A lymphocyte that fights off viral infections and tumors, also known as NK cells.
Neuroglial cell Cell of the supporting tissue of CNS and retina of the eye.
Null cell A lymphocyte exhibiting the features of neither a T cell nor a B cell.
Odontoblast cell A cell producing dentine.
Olfactory cell A special cell of the olfactory mucosa.
Osteoblast cell A mesodermal cell concerned with the production of bone matrix.
Osteocyte cell A cell found in bone matrix, concerned in its metabolic activity.
Oxyntic cell A parietal cell found in mucosa of the stomach concerned with secretion of hydrochloric acid.
Parent cell Mother cell.
Pigment cell Any cell containing pigment granules.
Plasma cell A cell derived from B lymphocytes concerned with the production of antibodies.
Prickle cell A cell having spine-like protoplasmic processes found in the stratum spinosum of the epidermis.
Purkinje cell A large cerebellar cortex neuron.
Pus cell A degenerated leukocyte found in the pus.
Quiescent cell A cell which replicates slowly.
Reticular cell A cell that can develop into one of the several types of connective tissue cells or into a macrophage, found in the spleen, bone marrow or lymphatic tissue.
Reticuloendothelial cell A macrophage or phagocytic cell.
Rod cell A long and narrow sensory retinal cell that is stimulated in dim light.

Segmented cell Neutrophil whose nucleus has two or more lobes.

Sensory cell A cell that on stimulation gives rise to nerve impulses that are conveyed to CNS.

Sickle cell An abnormal erythrocyte having shape like a sickle signet.

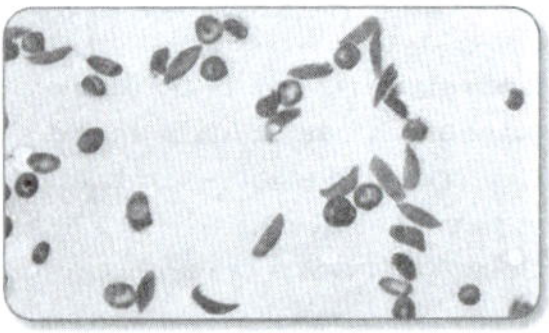

Sickle cells in peripheral blood smear

Ring cell A vacuolated cell with the nucleus at a side, often found in mucin secreting adenocarcinoma.

Smudge cell Cell with a large, ovoid nucleus filled with a granular amphophilic to deeply basophilic mass of an indistinct nuclear membrane, seen in adenovirus-infected cells.

Somatic cell Body cells of different shapes and functions that possess two sets of chromosomes (diploid).

Squamous cell A flat scale-like epithelial cell.

Stellate cell A star-shaped cell with processes extending from it.

Stem cell A cell capable of differentiation and self-renewal.

Stipple cell An RBC containing small basophilic staining dots, found in lead poisoning, malaria, severe anemia and leukemia.

Suppressor T cell A type of T lymphocyte that inhibits CD 4 + and B cell activity.

T cell A lymphoid cell from the bone marrow that migrates to the thymus gland where it matures as a differentiated lymphocyte. These cells are antigen-specific responding to an antigen processed by a macrophage and are identified by surface protein markers called cluster of differentiation (CD).

Target cell An erythrocyte with a rounded central area surrounded by lightly stained clear ring which in turn is encircled by a dense ring of peripheral protoplasm.

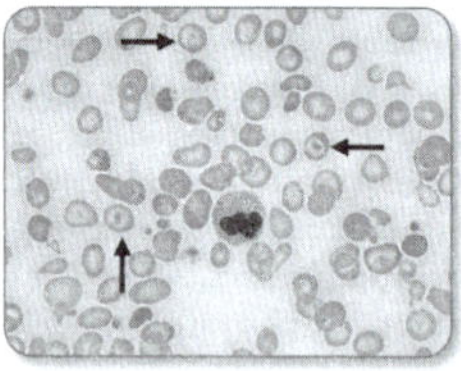

Target cells in blood smear

Tart cell A phagocytic cell that has ingested unaltered nuclear material of cells.

Totipotent cell An undifferentiated embryonic cell.

Undifferentiated cell A cell without any change into a mature cell of any type.

Wandering cell A macrophage capable of ameboid movement.

Zymogenic cell Enzyme producing chief cell of the gastric glands.

Cell adhesion molecule A cell surface protein that is used to connect to each other; CAM.

Cell body (*perikaryon*) Contains the nucleus and organelles responsible for the metabolism and gene expression that supports cell survival.

Cell cycle control system A system of regulatory proteins that governs progression through the cell cycle.

Cell division The process by which a single parent cell splits to form new cells or daughter cells.

Cell mediated immune response Activation of specific cells to launch an immediate response against an invading microbe.

Celsius centigrade scale (*sel'se-us*) A temperature scale on which the boiling point of water is 100° and the freezing point is 0°. This centigrade scale is named after Anden Celsius, Swedish astronomer.

Cellulitis (*set-u-li'tis*) Inflammation of the skin and the tissues beneath from a bacterial infection. It may be localized or spreading through the tissues.

Cellulose (*sel'u-los*) A polysaccharide that forms plant fiber though it does not give any nutrients, it stimulates peristalsis of intestines.

Cement (*se'ment*) A substance that hardens into a firm mass when prepared appropriately.

Cementocyte (*se-men'to-sit*) An entrapped cementoblast forming part of the cementum.

Cementoma (*se'men-to'ma*) Benign jaw tumors that originate from periodontal ligament elements.

Cement (cement) (*se'ment*) A substance that hardens into a firm mass when prepared appropriately.

Cementification (*se-men'ti-fi-ka'shun*) The process by which cementum of a tooth is formed.

Center (*sen'ter*) The mid-point of a body; a group of nerve cells within CNS that controls specific activity or function; a service facility in a particular field.

Central core myopathy An autosomal dominant myopathy causing hypotonia in infancy and non-progressive proximal muscle weakness.

Central line A venous access device inserted into and kept in the vein. It provides a route for administration of fluid and medicines and an access to the heart to obtain information about pressures in venous circulation.

Centers for disease control Prevention: US based public health agency meant to improve the health of people.

Central nervous system (CNS) Made up of the brain and the spinal cord. It is body's processing center.

Centrencephalic (*sen'tran-sa-falik*) The inference that the abnormal tissue in this disorder lies deep within the center of the brain, at the level of the brainstem reticular formation.

Centriacinar emphysema (*sen'tri-as'i-nar*) A chronic lung condition that damages the upper lobes of the respiratory passages.

Centrifugal (*sen-trif-u-gal*) Away from the center.

Centrifuge (*sen-tri-fuj*) A device that spins test tubes at high speeds, allowing heavy particles in the liquid to settle at the bottom and lighter liquid to go to the top.

Centriole (*sen'tre-ol*) A minute organelle consisting of a hollow cylinder, closed at one end and open at the other. It is found in the center of a cell. It divides into two daughter centrioles before mitosis and migrates to opposite poles of the cell during mitosis.

Centripetal (*sen-tripe-tal*) Toward the center.

Centromere (kinetochore) (*sen'tro-mer*) A constricted region of a chromosome and joining point of two chromatids.

Centrosome (centrosphere) (*sen'tro-som*) A region of the cytoplasm of a cell lying near the nucleus containing centrioles.

Centrosphere (*sen'tro-sfer*) The cytoplasm of the centrosome.

Centrum (*sen'trum*) Any center; the body of a vertebra.

Cephalad (*sef'a-lad*) Toward the head.

Cephalexin (*sef'a-lek'sin*) A first generation cephalosporin used to treat certain susceptible bacterial infections.

Cephalhematoma (*sef'al-he'ma-to'ma*) A mass of clotted blood located between the periosteum and the skull of a newborn. Characteristically limited to one skull bone.

Cephalhydrocele (*sef-al-hi'dro-sel*) An accumulation of serous or watery fluid under the pericranium.

Cephalic (*se-fal'ik*) Cranial; superior in position.

Cephalic index Cranial capacity obtained by dividing the maximal length of the head into the maximum breadth of the head by 100.

Cephalin A phospholipid with the phosphatidyl-ethaholamine. It helps to restore and maintain the natural barrier function of the upper most layer of the skin.

Cephalocele (*sef'a-lo-sel*) A herniation of cranial contents through a defect in the skull.

Cephalogram (*sef'a-lo-gram*) A radiograph of the head especially for orthodontic purposes.

Cephalometry (*sef'a-lom'e-tre*) Measurement of the head.

Cephalosporin A group of antibiotics derived from a fungus that has a wide range of activity against many important gram-positive and gram-negative bacteria and are of value for treatment of serious infections. The historical classification is by generations (first to fourth).

Cephalothin sodium Known as Cefalotin, is a broad spectrum antibiotic used for the treatment of bacterial infections such as skin infections, infection of UTI, bone and lower respiratory tract.

Cephamycin (*sefa-mi'sin*) Naturally occurring family of β-lactam cephalosporin-type antibiotics having a 7-methoxy group and possessing marked resistance to the action of beta-lactamases from gram-positive and gram-negative organisms.

Cercaria (*ser-ka're-a*) Pl. **cercariae**. A free swimming state in the development of a fluke.

Cerclage (*ser-klazh*) Encircling tissues with a ligature.

Cerebellum (*ser-e-bel'um*) Little brain. The region of the back of the brain concerned with the maintenance of posture and balance and the coordination of movement. It consists of two lateral hemispheres united by a narrow middle portion, the vennis.

Cerebral (*ser-e-br'al*) Pertaining to the cerebral hemisphere.

Cerebral angiography Radiologic examination of the blood vessels of the brain after injection of a contrast medium.

Cerebral cortex The outer surface of the brain concerned with mental functions, voluntary movement and sensation.

Cerebral dominance Left cerebral hemisphere is dominant in 90 – 95% of individuals and are right handed.

Cerebral embolism Blockage of one of the arteries to the brain by an embolus.

Cerebral gigantism An autosomal dominant disease with rapid early growth without endocrinopathy, accelerated bone maturation or precocious puberty.

Cerebral hemorrhage Rupture of a sclerosed or diseased blood vessel in the brain.

Cerebral hemisphere One of the halves of cerebrum.

Cerebral palsy Disorders of movement and posture caused by brain damage that occurs before birth, during birth or in early life.

Cerebral aqueduct (aqueduct of sylvius) A component of the brain's ventricular system, and it functions as a canal through which CSF flows, and joins the 3rd and 4th ventricles of the brain.

Cerebral cortex The layer of gray matter covering the entire surface of cerebral hemisphere. There is a laminar organization of its cellular and fibrous components.

Cerebral hemisphere One of the halves of cerebrum.

Cerebral hemorrhage Rupture of a sclerosed or diseased blood vessel in the brain.

Cerebral palsy Disorders of movement and posture caused by brain damage that occurs before birth, during birth or in early life.

Cerebral tumor Cancerous or non-cancerous mass or growth of abnormal cells in the brain.

Cerebration (*ser'e-bra'shun*) Activity of the mental processes; thinking.

Cerebroside (*ser'o-bro-sid*) A lipid present in nerve and other tissues.

Cerebrospinal fever (spotted fever) Meningococcal meningitis with acute onset of fever, headache, neck rigidity, vomiting and photophobia.

Cerebrospinal fluid (CSF) The fluid flowing inside and around the brain and spinal cord that provide support and nutrition. It is formed in the cerebral ventricles by an active secretion from choroid plexus and it passes through the interventricular foramen to the third ventricle and then through a median and two lateral foramina to subarachnoid space. It is absorbed into intracranial venous sinuses over the convexity of the cerebral hemisphere through the arachnoid villi.

Cerebrovascular disease Any disease affecting suddenly an artery that supplies blood to the brain.

Cerebrum (telencephalon) (*ser'e-brum*) The largest and most developed part of the brain. It performs the sensory and motor functions and various mental activities. It is derived from telencephalon and includes mainly cerebral hemisphere, (cerebral cortex and basal ganglia).

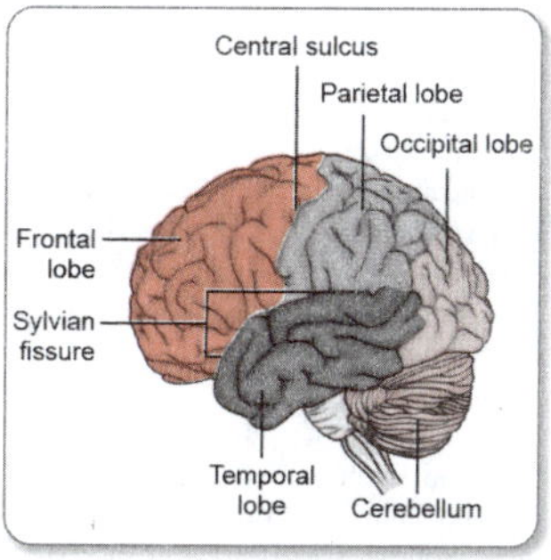

Cerebrum

Ceruloplasmin (*se'ru'lo-plaz'min*) A glycoprotein carrying copper in the blood.

Cerumen (earwax) (*se-ru'men*) Ear wax. A substance secreted by the glands at the outer third of the ear canal.

Cervical (*ser'vi-kal*) Pertaining to or in the region of the neck; pertaining to the cervix of an organ such as the cervix uteri.

Cervical cap A flexible thimble-shaped device providing a covering to uterine cervix as a contraceptive.

Cervical dysplasia Changes in the cells on the surface of the cervix, that is considered precancerous.

Cervical factor Any quality in the mucus produced by the cervix that is hostile to the sperm, and causes inhibition of fertility.

Cervical incompetence Abnormal weakness of the cervix that can cause recurrent hemorrhage.

Cervical mucus method A method of family planning that is based on observing changes in the mucus secreted by the cervix to determine the time of ovulation.

Cervical nerve A nerve in the first eight pairs of spinal nerves.

Cervical osteoarthritis A degenerative condition of the joints between the bones in the neck causing neck pain and stiffness.

Cervical plexus A network of first four cervical nerves that supplies parts of the face, neck, shoulder and chest, and diaphragm.

Cervical rib Accessory cervical rib.

Cervical rib syndrome Compression of the brachial plexus by a cervical rib causing pain, and parasthesias of the hand, neck, shoulder or arms.

Cervical ripening Softening and dilatation of the uterine cervix in preparation for childbirth.

Cervical spine The uppermost part of the vertebral column consisting of seven vertebrae.

Cervical spondylosis Disk degeneration with associated osteophyte formation and osteoarthritis of cervical vertebral joints.

Cervical stitch A surgical stitch that is tied like a downstring around a weakened cervix to prevent recurrent miscarriage.

Cervical vertebra One of the first seven bones of the vertebral column.

Cervical cancer (cervical carcinoma) Cancer that starts in the cells of the cervix.

Cervical intraepithelial neoplasia (CIN) Abnormal changes of the cells that line the cervix. CIN is not a cancer but can change to cancer if not treated.

Cervical smear (Papanicolaou (Pap) test) A specimen of tissue removed from the cervix for examination under a microscope to detect cell abnormalities; pap smear.

Cervical vertebrae Consists of 7 stacked bones in the neck region C. First vertebrae C1 is atlas, is ring shaped and begins at the base of the skull. Second-C1 is axis; C3-C7 are more classic vertebrae.

Cervicitis (*ser-vi-si'tis*) Inflammation of the cervix uteri.

Cervix (*ser'viks*) The neck or a part of an organ resembling a neck; cervix of uterus.

Cervix uteri The neck of the uterus. It is the small cylindrical lowest part of the uterus extending from the internal os to the external os, and protruding into the vagina. It separates the body of the uterus from the vagina. The menstrual flow and fetus escape through this canal.

Cervix vesicae Neck of the urinary bladder.

Cesarean section Removal of fetus from the gravid uterus by the abdominal route after 28th week of gestation.

Cesarean hysterectomy Cesarean section immediately followed by hysterectomy.

Cesium-137 A radioisotope used in Geiger-Muller counter and in radiation therapy.

Cestode (*ses'tod*) A tapeworm belonging to cestoda family.

Cetirizine (*se-tir'i-zen*) A selective Histamine-1 antagonist drug used in allergic rhinitis and chronic urticaria.

Cetylpyridinium chloride (*se'tal-pir'i-dine-am*) A compound used to reduce plaque and gingivitis, as well as whiten teeth.

CFTR gene Cystic fibrosis transmembrane conductance regulator gene.

Chaddock's reflex (*chad'oks*) Extension of big toe on stroking the outer edge of the dorsum of the foot and is present in pyramidal tract lesions; flexion of the wrist and fanning of the fingers on pressing the tendon of palmaris longus muscle, named after Charles Chaddock, US neurologist.

Chagas' disease (*chag' as*) American trypanosomiasis named after Carlos Chagas, Brazilian physician.

Chalazion (meibomian cyst) (*ka-la'ze-on*) A small hard cyst developing on the eyelids. It is due to distension of a meibomian gland with secretions.

Chalicosis (*kal-i-ko'sis*) A pulmonary disorder occurring among stonecutters that is caused by inhalation of stone dust.

Chancre (*shang'ker*) A painless sore usually on the genitals, that develops during the primary syphilis.

Hunterian chancre Primary syphilitic ulcer, a true ulcer which is hard ovoid with sloping edges, a blood-stained discharge, named after John Hunter, London surgeon.

Chancroid (*shang'kroyd*) A sexually transmitted disease caused by *Haemophilus ducreyi* that produces multiple, irregular tender ulcers on the genitals with tender unilateral, matted suppurative regional lymph nodes; erythromycin or co-trinioxazole are useful in the treatment.

Charcot-Leyden crystals Protein crystals in situations of fragmentation of eosinophils, in bronchial secretion of asthmatics and in stools in certain intestinal parasitic infestation.

Charcot-Marie-Tooth disease (peroneal muscular atrophy) Peroneal muscular atrophy named after Jean Charcot, Pierre Marie, French neurologists and Howard Tooth, British physician.

Charcot's joint (*shar-koz*) A painless disorganization of joints marked by hypermobility, encountered in tabes dorsalis, syringomyelia, or injury, named after Jean Charcot, French neurologist.

Charnley clamps An apparatus used to encourage arthrodesis between the ends of two bones on either side of a joint.

Cheiloplasty (*ki'lo-plas"te*) Plastic surgery to repair lip defects.

Cheiropompholyx (*ki'ro-pom'fo-liks*) Blistering condition of hands and feet, related to excessive sweating.

Cheiroplasty (*ki'ro-plas"te*) Plastic surgery on the hand.

Cheirospasm Spasm of the muscles of the hand as in writer's cramp.

Chelating agent A chemical used in the treatment of poisoning by metals such as lead, arsenic and mercury.

Chemoreceptor (*ke'mo-re-sep'ter*) A sense organ or sensory nerve ending sensitive to stimulation by chemical substances, such as oxygen receptors in carotid body.

Chemosis (*ke-mo-sis*) Edema of the conjunctiva producing a pronounced ring around the cornea.

Chemotaxis (*ke'mo-tak'sis*) The movement of additional white blood cells to the site of inflammation in response to the chemical mediators released by neutrophils, monocytes and injured tissue.

Chemotherapy (*ke'mo-ther'a-pe*) Treatment of disease by chemical agents most of which are toxic to cells undergoing division and to induce tumor cell lysis.

Combination chemotherapy Use of two or more drugs simultaneously in order to enhance their effectiveness or to prevent development of drug resistance.

Chest Thorax; the part of the body between the neck and diaphragm encased by ribs. It is divided into various regions as supraclavicular, suprasternal, clavicular, infraclavicular, mammary between the 3rd and 6th costal cartilages, inframammary between the 6th rib and the costal arch, sternal, axillary, infra-axillary, suprascapular, scapular, interscapular and infrascapular regions.

Alar chest A long flat chest with scapulae standing prominently like wings on either side.

Barrel-shaped chest Increase in anteroposterior diameter of the chest. The ribs are horizontal. The spine is unduly concave forward and sternum is prominently arched, the chest appears circular and the subcostal angle is greater than 90° encountered in chronic airflow obstruction.

Chest physiotherapy A rehabilitation programme consists of postural drainage, cough facilitation, breathing exercises, clapping and vibration over the affected areas of the lungs.

Elliptical chest Bilaterally symmetrical chest with its transverse diameter being greater than the posteroanterior diameter in the ratio of 7:5. The subcostal angle is <90°.

Flail chest An unstable chest moving paradoxically following multiple fractures.

Flat chest A shield-like chest with posteroanterior diameter being markedly decreased resulting in an increase in the transverse diameter.

Funnel chest Pectus excavatum, a funnel-like depression of the lower two-thirds of the sternum with prominent costochondral junctions junctions.

Pigeon chest Pectus carinatum; the sternum is bulged forward especially in its upper part. The ribs slope into meet the sternum on either side, losing their curvature. Chest appears triangular.

Rachitic chest Abnormalities of chest such as pigeon chest, funnel chest, Harrison's groove and rickety rosary, noted in those suffered from rickets and respiratory diseases in childhood.

Chiasma (*ki-az'ma*) A decussation or crossing.

Optic chiasma An X-shaped crossing of the optic nerve fibers originating from the nasal half of the retina. Beyond this point in the brain the fibers travel in optic tracts.

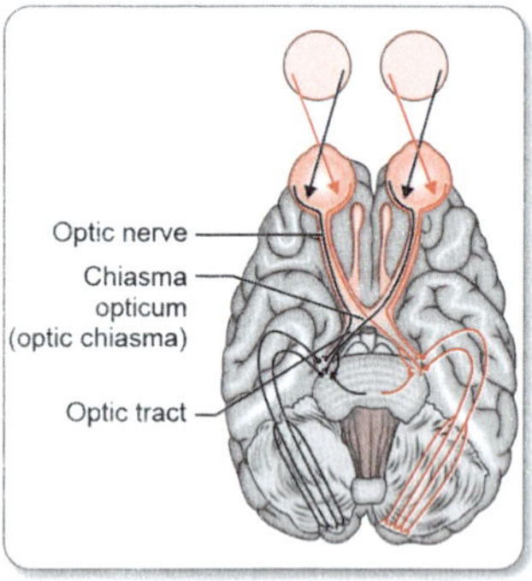

Optic chiasma

Chickenpox *(chik'en-poks)* Varicella; highly contagious disease caused by varicella zoster virus. It affects children. Rash appears on the second day of illness on the trunk, then spreads to the face and limbs. Macules are noted first which within a few hours become papular, then vesicular and within 24 hours pustular. They dry up in few days to form scabs. As the spots appear in crops, the lesions of all stages of development can be seen in any area at the same time.

Chiclero ulcer A form of leishmaniasis of the skin caused by Leishmania tropica maxicana. Ulcerating lesion on the earlobe is formed.

Chiggers (*chig'ers*) The six legged red larva of mites of the family *Trombiculidae*. Some species spread scrub typhus.

Chigoe (*chig'o*) A tropical flea, *Tunga penetrans*, the female of which lives on or burrows into the skin of its host, which includes humans.

Chikungunya (*chik'un-gun'ya*) An acute alpha-virus infection transmitted by Aedes mosquitoes producing a dengue-like fever.

Chilblain (*chil'blan*) A cutaneous injury from exposure to cold or damp climate producing localized itching, swelling and painful erythema. The common sites are fingers, toes and ears.

Child abuse Physical, emotional and sexual injury to a child.

Childbirth The process of giving birth to a child.

Chimerism (*ki-mer'ism*) The presence in a person of cells that are genetically different as they are derived from two different fertilized ova. It does not cause any ill health.

Human chimerism Migration of fetal cells into the blood of the mother during pregnancy; the two-way migration of cells between transplanted organs and their recipients.

Chiropody (podiatry) (*ki-rop'o-de*) Treatment of foot disorders.

Chiropractice A system of health care based on the concept that the nervous system is the single most important determinant of a person's state of health.

Chirospasm (*ki'-ro-spasm*) Writers' cramps; a spasm of hand muscles.

Chlamydiae (*kla-mid'e-ae*) Small gram-negative organisms that only grow inside the cells. Unlike viruses they possess both DNA and RNA in their structure. They have a cell wall and divide by binary fission. There are three species such as *Chlamydia 'pneumoniae'*, *C. psittaci* and *C. trachomatis*.

Chlamydiae pneumoniae A human pathogen that makes a person to person spread. It presents with sinusitis, pharyngitis, laryngitis and pneumonia. It is sensitive to tetracyclines and macrolides.

Chlamydiae psittaci A human infection is related to exposure to birds. It pursues a low-grade course with malaise, high fever, cough and muscular pains.

Chlamydiae trachomatis Causative agent of trachoma.

Chloasma (melisma) (*klo-az'ma*) Melasma; presence of brown macules often seen symmetrically over the cheeks and forehead, mostly in women. May occur spontaneously or in association with pregnancy and oral contraceptive pill.

Chloasma gravidarum Pigmentation over cheeks, forehead and around the eyes during pregnancy.

Chloracne (*klor-ak'ne*) A rare skin condition caused by certain toxic halogenated aromatic hydrocarbon chemicals, including the dioxins.

Chloral hydrate A colorless crystalline substance used as a sedative and hypnotic.

Chlorambucil (*klo-ram'bu-sil*) An alkylating cytotoxic agent used in chronic lymphatic leukemia and lymphomas.

Chloramphenicol (*klo'ram-fen'i-kol*) The only naturally occurring broad spectrum antibiotic containing nitrobenzene indicated in infections due to *Salmonella typhi, S. paratyphi, H. influrrizae* infections.

Chlorcyclizine (*klor-si'kli-zen*) H_1 histamine receptor antagonist.

Chlordiazepoxide (*klor'di-az'e-pok'sid*) A benzodiazepine derivative used in the treatment of anxiety disorders and alcohol withdrawal syndrome.

Chlorhexidine (*klor-heks'i-den*) An antiseptic used to sterilize for surgeries and in healthcare practice, to reduce pocket depth in periodontitis, and to treat gingivitis.

Chloride shift Exchange of plasma chlorides with red cell bicarbonate in tissues producing CO_2.

Chlorination (*klo'ri-na'shun*) Addition of chlorine and its compounds in a concentration of 1 part per million to the water to kill the bacteria.

Chlorine (*klo'ren*) A highly irritating gas, atomic number 17.

Chlorobutanol (chlorbutol) is an alcohol based preservative, without surfactant activity. It is a preservative sedative, hypnotic and weak local anesthetic. It has antibacterial and antifungal properties.

Chloroform (*klo'ro-form*) $CHCl_3$ colorless liquid with ethereal odor, used as solvent. Earlier, it was used at an inhalation anesthetic.

Chloroguanide (Proguamil) is used to treat and prevent malaria.

Chloroma (*klor-o'ma*) A malignant green colored tumor arising from myeloid tissue; green cancer.

Chlorophenothane (DDT); A colorless insecticide that is poisonous to humans and animals.

Chlorophyll (*klor'o-fil*) Any of green magnesium complex of the phorbin derivative found in photosynthetic plants.

Chloroprocaine (*klor'o-pro'kan*) A local anesthetic agent indicated for intrathecal injection in adults for the production of subarachnoid block, spinal anesthesia, or ocular surface anesthesia.

Chloropsia (*klor-op'se-a*) A defect of vision in which objects appear green.

Chloroquine (*klor'o-kwin*) An antimalarial drug used to treat susceptible infections with *P. vivax, P. malariae, P. ovale,* and *P. falciparum*. It is also used for second line treatment for rheumatoid arthritis.

Chloroquine resistant malaria Falciparum malaria increasingly resistant to the previously effective chloroquine.

Chlorosis (*klo-ro'sis*) Green sickness, Virgin's disease; iron deficiency anemia named for the yellow-green skin pallor in young females, associated with koilonychia.

Chlorothen (chloropyrilene) Antihistamine and anticholinergic.

Chlorothiazide (*klor"o-thi'a-zid*) A thiazide diuretic used to treat hypertension and edema in congestive heart failure, hepatic cirrhosis, and corticosteroid and estrogen therapy.

Chlorotrianisene (Brand name 'Tace'); a nonsteroidal estrogen, used to treat symptoms of menopause, deficiency in ovary function and in rare cases, prostate cancer.

Chloroxylenol An antiseptic and disinfectant agent used for skin disinfection and surgical instruments.

Chlorphenesin (*klor-fen'e-sin*) A topical antifungal agent.

Chlorpheniramine (*klor'fen-ir'a-men*) A pyridine derived antihistaminic preparation.

Chlorproguanil Antimalarial drug.

Chlorpromazine (*klor'pro'ma-zen*) A phenothiazine derivative used as a tranquilizer and as an antiemetic.

Chlorpropamide (*klor'pro'pa-mid*) An oral sulphonyl-urea, long acting hypoglycemic agent used in the treatment of noninsulin dependent diabetes mellitus.

Chlorprothixene A typical antipsychotic drug of thioxanthine class. It has a low antipsychotic potency.

Chloruria (*klo-rur'ea*) Excretion of excess chlorides in the urine.

Chlortetracycline (*klor'te-tra-si'klen*) Original tetracycline, relatively unstable antibiotic active against a wide range of microorganisms.

Chlorthalidone (*klor-thal'i-don*) An orally effective diuretic.

Choana (*ko-a'na*) Funnel-shaped cavity or infundibulum.

Choke urethrogram Micturition against external pressure with contrast in the bladder to improve urethrogram picture.

Cholagogue (*ko'la-gag*) A substance that stimulates contraction of gallbladder to promote bile flow.

Cholangiocarcinoma (*ko-lan'je-o-kar'si-no-ma*) An adenocarcinoma arising from the epithelium of the intrahepatic bile ducts.

Cholangiography (*kol-an'je-og'ra-fe*) Radiography of the bile ducts after they have been filled with a contrast medium.

Cholangiolitis (*kol-aan'je-o-lit'is*) Inflammation of the cholangioles.

Cholangioma (*ko-lan'je-o'ma*) A tumor of a bile duct.

Cholangitis (*kol-an'ji-tis*) Inflammation of common bile duct.

Cholecalciferol (*kol'e-kal-sef'er-ol*) Vitamin D2 and substance obtained from the diet or synthesized in the skin on irradiation of 7-dehydrocholesterol.

Cholecyst (*ko'le-sist*) The gallbladder.

Cholecystectomy (*ko'le-sis-tek'ta-me*) The surgical removal of the gallbladder.

Cholecystenterostomy (*ko'le-sis'ten-ter-os'to-me*) Surgical creation of a new communication between the gallbladder and intestine.

Cholecystitis (*ko'le-sis'ti-tis*) Inflammation of the gallbladder.

Cholecystoduodenostomy (*ko'le-sis-to-du'o-de-nos'to-me*) Surgical anastomosis of the gallbladder and duodenum.

Cholecystogastrostomy (*ko'le-sis-to-gas-tros'to-me*) Surgical anastomosis between the gallbladder and stomach.

Cholecystography (*ko'le-sis'tog-ra-fe*) Radiographic study of the gallbladder after oral administration of a cholecystopaque.

Cholecystokinin (pancreozymin) (*ko'le-sis'to-ki-nin*) A polypeptide substance secreted in the small intestine that stimulates gallbladder contraction and secretion of pancreatic enzymes.

Cholecystotomy (*ko'le-sis-to'to-me*) Formation of an opening through the abdominal wall into the gallbladder, usually done for drainage and to remove gallstones.

Choledochal (*ko'le-do'kal*) Pertaining to the common site duct.

Choledocholithiasis (*ko-led'o-ko-li-thia-sis*) Stone in the common bile duct.

Choledochotomy (*ko'le-do-koto-me*) Incision into the common bile duct.

Cholelithiasis (*ko'le-li-thi'a-sis*) The presence or formation of gallstones.

Cholelithotomy (*ko'le-li-thot'o-me*) Surgical incision of the biliary tract for removal of gallstone.

Cholera (*kol'er-a*) A severe acute gastrointestinal infection caused by *Vibrio cholera*. It is transmitted through infected drinking water contaminated by stool or vomit of patients with cholera. *Cholera vibrios* multiply in the lumen of small intestine and are not invasive. They adhere to the intestinal mucosa and secrete a powerful exotoxin which by stimulation cAMP results in outpouring of fluid. It presents with severe diarrhea without pain followed by vomiting of sudden onset. Later, there is passage of rice water material consisting of clear fluid with flecks of mucus. There is severe dehydration with muscular cramps. The skin becomes cold and clammy and wrinkled. The eyes are sunken. There is fall in blood pressure and pulse becomes and imperceptible and urine output diminishes. There is rapid improvement by replacement of water and electrolytes.

Choleresis (*kol'ler'e-sis*) The secretion of bile by the liver.

Choleretic (*ko'ler-et'ik*) Stimulating the bile production by the liver; an agent stimulating production of bile.

Cholestasis (*ko'le-sta'sis*) Obstruction to the flow of bile inside the liver, adj. **cholestatic**.

Cholesteatoma (*ko'le-ste'a-to-ma*) A mass of keratinized squamous epithelium and cholesterol in the middle ear from chronic otitis media; an epidermoid cyst arising in CNS.

Cholesterol (*ko-les'ter-ol*) The most abundant steroid in animal tissues that is precursor of bile acids and steroid hormones and a key constituent of cell membranes. Most is synthesized in the liver, but some is absorbed from dietary sources, found in food rich in animal fat. It circulates in the plasma complexed to proteins of various densities. It can accumulate or deposit abnormally and plays an important role in the pathogenesis of atheroma in the arteries.

Cholesterosis (*ko-les'ter-o'sis*) Characterized by mucosal villous hyperplasia with excessive accumulation of cholesterol esters within epithelial macrophages.

Cholestyramine (*ko'les-sti'ra-min*) A bile acid sequestrant used as an adjunct in the reduction of elevated serum cholesterol in patients with primary hypercholesterolemia, and for the relief of pruritus associated with partial biliary obstruction.

Cholic acid (cholalic acid) (*kol'ik*) One of the primary bile acids, usually exist conjugated with glycine or taurine. It helps in fat absorption and cholesterol excretion.

Choline (*ko'len*) A quaternary amine; a member of B-vitamin complex.

Cholinergic (*ko'lin-er'jik*) Relating to nerve fibers that employ acetyl choline as their neurotransmitter.

Choline salicylate Anti inflammatory pain reliever agent, related to aspirin.

Cholinesterase (*ko'lin-es'ter-as*) An enzyme that catalyzes the hydrolysis of the acyl group from different esters of choline.

Choluria (*kol'u're-a*) Presence of bile in the urine; discoloration of the urine with bile pigments. adj. **choluric**.

Chondralgia (*kon-dral'jia*) Pain in the region of a cartilage.

Chondrectomy (*kon-drek'to-me*) Surgical removal of a cartilage.

Chondrin A bluish-white gelatin like substance that forms the matrix of cartilage. Chondrin is made up of 2 proteins chondroalbutnoid and chondromucoid.

Chondriosome An organelle containing enzymes responsible for producing energy.

Chondroangioma (*kon"dro-an"je-o'ma*) A benign mesenchymoma containing cartilaginous and angiomatous elements.

Chondroblast (*kon'dro-blast*) An immature cartilage producing cell.

Chondroblastoma (*kon'dro-blas-to-ma*) A benign tumor arising in the epiphyses of long bones of adolescents, consisting of highly cellular tissue resembling fetal cartilage.

Chondrocalcinosis (*kon'dro-kal'si-no'sis*) Calcification of cartilage.

Chondroclast (*kond'ro-kla'st*) A cell concerned in the absorption of cartilage.

Chondrocranium (*kon'dro-kra'ne-um*) The cartilaginous cranial structures of the fetus.

Chondrodysplasia (chondro-osteodystrophy, chondrodystrophy, Morquio-Brailsford disease) *(-dis-pla'zah)* A disturbance in the development of epiphyseal cartilage of the long bones resulting in arrested growth of the long bones and dwarfism.

Chondrodystrophy *(-dis'tro-fe)* A disorder of cartilage formation. Also known as chondrodystrophia.

Chondropathy *(kon'drop'a-the)* Disease of cartilage.

Chondroitin sulphate *(kon-dro'i-tin)*A glycosaminoglycan found in the ground substance of the connective tissue particularly cartilage, bone, blood vessels and cornea.

Chondroma *(kon-dro'ma)* A nonmalignant tumor of cartilage cells on the surface of or inside the bones.

Chondromalacia *(kon'dro-ma-la'shea)* Softening of the cartilage.

Chondro-osteodystrophy A rare developmental familial disorder, characterized by skeletal abnormalities such as dwarfism and generalized body dermities.

Chondrosarcoma *(kon'dro-sarcoma)* A malignant growth of cartilage that usually affects the long bones, the pelvis and the clavicle.

Chondrosternoplasty *(kon"dro-ster'no-plas"te)* The surgical treatment of malformations of the sternum.

CHOP A chemotherapeutic regimen used for treatment of lymphoma consisting of cyclophosphamide, adreomycin, oncovin and prednisone.

Chorda *(kor'da)* A tendinous or cord-like structure. pl. **chordae**.

Chorditis *(kor-dit'is)* Inflammation of the vocal or the spermatic cords.

Chordoma *(kor-do'ma)* A malignant tumor arising from the embryonic remains of the notochord, appears most commonly in fifth and sixth decade in sacrococcygeal region.

Chorea *(kor-e'ah)* Irregular, purposeless, arrhythmic and asymmetric movements variable in type and location that constantly change in form and affecting different parts of the body at irregular intervals.

Chorea gravidarum Choreiform movements appearing in first trimester of pregnancy.

Huntington's chorea A progressive disorder noted in middle age with an autosomal dominant inheritance, choreoathetosis and dementia.

Senile chorea Chorea occurring in elderly age group.

Sydenham chorea Chorea occurring as a manifestation of rheumatic fever.

Choriocarcinoma *(kor'e-o-kar'si-no-ma)* A rare malignant tumor that develops inside the uterus from the placenta.

Chorioepithelioma (choriocarcinoma) *(kor'e-o-ep'i-thele-o'ma)* A malignant tumor, predisposed to early metastasis, and occurring not infrequently among women of childbearing age.

Chorion *(ko're-on)* The outermost of the two membrane layers containing the amniotic fluid and the fetus. It gets attached to the placenta.

Chorionic gonadotropin (human chorionic gonadotropin, hCG) Human chorionic gonadotropin.

Chorionic villus sampling (CVS) A prenatal diagnostic procedure in the ninth to 11th week of pregnancy under guidance of ultrasound scanning in which fetal cells are obtained from the placenta and studied for genetic abnormalities.

Choroid *(ko'roid)* The middle vascular structure of the eye situated between the sclera and the retina, adj. **choroidal**.

Choroid plexus A secretory tissue responsible for producing CSF in the brain.

Choroiditis *(ko'roi-dit'is)* An inflammation of the choroid.

Christmas disease A rare inherited coagulation abnormality; it is also called hemophilia B disease, bears the surname of child in whom the disorder was recognized first.

Chromaffin (*kro-maf'in*) Denoting granules or vesicles containing adrenaline and noradrenaline, and the secretory cells of the adrenal medulla in which they are found.

Chromate- (chromate-) (*kro'mat*) Any salt of chromic acid.

Chromatid One of the two identical halves of a chromosome that has been replicated in preparation for cell division.

Chromatin (*kro'ma-tin*) The materials inside cells consist of DNA and protein from which chromosomes are formed.

Chromatography (*kro'ma-tog'ra-fe*) A laboratory technique in which mixtures of complex molecules are separated along a gradient of pressure or solubility between liquid or gas and solid or liquid phase. The molecules are separated by absorption, gel filtration, ion exchange or partitioning.

Chromatolysis (*kro-ma-tol'i-sis*) Disintegration of the granules of chromophil substance, as in Nissl bodies of a neuron, which may occur after exhaustion of the cell or damage to its peripheral process.

Chromatophore (*-for*) Any pigmentary cell; color producing plastid.

Chromatopsia (*kro'ma-top'se-a*) A visual defect in which colorless objects appear to be tinged with color.

Chromomycosis (chromoblastomycosis) (*kro'mo-mi-ko'sis*) A chronic granulomatous infection of the skin and subcutaneous tissue caused by several different dematiaceous fungi.

Chromosome Thread-like structures inside the nuclei of cells that consist of one or more (23 in humans) usually paired, very long DNA molecules that are associated with RNA and histones, and the complete complement of chromosomes contain the complete genetic information present in a living organism.

Bacterial artificial chromosome A chromosome-like structure, constructed by geneticengineering, that is used as a vector to clone DNA fragments of genome in cells of the bacterium *Escherichia coli.*

Chromosome abnormality An abnormality in the number or structure of chromosomes inside a person's cells, that can cause series of birth defects.

Chromosome analysis A laboratory procedure in which cells of fetal origin are obtained either in the first trimester by chorionic villus biopsy or later in

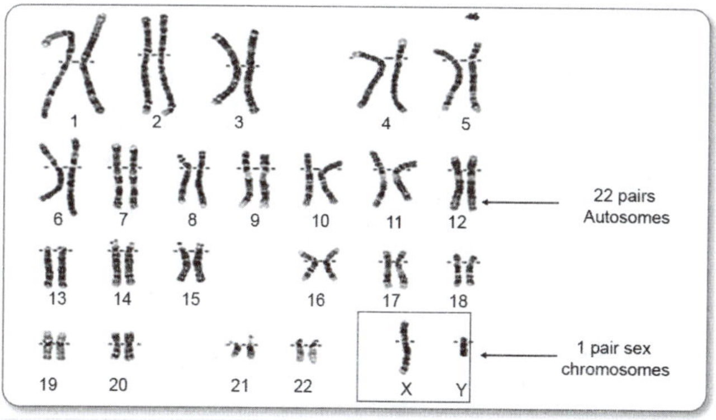

Chromosomes

pregnancy by amniocentesis and grown in a tissue culture medium to detect major chromosomal defects.

Chromosome banding A technique for identifying chromosome pairs and analyzing regions within chromosomes.

Chromosome breakage syndromes A group of inherited disorders in which the chromosomes have an increased fragility as in ataxia—telangiectasis, Fanconi syndrome. They exhibit an increased susceptibility to certain malignancies.

Chromosome condensation Compaction of entire chromosomes in preparation for cell division.

Chromosome replacement therapy A cytosurgical procedure that extracts existing chromosomes from a particular diseased cell and insert new ones in their place in that same cell.

Human artificial chromosome HAC, a vector used to transfer or express large fragments of human DNA.

Chronaxy (*kro'nak-se*) Minimum time required to stimulate a structure such as a neuron with a constant current twice the threshold voltage.

Chronic (*kron'ik*) A disorder that is persisting for a long time.

Chronic active hepatitis A type of hepatitis characterized by progressive inflammation and destruction of liver cells; it leads to cirrhosis of the liver.

Chronic fatigue syndrome (CFS) A severe disabling illness characterized by a self-reported persistent or relapsing fatigue of ≥6 consecutive months duration accompanied by infections, rheumatologic and neuropsychiatric symptoms, which are not attributable to other known conditions and a symptom complex.

Chronic granulomatous diseases (CGD) A heterogeneous group of immune system defects characterized by recurrent and potentially fatal pyogenic infections of early onset. The neutrophils though ingest pathogens fail to produce superoxide and related microbial oxygen intermediates.

Chronic obstructive pulmonary disease COPD diffuse obstruction involving structural and functional changes in the parenchyma and also in the large and small airways. The airway obstruction is constant or makes slow progress and exists without a specific cause such as bronchiectasis, cystic fibrosis or obliterative bronchiolitis or localized disease in upper airways.

Chronic prostatitis/chronic pelvic pain syndrome A type of prostatitis characterized by chronic genitourinary pain that may be associated with urinary and sexual dysfuncntion.

Chronopharmacology (*kron'o-far'ma-kol'oje*) A branch of chronobiology concerned with effect of drugs on times of biologic rhythm.

Chrysops (*kris'ops*) Genus of bloodsucking insects considered pests to humans and cattle. They are large flies with large brightly-colored compound eyes, and large clear wings with dark bands.

Chrysotherapy (*kris'o-ther'a-pe*) Treatment (of rheumatoid arthritis) by injection of gold salts, called also aurotherapy.

Chyle (*kil*) A milky fluid taken up by the lacteals from intestine during digestion. It consists of lymph and chylomicrons in a stable emulsion, carried by the lymphatic system *via* the thoracic duct into the circulation.

Chylomicron (*-mi'kron*) A class of lipoproteins that transport exogenous cholesterol, triglycerides and several apolipoproteins to tissues after meals.

Chyluria (*kil-ur'e-a*) The passage of chyle in the urine, giving a milky appearance.

Chyme (*kim*) The semidigested food passed from the stomach into the duodenum.

Chymopapain (*ki'mo-pa-pan'*) A proteolytic enzyme derived from papaya latex, used as a meat tenderizer and in nucleolysis medicine.

Chymotrypsin (*-trip'sin*) A serine proteinase produced in intestine by activation of chymotrypsinogen by trypsin.

Chymotrypsinogen (*-trip'sin'o-jen*) The precursor of chymotrypsin and converted to chymotrypsin by the action of trypsin.

Cicatrix (*sik'a-triks*) A scar, pl. **cicatrices**.

Cidofovir (*si-dofo-vir*) A nucleoside analogue and is active against herpes cytomegalovirus (CMV) retinitis infection.

Cilastatin (*si'la-stat'in*) A renal dehydropeptidase inhibitor used to prevent degradation of imipenem. Both medications are used together to treat a variety of infections.

Ciliary body A part of the middle layer of the wall of the eye.

Cilium (*sil'e-um*) Singular of cilia.

Cimetidine (*si-met'i-den*) An antagonist to H_2 receptors which inhibits gastric acid secretion and used to treat peptic ulcer.

Cimex (*si'meks*) A genus of insects in the family Cimicidae, commonly known as bed bugs.

CIN Cervical intraepithelial neoplasia.

Cinchona (*sin-ko'na*) The dried bark of the root and stem of various species of cinchona; it is the source of quinine and quinidine and cinchonine and cinchonidine.

Cinchonism (*sin'ko-nizm*) Toxic manifestation of cinchona characterized by flushed skin, tinnitus, blurred vision, dizziness, nausea, vomiting and diarrhea. Very high levels of cinchona exhibit skin rashes, somnolence, blindness and marked hypotension.

Cineangiocardiography (*sin'e-an'je-o-kar-de-og'ra-fe*) Motion pictures of the passage of a contrast medium through chambers of the heart and blood vessels.

Cingulectomy (*sin'gu-lek'to-me*) Electrolytic destruction of the anterior cingulate gyrus and corpus collosum.

Cingulum (*sing'gu-lum*) An anatomical band or encircling ridge. pl. **cingula**.

Ciprofloxacin (*sip'ro-flok'sa-sin*) A synthetic fluoroquinolone antibiotic effective against many gram-positive and gram-negative organisms.

Circle of Willis A ring of blood vessels at the base of the brain.

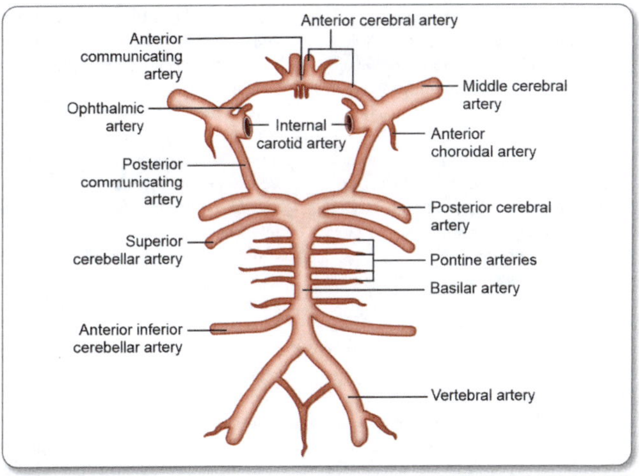

Circle of Willis

Circulatory system Made up of blood vessels that carry blood away from and towards the heart.

Circumcision (*serk'um-siz'un*) Surgical removal of the foreskin of the penis.

Circumduction (*-duk'shun*) Circular movement of the limb or of the eye.

Circumflex nerve One of the 5 peripheral nerves that run through the shoulder.

Circumoral Pertaining to the area of the face around the mouth.

Circumstantiality (*serk'um-stan'she-al'it-e*) *psy* A disturbance in the thought process in which one makes an unnecessary elaboration of many trivial details. Also known as circumstantial speech.

Cirrhosis (*si-rosis*) Progressive and widespread necrosis of liver cells associated with inflammation and fibrosis leading to loss of normal liver architecture. There is distortion and loss of normal hepatic vasculature with the development of portal systemic shunts and formation of nodules due to proliferation of surviving hepatocytes. The condition makes a gradual onset with anorexia, dyspepsia, reduction in liver size, mild jaundice, ascites and signs of liver cell failure and portal hypertension.

Alcoholic cirrhosis Cirrhosis developing in chronic alcoholism, which initially is associated with hepatomegaly due to fatty change and later by contraction of the liver.

Biliary cirrhosis Cirrhosis due to biliary obstruction which may be primary resulting from destruction of intrahepatic bile ducts or secondary to large duct biliary obstruction.

Cardiac cirrhosis An extensive fibrotic reaction within the liver due to prolonged congestive heart failure; pseudocirrhosis.

Laennec's cirrhosis Portal cirrhosis, named after Rene Laennec, a French physician and inventor of the stethoscope.

Micronodular cirrhosis Presence of regenerating nodules of 1 mm in diameter involving every lobule, surrounded by thick fibrous septa tends to evolve into macronodular cirrhosis.

Macronodular cirrhosis Nodules of variable size with many more than 3 mm in diameter and connective tissue septa varies in thickness.

Portal cirrhosis A chronic disease of liver where the normal liver lobules are replaced by small regenerating nodules separated by fibrous tissue strands.

Postnecrotic cirrhosis Necrosis of whole lobules with collapse of reticular framework resulting in large scars, that may follow viral or toxic necrosis, adj. **cirrhotic**.

Cirsoid (*ser'soid*) Resembling a varix.

Cisplatin (*sis'plat-in*) A platinum chemotherapeutic agent with antitumor activity. It binds DNA and interferes with DNA synthesis.

Cisterna (*sis-ter'na*) Cistern.

Cisterna basalis Interpeduncular cistern, dilatation of the subarachnoid space in front of the pons, where arachnoid membrane stretches across the two temporal lobes.

Cisterna chyli A dilated part of the thoracic duct at its origin in lumbar region into which the intestinal trunk and two lumbar lymphatic trunks open.

Cisterna magna Cerebellomedullary cistern, the largest of the subarachnoid cisterns between the cerebellum and medulla oblongata.

Terminal Cisterna's Pairs of transversely oriented tubules of the sarcoplasmic reticulum occurring at regular intervals in skeletal muscle fibers.

Cistron (*sis'tron*) The smallest unit of genetic material that must be intact to function as a transmitter of genetic information; gene.

Citric acid (*sit'rik*) A tricarboxylic acid obtained from citrus fruits and functions as a key intermediate in intermediate metabolism.

Citrobacter (*sit'ro-bak'ter*) A genus of gram-negative coliform bacteria in the family *Enterobacteriaceae* which is a relatively common opportunistic pathogen in humans. The most common species are *Citrobacter freundii* and *Citrobacter koseri* formerly referred to as *Citrobacter diversus*.

Citrulline (*sit-rul-en*) An amino acid formed from ornithine in the course of urea cycle, which gets converted into arginine. It is also a product in nitric oxide biosynthesis.

Citrullinemia (*sit-rul'in-e'me-a*) An autosomal recessive disorder characterized by the accumulation of ammonia and other toxic substances in the blood due to malfunction of the urea cycle; excess of citrulline in the blood.

Clamp (*klamp*) A surgical device for compressing a part or structure.

Clarithromycin (*kal-rith'tro-mi'sen*) A macrolide antibiotic effective against a wide range of gram-positive and gram-negative organisms.

Clasmocyte A macrophage. They play a role in nonspecific local cutaneous immunity to staphylococcus.

Clasp (*klasp*) A device to hold something. ***Clasp knife spasticity*** In pyramidal lesions there is hypertonia offering increased resistance to passive movement. The resistance is greatest at the initial phase of movement and then suddenly it gives way during the latter phase. It is best appreciated in the flexor muscles of the upper limb and the extensor muscles of the lower limb.

Claudication (*klaw'di-ka'shun*) Limping. ***Intermittent claudication*** Attacks of pain and lameness brought on by walking chiefly in the calf muscle and the condition is seen in occlusive arterial disease.

Claustrophobia (*-fo'be-a*) Intense fear of closed places or crowded areas.

Claustrum (*claws'trum*) One of the four basal nuclei in each cerebral hemisphere, there is a thin layer of gray matter separated from the lentiform nucleus by a layer of white matter.

Clavicle (*klav'i-kl*) The collar bone. *see* Table of bones. adj. **clavicular**.

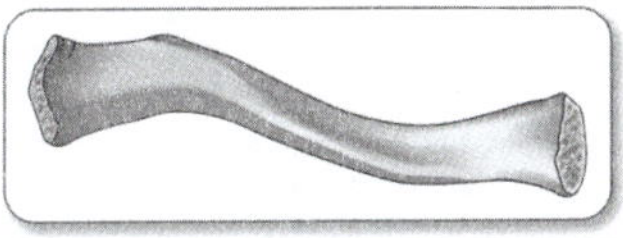

Clavicle

Clavus (*kla'vus*) A corn caused by pressure over a bony prominence.

Claw foot (*klaw'foot*) A high arched foot with the toes hyperextended at the metacarpophalangeal joints and flexed at the distal interphalangeal joints.

Claw hand Atrophy of the interosseous muscles of hand with hyperextension at the metacarpophalangeal joints and flexion at the interphalangeal joints.

Clearance (renal clearance) (*kler'ans*) The act of removal of something from some place; removal of a substance from blood. ***Creatinine clearance*** Measurement of the clearance of endogenous creatinine, used to measure glomerular filtration rate. ***Inulin clearance*** Determination of rate of filtration through the glomeruli by use of inulin that filters freely with water and it is neither excreted nor reabsorbed through tubules.
Mucociliary clearance The clearance of mucus and foreign bodies from the airways by ciliary beating.

Cleavage (*klev'aj*) Division into distinct parts.

Cleft palate A birth defect characterized by a gap in the roof of the mouth, often associated with cleft lip.

Cleidocranial dysplasia (*kli'do-kra'ne-al*) A disorder involving the abnormal development of bones in the skull and collar (clavicle) area.

Clemastine (*klem'as-ten*) An antihistamine with sedative and anticholinergic effects used to treat the symptoms of allergic rhinitis.

Clemizole H1 receptor antagonist, thereby preventing the interaction between histamine and H1 receptor and inhibiting H1-mediated signaling.

Client-centered therapy (Rogerian therapy) A form of psychotherapy, developed by Carl Rogers, is a nondirective techniques so client can act as equal partners in the talk therapy process.

Climacteric (*kli-mak'ter-ik*) The time span during which a woman moves from her reproductive to nonreproductive years.

Clindamycin (*kl'in-da-mi-sin*) A semi-synthetic derivative of lincomycin active against gram-positive organisms.

Clinic (*klin'ik*) An institution where medical instruction is given to the medical students by means of demonstration of physical signs in a patient; an institution where ambulator patients are taken care of.

Clitoridectomy (*klit'o-ri-dek'to-me*) Excision of the clitoris.

Clitorimegaly (*-meg'a-le*) Enlargement of clitoris; seen in excessive levels of androgenic hormones.

Clitoris (*klit'o-ris*) A small sensitive female genital organ, partly enclosed in the labia, that swells in response to sexual stimulation.

Clitoroplasty (*klit'o-ro-plas"te*) The surgical creation of a clitoris, to repair female genital mutilation or as part of sex reassignment surgery.

Clivus (*kli'vus*) A downward sloping surface; the sloping surface in the posterior cranial fossa from the dorsum sellae to the foramen magnum.

Cloaca (*klo-a'ka*) An endodermal chamber in early embryos, into which the hindgut and allantois empty.

Clofibrate (*klo-fi'brat*) An antihyperlipidemic agent to reduce serum lipids.

Clomipramine (*klo-mip'ra-men*) A tricyclic antidepressant used in the treatment of obsessive-compulsive disorder and disorders with an obsessive-compulsive component, such as depression, schizophrenia, and Tourette's disorder.

Clomocycline A tertacycline antibiotic prescribed by for treatment of acne.

Clonazepam (*klo-naz'a-pam*) A long-acting benzodiazepine with intermediate onset commonly used to treat panic disorders, severe anxiety, and seizures.

Clone (*klon*) An exact copy; often applied to a group of identical genes or a group of genetically identical cells or organisms.

Clonic (*klo-nic*) Period of shaking or jerking part of body.

Clonidine (*klo'no-den*) An antihypertensive agent that stimulates adrenergic receptors in the brain leading to a decrease in sympathetic outflow.

Clonogenic (*klo'no-jen'ik*) Arising from or consisting of a clone.

Clonorchiasis (*klo'nor-ki'a-sis*) A disease caused by infection with the liver fluke *Clonorchis sinensis*.

Clonus (*klo'nus*) Rhythmic contraction and relaxation of the muscles from a sustained stretch of the tendon in a pyramidal lesion.

Ankle clonus While a patient is lying supine, the hip and knee are semi-flexed. The leg is held parallel to the bed giving support to the hip. The forepart of the foot is grasped and pushed suddenly backward and the pressure is maintained. Clonus is exhibited by sustained repetitive flexion and extension of foot due to the contraction of the calf muscles, in presence of a pyramidal lesion.

False clonus An unsustained clonus noted in individuals who are tense or anxious. Clonus tends to diminish and becomes irregular.

Patellar clonus While the knee is kept in extension, the patella held at its lateral borders is pushed downward suddenly and the pressure is maintained. Clonus is revealed by repetitive jerky contractions and relaxation of quadriceps which pulls the patella upward.

True clonus A sustained clonus that increases by dorsiflexion of foot.

Wrist clonus Elicited by suddenly hyperextending the wrist and maintaining the stretch on long flexors and the hand.

Clopidogrel (*klo-pid'o-grel*) An antiplatelet agent used to prevent blood clots in peripheral vascular disease, coronary artery disease, and cerebrovascular disease.

Clopamide A diuretic drug that is used to treat hypertension and edema

Clorazepate (*klor-az'a-pat*) A benzodiazepine that is used to treat anxiety disorders, partial seizures, or alcohol withdrawal symptoms.

Clostridium (*klos-trid'e-um*) A genus of anaerobic spore-forming, motile bacteria belonging to bacillaceae. They are found in soil and intestinal tract, pl. **clostridia**.

Clotrimazole (*klo-trim'a-zol*) An imidazole derivative used as an antifungal agent.

Clotting factor One of several substances in the blood that are needed for blood to clot.

Clotting time The test measures the time taken for blood vessel constriction and platelet plug formation to occur. The expected range of clotting time is 4–10 minutes.

Cloxacillin (*klok'sa-sillin*) A semisynthetic penicillin useful in the treatment of infections due to staphylococcal penicillinase-positive organisms.

Clubbing (*klub'ing*) Proliferation of soft tissues, especially nail beds affecting the fingers and toes. There is thickening of the terminal part of the digits and the nails are abnormally curved.

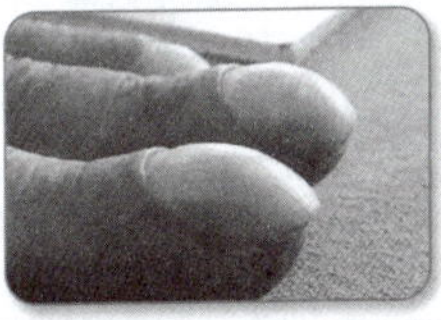

Clubbing

Clubfoot (talipes) (*klub'foot*) A congenital deformity in which the affected foot appears rotated internally at the ankle. *see* Talipes.

Clumping (*klump'ing*) The aggregation of particles.

Clutton's joint Symmetrical arthrosis of knee joints, in congenital syphilis, named after Henry Clutton, British surgeon.

Clyster (*klis'ter*) An enema.

CML Chronic myeloid leukemia.

Coagulant (*ko-ag'u-lant*) An agent that causes or stimulates coagulation, especially of blood.

Coagulase (*-las*) An antigenic substance especially that produced by staphylococci, may be related to the formation of thrombus.

Coagulation (*ko-ag'u-la'shun*) The conversion of blood into a jelly-like clot; transformation of a sol into a semi-solid mass.

Blood coagulation The sequential process by which different coagulation factors or blood interact to result in the formation of clot.

Disseminated intravascular coagulation (DIC) A hemorrhagic condition which occurs following an uncontrolled activation of clotting factors and fibrinolytic enzymes throughout small blood vessels.

Electric coagulation Destruction of tissues by application of electric current.

Coagulum (*ko-ag'u-lum*) A clot or a curd; a soft insoluble mass formed when a solution undergoes coagulation.

Coalescence (*ko'a-les'ens*) The fusion of parts.

Coarctation (*ko-ark-ta'shun*) A constriction, narrowing or stricture.

Aortic coarctation Obstruction of the aorta in the region of the ductus arteriosus or ligamentum arteriosum just distal to the left subclavian artery. It is characterized by absence or delay of the femoral pulses, presence of high blood pressure in upper limbs, low blood pressure in the lower limbs and cardiac abnormalities.

Reversed coarctation Aortoaortitis with absence of pulse in upper limbs and hypertension in lower limbs; Takayasu's disease.

Cobalamin (*ko-bal'a-min*) A compound containing the substituted ring and nucleotide structure characteristic of vitamin B_{12}.

Cobalt (*co'ba-lt*) A metallic element and a constituent of vitamin B_{12}.

Cocaine (*ko-kan*) An alkaloid obtained from the leaves of *Erythroxylon coca* or by synthesis from egonine. It has topical anesthetic activity and pronounced psychotropic effects. Its abuse leads to addiction.

Cocainism Habituation to cocaine.

Cocarcinogen (*ko-kar-sin'o-jen*) A substance that by itself cannot cause cancer, but increases the activity of a cancer causing substance consisting of large pieces; rough, not smooth.

Coccidioidomycosis (*kok-sid'e-oi'do-mi-ko'sis*) A disease caused by *Coccidioides immitis* with lesions evolving like pulmonary tuberculosis, restricted to semi-desert areas of south-western US.

Coccobacillus (*kok'o-ba-sil'us*) Pl. **coccobacilli**. A short, thick bacterial rod having a shape of an oval or slightly elongated coccus.

Coccus (*kok'us*) Pl. **cocci**. A round, spheroid or oval bacterium; adj. **coccal**.

Coccygodynia (*kok"si-go-din'e-a*) Pain in the coccyx and neighboring region.

Coccyx (*kok'siks*) The small bone at the end of the vertebral column in humans, formed by the fusion of four rudimentary vertebrae.

Cochlea (*kokle-a*) A coiled structure in the inner ear; the organ responsible for hearing. It translates the sound vibrations into the electrical nerve impulses and transmits them to the brain *via* the auditory nerve.

Cochlear implant A device to treat deafness, consisting of electrodes implanted inside the cochlea to transmit sound generated nerve impulses to the brain.

Cochlear nerve The 8th cranial nerve (vestibulocochlear) carries auditory sensory information from the cochlea of the inner ear directly to the brain.

Cocoon syndrome A lethal inherited condition characterized by multiple fetal malformations such as defective face and seemingly absent limbs, which are bound to the trunk and encased in a tight, abnormally thick and adhesive skin and the fetuses are spontaneously aborted.

Codeine (*ko'den*) A narcotic alkaloid obtained from opium or prepared from morphine; acts as an analgesic and antitussive.

Codon (*cod'on*) A three nucleotide sequence of DNA or RNA that specifies a single amino acid.

Coenzyme (*ko-en'zim*) Dialysable and relatively heat stable organic substance of low molecular weight that enhances or necessary for the action of enzymes.

Coenzyme A A coenzyme containing pantothenic acid, involved in transfer of acyl groups, especially in transacetylations.

Cofactor (*ko'fak-tor*) An element essential for enzyme action, such as heme, coenzymes and magnesium ions; a substance that works in combination with something else to bring shout a certain effect.

Cognitive behavioral therapy A psychotherapy with an aim to find the patterns of thinking that underlie a disorder and the ways to reinforce those thoughts.

Coitus (sexual intercourse, copulation) *(ko'i-tus)* Sexual union between male and female by insertion of the penis into the vagina.

Coitus reservatus Coitus in which ejaculation is delayed or suppressed.

Coitus interruptus A method of voluntary fertility control where male withdraws before ejaculation thereby preventing deposition of semen into the vagina.

Colchicine (*kol'chi-sin*) An alkaloid from *Cochicum autumnale*, used in the treatment of gout.

Cold (common cold) Catarrhal disorder of the upper respiratory tract; low temperature; the opposite of hot; spiritless; indifferent.

Cold abscess Focal, well-circumscribed abscess without usual signs of inflammation, seen in paravertebral tuberculous cold abscess.

Cold agglutinin disease An immune disorder characterized by IgM autoantibodies that agglutinate red blood cells at very low temperatures.

Cold chain A system of storage and transport of vaccines at low temperature from the manufacturer to the actual vaccination site.

Cold hypersensitivity Exaggerated response of autonomic nervous system to low, environmental temperature characterized by bradycardia and a local wheal-and-flare reaction.

Cold nodule A focus of reduced radioisotope uptake on a ^{131}I or 99m Tc scintillation scan of thyroid, seen in cystic or solid nonfunctional thyroid swellings.

Cold pack Covering a patient or an area in towel dipped in cold water and used to reduce fever, pain or swelling.

Cold pressor test A test to measure blood pressure response to the immersion of one hand in ice cold water.

Cold stress Hypothermia.

Common cold Acute illness of short duration presenting as an acute inflammation of the upper respiratory passages and it is frequently due to rhinoviruses. It is characterized by nasal irritation, nasal stuffiness, sneezing, sore throat, conjunctival irritation and watery nasal discharge, usually afebrile.

Feverish cold Infection from rhinovirus, adenovirus and influenza virus associated with fever, weakness and profound prostration.

Cold sore (herpes simplex) Infection by herpes simplex virus on the lips and adjoining skin; herpes labialis.

Colectomy (*ko-lek'to-me*) Surgical removal of a part or whole of the colon.

Colestipol (*ko-les'ti-pol*) An FDA-approved bile acid sequestrant; antihyperlipidemic drug used for the treatment of primary hypercholesterolemia.

Colic (*kol'ik*) Painful spasm in any hollow organ or tubular structure; pertaining to the colon.

Biliary colic Colic due to passage of gallstones along the bile duct.

Infantile colic Paroxysms of pain with crying and irritability occurring in infants.

Intestinal colic Severe abdominal pain.

Lead colic Severe abdominal pain due to lead poisoning.

Menstrual colic Dysmenorrhea.

Renal colic Pain in the lumbar region radiating over to the abdomen into the groin associated with the passage of renal calculi.

Uterine colic Severe colic arising in the uterus during menstrual period.

Coliform bacteria Motile or non-motile Gram negative, non-spore forming bacilli that possess β-galactosidase to produce acid and gases under optimum conditions.

Colistin (*ko-lis'tin*) An antibiotic effective against some gram-negative microorganisms, especially pseudomonas, that are resistant to other antibiotics.

Colitis (*ko-li'tis*) Inflammation of the colon.

Amoebic colitis Colitis due to *Entamoeba histolytica*.

Antibiotic associated colitis Antibiotic-induced diarrhea.

Granulomatous colitis Granulomas involving the colon giving rise to colitis.

Ischemic colitis Acute vascular insufficiency of the colon in the territory of inferior mesenteric artery giving rise to pain in left iliac fossa, bloody diarrhea and abdominal distension.

Mucous colitis Irritable bowel syndrome.

Pseudomembranous colitis Colitis associated with antibiotic therapy, usually due to a toxin produced by Clostridium difficile, characterized by formation of pseudomembrane on the mucosa of the colon with diarrhea, passage of blood and mucus, abdominal pain and fever.

Radiation colitis Colitis developing from radiation therapy.

Ulcerative colitis A form of inflammatory bowel disease, it causes swelling, ulcerations and loss of function of the large intestine.

Collagen (*kol'a-jen*) The protein substance of white fibers of connective tissue, cartilage and bone. It contains glycine, alanine, proline and hydroxyproline. adj. **collagenous**.

Collagen vascular diseases A group of disorders characterized by arthropathies, immune complex deposition, renal involvement and partial or temporary response to corticosteroids.

Collar bone Clavicle.

Collateral (*ko-lat'er-al*) Accessory or subsidiary to main thing; a side branch of a vessel or nerve accompanying side by side.

Collateral blood vessels Tiny, latent vessels that may spontaneously enlarge and become functional.

Collateral damage An undesired, but unavoidable comorbidity associated with a treatment modality.

Collateral circulation Maintenance of blood flow in small anastomozing channels when main vessel is obstructed.

Colles' fracture Named after Abraham Colles, Irish surgeon, 1773–1843. Fracture of the lower end of the radius at the wrist following a fall on the outstretched hand. Typically, it produces the 'dinner fork' deformity. Smith's fracture is a fracture of lower end of radius with forward displacement of lower segment.

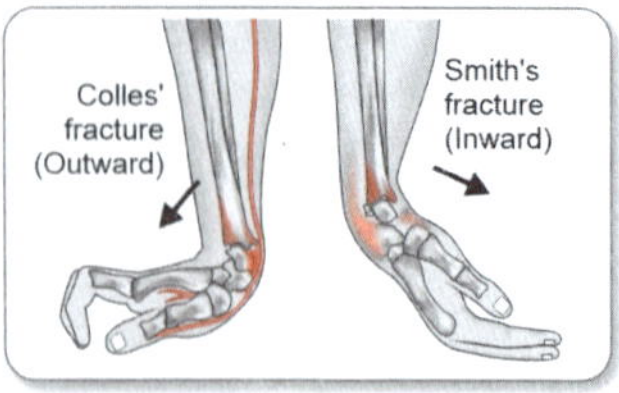

Colles' fracture and Smith's fracture

Colliculus (*kol-lik'u-lus*) Pl. **colliculi**. A small eminence above the surrounding parts.

Seminal colliculus An elevated portion of male urethral crest upon which open the prostatic utricle and two ejaculatory ducts.

Collodion (*ko-lo'de-on*) A liquid prepared by dissolving pyroxylin in ether and alcohol, which on evaporation gives a glossy, contractile film. It is applied topically to the skin on wounds, cuts and abrasions, and to hold surgical dressings in place and to keep medications in contact with the skin.

Collyrium (*ko-lir'e-um*) A medicated eyewash.

Coloboma (*kol'o-bo'ma*) Any defect of the eye. It may affect the choroid, ciliary body, eyelid, iris, lens, optic nerve or retina. It may be congenital, pathological or surgical.

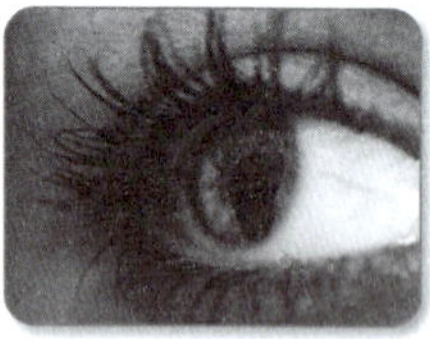

Coloboma

Colon (*ko'lon*) The division of large intestine extending from cecum to the rectum. It is 1.5 m long and it mixes the intestinal contents. No digestive enzymes are secreted by colon. As more water is absorbed in the colon, the contents get dehydrated. adj. **colonic**.

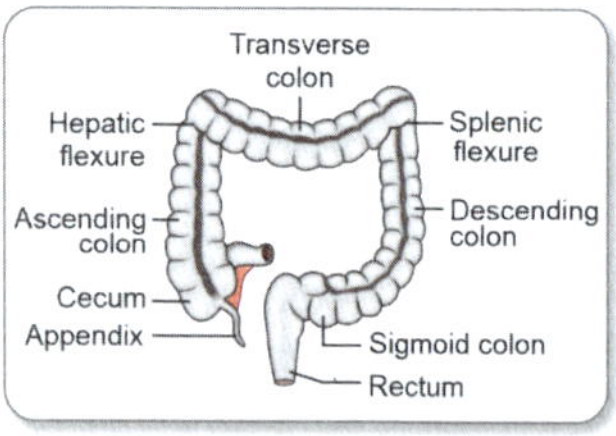

Structure of colon

Ascending colon The portion of the colon between cecum and the right colic flexure.

Descending colon The part of the colon extending from left colic flexure to the sigmoid colon.

Iliac colon The part of the descending colon lying between the crest of left ilium and the pelvic brim.

Irritable colon A functional disorder characterized by abdominal pain associated with defecation and it develops in response to psychological factors, altered gastrointestinal motility and increased sensitivity to intestinal distension.

Sigmoid colon Colon having an S-shaped curve found in the pelvis and it extends from descending colon to the rectum.

Spastic colon Irritable bowel syndrome.

Transverse colon The part of large intestine extending transversely across the abdomen between the right and left colic flexures.

Colonic irrigation Colonic wash by injection of a large amount of fluid into the colon through a tube.

Colonoscopy (*ko'lon-us'ko-pe*) Visualization of the large intestine using a colonoscope.

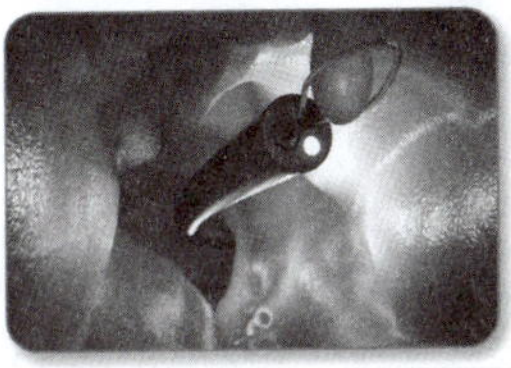

Colonoscopy

Colony (*kol'o-ne*) A growth of microorganisms in a culture media; a group of cells.

Colony stimulating factor-1 CSF-1, a serum protein that promotes the differentiation of monocytes.

Color blindness Inability to distinguish certain colors, and occurs as a genetically determined condition.

Colorimeter (*ku'lor-im'e-ter*) An instrument for measurement of the intensity of color in a fluid such as amount of hemoglobin in the blood.

Colostomy (*ko-los'to-me*) The surgical creation of an opening of a portion of the colon through the abdominal wall to its outside surface.

Colostrum Breast fluid secreted in the first 2 to 3 days after birth. It is a thin yellowish fluid rich in protein and other nutrients for the needs of the body and it contains anti-infective factors which protect the baby against infections.

Colpocoele (*kol'po-sel*) Herniation into the vagina.

Colpocytogram (*kol'po-si'to-gram*) A differential listing of the cells observed in smears from the vaginal mucosa.

Colporrhaphy (*kol-por'a-fe*) A surgical procedure to repair pelvic organ prolapse such as cystocele or rectocele.

Colpoperineorrhaphy (*kol'po-per'in-e-or-ra-fe*) Surgical repair of the perineal tear in the vagina.

Colposcope (vaginoscope) (*kol'po-scop*) An endoscope for visualization of tissues of the vagina and cervix through a magnifying lens.

Colposuspension (*kol'po-sus'pen-shun*) Suspension of the anterior vaginal wall at the level of the bladder neck in women with stress incontinence.

Colpotomy (*kol-pot'o-me*) An incision into the wall of the vagina.

Colpoxerosis (*kol'po-ze-ro'sis*) A condition in which the vagina is unusually dry.

Columella (*kol'u-me-la*) The strip of skin running from the tip of the nose to the upper lip, which separates the nostrils; a small column; a portion of the sporangiophore on which the spores develop.

Column (*kol'um*) A pillar or cylindrical supporting structure.

Anal column Vertical folds of the mucous membrane in the upper half of the anal canal.

Anterior column The anterior or ventral portion of the gray matter on either side of the spinal cord that appears like a horn in transverse section.

Column of Bertin Renal column.

Column of Burdach Fasciculus cuneatus of the spinal cord.

Clarke's column Collection of large cells in the posterior gray column of the spinal cord extending from the eighth cervical segment to the third or fourth lumbar segment.

Column of Gall Gray columns of the anterior, posterior and lateral masses of gray matter extending longitudinally through the lateral half of the spinal cord.

Column of Gowers The tract of ascending fibers anterior to direct cerebellar column and on the lateral surface of the spinal cord.

Column of Morgagni Anal column.

Gray column The longitudinally oriented anterior and posterior horns of gray matter of spinal cord.

Lateral column Lateral portion of the gray matter of spinal cord projecting into the lateral funiculus or white matter between the roots of the spinal nerves on either side especially marked in the thoracic region.

Posterior column Posterior or dorsal portion of gray matter of the spinal cord; palato-pharyngeal arch.

Rectal columns Anal columns.

Renal column The inward extension of the cortical material of kidney separating the pyramids of the kidney.

Spinal column Vertebral column.

Vertebral column Spinal column.

Coma (*ko'ma*) Profound degree of unconsciousness with an unarousable psychological unresponsiveness in which the subjects lie with eyes closed. adj. **comatose**.

Coma vigil Coma in which the patient appears to be in sleep but ready to be aroused.

Diabetic coma Coma due to severe diabetic ketoacidosis.

Hepatic coma Coma accompanying hepatic encephalopathy noted in advanced cirrhosis, fulminant hepatitis or poisoning.

Irreversible coma Brain death.

Metabolic coma Coma resulting from metabolic abnormalities.

Uremic coma Coma due to disturbances in kidney function with retention of metabolic end products.

Comedo (*kom-e-do*) Pl. **comedos, comedones**. A plug of sebaceous material and epithelial debris in the pilosebaceous orifice.

Closed comedo White head; comedo appearing as a papule from which the contents are not easily expressed as the orifice is narrow.

Open comedo Blackhead; a comedo with a dilated orifice from which the debris can be easily expressed.

Commensal (*ko-men'sal*) An organism living on or within another organism and deriving benefit and host is not harmed.

Comminuted fracture A bone that is broken in at least two places.

Commissure (*kom'i-shur*) A bundle of nerve fibers passing from one side to another in the brain or spinal cord; a site of union of corresponding parts such as the sites of junction between adjacent cusps of heart valves; angle or corner of the eye, lips or labia.

Anterior cerebral commissure A band of fibers that pass through lamina terminalis connecting the two cerebral hemispheres.

Anterior gray commissure The commissure lying in front of the central canal of the spinal cord.

Anterior white commissure The band of fibers lying in front of the central canal and the anterior gray commissure of the spinal cord.

Commissure of cerebral hemispheres Corpus callosum.

Hippocampal commissure A thin sheet of fibers connecting the medial margins of the crura of the fornix.

Posterior cerebral commissure A thin band of white matter just above the midbrain connecting superior colliculi.

Posterior gray commissure The gray commissure lying behind the central canal of the spinal cord and connecting both halves of the spinal cord.

Supra optic commissure Commissure crossing the midline of the brain dorsal to the caudal border of optic chiasma.

Communicable disease (contagious disease, infectious disease) An illness due to a specific infectious agent or its toxic products capable of being directly or indirectly transmitted from man to man or from the environment to man.

Communication A joining structure in anatomy such as tendons and nerves.

Community medicine The practice of medicine concerned with groups or populations rather than with individual patients.

Comparative mortality figure The expected number of deaths in standard population compared with those observed.

Compatibility Suitability of mixing or taking without any adverse effects, as drugs; ability of two persons or groups living in harmony.

Compensation (*kom'pen-sa'shun*) Making up for any defect as in valvular defect; a mechanism by which a person tries to make up for real or imagined physical and psychologic deficiencies.

Complement (*kom'ple-ment*) Globulins found in varying proportion in the serum. They have been named as Clq, Clr, Cls and C_2 to C_9. The complement system is activated sequentially when antibody attaches to antigen components on the cell surface. Some microbial polysaccharides activate an alternate pathway bypassing the initial complement components, and it does not require specific antibodies.

Complement fixation A test to determine occurrence of antigen-antibody disorder by using complement.

Complex (*kom'pleks*) A combination of ideas, feelings, thoughts and perceptions; a composite of chemical or immunological structure; an entity consisting of three or more interrelated components; an electrocardiogram showing atrial or ventricular systole; a group of related structures.

AIDS dementia complex Affective disorders with depression in HIV infection.

AIDS related complex ARC patients exhibiting symptoms but do not have AIDS-defining condition. These patients are relatively immunosuppressed.

Antigen-antibody complex A complex formed by binding of antigen to antibody.

Atrial complex P wave in ECG representing atrial electrical activity.

Eisenmenger's complex Increased pulmonary flow due to an initial left-to-right shunt causes severe pulmonary hypertension and reversal of the shunt with central cyanosis and digital clubbing.

Ghon's complex Primary complex.

Golgi complex A complex cellular organelle consisting of flattened saccules, vesicles and vacuoles lying adjacent to the nucleus and are concerned with formation of secretory products.

Immune complex Antigen combined with a specific antibody to which complement may also be fixed.

Inferiority complex A feeling of inferiority causing shyness or timidity or as a compensatory reaction in aggressiveness or exhibitionism.

Primary complex Lesions of primary tuberculosis consisting of a subpleural focus of infection with hilar lymph node involvement.

QRS complex The main deflection in ECG representing ventricular depolarization.

Superiority complex An increased conviction of one's own superiority.

Symptom complex Clinical manifestations.

Ventricular complex The QRST complex in ECG.

Complication The development of a fresh symptom in a proportion of those suffering from a particular disease and which deteriorates the clinical condition of the patient further.

Compress (*kom'pres*) A pad of gauze or other material applied with pressure. It may be hot or cold; wet or dry.

Compressed air illness (Caisson disease) Decompression sickness.

Compulsion (*kom-pul'shun*) Uncontrollable impulse to perform an act repetitively.

Computed tomographic angiography A diagnostic study in which a contrast substance is injected into the circulation and its movement is tracked by a tomographic X-ray device.

Conation (*ko-na'shun*) An initiative, drive and an impulse to act.

Conception (*kon-sep'shun*) A mental process of forming an idea; the union of sperm and ovum; fertilization.

Conceptus (*kon-sep'tus*) The products of conception.

Concha (*kong'ka*) Pl. **conchae**. The outer ear; pinna; one of the three nasal conchae.

Concha auriculae The hollow of the auricle of the external ear between the anterior portion of the helix and antihelix.

Nasal concha A thin bony plate with curved margins projecting from the lateral wall of nasal cavity, and separating the middle from inferior meatus (inferior), the superior from middle meatus (middle) and superior meatus from the sphenoethmoidal recess (superior).

Sphenoidal concha One of the two curved plates forming the roof of the nasal cavity.

Concordance (*kon-kor'dans*) Occurrence of a given trait in both members of a twin pair; agreement; harmony.

Concretion (*kon-kre'shun*) Formation of solid material; a calculus.

Concussion (*kon-kush'un*) Transitory loss of consciousness, accompanied by a variable period of amnesia for events before and after the injury as a result of head trauma.

Condenser (*kon-den'ser*) An apparatus used to cool a gas to a liquid or a liquid to a solid; an instrument to pack material into a cavity of a tooth; a lens on a microscope used to supply the illumination required for visibility of the specimen under observation.

Conditioning (*kon'dish'un-ing*) Improvement of the physical capability of a person; a change in the behavior due to an influence of the environment.

Condom (French letter, rubber) (*kon'dom*) A sheath or covering used to reduce the probability of pregnancy and sexually transmitted disease. Male condom: A thin rubber covering made to fit over a man's erect penis. it is also called rubbers, sheaths, skin, made of thin latex rubber, some condoms are coated with a dry lubricant or with spermicide.

Female condom A thin, transparent, soft plastic sheath inserted into a woman's vagina.

Conduct disorder *psy* A repetitive and persistent pattern of behavior in which the basic rights of others are violated or major age-appropriate rules of society are broken.

Condylarthrosis (condyloid joint) (*kon'dil-ar-thro'sis*) A joint formed by condylar surfaces.

Condyle (*kon'dil*) Pl. **condyles**. The rounded articular surface at the end of a bone.

Condyloma (*kon'di-lo'ma*) A wart-like growth on the skin.

Condyloma accuminatum An epithelial proliferation like a 'cauliflower' induced by human papilloma viruses of low malignant potential.

Confabulation (*kon-fab'u-la'shun*) Unconscious filling of gaps in memory by imaginary experiences that patient believes but that have no basis at all.

Confection (*kon-fek'shun*) A pharmaceutical preparation consisting of a drug mixed with a sweetener.

Confluence A flowing or running together; a joining.

Congenital (*kon-jen'i-tal*) Present at birth.

Congestion (*kon-jes'chun*) An abnormal amount of fluid in a part or organ.

Active congestion Congestion due to an increased blood flow to a part.

Hypostatic congestion Congestion due to pooling of venous blood in a dependent part.

Passive congestion Congestion due to stagnation of blood.

Pulmonary congestion Engorgement of the pulmonary vessels with transudation of fluid into alveolar and interalveolar spaces.

Coniine Poisonous chemical compound found in hemlock and other plants. It affects the motor nerves, causing paralysis and asphyxia.

Conization (*ko'ni-ze'shun*) Removal of a cone-shaped section of tissue from the cervix for diagnosis or treatment; cone biopsy.

Conjugate (conjugate diameter, true conjugate) (*kon'ju-gat*) Paired or joined; a product of chemical conjugation; a conjugate diameter of the pelvic inlet, the distance from the premontory of the sacrum to the upper edge of the pubic symphysis.

Conjugation (*kon'ju-ga'shun*) The union of two unicellular organisms or of the male and female gametes; the combination by which the biologic effects of some chemical substances are terminated; transfer of genetic material from a donor bacterial strain to a receptor strain.

Conjunctiva (*kon'junk-ti'va*) The delicate mucous membrane covering the anterior surface of the eyeball and lining the eyelids.

Bulbar conjunctiva Covering of the anterior eyeball.

Palpebral conjunctiva Cover of the undersurface of the eyelids. adj. **conjunctival**.

Conjunctiva reflex Closure of the eyelids on touching the conjunctiva with a wisp of cotton and it gives information on integrity of the upper cervical sensory neurons.

Conjunctivitis (pink eye) (*kon-junk'ti-vi'tis*) Inflammation of the conjunctiva.

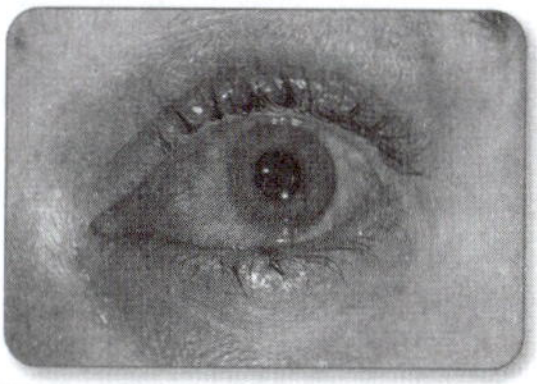

Conjunctivitis

Acute contagious conjunctivitis Acute epidemic conjunctivitis. Pink eye, highly contagious condition with intense hyperemia and profuse mucopurulent discharge, caused by *Haemophilits aegypticus*.

Acute hemorrhagic conjunctivitis A contagious viral infection characterized by pain, swollen eyelids, hyperemia and subconjunctival hemorrhage.

Allergic conjunctivitis A conjunctival reaction to a substance causing an allergic reaction.

Catarrhal conjunctivitis Conjunctivitis due to bacteria, foreign bodies or *Chlamydia trachomatis*.

Gonococcal conjunctivitis Intensely swollen, congested conjunctiva, profuse purulent discharge and swollen eyelids caused by *Neisseria gonorrhoeae*.

Granular conjunctivitis Acute contagious inflammatory conjunctivitis with granular elevations on the lids that ulcerate and scar.

Phlyctenular conjunctivitis Marked nodules that may ulcerate.

Vernal conjunctivitis Conjunctivitis occurring in spring.

Connective tissue Tissue that supports, protects and gives structure to other tissues and organs in the body.

Consanguinity (*kon'san-gwin'i-te*) A state of close genetic relationship and marriage between close blood relatives, associated with an increased risk in offspring of traits controlled by recessive genes and those determined by polygenes.

Conservative treatment Wide range of therapies that do not involve surgery.

Consolidation (*kon-sol-i-da'shun*) The process of becoming solid, especially in pneumonia from an acute inflammatory exudate into the alveolar spaces. It is characterized by dull percussion note and tubular breathing.

Constipation (*kon'sti-pa'shun*) Infrequent passage of hard stools, often-associated with straining, a sensation of incomplete evacuation.

Constrictor (*kon-strik'tor*) That which constricts or draws together; a muscle action to narrow a canal as a sphincter.

Consumption (*kon-sump'shun*) Using of something; wasting of the tissues of body, usually tuberculosis.

Consumption coagulopathy Disseminated intravascular coagulation.

Contact (*kon'takt*) Touching of two bodies; an individual who has been exposed to a contagion.

Contact dermatitis A disorder of skin as a result of the skin coming in contact with irritants which cause an altered state of sensation and morphologic changes.

Contact inhibition Ability of a tissue, on reaching its mature size, to suppress additional growth.

Contact lens A transparent device that fits over the cornea or part of the cornea to bring changes in refractive ability of the cornea or lens of the eye.

Contact range A funnel-shaped depression of the skin with marginal abrasion and bruising of epidermis caused by a zero range gun shot wound.

Contact surface A proximal tooth surface.

Contact therapy Therapy using contact with the parts of the body that feel tense, stuck or sore.

Contagious disease The disease that spreads from person to person in several ways such as flue and colds.

Continuous Joined together; without interruption.

Continuous ambulatory peritoneal dialysis (CAPD) A maintenance system of peritoneal dialysis wherein an indwelling catheter allows fluid to drain into and out of peritoneal cavity.

Continuous cycling peritoneal dialysis (CCPD) A dialysis method in which the patient is attached to an automatic cycler for short exchanges while sleeping.

Continuous murmur Murmur due to the continuous flow of blood through an abnormal communication from a high pressure to a region of low pressure with a large pressure gradient between the two regions.

Contra- Prefix indicating opposite or against.

Contraception (*kon'tra-sep'shun*) Prevention of conception or impregnation.

Contraction (*kon-trak'shun*) A shortage or shrinkage; increase in tension.

Contracture (*kon-trak'chur*) Fibrosis of connective tissue in skin, fascia, muscle or a joint capsule that hinders normal mobility of the related tissue or structure.

Contraindication (*kon'tra-in-di-ka'shun*) Any condition or circumstance that renders a particular mode of treatment improper or inadvisable.

Contralateral (*kon'tra-later-al*) Occurring on the opposite side.

Contrecoup (*kawn-tra-ku*) An injury as in the skull or brain occurring at a site opposite to the point of impact.

Controlled Substances Act The statute establishing federal US drug policy under which the manufacture, importation, possession, use, and distribution of certain substances is regulated.

Contusion (*kon-tu'zhun*) A bruise; an injury without a break in the skin.

Conus arteriosus The anterior part of the right ventricle which terminates in the pulmonary artery.

Conus medullaris The cone-shaped lower end of the spinal cord.

Convergence (*kon-ver'jens*) Movement of two objects toward a common point as in turning the eyes medialward.

Conversion (*kon-ver'zhun*) Changing from one form to another; correction of fetal position during labor; *psy* transformation of emotional conflicts into physical symptoms without any organic basis.

Conversion disorder A syndrome characterized by a loss or distortion of neurologic function not fully explained by organic disease and it presents with gait disturbance; dissociative disorder.

Conversion symptom Common presentation of conversion disorder are gait disturbances, loss of function in the limbs, aphonia, pseudoseizures, sensory loss and blindness.

Convolution (*kon'vo-lu'shun*) A rolling of an organ by infolding upon itself; a gyrus, one of the many folds on the surface of cerebral hemisphere.

Convulsion (*kon-vul'shun*) An involuntary muscular spasms of voluntary muscles occurring in paroxysms; seizure.

Clonic convulsion A convulsion in which muscles contract and relax alternately.

Febrile convulsion Convulsions associated with high fever especially in infancy and early childhood.

Hysterical convulsion Convulsions noted in hysteria.

Mimic convulsion Facial muscle spasm.

Puerperal convulsion An eclamptic convulsion in pregnancy or puerperium.

Salaam convulsion A nodding spasm.

Tonic convulsion Sustained muscle contraction.

Cooley's anemia Thalassemia major, named after Thomas Cooley, US pediatrician.

Coomb's test In acquired hemolytic anemia, antibodies are formed against red cell antigens and cause inappropriate destruction of red blood cells. The presence of antibody on red cells is established by direct antiglobulin test using an antihuman globulin antiserum which causes agglutination of erythrocytes (direct test) and when antibodies are present in the serum they have to get attached to red cells with appropriate antigen before they can be detected (indirect test) named after R. Coomb, British immunologist.

Coprolalia (*kop'ro-la'le-a*) Use of obscene language.

Coprolith (*kop'ro-lith*) A hard mass of inspissated fecal material.

Coproporphyrin (*kop'ro-por'fir-in*) One of two porphyrin compounds found normally in the urine and feces as a decomposition product of bilirubin.

Copulation (*kop'u-la'shun*) Sexual intercourse.

Cor The heart; relating to the heart.

Cor bovinum Markedly, enlarged heart due to hypertrophied or dilated left ventricle.

Cor triatriatum heart With three atrial chambers with pulmonary veins emptying into an accessory chamber above the true left atrium.

Coracoid (*kor'a-koyd*) Scapular process shaped like a crow's beak.

Cord (*kord*) Any long cylindrical, firm structure.

Cordectomy (*kor-dek'to-me*) Surgical removal of a cord as of a vocal cord.

Cordocentesis (*cor'do-sen-te'sis*) A procedure for delivering a blood transfusion to a fetus that involves threading a fine needle through a pregnant woman's abdomen and into the umbilical cord with the aid of ultrasound imaging.

Cordotomy (*kor-dot'o-me*) Division of lateral spinothalamic tracts of the spinal cord.

Corectopia (*kor-ek-to'pe-a*) Eccentric location of the pupil instead of being in the center of the iris.

Corium (*ko're-um*) Pl. **coria**. The dermis, layer of skin deep to the epidermis, the superficial thin layer interdigitates with the epidermis and the deeper thick layer of dense irregular connective tissue, contains blood vessels, nerves, nerve endings and glands.

Corn (*korn*) A horny induration and thickening of the skin caused by friction and pressure.

Hard corn Located on the outside of little toe or the anterior surface of other toes.

Soft corn Located between the toes, kept soft by moisture.

Cornea (*kor-ne'a*) The transparent circular anterior part of the eye, whose curvature is greater than that of other parts of the eye, hence, functions as a refractive medium. It continues at its periphery with the sclera. adj. **corneal**.

Conical cornea Keratoconus.

Cornea reflex Reflex dependent on integrity of the ophthalmic branch of trigeminal nerve and the facial nerve with center at pons. It is tested by an elongated wisp of cotton brought from the side, touching the lateral edge of the cornea. It causes blinking of both eyes.

Cornea transplant/graft Implantation of a cornea from a healthy donor eye.

Cornification (*kor'ni-fi-ka'shun*) Keratinization.

Cornu (*kor'nu*) Pl. **cornua**. Any structure resembling a horn.

Cornu ammonis The hippocampus major of the brain.

Cornu anterius The anterior horn of the lateral ventricle of the brain; anterior gray column of the spinal cord in cross section.

Cornu cutaneum A horn-like appearance in the lateral ventricle of the brain.

Cornu inferius The inferior horn of the lateral ventricle of the brain.

Cornu posterius The posterior horn of the lateral ventricle of the brain; the posterior gray column of the spinal cord in cross section.

Corona (*ko-ro'na*) A structure resembling a crown.

Corona capitis The crown of the head.

Corona dentis The crown of a tooth.

Corona glandis The prominent posterior border of the glans penis.

Corona radiata The radiating fibers from internal capsule to every part of the cerebral cortex.

Coronary (*kor'o-na-re*) Resembling or relating to a crown; encircling, referring to the arteries of the heart.

Coronary angiography Procedure useful to detect stenosis and guide revascularization procedures in patients with coronary artery disease, and the procedure is accomplished by cannulating the right femoral or brachial artery.

Coronary artery bypass surgery CABG, surgical establishment of a shunt that enables blood to travel from the aorta to a branch of coronary artery at a point past obstruction. The reversed segments of saphenous vein or internal mammary arteries are used to bypass the obstruction.

Coronary stent A piece of coated metallic 'scaf-folding' that can be sent on a balloon and used to dilate a stenosed vessel after coronary angioplasty.

Coronary thrombosis Occlusion of one or more of the coronary arteries by a thrombus.

Coronal Relating to the frontal plane that passes through the long axis of the body.

Coronal suture The transvers suture in the skull separating the frontal bone from the parietal bones.

Corona radiata A white matter sheet that continues inferiorly as the internal capsule and superiorly as the centrum semiovale.

Coronary angioplasty (balloon angioplasty) Undertaken by passing a fine guidewire across a coronary stenosis under radiographic control and using it to position a balloon which is then inflated to dilate the stenosis.

Coronary thrombosis Occlusion of one or more of the coronary arteries by a thrombus.

Coroner (*kor'o-ner*) A person to investigate and provide official interpretation regarding the manner and possible cause(*s*) of deaths occurring suddenly, violently, without natural cause, with conflicting findings between stated cause and postmortem findings and foul play.

Coronoidectomy (*kor'o-noy-dek'to-me*) Surgical removal of the coronoid process of the mandible.

Corticosterone (*kor'ti-kos'te-ron*) A natural corticoid from the adrenal cortex that induces glycogen deposition in the liver, retention of sodium and excretion of potassium.

Cor pulmonale A heart affected secondarily to pulmonary disease resulting in right ventricular hypertrophy.

Acute cor pulmonale Develops when pulmonary embolus is sufficiently massive to obstruct more than two-thirds of pulmonary circulation. There is obstruction to the right ventricular outflow.

Chronic cor pulmonale Hypertrophy of the right ventricle resulting from diseases affecting the function and/or the structure of the lung except when these pulmonary manifestations are the result of diseases that primarily affect the left side of the heart, or of congenital heart disease.

Corpus (*kor'pus*) Pl. **corpora**. A human body consisting of head, neck, trunk and limbs; any body or mass; the principal part of any organ or body.

Corpus amygdaloideum A rounded mass of gray matter in the anterior portion of temporal lobe of the cerebrum.

Corpus amylacea One of a number of small ovoid bodies resembling a grain of starch found in nervous tissue, prostate and lungs.

Corpus cavernosum clitoridis One of the two columns of erectile tissue in the body of clitoris.

Corpus cavernosum penis One of the two parallel columns of erectile tissue forming the dorsal part of the penis.

Corpus ciliaris Ciliary body.

Corpus coccygeum Coccygeal body.

Corpus delicti *for* Body of evidence which denotes homicide.

Corpus geniculatum The medial and lateral geniculate body lying in the thalamus.

Corpus hemorrhagicum Corpus luteum containing a blood clot.

Corpus mamillare Mamillary body protruding into the interpeduncular fosssa from hypothalamus.

Corpus quadrigemina Quadrigeminal bodies.

Corpus spongiosum penis The medial column of erectile tissue located between and the ventral to the two corpora cavernosa of the penis.

Corpus ventriculi Body of the stomach.

Corpus vitreum Vitreous.

Corpus albicans A white fibrous tissue replacing the regressing corpus luteum in the ovary.

Corpus callosum An arched mass of white matter in the longitudinal fissure composed of nerve fibers interconnecting the cortical hemispheres.

Corpus luteum Small yellow endocrine body formed in the ovary at the site of ruptured ovarian follicle following ovulation.

Corpus luteum Small yellow endocrine body formed in the ovary at the site of ruptured ovarian follicle following ovulation.

Corpuscle (*kor'pus-el*) Any small mass; a blood cell; an encapsulated nerve ending. adj. **corpuscular**.

Blood corpuscle A red or white blood cell.

Corneal corpuscle Star-shaped connective tissue cell found between the laminae of fibrous tissue in the cornea.

Genital corpuscle An encapsulated sensory nerve ending found in the skin of external genitalia and nipple.

Ghost corpuscle Achromocyte.

Golgi-Mazzoni corpuscle An encapsulated sensory nerve ending in the skin of the finger tips.

Hassall's corpuscle Flat epithelial cells arranged around a granular nucleated cell found in the medulla of thymus.

Lamellated corpuscle Large encapsulated nerve ending found throughout the body. Also called pacinian corpuscle.

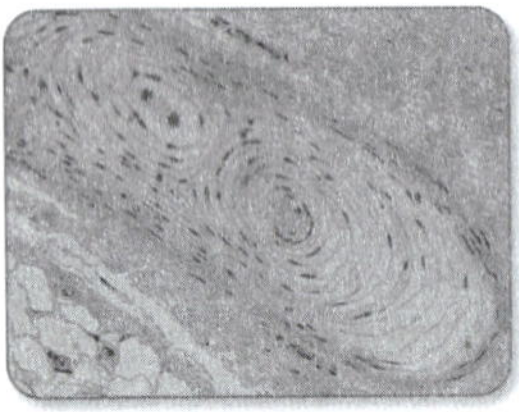

Pacinian corpuscle

Lymph corpuscle A lymphocyte.

Malpighian corpuscle Renal corpuscle.

Meissner's corpuscle Tactile corpuscle.

Red corpuscle Erythrocyte.

Ruffinis corpuscle Ovoid capsule with sensory nerve endings in subcutaenous tissues of the fingers.

White corpuscle Any type of leukocyte.

Corpus striatum A striate body consisting of caudate and lentiform nuclei in the cerebral hemisphere.

Correlation (*kore-la'shun*) A statistical index of the relationship between variables.

Cortex (*kor'teks*) Pl. **cortices**. The outer part of an organ as distinguished by inner medulla.

Adrenal cortex The outer larger part of the adrenal gland consisting of three zones: zona glomerulosa, zona fasciculata and zona reticularis, secreting corticosteroids and androgens.

Auditory cortex Auditory area in cerebral cortex.

Cerebellar cortex The thin layer of gray matter in the surface of cerebellum that contains Purkinje's cells.

Cerebral cortex The layer of gray matter covering the entire surface of cerebral hemisphere. There is a laminar organization of its cellular and fibrous components.

Motor cortex The region of cerebral cortex influencing the movements of the body.

Renal cortex The part of the kidney containing the glomeruli and the proximal and distal convoluted tubules.

Sensory cortex Cerebral cortex refelecting to somatic, sensory, auditory, visual and olfactory regions.

Corticosteroid (corticoid) (*kor'ti-ko-ster'oyd*) Any of the steroids produced by the adrenal cortex or any synthetic equivalents. They are classified into two major groups based on their biologic activity: Glucocorticoids involved in carbohydrate metabolism, increased gluconeogenesis and increased protein catabolism. It is also involved in immunomodulation and regulation of blood pressure, and mineralocorticoids concerned with the regulation of electrolyte and water balance used in hormone replacement therapy, as anti-inflammatory agents to suppress immune response and for suppression of ACTH secretion.

Corticosterone (*kor'ti-kos'te-ron*) A natural corticoid from the adrenal cortex that induces glycogen deposition in the liver, retention of sodium and excretion of potassium.

Corticotropin (*kor'ti-ko-tro'pin*) **corticotrophin** (*-tro'fin*) Adrenocorticotropic hormone secreted by the anterior pituitary gland having a stimulatory effect on adrenal cortex.

Cortisol (*kor'ti-sol*) Major glucocorticoid in humans whose levels are highest in the morning on waking and lowest in the middle of the night. The level increases during stress and illness. 95% is bound to protein (cortisol-binding globulin) and free fraction is biologically active and it acts through glucocorticoid receptors.

Cortisone (*kor'ti-son*) A natural glucocorticoid secreted by the adrenal cortex and also prepared synthetically. It becomes active on conversion to cortisol. It is used as an anti-inflammatory, and immunosuppressive agent and for adrenal replacement therapy.

Cor triloculare A rare congenital cardiac anomaly in which there is complete absence of interatrial septum and resultant single large atrial chamber with both pulmonary veins and superior vena cava draining into the common chamber.

Corynebacterium (*ko-ri'ne-bak-te're -um*) A genus of non-motile rod-shaped gram-positive bacteria belonging to the family of Corynebacteriaceae. The important species is *C. diphtheria* and it causes diphtheria.

Coryza (cold in the head) (*ko-ri'za*) An acute catarrhal inflammation of nasal mucous membrane with profuse nasal discharge; acute rhinitis.

Costal (*kos'tal*) Pertaining to a rib.

Costal cartilage Flexible cartilage that connects ribs to the sternum.

Costalgia (*kos-tal'je-a*) Pain in the costal muscles; also called pleurodynia.

Costive bone Having constipation.

Costochondritis Inflammation of costochondral junctions presenting with dull localized pain and tenderness over the costochondral junctions.

Cotrimoxazole (*Co'tri-moks'a-zol*) An antibiotic consisting of a mixture of trimethoprim and sulfamethoxazole (a sulfa drug), used especially to treat infections of the urinary tract and lungs (as in AIDS).

Cotyledon (*kot'i-le'don*) A subdivision of the uterine surface of the placenta.

Cotyloid (*kot'i-loyd*) Cup-shaped, relating to acetabulum.

Cough (*kawf*) A protective reflex mechanism induced reflexly or consciously to get rid of foreign material or accumulated secretions in the airways.

Hacking cough A short, frequent, shallow cough.

Pharyngeal cough Short and dry irritative cough accompanied by pain behind jaw or in the neck.

Productive cough Accompanied by expectoration of sputum.

Wet cough Productive cough.

Coumarin (*ku'ma-rin*) One of the natural or synthetic compounds containing dicumarol that inhibits hepatic synthesis of vitamin K-dependent coagulation factors.

Counterextension (*kown'ter-eks-ten's hun*) Traction in a proximal direction offering resistance to extension.

Counterirritant (*kown'ter-ir'i-tant*) An agent that causes irritation or inflammation of the skin to relieve symptoms of a deep-seated inflammatory process.

Countertraction (*kown'ter-trak'shun*) Traction opposed to another traction used in the reduction of fracture.

Cowper's glands (bulbourethral glands) Bulbourethral glands situated on either side of the membranous urethra, that secrete fluid into the urethra during sexual stimulus, named after William Cowper, English surgeon.

Cowpox (*kow'poks*) A mild eruptive skin disease caused by vaccinia virus, affects the udder and teats of cows and may be transmitted to man by inoculation and contact.

COX 2 Cyclooxygenase-2.

Coxa (*kok'sa*) The part of the body lateral to and including the hip joint.

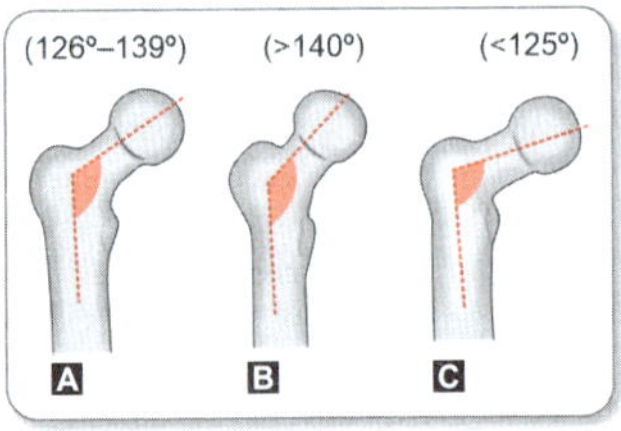

A. Normal, B. Coxa valga and C. Coxa vara

Coxiella (*kok'se-el'la*) A genus of bacteria of the order Rickettsiales, named after Herald Cox, US bacteriologist; *C. burnetii* is responsible for Q fever.

Coxsackievirus (*kok-sake-virus*) A family of picornaviruses named after a city in New York State, which may produce herpangina, aseptic meningitis, epidemic pleurodynia, acute non-specific pericarditis and myocarditis.

Crab louse Pubic louse.

Cradle (*kra'dl*) A light weight frame placed over part of bed for protection of injured parts, or for application of heat or cold.

Cradle cap Thick yellow scales occurring in patches over the scalp in infants.

Cramp (*kramp*) A painful spasmodic muscular contraction, often noted during or after exercise.

Crani- (cranio-) Combining word for skull.

Cranial nerves Set of 12 paired nerves emerging from the brain that innervate the head, neck, thorax and abdomen.

Craniomalacia (*-ma-la' she-a*) Markedly soft bones of the skull.

Craniopagus (dicephalus) twins Conjoined twins who are fused at the cranim.

Craniopharyngioma (*kra'ne-o-fa-rin'je-o'ma*) A tumor arising from cell rests derived from the hypophyseal stalk or Rathke's pouch. There is raised intracranial tension and calcium deposits.

Cranioschisis (*kra'ne-os'ki-sis*) Congenital malformation with incomplete closure of the cranium.

Craniostenosis (*-ste-no'sis*) Deformity of the skull caused by premature closure of the cranial sutures.

Craniotomy (*kra'ne-ot'o-me*) Any operation on the cranium; an operative procedure to decrease the size of the head of a dead fetus to facilitate delivery.

Cranium (*kra'ne-um*) The skeleton of head that includes all the bones of the head except mandible, and it acts as a vault to contain brain.

Creatinase (creatine kinase) (ck) An enzyme that catalyzes the phosphorylation of creatine by ATP to form phosphocreatine. It occurs in three isozymes specific to brain (CK-BB), cardiac muscle (CK-MB) and skeletal muscle (CK-MM).

Creatine (*kre'a-tin*) An amino acid occurring in vertebrate tissues.

Creatinine (*kre-at'i-nin*) The final product of creatine catabolism.

Creatinuria (*kre-a-tin-nu're-a*) Excretion of increased amount of creatine in urine.

Creatorrhea (*kre-a-to-re'a*) Presence of muscle fibers in the stools in chronic pancreatitis, demonstrable by microscopy.

Crede's method (*kra-daz*) A technique to expel placenta wherein downward pressure is applied on the uterus through the abdominal wall. Such a technique is also adapted to empty a flaccid bladder, named after Karl Crede, German gynecologist.

Creeping eruption (larva migrans) A skin infection caused by hook-worms and is characterized by severe itching, blisters, redness and rash.

Crenation (*kren-a'shun*) Abnormal notching in the edge of an erythrocyte.

Crepitation (rale) (*krep'i-ta'shun*) Crackles; the discontinuous explosive sounds heard in either phases of respiratory cycle, may be fine or coarse.

Coarse crepitation Low pitched, loud adventitious sounds appear bubbling in bronchiectasis.

Fine crepitation Crackles, sounds simulated by rubbing of a lock of hair between the thumb and finger near ear. They may be heard either in early (widespread airflow obstruction) or late (restrictive lung diseases) inspiration and also during expiration.

Post-tussive crepitation A deep inspiration after coughing, often heard over minimal lesions of tuberculosis or cavities.

Crepitus (*krep'i-tus*) A grating sensation felt by hand kept on knee joint when it is moved passively as in osteoarthropathy; a crackling sensation felt on palpation of the skin in subcutaneous emphysema or in gas gangrene.

Cresol (*kre'sol*) Yellow-brown liquid from coal tar, used as a disinfectant.

Crest (*krest*) A ridge, or an elongated prominence especially on a bone.

Cretinism (*kret'in-izm*) A congenital condition due to lack of thyroid hormone causing arrest of physical and mental development.

Endemic cretinism Nervous cretinism noted in Himalayas. Intellectual functions are impaired and there is hearing defect.

Myxedematous cretinism A sporadic type of cretinism.

Sporadic cretinism Occurs from dysgenesis of thyroid gland, inadequate hormone synthesis due to enzyme defect and damaged gland.

Crib death (cot death, sudden infant death syndrome) Sudden infant death syndrome.

Cribriform (*krib'ri-form*) Containing multiple perforations; sieve-like histological pattern, in which sheets of epithelial cells are punctuated by gland-like space.

Cricoid cartilage Signet ring-shaped lowermost cartilage of the larynx.

Cri du chat syndrome A chromosomal disorder wherein a piece of chromosomal material is missing from a particular region of chromosome 5 and presents with unusual facial features, hypotonia, microcephaly, mental retardation and cat-like cry; chromosome-5 deletion syndrome, cat cry syndrome.

Crigler-Najjar jaundice A recessive defect of bilirubin conjugating enzyme in the liver leading to unconjugated hyperbilirubinemia.

Crinophagy (*krin-of'a-je*) Elimination of excess granules by lysosomes.

Crisis (*kris'sis*) Any acute exacerbation of a clinical condition.

Addisonian crisis Acute adrenocortical insufficiency.

Dietl's crisis Paroxymal attacks of lumbar and abdominal pain due to kinking of ureter in persons with wandering kidney.

Identity crisis A disorientation concerning one's sense of self and role in society, occurring acutely.

Sickle cell crisis Recurrent acute symptoms in patients with sickle cell anemia due to vascular occlusion or hemolysis.

Thyrotoxic crisis Thyroid storm, aggravation of symptoms of thyrotoxicosis following surgery, shock or thyroidectomy.

Crohn's disease Regional ileitis; common sites of involvement are terminal ileum, right side of colon; entire wall of bowel is edematous and thickened; deep ulcers occur like linear fissures and are patchy. Presents with bloody diarrhea, passage of mucus and constitutional symptoms, named after B Crohn, US physician.

Cromolyn (*kro'mol-in*) A kellin compound that acts on tissue mast cell and stabilizes its cell membrane and prevents its degranulation, thus of release of histamine and other tissue mediators involved in asthmatic attack. It is used as a prophylactic.

Crossbite (*kros'bit*) An abnormal relation of one or more teeth of upper and lower jaw due to deviation of teeth or to abnormal position of jaw.

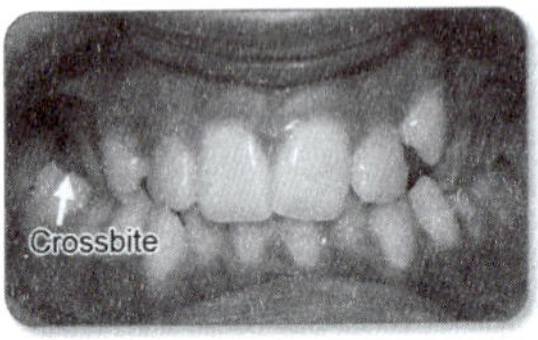

Crossbite

Crossing-over (*kros'ing o'ver*) Exchange of lengths of DNA between members of each chromosome pair during prophase of first meiotic division.

Crotamiton (*krot'a-mi'ton*) A light yellow oily liquid useful in scabies.

Croup (*kroop*) Laryngotracheobronchitis in infants and young children by para-influenza virus.

Crown (*krown*) Corona; the part of teeth covered with enamel.

Crowning (*krown'ing*) First sight of vertex at vulva during labor.

Crude rate Simple enumeration of cases, death, etc. in a population without making any adjustment for nature of population.

Crural (*kroor'al*) Relating to the thigh or leg.

Crus (*krus*) The leg, the part between the knees and the ankle; any structure resembling a leg, as elongated masses or a pair of diverging bands.

Cryanesthesia A technique wherein peripheral nerves are destroyed by extreme cold to achieve pain relief.

Cryesthesia (*-es-the'zhah*) Subjective sensation of cold; sensitivity to cold.

Cryobank (*kri'o-bank*) A place for storage of biological tissues at very low temperatures.

Cryoglobulin (*-glob'u-lin*) Precipitation of plasma protein especially IgM-IgG complex when cold.

Cryoprecipitate (*-pre-sip'i-tat*) A soluble material from plasma getting precipitated on cooling, and the material is rich in factor VIII.

Cryoprobe (*kri-o-prob*) An extremely cold instrument used in cryosurgery.

Cryostat (*kri'o-stat*) Refrigerator working at temperatures below freezing.

Cryosurgery (*kri'o-ser'jer-e*) Treatment by local freezing.

Crypt (*kript*) A pit-like depression; a recess in tubule.

Crypt of Lieberkuhn A tubular gland of intestine concerned with secretion of intestinal juice.

Tonsillar crypt A deep invagination of the stratified epithelium and substances of tonsils.

Crypt- (crypto-) Combining word for concealed; crypt.

Cryptococcosis (torulosis) (*krip"to-ko-ko'sis*) A pulmonary or disseminated infection acquired by inhalation of soil contaminated with the encapsulated yeasts *Cryptococcus neoformans* or *C. gattii*. Symptoms are those of pneumonia, meningitis, or involvement of skin, bones, or viscera; it is characterized by granulomatous lesion of the lung, bones, brain and meninges. Immunocompromised persons are at special risk. Amphotericin B and flucytosine are useful in the management.

Cryptococcus (*-kok'us*) A genus of yeast-like fungi that reproduces by budding: *C. neoformans* is a ovoid and thick-walled. It contains a mucinous capsule with large amounts of polysaccharide demonstrable by India ink.

Cryptomenorrhea (*krip'to-men'ore-a*) Absence of menstrual flow.

Cryptophthalmos (*krip'tof-thal'mos*) Congenital absence of eyelids.

Cryptorchidism (cryptorchism) (*krip-tor'ki-dizm*) The absence of at least one testicle from the scrotum.

CSF 1 Colony-stimulating factor 1.

CS gas 2-chlorobenzalmalononitrile, a cyanocarbon, is a tear gas used to control riots.

CT scanner Computed tomography scan is an imaging that uses X-rays to create detailed images of the body.

Cubital (*ku'bi-tal*) Relating to the elbow or to the ulna.

Cuboid bone One of the 7 tarsal bones of the foot.

Culdoscope An instrument, used to visualize female pelvic organs and is introduced through the vagina.

Culex (*ku'leks*) A genus of mosquitoes belonging to the family of Culicidae which transmit diseases to man.

Culicide (*ku'li-sid*) An agent that destroys mosquitoes.

Culture (*kul'cher*) Growth of microorganisms on or in a media; a mass of microorganisms on or in a medium.

Cuneiform bones Wedge shaped bones.

Cuneus (*ku'ne-us*) Pl. **cunei**. Region of the medial aspect of the occipital lobe on either side of cerebral hemisphere bounded by parieto-occipital and calcarine fissures.

Cuniculus (*ku-nik'u-lus*) A burrow of itch mite in the epidermis.

Cupola (*ku'pa-la*) Cupula.

Cupping (*kup'ing*) Occurrence of a cup-shaped excavation; application of cupping glass.

Cupula (*ku'pu-la*) A dome-like structure closing ampulla of semicircular canals.

Curare (*ku-ra're*) An extract of *Strychnos toxifera* that produces paralysis of skeletal muscles by blocking transmission at the myoneural junctions.

Curet (*ku-ret*) A spoon-shaped surgical instrument for the removal of tissue from the walls of body cavities.

Curettage (curettement) (*ku're-taz*) Scraping, usually of the interior of a cavity or tract to obtain material for tissue diagnosis and to remove abnormally looking tissues.

Curie (*ku're*) Radioactivity unit, named after Pierre and Marie Curie, French scientists.

Curschmann's spirals (*kursh'manz*) Twisted strips of cell debris in the sputum of asthmatic patients, named after G Curschmann, German physician.

Cushing's syndrome A syndrome caused by pituitary-dependent bilateral adrenal hyperplasia, ectopic ACTH production, iatrogenic (ACTH and glucocorticoid therapy), adrenal adenoma, and adrenal carcinoma characterized by moon face, psychosis, acne, plethora, centripetal obesity, hypertension, striae, osteoporosis, bruising, hyperglycemia, peptic ulcer, menstrual disturbances, tendency to infection and poor wound healing.

Cusp (*kusp*) A leaflet of one of the heart's valves; a conical elevation arising on the surface of a tooth.

Cutaneous (*ku-ta'ne-us*) Pertaining to the skin.

Cuticle (*ko'ti-k'l*) Epidermis; an outer thin layer.

Cutis (*ku'tis*) Skin; protective covering of the body consisting of epidermis and dermis.

Cyanide (*si'a-nid*) A chemical compound that contains a C≡N functional group, that can kill people.

Cyanocobalamin (*-ko-bal'a-min*) Vitamin B_{12}, a complex of cyanide and cobalamin, used in the treatment of pernicious anemia.

Cyanopsia (*si'a-nop'se-a*) A condition where all objects appear blue; it may be temporarily seen following cataract extraction.

Cyanosis (*si'a-no'sis*) Bluish discoloration of the skin and mucous membranes due to presence of excess amounts of reduced hemoglobin in the arterial blood. Cyanosis becomes visible when the amount of reduced hemoglobin exceeds 5 g/dL.

Central cyanosis Occurs due to mixing of arterial and venous blood at the level of heart or great vessels and to defective oxygenation in the lungs. The central parts such as tongue and peripheral parts such as nail beds, tip of the nose, finger and toes are cyanosed. The extremities are warm.

Differential cyanosis Occurrence of Eisenmenger's reaction in a patent ductus arteriosus, causes cyanosis in the lower limbs with sparing of upper limbs.

Peripheral cyanosis Extremities such as tips of the fingers and toes, nail bed and tip of the nose are cyanosed. It is caused by excess extraction of oxygen by the tissues from capillaries, which is secondary to impaired circulatory state either due to reduction in cardiac output or vasospasm. The extremities are cold to feel.

Regional cyanosis Noted in Raynaud's disease, arterial occlusion and thrombophlebitis.

Cybernetics (*si'ber-net'iks*) A comparative study of computers and nervous system; the science of control and communication.

Cyclitis (*si-klit'is*) Inflammation of ciliary body.

Cyclizine (*si'kli-zin*) Antihistamine with sedative effect chiefly used in motion sickness.

Cyclobenzaprine (*si''klo-ben'za-pren*) A centrally acting skeletal muscle relaxant structurally related to tricyclic antidepressants.

Cyclodialysis (*si'klo-di-al'i-sis*) Creation of a communication between the anterior chamber and suprachoroidal space to decrease intraocular tension in glaucoma.

Cyclomethycaine A local anesthetic.

Cyclopentolate Used to dilate the pupil while eye examination.

Cyclophoria (*si'klo-for'e-a*) Tendency of the eyes to rotate around their anteroposterior axis due to weakness of oblique muscles.

Cyclophosphamide (*si'klo-fos'fa-mi-de*) Alkylating cytotoxic agent.

Cycloplegia (*si'klo-ple'je-a*) Paralysis of ciliary muscle and accommodation.

Cyclopropane (*si'klo-pro'pan*) A highly flammable, explosive, colorless gas that was once in wide use as an anesthetic but has been mostly replaced by less flammable gases.

Cycloserine (*si'klo-se'ren*) A weak bacteriostatic antituberculosis agent that acts by inhibiting the D-alanine enzymes leading to defective cell wall synthesis.

Cyclosporine (*si'klo-spor'en*) An agent obtained from a soil fungus used to suppress the rejection of allografts.

Cyclothymia (*si'klo-thi'me-a*) Alternating between maniac and depressive maniac and depressive phase.

Cyclotron (*si'klo-tron*) An apparatus for accelerating protons or deuterons or high energies. It is done by rotation between magnets.

Cyesis (*si-e'sis*) Pregnancy.

Cyproheptadine Powerful antagonist of histamine and 5-hydroxytryptamine.

Cyproterone An antiandrogen. It suppresses the action of testosterone on tissues.

Cyrtometer (*sir-tom'e-ter*) An instrument to measure curved surfaces of the body.

Cyst (*sist*) A swelling containing fluid or semisolid material, which is lined by epithelium, endothelium or granulation tissue. It may be true or false; stage in the life cycle of some parasites during which they are enveloped in a protective wall.

Congenital cyst May arise from the fetal remnants of buried epithelium along the lines of fusion (sequestration dermoid) or from collection of fluid in an ectodermal tube (tubuloembryonic or tubulodermoid) or from remnants of embryonic tubules and ducts.

Cyst lens A transparent device that fits over the cornea or part of the cornea to bring change in refractive ability of the cornea or lens of the eye.

Degenerative cyst A false cyst occurring due to collection of fluid in the center of a degenerating tumor from hemorrhage or necrosis.

Distension cyst Cyst occurring from dilatation of acini as in thyroid gland or from distension of the follicles as in ovary.

Dental cyst Occurs in connection with a carious tooth, epithelial in origin and produces an elevation of the alveolus especially in the upper jaw and contains sterile, clear fluid with cholesterol crystals.

Exudation cyst Cyst occurring due to exudation of fluid in a normal anatomical space which is lined by endothelium as in hydrocele of tunica vaginalis, or a false cyst due to encysted collection of exudate.

False cyst Pseudocyst devoid of an epithelial lining which usually contains exudative or degenerative fluid as in pseudocyst of pancreas, or cystic degeneration of the tumor.

Ganglionic cyst A localized round cystic swelling occurring in relation to a tendon sheath or a joint capsule, contains gelatinous fluid under tension.

Hemorrhagic cyst A cyst resulting from a resolving hematoma of muscle and is lined by endothelium, contains straw-colored fluid.

Infestation cyst Cyst occurring in any organ of the body but commonly in liver as hydatid cyst.

Mesenteric cyst A spherical smooth, soft or firm swelling along the course of the mesentery.

Neoplastic cyst Benign or malignant cystadenoma of ovary or cystic teratoma of ovary and testis.

Parasite cyst Infestation cyst.

Retention cyst Cyst occurring due to accumulation of secretion common in the scalp, face and scrotum.

Sebaceous cyst An epidermal cyst containing desquamated cells due to obstruction of duct of the sebaceous gland. The obstructed opening is seen as a blue spot (punctum) which is fixed to the skin.

True cyst A cyst usually lined by epithelium, endothelium or granulation tissues, containing fluid that may be watery, serous, mucus, blood stained or seropurulent.

Thyroglossal cyst An elongated swelling along the course of the thyroglossal tract in the upper neck that moves up on protrusion of the tongue.

Urachal cyst An immobile swelling of variable size in the hypogastrium deep to the abdominal muscles developing from the persistence of middle segment of urachus (remnant of allantois extending from the urinary bladder to the umbilicus).

Cyst- (cysto-) Combining word for cyst, sac, bladder.

Cystadenoma (*sis-tad'e-no-ma*) A benign tumor derived from glandular epithelium, containing cystic accumulations of retained secretions.

Cystalgia (*sis-tal-jea*) Pain in the bladder.

Cystectomy (*sis-tek'to-me*) Removal of cyst or bladder.

Cysteine (*sis'te-en*) Sulfur-containing amino acid derived from methionine in the body.

Cystic (*sis'tik*) Relating to a cyst; containing cysts; relating to bladder.

Cystic fibrosis CF, an autosomal recessive genetic disease characterized by a defect in electrolyte transport in the airway lumen and an increase in reabsorption of sodium from the airway lumen leading to a decrease in water content and an increase in viscosity of airway secretions. It is responsible for thick and poorly cleared inspissated airway secretion, impaired mucociliary clearance, chronic bacterial infections, bronchiectasis, and progressive respiratory failure. Lung is predominantly involved and there is also involvement of epithelial tissues of pancreas, sweat duct and gastrointestinal tract.

Cystic hygroma The only brilliantly translucent swelling of the neck, a lymph cyst occurring in early childhood, that can be reduced in size by steady pressure.

Cystic duct A tube that carries bile from the gallbladder.

Cysticercosis (*sis'ti-ser-ko'sis*) Disease caused by encystment of cysticercus larvae of *Taenia solium* in the subcutaneous tissue, skeletal muscles and brain. They present with pea-like ovoid bodies under the skin or epileptic fits. Praziquantel and albendazole are used in the treatment.

Cysticercus (bladderworm) (*sis'ti-ser'kus*) Larval form of *Taenia solium*.

Cystic fibrosis Fibrocystic disease of the pancreas, mucoviscidosis

Cystine (*sis'ten*) An oxidation product of cysteine.

Cystinosis (*sis'ti-no'sis*) A hereditary disorder of early childhood characterized by deposits of cystine crystals throughout the body due to abnormality in the metabolism of cysteine. It is accompanied by aminoaciduria, glycosuria, polyuria and vitamin D-resistant rickets.

Cystinuria (*sis'ti-nu're-a*) A defect in renal tubular function associated with excess excretion of cystine in the urine.

Cystitis (*sis-tit'is*) Inflammation of the bladder.

Cystotomy (*sis-tit'o-me*) Surgical incision of a cavity; incision into the lens capsule.

Cystocele (*sis'to-sel*) Herniation of urinary bladder into the vagina.

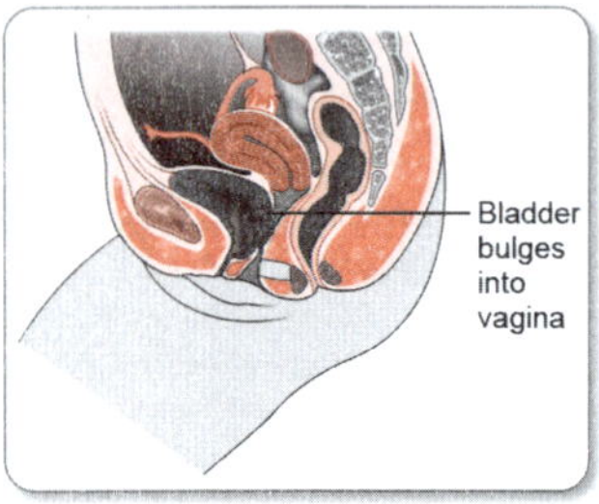

Cystocele

Cystography (*sis-tog'ra-fe*) Radiography of the bladder after injection of a radiopaque substance.

Cystolithiasis (*sis'to-li-thi'a-sis*) Presence of a vesical calculus.

Cystometer (*sis-tom'e-ter*) A device useful in the study of bladder function such as its capacity, intravesical pressure and residual urine.

Cystopexy (vesicofixation) (*sis'to-pek'se*) Surgical attachment of gallbladder or of urinary bladder to the abdominal wall or other supporting structures.

Cystoplasty (*sis'to-plas'te*) Surgical repair of a defect in the urinary bladder.

Cystosarcoma (*sis-to-sar-ko'ma*) A sarcoma containing cysts or cyst-like foci.

Cystoscopy (*sis-tos'ko-pe*) Endoscopy of the urinary bladder *via* the urethra.

Cystostomy (*sis-tos'to-me*) Suprapubic drainage of bladder, by farming a surgical opening into the urinary bladder.

Cystotomy (*sis-to'to-me*) A surgical incision into the urinary bladder.

Cytarabine (*si-tar'ah-ben*) An antimetabolite inhibiting DNA synthesis.

Cytidine (*si'ti-den*) A purine nucleoside consisting of cytosine and ribose, a constituent of RNA.

Cytochemistry (*si'to-kem'is-tre*) Study of intracellular distribution of chemical compounds and their activities.

Cytochrome (*si'to-krom*) A class of hemoprotein found in the mitochondria that transport electron and/or hydrogen.

Cytochrome oxidase An enzyme complex containing cytochrome and copper found in the mitochondria.

Cytogenetics (*-je-net'iks*) The branch of genetics concerned with the structure and function of the cells, with special reference to the chromosomes.

Cytokinesis (*si'to-ki-ne'sis*) Changes that occur in the the protoplasm of a cell during cell division.

Cytology (*si-tol'o-je*) The study of a cell.

Exfoliative cytology Examination for diagnosis, of the cells denuded from a lesion and recovered from the sediment of exudate, secretions or washings from the tissue.

Cytolysis (*si-tol'i-sis*) Dissolution of a cell.

Cytomegalovirus (CMV) (*sit'o-meg'a-lo-vi'rus*) (CMV) A herpes virus that inhabits salivary glands, causes characteristic giant cells with large intranuclear inclusion. It is transmitted from mother with a latent infection to her fetus either transplacentally or at the time of birth, or by blood transfusion.

CMV infection CMV infection may be congenital (hepatosplenomegaly, encephalitis, mental retardation) or acquired in immunocompetent (asymptomatic, mononucleosis-like illness) in immunosuppressed (retinitis, pneumonia, enteritis) individuals.

Cytometer (*si-tom'e-ter*) An instrument for counting and measuring cells.

Cytomorphosis (*si'to-mor-fo'sis*) The changes in form of a cell as it develops.

Cytopenia (*si'to-pe'ne-a*) Decrease in the number of cellular elements in the blood.

Cytophotometry Used for cell counting, sorting, characterization along with microorganism or biomarker detection.

Cytoplasm (*sit'o-plazm*) The protoplasm of a cell.

Cytoplasmic inheritance Inheritance of organelle DNA in the offspring from the parent's DNA.

Cytosine (*si'to-sen*) A pyrimidine base condensed with ribose or deoxyribose to form the nucleosides, cystidine and doxycystidine in the nucleic acids.

Cytosome (*si'to-som*) The cell body exclusive of its nucleus.

Cytotoxic drug Inhibits cell division and in this way cause cancer cells to die.

Cytotrophoblast (*si'to-trof'o-blast*) The inner layer of the trophoblast.

D

Dabigatran (*de-big'e-tran*) New class of antithrombotic drug known as direct thrombin inhibitors, used to prevent clots.

Dacarbazine (*da-kahr'ba-zen*) An antineoplastic agent used to treat malignant melanoma and Hodgkin's disease.

Daclizumab (*da-kliz'u-mab*) A monoclonal anti-CD25 antibody that blocks the interleukin-2 receptor which is used to treat relapsing forms of multiple sclerosis.

Dacryoadenitis (*dak-re-o-ad-e-ni-tis*) Inflammation of the lacrimal gland.

Dacryocystitis (*dak're-o-sis'ti'tis*) Inflammation of the lacrimal sac caused by obstruction of the nasolacrimal duct. It is associated with excessive tears, redness and swelling in the area of lacrimal sac. It requires hot compresses, antibiotic therapy and incision and drainage of the sac.

Dacryocystorhinostomy (*dak're-o-sis'to -ri-nos'to-me*) Creation of a fistula between lacrimal sac and nasal cavity for lacrimal duct obstruction.

Dacryocystocele (*dak're-o-sis'to-sele*) Benign cyst or mass formation due to obstruction in nasolacrimal gland.

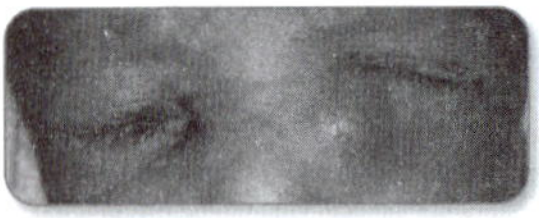

Dacryocystocele

Dacryocystotomy (*dak're-o-sis-tot'o-me*) Incision of the lacrimal sac.

Dacryops (*dak-re-ops*) A watery state of the eye.

Dactinomycin (*dak"ti-no-mi'sin*) An actinomycin used to treat various cancers.

Dactyl- (*dak'til*) A digit, a finger or toe.

Dactylitis (*dak'til-itis*) Inflammation of a digit.

Tuberculous dactylitis Commonly involves metacarpals or phalanges and bone which are enlarged as fusiform swelling due to thickened and raised periosteum and there is destruction of original bone.

Syphilitic dactylitis There is infiltration of the bones of hands or foot with syphilitic granulation tissue which may undergo central necrosis.

Dactylology (*dak"ti-lol'a-je*) Hand and finger movements for communication.

Dagger sign Ossification of the posterior longitudinal ligament with spinal cord compression due to a dense vertical ossified plaque at the posterior margin of the vertebral body and intervertebral discs, noted in cervical spine or upper thoracic spines.

Dale's reaction An *in vitro* test for anaphylactic sensitization in a guinea pig named after Sir Henry Dale, British physiologist.

Dallas criteria Standards for the diagnosis of myocarditis from endomyocardial biopsy. Subdivided as no myocarditis, borderline myocarditis or lymphocytic myocarditis established by a group of cardiac pathologists in Dallas.

Darier's disease (*dar-e-az*) A rare hereditary disorder characterized by wart-like blemishes on the body that coalesce into plaques and are found on the scalp, face, neck, trunk and axillae, named after J Darier, French dermatologist.

Darling's disease Histoplasmosis named after Samuel Darling, Panama physician.

DASH Dietary approaches to Stop Hypertension, a low-fat, low-cholesterol diet plan with a low sodium-content, that lowers blood pressure.

Deltonism Color blindness.

D and C Dilatation and curettage, dilatation of the uterine cervix and scrapping of the endometrium of uterus with a curette.

Dandruff (scurf) (*dan'druf*) An excess amount of scaly material composed of dead keratinized epithelium shed from scalp.

Dapsone (*dap'son*) 4, 4-diammodiphenyl sulfone (DDS) compound used in treatment of leprosy and dermatitis herpetiform.

Dark adaptation The time required for the retina to get adapted to low illumination alter exposure to bright light.

Day blindness Hemeralopia, inability to see clearly in a bright light.

Davis gag Clamp to hold mouth wide open especially for tonsillectomy.

DDT (chlorophenothane, dicophane) Dichloro-diphenyl-trichloroethane, a highly hepatotoxic and potentially neurotoxic insecticide. It is effective against a wide variety of insects such as flea, fly, louse, mosquito, bedbug and cockroach.

Dead space Non air exchanging space of the portion of a syringe's tip and needle that contains medication that cannot be administered.

Alveolar dead space Noted in ventilation and perfusion imbalance wherein there is ventilation of alveoli which are not perfused or inadequately perfused with blood or hyperventilation of alveoli with normal perfusion resulting in diminished volume of air available for gas exchange.

Anatomical dead space The air in the conducting system from nose to the bronchioles that does not participate in the gas exchange and considered wasted ventilation.

Physiologic dead space The tidal volume which does not participate in gas exchange. It includes anatomical and alveolar dead spaces.

Deafness (*def'nes*) Loss of sense of hearing either completely or partially.

Deamination (*de-am'i-na'shun*) Removal of the amino group.

Death (*deth*) The cessation of life. A person is dead if there is irreversible cessation of circulatory and respiratory functions or irreversible cessation of all functions of brain, including the brain stem.

Black death Bubonic plague.

Brain death Irreversible brain damage with unresponsiveness to all stimuli, absence of all spontaneous muscle activity.

Cot death, crib death Sudden infant death syndrome.

Death certificate Certificate giving the immediate cause of death and the underlying cause of death which initiated the train of morbid events leading directly to death. It also contains record of any significant associated diseases.

Death rate The number of deaths per 1000 population per year in a given community. Indicative of the rate at which people are dying.

Death rattle A sound characteristic of end-stage lung disease, wherein the clearance of large airway secretions becomes impossible.

Death star A pattern of the round aggregates of malignant cells obtained from fine needle aspiration biopsies from breast cancer and it implies poor prognosis.

Death trance *For* Obvious absence of apparent signs of life which cannot be determined by ordinary clinical tests due to suspended state of activity of heart, lungs, brain, etc., associated with a state of insensibility or loss of voluntary power; suspended animation.

Neonatal death The death of a liveborn infant during the period that commences at birth and ends 28 completed days after birth.

Perinatal death The death of a fetus weighing at least 500 g or the death of an infant during the first week of life.

Debt (*det*) Deficit.

Oxygen debt Oxygen requirement following a strenuous exercise to oxidize the excess LICGC acid and to replenish depleted stores of ATP.

Debridement (*da-bred-men't*) Surgical removal of foreign material and/or devitalized, infected taste and all foreign materials from a wound surface or burn. It facilitates exposure of healthy tissue and prompts healing process.

Debrisoquine Antihypertensive drug similar to quanethidine.

Decadron Corticosteroid similar to a natural hormone produced by the adrenal glands; used to treat disorders of skin, arthritis, blood, kidney, eyes and intestine.

Decalcification (*de'kal-si-fi-ka'shun*) Loss of calcium salts from bones or teeth.

Decannulation (*de-kan'nu-la'shun*) The removal of a cannula.

Decapitation (*de-kap'i-ta'shun*) The separation of the head from the body; beheading; separation of the head from the shaft of the bone.

Decapsulation (*de-kap"su-la'shun*) Removing the capsule or protective layer.

Decay (*de-ka'*) Decomposition of organic matter; radioactive disintegration of an atom.

Decerebration (*de-ser-e-bra'shun*) Removal of a portion of the brain.

Decibel (DB) (*des'i-bel*) A unit to measure the ratio of two powers such as electric or acoustic powers equal to one-tenth of a bel, db, dB.

Decidua (*de-sid'u-a*) The endometrium of the uterus which undergoes modification preparing for and during pregnancy and it gets cast off at the time of parturition or during menstruation.

Decidua basalis The layer immediately external to the embryo constituting the maternal vascular socket.

Decidua capsularis The layer that covers the endometrium around the remainder of non basalis portion of embryonic sac.

Decidua parietalis That portion of the decidua seen at the fallopian tube junction with the endometrium.

Deciduoma (*de-sid'u-o'ma*) A uterine tumor containing decidual tissue.

Deciduous teeth Primary dentition which is replaced by permanent teeth.

Declive (*de-kliv'*) A slanting surface.

Decomposition (*de-kom-po-zish'un*) Decay, putrefactive process; reducing a compound to its simpler constituents with decompression technique to readjust an individual to normal atmospheric pressure after exposure to high pressures.

Decomposition laminectomy Removal of spine and laminae on either side so as to allow the spinal cord to move backward.

Decomposition sickness A painful, sometimes fatal, disorder that results from formation of gas bubbles in body tissues; this is especially noticed when a diver ascends too rapidly to the surface.

Decompression (*de"kom-presh'un*) A reduction in pressure around someone or something.

Decompression sickness Occurs when rapid pressure reduction (like in a dive) causes gas previously dissolved in blood or tissues to form bubbles in blood vessels. Symptoms include pain, neurologic symptoms or both.

Decongestant (*de-kon-jes'tant*) An agent that relieves congestion or swelling.

Decortication (*de-kor'tika'shun*) Removal of the cortical substance.

Pulmonary decortication Removal of the thickened pleura.

Renal decortication Removal of renal capsule.

Decubitus (*de-ku'bi-tus*) Lying down, recumbent or horizontal position.

Decubitus ulcer A pressure sore resulting from ulceration of the skin occurring in persons confined to bed for a long period of time.

Decussation A crossing of structures in the form of an X.

Defecation (*def-e-ka'shun*) The elimination of feces through the anus.

Defecation syncope Syncope occurring during or immediately after defecation.

Defecography (*def'a-kog'ra-fe*) A fluoroscopic technique to evaluate pelvic floor prolapse.

Defense mechanism An unconscious psychological operation used by the ego, to decrease internal stress, ultimately.

Deferent (*def'er-ent*) Conveying something away from or downward.

Deferoxamine Chelating agent used to remove excess iron.

Defervescence (*def'er-ves'ins*) Bodily defenses begin to take an upper hand over the infecting agent and the patient begins to feel better. It marks the subsidence of fever.

Defibrillation (*de-fib'ril-a'shun*) Giving a brief electric shock to the heart to reverse some types of irregularities in the rhythm.

Defibrination (*de-fi'bri-na'shun*) The removal of fibrin from the blood.

Defibrination syndrome Persistent bleeding as the blood fails to clot. It may be associated with circulatory collapse and it requires restoration of fibrinogen level to a safe level.

Deficiency (*de-fish'en-se*) A shortage; lack.

Deficiency disease Any clinical condition that results from the inadequate availability of an essential nutrient such as proteins, vitamins or minerals.

Deflorescence Disappearance of an eruption of the skin.

Degeneration (*de-jen'er-a'shun*) Deterioration or an impairment of an organ or part of the body.

Deglutition (*de'glu-tish'un*) The act of swallowing.

Dehiscence (*de-his'ens*) Rupture of a wound closure, separation of a surgical incision.

Dehumidifier (*de'hu-mid'i-fi'er*) A device for removing moisture from air.

Dehydration (*de'hi-dra'shun*) A dangerous fall in water content of body or tissues.

Dehydration fever Raised temperature in a neonate due to inadequate fluid intake especially at high ambient temperature.

Dehydrogenase (*de-hi-droj'e-nas*) An enzyme that catalyzes the oxidation of a specific substance.

Déjà vu Illusion of visual recognition in which a new situation is incorrectly considered a repetition of a previous event.

Dejan syndrome Pain and anesthesia in cheek, exophthalmos and diplopia indicating a lesion of the floor of orbit, named after M.C. Dejans, French ophthalmologist.

Dejerine sign (*de'zher-en*) Nerve root pain that increases on coughing named after Joseph Dejerine, French neurologist.

Delta sign A filling defect in cerebral venous sinus thrombosis seen by CT.

Delta wave The slowest of the four brain waves; *ECG* a slow upstroke of the QRS wave in a background of short PR interval in ECG of WPW syndrome.

Deletion (deficiency) (*de-le'shun*) Loss of genetic material from a single base for RNA or base pair for DNA to a large piece of chromosome.

Deletion syndromes Hereditary disease complexes due to the loss of major chromosome segments.

Delhi boil Oriental sore infestation by *Leishmania tropica* results in an indurated papule on face or hand which breaks down to form an indolent ulcer and on healing an ugly pigmented scar.

Delirium (*de-lir'e-um*) A delirious state due to physical illness.

Puerperal delirium The mental manifestation of a severe toxic infection such as puerperal sepsis. It is characterized by confusion, drowsiness alternating with excitement and visual illusions and hallucinations.

Delirium tremens A state of confusion accompanied by trembling and hallucinations noted in chronic alcoholics when they abstain drinking.

Delivery (*de-liv'er-e*) Childbirth; making available of health services to those who need it.

Abdominal delivery Delivery of an infant through an incision made into intact uterus through abdominal wall.

Breech delivery Delivery of an infant in breech presentation.

Forceps delivery Extraction of a child from maternal passages by application of forceps to the child's head.

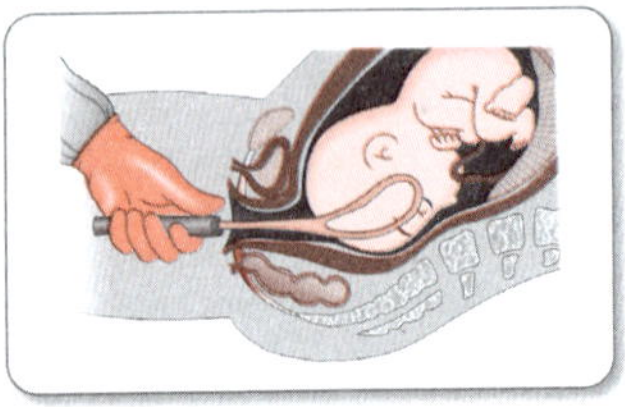

Forceps delivery

Postmature delivery Delivery of a postmature infant.

Postmortem delivery Birth of a child after death of the mother.

Premature delivery Birth of a premature infant.

Spontaneous delivery Birth of an infant without any aid.

Vaginal delivery Delivery of an infant through the normal opening of the uterus and vagina.

Deltoid (*del'toid*) A triangle-shaped.

Deltoid ligament Internal ligament of ankle joint.

Deltoid muscle A large triangular muscle covering the shoulder prominence.

Deltoid ridge Ridge on humerus where deltoid muscle is attached.

Delusion (*de-lu'zhun*) False belief based on incorrect inference about external reality. It is not consistent with patient's intelligence and cultural background.

Bizarre delusion An absurd, very strange false belief.

Delusion of accusation False feeling of remorse and guilt.

Delusion of control False feeling that one's will, thoughts or feelings are controlled by external forces.

Paranoid delusion Delusions of persecution and delusions of references, control and grandeur.

Somatic delusion False belief involving functioning of one's body.

Systematized delusion False belief or beliefs united by a single event or theme.

Demeclocycline A tetracycline antibiotic used to treat a wide variety of susceptible bacterial infections.

Dementia (*de-men'shea*) The loss of cognitive functioning—thinking, remembering, and reasoning, to such an extent that it interferes with a person's daily life and activities.

Demography (*de-mog'ra-fe*) The scientific study of human population especially the changes in population size, the composition of the population and distribution of population in space.

Demulcent Soothing agent.

Demyelination (*de-mi'e-li-na'shun*) Destruction of myelin from the sheath of the nerve fibers.

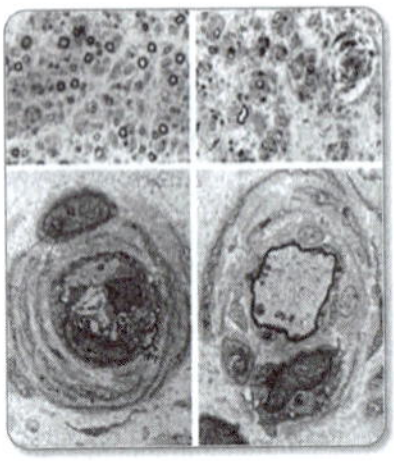

Demyelinating polyradiculoneuropathy histopathology.

Denaturation (*de-na'chur-a'shun*) Alteration of proteins by moderate heat that leads to loss of function.

Dendrite (*den'drit*) A short thread-like extension of a neuron which conducts impulses received from the terminal of other neurons.

Dendritic ulcer Herpetiform corneal ulcers seen in the autosomal recessive tyrosinemia.

Denervation (*de"ner-va'shun*) Excision or blocking of a nerve supply.

Dengue (breakbone fever) (*deng'ge*) Breakbone fever derived from Spanish language; a flavi viral infection (group B virus) carried, by aedes mosquito. It is characterized by abrupt onset of fever, malaise, headache, severe backache, conjunctival suffusion and a morbilliform rash. The fever is biphasic. Convalescence is protracted. Treatment is symptomatic.

Dengue hemorrhagic fever A severe form of dengue fever associated with spontaneous hemorrhage into the skin, epistaxis, hematemesis and melena and hypotension.

Dengue shock syndrome More severe form of dengue with vascular leakage. There is rapid onset of circulatory failure.

Dens (*denz*) A tooth; the odontoid process of the axis.

Dens in dente A malformed tooth with invaginated outer enamel epithelium of the odontogenic germ layer; *dens invaginus.*

Densitometer (*den'si-tom'e-ter*) An instrument that measures bacterial growth; an instrument that measures the optical density of a radiograph.

Dental (*den'tel*) Relating to teeth.

Dental arch Arch formed by the cutting and chewing surface of the teeth.

Dental disk A thin circular piece of paper cloth charged with abrasive powder for cutting or polishing teeth and fillings.

Dental fossa Thread or tape used for cleaning and removing plaques between teeth and testing for defects in the teeth.

Dental pulp Narrow cover of tooth, of vascular connective tissue with nerve fibers and odontoblasts.

Dental caries A pathologic process of localized destruction of the tooth.

Dental floss A cord of thin filaments used for intradental cleaning.

Dental nerve A sensory branch of the mandibular nerve, which is itself the third branch of the trigeminal nerve.

Dentate (*den'tat*) Notched.

Dentate nucleus Largest cerebellar nucleus.

Dentifrice (*den'ti-fris*) A paste, liquid, gel or powder for cleaning teeth.

Dentine (dentin) (*den'tin*) Hard dense bony tissue forming the bulk of a tooth, beneath the enamel. It surrounds the pulp chamber, covered by enamel in the crown and cementum in the root area.

Dentinogenesis (*den"ti-no-jen'e-sis*) The formation of dentin, a substance that forms the majority of teeth.

Dentist (*den'tist*) A person practicing dentistry.

Dentistry (*den'tis-tre*) The science concerned with the prevention, diagnosis and treatment of diseases of teeth and gums.

Dentition The type, number and arrangement of teeth in the dental arch.

Denture (prosthesis) (*den'chur*) A partial or complete set of artificial teeth set.

Denture mouth Chronic atrophic candidiasis.

Denver classification The classification of human chromosomes on the basis of size and centromere position; the 23 pairs of chromosomes are classified in 7 groups in order of decreasing.

Denys-Drash syndrome A constellation of nephropathy with ambiguous genitals and bilateral Wilm's tumor.

Deossification (*deos'i-fi-ka'shun*) Loss or removal of mineral matter from bone.

Deontology (*de'on-tol'o'je*) Medical ethics.

Deoxycholic acid A bile acid that lacks a hydroxyl group on C-7 and a free bile acid that is derived from the loss of an oxygen atom from bile acid.

Deoxycorticosterone A C-21 steroid hormone synthesized by zona fasciculata and zone glomerulosa it is a precursor for the synthesis of cortisol and aldosterone.

Deoxyribonuclease (*de-ok'se-ri'bo-nu'kle-as*) **(DNase)** An enzyme that depolymerizes DNA.

Deoxyribonucleic acid (*de-okse-ribo-nu-kle'ik*) **(DNA)** A complex nucleic acid consisting of deoxyribose, phosphoric acid and four bases (two purines—adenine and guanine and two pyrimidines—thymine and cytosine) which are arranged as two long chains that twist around each other to form a double helix. It forms the chemical basis of heredity and carries genetic information for all organisms except RNA viruses.

Dependence (drug dependence) (*de-pen'dens*) Substance abuse. A psychological compulsion for a person to use a substance such as narcotic on a chronic and repeated basis.

Depersonalization *psy* A dissociative symptom in which the patient feels that his or her body is unreal, is changing or is dissolving.

Depilatory (*da-pil'a-tor"e*) A substance used for removing unwanted hair from the human body.

Depolarization (*de-polar-i-za'shun*) Reversal of normal potential across cell membrane, leading to inflow of sodium.

Depolymerization (*de-po"li-mer-i'-za'shun*) To decompose (macromolecules) into simpler compounds (such as monomers).

Depressant An agent that decreases the level of a body function or nerve activity.

Depression (*de-presh'un*) Psychopathologic feeling of sadness; a hollow region; a decrease in vital functions.

Depressor (*de-pres'er*) An instrument for drawing down a part of the body.

Tongue depressor Device used to bring down the tongue, to facilitate visual examination of the throat.

Dequalinium Quaternary ammonium-cation antimicrobial used to treat common infections of the mouth and throat and vaginal candidiasis.

Derealization (*d'real'i-zashun*) An alteration in the perception or experience of the external world that it seems strange or unreal.

Dereism (*de're-izm*) *psy* Mental activity not concordant with logic or experience.

Dermacentor (*der'ma-sentor*) A genus of ticks in the family Ixodidae, the hard ticks, primarily responsible for maintenance of sylvatic disease cycle and transmission to animals and humans in the United States.

Dermal (*der'mal*) Relating to skin and especially to the dermis.

Dermanyssus (*der"ma-nis'us*) A genus of mites in the family Dermanyssidae, comprising a number of blood-sucking mites that are parasitic on birds.

Dermatitis (*der'ma-ti'tis*) Inflammation of the skin characterized by itching, redness and various skin lesions.

Actinic dermatitis Reaction of skin to sunlight or X-rays.

Atopic dermatitis An allergic disorder of the skin where the patient inherits an increased tendency of getting sensitized to various antigens in his environment.

Contact dermatitis Allergic reaction of the skin mediated by delayed hypersensitivity to a substance which comes in contact with the surface of the skin.

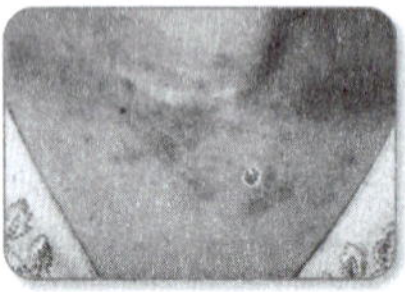

Contact dermatitis

Dermatitis artifacta Factitial dermatitis, which self-limits..

Dermatitis herpetiformia A chronic inflammatory condition characterized by erythema, papules, vesicles, and pustules. These lesions may coalesce and produce itching and burning sensation.

Dermatitis medicamentosa A skin eruption due to medicinal preparation ingested or applied.

Dermatitis verrucosa A chronic fungal infection of the skin manifesting with wartlike nodules.

Diaper dermatitis Irritation of the skin in contact with a diaper such as soap, powder, urine and feces.

Exfoliative dermatitis An erythematous condition characterized by erythema and scaling.

Photo contact dermatitis Application of photo sensitizer substance to the skin and subsequent exposure to sunlight resulting in skin lesions.

Seborrheic dermatitis An inflammation of the sebaceous glands manifesting in the form of diffuse scaling and erythema.

Stasis dermatitis Impaired circulation resulting in eczema of the legs.

Dermatobia (*der"ma-to'be-a*) Large tropical American fly; parasitic on humans and other mammals.

Dermatofibrosarcoma protuberans (DFSP) is a rare type of skin cancer that starts in your skin's middle layer (the dermis).

Dermatoglyphics (*der"ma-to-glifiks*) The study of skin markings or patterns on fingers, hands, and feet, and their application, especially in criminology.

Dermatology (*der'ma-tol'o-je*) The medical specialty of the skin and its diseases.

Dermatome (*der'ma-tom*) An area of skin in which sensory nerves derive from a single spinal nerve root.

Dermatomyositis (*der'ma-to-mi'o-si'tis*) An auto-immune disease in which skeletal muscle is damaged by a non suppurative inflammatory process dominated by lymphocytic infiltration. There is heliotrope (lilac) discoloration of the eyelids, erythematous rash over the face, neck and upper part of the body. The condition may coexist with other connective tissue disorders.

Dermatophagoides (*der'ma-tof'a-goi'des*) Mites found in house dust live on human skin scales and are concentrated on a bedding and mattresses especially in damp places. *D pteronyssinus* and *D culinae* are important examples which can provoke asthma.

Dermatophyte (*der'ma-to-fit's*) Fungi that live on keratinous structures and can infect the epidermis, the hair and nails. Those responsible for human infections belong to three genera—*Microsporan*, *Trichophyton* and *Epidermophyton*.

Anthropophilic dermatophytes Dermatophytes living only on the humans.

Geophilic dermatophytes Dermatophytes thriving in the soil.

Zoophilic dermatophytes Dermatophytes infecting animals.

Dermatophytosis (*der"ma-to-fi-to'sis*) A skin condition caused by dermatophyte fungus.

Dermatoplasty (*der'ma-to-plas'te*) Transplantation of living skin to cover cutaneous abnormality caused by injury, operation or disease.

Dermatosis (*der'ma-to-'sis*) Pl. **dermatoses**. Any disease of the skin in which inflammation may not be a feature.

Dermis (corium) (*der'mis*) The layer of the skin lying below the epidermis; true skin. It is composed of fibrous connective tissue composed of collagen and elastin. It consists of numerous capillaries, lymphatics and nerve endings. The hair follicles, sebaceous glands and sweat glands and their ducts are hidden in dermis.

Dermographia A form of urticaria due to allergy.

Dermoid (*dur'moid*) A cyst lined by an epidermis containing various epidermal appendages. Such lesions are found along embryonal fusion planes such as lateral third of eyebrows, nose and scalp. They can be inflamed and infected necessitating excision.

Dermoid cyst (dermoid) The most common orbital/periorbital tumors found in pediatric population; simple, skin-lined cyst under the skin.

Dermoidectomy (*der"moid-ek'te-me*) Excision of a dermoid cyst.

Descemet's membrane Basement membrane of endothelium lining posterior surface of cornea named after Jean Descemet, French anatomist.

Desensitization A therapeutic modality that attempts to reduce IgE-mediated hypersensitivity to various substance by administering ever increasing amounts of an antigen to form blocking antibodies.

Deserpidine An alkaloid obtained from a plant of the genus Rauvolfia (R. canescens) that is structurally related to reserpine, blocks adrenergic neurons, and is used especially as an antihypertensive and sometimes as a tranquilizer.

Desipramine A tricyclic antidepressant, used for symptomatic relief in a variety of depressive states.

Desjardin's forceps Forceps for removing the stones from bile ducts, named after Abel Desjardin French surgeon.

Desmopressin Vasopressin.

Desmosome An area of close contact and attachment between epithelial cells.

D'Espine's sign (*des-penz*) Normally whispering pectoriloquy is heard on the back up to T4 spine due to trachea. It may be heard to lower down due to enlarged lymph nodes named after Jean d'Espine, French physician.

Desoximetasone (*des-ok"si-met'a-son*) A fluorinated, high-potency corticosteroid, used to treat inflammatory and pruritic corticosteroid-responsive dermatoses.

Desquamation Abnormal shedding or an accumulation of stratum corneum in perceptible flakes.

Detached retina An emergency situation in which a thin layer of tissue (the retina) at the back of the eye pulls away from its normal position.

Detoxication (detoxification) Removal of a toxic excess of any agent, including overdosage of a therapeutic agent, drug of abuse or toxic agent (pesticides) and heavy metals from the body by inducing vomiting, administrating activated charcoal, dialysis or metabolic interference.

Detrition (*de-trish'un*) To become impaired in quality, functioning, or condition.

Detrusor Thruster down or out.

Detumescence (*de'tu-mes'ens*) Subsidence of a swelling; subsidence of swelling of erectile tissue of genitalia (penis or clitoris) following erection.

Deuteranopia (*du"ter-e-no'pe-a*) A disorder of the eyesight in which the retina does not respond to green.

Deutoplasm Comprises the food particles stored in the cytoplasm of an ovum or a cell.

Developmental disorder Impairments in a child's physical, cognitive, language or behavioral development.

Deviance A variation in the accepted norm.

Deviation To move steadily away from an accepted norm.

Ulnar deviation A hand deformity, in which the swelling of the metacarpophalangeal joints causes the fingers to become displaced to the ulnar side. Seen in chronic rheumatoid arthritis and lupus erythematosus.

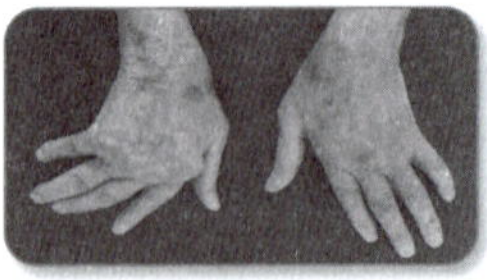

Ulnar deviation and ulnar drift

Devic's disease Neuromyelitis optica, named after M.E. Devic, French neurologist.

Devitalization (*de-vital-iza'shun*) The deprivation of vitality of life.

Dexamethasone Synthetic glucocorticoid with minimal mineral activity.

Dexamethasone suppression test Dexamethasone suppresses production of cortisone in low doses in normal, and in moderate doses in Cushing's disease. But it fails to suppress cortisone secretion in adrenal tumors or ectopic ACTH.

Dextran (*dek'stran*) A high molecular weight, branched-chain polysaccharide polymer of glucose.

Dextrin (*dek'strin*) Partially hydrolyzed starch or glycogen.

Dextrinosis (*dek"stri-no'sis*) An autosomal recessive metabolic disorder due to deficient expression of amylo-1,6-glucosidase (one part of the glycogen debranching enzyme system). The clinical course of the disease is similar to that of glycogen storage disease type 1, but milder.

Dextroamphetamine A sympathomimetic agent used in the treatment of attention deficit hyperactivity disorder (ADHD) and narcolepsy.

Dextrocardia (*dek'stro-kar-de-ah*) Abnormal location of the heart on the right side of the chest.

Mirror-image dextrocardia Dextrocardia with concomitant situs inversus of the abdominal organs.

Dextromethorphan A levorphanol derivative and codeine analog commonly used as a cough suppressant and also a drug of abuse.

Dextrose (*dek'stros*) Glucose, a simple sugar of the monosaccharide group.

Dextrothyroxine A thyroid hormone used to treat hyperlipidemia.

Dhobie itch Contact dermatitis associated with the use of laundry marking fluids.

Diabetes (*di'a-be'tes*) A term applied to diseases marked by an increased amount of urination, usually refers to diabetes mellitus.

Brittle diabetes A condition exhibiting frequent episodes of hypoglycemia followed by hyperglycemia necessitating constant adjustment of dietary intake and insulin dosage.

Bronzed diabetes Damage to several organs from excess iron deposition with features of diabetes mellitus associated with leaden-grey skin pigmentation; hemochromatosis.

Chemical diabetes Altered glucose metabolism without obvious features of diabetes mellitus.

Diabetes insipidus A condition characterized by persistent excretion of excessive quantities of dilute urine, and thirst. These are of two types as Cranial (deficient production of ADH due to a genetic defect or lesions of hypothalamus on high stalk or idiopathic) and Nephrogenic (renal tubules are unresponsive to ADH, as in genetic defect, hypokalemia, hypercalcemia, lithium or heavy metals poisoning) diabetes insipidus.. Cranial type is treated with desamino desaspartate-arginine vasopressin and peripheral type with thiazide diuretics.

Diabetes mellitus A metabolic disorder characterized by disturbances in carbohydrate, lipid and protein metabolism. These metabolic derangements result from a combination of insulin deficiency and/or insulin resistance and lead to a variety of acute and chronic complications.

Endocrine diabetes Diabetes mellitus associated with diseases affecting pituitary, thyroid or adrenal cortex.

Fibrocalculous pancreatic diabetes (FCPD) Diabetes mellitus associated with presence of stones in the pancreatic duct and its main branches. Consumption of tapioca (*cassava*) rich in cyanoglucosides leads to diabetes mellitus especially in Kerala, India.

Gestational diabetes Onset or first recognition of diabetes mellitus during pregnancy, most commonly during the third trimester. They exhibit insulin resistance and impaired insulin secretion.

Insulin dependent diabetes (IDDM) Diabetes mellitus usually having its onset before the age of 30 in which the essential abnormality is related to absolute insulin deficiency whose pathogenesis is due to genetic, environmental or immunological factors.

Juvenile onset diabetes Type 1 diabetes.

Latent diabetes Diabetes mellitus manifesting during times of stress such as pregnancy, obesity, infections or trauma.

Malnutrition related diabetes (MRDIVI) Young persons with age of onset of diabetes mellitus below 30 years and evidence of past or present malnutrition. It includes protein deficient diabetes mellitus and fibrocalculous pancreatic diabetes.

Maturity-onset diabetes of the young (MODY) NIDDM with age of onset <25 years. It has an autosomal mode of inheritance.

Noninsulin dependent diabetes (NIDDM) Diabetes with resistance to ketoacidosis in the absence of hepatic production of glucose and resistance to the action of insulin in muscle.

Type I diabetes All causes of diabetes that result from destruction of the pancreatic beta cells. This may be immune mediated or idiopathic. Immune mediated type I diabetes mellitus (IDDM or juvenile onset diabetes) is caused by an autoimmune cell-mediated destruction of pancreatic beta cells. Idiopathic type is characterized by insulinopenia without any evidence of autoimmune beta-cell destruction.

Type II diabetes All forms of diabetes that are characterized by the combination of insulin resistance and deficient secretion of insulin. This condition previously known as NIDDM, has a strong genetic disposition, typically has its onset later in life and is associated with insulin resistance syndrome (dyslipidemia, hypertension, atherosclerotic cardiovascular disease).

Diaclast A surgical instrument used for the destruction of the skull of a fetus. The procedure enables a dead fetus to be delivered through the birth canal.

Diagnosis (*di'ag-no'sis*) The determination of nature of a disease based on signs and symptoms.

Antenatal diagnosis Determination of health status of a fetus.

Clinical diagnosis Identification of a disease by history and physical signs, and laboratory studies.

Community diagnosis The pattern of disease in a community described in terms of the important factors which influence this pattern.

Cytologic diagnosis Identification of a disease based on cells present in body tissues or exudates.

Pathologic diagnosis Identification of an illness based on structural lesions.

Physical diagnosis Recognition of disease by physical examination.

Preimplantation genetic diagnosis Technique for evaluating the genes of an embryo that has undergone in vitro fertilization before it is implanted in the uterus.

Radiologic diagnosis Recognition of a disease by interpretation of radiographic findings.

Serologic diagnosis Identification of a disease through serologic test.

Diagnosis related group (DRG) A system to categorize patients with similar clinical diagnoses to control hospital cost and determine pay or reimbursement rates.

Diakinesis (*di'a-ki-ne'sis*) The homologous chromosomes becoming thick and short in the final stages of cell division.

Diaphysis (*di'ah-f'i-sis*) The shaft of a long bone.

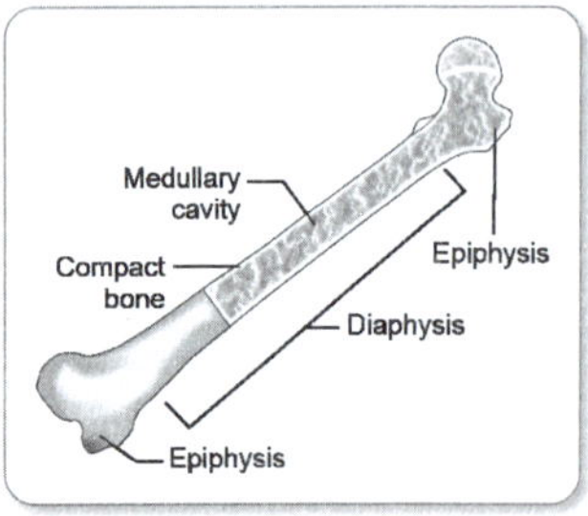

Diaphysis

Dialyzer (*di'a-liz"ar*) An apparatus in which dialysis is carried out.

Diamophine A substance made from morphine. It is illegal and very addictive drug. Used to manage severe pain.

Diapedesis (*di'a-pe-de'sis*) The passage of blood or any of its cells through the pores of blood vessels.

Diaper rash A form of dermatitis that looks like patches of inflamed skin on the buttocks, thigh and genitals.

Diaphoresis Referred to as excessive or profuse perspiration or sweating which may be due to associated medical conditions and might be induced as a side effect of a drug substance.

Diaphoretic (sudorific) (*di'a-for-et'ik*) An agent that causes sweating.

Diaphragm (*di'af-fram*) The muscular membranous structure separating

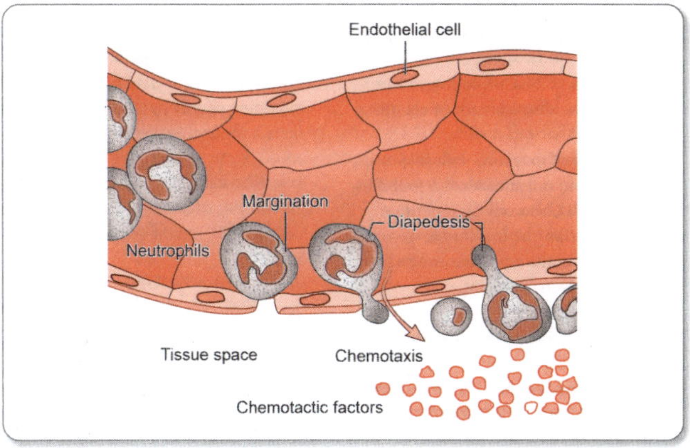

Diapedesis: Cell migration

thorax and abdominal cavity; any dividing membrane; a soft rubber cap that covers the uterine cervix and used for contraceptive purpose; an apparatus located beneath the opening in the stage of microscope and permitting the amount of light passing through the object.

Slit-pore diaphragm The gap between adjacent foot processes in the glomerulus.

Diaphysial aclasis Hereditary condition or may be due to genetic mutation; characterized by the development of multiple osteochondromas.

Diaphysitis (*di"-fiz-i'tis*) The main or midsection (shaft) of a long bone.

Diarrhea (*di'ah-re'ah*) Abnormal frequent passage of loose stools.

Chewing gum diarrhea An osmotic diarrhea caused by excessive intraluminal sorbitol in chewing gum.

Dysenteric diarrhea Diarrhea due to dysentery characterized by passage of blood and mucus.

Fatty diarrhea Diarrhea with stools containing undigested fat.

Infantile diarrhea Diarrhea in infants with increased frequency and amount of stools with change of color and consistency and signs of dehydration.

Mucous diarrhea Diarrhea with mucus.

Osmotic diarrhea Diarrhea caused by retention of osmotically active solutes in the small intestine which facilitates the fluid to be drawn into the intestinal lumen.

Secretory diarrhea A large volume of fecal output from abnormalities of the movement of fluid and electrolytes into the intestinal lumen.

Summer diarrhea Diarrhea occurring in children during summer.

Traveler's diarrhea Diarrhea experienced by travelers who move from an area in which organisms that commonly cause diarrhea are endemic.

Diarthrosis (synovial joint) Joint with synovial cavity.

Diaschisis (*di-as'ki-sis*) A loss of function within a region distant to the site of the lesion and results from deafferentation of neurons as a result of axon damage caused by stroke.

Diastase (*di'a-stas*) The separation of an epiphysis from the long bone to which it is normally attached without fracture of the bone.

Diastole (*di-as'to-l*) Rhythmic relaxation of the heart chambers during which time they fill with blood.

Diastolic gallop The triple rhythm produced by the development of the third heart sound.

Diastolic gallop shock Palpable pulmonary component of second sound in presence of pulmonary hypertension.

Diathermy (*di'ah-therme*) Local generation of heat in the body tissues by a high frequency electric current.

Diathesis (*di'ath'i-sis*) An inherited or congenital bodily predisposition to a disease.

Diazepam (*di-az'e-pam*) A long-acting benzodiazepine with rapid onset, commonly used to treat panic disorders, severe anxiety, alcohol withdrawal, and seizures.

Diazoxide Direct acting vasodilator antihypertensive used intravenously in hypertensive crisis.

Dibenzazepine (*di-ben-zaz'a-pen*) An antipsychotic drug used in treatment-resistant schizophrenia and to decrease suicide risk in schizophrenic patients.

Dibucaine (*di'bu-kan*) A topical anesthetic, produces numbness for a short period of time by stopping nerves from sending pain impulses to the brain.

DIC Disseminated intravascular coagulation.

Dicephalus (*di-sefa-las*) Having two heads.

Dichloralpheazone (*dl'klor-al-fena-zon*) A sedative composed of chloral hydrate and phenazone. It is typically found in combination products Nodolor and Midrin containing isometheptene and acetaminophen used for the relief of tension and vascular headaches.

Dichlorophen An anticestodal, fungicide, germicide, and antimicrobial agent; used in combination with toluene for the removal of parasites.

Dichlorphenamide (*di"klor-fena-mid*) A carbonic anhydrase inhibitor used for the management of open-angle and secondary glaucoma, as well as acute angle-closure glaucoma in delayed preoperative setting requiring a reduction in intraocular pressure.

Dichromatic (*di'kro-mat'ik*) Having or consisting of only two colors.

Dick test A test to determine the susceptibility or immunity to scarlet fever following injection of the erythrogenic toxin from streptococcus, named after George Dick and Glady Dick, US bacteriologists.

Diclofenac (*di-klo'fen-ak*) A nonsteroidal anti-inflammatory drug (NSAID), used to treat the signs and symptoms of osteoarthritis and rheumatoid arthritis.

Dicloxacillin (*di-kloks-sil'in*) A semisynthetic penicillinase-resistant penicillin.

Dicrotism (*di'kro-tiz-m*) Having a double beat.

Dictyoma A rare tumor arising from primitive medullary epithelium in the ciliary body of the eye.

Dicumarol (*di-ku'ma-rol*) An anticoagulant that acts in the liver to impair synthesis of vitamin K dependent coagulation factors including prothrombin. It is used in the prophylaxis and treatment of intravascular thrombosis and in postoperative thrombophlebitis, pulmonary embolism, and acute coronary thrombosis.

Dicyclomine (*di-si'klo-men*) A muscarinic M1, M3, and M2 receptor antagonist as well as a noncompetitive inhibitor of histamine and bradykinin used to treat spasms of the intestines seen in functional bowel disorder and irritable bowel syndrome.

Dieldrin (*di-eldrin*) Closely related to aldrin, which reacts further to form dieldrin. It has been linked to health problems such as Parkinson's, breast cancer, and immune, reproductive, and nervous system damage. It is also an endocrine disruptor, acting as an estrogen and antiandrogen, and can adversely affect testicular descent in the fetus if a pregnant woman is exposed to it.

Diencephalon (*di-en-sef'a-lon*) Midline structure from which cerebral hemispheres arise.

Dienestrol (*di'en-es'trol*) Synthetic estrogen.

Diet (*di'et*) Bodily nourishment.

Dietary fiber (roughage) Skeletal remains of plant cells including cellulose and cell wall polymers that are resistant to digestion by enzymes in man.

Dietetics (*di'atet'iks*) The study of diet in relation to health and diseases.

Diethylstilbesterol A synthetic estrogen that is more potent than natural estrogens.

Diethylpropion An appetite suppressant used for the short term treatment of exogenous obesity in addition to calorie restriction.

Dietl's crisis (*de'tiz*) Relief of pain and disappearance of swelling on drinking large quantity of water in intermittent hydronephrosis due to reflex polyuria named after Jozef Dietl, Polish physician.

Differential leukocyte count (differential blood count) the percentage of each type of WBC present in blood. A differential can detect immature WBCs and abnormalities.

Diflunisal (*di-flu'ni-sal*) An NSAID used to treat mild to moderate pain, inflammation, osteoarthritis, and rheumatoid arthritis.

Digestion (*di-jes'shun*) To break up food into simpler, assimilable compounds.

Digitalis (*dij'i-tal'is*) A preparation from dried leaves of *Digitalis purpura*. It has a positive inotropic and negative chronotropic effect on heart. It reduces the heart rate which is useful in atrial fibrillation and atrial flutter. It increases cardiac output with secondary increase of renal flow and glomerular filtration rate.

Digitalization (*diji'i-tal-i-za'shun*) Administration of sufficient amount of digoxin to have its effect, can be achieved by intravenous route.

Digitoxin (*dij-i-tok'sin*) A cardiac glycoside used as a heart stimulant.

Digoxin (*di-jok'sin*) Commonly used cardiac glycoside, used in cardiac failure, atrial fibrillation and flutter.

Dihydralazine Antihypertensive drug; works by combating the effects of adrenaline and by expanding the blood vessels so as to enable smoother flow of blood by reducing the pressure.

Dihydroergotamine (*di-hi'dro-er-gota-min*) A vasoconstrictor useful in migraine.

Diiodotyrosine A precursor in the production of thyroid hormone, that results from iodization of monoiodotyrosine at the other meta- position on the phenol ring.

Dilaceration (*di-las"r-a'shun*) The result of a developmental anomaly in which there has been an abrupt change in the axial inclination between the crown and the root of a tooth.

Dilation Expansion of organ, orifice or vessel.

Dilation and curettage (D and C) Dilatation and curettage, dilatation of the uterine cervix and scrapping of the endometrium of uterus with a curette.

Dilator An instrument for dilating muscles or for stretching cavities or openings.

Diloxanide Drug used to treat amoebic infections.

Diltiazem An antihypertensive and vasodilating agent that works by relaxing the vascular muscle and reducing blood pressure.

Dimenhydrinate (*di'men-hi'dri-nat*) An antihistamine indicated for the prevention and treatment of nausea, vomiting, or vertigo of motion sickness. It has a short duration of action of 4–8 hours.

Dimercaprol (*di-mer-kap'rol*) An antidote in poisoning from heavy metals such as arsenic, gold and mercury.

Dimethyl sulfoxide (DMSO) (*di-meth'il-sul-fok'sid*) An organosulfur compound with the formula $(CH_3)_2SO$. This colorless liquid is the sulfoxide most widely used commercially.

Dinner fork deformity Deformity of the hand in Colles' fracture.

Diopter (*di-op'ter*) The unit (d) used to designate the refractive power of a lens.

Dioptometer (*di-op-tom'i-tre*) An instrument for measuring refraction and accommodation of the eye.

Dipeptidase (*di-pep'ti-das*) An enzyme that catalyzes the hydrolysis of dipeptides to amino acids.

Dipeptide (*di-pep'tid*) A protein obtained by hydrolysis of the proteins.

Diphenhydramine H_1-receptor blocking antihistamine.

Diphenoxylate (*di'fen-ok-si-lat*) A smooth muscle relaxant used with atropine to treat diarrhea.

Diphosphonate A drug or substance used to treat hypercalcemia (abnormally high blood calcium) and bone pain caused by some types of cancer.

Diphtheria (*dif-ther'e-a*) An acute contagious disease caused by *Corynebacterium diphtheritic*. It spreads by droplet infection. The organisms remain localized at the site of infection-upper respiratory tract. The serious consequences are from the absorption of a soluble exotoxin. The disease begins insidiously and presents with membranous tonsillitis, nasal or laryngeal infection. It may lead to complications due to damage to the heart muscle or nervous system with features of laryngeal obstruction or paralysis, myocarditis and peripheral neuropathy. The condition is treated by administration of antitoxin and penicillin. Prevented by active immunization.

Diphtheroid (*dif'ther-oid*) Resembling diphtheria; a false membrane not due to the diphtheria bacillus.

Diphyllobothrium (*di-filo-both're-um*) A genus of tapeworms which can cause diphyllobothriasis in humans through consumption of raw or undercooked fish. The principal species causing diphyllobothriasis is D. latum, known as the broad or fish tapeworm, or broad fish tapeworm. D. latum is a pseudophyllid cestode that infects fish and mammals.

Diplacusis A hearing disorder in which the same sound is perceived differently between the two ears in intensity, pitch and tonality.

Diplegia (*di-ple-je-a*) Paralysis of corresponding parts of both sides of the body.

Diplococcus (*dip'lo-kok'us*) Spherical gram- positive bacteria joined together in pairs; former name for a genus for bacteria of tribe *streptococceae*; *Streptococcus pneumoniae* is an example. pl. **diplococci**.

Diploe (*dip'lo-e*) Spongy bone with a limited marrow cavity between the two tables of the cranial bones.

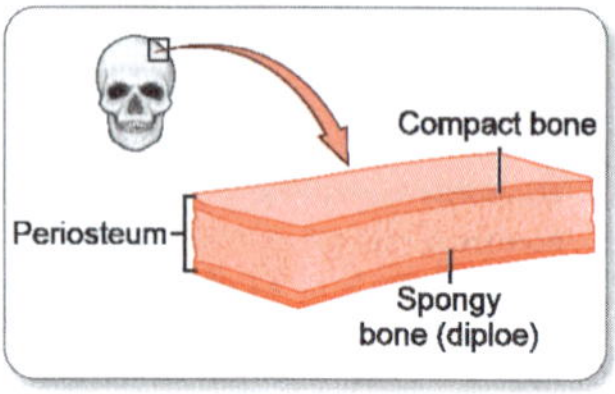

Diploe

Diploid (*dip'loid*) Having two sets of chromosomes in the somatic cells.

Diplopia (*di-plo'pea*) Double vision.

Diplotene Refers to the fourth stage of Meiosis Prophase I. This stage is characterized by chiasmata formation and the start of desynapsis.

Diprosopus A rare, life-threatening developmental defect during embryogenesis, and a sub-type of conjoined twins; characterized by partial or complete duplication of the facial structures on a single head, neck, trunk and body.

Dipsesis The passage of blood cells through the unruptured wall of a blood vessel into the surrounding tissues.

Dipsomania An insatiable uncontrollable desire for alcoholic drinks.

Diptera (*dip'ter-a*) Insects characterized by sucking or piercing mouth parts and a pair of wings; flies and mosquitoes are examples.

Dipylidium (*dipi"-lid'e-um*) A genus of taenioid tapeworms including the common dog tapeworm (D. caninum) that is a cosmopolitan parasite of dogs, cats, and other carnivores and occasionally infests humans.

Dipyridamole An antiplatelet agent, which in combination with aspirin reduces thrombosis in patients with thrombotic diseases. It inhibits embolization from prosthetic valves.

Disability (*dis'a-bil'i-te*) Any restriction or lack of ability to perform an activity in the manner or within the range considered normal for a person.

Disability limitation Preventing or halting the transition of the disease process from impairment to handicap when a patient reports late in the pathogenesis phase.

Disability prevention Reduction of the occurrence impairment by immunization (primary), by treatment (secondary) and by preventing the transition of disability into handicap (tertiary).

Disaccharide (*di-sak'i-rid*) A carbohydrate containing two monosaccharides.

Disarticulation (*dis'ar-ti-ku-la-shun*) Separation of the bones at the joint.

Disease (*di-zez*) Without ease, a physiological/psychological dysfunction resulting from a complex interaction between man, agent and the environment.

Acute disease A disease with a rapid onset and relatively of short duration.

Autoimmune disease A disease produced when the body's normal tolerance of antigens on its own cells disappears.

Chronic disease A disease with a slow onset and lasting for a long duration.

Chronic obstructive pulmonary disease (COPD) A disease state characterized by the presence of air-flow obstruction due to chronic bronchitis or emphysema, the air-flow obstruction is generally progressive.

Communicable disease A disease in which the causative organism is transmissible from one person to another either directly or indirectly.

Congenital disease A disease that is present at birth.

Connective tissue disease A group of diseases that affect connective tissue. It includes muscle, cartilage, tendons, vessels, skin and ligaments.

Contagious disease An infectious disease readily transmitted from one person to another.

Deficiency disease A disease resulting from inadequate intake or absorption of essential dietary factors.

Degenerative disease A disease resulting from deterioration of tissues and organs.

Degenerative joint disease Osteoarthritis.

Demyelinating disease A disorder of nerve fibers due to destruction of their myelin sheath.

Endemic disease A disease present continuously in a community and it may recur frequently.

Epidemic disease A disease affecting a large number of persons in a community at the same time.

Epizootic disease An epidemic affecting animals of a particular region, usually in a short period of time.

Extrapyramidal disease Degenerative disease of nervous system involving the extrapyramidal system and basal ganglion of the brain. Parkinsonism is a classic example.

Familial disease A disease occurring in several members of the same family.

Focal disease A disease confined to a specific area such as tonsils, adenoids or a boil.

Foot and mouth disease A viral disease noted in cattle and horses, that is rarely transmitted to humans.

Functional disease A disease in which no anatomic changes can be seen to account for the symptomatology.

Heavy chain disease A group of diseases. involving serum immunoglobulins.

Hereditary disease A disease due to genetic factors transmitted from parent to offspring.

Hookworm disease Ankylostomiasis.

Hydatid disease The disease produced by larval stage of *Echinococcus granulosus*.

Iatrogenic disease A disease produced by medical or surgical intervention.

Idiopathic disease A disease for which no causative agent can be recognized.

Infectious disease Any disease caused by growth of pathogenic organisms in the body.

Intercurrent disease A disease developing during the course of another, unrelated disease.

Iron storage disease Hemochromatosis.

Lysosomal storage disease A disease caused by deficiency of specific lysosomal enzymes that normally degrade glycoproteins, glycolipids or mucopolysaccharides, and such substances accumulate in lysosomes.

Malignant disease Cancer; a disease not necessarily making rapid progress and is life threatening.

Metabolic disease A disease occurring from under-production or overproduction of substances needed by the body in the metabolic process.

Mixed connective tissue disease A connective tissue disorder-exhibiting features of SLE, progressive systemic sclerosis and polymyositis.

Motor neuron disease A progressive neurological disorder that presents with both lower motor neurons (anterior horn cells that project from the brainstem and the spinal cord to the muscle) and upper motor neuron signs (neurons that project to the brainstem and spinal cord from higher cortical centers) (*see figure*).

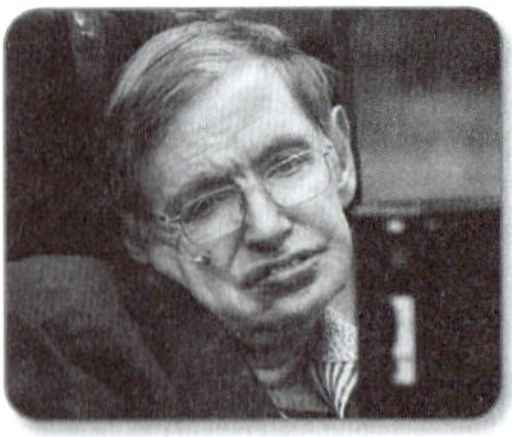

Motor neuron disease

Natural history of disease The way in which a disease evolves over time from earliest stage of its prepathogenesis phase to termination as recovery, disability or death in the absence of treatment or prevention.

Occupational disease A disease resulting from factors associated with occupation.

Organic disease A disease resulting from anatomical alteration in an organ or tissue of the body.

Pandemic disease A widespread epidemic affecting the population of several countries as in influenza.

Parasitic disease A disease resulting from the growth and development of parasites in or on the body.

Psychosomatic disease An organic disease caused or exacerbated by psychological factors.

Reactive airway disease Persistence of airway reactivity after acute exposure to respiratory irritants.

Restrictive lung disease Any chest disease that results in a reduced lung volume.

Secondary disease A disease caused by another condition such as obesity.

Self-limited disease A disease that recedes of its own.

Storage disease A disorder involving abnormal deposition of a substance in body tissues.

Subacute disease An intermediate between acute and chronic disease.

Systemic disease A generalized disease.

Venereal disease A disease acquired through sexual contact.

Disimpaction The process of separating the broken ends of a bone when they have been forcibly driven together due to a fracture.

Disinfectant A substance which destroys harmful microbes with the object of preventing transmission of diseases.

Disinfection (*dis-in-fek'shun*) The destruction of infectious agents by direct exposure to chemical or physical agents.

Concurrent disinfection Application of disinfection measures as soon as possible after the discharge of infectious material from the body of an infected person or after soiling of articles with such infectious discharges.

Prophylactic disinfection Disinfection to prevent acquiring infectious agents like chlorination of water, pasteurization of milk and hand washing.

Terminal disinfection Application of disinfection measures after the death of the patient or after moving the patient to the hospital.

Disinfestation (*dis'in-fes-ta'shun*) Killing of infested insects and parasites.

DISH (*dish*) diffuse idiopathic skeletal hyperostosis.

Disintegrative psychosis A rare condition characterized by late onset of developmental delays in language, motor skills and social function.

Disjunction (*dis-junk'shun*) Separation of homologous pairs of chromosomes during anaphase of the first meiotic division.

Diskitis (*dis-ki'tis*) An inflammation of the vertebral disk space often related to infection.

Diskography (*dis-kog'ra-fe*) The injection of radiopaque dye into the IVD. This technique is useful as an adjunct in the evaluation of symptomatic disorders of the disc.

Dislocation (luxation) (*dis'lo-ka'shun*) Displacement of a limb or organ from the normal position.

Joint dislocation Total displacement of articular surfaces causing a loss of apposition between them. The dislocation may occur spontaneously at any joint in consequence of a structure defect or of destructive disease, or trauma.

Dismemberment (*dis-mem'bar-ment*) To cut off or disjoin the limbs, members, or parts of.

Disoma A double-bodied fetus with a single head.

Disomy The inheritance of both haploid chromosomes from one parent.

Disopyamide (*di"so-pi'a-mid*) A class 1A antiarrhythmic agent used to treat life-threatening ventricular arrhythmias.

Disorientation (*dis-or'ie-enta'shun*) Loss of sense of direction or location; a state of mental confusion as to time, place or person.

Dispensary (*dis-pen'ser-e*) Any place where drugs and medicines are dispensed.

Displacement (*dis-plas'mant*) The act of displacing or the condition of being displaced.

Dissection (*di-sek'shun*) The act of dissecting.

Disseminated (*di-sem'i-nat"ed*) Widely dispersed in a tissue, organ, or the entire body.

Disseminated intravascular coagulation (DIC) A consumptive coagulopathy, noted in critically ill patients and often heralds the onset of multiorgan failure. It is characterized by an increase in prothrombin time, partial thromboplastin time and fibrin degradation products and a fall in platelets and fibrinogen. There is either widespread bleeding from vascular access points or widespread microvascular and even macrovascular thrombosis. It is treated with fresh frozen plasma, platelets and low dose heparin.

Disseminated sclerosis A chronic progressive nervous disorder involving loss of myelin sheath around nerve, fibers; also known as multiple sclerosis.

Dissociation (*dis-so'se-a'shun*) Separation; ability to move one body segment independently of another; not going together; *psy* the breaking off of normal thought processes from consciousness.

Distal (*dis'-t'l*) Farthest from a point of reference.

Distichiasis (*dis"ti-ki'a-sis*) A congenital or acquired condition where eyelashes arise from the meibomian glands on the posterior lamella of the eyelid margin.

Disulfiram (*di-sul'fi-ram*) An alcohol antagonist used to support the treatment of chronic alcoholism by producing an acute sensitivity to ethanol (drinking alcohol).

Diuresis (*di"u-re'sis*) Excessive production of urine; polyuria.

Diuretic (*di'u-ret'ik*) Agent that increases amount of urine.

Diverticular disease Diverticular disease condition that occurs when small pouches, or sacs from and push outward through weak spots in the well of colon.

Diverticulitis (*di'ver-tik'ul'it-is*) Inflammation of a diverticulum.

Diverticulosis (*di'ver-tiku-lo'sis*) Diverticula in the colon develop in individuals who are on a life long refined diet with relative deficiency of fiber and symptoms are result of associated constipation or spasm, generally asymptomatic.

Diverticulum (*di'ver-tik'u-lum*) A sac-like protrusion of mucosa covered by peritoneum from a tubular organ, most common in the sigmoid and descending colon and is acquired. pl. **diverticula**; *Meckel diverticulum.*

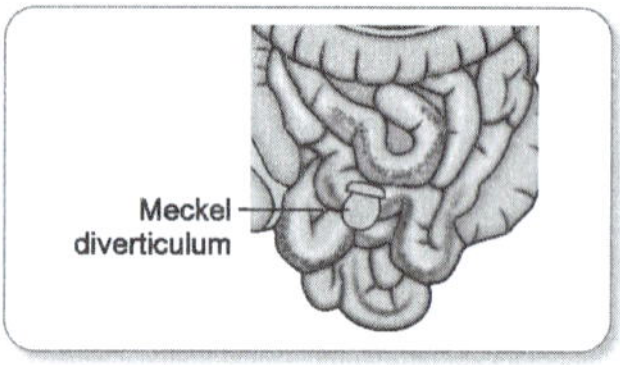

Meckel diverticulum

Division A process of splitting a specific amount into equal parts.

Dizygotic twins The twins resulting from the fertilization of two separate eggs with two different sperms during the some pregnancy.

DMD Duchenne muscular dystrophy.

DMARD Disease-modifying antirheumatic drugs.

DNA Deoxyribonucleic Acid.

DNA finger-print A distinctive pattern of bands formed by repeating sequences of base pairs of satellite DNA which are different in every individual.

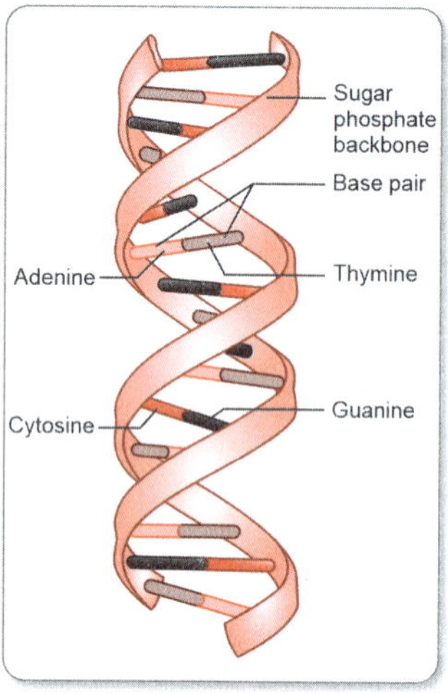

DNA

DNA gyrase An essential bacterial enzyme that catalyzes the ATP-dependent negative super-coiling of double-stranded closed-circular DNA.

DNA helicase An enzyme that separates and unwinds the two DNA strands in preparation for replication or transcription.

DNA library A collection of DNA fragments that are cloned into plasmids or viral genomes.

DNA ligase An enzyme that joins two DNA strands together to make a continuous DNA molecule.

DNA methylation The addition of a methyl group to DNA at the 5-carbon of the cytosine pyrimidine ring that precedes a guanine.

DNA methyltransferases Family of enzymes that catalyze the transfer of a methyl group to DNA using S-adenosyl methionine as the methyl donor.

DNA microarray A technology that is used to study many genes or other sequences at once.

DNA polymerase A type of enzyme that is responsible for forming new copies of DNA, in the form of nucleic acid molecules.

DNA primate An enzyme that synthesizes a short strand of RNA that serves as a primer for DNA replication.

DNA probe Labelled segment of single-strand DNA of known type used to identify similar sequences on DNA chain.

DNA repair capacity Ability of natural cellular processes to repair damages that occur in DNA.

DNA sequencing The process of determining the exact order of the bases-A,T,C and G- in a piece of DNA.

DNA topoisomerase Enzymes that control the topology of DNA in all cells. There are two types, I and II, classified according to whether they make transient single- or double-stranded breaks in DNA.

Mitochondrial DNA DNA founding mitochondria; mDNA.

Docusate (*dok'u-sat*) Any of several laxative salts and especially the sodium salt used to soften stools in the treatment or prevention of constipation.

Dolichocephaly (*dol'i-ko-se-fal-e*) Long head.

Doll's eye sign Movement of the eyes in a direction opposite to a sudden movement of the head caused by a lesion in the central mechanism for voluntary eye movement.

Dolor (*do'lor*) Pain, one of the cardinal signs of inflammation.

Dolorimeter (*do'lor-im'e-ter*) An instrument used to measure pain threshold and pain tolerance.

Dominant A trait expressed in individuals who are heterozygous for a particular gene.

Donor One who donates tissue, an organ, blood or blood products.

DOPA 3, 4 dihydroxy phenylalanine produced by exudation of tyrosine. It is a precursor of catecholamines and melanin.

Dopamine A sympathomimetic agent which is the immediate metabolic precursor of norepinephrine and epinephrine. Useful in treatment of shock with oliguria and low or normal peripheral vascular resistance, also useful in the treatment of cardiogenic and septic shock.

Dorsal (*dor'sal*) Relating to the back.

Dorsiflexion Movement of a part at a joint to bend the part toward the dorsum.

Dorsoventral (*dor"so-ven'tral*) Relating to both the dorsal and ventral sides; extending from the back to the belly.

Dorsum The posterior surface or back of a part.

Dose (*dos*) The amount of medicine or radiation to be administered at one time.

Bolus dose An amount of medicine given intravenously rapidly at the beginning of treatment.

Booster dose An additional dose of an immunizing agent to increase the protection afforded by original series of injections.

Cumulative dose Amount of drug present in the body after repeated exposure; total dose resulting from repeated exposure to radiation.

Divided dose Fractional portions of drug administered at short intervals.

Fatal dose A dose resulting in death.

Infective dose The amount of microorganisms that will cause disease.

Loading dose Initial administration of a drug in doses that exceeds the elimination rate of the drug from the body.

Maintenance dose The dose required to maintain the desired effect.

Maximum dose The largest dose that is safe to administer.

Minimum dose The smallest effective dose.

Therapeutic dose The dose required to produce desired effect.

Toxic dose A dose that causes signs and symptoms of drug toxicity.

Dosimeter A device to used to measure the absorbed dose of ionizing radiations.

Dosimetry (*do'sim'e-tre*) Measurement of doses.

Double (*dub'l*) Twofold.

Double blind Relating to, or being an experimental procedure in which neither the subjects nor the experimenters know which subjects are in the test and control groups during the actual course of the experiments.

Double cortex syndrome A genetic defect with presence of a band of gray matter within the subcortical white matter presenting with mental retardation and epilepsy.

Double vision Two images of an object seen at the same time.

Double J stents Also known as ureteral stenting is a thin tube inserted into the ureter to prevent or treat obstruction of the urine flow from the kidney.

Double uterus (Uterus didelphys) a rare condition where a woman has two uteruses. It is a congenital abnormality.

Double vision Two images of an object seen at the same time.

Douche (*doosh*) A stream of liquid directed into a cavity of body.

Down's syndrome (*downz*) A chromosomal abnormality having three chromosomes instead of normal two in the pair no. 21 (47XY) resulting in many congenital defects described by an English physician John Down; mongolism. It is characterized by dwarfed physique, low set ears, a flat nose, short broad hands with a single palmar crease, a sloping forehead and small ear canals.

Doxepin (*dok'sa-pin*) A psychotropic agent used for the treatment of depression, anxiety, manic-depressive disorder, and insomnia.

Doxorubicin An antineoplastic antibiotic effective in acute leukemias and malignant lymphomas and is administered intravenously. Myelosuppression is a major complication.

Doxycycline An antimicrobial agent belonging to tetracycline group has antimicrobial activity against aerobic and anaerobic, gram-positive and gram-negative bacteria especially useful in diseases caused by rickettsia, mycoplasma and chlamydiae.

DPT vaccine Diphtheria, pertussis and tetanus vaccine used to immunize infants against three infectious diseases such as diphtheria, pertussis and tetanus.

Dracunculosis (*dra-kun'ku-lo'sis*) dracantiasis, dracunculiasis infection acquired by ingesting a small crustacean, cyclops which inhabits step wells and ponds and which contain infective larval stages of *D. medinensis*. They penetrate intestinal wall and migrate, through connective tissue. The fully mature female surfaces under skin to discharge its larvae externally. Symptoms are painful vesicle, ulcer, cellulitis usually on leg and secondary infection. The disease has been eradicated.

Drain (*dran*) Provision of exit for the fluid.

Drainage (*dran'ij*) The free flow or withdrawal of fluids from a wound or cavity.

Drainage angle The tiny channel through which fluid leaves the eyeball.

Drainage tube A device for allowing escape of fluid, pus, serum from a wound.

Draw sheet A rubber or plastic sheet to protect the mattress and bed sheet from drainage and soilage.

Drawer's sign Useful in the diagnosis of tear of cruciate ligaments when the patient lying on the back with the knee to be tested flexed the upper end of tibia which is grasped and pushed backward and pulled forward and a free movement of tibia over the lower end of the femur. There is abnormal mobility of tibia on femur in tear of cruciate ligaments which can even be demonstrated on the extended knee.

Drepanocyte (sickle cell) Formed as a result of the presence of hemoglobin S in the red cell.

Drepanocytosis Sickle cell disease, an inherited blood disorder that affects hemoglobin.

DRESS syndrome Drug rash with eosinophilia and systemic symptoms; a severe form of cutaneous drug reaction characterized by fever, skin rash, lymphadenopathy, hematological abnormalities, and internal organ involvement.

Dressing (*dres'ing*) Bandage applied to a wound or lesion to prevent external infection.

Drip (intravenous drip) Slow injection of a solution into a vein a drop at a time.

Drocode Trade name for drug dihydrocodeine.

Dromograph (*dromo-graf*) An instrument for measuring changes in volume within an organ or whole body.

Dromostanolone A synthetic androgenic anabolic steroid and is approximately 5 times as potent as natural methyltestosterone.

Dropsy (*drop'se*) Hydrops; generalized accumulation of fluid in the body.

Drosophila A genus (Drosophila) of fruitflies used in genetic research.

Drug Substance used as medicine, narcotic or hallucinogen.

Drug abuse Self-administration of a drug for non-medical reasons in quantities and frequencies which may impair an individual's ability to function effectively and which result in social, physical or emotional harm.

Drug addict A person exhibiting psychological dependence with an over-powering desire to take the drug and obtain it by any means.

Drug addiction A state of periodic or chronic intoxication detrimental to the individual and society produced by the repeated intake of habit forming drugs.

Drug resistance Situation where patient fails to show response to chemotherapy. It may be primary when the patient has been infected with organisms that are resistant to one or more drugs; or secondary wherein the infection is acquired either from a patient who has received inadequate chemotherapy or from a naturally resistant organism (wild strain).

Drug synergism Enhancement of a drug effect as a result of the presence of additional drugs within the system.

Drug tolerance Progressively decreased sensitivity to a drug that a person has taken repeatedly requiring high doses to produce the desired effect.

Drug withdrawal Symptoms experienced by a person on stopping the drug on which he or she had become physically dependent.

Drug dependence A state of psychic and sometimes also physical resulting from the interaction between an individual and a drug characterized by behavioral and other responses that always include a compulsion to take the drug on a continuous or periodic basis.

Dry socket *dent* A painful condition following tooth extraction in which a blood clot does not properly fill the empty socket, leaving the bone underneath exposed to air and food.

Duchenne dystrophy A genetic disorder characterized by progressive muscle degeneration and weakness due to alterations in the proteins; most severe form of inherited muscular dystrophies.

Duke's criteria Clinical criteria described by Duke University, North Carolina US for or the diagnosis of infective endocarditis that includes the major criteria of a positive blood culture, and evidence of valvular disease, and minor criteria of fever and evidence of embolism.

Duct (*dukt*) A tube to convey the products of a gland to another part of the body.

Alveolar duct A branch of respiratory bronchiole that leads to the alveolar sacs. The duct contains alveoli in their walls.

Biliary duct A canal that carries bile.

Bile duct The duct that carries bile and pancreatic juice to the duodenum. It is formed by the union of the cystic duct of the gallbladder and the hepatic duct of the liver and is joined by the pancreatic duct.

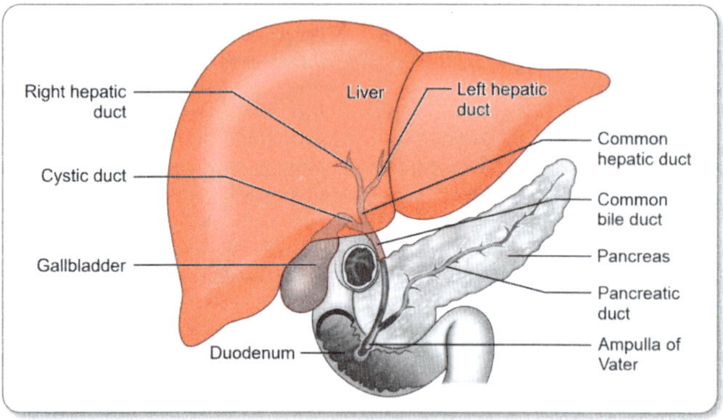

Biliary duct

Cystic duct The secretory duct of gallbladder.

Efferent duct One of a group of small tubes from the testis, and lie within the epididymis.

Ejaculatory duct The duct conveying semen from the vas deferens and seminal vesicle to the urethra.

Hepatic duct A duct receiving bile from liver and carrying it to the common bile duct.

Interlobular duct A duct passing between lobules within a gland.

Lacrimal duct One of two short ducts (inferior and superior) that conveys tears from the lacrimal lake to the lacrimal sac. They open on the margin of upper and lower eyelids.

Lactiferous duct One of the several ducts draining the lobes of the mammary gland. They open in a slight depression in the tip of the nipple.

Lymphatic duct One of the two main ducts conveying lymph to the blood stream. The right lymphatic duct drains lymph from the region above the diaphragm and discharges into the right subclavian vein.

Mesonephric duct An embryonic duct connecting the mesonephros with the cloaca.

Mullerian duct One of the bilateral ducts in the embryo that forms the uterus, vagina and fallopian tubes named after Johannes Muller, German physiologist.

Nasolacrimal duct A duct that conveys tears from the lacrimal sac to the nasal cavity. It opens beneath the inferior nasal cavity.

Pancreatic duct A duct that conveys pancreatic juice to the duodenum called Wirsung's duct, named after Johann Wirsung, German physician.

Parotid duct A duct carrying secretions from the parotid gland to the oral cavity. It opens opposite the second upper molar tooth also called Stensen's duct, named after Niels Stensen, Danish physician.

Prostate duct One of about 20 ducts that discharge prostatic secretions into the urethra.

Semicircular duct One of the three (anterior, posterior and lateral) membranous tubes forming a part of the membranous labyrinth of the inner ear. They are present within the semicircular canal's.

Skene's duct One of the two blend ducts of Skene's gland that open either side of the urethral orifice of women, named after Alexander American, gynecologist.

Sublingual duct Any of the secretory ducts of sublingual gland also called Bartholin duct, named after Casper Bartholin Jr., Danish anatomist.

Submandibular duct A duct of the submandibular gland that opens on a papilla at the side of frenum of the tongue, also called Wharton's duct, named after Thomas Wharton, British anatomist.

Thoracic duct Lymphatic duct draining the left side of the body above the diaphragm and all of the body below the diaphragm and it opens into the left subclavian vein.

Utriculosaccular duct A narrow tube arising from the utricle connecting it into the saccule and open into the endolymphatic duct of the inner ear.

Vitelline duct A narrow duct, in the embryo connecting yolk sac with the intestine.

Ductless gland Gland lacking an external duct; endocrine gland.

Ductile (*duk'til*) (of a metal) Able to be drawn out into a thin wire.

Ductus (*duk'tas*) A duct or walled passageway suitable for the conveyance of air or, more often in the body, liquids.

Ductus arteriosus A vessel leading from the bifurcation of the pulmonary artery to the aorta just distal to the left subclavian artery. Normally the vascular channel closes immediately after birth.

Dumdum fever Also called kala-azar is a chronic, potentially fetal parasitic disease due to Leishmania donovani.

Dumping syndrome Post-gastrectomy syndrome.

Early dumping syndrome In patients with gastrectomy, rapid gastric emptying leads to distension of the proximal small intestine. There is abdominal discomfort and diarrhea after eating and vasomotor features such as flushing, palpitations, sweating, tachycardia and hypotension. The patients should avoid large meals with high carbohydrate.

Late dumping syndrome Symptoms develop 90–180 minutes after eating. There is reactive hypoglycemia from exaggerated release of insulin causing mental confusion.

Duodenal ulcer Ulcer in the first part of the duodenum. The patients have a greater number of parietal cells and a tendency to higher gastric acid secretion, noted in age group 20–40 years. Presents with pain on an empty stomach with a clock-like regularity with relief on food intake.

Duodenoscope (*du"o-de'no-skop*) Specialized endoscopes or flexible, lighted tubes that are threaded through the mouth, throat, and stomach into the top of the small intestine (duodenum).

Duodenoscopy (*du'o-de-nos'ko-pe*) Inspection of the duodenum with an endoscopic.

Duodenostomy (*du'od-e-nos'to-me*) Surgical creation of a permanent opening into the duodenum through the wall of abdomen.

Duodenum (*duo-de'num*) The first part of the small intestine shaped like a horse shoe, between the stomach and jejunum. It is 20–28 cm long. It receives the hepatic and pancreatic secretions through a common bile duct at the ampulla of Vater, named after Abraham Valet. German anatomist.

Dupuytren's contracture (*du-pwe-tranz*) Thickening and contracture of palmar fascia, typically affects the ring finger and may involve years later incompletely, little finger. The finger resists extension, described by Baron Dupuytren, French surgeon.

Dura (dura mater, pachymeninx) A tough fibrous white membrane forming the outermost of the three coverings of the brain and spinal cord.

Dural (*du'ral*) Relating to or affecting the dura mater.

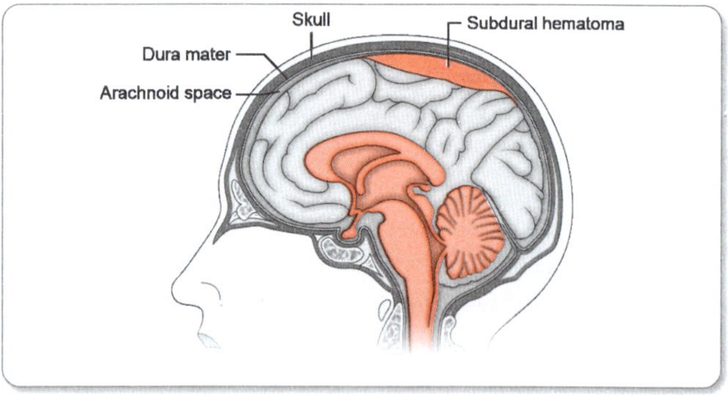

Dura mater

Dwarfism *(dwarf'izm)* Failure to attain full growth potential.

Dynamometer *(di'na-mom'e-ter)* A device for measuring muscular strength or magnifying power of a lens.

Dyne *(din)* A unit of force equal to 10^{-5} Newton. The force needed for imparting an acceleration of 1 cm/sec to a gram mass.

Dyphylline A theophylline derivative used to treat asthma, bronchospasm, and COPD.

Dysarthria *(dis-ar'thre-a)* Difficulty in articulation of speech.

Dysacusis *(dis'a-kusis)* Discomfort caused by loud noise; a condition in which sound produces discomfort.

Dysbarism *(dis'bar-iz-m)* Any adverse medical condition that results from changes in ambient pressure.

Dyschezia *(dis-ke'ze-a)* Difficult or painful defecation.

Dyschondroplasia *(dis'kon-dro'pla'ze-a)* A congenital condition where masses of unossified cartilage persist within the metaphysis of certain long bones and the growth of the bone is retarded; multiple chondromatosis.

Dyscrasia *(dis'kra-zea)* A morbid condition.

Dysdiadochokinesia *(dis'di-ad'o-ko-ki-ne-se-a)* Inability to make alternate movements in rapid succession.

Dysentery *(dis'in-te're)* Frequent watery stools with blood and mucus accompanied by abdominal pain.

Amoebic dysentery Infection of intestine by *Entamoeba histolytica* presents with bloody motions, lower abdominal pain, the motions have more stool, less blood. Stools reveal presence of amoebic trophozoites.

Bacillary dysentery Shigellosis, named after Kiyoshi Shiga, Japanese physician, is an infection of intestine by bacteria of shigella, such as *S. dysenteriae. S. boydii. S. flexneri* and *S. sonnei*, characterized by abrupt onset of fever, malaise, abdominal pain, bloody diarrhea with mucus and fecal urgency.

Balantidial dysentery Dysentery caused by ciliate protozoa, *Balantidium coli.*

Dysesthesia *(dis'es-the'ze-a)* Abnormal sensations experienced in the absence of stimulation.

Dysgenesis *(dis-jen'i-sis)* Defective embryonic development.

Gonadal dysgenesis A disorder due to failure of ovaries to respond to pituitary gonadotrophins resulting in amenorrhea, short suture and failure of sexual maturation.

Dysgerminoma (germinoma, gonocytoma) *(dis-jerm'in-o-ma)* A rare malignant ovarian tumor originating from primordial germ cells of the sexually undifferentiated embryonic gonad.

Dysgraphia (*dis-graf'e-a*) Inability to write coherently, as a symptom of a neurological condition or as an aspect of a learning disability.

Dyshidrosis (dysidrosis) (*dis'hi-dro'sis*) An abnormality of sweat production.

Dyskinesia A movement disorder after chronic exposure to dopamine receptor antagonists characterized by stereotyped orolingual and masticatory movements such as lip smacking, lip pursing, tongue protrusion, licking and chewing.

Dyslalia (*dis-la'le-a*) Impaired speech due to defective speech organs.

Dyslexia (*dis-lek'se-a*) A learning disability wherein the individual experiences difficulty with written symbols.

Dyslogia Impaired ability to express ideas verbally.

Dysmenorrhea (*dis'men-or-e'a*) Pain or discomfort experienced just before or during menstrual periods.

Dysmorphophobia A mental disorder defined by an overwhelming preoccupation with a perceived flaw in one's physical appearance.

Dysostosis (*dis'os-to-sis*) Defective bone formation.

Dyspareunia (*dis'pa-ru'ne-a*) Pain or discomfort in vaginal or pelvic area experienced by a woman during sexual intercourse.

Dyspepsia (Indigestion) (*dis-pep'se-a*) Indigestion. Often a symptom of other diseases and characterized by vague abdominal discomfort, a sense of fullness after eating, eructation, nausea, vomiting and loss of appetite.

Dysphagia (*dis-fa'je-a*) Difficulty in swallowing.

Dysphagia lusoria Dysphagia from pressure exerted on esophagus by an anomalous subclavian artery.

Dysphagia paralytica Dysphagia due to paralysis of pharyngeal or esophageal muscles.

Dysphasia (*dis-fa'zea*) Impairment of coordination in speech and inability to arrange words in their proper order.

Dysphemia Speech disorder characterized by stammering or stuttering and usually has a psychological basis.

Dysphonia (*dis-fo'ne-a*) Difficulty in speaking due to a physical disorder of the mouth, tongue, throat, or vocal cords.

Dysplasia (alloplasia, heteroplasia) (*dis-pla'zea*) A defective growth of tissues; a histologic lesion with premalignant potential.

Dysplasia associated lesion or mass (DALM) Presence of dysplasia histologically and a mass by endoscopy as in adenocarcinoma of colon with ulcerative colitis.

Dyspnea (*disp-ne'a*) Difficulty or labored breathing and is a subjective complaint.

Acute dyspnea Sudden onset of shortness of breath from pulmonary edema, asthma, spontaneous pneumothorax, pulmonary embolism, ARDS, pleural effusion, or injury to chest wall and intrathoracic structures.

Chronic dyspnea Progressive breathlessness is a feature of left ventricular failure, diffuse interstitial fibrosis, COPD, asthma, pleural effusion, and pulmonary thromboembolic disease.

Dyspraxia (*dis-prak'se-a*) Impaired functioning of an organ or a part.

Dyssynergia (asynergia) Any disturbance of muscular coordination, resulting in uncoordinated and abrupt movements.

Dystocia (*disto-se-a*) Difficult childbirth.

Dystonia (*dis-to'ne-a*) Rigidity of muscles causing painful spasms or abnormal movement patterns.

Dystrophia myotonica Progressive muscle wasting and weakness; characterized by prolonged muscle contraction (myotonia) and the affected person is not able to reflex certain muscles after use.

Dystrophy (dystrophia) (*dis'trof-e*) Progressive changes caused by faulty nutrition. Also known as dystrophia.

Dysuria (dis-u-re-a) Difficulty or pain in urination.

E

Ear The organ of hearing and balance. It consists of the external, middle and internal ear. The external ear has the skin covered cartilaginous auricle and the external auditory canal. They form a funnel directing sound waves toward the tympanic membrane or ear drum. On the other side of the ear drum is the air-filled middle ear. It contains three very small bones, the malleus, incus and stapes which transmit the vibrations caused by the sound waves reaching the tympanic membrane to the oval window of the inner ear. The inner ear consists of two separate organs. The vestibular apparatus providing the sense of balance and the organ of Corti which translates the vibrations received from the middle ear into nerve impulses which are interpreted by the brain cells as specific sounds.

Bladder ear *uro* Transient bilateral extraperitoneal herniation of the bladder in infants.

Ear drops A topical liquid medication for the local treatment of infection of the lining of external auditory canal or impacted cerumen.

Ear oximeter A device helping to measure the level of saturated hemoglobin in the blood.

Ear speculum A short funnel-shaped tube attached to an otoscope for examination of the ear canal.

Ear ache (*er'ak*) Pain in the ear.

Ear drum A thin oval membrane separating the middle ear from external ear that transmits sound waves.

Ear wax A waxy secretion produced by sweat glands in the external ear canal, cerumen.

Eburnation (*eb'ur-na'shun*) Ivory-like appearance of weight-bearing joints with erosion of cartilages, leaving polished, sclerotic bone as the new articular surface.

Ecbolic (*ek-bol'ik*) A drug or agent that hastens labor or abortion.

Ecchondroma (*ek-on-dro'ma*) Overgrowth of cartilage on a normally situated cartilage.

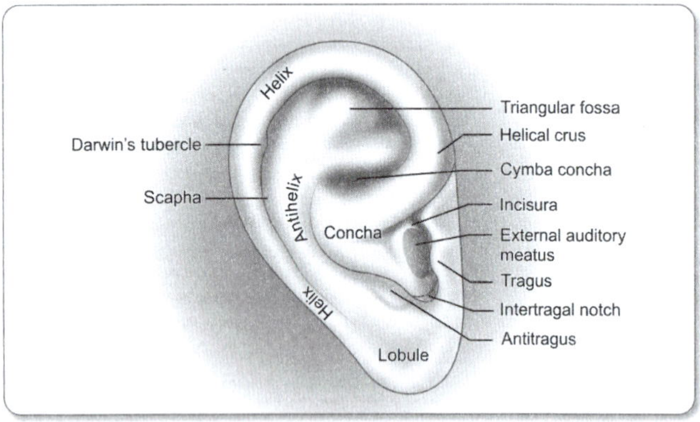

External ear

Ecchymosis (*ek-i-mo'sis*) A purplish discoloration from extravasated blood into the skin or mucous membrane. It follows bleeding from a large vessel.

Eccrine (*ek'rin*) Exocrine secretion by cells which remain intact.

Eccrine gland Sweat glands found in the corium of the skin. They secrete outwardly through a duct to the surface of the skin. They promote cooling by evaporation of their secretions.

Ecdemic Of relating to a disease that originates outside the locality or country.

ECG Electrocardiogram or graph.

Echinococcosis (*e-ki'no-kok-a'sis*) Echinococcal infestation, hydatid disease.

Echinococcus (*e-ki'no-kok'us*) A small tapeworm whose larval infection forms hydatid cysts.

Echinococcus granulosus *Taenia echinococcus.* By handling a dog or drinking contaminated water, man may ingest eggs. The embryo liberated from the ovum in small intestine reaches the liver, sometimes lung and the resultant cyst grows slowly.

Echinococcus multilocularis Tapeworm producing multilocular hydatid cysts.

Echoacousia The subjective experience of hearing echoes after normally heard sounds.

Echocardiography (*ek'o-kar'de-og'ra-fe*) A two-dimensional imaging technique using Doppler ultrasonography that provides information on pressure differences and blood flow in the heart and great vessels. The blood flowing through the heart produces sound, some of which is reflected back by each acoustic interface the blood encounters (Doppler effect) which is received by a transducer; the time elapsed between the sound transmission to the time that the echo is received is converted to a display and there is production of an imaging plane with construction of two-dimensional echocardiogram which is useful in evaluating cardiovascular disorders.

Echoencephalogram (*ek'o-en-sef'a-lo-gram*) Recording of the ultrasonic echoes of the brain, useful in determining the cause of shift in midline structures of the brain.

Echography (*a-kog'ra-fe*) Medical examination of the internal structures of the body by means of ultrasound.

Echokinesis (*ek"o-ki-ne'sis*) The compulsion or the act of imitating movements of others.

Echolalia (*ek'o-lale-a*) The repetition by a person of words or phrases spoken by others. It may be spoken with a mocking or staccato intonation.

Echopraxia (echokinesis) Repetition or imitation of another person's gestures, involving the exact imitation of the provoking person's movements, facial and oral expression, and sometimes even of words and sentences spoken in foreign languages.

Echotomography Tomography imaging by detecting acoustic (usually ultrasonic) reflections from variations in emission of sound waves; ultrasonography.

ECHO virus Enteric cytopathic human orphan virus associated with enteric disease in humans; produces cytopathic effects in cell cultures.

Eclabium (*ek-la'be-um*) Eversion of a lip or lips.

Eclampsia (*e-klamp'se-a*) Toxemia of pregnancy noted in late pregnancy, labor or the immediate puerperium, characterized by convulsions, hypertension albuminuria, hypoproteinemia, raised blood urea nitrogen, hemoconcentration and sodium retention with edema.

Ecology (bionomics) (*e-kol'o-je*) Biological science concerned with the inter-relationship between organisms and environment.

Ecology of health Health as a state of dynamic equilibrium between man and his environment.

Ecraseur A surgical instrument having a chain or wire loop; used to encircle and severe a projecting mass of tissue by gradual tightening of chain or loop.

Ecstasy (*ek'sta-se*) A feeling of intense rapture.

ECT Electroconvulsive therapy; electric shock treatment.

Ectasia (ectasis) A dilation of ducts with loss of elastin in duct inflammatory cells, especially plasma cells, around duct walls.

Ecthyma (*ek-thi'ma*) A pyogenic infection of the skin with ulcers covered by adherent crusts.

Ectoderm (*ek'to-derm*) The outermost germ layer of cells in the embryo. It gives rise to epidermis, teeth, tongue, palate, salivary glands, anogenital region, hypophysis, nervous system and sensory organs such as eyes, ears and nose.

Ectomorphy (*ek'to-mor"fe*) Characterized by having a thin body build, relative prominence of structures developed from the embryonic ectoderm.

Ectoparasite (*ek'to-par'a-sit*) A parasite that lives on the surface of the host's body.

Ectopia (*ek-to'pe-a*) Congenital displacement or of malposition of any organ or part of the body.

Ectopia lentis Displacement of lens of the eye.

Ectopia vesicae Extroversion of the bladder.

Ectopic beat Extrasystoles.

Ectopic hormone A hormone is considered ectopic if there is an abnormal endocrine function demonstrable by biochemical and clinical evidence and coexistence of a tumor. It is considered a paraneoplastic syndrome.

Ectopic pregnancy (extrauterine pregnancy) The implantation of an embryo in sites anywhere outside the uterus not designed to accommodate the massive vascular supply needed by a growing fetus.

Ectoplasm Viscous, clear outer layer of the cytoplasm in amoeboid cells.

Ectrodactyly (*ek'tro-dac'tili*) Malformation consisting of split hands and feet.

Ectromelia (*ek'tro-me'le-a*) Congenital absence of one or more limbs.

Ectropion (*ek-tro'pe-on*) The abnormal eversion of the margin of a part especially of an eyelid.

Eczema (*ek'ze-ma*) A superficial inflammation affecting the epidermis which manifests in redness, itching, weeping, oozing and crusting.

Asteatotic eczema 'Crazy paving' pattern of fine fissuring on an erythematous background in the legs in elderly with dry skin.

Atopic eczema A generalized and prolonged hypersensitivity to common environmental antigens. The individuals exhibit a genetic predisposition to form excessive IgE.

Discoid eczema Discrete coin-shaped lesions of eczema on the limbs of young one.

Dyshidrotic eczema Recurrent vesicles and bullae over palms, palmar surface of the fingers and soles, that are very itchy.

Gravitational eczema Eczema on the legs and is often associated with signs of venous insufficiency; stasis eczema.

Irritant eczema Detergents, alkalis, acid and solvents producing reaction at the site of contact.

Napkin eczema Eczema in babies due to irritant ammoniacal urine and feces.

Seborrheic eczema Eczema unrelated to seborrhea, affects the scalp, ears, central face and nasolabial folds.

Edema (*e-de'ma*) Accumulation of fluid in subcutaneous tissue due to extracellular volume expansion. There is swelling of tissues which can be demonstrated by pressing lightly with the thumb over a bony prominence.

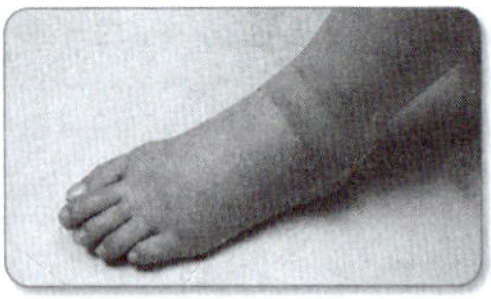

Edema of foot

Dependent edema Edema over the dorsum of the feet, around the ankles.

Nonpitting edema Occurs in lymphatic obstruction, myxedema and systemic sclerosis.

Pitting edema On pressure, a pit appears for a while, noted in heart failure, nephrotic syndrome, cirrhosis of the liver, and hypoproteinemia.

Sacral edema Edema over the sacrum in those confined to bed from gravitational effect.

Unilateral edema Edema in venous or lymphatic obstruction in one limb.

Edentulous (*e-dent'u-lus*) Without teeth edge, a border at which a surface ends.

Edrophonium A readily reversible acetylcholinesterase inhibitor; prevents breakdown of the neurotransmitter acetylcholine and acts by competitively inhibiting the enzyme acetylcholinesterase (at the neuromuscular junctions).

EDTA (ethylenediamine tetraacetic acid) Ethylene diamine tetra acetic acid. A chelating agent that binds substances like calcium, lead, magnesium and arsenic. It is used to treat lead and other heavy metal intoxication. It is added to specimen tubes in the laboratory to transport specimens.

EEG (electroencephalogram) Electroencephalogram.

Efferent Conveying from a center.

Efferent nerve A nerve that conveys impulses away from the brain or spinal cord to muscles or glands.

Effleurage (*e-fler-ahzh'*) A light friction technique used to encourage the lymphatic system to flow starting at the bottom of the limb and pushing back toward the heart.

Effusion (*e-fu'zhun*) The escape of a fluid into a cavity or space.

Egg cell Female reproductive cell, ovum; gamete.

Ego (*e'go*) The conscious sense of the self.

Egophony An auscultatory finding due to a change in the quality (timbre) of the voice.

Eidatic images (*i-det'ik*) Visual memories of almost hallucinatory vividness.

Eikonometer (*i"ko-nom'e-ter*) An instrument used to measure aniseikonic errors. It measures the rotations of the observed field affected by binocular perception only.

Eisenmenger syndrome (*i'zen-meng'erz*) A condition that develops when increased pulmonary flow due to an initial left-to-right shunt produces severe pulmonary hypertension and reversal of the shunt. On establishment, the raised pulmonary resistance is irreversible. There is development of central cyanosis and digital clubbing. ECG shows right ventricular hypertrophy, coined after Victor Eisenmenger, German physician.

Ejaculation (*e-jak'u-la'shun*) A sudden act of expulsion; an abrupt exclamatory utterance; the release of semen from penis at orgasm.

Electro-ejaculation A technique for inducing ejaculation by direct electrical stimulation of the efferent nerves innervating the seminal vesicles and the terminal vas.

Retrograde ejaculation Failure of reflex closure of the internal urethral sphincter enabling backward ejaculation.

Premature ejaculation Persistent or recurrent ejaculation with minimal sexual stimulation that occurs before, during or shortly after penetration and before person wishes it.

Elastic cartilage Yellow cartilage seen in external ears, epiglottis and pharynx.

Elastic tissue Connective tissue with elastic fibers.

Elastin (*e-las'tin*) A fibrous protein similar to collagen, this rubbery substance is found in arterial walls, vocal cords, alveolar septa and ligaments.

Elastosis (*e-las-to'sis*) Local overgrowth of elastic tissue.

Elation (exaltation) (*e-la'shun*) Joyful emotion.

Electroanesthesia A weak, nonpainful electrical current which is delivered to the specific body site these electrical impulses confuse the transfer of pain along the nerve pathways.

Electrocardiogram (ECG) (*e-lek'tro-kar'de-o-gram*) A graphic record of the electric current produced by the excitation of the cardiac muscle; ECG, EKG.

Electrocardiography Producing graphic records of the electrical activity of the heart muscle.

Ambulatory electrocardiography Recording of the electrical activity of the heart over extended period with the patient engaged in all routine activities.

Dynamic electrocardiography Ambulatory electrocardiography.

Exercise electrocardiography The recording of the electrical activity of the heart while the individual is subjected to the stress of graded exercises performed by bicycle ergometer or the treadmill.

Electrocardiophonography Detects and records heart sounds, the sounds made by the various cardiac structures pulsing and moving blood. This method is a visual representation on a chart of a cardiac sound.

Electrocautery (galvanocautery) (*e-lek'tro-kaw'ter-e*) A platinum wire which when heated by an electric current cauterizes the tissue.

Electrocoagulation A procedure that uses heat from an electric current to destroy abnormal tissue, such as a tumor or other lesion.

Electroconvulsive therapy (ECT, Electroshock) (ECT) *psy* Iatrogenic induction of generalized tonic-clonic seizures for treating depression.

Electrodesiccation (*e-lek"tro-des"i-ka'shun*) A fast and simple office-based procedure that uses electric current delivered *via* a needle-shaped electrode to superheat the skin in pinpoint precise areas.

Electroencephalogram (EEG) (*e-lek'tro-en-sef' a-lo-gram*) a graphic record of the electrical activity of the brain.

Electroencephalography The recording and study of the electrical activity of the brain.

Electromyographyy (*e-lek"tro-ki-mog're-fe*) The photography on X-ray film of the motion of heart or other structures using an electromyograph.

Electrolyte (*e-lek'tro-lit*) A solution that conducts electricity; an ionized salt in the blood, tissue fluids and cells, which include sodium, potassium and chlorine.

Electromyography (*e-lek'tro-mi-og'ra-fe*) Recording and study of the electrical activity in muscle.

Electronarcosis Electric stunning or electrostunning, produced by passing an electric current through the brain.

Electron microscope Bean of electrons and their wave-like characteristics are used to magnify image under observation.

Electroneurography (*e-lek"tro-nu-rog're-fe*) An objective test that measures evoked compound muscle action potentials using skin electrodes.

Electroneuromyography (*e-lek"tro-nur"o-mi-og're-fe*) A technique that uses surface electrical probes to obtain electrophysiological readings from nerve and muscle cells.

Electronic fetal monitoring Use of electronic or pressure sensitive devices for the measurement of the fetal heart rate and woman's uterine contractions during labor.

Electro-oculogram (*e-lek'tro-ok'u-lo-gram*) A graphic recording of the movement of the eyes; EOG.

Electrophoresis (*e-lek-tro-for-e'sis*) The motion of the colloid particles suspended in a liquid under the influence of an applied electric field, useful in identification of proteins.

Electroretinography A diagnostic tool to measure the electrical activity of the retina in response to a light stimulates. It measures the electrical response of the retina to light.

Electroshock (*e-lek'tro-shok*) Denoting or relating to medical treatment by means of electric shocks.

Electrosurgery (*e-lek"tro-sur'jer-e*) A technique often used in surgery to control bleeding and to rapidly dissect soft tissue in surgery.

Electrotherapy (*el'ek-tro'the-ra-pi*) Treatment procedures that use electromagnetic energy either by direct application to the body or by placing the relevant part of the body in an electromagnetic field.

Elephantiasis (*el'e-fan-ti'a-sis*) Cutaneous induration due to lymphatic obstruction. It may occur in legs or scrotum due to filariasis, in the penis and scrotum due to lymphogranuloma venereum or in the arms following axillary lymph node dissection in radical mastectomy.

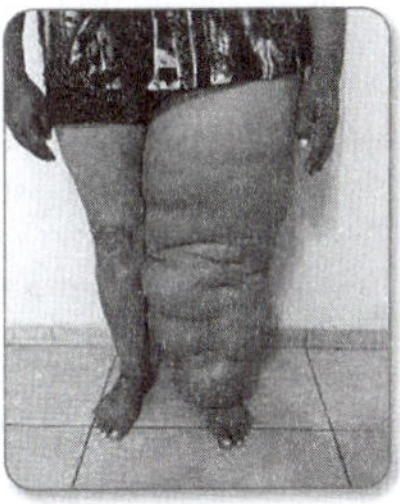

Elephantiasis

Elevator An instrument for elevating tissues.

Elevator neuromatosa Neurofibromatosis associated with deep, diffuse and massive lesions causing broad-based hanging of tissue filled with neurofibromas.

Elevator nostra Pseudoelephantiasis; an inflammation, edema or obstruction of the scrotal lymphatics in temperate climate due to non-filarial infections such as granuloma inguinale, lympho-granuloma venereum, syphilis, tuberculosis or streptococcal infections.

Elevator testicle Migrating testicle that is highly mobile in the inguinal canal and it may even migrate into the abdominal cavity.

Elfin facies syndrome An idiopathic hypercalcemic disorder with possibly hypovitaminosis D exhibiting a characteristic face such as small mandible, prominent maxilla, an upturned nose, depressed nasal bridge, anteverted nares, medial eyebrow flare, a 'cupid's bow' upper lip, short palpebral fissures, carious peg teeth. It is associated with feeding difficulties, failure to thrive, supravalvular aortic stenosis and septal defect.

Elimination The act of expulsion, zero disease in a defined geographic area as a result of deliberate efforts, and control measures needed to prevent reestablishment of transmission.

ELISA Enzyme-linked immunosorbent assay.

Ellis's curve (*el'i-sez*) The level of dullness in pleural effusion, is highest in the axillary region from which it slopes down in front and back assuming an S-shape, named after Calvin Ellis, US physician.

Elixir A substance, usually a liquid, with a magical power to cure, improve or preserve something.

Elliptocytosis (*e-lip"to-si-to'sis*) An inherited heterogeneous red blood cell (RBC) disorder, characterized by elongated, oval, or elliptical-shaped red blood cells on the peripheral blood smear.

Elutriation A process for separating lighter particles from heavier ones using a vertically-directed stream of gas or liquid.

Emaciation A wasting of the body.

Emasculation (*e-mas"ku-la'shun*) The act of castrating (removing the male sexual parts of) a man or male animal, or removing the male parts of a plant.

Embalming (*em'balm'ing*) The treatment of a dead body with preservatives and antiseptics so as to preserve it.

Embedding (*em-bed'ing*) The process by which a piece of tissue is placed in paraffin, it is used to cut into thin section for microscopic examination.

Embolectomy (*em"bo-lek'to-me*) Surgical removal of an embolus from a blood vessel.

Embolism (*em'bo-lizm*) The sudden obstruction of an artery by a clot or foreign material which has been brought by circulation from a different side.

Air embolism Presence of gas in the coronary of cerebral arteries and 100 mL of gas can kill a person. There is bubbling where the organ is opened under water during autopsy.

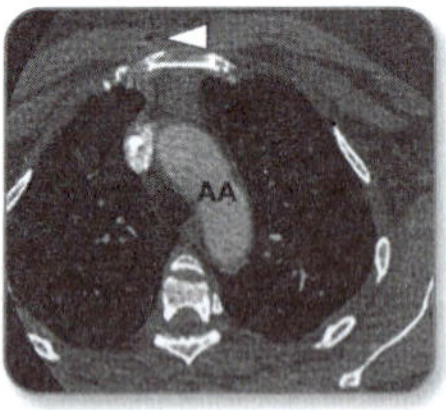

Air embolism

Amniotic fluid embolism Embolism of amniotic fluid through communication in the maternal circulation.

Fat embolism Long bone fractures lead to the entry of fat into the lungs causing ARDS, and to the brain causes coma.

Nitrogen embolism Noted in divers who surface too rapidly where the nitrogen boils in the vessels causing joint and abdominal pain.

Paradoxical embolism An embolus that migrates in the direction opposite to the blood flow, a complication of right-to-left shunt in congenital heart disease, especially through a patent foramen ovale.

Pulmonary embolism Condition associated with the obstruction of pulmonary artery by thrombus arising from an extrapulmonary source. It occurs as a potential lethal complication of deep vein thrombosis in the legs or pelvis.

Embolus (*em'bo-lus*) A clot or other material carried by the blood stream and impacted in some part of the vascular system.

Embrasure (*em-bra'zher*) *dent* A space continuous with an interproximal space, produced by curvatures of teeth in contact in the same arch, it provides a passage through which food escapes from the occlusal surfaces during mastication.

Embrocation A liquid for rubbing on the body to relieve pain from sprains and strains.

Embryo (*em'bre-o*) The entity prior to the time at which all organs are developed, at about the eighth week after conception.

Embryopathy (*em'bre-op'a-the*) Developmental anomalies from interference with normal embryonic development.

Embryoplastic (*em"bre-o-plas'tik*) Embryogenic.

Embryology The science dealing with the study of development of the individual during the embryonic stage.

Embryotomy (*em'bre-ot'o-me*) The dismemberment of the fetus in the uterus or vagina.

Embryotoxicity (*em"bre-o-tok-sis'i-te*) The state of being toxic to embryos.

Emesis (*em'e-sis*) Vomiting; act of vomiting.

Emetic (*e-met'ik*) An agent that induces vomiting.

Emetine (*em'e-ten*) Alkaloid from ipecacuanha root, used as amebicide and emetic.

Emigration The escape of leukocytes through the walls of small blood vessels; departure from a place of abode, natural home, or country for life or residence elsewhere.

Eminence A prominence; projection.

Emissary vein A small vein that pierces the skull. It carries blood from the sinuses within the skull to the veins outside it.

Emission (*e-mish'un*) A discharge.

Emmenagogue (*em'me-na-gog*) A substance that encourages menstrual flow.

Emmetropia (*em'e-tro'pe-a*) Normal refraction of the eye.

Emollient (*e-mol'yent*) Having softening or soothing effect.

Emotion (*e-mo'shun*) A mental state experiencing joy, sorrow, fear, hate, love or the like.

Empathy (*em'pa-the*) Ability to see the world from the client's perspective.

Emphysema (*em'fi-se'ma*) Inflation, abnormal distension of an organ or part.

Centriacinar emphysema Destruction of the wall of respiratory bronchioles of the first or second order and of peribronchiolar alveoli and the alveolar duct and they are converted into abnormal airspaces. Changes seen in men and associated with chronic bronchitis and cigarette smoking.

Distal acinar emphysema Predominant involvement of distal part of the acinus, alveolar ducts and sacs in emphysematous changes.

Emphysema lung Abnormal permanent enlargement of the airspaces distal to the terminal bronchioles accompanied by destructive changes of the alveolar walls and without fibrosis.

Mediastinal emphysema Air inside the mediastinal space following chest injury or secondary to rupture of an emphysematous bulls, usually associated with surgical emphysema. There is pain or feeling of tightness over the sternum.

Panacinar emphysema Destruction of the wall of alveolar ducts and alveoli and there is involvement of all components of the acinus in a uniform manner, commonly associated with alpha-I antiprotease deficiency.

Senile emphysema With age, there is thinning of the alveolar walls resulting in the enlargement of alveoli and bronchioles, not associated with airway obstruction.

Subcutaneous (surgical) emphysema A crackling sound and crepitus due to displacement of gas bubbles or air in the subcutaneous tissue or in the underlying muscles.

Empirical (*em-pir'i-k'l*) Based on experience.

Empyema (Pyothorax) (*em'pi-e'ma*) A collection of pus in a body cavity.

Empyema necessitans A swelling in the side of the chest in conditions of empyema which exhibits an impulse on coughing.

Empyema thoracis A collection of suppurative material in the pleural space characterized by opaque appearance, foul odor or demonstration of organisms in Gram stain.

Emulsion (*e-mul'shen*) A preparation of one liquid distributed in small globules in another liquid.

Enalapril An angiotensin-converting enzyme inhibitor with a vasodilator activity useful in improving hemodynamic indices and the symptoms of congestive heart failure.

Enamel (*e-nam'el*) White, hard calcareous substance that covers and protects the corner of a tooth.

Enanthema (*en-an'thema*) An eruption upon a mucous membrane.

Enarthrosis (*en'ar-thro'sis*) Ball and socket joint.

Encapsulated Enclosed within a capsule.

Encephalin A variant of enkephalin which has similar effects to morphine.

Encephalitis (*en-sef'a-li'tis*) Inflammation of the substance of the brain.

Japanese B encephalitis Caused by a specific arbovirus, transmitted to man by bite of infected culicine mosquitoes (Culex tritaeniorhynchus) and the reservoir of infection is pigs. Children are more prone and may present with febrile headache type, meningitic type and encephalitic type with severe headache, fever, vomiting, twitching, muscular rigidity, convulsions, carries high mortality and corticosteroids are useful.

Encephalocele (*en-sef'a-lo-sel*) A gap in the skull leading to hernia of the brain.

Encephalography (*en-sef'a-log'ra-fe*) The branch of medical science concerned with taking and analyzing X-ray photographs of the brain.

Encephaloid (*en-sef'e-loid*) Resembling the material of the brain.

Encephalolith (*en-sef'e-lo-lith"*) Calculi in brain.

Encephalomyelitis (*en'sef'a-lo-mi'el-i-tis*) Inflammation of the brain and spinal cord.

Acute demyelinating encephalomyelitis May develop in association with viral diseases (measles, chickenpox, mumps) or follow vaccination against rabies. There is massive and widespread demyelination of white matter and is probably caused by immunologic damage. It presents with headache, vomiting, fever, clouding of consciousness, meningeal irritation, convulsions and coma, flaccid paralysis of limbs and cranial nerve palsies. Treatment is supportive.

Encephalomyelopathy (*en-sef'a-lo-mi'el-op'a-the*) Any disease of the brain and spinal cord.

Encephalomyocarditis (*en-sef"a-lo-mi"o-kahr-di'tis*) An acute febrile disease especially of swine and some nonhuman primates caused by a picornavirus and marked by degeneration and inflammation of skeletal and cardiac muscle and lesions of the central nervous system.

Encephalon (*en-sef'al-on*) The brain.

Encephalopathy (*en-sef'a-lop'a-the*) Any disorder of the brain that involves widespread destruction or degeneration of brain tissue.

Enchondroma (*en'kon-dro'ma*) A benign hypertrophy of a cartilage arising in the metaphysis of a bone.

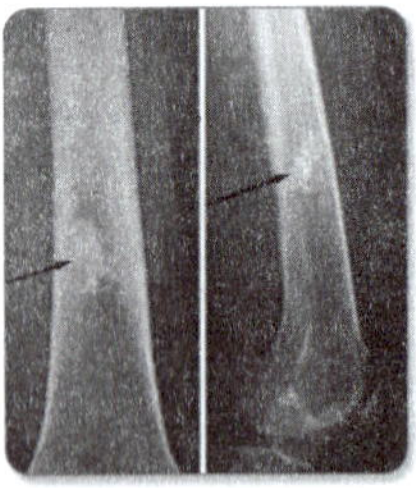

Enchondroma of knee (PA view and lateral view)

Encopresis (*en'co-pres'is*) Fecal incontinence.

Encysted (*en-sist'ed*) Enclosed in a sac or cyst.

Encysted effusion Collection of fluid which is walled off in the pleural space.

Endarterectomy (*end'ar-ter-ekto-me*) Surgical removal of the thickened, atheromatous *tunica intima* of an artery to restore normal blood flow.

Endarteritis (*end-ar-ter-itis*) An inflammation of the innermost layer of an artery.

End-artery The artery having no anastomosis.

Endemic (*en-dem'ik*) Constant existence of a disease or infectious agent in a locality at all times, without importation from outside.

Endemic goiter Thyroid swelling in areas of iodine deficiency.

Endocarditis (*en'do-kar-di'tis*) Infection of the endocardium and heart valves.

Infective endocarditis Caused by bacteria.

Nonbacterial endocarditis Sterile platelet or fibrin thrombi on damaged cardiac valve. There is sterile emboli, negative blood culture and valvular vegetations in chronically ill-patient, requires anticoagulants.

Endocardium The serous membrane that lines the cavities of the heart.

Endocervix (*en'do-ser'viks*) The mucous membrane lining uterine cervical canal.

Endochondral (*en'do-kon'dral*) Occurring within cartilage.

Endocrine gland (ductless gland) A gland that secretes hormones directly into the bloodstream.

Endocrinology (*en'do-krin-ol'o-je*) Branch of medical science dealing with the endocrine glands and their secretions.

Endoderm (*en'do-derm*) The innermost of the embryo's primary germ layers. It develops into the lining of the mouth, pharynx, gastrointestinal and respiratory tracts, liver, gallbladder and pancreas.

Endodermal sinus tumor An ovarian tumor of female children and adolescents characterized by a large tumor mass composed of a meshwork of cuboidal cells recapitulating the embryonic yolk sac and elevated levels of alpha-fetoprotein; yolk sac tumor.

Endodontics (*en'do-don-tik's*) The branch of dentistry concerned with disorders affecting the dental pulp and root.

Endogenous (*en-doj'e-nus*) Originating within; arising from inside the body.

Endolymph (*en'do-limf*) The fluid within the membranous labyrinth of the ear.

End of life care Multi-dimensional and multi-disciplinary physical, emotional and social care of patients with terminal illness.

Endolymphatic duct A small epithelial-lined channel, part of the membranous labyrinth that passes through the vestibular aqueduct in the bony labyrinth of the petrous temporal bone.

Endometriosis (*en'do-me-tre-o'sis*) A disorder in which fragments of uterine mucous membrane occur in locations outside the uterus.

Endometritis (*en'do-me-tri-tis*) Inflammation of the endometrium.

Endometrium (*en-do-me'tre-um*) The mucous membrane lining the inner surface of the uterus. It increases in thickness during each menstrual cycle and is shed during menstruation.

Endomorphic Having a heavy rounded body build often with a marked tendency to become fat.

Endomyocarditis (*endo-mi"o-kar-di'tis*) Inflammation of the heart muscle and the inner lining of the heart.

Endomysium (*endo-mis'e-um*) Within the fasciculus, each individual muscle cell, called a muscle fiber, is surrounded by connective tissue.

Endoneurium (*en"do-nur'e-um*) A layer of delicate connective tissue around the myelin sheath of each myelinated nerve fiber in the peripheral nervous system.

Endoparasite A parasite living within the body of the host.

Endopeptidase (*en'do-pep'ti-das*) An enzyme which breaks peptide bonds other than terminal ones in a peptide chain.

Endoplasm (*en'do-plaz"en*) The central portion of the cytoplasm of a cell.

Endoplasmic reticulum (ER) Cytoplasm membrane that holds ribosomes.

End-organ Large encapsulated ending of the sensory nerves.

Endorphins (*en-dor'fins*) Endogenous opioid peptides such as endorphin, leu-encephalin, met-encephalin and dynorphin produced in the brain that help in controlling response to pain and stress and improve mood.

Endoscope (*en'do-skop*) Slender tubular lighted viewing instrument to examine the interior of a hollow viscus or a body cavity.

Endoscopic Retrograde Cholangio Pancreatography (ERCP) A procedure in which flexible endoscope is inserted through the ampulla of Vater with the injection of radio contrast material to delineate the bile and pancreatic ducts.

Endosteum (*en-dos'te-um*) The membranous lining of the medullary cavity of a bone.

Endothelin One of several peptides obtained from the vascular endothelium, most powerful vasoconstrictor causing prolonged pressor response, stimulating aldosterone release and inhibition of renin release.

Endothelioma (*en'do-the-le-o'ma*) A tumor originating from the endothelium.

Endothelium (*en'do-the'le-um*) The single layer of flattened cells lining the cavities of the heart, and of the blood and lymphatic vessels and the serous cavities of the body.

Endothermic (*en'do-thermik*) Taking place or being formed by absorbing heat.

Endotoxin Toxin present within the bacterial cell of gram-negative bacteria which is liberated when the microorganism dies and disintegrates. It is a heat-stable lipopolysaccharide which induces release of pyrogens from neutrophils, potentially causing hemorrhagic shock and altering resistance to infection.

Endotracheal tube A narrow plastic tube surrounded by an inflatable cuff that is introduced through the mouth or nose into the trachea to maintain breathing in an unconscious or anesthetized person.

Endourology (*en"do-yur-olo-je*) A minimally invasive technique in which small telescopes and lasers are used to treat tumors, strictures, or congenital anomalies of the bladder, ureter, and kidney.

End-plate A flattened discoid expansion at the neuromuscular junction where a myelinated motor nerve fiber joins a skeletal muscle fiber.

Enema (*en'e-ma*) The introduction of a liquid into the rectum, to stimulate bowel activity.

Air contrast enema An enema in which thick barium sulfate and air are introduced simultaneously to obtain multiple radiographs of the colon.

Barium enema Introduction of barium sulfate to visualize colon.

Cleansing enema An enema containing soap water to empty the colon.

Nutrient enema An enema containing predigested food material.

Retention enema A small amount of solution (100–200 mL) administered to provide medication, which will not stimulate nerve endings.

Enervation A section of a nerve.

Engagement Descent of the fetus head into the mother's pelvis; entry of the fetal head or presenting part into the pelvis prior to delivery.

Engram (*en'gram*) A physical change or memory trace made on the central nervous system of an organism as a result of experience or the repetition of stimuli.

Enophthalmos (*en'of-thal'mos*) A backward displacement of the eyeball into the orbit.

Ensiform cartilage Sword-shaped; xiphoid.

Entamoeba (*en'ta-me'ba*) A genus of amebae. ***E coli*** common non-pathogen of gut ***E. hartmanni*** small ameba related to ***E histolytica*** but nonpathogenic ***E histolytic*** passes its life cycle in one host-human being. Cysts reach intestine where encystation occurs as the wall is digested by trypsin. Some mature and burrow their way into submucosa of large and small intestine and cause amebic ulcers. Some of them enter the portal radicals and reach liver and cause amebic hepatitis with or without ulcer formation. It may rarely metastasize to lungs or brain. Amebae are passed in the stools as cysts.

Enteral (*en'ter-al*) Within, by way of or referring to the small intestine.

Enteralgia (*en"ter-al'je-a*) Pain in the intestines.

Enterectomy (*en'ter-ek'to-me*) Resection of a portion of the intestine.

Enteric (*en'ter'ik*) Relating to the small intestine.

Enteric coated A special coating applied to the tablets whose contents are released only in the intestine; one that is designed to temporarily withstand attack by stomach acid, so that it does not dissolve in the stomach but allows release of the medication in the intestine.

Enteric fever Typhoid and paratyphoid fever.

Enteritis (*en'ter-i'tis*) The inflammation of the intestines.

Enteroanastomosis (*en'ter-o-an-as'to-mo'sis*) Formation of an anastomosis between two portions of the intestine.

Enterobiasis (oxyuriasis) (*en'ter-o-bi'a-sis*) Infestation of the intestines by nematodes of the genus *Enterobius*.

Enterobius (Oxyuris) (*en'ter-o'be-us*) A genus of intestinal nematodes

Enterobius vermicularis Pinworm, thread worm; or seat worm common small nematode of caecum gravid female migrates to anus to lay eggs, which after ingestion hatch in duodenum.

Enterocele (*en'ter-o-sel*) A protrusion of the small intestines and peritoneum into the vaginal canal.

Enterocentesis (*en"ter-o-sen-te'sis*) A procedure that involves puncturing the intestine to withdraw fluid or gas.

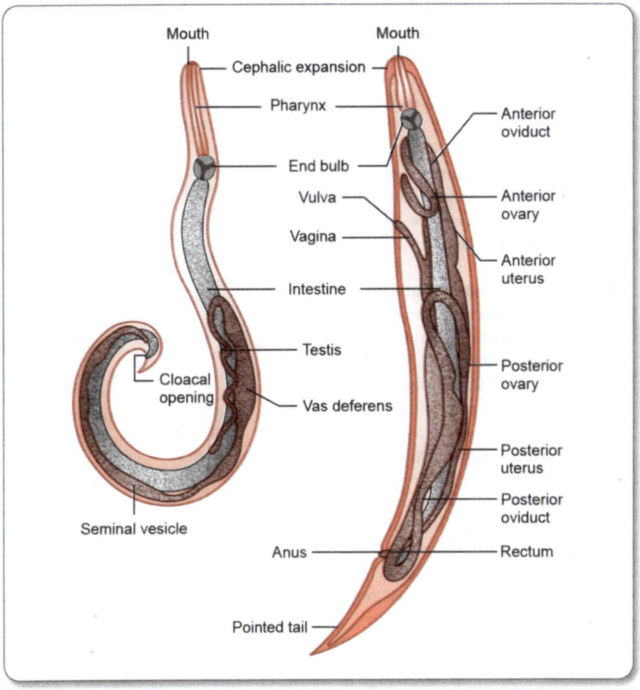

Enterobius vermicularis

Enterocolitis (*en'ter-o-ko-li'tis*) Inflammation of the small intestine and colon.

Enterogastrone (*en'ter-o-gas'tron*) A hormone secreted by the intestinal mucosa which controls the emptying of food from the stomach into the duodenum by depressing gastric motility and secretion.

Enterogenous (*en'ter-oj'e-nus*) Originating within the small intestine.

Enterohepatic (*en'ter-o-he-pat'ik*) Pertaining to the intestines and liver.

Enterokinase An enzyme in the intestinal juice that converts inactive trypsinogen into active trypsin.

Enterolith (*en'ter-o-lith*) An intestinal calculus.

Enteromegaly (*en'ter-o-meg'a-le*) Enlargement of the intestine.

Enteropathy (*en'ter-op'a-the*) Any disease of the intestine.

Enteropeptidase (*en"ter-o-pep'ti-das*) An enzyme secreted from the brush border of the small intestine, also in response to secretin and CCK.

Enteropexy (*en'ter-o-pek'se*) Surgical fixation of the intestine to the abdominal wall.

Enteroptosis (*en'ter-op-to'sis*) Downward displacement of the intestines in the abdominal cavity.

Enterorrhaphy (*en'ter-or'a-fe*) Repair of the intestine.

Enterospasm A painful, intense contraction of the intestine.

Enterostomy (*en'ter-os'to-me*) The making of an artificial opening into the intestine which opens into the abdominal wall.

Enterotomy Surgical incision into an intestine. It is done to remove an obstruction or foreign body from the intestine.

Enterotoxemia (*en"ter-o-tok-se'me-a*) A systemic disease of livestock, caused by intestinal toxins of the bacterium Clostridium perfringens, characterized by diarrhea and convulsions, and usually rapidly fatal.

Enterotoxin (*en'ter-o-tok'sin*) A toxin arising in the intestine; a toxin specific for the cells of intestinal mucosa.

Enterovirus (*en'ter-o-vi"rus*) A virus that enters the body through the gastrointestinal tract and thrives there, often moving on to attack the nervous system; virus infecting the gastrointestinal tract, belonging to genus of picornaviruses which includes polio-, coxsackie- and echoviruses.

Enthesis (*en'the-sis*) The site of attachment of a muscle or ligament to bone.

Enthesopathy Inflammation at the zone of a ligament's insertion into the bone often encountered in HLA-B27-linked ankylosing spondylitis.

Entoptic phenomena Visual perceptions arising from the sources within the eye rather than the outside world.

Entropion (*en-tro'pe-on*) A turning inward of an edge or margin such as eyelid margins.

Enucleation (*e-nu'kle-a'shun*) The removal in *toto* from its enveloping capsule, sac or covering.

Enuresis (*en'u-re-sis*) Involuntary discharge of urine; bed-wetting.

Environment The aggregate of surrounding things; conditions which have influence on existence or development.

Enzootic (*en'zu-t'ik*) An endemic occurring in animals.

Enzygotic (*en"zi-got'ik*) Peculiar to or constantly present in a locality.

Enzyme (*en'-zim*) A complex organic substance having capacity to accelerate or promote chemical changes in a substrate. The examples are oxidoreductases (catalyze oxidation/reduction), transferase (catalyze transfer of one molecular species to another), hydrolase (catalyze hydrolytic cleavage), lyase (catalyze removal or addition of a group to a double bond), isomerase (catalyze intramolecular rearrangement) and ligase (catalyze a reaction that joins two molecules).

Enzyme blocker A drug that inhibits the action of an enzyme.

Enzyme induction Stimulation of increased production of an enzyme.

Enzyme replacement therapy Any of therapeutic modality in which a congenitally defective enzyme is administered, by coupling the enzyme to a carrier molecule or by introducing the gene into the recipient.

Enzyme therapy Supplementation of an enzyme such as streptokinase, tissue plasminogen activator or serine protease.

Restriction enzyme A chemical that snips a specific point on a DNA molecule.

Eosin (*e'o-sin*) A red colored synthetic dye used to stain tissues for microscopic examination.

Eosinopenia (*e'o-sin-o-pe'ne-a*) An abnormal decrease in the number of eosinophils in the blood.

Eosinophil (*e'o-sin'o-fil*) A granular leukocyte with a bilobed nucleus and cytoplasm containing coarse round granules. It forms less than 3% of the circulating leukocytes. There is marked affinity for acidic dyes. The granules in mature eosinophils are heterogeneous in their densities. The core of the granules contains the highly toxic cationic proteins.

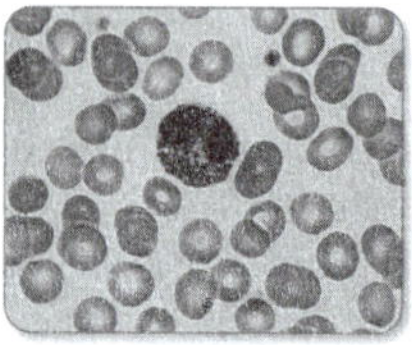

Eosinophil

Eosinophilia (*e'o-sin-o-fil'e-a*) An abnormal increase in the number of eosinophils in the blood and it may develop in a variety of conditions (*see* **Table**).

Eparterial (*ep'ar-te're-al*) Over an artery.

Ependyma (*ep-en'di-ma*) A membrane lining the ventricles of the brain and the central canal of the spinal cord.

Ependymoma (*ep-en'di-mo'ma*) A tumor arising from ependymal cells.

Ephebiatrics (hebiatrics) (*e-fe"be-at'riks*) Branch of medicine that deals especially with the diagnosis and treatment of diseases and problems peculiar to youth.

Ephedrine A sympathomimetic agent, used as a bronchodilator.

EPI- Expanded program of immunization.

Epiblepharon A condition in which the eyelid pretarsal muscle and skin ride over the eyelid margin to form a horizontal fold of tissue that causes the cilia to assume a vertical position.

Epicanthus (epicanthic fold) (*ep"i-kan'thes*) A vertical fold of skin on either side of the nose which sometimes covers inner canthus.

Epicardia (*ep'i-kard'e-a*) The abdominal portion of the esophagus.

Epicardium (*ep"i-kar'de-em*) The inner serous layer of the pericardium on the surface of the heart.

Epicondyle (*ep-i-kon'di'l*) Either of the bony eminences above its condyles at the distal end of the humerus.

Epicranium The soft tissue covering of the cranium.

Epicritic (*ep-i-krit'ik*) Discriminative responsiveness to small variations of touch or temperature stimuli.

Epidemic (*ep'i-dem'ik*) Affecting a large number of persons in a community at the same time suddenly by disease, or specific health-related behavior such as smoking or other health-related events such as traffic accidents.

Epidemic dropsy Contamination of mustard oil with argemone oil. The

Table: Conditions associated with peripheral blood eosinophilia

1. Allergic diseases	• Bronchial asthma • Aspirin-sensitive asthma • Bronchopulmonary aspergillosis • Allergic angiitis and granulomatosis • Atopic dermatitis • Allergic urticaria • Drug hypersensitivity
2. Parasitic infestation	• Tropical pulmonary eosinophilia • Loeffler's syndrome • Helminthic infestations • Visceral larva migrans
3. Respiratory disorders	• Chronic eosinophilic pneumonia • Acute eosinophilic pneumonia
4. Lymphoreticular and neoplastic conditions	• Hodgkin's disease • Chronic myeloid leukemia • Eosinophilic leukemia • Ovarian carcinoma
5. Miscellaneous conditions	• Hypereosinophilic syndrome • Selective IgA deficiency • Addison's disease • Eosinophil-myalgia syndrome

toxic alkaloid, sanguinarine from argemone oil interferes with the oxidation of pyruvic acid which accumulates in the blood. The condition presents with sudden bilateral swelling of legs, diarrhea, dyspnea, glaucoma and cardiac failure. On addition of nitric acid to a sample of oil in the test tube and shaking, there is appearance of brown or orange-red color in the presence of argemone oil.

Epidemic investigation Investigation to define the magnitude of the epidemic outbreak, to determine the factors responsible and to identify the cause, source of infection and modes of transmission, to determine measures to control the epidemic and to make recommendations to prevent recurrence.

Epidemiology (*ep'i-de-me-ol'o-je*) The branch of medical science concerned with the study of the distribution and determinants of health-related states or events in specified populations and the application of this study to control health problem.

Epidermis (*ep'i-der'mis*) The thin outermost nonsensitive nonvascular layer of the skin.

Epidermoid (*ep'i-der'moyd*) Resembling epidermis.

Epidermoid cyst Cyst lined by squamous epithelium.

Epidermoid pearl A compact round cluster of curved and flattened keratinocytes seen in well-differentiated squamous cell carcinoma.

Epidermolysis (*ep'i-der-mol'i-sis*) A loosened state of the epidermis.

Epidermophyton (*ep"i-der-mofi-ton*) A genus of fungi which grows on the epidermis and is responsible for athlete's foot and dhobi itch.

Epidiascope An optical projector, or episcope which is capable of giving images of both opaque and transparent objects.

Epididymis (*ep'i-did'i-mis*) The elongated coiled tube at the back of each testis in which sperms mature, and develop their swimming capabilities.

Epididymitis (*ep'i-did'i-mi'tis*) Inflammation of the epididymis.

Epididymo-orchitis (*ep'i-did'im-o-or-ki'tis*) Inflammation of the epididymis and testis.

Epididymovasostomy (*ep"i-did"-mo-va-sos'to-me*) A complex surgical procedure, also known as Vasoepididymostomy and is done to reverse a vasectomy or treat an obstruction.

Epidural (extradural) Situated upon or outside the dura.

Epidural anesthesia Injection of anesthetic into the epidural spaces to block the nerves for pain relief.

Epidural hemorrhage Bleeding between dura mater and the inner surface of the skull.

Epidural space The space outside the dura mater of the brain and spinal cord.

Epigastrium (*ep'i-gas'tre-um*) The upper and middle portion of the abdomen lying over the stomach.

Epigastrocele (*ep'i-gas'tro-sel*) Hernia of the epigastric region.

Epiglottis (*ep'i-glot'is*) The flap of cartilage structure behind the tongue that covers the entrance to the larynx and helps to prevent food or liquid from being inhaled.

Epiglottitis Inflammation of the epiglottis.

Epilation (*ep-i-la'shun*) The removal of hair by the roots.

Epilepsy (*ep'i-lep'se*) A disorder of the brain caused by abnormal electrical activity, characterized by seizures and is a symptom rather than a disease itself.

Childhood absence epilepsy Frequent and brief loss of consciousness in childhood.

Juvenile absence epilepsy Less frequent loss of consciousness than childhood absence epilepsy.

Juvenile myoclonic epilepsy Generalized tonic-clonic seizures with loss of consciousness and morning myoclonus in the age group of 15–20 years.

Partial epilepsy Partial seizures may arise from any disease of cerebral cortex and frequently generalize. The condition implies presence of focal cerebral pathology.

Primary generalized epilepsy Idiopathic epilepsy with onset in childhood or adolescence. There is no structural abnormality and greater genetic predisposition is present.

Secondary generalized epilepsy Generalized epilepsy may arise from spread of partial seizures. It is due to structural disease or secondary to drugs or metabolic disorders.

Epileptogenic *(ep'i-lep-to-jen'ik)* Producing epileptic attacks.

Epiloia *(ep'i-loy'a)* Tuberous sclerosis.

Epimenorrhagia Too frequent and too excessive menstruation.

Epimenorrhea Abnormally frequent menstruation.

Epimysium *(ep"i-mis'e-em)* The dense connective tissue that surrounds the entire muscle tissue.

Epinephrine (adrenaline) *(ep'i-nef'rin)* Also called adrenaline, a hormone produced by the adrenal glands. It accelerates heart rate and blood flow, improves breathing and helps the body to cope with demands of exercise.

Epineural *(ep'i-nu'ral)* Situated upon a neural arch.

Epineurium *(ep'i-nu're-um)* The connective tissue covering of a peripheral nerve.

Epiphenomenon *(ep'i-fe-nom'e-non)* An accidental occurrence during the course of any disease; an additional condition or symptom in the course of a disease, not necessarily connected with the disease.

Epiphora *(e-pif'o-ra)* An abnormal overflow of tears down the cheeks due to stricture of the lacrimal duct.

Epiphysis *(e'pif'i-sis)* Either of the two growing wider ends of the long bones of the upper or lower extremities.

Epiphysitis *(e-pif'i-si'tis)* Inflammation of an epiphysis.

Epiploon *(e-pip'lo-on)* The omentum.

Epirubicin *(ep"i-roo'bi-sin)* An anthracycline topoisomerase II inhibitor used as an adjuvant to treating axillary node metastases in patients who have undergone surgical resection of primary breast cancer.

Episiotomy *(e-pis'e-ot'o-me)* Planned surgical incision of the perineum to enlarge the vaginal opening for obstetrical purposes during the birth process; surgical incision of the vulva to facilitate childbirth.

Epispadias *(ep'i-spa'de-as)* A congenital defect wherein the urethra opens on the dorsum of the penis, rather than at its tip.

Episioplasty *(e-piz'e-o-plas'te)* Surgical repair of the vulva.

Episiorrhaphy The suturing of the labia majora.

Episiostenosis *(e-piz"e-o-ste-no'sis)* Narrowing of the vulvar opening.

Epispadias *(ep'i-spa'de-as)* A congenital defect wherein the urethra opens on the dorsum of the penis, rather than at its tip.

Epistasis *(e-pis'ta-sis)* A circumstance where the expression of one gene is modified (e.g., masked, inhibited or suppressed) by the expression of one or more other genes.

Epistaxis *(ep'i-stak'sis)* Hemorrhage from the nose; nose bleed.

Epithalamus *(ep'i-thal'a-mus)* The region above and behind the thalamus.

Epithelioma *(ep'i-the'le-oma)* Any tumor derived from epithelium.

Epithelium *(ep'i-the'le-um)* The covering of the internal and external surfaces of the body.

Epitrichium (periderm) The outermost layer of the epidermis in most mammalian fetuses, usually disappearing before birth.

Epituberculosis Collapse of middle lobe occurring from enlarged glands in tuberculosis. The lobe re-expands following subsidence in the size of the glands. It may lead to stricture of the bronchi.

Eponychium *(ep"o-nik'e-um)* The thickened layer of skin at the base of the fingernails and toenails.

Eponym *(ep'o-nim)* Any syndrome, lesion, clinical sign diagnostic or treatment procedure that bears the name of the author who first described the entity or less commonly the name of the index patient in whom the lesion was first described or the place where the disease entity was recognized.

Epoophoron (*epö-ofö-ron*) A vestigial structure consisting of mesonephric tubes associated with the ovary; a remnant of the mesonephric duct that can be found next to the ovary and fallopian tube.

Epstein-Barr virus (EBV) A DNA herpes virus associated with aplastic anemia, infectious mononucleosis, Burkitt's lymphoma, hairy cell leukemia histiocytic sarcoma in renal transplantation and immune compromise, named after MA Epstein, British physician and YM Barr, Canadian physician.

Eptifibatide (*ep"ti-fibe-tid*) A platelet aggregation inhibitor indicated for treatment of acute coronary syndrome (ACS) managed medically or with percutaneous coronary intervention (PCI), and treatment of patients undergoing PCI (including intracoronary stenting).

Epulis (*ep-u'lis*) A growth on the gingiva.

Erb's paralysis Paralysis of the group of shoulder and arm muscles involving the cervical roots of fifth and sixth spinal nerves. The arm hangs down with the hand turned backward, with loss of normal movements, named after Wilhelm Erb, German neurologist.

ERCP Endoscopic retrograde cholangiopancreatography.

Erectile (*e-rek'til*) Ability to erect.

Erectile dysfunction Inability to achieve erection.

Erection Becoming rigid and distended.

Erepsin (*e-rep'sin*) A group of enzymes in the small intestine which catalyze hydrolysis of partially digested proteins.

Erg A human oncogene located in chromosome 21.

Ergocalciferol (*er"go-kal-sif'er-ol*) A synthetically pure form of vitamin D_2 currently used in the prevention and treatment of vitamin D deficiency.

Ergograph (*er-go-graf*) An instrument that records the amount of work done when muscle contracts.

Ergonomics (*er"go-nom'iks*) An applied science concerned with designing and arranging things people use so that the people and things interact most efficiently and safely; called also biotechnology, human engineering, human factors.

Ergonovine (ergometrine) (*er"go-no'vin*) An ergot alkaloid used for the treatment of postpartum hemorrhage and postabortion hemorrhage in patients with uterine atony.

Ergosterol Precursor of vitamin D_3.

Ergot (*er'got*) A fungus whose derivatives are used to make the uterus contract after childbirth or in the treatment of migraine.

Ergotamine An alpha-1 selective adrenergic agonist vasoconstrictor used to treat migraines with or without aura and cluster headaches.

Ergotism (*er'go-tizm*) Poisoning from excess of ergot. It presents with vomiting, abdominal cramps, excessive thirst, profound weakness, diarrhea and dilated pupils.

Erogenous (*er-oj'e-nus*) Arousing erotic feelings.

Erogenous zone Any part of the body, touching or stroking of which can cause sexual excitement.

Erotism (*er'o-tiz"m*) A state of sexual arousal or anticipation.

Erosion (*e-ro'shun*) An eating away; ulcerate.

Erotogenic (*e-ro'to-jen'ik*) Producing erotic excitement.

Erotomania Excessive sexual desire.

Eructation (*e-ruk-ta'shun*) Belching.

Eruption (*e-rup'shun*) Breaking out as in the emergence of a new tooth or the sudden appearance of a skin rash.

Erysipelas (*er'i-sip'e-las*) A contagious disease of skin and subcutaneous tissue with diffuse deepened inflammation due to infection with *Streptococcus pyogenes*. It has an acute onset of fever, malaise, skin lesions with cellulitis, brawny induration and a butterfly rash on the face.

Erysipeloid (erythema serpens) (*er-i-spi'e-loyd*) An infection by microaerophilic gram-positive *Erysipelothrix rhusiopathiae* noted in persons handling animal products. It is associated with sharply-demarcated red maculopapular lesions of the hands.

Erysipelothrix (*er"i-sip'e-lo-thriks"*) Any of several rod-shaped, facultatively anaerobic bacteria of the genus Erysipelothrix, often forming long filaments and occurring as parasites on mammals, birds, and fish.

Erythema (*er'i-the'ma*) Abnormal redness of the skin due to congestion of the capillaries.

Erythema gyratum Dusky red macular itchy rash over face, trunk and limbs noted in lung cancer.

Erythema multiforme A macular eruption with dark red papules, vesicle, on the extremities, which may appear as rings, patches, elevations or figures, occurs as immune reaction to antigens.

Erythralgia (*er'i-thral'je-a*) A condition characterized by pain and redness of the skin.

Erythrasma (*er"e-thraz'ma*) A skin condition caused by the normal skin bacteria Corynebacterium minutissimum.

Erythremia (*er"e-thre'me-a*) A condition characterized by the excess production of red blood cells. *see* Polycythemia vera.

Erythrityl Tetranitrate: A drug used for the treatment of angina pectoris, chest pain caused by reduced blood flow to the heart. It has vasodilator properties.

Erythroblast (*e-rith'ro-blast*) Immature red blood cell, nucleated red cell.

Erythroblastopenia (*e-rith'ro-blas"to-pen'ie-a*) A deficiency in bone marrow erythroblasts.

Erythroblastosis (*e-rith'ro-blas-to'sis*) Erythroblastemia.

Erythroblastosis fetalis A hemolytic disease of newborn characterized by anemia, jaundice, hepatosplenomegaly and edema.

Erythroclasis Fragmentation of the red blood cells.

Erythrocyanosis (*e-rith"ro-si"e-no'sis*) Discoloration on the legs that has a bluish or purple hue.

Erythrocyte (red blood cell) (*e-rith'ro-sit*) Red blood cell or corpuscle.

Erythrocytic (*e-rith'ro-sit'ik*) Pertaining to erythrocytes.

Erythrocytorrhexis (*e-rith"ro-si"to-rek'sis*) Rupture of a red blood cell.

Erythroderma (exfoliative dermatitis) (*e-rith'ro-der'ma*) Abnormal redness of the skin over a wide area.

Erythrodontia (*e-rith'ro-don'she'a*) Reddish brown pigmentation of the teeth.

Erythrogenesis (*e-rith'ro-jen'e-sis*) Production of erythrocytes.

Erythrokeratodermia (*e-rith"ro-ker"a-to-der'me-e*) An autosomal dominant skin disease characterized by transient and variable noninflammatory erythema and hyperkeratosis.

Erythromelalgia (*e-rith'ro-mel'al-gia*) Red, painful extremities.

Erythromycin A macrolide antibiotic that binds to ribosomal subunits of bacteria and suppresses protein synthesis, used in treatment of respiratory infections, and in infections where patient is sensitive to penicillin.

Erythron (*er'i-thron*) The red blood cells and their precursors in the bone marrow.

Erythropenia (*e-rith"ro-pe'ne-a*) The presence of decreased number of erythrocytes in the blood, as occurs in some forms of anemia.

Erythropoiesis (erythrogenesis) (*e-rith'ro-poy-e'sis*) The production of erythrocytes.

Erythropoietin (*e-rith'ro-poy'e-tin*) A hormone that stimulates red blood cell production in the bone marrow. It is a glycoprotein growth factor produced by cells adjacent to the proximal renal tubules in response to hypoxia.

Erythroprosopalgia (*e-rith"ro-pros"o-pal'jea*) A distinctive syndrome of headaches, also known as cluster headache or migrainous neuralgia.

Erythropsia A defect of vision in which objects appear red.

Eschar (*es'kar*) A slough produced by a thermal burn or a corrosive application or by gangrene.

Escharotic (*es"ka-rot'ik*) Producing an eschar, as a medicinal substance.

Escherichia (*esh-er-ik'e-a*) Gram-negative microorganisms of the family Enterobacteriaceae.

Escherichia coli Gram-negative nonspore forming motile bacilli found in the alimentary tract. They are normally nonpathogenic, may be responsible for urinary tract infection.

Esmolol (*es'mo-lol*) A cardioselective beta-adrenergic blocker used for the short-term control of ventricular rate and heart rate in various types of tachycardia, including perioperative tachycardia and hypertension.

Esophageal ulcer A distinct break in the margin of esophageal mucosa, caused by gastroreflux disease or from severe sustained esophagitis from other causes.

Esophagitis (*e-sof"e-ji'tis*) The irritation and inflammation of the lining of your esophagus or food pipe; inflammation of the esophagus secondary to reflux. Typical symptoms are heart burn, retrosternal pain and vomiting.

Esophagocele (*e-sofa-go-sele*) A hernia of the mucous membrane of the esophagus through its walls.

Esophagocoloplasty (*e-sofa-go-ko'lo-plaste*) Excision of a portion of the esophagus and its replacement by a segment of the colon.

Esophagostomy (*e-sofe-got'o-me*) Surgical creation of an artificial opening into the esophagus. Also known as esophagotomy.

Esophagus (*e-sof'a-gus*) Muscular tube connecting the pharynx to the stomach. It is 25 cm long extending from cricopharyngeal sphincter at the level of the sixth cervical vertebra to the gastroesophageal junction.

Barrett's esophagus Metaplasia of the normal squamous epithelium of the esophagus to form columnar epithelium as a consequence of chronic gastroesophageal reflux.

Corkscrew esophagus Classical finding of diffuse esophageal spasm in barium studies reflecting abnormal contractions compartmentalization and curling of esophagus.

Esophagogastroduodenoscopy (*e-sofa-go-gastro-duo-den-osko-pe*) Also known as EGD or upper endoscopy. A procedure that enables the examiner (usually

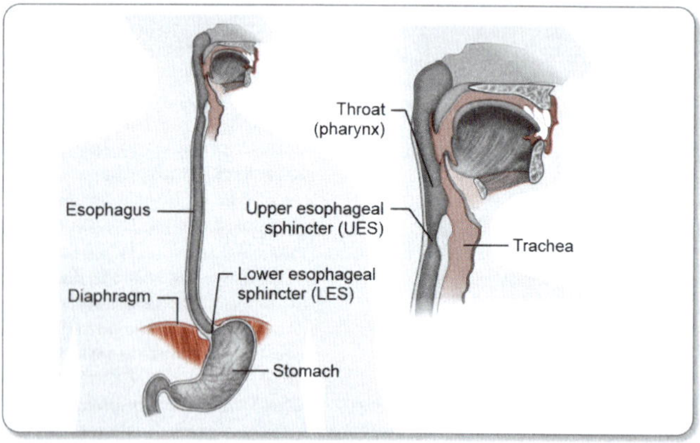

Esophagus in GIT

a gastroenterologist) to examine the esophagus (the swallowing tube), stomach, and duodenum (the first portion of small bowel) using a thin flexible tube (a "scope") that can be looked through or seen on a TV monitor.

Esophagogastrostomy *(e-sofa-go-gastros'to-me)* The surgical formation of an artificial communication between the esophagus and the stomach.

Esophagojejunostomy *(e-sofa-go-je"junos'to-me)* The surgical formation of an artificial communication between the esophagus and the stomach.

Esophagoscopy *(e-sof"e-gos'ko-pe)* Examination of the esophagus by means of an esophagoscope; endoscopic examination of upper gastrointestinal tract.

Esophagostomiasis *(e-sof'a-go-sto-mi'a-sis)* A genus of nematode *oesophagostomum* causing infection of a human or other animals.

Esophoria *(es"o-fo're-a)* A latent tendency for the eyes to turn involuntarily inward.

Esotropia *(es-o-tro'pe-a)* A cross-eye wherein one of the eyes is directed inward.

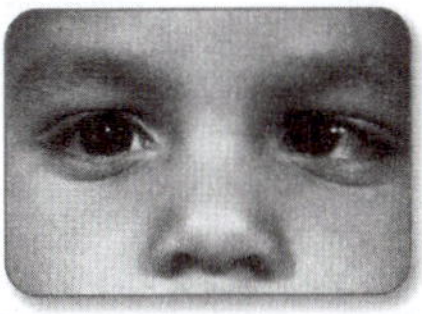

Infantile esotropia

Espundia (mucocutaneous leishmaniasis) Serious clinical form of leishmaniasis that is due to inflammation of upper respiratory passage mucosa.

ESR Erythrocyte sedimentation rate. A test that measures the rate at which red cells in the venous blood mixed with sodium citrate settle to the bottom of a special tube. It is a nonspecific indicator of inflammation. It is raised in collagen vascular diseases, neoplasia anemia, pregnancy and is decreased in polycythemia, microcytosis and in sickle cell anemia.

Essence *(es'ens)* The most significant element, quality, or aspect of a thing or person.

Essential Idiopathic; indispensable.

Essential amino acids A group of eight amino acids—isoleucine, leucine, lysine, methionine, phenylalanine, threonine, tryptophan and valine—that are essential for normal growth and development. A negative nitrogen balance is produced in their absence. Premature infants need histidine, arginine and cystine.

Essential hypertension Primary hypertension where an etiology of hypertension is not established and it accounts for 95% of cases of hypertension.

Essential thrombocythemia Primary myeloproliferative disorder with raised platelet count exhibiting features like polycythemia vera and splenomegaly.

Essential thrombocytopenia Low platelet count with clinically significant bleeding.

Essential amino acid A group of eight amino acids—isoleucine, leucine, lysine, methionine, phenylalanine, threonine, tryptophan and valine—that are essential for normal growth and development. A negative nitrogen balance is produced in their absence. Premature infants need histidine, arginine and cystine.

Essential fatty acid Fatty acids that humans cannot synthesize. They include linoleic acid and linolenic acid.

Esterase *(es'ter-as)* An enzyme that accelerates the hydrolysis or synthesis of esters.

Estradiol *(es-tra'de-ol)* An estrogenic steroid used to treat vasomotor symptoms of vulvar and vaginal atrophy in menopause, hypoestrogenism, prevention of postmenopausal osteoporosis, treatment of breast cancer, and advanced androgen-dependent carcinoma of the prostate.

Estriol (*es'tre-ol*) A weak estrogen used to treat vaginal dryness and estrogen deficiency conditions, such as vaginitis and vulvar itching.

Estrogen (*es'tro-jen*) A female steroid/sex hormone that is produced by the ovaries and, in lesser amounts, by the adrenal cortex, placenta and male testes.

Designer estrogens Substances capable of mimicking estrogen effects at some receptors but not at others.

Estrogen replacement therapy Hormone replacement therapy effective for menopausal symptoms and prevents osteoporosis. It may have benefit for coronary artery disease, with a small increase in risk of breast and endometrial cancer.

Estrone (*es'tron*) A natural estrogenic hormone that is a ketone $C_{18}H_{22}O_2$ found in the body chiefly as a metabolite of estradiol, that is also secreted especially by the ovaries, and that is used to treat various conditions (such as ovarian failure and menopausal symptoms) relating to estrogen deficiency.

Ethacrynic acid (*eth"a-krin'ik*) A diuretic used to treat ascites and edema in congestive heart failure, liver cirrhosis, and renal disease.

Ethambutol (*e-tham'bu-tol*) A synthetic antituberculosis bacteriostatic agent, gets absorbed rapidly and completely on oral administration, attains peak serum concentrations in 2 – 4 hours after ingestion and is excreted essentially through the kidneys, nonallergic and rarely may cause retrobulbar neuritis.

Ethanol (ethyl alcohol) (*etha-nol*) Ethyl alcohol.

Ether (*ether*) Any organic compound in which an oxygen atom links with carbon chains, used as an anesthetic.

Ethical committee A body to ensure protection of the dignity, rights, safety and well-being of the research participants.

Ethinylestradiol An estrogen used in birth control pills in combination with progestins.

Ethionamide (*e-thi'on-am'id*) A potent bactericidal anti-tuberculosis agent, that diffuses well in tissues and CSF. It produces most unpleasant gastrointestinal side effects, used as a reserve drug.

Ethmoidal bone A sieve-like spongy bone that forms the roof of the nasal fossae and part of the floor of the anterior cranial fossa. It permits the passage of olfactory nerves to the brain.

Ethnology (*eth-nolo-je*) The branch of anthropology that deals with the study of the origin and descent of human races and ethnic groups and their distribution and relationships.

Ethnopharmacology (*eth"no-far"ma-kol'o-je*) The study of medicines derived from naturally occurring substances like plants and fungi that have been traditionally used by specific groups of people for medicinal purposes.

Ethopropazine (*eth"o-pro'pa-zen*) An antidyskinetic phenothiazine used to treat the symptoms of Parkinson's disease.

Ethosuximide (*eth"o-suk'si-mid*) An anticonvulsant, $C_7H_{11}NO_2$, used in medicine to treat certain kinds of epilepsy, especially petit mal.

Ethotoin (*eth'o-to"in*) A hydantoin antiepileptic used to control tonic-clonic and complex partial seizures.

Ethylenediamine (*eth'il-en-di'a-men*) An alkane-alpha, omega-diamine in which the alkane is ethane, acts as a GABA agonist. It is derived from a hydride of an ethane, used as a building block for the production of many other chemical products.

Ethynodiol (*e-thi"no-di'ol*) A progestational agent used, as the diacetate salt, in combination with an estrogen component as an oral contraceptive.

Etiology (aetiology) (*e"te-ol'o-je*) The cause or causes of a disease.

Etoglucid A drug used in chemotherapy. It is an epoxide compound.

Etomidate (*e-tom'i-dat*) A short-acting intravenous anesthetic indicated for the induction of anesthesia and supplementation of subpotent anesthesia during short operative procedures.

Etoposide A semisynthetic chemotherapeutic agent obtained from podophyllotoxin. It inhibits nucleoside transport and mitochondrial electron transport. It is active against monocytic leukemia, lymphoma, small cell carcinoma and testicular tumor.

Eubacterium (*u"bak-te're-am*) Any of the bacteria excluding those included in the archaebacteria or the archaea.

Eucalyptol (*u"ke-lip'tol*) Naturally produced cyclic ether and monoterpenoid. Eucalyptol is an ingredient in many brands of mouthwash and cough suppressant. It controls airway mucus hypersecretion and asthma *via* anti-inflammatory cytokine inhibition. Eucalyptol is an effective treatment for nonpurulent rhinosinusitis. Eucalyptol reduces inflammation and pain when applied topically. It kills leukemia cells in vitro.

Euchromatin (*u-kro'ma-tin*) Nuclear chromatin that is maximally uncoiled, seen in interphase.

Eucrasia (*u-kra'se-a*) A state of health.

Eugenics (*u-jen'iks*) The study of hereditary characteristics of future generation through selective breeding.

Eumenorrhea Normal menstruation.

Eupepsia (*u-pep'se-a*) Good digestion.

Euphoria (*u-for'e-a*) A feeling or state of intense elation.

Euplastic (*u-plas'tik*) Readily becoming organized; adapted to the formation of tissue as in embryonic development or wound healing.

Euploidy (*u-ploy'de*) The state of having a balanced set or sets of chromosomes in any number.

Eustachian canal (*u-sta'she-an*) *Tuba audititva*, tube that connects the middle ear cavity to the nasopharynx, 3–4 cm long and lined with mucous membrane, named after an Italian anatomist, Bartolomeo Eustachi.

Euthanasia (*u-tha-na'ze-a*) Mercy killing; painlessly putting to death persons suffering from incurable conditions or diseases.

Direct euthanasia Process of inducing death, often through the injection of a lethal drug.

Indirect euthanasia Process of allowing a person to die by disconnecting life support systems or withholding lifesaving techniques.

Euthyroid (*u-thi'royd*) Normally functioning thyroid.

Evacuator (*e-vak'u-a-tor*) An instrument to remove fluid or small particles from a body cavity.

Evagination (*e-vaj-i-na'shun*) An outpouching of a layer or part.

Eversion (*e-ver'zhun*) A turning outward; a turning inside out.

Evisceration (*evi'ser-a'shun*) Removal of eye contents; extrusion of the viscera or internal organs.

Euvolemia (*u-vo-le'me-a*) The state or condition of having normal volume of blood or fluids in the body.

Evans syndrome A clinical condition characterized by immune thrombocytopenia and autoimmune hemolytic anemia with no known underlying cause, described by Evans and colleagues in 1951.

Evulsion (*e-vul'shun*) Extraction by fork.

Ewing's tumor A cancerous bone tumor affecting children, named after James Ewing, US pathologist.

Exaltation State of extreme happiness.

Exanthem (*ekz-an-the'm*) The eruption; rash. pl. **exanthemata**.

Excavator (*eks'ka-vator*) A form of scoop or gouge for surgical use.

Exchange transfusion A therapeutic procedure to reduce immunotoxins in the neonate, wherein the donated blood is infused in exchange for most of an infant's circulating blood. Exchange transfusion is useful in hemolytic disease of new born and neonatal hyperbilirubinemia.

Excipient (*ek-sip'e-ent*) A vehicle; an inert substance added to make a suitable consistency.

Excise (*ek-siz'*) To cut out entirely.

Excitation An act of stimulation or irritation.

Excoriation (*eks-ko-re-a'shun*) A superficial wound in a body surface by deep scratching.

Excrescence (*eks-kres'ens*) Any abnormal outgrowth.

Excreta (*eks-kre-ta*) Waste product excreted from the body, including feces, urine and sweat.

Excreta disposal Proper disposal of human excreta by sanitary latrines, water carriage system and sewage treatment to prevent soil pollution, water pollution, contamination of foods and propagation of flea.

Excretion (*eks-kre'shun*) The act of elimination of waste products from individual cells, tissues, organs of the body.

Exemestane (*ek"se-mes'tan*) A steroidal aromatase inhibitor that suppresses the synthesis of estrogen, a hormone that acts as a growth factor for breast cancer cells.

Exenteration (*ek-sen"ter-a'shan*) A medical procedure involving an incision with instruments; performed to repair damage or arrest disease in a living body.

Exercise A physical or mental activity undertaken to maintain, restore or increase normal capacity.

Aerobic exercise Submaximal, rhythmic, repetitive exercise of large muscles during which the required energy is supplied by inspired oxygen.

Closed-chain exercise Exercise in which the distal end of the segment is fixed to a supporting surface, as the trunk and proximal segments more over the fixed point.

Eccentric exercise Overall lengthening of the muscle due to tension and contraction to control motion against the resistance of an outside force.

Exercise duration The total number of days, weeks or months during which an exercise program is performed.

Exercise frequency The number of times exercise is performed within a day or within a week.

Exercise induced asthma Exercise can initiate or exacerbate bronchospasm.

Exercise load The amount of weight used as resistance during an exercise.

Exercise prescription Individualized exercise program involving the duration, frequency, intensity and - mode of exercise.

Exercise stress test Monitor the heart rate during vigorous exercise usually while a person walks on a exercise treadmill or rides an exercise cycle.

Isokinetic exercise A form of active-resistance exercise in which the speed of movement of the limb is controlled by a preset rate-limiting device.

Isometric exercise A form of static exercise in which tension develops in the muscle but no mechanical work is performed.

Isotonic exercise A form of dynamic exercise involving concentric or eccentric muscular contractions that result in movement of a joint or body part against a constant load.

Muscle-setting exercise A form of isometric exercise but not performed against any appreciable resistance, and gentle static muscle contractions are used to maintain mobility between muscle fibers and to decrease muscle spasm and pain.

Open-chain exercise Exercise in which a distal segment of the body moves freely in space.

Pendulum exercise Self mobilization technique that uses the effects of gravity.

Progressive resistance exercise An approach to exercise whereby the load or resistance to the muscle is applied by some mechanical means and is quantitatively and progressively increased over time.

Pumping exercise Active repetitive exercise, usually of ankle or wrist, performed to maintain or improve circulation in the extremities.

Resistance exercise Any form of active exercise in which a dynamic or static muscular contraction is resisted by an outside force.

Short-arc extension exercise Active or active-resisted extension of a joint through the final degree of the range of motion, most often applied to the knee from 35° flexion to full extension.

Stabilizing exercise A form of exercise designed to develop control of proximal areas of the body in a stable, symptom-free position in response to fluctuating resistance loads.

Exercise stress test An electrocardiogram that is done while a person exercises on a treadmill or stationary bicycle.

Exflagellation (*eks'flaj-e-la'shun*) Formation of flabelliform gametes.

Exfoliation (*eks'fo-le-a'shun*) A shedding of the scales from a surface.

Exhalation (expiation) (*eks'ha-la'shun*) The act of breathing out.

Exhibitionism Exposure of the body or genitals to attract sexual interest.

Exocrine gland A gland where secretion reaches an epithelial surface either directly or through a duct.

Exocytosis (*eks'o-si-to'sis*) The discharge of particles from a cell.

Exoenzyme (*ek"so-en'zim*) Also known as extracellular enzyme, an enzyme that is secreted by a cell and functions outside of that cell.

Exoerythrocytic (*ek'so-e-rith'ro-si'tik*) Outside the erythrocyte.

Exfoliation (*eks'fo-le-a'shun*) A shedding of the scales from a surface.

Exhalation (expiration) (*eks'ha-la'shun*) The act of breathing out.

Exhibitionism Exposure of the body or genitals to attract sexual interest.

Exocrine gland A gland where secretion reaches an epithelial surface either directly or through a duct.

Exoenzyme (*ek"so-en'zim*) Also known as extracellular enzyme, an enzyme that is secreted by a cell and functions outside of that cell.

Exoerythrocytic (*ek'so-e-rith'ro-si'tik*) Outside the erythrocyte.

Exogenous (*eks-oj'e-nus*) Growth arising from outside the body.

Exomphalos (*eks-om'fa-lus*) Hernia of the abdominal viscera into the umbilical cord.

Exopeptidase (*ek"so-pep'ti-das*) An enzyme that catalyzes the cleavage of the terminal (last) or next-to-last peptide bond from a polypeptide or protein, releasing a single amino acid or dipeptide.

Exophoria (*ek-so-for'e-a*) An outward deviation of the eyes.

Exophthalmic goiter (Graves' disease) Oversecretion of thyroid hormone, characterized by protruding eye balls weight loss and increase in BMR.

Exophthalmometry (*ek"sof-thal-mom'e-tre*) Measurement of the extent of protrusion of the eyeball in exophthalmos.

Exophthalmos (*eks'of-thal'mos*) Abnormal protrusion of the eyeball.

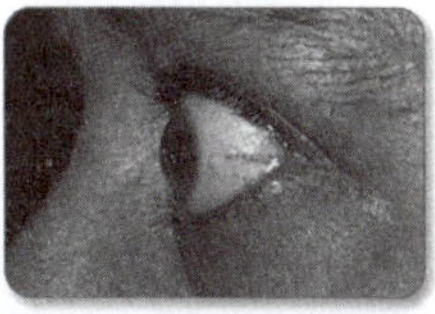

Exophthalmos (bulging eyes) and lid retraction in Grave's disease

Exosmosis (*ek"sos-mo'sis*) Osmosis toward the outside of a cell or vessel.

Exostosis (*eks'os-to'sis*) A bony growth projecting outward from the surface of a bone.

Exothermic (*ek"so-ther'mik*) Involving the release or loss of heat.

Exotic (*eg-zot'ik*) Of foreign origin; diseases which are imported into a country in which they do not otherwise occur.

Exotoxin (*eks'o-toks'in*) A toxic substance formed by a microorganism that is found outside the bacterial cell.

Exotropia (*eks'o-tro'pe-a*) A cross-eye in which one eye is directed outward in relation to the other eye; external squint.

Expectorant (*ek-spek'to-rant*) Agent promoting the coughing up of the secretions.

Expectoration (*ek-spek'to-ra'shun*) Sputum; the act of coughing up and spitting.

Expiration (*eks'pi-ra'shun*) The act of breathing out; death.

Expiratory reserve volume (ERV) Air that can be expired forcibly from the end of tidal expiration.

Explant (*eks-plant'*) To transfer tissue from the body and place it in a culture medium for growth.

Exploration To examine.

Exposure The act of laying open; amount of radiation delivered over a given area.

Exsanguination (*ek-san'gwin-a'shun*) Loss of blood due to hemorrhage.

Exsiccation (*ek"si-ka'shun*) To remove moisture from.

Exstrophy (*eks'tro-fe*) The turning inside out of an organ. It occurs as a developmental defect involving the bladder.

Exsufflation The removal of material from a body cavity (especially lungs) by strongly forced expiration of air.

Extended release (*ek-stend'ad-re-les'*) Designed to slowly release a drug in the body over an extended period of time especially to reduce dosing frequency.

Extension (*eks-ten'shun*) A joint movement to straighten two adjoining bones.

Extensor That which extends.

Extensor muscle Any muscle that produces extension of a joint when it contracts.

Exteriorization To bring out of the body (as for surgery).

Exteroceptor (*eks'ter-o-sep'tor*) A sensory nerve terminal that is stimulated by the immediate external environment.

Extinction Disappearance of a conditioned response.

Extirpation (*eks-tir-pa'shun*) Complete removal.

Extracellular (*eks'tra-sel'u-lar*) Outside a cell or cells.

Extracochlear implant Implantation of hearing aid with electrode in middle ear usually on round window.

Extracorporeal (*eks'tra-kor-por'e-al*) Situated outside the body.

Extract (*eks-trakt*) A concentrated preparation consisting of active constituents.

Extraction Preparation of an extract.

Extractor An instrument for removing foreign bodies.

Extradural (*eks-tra-du'ral*) Situated outside the dura mater.

Extradural anesthesia Injection of an anesthetic into the space in the spinal canal outside the dura mater to cause loss of sensation in part of the body.

Extradural hemorrhage Bleeding from meningeal vessel involved by skull fracture, characteristically there is recovery following injury, clear interval and relapse as hematoma enlarges.

Extraembryonic coelom (exocoelom) Cavity that contains the chorion (in embryo).

Extraocular muscle A muscle attached to the eyeball that controls eye movement and coordination.

Extrapleural Outside the pleural cavity.

Extrapyramidal lesion Lead pipe or cog wheel rigidity, poverty of movement from rigidity, involuntary movements, absence of emotional movements and normal reflexes as in Parkinsonism.

Extrasensory perception (ESP) Perception that occurs independently of the known sensory processes; also known as a sixth sense, and is a claimed paranormal ability.

Extrasystole (*eks'tra-sis'to-le*) A premature contraction of the heart.

Extrauterine (*eks'tra-u'ter-in*) Outside the uterus.

Extravasation (*eks-trav'a-sa'shun*) A discharge from a vessel into the tissues.

Extraversion (*eks"tra-vur'zhan*) An aspect of a personality that is often characterized by expressive and outgoing patterns of behavior.

Extraversion (*eks"tra-vur'zhan*) An aspect of a personality that is often characterized by expressive and outgoing patterns of behavior.

Extrinsic (*eks-trin'sik*) Coming from outside.

Extrinsic allergic alveolitis A hypersensitivity reaction occurring at the peripheral gas exchanging parts of the lungs in response to repeated inhalation of antigens contained in finely particulate organic dust of wide variety and other agents by a susceptible individual.

Extrinsic atopic asthma Commonly seen in children and young adults due to known external allergens. There is an inborn ability to produce reaginic (IgE) antibodies in large amount very easily to substances of every day exposure in life.

Extrovert A person whose interest is turned outward toward external values.

Exudation (*eks'u-da'shun*) The escape of fluid from the blood vessel due to inflammatory, infectious, connective tissue or neoplastic process.

Eye The organ of vision; oculus. It is contained in a bony cavity (orbit) embedded in the orbital fat and innervated by one of a pair of optic nerves. The eyeball consists of three layers: (i) the **inner retina** containing the photo receptors — rods and cones, (ii) the middle uvea consisting of **choroid**, ciliary body and iris and (iii) the outer **sclera and cornea**. It has two cavities: (i) smaller anterior cavity in front of the lens, which is further divided by the iris into an anterior chamber and (ii) a posterior chamber cavity both filled with aqueous (watery) humor. There is a larger posterior chamber behind the lens containing jelly-like vitreous humor. The lens is behind the iris, held in place by the ciliary body and suspensory ligaments. The visible part of the sclera is covered by the conjunctiva, a thin membrane that continues as a lining of the eyelids. The cornea is transparent. Six extrinsic ocular muscles (superior, inferior, medial and lateral rectus muscles and the superior and inferior oblique muscles) move the eyeball in all directions.

Eye cup (*i'kup*) A device for applying eyewash to the eye, consisting of a cup or glass with a rim shaped to fit snugly around the orbit of the eye.

Eye glasses (*i'glas-az*) The lenses of which have been made specifically to match the wearer's defects of vision.

Eye rolling Rhythmic eye movements accompany rotation of the head.

Eye worm *Loa loa.*

Eyeball The globe of the eye.

Eyebrow A transverse elevation at the junction of forehead and the upper eyelid covered by hair.

Eye ground The fundus of the eye.

Eye lash Hair at the edge of the eyelid.

Eyelid Either of the two movable folds that protect the anterior surface of the eyeball.

Eyepiece The lens of the microscope near the eye of the user, that seems to further magnify the image produced by the objective.

Eyestrain (*i'stran*) Also known as asthenopia, caused by long periods of activity involving eye focus that manifests through nonspecific symptoms such as fatigue, pain in or around the eyes, blurred vision, headache, and occasional double vision.

Ezetimibe (*eze-ti'mib*) A selective cholesterol and related phytosterols absorption inhibitor from small intestine.

Ezogabine An antiepileptic agent used as an adjuvant treatment of partial-onset seizures.

F

Fab Fragment antigen binding, refers to either of two segments of the IgE molecule.

Fabry's disease (*fa'brez*) A genetic disorder inherited as a recessive X-linked trait due to deficiency of the lysosomal alpha galactosidase. It results in accumulation of a glycolipid in the kidneys and other organs causing impairment in their function, named after Fabry, German physician.

Face-bow (*fas'bo*) A device to measure the relationship of the maxillae to the temporomandibular joints, which is necessary for the fabrication of dental casts.

Facet (*fas'et*) A small smooth surface of a bone for articulation.

Facial nerve Seventh cranial nerve, a mixed nerve supplying all the muscles of facial expression except levator palpebrae superioris and submandibular and sublingual salivary glands, and carrying taste sensation from the anterior two-thirds of the tongue.

Facies (*fa'she-ez*) Expression or appearance of the face; surface or face of any structure.

Hippocratic facies Sunken eyes and cheeks, parched dry skin, pinched nose; seen in severe dehydration and wasting diseases.

Leonine facies Face with flat nose, thick skin with nodules and thinning of the eyebrows.

Mask-like facies Expressionless and immobile face and infrequent blinking seen in Parkinsonism.

Mongoloid facies Stupid look, epicanthic folds, slanting eyes and broad flat nose seen in Mongolism.

Moon facies Round face with flushed skin, prominent cheeks, acne and hirsutism noted in Cushing's syndrome.

Nephritic facies Pale puffy face, swollen eyelids noticeable more in the morning in acute glomerulonephritis and nephrotic syndrome.

Facelift (*fas'lift*) A plastic surgery to eliminate wrinkles.

Facial (*fa'shel*) Relating to the face.

Facial angle Degree of protrusion of the lower face.

Facial diplegia Bilateral paralysis of various muscles of the face.

Facial paralysis Paralysis affecting muscles of the face.

Facial spasm An involuntary contraction of the facial muscles on one side of the face.

Facial tic Repetitive spasmodic and involuntary contraction of groups of facial muscles.

Facilitation (*fa-sil'i-ta'shun*) Reinforcement of an action or process.

Factitious (*fak'tish-es*) Self-induced; artificially produced.

Factitious dermatitis A skin rash caused by the patient for secondary gain; dermatitis artefacta.

Factitious disorders Conditions characterized by disease symptoms caused by deliberate efforts of a person to gain attention.

Factor (*fak'ter*) A contributory cause; an essential element; a gene; a coagulation factor; physiologically active material.

Facultative (*fak'ul-ta-tiv*) Not obligatory; able to live under different environmental conditions.

FAD (flavin adenine dinucleotide) Flavin adenine dinucleotide.

Faget's sign (*fa'jet*) A constant pulse with a raising temperature as in yellow fever, described by an American physician, Jean Faget.

Fainting Suddenly loosing consciousness for a few seconds.

Falciform ligament Triangular ligament attached to the sides of sacrum and coccyx.

Fallopian tube (oviduct, uterine tube) Either of a pair of funnel-shaped ducts opening at one end into uterus and at the other end at the peritoneal cavity over the ovary, named after an Italian anatomist, Gabriele Fallopio. It serves as a passage for ovum from ovary to the uterus and spermatozoa from uterus toward ovary.

Falloposcopy *(fa-lo-pos'ko-pe)* A micro-endoscopic technique that uses a trans-vaginal approach to visualize human blood vessels from the uterosalpinx ostium to the fimbriae.

Fallot's tetralogy A rare conditon caused by a combination of four heart defects that are present at birth.

Falx (falx cerebri) *(falks)* A sickle-shaped structure. pl. **falces**.

Falx cerebelli A fold of dura mater forming a vertical partition between the hemispheres of the cerebellum.

Falx cerebri A fold of dura mater lying in the longitudinal fissure separating the two cerebral hemispheres.

Falx inguinalis A conjoint tendon forming the origin of the transversus abdominis and internal oblique muscles.

Falx ligamentosa The broad ligament of the liver.

Famciclovir *(fam-si'klo-vir)* A nucleoside analog DNA polymerase inhibitor indicated for the treatment of herpes labialis and genital herpes and the treatment of herpes zoster in healthy and HIV-infected patients.

Familial *(fa-mil'e-al)* A characteristic condition or disease occurring in some families and it is usually but not always hereditary.

Familial disease Follows one of the several possible inheritance patterns: autosomal dominant, autosomal recessive, X-linked recessive, X-linked dominant, polygenic, multifactorial, chromosomal, mitochondrial or non-genetic.

Familial hypercholesterolemia An inherited disorder transmitted as a dominant trait, and characterized by hypercholesterolemia, tendinous xanthomas and early evidence of athero-sclerosis, especially of the coronary arteries.

Familial mediterranean fever An inherited disorder presenting with fever, abdominal pain, chest pain and rash. Some may develop amyloidosis. The disease is self-limited.

Familial megaloblastic anemia Anemia due to the absence of intrinsic factor, with onset in infancy.

Familial periodic paralysis Attacks of flaccid paralysis of limbs often associated with hypokalemia.

Familial polyposis Presence of multiple polyps in the colon and rectum inherited as an autosomal dominant condition and it exhibits high malignancy potential.

Familial spinal muscular atrophy Progressive atrophy of the skeletal muscle from degeneration of anterior horn cells of the spinal cord.

Famotidine *(fam-oti-din)* H_2 receptor blocking antihistamine used to reduce gastric acid.

Fanconi syndrome Inborn defect of transport mechanism in the proximal renal tubule presenting with renal glycosuria, aminoaciduria, proteinuria and excessive urinary losses of phosphate, bicarbonate, potassium and water in various combinations.

Fantasy (phantasy) *(fan'ta-se')* *psy* A mechanism of creating an unusual thing or scene in the mind.

Farad *(far'ad)* Unit of electrical capacitance, the ability of a body to store an electrical charge.

Faradism *(far'a-dizm)* Use of an interrupted current to stimulate muscles and nerves.

Farcy *(fahr'se)* A form of melioidosis that usually affects the skin and lymphatic vessels of horses and mules.

Farmer's lung An allergic alveolitis caused by inhalation of moldy hay containing *Actinomyces micropolyspora* and *Themoactinomyces vulgaris*.

Farsightedness A refractory error wherein the parallel rays come to a focus behind the retina with accommodation completely relaxed. It allows individuals to see distant objects clearly but not near objects; hyperopia.

Fascia *(fashe-a)* Fibrous tissues that enclose and connect the muscles and also the body beneath the skin. pl. **fasciae**.

Deep fascia Fascia enclosing and binding muscles.

Fascia bulbi A thin membranous socket that envelops the eyeball from the optic nerve to the ciliary region and allows the eyeball to move freely.

Superficial fascia Fibrous membranous covering that unites the skin with underlying tissues.

Fasciculation *(fa-sik'u-la-shun)* A localized uncoordinated, uncontrollable muscular twitching; formation of fascicles.

Fasciculus (fascicle) *(fa-siku-lus)* A small bundle of muscles, tendons or nerve fibers.

Fasciitis *(fase-i-tis)* An inflammation of the connective tissue caused by infection, injury or an autoimmune reaction.

Fasciola *(fa-si'o-la)* A genus of flukes belonging to the class Trematodes.

Fasciola hepatica A species of flukes infesting liver; liver fluke miracidia penetrates a fresh water snail and then encysts on water cress before being eaten by sheep or man.

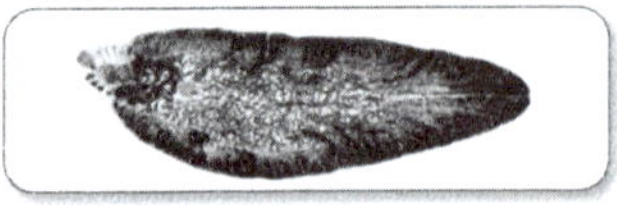

Fasciola hepatica

Fascioliasis *(fase-o-li'a-sis)* Infection with the liver fluke, *Fasciola hepatica*. It presents with upper abdominal pain, fever, chills, hepatomegaly and occasionally jaundice. Eggs are demonstrable in stools. Bithionol is effective in the treatment.

Fascioplasty *(fash-e-o-plas'te)* Plastic surgery of fascia.

Fasciotomy *(fashe-o-tome)* Surgical incision into an area of fascia to relieve pressure on muscles.

Fasciolopsiasis *(fase-o-lop-si'a-sis)* Intestinal infection due to fluke *Fasciolopsis buski* characterized by diarrhea, abdominal pain and anorexia, and treated by praziquantel.

Fasciolopsis *(fase-o-lop-sis)* A genus of trematodes, also known as giant intestinal flukes. Causes pathological condition fasciolopsiasis.

Fastigium *(fas-tije-um)* Summit; highest point in the course of a fever.

FAST Scan Focused assessment with sonography in trauma.

Fat *(fat)* A substance composed of lipids or fatty acids; adipose tissue of the body.

Fat boy syndrome Narcolepsy in obese males, description found in Charles Dicken's novel, Pickwick papers.

Fat embolism Blocking of an artery in the brain by a fat embolus following a fracture of long bone.

Fat necrosis Local breakdown of fat by liberated lipolytic enzymes.

Fatigue *(fa-tig)* A state of exhaustion; loss of ability of tissues to respond to stimuli.

Fatigue fever Occurrence of fever and muscle pain after exhaustion.

Fatigue fracture Any fracture resulting from excessive physical activity.

Fatty acid A hydrocarbon in which one of the hydrogen atoms has been replaced by a carboxyl (COOH) group.

Essential fatty acid An unsaturated fatty acid that cannot be synthesized in the body and is essential to maintain health.

Free fatty acid Nonesterified fatty acid which leaves the cell to be transported for use in another part of the body.

Omega 3 fatty acid Fatty acid used to reduce very low density lipoproteins and chylomicrons in plasma.

Omega 6 fatty acid Linoleic and arachidonic acids.

Saturated fatty acid Acids with single bonds in their carbon chain. It includes palmitic and stearic acids.

Unsaturated fatty acid Acids with one, two or three bonds in the carbon chain. It includes oleic, linolenic, linoleic and arachidonic acids.

Fatty degeneration Deterioration of the cells of the body, accompanied by the formation of fat globules within the diseased cells.

Fauces *(faw'sez)* Space between the mouth cavity and the oral pharynx. It is bounded by the soft palate, base of the tongue and the palatine arches.

Favism *(fa'vizm)* An acute hemolytic anemia caused by ingestion of bean or inhalation of the pollen of *Viscia faba* plant and is seen in persons with an inherited deficiency of the enzyme glucose-6-phosphate dehydrogenase.

Favus *(fa'vus)* A fungal infection of the scalp by *Trichophyton schoenleinii* wherein yellowish crusts occur to callused patches on the scalp.

FDA Food and Drug Administration.

Fear Fright, anxiety resulting from consciously recognized and realistic danger.

Febricula *(feb'ri-cula)* Minor episode of fever.

Febrifuge *(feb'ri-fuj)* An agent that reduces body temperature; antipyretic.

Febrile *(fe'bril)* Feverish.

Febrile convulsions Occurrence of convulsions with fever in the age group of six months to two to three years.

Fecal fistula Fistula between large intestine and exterior.

Fecalith *(fe'ka-lith)* A hard impacted mass of feces, a fecal concretion.

Feces *(fe'sez)* Stools, excreta. It is body waste consisting of food residue, bacteria, mucus and epithelium, discharged from the bowel through the anus. adj. **fecal**.

Feculent vomit Vomiting distinguished by fecal odor noted in late intestinal obstruction.

Feeble-minded Mentally defective who requires care but capable of most simple activities.

Feedback *(fed'bak)* The return of information; influence of the output or result of a system on the input or stimulus.

Negative feedback The result of the process reverses or shuts off the stimulus.

Positive feedback The result of the process intensifies the stimulus.

Fehling's test A test used to differentiate between ketone functional groups and water soluble carbohydrates. It is used to estimate or detect reducing and non-reducing sugars.

Felon *(fel'on)* An extremely painful suppurative abscess involving the distal phalanx of a finger.

Female athletic triad A combination of disorders frequently found in female athletes that includes disordered eating, osteoporosis and oligo- or amenorrhea.

Feminization *(fem'i-ni-za'shun)* The development of female secondary characteristics in the male.

Femoral *(fem'or-al)* Pertaining to femur or thigh bone.

Femoral canal Space behind inguinal ligament between femoral vein and edge of pectineal ligament.

Femoral hernia A protrusion of extraperitoneal fat, peritoneum and occasionally the abdominal contents through the femoral canal; strangulation is more common.

Femoral ring Upper end of the femoral canal. It is bounded anteriorly by the inguinal ligament, posteriorly by pectineus, medially by the concave margin of lacunar ligament and laterally by septum separating it from femoral vein.

Femoral vein Continuation of the popliteal vein toward the external iliac vein.

Femoral artery Artery that begins at the external iliac artery and ends behind the knee as the popliteal artery.

Femoral nerve Nerve in thigh that supplies skin on the upper thigh and inner leg and the muscles that extends the knee. It is largest branch of lumbar plexus.

Femoral triangle (scarpa's triangle) A triangular depression on the front of upper third of the thigh immediately below the inguinal ligament bounded laterally by the sartorius, medially by the adductor longus and inguinal ligament forms the base.

Femur (thigh bone) *(fe'mer)* Thigh bone which extends from the pelvis to the knee and is the longest and strongest bone in the skeleton.

Fenestra *(fen-es'tra)* Window-like; an aperture often closed by a membrane.

Fenestra cochleae The round opening leading into the cochlea, closed by secondary tympanic membrane.

Fenestra ovale Fenestra vestibuli.

Fenestra rotunda Fenestra cochleae.

Fenestra vestibuli An oval opening on the inner wall of the middle ear holding foot of stapes leading to vestibule.

Fenestration *(fen'es-tra'shun)* A surgical procedure wherein an opening is created to gain access to a cavity within an organ or a bone.

Fenfluramine *(fen'floor'e-men)* An amphetamine analog that acts to release serotonin and, to a lesser extent, dopamine from nerve terminals in the brain.

Fenoprofen *(fen"o-pro'fen)* An anti-inflammatory analgesic used to treat mild to moderate pain in addition to the signs and symptoms of rheumatoid arthritis and osteoarthritis.

Fentanyl *(fen'ta-nal)* A synthetic opioid that is up to 50 times stronger than heroin and 100 times stronger than morphine.

FER Forced expiratory ratio.

Fermentation *(fer'men-ta'shun)* An oxidative decomposition of complex substance by the action of enzyme or ferments produced by bacteria, molds and yeast.

Fernandez reaction Rapid erythematous response to lepromin.

Ferritin *(fer'i-tin)* A form in which iron is stored in the tissues of the body. It is an iron-phosphorous-protein complex.

Fertility rate Live births per 1000 women between 15 and 44 years.

Fertilization *(fer'ti-li-za'shun)* The union of male and female gametes to form a zygote from which the embryo develops.

In vitro fertilization (IVF) Technique enabling pregnancy in infertile women. Following drug-induced follicle-maturation, a sample of ova and follicular fluid is removed and mixed with the partner's sperm and incubated. The resulting zygote is introduced into the woman's uterus for implantation.

Festination *(fes"ti-na'shan)* An involuntary quickening of gait.

Fetal surgery An operation performed to correct defects before an infant is born.

Fetal alcohol syndrome A cluster of birth defects that includes abnormal facial features and mental retardation caused by the mother's consumption of alcoholic beverages during pregnancy.

Fetishism *(fet'ish-izm)* Erotic stimulation following contact with non-living objects such as dress or a braid of hair.

Fetography *(fe'to-graph-e)* X-ray of fetus following intra-amniotic injection of lipid-soluble contrast medium.

Fetor *(fe'tor)* Very offensive odor.

Fetor hepaticus Musty odor due to mercaptans from excess circulating methionine encountered in hepatic coma.

Fetor oris Halitosis.

Fetoprotein *(fe'to-pro'ten)* A fetal protein and it may be found in adults.

Fetoscopy A procedure to observe fetus inside the uterus using a fetoscope.

Fetus *(fe'tus)* The developing human form in uterus from the end of the eighth week after fertilization until birth.

Fetus-in-feto Rudimentary twin born as appendage attached to otherwise normal infant.

Fetus papyraceous Remains of death of one twin early in monovular pregnancy being flattened against membranes.

Feulgen reaction/staining Used for the quantitative determination by DNA.

Fever (pyrexia) *(fe'ver)* An abnormal elevation of the body temperature to above 37.7°C in a resting person; pyrexia.

Continuous fever Temperature remains elevated for many days without showing much fluctuation as in typhoid, urinary tract infection, subacute infective endocarditis and brucellosis.

Drug fever Prolonged fever 1–3 weeks after starting of a drug.

Filarial fever Acute episodic adenolymphangitis in filariasis.

Fever of unknown origin An illness associated with prolonged fever whose diagnosis is not established after one week of hospital investigation.

Intermittent fever Temperature rises to a variable height and touches normal level for several hours daily as in malaria, sepsis and abscess.

Irregular fever Temperature exhibiting marked variability.

Jail fever Epidemic louse-borne typhus.

Quartan fever Paroxysm of intermittent fever noted on every fourth day.

Quotidian fever Paroxysm of intermittent fever noted on every day.

Relapsing fever Febrile state for several days alternating with variable periods of apyrexia as in Hodgkin's disease, relapsing fever, dengue fever and brucellosis.

Remittent fever Temperature exceeding 2°C in a day without touching normal as in tuberculosis, malaria or sepsis.

Rose fever Allergic rhinitis.

Saddle back fever Initial fever of 2–3 days, then a remission for 2 days followed by reappearance of fever as in dengue fever.

Tertian fever Paroxysm of intermittent fever noted every third day.

Undulant fever Brucellosis.

War fever Epidemic louse-borne typhus.

Fiber *(fi'ber)* A thread-like element; an elongated thread-like structure; a slender cellulose structure.

Afferent fiber A nerve fiber carrying sensory impulses from receptors in the periphery to CNS.

Circular fiber Collagen bundles surrounding a tooth.

Dietary fiber The food components such as cellulose, hemicellulose, lignin and pectin that resist chemical digestion.

Efferent fiber A nerve fiber carrying motor impulses from CNS to effector organ.

Motor fiber Axons of motor neurons innervating skeletal muscles.

Muscle fiber A muscle cell found in striated, smooth and cardiac muscle.

Myelinated fiber A nerve fiber whose axon or dendrite is surrounded by a myelin sheath.

Nerve fiber A neuron.

Postganglionic fiber The axon of a postganglionic neuron that passes from an autonomic ganglia to a visceral effector.

Purkinje fiber Any of the atypical muscle fibers lying beneath the endocardium. It is part of impulse-conducting system of the heart.

Unmyelinated fiber A nerve fiber that lacks a myelin sheath.

Fiber optics The science of transmitting data, voice and images by the passage of light through thin, transparent fibers. Used in fiberoscopes like endoscopy.

Fiberoscope *(fi'ber-skop)* A flexible instrument having an inner shaft combined with light conveying thin, flexible fibers to visualize internal structures.

Fibril *(fi'bril)* A small fiber; a very small filamentous structure.

Fibrillation *(fi'bril-a'shun)* Involuntary recurrent inefficient contraction of muscle fibers; formation of fibrils.

Atrial fibrillation Arrhythmia wherein the atria beat rapidly, chaotically and ineffectively. Ventricles respond at irregular intervals resulting in an irregularly irregular pulse.

Ventricular fibrillation Arrhythmia producing rapid ineffective uncoordinated movement of ventricles, failing to produce a pulse. ECG shows chaotic, bizarre, irregular complexes.

Fibrin *(fi'brin)* An insoluble protein produced by action of thrombin on fibrinogen. It helps to plug and seal damaged blood vessels.

Fibrin degradation product Substance produced when plasmin lyses either fibrin or fibrinogen.

Fibrin split products The materials produced when fibrin in a blood clot is digested by plasmin.

Fibrinogen *(fi-brin'o-jen)* A plasma protein essential for blood clotting which is converted into fibrin by thrombin in the presence of calcium ions.

Fibrinogenopenia *(fi-bri"no-jeno-penia)* A deficiency of fibrin or fibrinogen or both in the blood.

Fibrinokinase Direct fibrinogenolytic enzymes which degrade fibrinogen into small fragments, rendering it unclottable by thrombin.

Fibrinolysin *(fi"bri-no-l'e-sin)* A proteolytic enzyme, produced in the blood from plasminogen, resulting in the breakdown of the fibrin in blood clots.

Fibrinolysis *(fi'brin-ol'i-sis)* A process of decomposition of fibrin.

Fibroadenoma *(fi'bro-ad'e-no'ma)* A benign tumor composed of dense epithelial and fibroblastic tissues.

Fibroblast *(fi'bro-blast)* Spindle-shaped undifferentiated cell in the connective tissue.

Fibroblastoma *(fi'bro-blas-to'ma)* A tumor derived from a fibroblast.

Fibrocartilage *(fi'bro-kahr'ti-laj)* A proportional mixture of cartilaginous and fibrous tissues, they are tough, very strong tissues found predominantly in the intervertebral disks and at the insertions of ligaments and tendons.

Fibrochondritis *(fi'bro-kon-dri'tis)* Inflammation of fibrocartilage.

Fibrocollagenous *(fi"bro-ko-laj'e-nus)* Comprising fibrous and collagenous components or substances; made up of fibers and collagen.

Fibrocystic disease of the pancreas A chronic debilitation of infancy and early life, characterized by disordered pancreatic function and chronic infections of the lung.

Fibrocyte *(fi'bro-sit)* Cells of hematopoietic origin directly contribute to tissue fibrosis in the body by producing collagen after injury, during disease, and during aging.

Fibroidectomy *(fi'broid-ek'to-me)* Also known as myomectomy, an operation to remove fibroids while preserving the uterus.

Fibrodysplasia *(fi'bro-dis-pla'se-a)* Abnormal development of fibrous tissues.

Fibroelastosis *(fi"bro-e"las-to'sis)* Persistent and increased thickening within the muscular lining.

Fibroepithelial polyp Benign tumors that usually occur in skin folds, such as axille, genital area or neck.

Fibroid *(fi'broyd)* A growth of muscular and fibrous tissues.

Fibroma *(fi'bro'ma)* A benign tumor made up of muscular and fibrous tissues growing in the wall of uterus.

Fibromyoma *(fi"bro-mi-o'ma)* Benign tumors that grow in the uterus.

Fibromyxosarcoma *(fi"bro-mik"so-sar-ko'ma)* A rare form of cancer that originates in connective tissues, starting in the arms and legs, but spreads into healthy tissues elsewhere in the body.

Fibronectin *(fi'bro-nek'tin)* An extracellular glycoprotein that exists in a soluble form in body fluids and in an insoluble form in extracellular matrix.

Fibroplasia *(fi'bro-pla'se-a)* Production of fibrous tissues as in wound healing.

Fibrosarcoma *(fi'bro-sar-ko'ma)* A sarcoma that contains connective tissues.

Fibrosis *(fi'bro'sis)* A proliferation of fibrous connective tissues.

Pulmonary fibrosis The lung tissue is replaced by fibrous tissue which may be the result of inflammatory processes.

Fibrositis *(fi'bro-si'tis)* An inflammation of fibrous connective tissue.

Fibroxanthoma *(fi"bro-zan-tho'ma)* An uncommon, pleomorphic, spindle cell cutaneous malignancy that most commonly presents as a solitary red or pink papule or nodule on the head or neck.

Fibrous dysplasia A chronic problem in which scar like tissue grows in place of normal bone.

Fibula *(fib'u-la)* The lateral long thin bone of the leg extending from the knee to the ankle articulating above with the tibia and below with the tibia and talus.

Field *(feld)* A specific area in relation to an object.

Field block Local anesthesia by infiltration of an anesthetic agent around a relevant area.

Field fever A form of leptospirosis occurring in agricultural workers.

High power field The portion of an object seen through the high-magnification lens of a microscope.

Low power field The portion of an object seen through the low magnification lenses of a microscope.

Field of vision The entire area that a person or animal is able to see when their eyes are fixed in one position.

FIGLU test (Formiminoglutamic acid) Used to identify vitamin B_{12} deficiency, folate deficiency and liver failure or liver disease.

Figo staging (Federation of gynecology and obstetrics) staging for cervical, cancer is based on the cancer's size, location and spread.

Filament A fine thread-like fiber.

Filaria *(fil-a're-a)* Nematode worm, examples are *Dracunculus medinensis, Loa loa* and *Wuchereria bancrofti.* pl. **filariae**, adj. **filarial**.

Filariasis A disease caused by filaria or microfilaria in the tissues of the body. The condition may remain asymptomatic with circulating microfilaria, or present with acute form exhibiting lymphatic inflammation with streaky tender lymphangitis and enlarged tender lymph nodes or chronic form with lymphatic obstruction resulting in lymphedema, hydrocele, and elephantiasis of the limbs.

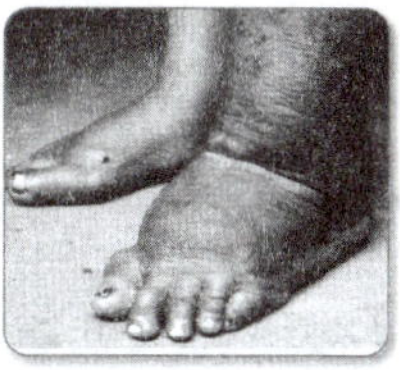

Filariasis

Filiform *(fil'i-form)* Having the form of a thread.

Filling *dent* Dental material that occupies the space remaining within a tooth after the decayed portion has been removed.

Filum *(fi'lum)* A thread-like structure; filament.

Fimbria *(fim'bre-a)* Border resembling a fringe-like structure.

Fimbriectomy *(fim"bre-ek'to-me)* A surgical procedure to remove the fimbrial and infundibular portions of the fallopian tube.

Fimbrioplasty *(fim'bre-o-plas"te)* A procedure that restores the integrity of the fallopian tubes, allowing infertile women to become pregnant.

Finger *(fing'gar)* One of the five digits of the hand.

Finger spelling A method of communication wherein the words are spelled out letter by letter and it is used by persons with impaired hearing.

Finger splint A padded strip of malleable metal used to immobilize a fractured finger.

Finger stick A technique for collecting a very small amount of blood from the fingertip region.

Mallet finger The terminal phalanx cannot be extended because insertion of the extensor tendon is torn.

Webbed finger Syndactylism where two or more fingers are webbed, which may involve skin, fibrous or bony region.

Whale finger Erysipeloid cellulitis of the fingers and hand due to infection from Erysipelothrix rhusiopnthiae.

Fingerprint An imprint made by the cutaneous ridges of the fleshy portion of the distal end of a finger.

First aid The immediate care that is given to an injured or ill person before treatment by medically trained person.

First intention healing Healing that occurs when wound edges are held or sutured together without the formation of granulation tissue.

First pass effect Drug effectively removed or inactivated in one passage through the liver.

Fish skin disease A skin disease characterized by increased horny layer and decreased secretions; ichthyosis.

Fission *(fish'un)* Process of splitting.

Fissure *(fish'ur)* A long, deep, narrow space in a surface; groove or a cleft on a body surface.

Fissure sealant A protective layer applied to the fissures in your teeth to prevent tooth decay.

Fistula *(fis'tu-la)* An abnormal passage from an internal organ to the body surface or between two internal organs.

Anal fistula A fistula near the anus; fistula in a'no.

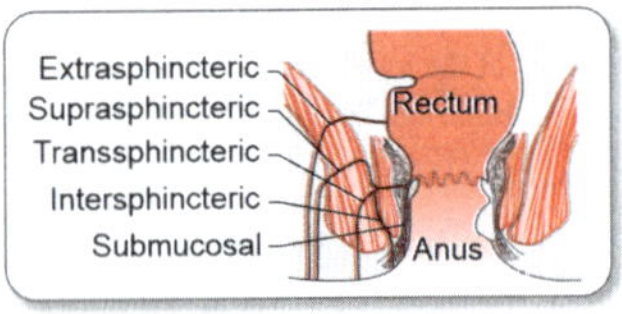

Anal fistula

Arteriovenous fistula A fistula between an artery and a vein.

Biliary fistula A fistula through which bile is discharged after an operation.

Blind fistula A fistula that is open at one end only.

Bronchopleural fistula An abnormal communication between the pleural space and a bronchial tube.

Caroticocavernous fistula Presence of pulsations and continuous bruit over the eyeball.

Cervical fistula An abnormal opening into uterine cervix.

Fecal fistula A fistula in which there is discharge of feces through the opening.

Fistula-in-ano Anterior fistula communicates directly with anal canal and the posterior fistula is always horseshoe in type entering the anal canal in the midline.

Horseshoe fistula A perianal fistula in which the tract goes around the rectum and communicates with the skin at one or many points.

Parotid fistula A fistula from the parotid gland to the skin surface.

Pilonidal fistula A fistula resulting from a pilonidal cyst.

Thyroglossal fistula A midline fistula above thyroid gland. The tract connects the skin to a persistent embryonic thyroglossal duct.

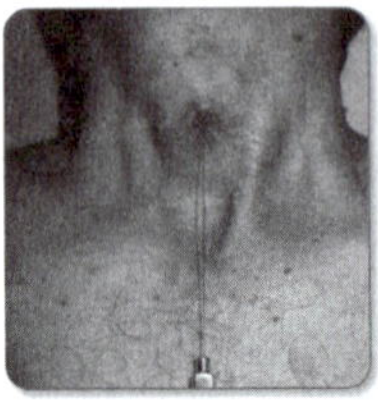

Thyroglossal fistula

Umbilical fistula A fistula between the umbilicus and gut due to nonclosure of the urachal duct.

Ureterovaginal fistula A fistula between the ureter and the vagina.

Vesicovaginal fistula A fistula between the bladder and vagina.

Vesicouterine fistula A fistula between the bladder and the uterus.

Fit Seizure; sudden attack of convulsion; a paroxysm; physical strength.

Fixation The act of holding in a rigid position; immobility; making the material adherent to the slide before staining; making a film-recorded image permanent.

Fixative (fixing agent) *(fi-k'sa-tiv)* A substance that makes rigid; a substance used to prepare microscopic slides or to preserve specimens.

Flaccid *(flak'sid)* Weak; soft.

Flaccid paralysis Paralysis marked by loss of muscle tone, loss of tendon reflexes, atrophy and degeneration of muscles due to lesions of lower motor neurons of the spinal cord.

Flagellate Protozoa of class Flagellata such as Giardia, Trichomonas; male gamete of malarial parasite.

Flagellum *(fla-jel'am)* A slender, hair-like structure composed of a complex arrangement of multiple proteins, lipids and other molecular components. Flagella are appendages responsible for propulsion and movement.

Flap *(flap)* A mass of partially detached tissue of an adjacent area; an uncontrolled movement.

Flap graft Whole skin grafts including subcutaneous tissue transferable as free grafts.

Tissue flap Section of tissue detached from its blood supply, moved to another part of the body and reattached by microsurgery to new blood supply pedicle of a section of tissue with its blood supply intact, which is maneuvered to another part of the body.

Flare *(flar)* A flush.

Nasal flare Dilatation of the nostrils during inspiration.

Flashback *psy* A recurrence of a memory, feeling or perceptual experience from the past.

Flat foot Abnormal flatness of the sole and the arch of the foot.

Flatulence *(flat'u-lens)* The presence of an excessive amount of air or gas in the stomach and intestine.

Flatus *(flat'us)* Air or gas in the intestine that is expelled.

Flatus tube A tube passed into the rectum to evacuate gas from the lower bowel through the anus. This is done to relieve intestinal flatulence.

Flat worm A worm belonging to the phylum Platyhelminthes.

Flavin *(flavin)* A ketone that forms the nucleus of certain natural yellow pigments like riboflavin.

Flavin adenine dinucleotide A coenzyme form of vitamin B_2 used in clinical conditions associated with vitamin B_2 deficiency.

Flavonoid *(fla'va-noid)* Any of a class of non-nitrogenous biological pigments, water-soluble phenolic compounds (having a –OH group attached to an aromatic ring) and are found in the vacuoles of plant cells.

Flea *(fle)* A small wingless, bilaterally compressed blood-sucking insect with a hard chitinous exoskeleton and covered with backwardly directed strong bristles, acts as a vector of bubonic plague and rickettsial disease.

Flea index The average number of fleas of all species per rodent.

Flexion *(flek'shun)* Bending or the condition of being bent, especially bending of a limb or joint.

Flexor *(fleks'or)* A muscle that brings two bones closer together.

Flexor spasm Involuntary painful flexion of the lower extremities in presence of spinal cord lesions.

Flexure *(flek'sher)* A fold or bend.

Floccillation *(flok'si-la'shun)* An aimless plucking at the bed clothes; carphologia.

Flocculation *(flok'u-la'shun)* Precipitation as fluffy particles.

Flocculus *(flok'u-lus)* A small size cerebellum lobe at the posterior border of the middle cerebellar peduncle anterior to the biventer lobule.

Flooding *(flud'ing)* An overflowing of water onto land that is normally dry.

Floppy infant Infant with poor muscular tone and/or response to stimulation of extremities caused by a variety of neuromuscular and musculoskeletal disorders.

Floppy valve syndrome Mitral valve prolapse.

Intestinal floppy valve syndrome Bacteria present in the intestines.

Flow cytometry A lab test used to analyze characteristics of cells or particles.

Flowmeter *(flo'me-ter)* A type of flow instrument that is used to indicate the amount of liquid, gas, or vapor moving through a pipe or conduit by measuring linear, non-linear, mass, or volumetric flow rates.

Floxuridine *(floks-ur'i-den)* An antimetabolite used as palliative management for liver metastases of gastrointestinal malignancy.

Fluctuation test A physical sign to demonstrate fluid in the knee joint. The knee is kept in extension and suprapatellar pouch is squeezed with the left hand toward knee joint and kept pressed. The sides of the joint are held between the thumb and index finger of the right hand. When they are pressed firmly an impulse is felt by the left hand in the presence of fluid.

Fludrocortisone Synthetic mineral corticosteroid, active orally.

Fluke *(fluk)* A parasitic worm belonging to the class Trematoda phylum Platyhelminthes; flatworm.

Flunisolide *(flu-nis'o-lid")* A corticosteroid often prescribed as treatment for allergic rhinitis.

Fluocinonide *(flu"-sin'o-nid)* A potent topical glucocorticoid used as an anti-inflammatory agent for the treatment of skin disorders such as eczema and seborrheic dermatitis.

Fluorescein staining Used to demonstrate loss of corneal epithelium. On instillation of a drop of 2% solution of fluorescein into the eye, the area devoid of epithelium takes a green stain.

Fluorescence *(flor-es'ents)* The light emitting property of certain substances when exposed to certain types of light radiation, usually ultraviolet light.

Fluorescence in situ hybridization (FISH) A molecular cytogenetic technique used as a diagnostic test in chronic myeloid leukemia and acute promyelocytic leukemia; a laboratory technique for detecting and locating a specific DNA sequence on a chromosome.

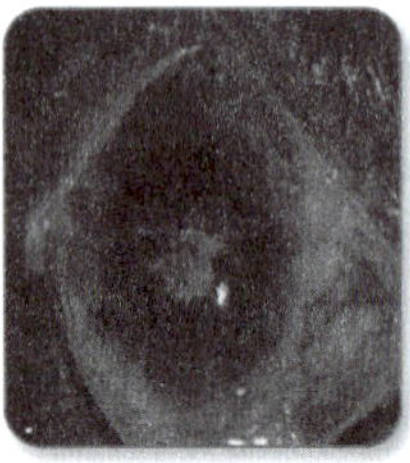

Fluorescence staining of epithelial keratitis after cataract surgery

Fluorochrome *(flur'o-krom)* Chemical molecules that have the ability to absorb light of a certain wavelength and then re-emit light at a longer wavelength.

Fluoridation *(flu'or-i-da'shun)* Addition of small amounts of fluoride to drinking water to reduce occurrence of cavities in the teeth.

Fluorometry *(flu-rom'e-tre)* A method of identifying and analyzing samples based on the light absorbed and then emitted from a sample.

Fluoride *(flor'-id)* A mineral that helps in mineralization, development and function of bones and teeth.

Fluoroscope *(flu'or-o-skop)* An instrument for visual observation of the body by X-ray.

Fluorosis *(flu-or-o'sis)* Excessive ingestion of fluorine and its compounds resulting in mottled, pitted enamel of tooth, chalky white discolored teeth and osteosclerosis.

Dental fluorosis Excess fluoride combines with calcium to form calcium fluorapatite making the teeth to become hypoplastic and later brown discoloration.

Skeletal fluorosis Excess deposition in the bones causes hyperostosis and irregular new bone formation along the attachment of ligaments, muscles, joint capsules and interosseous ligaments. There can be compressive radiculomyelopathy. The bones give a structureless marble white appearance.

Fluorouracil Pyrimidine antimetabolite, blocking DNA synthesis used in the treatment of cancer.

Fluoxetine *(flu-ok'sa-ten)* A selective serotonin reuptake inhibitor used to treat major depressive disorder, bulimia, OCD, premenstrual dysphoric disorder, panic disorder, and bipolar I.

Fluphenazine *(flu-fen'a-zen)* A trifluoro-methyl phenothiazine derivative intended for the management of schizophrenia and other psychotic disorders.

Flurazepam *(flu-raz'a-pam)* A benzodiazepine used for insomnia.

Flurbiprofen *(flur-bi'pro-fen)* A nonsteroidal anti-inflammatory drug (NSAID) used to relieve symptoms of arthritis (osteoarthritis and rheumatoid arthritis), such as inflammation, swelling, stiffness and joint pain.

Flush *(flush)* Blush, sudden redness of the skin, irrigation of a cavity with water.

Hot flush Flush accompanied with a sensation of heat, noted during menopause or neuroses.

Malar flush A bright flush over the malar region and cheek seen in febrile diseases and mitral stenosis.

Fluspirilene Antipsychotic drug used in schizophrenia; it is administered intramusculary.

Flutter Tremulousness; rapid abnormal but rhythmic contractions.

Atrial flutter Rapid atrial contraction due to intra-atrial reentry; ECG a regular undulating baseline (flutter or F waves) resulting in a saw-tooth appearance. They appear at a regular rate of 250–350 min.

Diaphragmatic flutter Rapid contraction of the diaphragm.

Flutter fibrillation Flutter waves exhibiting some irregularity.

Ventricular flutter Ventricular contractions of the heart at 250 per minute.

Flux *(fluks)* An excessive flow or discharge from an organ or cavity of the body.

FMN (flavin monoucleotide) Flavin mononucleotide.

Foam test The presence of bile is recognized by shaking the freshly voided urine. The froth gives yellow color in the presence of bile pigment.

Focal distance The distance between the plane of the sensor and the optical center or nodal point of the lens.

Focus Site of convergence or divergence of rays; local small area of infection; any visible small patch of lesion.

Folic acid (pteroylglutamic acid) *(fo'lik)* A member of vitamin B complex, essential in synthesis of amino acids and DNA and red cell maturation, whose deficiency results in megaloblastic anemia.

Folie a deux (communicated insanity) Communicated emotional illness between two persons.

Folinic acid (leucovorin) An active form of folic acid.

Folium *(fo'le-am)* One of the leaflike subdivisions of the cerebellar cortex.

Follicle *(fo'le-kel)* A small pouch-like depression or cavity.

Follicle-stimulating hormone (FSH) Hormone produced by the anterior pituitary in response to gonadotropin-releasing hormones (GnRH) from the hypothalamus. FSH plays a role in sexual development and reproduction in males and females.

Folliculitis *(fo-lik'u-li'tis)* Inflammation of hair follicle.

Fomentation *(fo'men-ta'shun)* A warm application.

Fonazine Antihistamine used to treat allergies such as hay fever; given orally sick effects include nausea, dry mouth, drowsiness, stomach pain, vertigo, diarrhea, mild headache.

Fontanel *(fon'ta-nel)* A soft membrane covering the space at the junction of the sutures on a baby's skull.

Food poisoning Occurrence of rapid onset of vomiting, profuse watery diarrhea and abdominal pain after ingestion of preformed bacterial toxins produced by *Staphylococcus aureus, Clostridium perfringens* type A and *Bacillus cereus* and organic and inorganic chemicals.

Foramen *(for-a'men)* A natural opening.

Aortic foramen Hiatus aorticus

Epiploic foramen Foramen omentale.

Jugular foramen The opening formed by the jugular notches on the temporal and occipital bones, for the transmission of various veins, arteries, and nerves.

Forceps *(for'seps)* An appliance to hold, treated both singular and plural.

Forebrain (prosencephalon) *(for'bran)* Region of the developing vertebrate brain.

Foregut *(for'gut)* The cephalic portion of embryonic alimentary tract.

Forensic medicine Branch of medical discipline which deals with the application of medical knowledge to the administration of law, branch of medical science dealing with legal aspects of health care.

Forequarter amputation A surgical procedure in which the upper extremity and a variable portion of the supporting shoulder girdle are amputated as in malignancy.

Foreskin *(for'skin)* Loose fold of skin covering the tip of the penis or clitoris.

Forewaters The fluid that comes out of vaginal opening when the bag (amnion) around the fetus bursts during labor.

Formaldehyde *(for-mal'de-hid)* A histologic fixative and disinfectant.

Formalin *(for-mah-lin)* Saturated solution of formaldehyde.

Forme fruste *(form-frust)* *(F)* An incomplete or atypical expression of a clinical entity or pathologic condition.

Formication *(for'mi-ka'shun)* A paresthesia wherein there is a sensation of ants running over the skin.

Formulary *(for'mu-lar'e)* Summary listing of recommended drugs, their uses and dosage.

Fornix *(for'niks)* An arch-shaped structure. pl. **fornices.**

Fossa *(fo'sa)* A depression on the surface of a bone.

Fovea *(fo.ve-ah)* Depressed central area of retina having cones only.

Foveola *(fo've'o-la)* Most depressed, and highly sensitive part of the fovea.

Fracture *(frak'cher)* Injury to a bone wherein the continuity of the bone is broken. It is characterized by pain and tenderness, deformity in the form of swelling, shortening or angulation and loss of function, other features like abnormal mobility at the site of fracture, crepitus and loss of transmitted movements though may be present, are not sought normally.

Avulsion fracture Two fragments of bone are pulled apart.

Burst fracture Caused by hyperflexion of the spine usually accompanied by compression, and fragments of arc pushed circumferentially.

Butterfly fracture If a bone is struck with a direct blow and when two break lines spread out obliquely from the point of contact of the blow producing a free-floating butterfly fragment between the two fractures.

Commuted fracture Occurrence of fracture when a large amount of energy is dissipated into bone. The bone breaks into fragments which may impact into each other or separate and become displaced.

Compression fracture If load applied along the length of a bone exceeds that of its strength, then it may collapse into itself.

Distraction fracture Avulsion fracture.

Galeazzi fracture A distal radius fracture with separation of the distal ulnar epiphysis rather than a true joint disruption.

Green stick fracture Occurrence of fracture in young people where bones are very flexible. They bend and then may buckle or partially break when over loaded.

Hangman's fracture A fracture of the pedicle of C_2 vertebra caused by hyperextension of the spine.

Jefferson fracture Fracture of the ring of Cl vertebra, usually caused by axial loading, named after Jefferson, English neurosurgeon.

Monteggia fracture Injury characterized by a dislocation of the radial head at the elbow together with a ulna fracture.

Partial fracture Greenstick fracture.

Pathological fracture Occurrence of fracture when the strength of bone is reduced by disease.

Shear fracture Shearing of the calcaneum into medial and lateral halves by the load of eccentrically placed talus.

Stress fracture Occurrence of fracture when bones are subjected to a very large number of load, none of which alone would be enough to break the bone but which means that the mechanical structure of the bone can gradually fatigue.

Teardrop fracture Fracture dislocation where part of the injury goes through the lower part of the vertebra and part of the injury is ligamentous.

Traumatic fracture Occurrence of fracture when an excessive load is applied to normal bone.

Wedge fracture Most common lower cervical spine fracture caused by hyperflexion of the spine where bone is compressed.

Fragile-X syndrome A sex chromosome abnormality presenting with mental retardation in males. It is associated with a 'fragile site' on the distal long arm of one X-chromosome and its inheritance is X-linked recessive.

Fragilitas ossium Osteogenesis imperfecta, characterized by recurrent fractures of long bones and blue sclera.

Frambesia (*fram-be-ze-a*) Yaws.

Framycetin Amnioglycoside antibiotic used to treat hemorrhoids, eye and ear infections and to reduce nasal carriage of staphylococus.

Fraternal (*fra-tur'nal*) Derived from two ova.

Freckle (*frek'al*) Asymptomatic small, circular brownish macules appearing early in life on the face, hands and forearm and is due to an abnormally large amount of melanin in the epidermis.

Freeze-drying Method of tissue protein preservation, freezing hesitation on gait initiation seen in well developed Parkinson's disease.

Freeze-etching The sublimation of surface ice under vacuum to reveal details of the fractured structure that were originally hidden.

Frei test (*fri*) Skin test for lymphogranuloma inguinale described by a German dermatologist, Wilhelm Frei.

Fremitus (*frem'i-tus*) Vibration perceptible on palpation.

Frenoplasty (*fre'no-plas"te*) Refers to a urological procedure where surgical alteration of the frenulum, a small fold of tissue which is located on the underside of the penis, is made.

Frenulum Median fold under tongue and other similar folds.

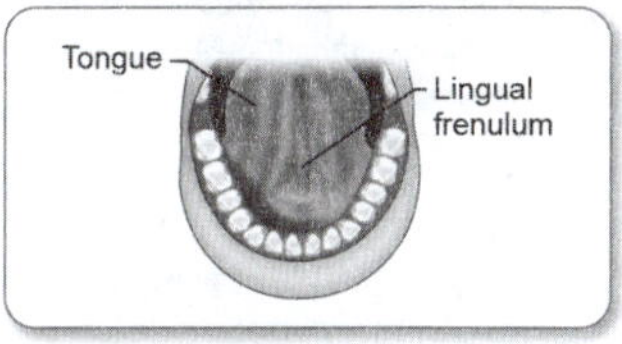

Frenulum of tongue

Frenum (frenulum) A restraining structure.

Freudian (*froi'de-an*) Relating to Sigmund Freud, the neurologist, psychiatrist, and founder of psychoanalysis, or to the theory and practice of psychoanalysis and psychotherapy developed by Freud. Freudian psychoanalysis concentrates on finding the roots of adult behavior in childhood conflicts.

Friction murmur (friction rub) An audible rapsy breathing sound, a medical sign present in some patients with pleurisy which affects the chest cavity.

Freiberg's disease *(fri'bergz)* Osteochondritis of the heads of the second and or third metatarsal bones characterized by pain, limitation of plantar flexion and broadening of affected foot, named after Frederick Freiberg, British orthopedic surgeon.

Friedman's curve A graph depicting the progress of labor, described by American obstetrician, Friedman.

Friedreich's ataxia *(fred'riks)* An autosomal recessive disorder characterized by progressive degeneration of dorsal root ganglia, spinocerebellar tracts, corticospinal tracts and cells of cerebellum. It develops in childhood with features of difficulty in walking, cerebellar dysarthria, ataxic weak limbs, absent deep tendon reflexes and extensor plantar response. There is loss of posterior column sensations, club foot, scoliosis and cardiac involvement.

Frigidity *(fri-jid'i-te)* Failure of a female to respond to sexual stimulus.

Frog face Long-standing angiofibroma of the intranasal cavities which may extend into the orbits to result in bilateral exophthalmos. It is associated with nasal congestion and a flat, croaking voice.

Frohlich's syndrome *(fro'liks)* Adiposogenital dystrophy, characterized by adioposity, delayed puberty, mental defect, and polydipsia, named after A. Frohlich, Austrian physician.

Froin syndrome *(frow'an')* Cerebrospinal fluid having yellow color, raised level of proteins and absence of an increased number of cells in spinal block, named after G. Froin, German physician.

Frontal Forehead.

Frontal bone The bone in the front of skull that forms the forehead.

Frontal lobe The largest part of the cerebrum that influences personality and mental activities.

Frontal sinus An accessory nasal sinus in the frontal bone.

Frostbite *(frost'bit)* A traumatic effect caused by freezing of body tissues from exposure to extreme cold for a long period of time. The peripheral parts of the body such as the tip of the nose, the external ears and the fingers and toes become numbed and white due to vasoconstriction.

Frottage *(fro'ta-j)* Pervert way of obtaining sexual pleasure by rubbing sexual organs against someone.

Frozen chest Pleural or parenchymal fibrosis causing immobilization of the chest.

Frozen shoulder A painful stiff shoulder secondary to periarthritis of the shoulder joint, a shoulder that becomes scarred and cannot move.

Fructose Monosaccharide obtained from honey and fruits.

Frusemide A thiazide loop diuretic.

Fructosuria (levulosuria) Presence of fructose in urine.

Fuchsin (magenta) *(fuk"sinz)* Red dyes of rosaniline group, named after L Fuchs, German botanist.

Fugue *(fug)* A state wherein an individual exhibits forgetfulness of a past event and takes a new identity.

Fulguration (electrodesiccation) *(ful'gu-ra'shun)* Destruction of living tissue by high frequency current.

Full house syndrome Familial focal facial dermal dysplasia (FFFDD), an autosomal dominant condition characterized by lesion devoid of hair with fingerprint-like puckering of the skin, especially at the temples. It is due to alternate bands of dermal and epidermal atrophy. The condition derives its name from a card game where a full house is three cards of one value and two of another.

Fulminating (fulminant, fulgurant) A condition that has a sudden onset is severe and is of short duration.

Fumigation *(fu'mi-ga'shun)* Disinfection of room by poisonous gases; use of poisonous gases or fumes to destroy living organisms.

Functional illness An unidentified illness in which no cause has been found for the symptoms.

Functional MRI A technique to map the functioning of human brain that is dependent on regional blood perfusion, blood volume and blood oxygenation that accompany the neuronal activity, fMRI.

Functional residual capacity (FRC) The gas volume in the lungs after a normal expiration. It is measured by a gas dilution method or body plethysmography.

Fundus Base.

Fungicide *(fun'ji-sid)* A substance that destroys fungus.

Fungoid *(fun'goid)* Caused by a fungus or fungi.

Fungus A parasitic plant lacking in chlorophyll. pl. **fungi**.

Fungus ball A tumor-like mass of fungi. The saprophytic form of Aspergillus species may colonize a pre-existing pulmonary cavity.

Funiculitis Any abnormal inflammatory condition of a cord-like structure of the body.

Funiculus *(fu-nik'u-lus)* A bodily structure suggesting a cord.

Funis *(fu'nis)* Cord-like structure.

Furcation *(far-ka'shun)* Something that is branched.

Furfuraceous *(fur"fu-ra'shas)* Covered with or character ized by scales that resemble bran.

Furor *(fu'ror)* A general outburst of enthusiasm, excitement, controversy, or the like.

Furosemide *(fu-ro'sa-mid)* A loop diuretic used to treat hypertension and edema in congestive heart failure, liver cirrhosis, renal disease and hypertension.

Furuncle *(fu'run-kl)* A localized suppurative condition occurring in a hair follicle.

Furunculosis *(fu-rung'ku-lo'sis)* Boils.

Fusiform *(fu'zi-form)* Tapering at both ends; spindle-shaped.

Fusion *(fu'zhan)* When two nuclei combine to form a new nucleus.

Fusion inhibitor An anti-HIV drug targeting the point where HIV locks to an immune cell.

Fusobacterium *(fu'zo-bak-te're-um)* A gram-negative anaerobic rod-shaped bacteria found in the oral cavity and bowel.

FVC Forced vital capacity.

F waves *ECG* The atrial flutter waves appear on the electrocardiogram with a 'sawtooth' pattern in leads II, III and avF and at a rate of 280–320/min; an undulation of the electromyogram that corresponds to time between the application of stimulus to the axon of the motor neuron and its return after propagation.

G

GABA Gamma-aminobutyric acid, a major inhibiting neurotransmitter widely distributed in brain.

GABA-ergic (*gab'a-er'jik*) The main inhibitory neurotransmitter system in brain circuits, pertain to or affects the neurotransmitter GABA, Gamma-Aminobutyric Acid.

Gabapentin (*gab'a-pen'tin*) An anticonvulsant medication primarily used to treat partial seizures and neuropathic pain.

Gait (*gat*) Style of walking.

Ataxic gait Patient walks on a broad and irregular base, keeping the feet widely apart and swinging the legs irregularly, simulating the gait of a drunken person, also called reeling gait of cerebellar ataxia.

Dancing gait Jerky involuntary movements which exaggerate during walking and the limbs are thrown apart as in chorea.

Festinating gait In Parkinsonism, the patient's head and body bent forward. The hips and knees are slightly flexed. The patient walks with quick short shuffling steps giving an impression of trying to catch up with the center of gravity.

Hemiplegic gait A spastic gait alphabet, with abnormality involving on one side in patients with residual hemiplegia or hemiparesis. The limbs are stiff, foot plantar flexed. The leg is dragged forward in semicircle first away from and then toward the body (circumduction) slowly.

High steppage gait In polyneuropathy, poliomyelitis and peroneal muscular dystrophy the patient raises the foot to overcome the foot drop and is brought down and the toes touch the ground first.

Hysterical gait An irregular bizarre type of gait altering from time to time.

Scissor gait In cerebral diplegia and lathyrism there is medial rotation of the legs which cross each other while walking.

Spastic gait The protein legs are stiff and are advanced slowly on a narrow base by dragging the feet. The foot is raised from the ground by tilting the pelvis and then the leg is swung forward. The foot makes an arc and the toes scrape the ground. This is seen in paraplegia in extension.

Stamping gait The patient in posterior column lesions walks by placing the feet wide apart. The feet are raised high and brought down suddenly with the heel slamming the floor.

Stuttering gait A walking disorder characterized by hesitancy that resembles stuttering; seen in some hysterical or schizophrenic patients as well as in patients with neurologic damage.

Trendelenberg gait An abnormal gait resulting from a defective hip abductor mechanism.

Waddling gait Oscillation of the body from side to side with each step as in pseudohypertrophic muscular dystrophy, congenital dislocation of the hip, osteomalacia and advanced pregnancy.

Galact- (galacto-) Combining word for milk.

Galactagogue (*ga-lak'ta-gog*) An agent that promotes the secretion and flow of milk.

Galactocele (*gah-lak'to-sel*) A cystic milk fission filled swelling in an obstructed milk duct in the breast.

Galactorrhea (*ga-lak'to-re'ah*) Production of breast milk not associated with childbirth. Sometimes, it may be a manifestation of a pituitary gland tumor.

Galactose (*ga-lak'tos*) A monosaccharide has the same chemical formula as glucose, i.e., $C_6H_{12}O_6$, found in the form of lactose in milk and yogurt, which is digested to galactose and glucose.

Gallbladder (*gawl'blad-er*) A small pear-shaped sac under the visceral surface of the right lobe of the liver that acts as a reservoir of bile secreted by the liver. It receives bile from the liver through hepatic duct and it contracts during digestion of fats allowing the flow of the bile through the common bile duct into the duodenum.

Gallbladder carcinoma A malignant condition affecting gallbladder presenting with anorexia, nausea, vomiting, weight loss, right upper abdominal pain, and jaundice. The gallbladder becomes palpable and it fails to concentrate radiopaque dye.

Hydrops gallbladder Distension of gallbladder due to impaction of a large stone in the cystic duct with persistent obstruction.

Porcelain gallbladder Long standing gallstone disease with deposition of calcium in the fibrotic gallbladder giving an egg shell appearance on a radiograph.

Gallium (*gal'e-um*) A rare metallic element, atomic number 31.

Gallium scan radio-scintillation imaging method using 67 Gallium citrate. On injection gallium binds to transferrin and any tissue that concentrates lactoferrin also concentrates gallium, used to stage lymphoma, lung cancer, hepatoma and metastasis.

Gallstone (*gawl-ston*) Calculus formed in the gallbladder or in a bile duct from the constituents of bile due to disturbances in cholesterol and bile pigment metabolism, infection, and biliary stasis.

Cholesterol gallstone Stones that are formed when the bile is supersaturated with cholesterol.

Gallstone ileus Obstruction of ileum by a gallstone passed from cholecystoduodenal fistula.

Galvanism (*gal'va-niz-am*) Generation of electricity by chemical means.

Galvanocautery Cautery by means of a knife or needle heated by a galvanic current.

Gambler's fallacy The erroneous belief that the outcomes of recent random events have some bearing on future random events: the Monte Carlo fallacy.

Gamete (*gam'et*) A mature male (spermatozoon) or female (ovum) reproductive cell.

Gamete intrafallopian transfer (GIFT) A technique of human fertilization for treating infertility wherein the male and female gametes are injected into

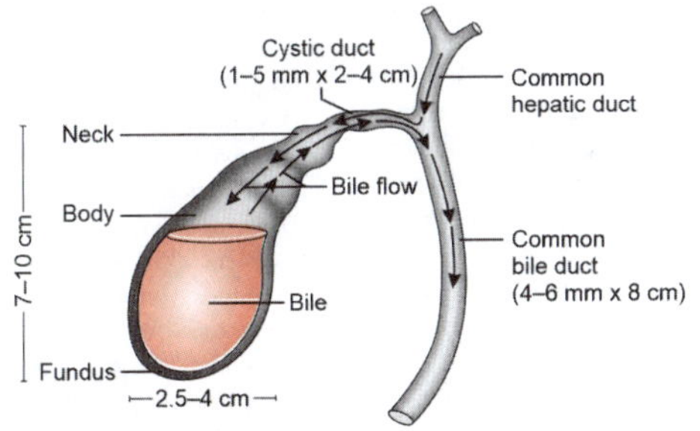

Gallbladder—anatomy

the fimbrian ends of the fallopian tubes through a laparoscope.

Gametocide (*gah-me'to-sid*) An agent that destroys the gametes or gametocytes, especially the malarial parasite.

Gametocyte (*gah-me'to-sit*) A cell that produces gametes (spermatocyte or oocyte).

Gametogenesis (*gah-mi'to-jen'esis*) Formation and development of gametes.

Gamma camera A device that produces an image of the distribution of radioactive material in a patient, who has been injected with small amounts of radioactive materials.

Gamma globulin (Ig) Gamma fraction of protein on electrophoresis of plasma.

Gamma rays High-energy short wavelength radiation emitted by radioactive materials.

Gamogenesis (*gam'o-jen'e-sis*) Sexual reproduction.

Gamma (*gam'ah*) Third letter of Greek alphabet, written as γ; symbol for the heavy chain of immunoglobulin G (IgG).

Ganglion (*gang'gle-on*) A mass of nerve cell collection situated outside the central nervous system; a cystic swelling developing on a tendon or an aponeurosis due to mucoid degeneration of tendinous tissue usually on the wrist. pl. **ganglia**.

Gangrene (*gang'gren*) Death and subsequent putrefaction of the tissues, such an occurrence is common in distal parts of lower extremities or internal organs.

Dry gangrene A condition caused by chronic occlusion of blood supply from a peripheral vascular disease that slowly progresses to severe tissue atrophy and mummification, seen in diabetes mellitus and atherosclerosis.

Gas gangrene A condition seen in open or poorly cleaned wounds infected by Clostridia group of organisms especially *C. welchii*, *C. septicum* and *C. oedematiens* that release histolytic enzymes produce gas and crepitus may be felt.

Vascular gangrene Moist gangrene occurring in the viscera.

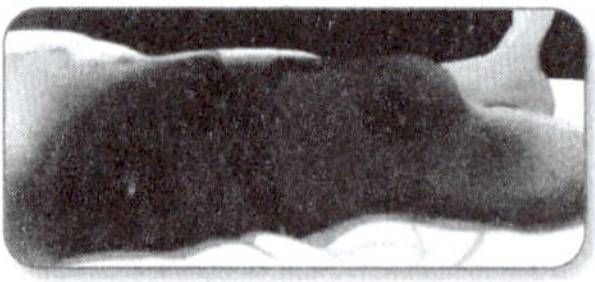

Gas gangrene due to Clostridium perfringens infection

Wet gangrene Condition caused by relatively acute vascular occlusion such as burns, injuries, thromboembolism and freezing. It results in liquefactive necrosis causing bleb and bullae formation violaceous discoloration.

Ganglioneuroma (*gang"gle-o-nu-ro'ma*) Tumors of the sympathetic nervous system that originate from neural crest sympathogonia, which are completely undifferentiated cells of the sympathetic nervous system. Along with neuroblastomas, ganglioneuromas and ganglioneuroblastomas are collectively known as neuroblastic or neurogenic tumors.

Ganglioside (*gang'gle-o-sid"*) Localized in the outer leaflets of plasma membranes and are integral components of cell surface microdomains with sphingomyelin and cholesterol from which they participate in cell-cell recognition, adhesion, and signal transduction.

Ganser's syndrome (*gan'zerz*) An unusual factitious disorder characterized by dissociative symptoms and absurd answers to direct questions, named after Sighert Ganser, a German psychiatrist.

Gargoylism (*gar'goi-izm*) Mucopolysaccharidosis. Hurler's syndrome.

Gas gangrene A condition seen in open or poorly cleaned wounds infected by Clostridia group of organisms especially *C. welchii*, *C. septicum* and *C. oedematiens* that release histolytic enzymes produce gas and crepitus may be felt.

Gasterophilus (*gas"ter-ofi-las*) A parasitic fly of genus from the family Oestridae commonly known as botfly that affects different types of animals, especially horses, but it can also act on cows, sheep, and goats.

Gastrectasia Dilatation of the stomach.

Gastrectomy (*gas-trek'to-me*) Surgical removal of the stomach either partially or totally.

Gastric (*gas'trik*) Pertaining to stomach.

Chronic gastric ulcer Single ulcer situated on the lesser curve within the antrum or at the junction between body and antral mucosa. It extends below to muscularis mucosa. It presents with recurrent abdominal pain sharply localized to the epigastrium, and is noted after food.

Gastric acid Digestive acid secreted by glands in the stomach.

Gastric analysis Analysis of gastric contents of the stomach for determination of amount of hydrochloric acid and for presence of blood, bile and bacteria.

Gastric carcinoma Stomach cancer, a disease of the old with features of recent onset of dyspepsia, vomiting, ulcer like pain, pain not relieved by food or antacids, easy satiety, weight loss and gastrointestinal bleeding. Majority of gastric cancers are adenocarcinomas.

Gastric digestion The phase of digestion that takes in the stomach. Pepsin hydrolyses proteins to peptones, and coagulates the milk.

Gastric erosion A break in the mucosa of the stomach.

Gastric inhibitory polypeptide A polypeptide hormone secreted by duodenum and jejunum that inhibits the motility and the secretion of gastric hydrochloric acid and pepsin.

Gastric lavage Stomach wash.

Gastric triangle An anatomic region defined by the junction of systemic and common bile duct superiorly, the junction of second and third segments of the duodenum inferolaterally and the neck and body of the pancreas medially. Most gastrinomas are located in this region.

Gastric ulcer Ulceration in mucosa.

Gastric glands Tubular glands that lie in the mucus membrane of the stomach well. These are of 3 types—pyloric, fundic and cardiac.

Gastric juice A mixture of digestive secretions (pepsin, hydrochloric acid, mucin, inorganic salts of the stomach) from stomach lining and it breaks down protein in food and destroys infectious organisms.

Gastrin (*gas'trin*) A polypeptide hormone secreted by the glands in the pyloric end of the stomach which stimulates the secretion of gastric acid and pepsin.

Fasting serum gastrin The test used to help detect excess production of gastrin and gastric acid. It is used to help diagnose gastrin-producing tumors called gastrinomas, Zollinger-Ellison (ZE) syndrome, and hyperplasia of G-cells.

Gastrinoma (*gas'tri-no'ma*) A gastrin secreting tumor of the pancreatic islet delta cells associated with Zollinger-Ellison syndrome.

Gastritis (*gas-trit'is*) Inflammation of the mucous membrane lining of the stomach.

Acute gastritis Acute and sudden irritation of the gastric mucosa due to ingestion of alcohol or poisons.

Atrophic gastritis Chronic gastritis with atrophied mucosa and glands.

***Autoimmune* gastritis** A chronic disease that affects the corpus-fundus of the stomach, is characterized by the development two types of autoantibodies: antiparietal cells antibodies and anti-intrinsic factor antibodies.

Chronic gastritis Prolonged inflammation of gastric mucosa.

***Helicobacter pylori* gastritis** Gastritis caused by infection of *H. pylori*.

***Stress* gastritis** Sores in the digestive tract that can cause stomach upset and lead to bleeding.

Gastrocele (*gas'tro-sel*) Hernial protrusion of the stomach.

Gastrocnemius (*gas'tro-sne'me-us*) The most superficial large muscle in the posterior part of the leg. It flexes the knee and plantar flexes the foot.

Gastrocolic reflex Physiological reflex that controls the motility of lower gastrointestinal tract following a meal.

Gastroduodenostomy (*gas'tro-du'o-den'os-to-me*) An anastomosis of upper part of the stomach and duodenum following excision of pylorus of the stomach.

Gastroenteritis (*gas'tro-en'ter-it-is*) Inflammation of the lining of the stomach and intestine because of infection.

Bacterial gastroenteritis A type of gastroenteritis caused by bacterial toxin.

Norwalk gastroenteritis A type of gastroenteritis caused by Norwalk virus.

Viral gastroenteritis A type of gastroenteritis caused by virus.

Gastroenterology (*gas'tro-en'ter-ol-ah-je*) Study of the alimentary tract and its diseases.

Gastroenterostomy (*gas'tro-en-tros'to -me*) Surgical anastomosis of the stomach to the intestine usually at the jejunum.

Gastrofiberscope (*gas"tro-fi-ber-skop*) A fiberscope for viewing the stomach.

Gastroileal reflex One of the tree extrinsic reflexes of GI tract; other two are gastrocolic and enterogastric.

Gastrolithiasis (*gas"tro-li-thi'a-sis*) Refer to inflammation due to some food or foreign body that can neither pass through the pylorus in time nor be digested, it stays in the stomach and gathers into a mass, or coagulates into a solid mass with gastric mucosa.

Gastrojejunostomy (*gas"tro-je-ju'no-sto-me*) Surgical anastomosis of the stomach to the jejunum that bypasses the duodenum to prevent gastric acid from irritating a duodenal ulcer.

Gastropexy Surgical attachment of stomach to the abdominal wall.

Gastroplasty (*gas"tro-plas'te*) A plastic operation of the stomach.

Ring gastroplasty A type of vertical banded gastroplasty in which the band is a plastic ring.

Vertical banded gastroplasty (VBG) A surgical treatment for morbid obesity in which the upper stomach near the esophagus is stapled vertically to create a small pouch along the inner curve of the stomach.

Gastroptosis (*gas"trop-to'sis*) Downward displacement of the stomach.

Gastrorrhea (*gas"tro-re'a*) Excessive secretion of gastric juice by the stomach (hyperchlorhydria) or mucus.

Gastroscope (*gas"tro-skop*) An endoscope utilized to visualize the interior of the stomach.

Gastrostaxis (*gas"tro-stak'sis*) A slow hemorrhage from the stomach, not explained by ulceration or erosion.

Gastrostomy (*gas"tros'to-me*) Surgical creation of an artificial opening into the stomach through the abdominal wall.

Gastrostomy feeding The introduction of a nutrient solution through a tube that has been inserted into the stomach through the abdominal wall.

Gastrotomy (*gas"trot'o-me*) Incision into the stomach.

Gastrula (*gas"troo-la*) An early embryonic stage formed by the invagination of the blastula. It consists of an outer ectoderm and inner mesoderm.

Gaucher's disease (*go"shaz*) A rare hereditary disorder of glucocerebroside metabolism characterized by widespread reticuloendothelial cell hyperplasia, leading to enlargement of the liver and spleen, bone damage and anemia, described by a French physician, Phillipe Gaucher.

Gauss (*gows*) A unit of magnetic flux density equal to 1 maxwell per square centimeter.

Gauze (*gawz*) A light, open meshed cotton fabric used in the bandages and dressings.

Gavage (*gah-vahzh'*) Forced feeding through the stomach tube.

Gel (*jel*) A colloid that is firm in consistency.

Agar gel A semisolid medium prepared from the seaweed agar.

Aluminum hydroxide gel A white viscous suspension of aluminum hydroxide used as an antacid.

Gelatin (*jel'a-tin*) A substance obtained by partial hydrolysis of collagen.

Gemfibrozil A fabric acid derivative having potent lipid-lowering effect.

Gemmule (*jem'ul*) A reproductive buds found in sponges and are involved in asexual reproduction.

Gene (*jen*) The basic functional unit of heredity located at a definite locus on a particular chromosome. It consists of deoxyribonucleic acid (DNA) which controls the cell function and reproduction.

Gene clone A molecular method of molecular biology that is used to make multiple exact copies or clones of a particular gene of interest.

Candidate gene A gene located in a chromosome region suspected of being involved in a disease, whose protein product suggests that it could be the disease gene in question.

Dominant gene A gene that expresses a trait without the assistance from its allele.

Gene amplification The increase in copy numbers of a gene and it is associated with cellular oncogenes in malignancy.

Gene diversity A variety of immune response that an antigen is capable of evoking.

Gene expression Transcription of a segment of DNA to mRNA and translation into a protein.

Gene mapping Determining the relative positions of genes on a chromosome and the distance between them.

Gene pod The sum total of genes, with all their variations, possessed by a particular species at a particular time.

Gene product A polypeptide encoded by a gene.

Gene promotion Activation of genes. It is facilitated by breaks in the ordered array of nucleosomes.

Gene rearrangement The shuffling of genetic material where the intervening sequences (introns) are recovered and exons are spliced together to form mRNA.

Gene splicing The use of micromanipulation methods to insert a portion of a gene from one species into a gene from another species enabling the altered gene to function differently.

Gene testing The study of genetic material to diagnose conditions caused by abnormalities of genes or chromosomes.

Gene therapy The introduction of normal genes into tissues expressing defective genes.

Gene tracking The study of DNA markers to establish the transmission pattern of a specific disease causing gene in a family.

Gene transfer Transfer of a gene from one animal to another to repair an inherited defect in the recipient.

Mutant gene An altered gene that functions differently than it did before its change.

Recessive gene A gene that does not express itself in presence of its dominant allele. A recessive trait may be apparent in phenotype only if both alleles are recessive.

Sex-linked gene A gene found within the X or Y chromosomes.

SRY gene Sex-determining region Y gene, found at the distal end of chromosome Y and its presence dictates development of testicles while its absence results in ovarian differentiation.

Structural gene A gene that determines the structure of polypeptide chains by having control on the sequence of amino acids.

Suicide gene A strategy to make cancer cells more vulnerable or sensitive to chemotherapy.

Tumor suppressor gene A gene that suppresses the growth of malignant cells.

X-linked gene A gene on X chromosome for which there is no corresponding gene on Y chromosome.

General adaptation syndrome A defense response of the body or the psyche to injury or prolonged stress. There is an initial phase of shock followed by a phase of adaptation by utilizing various defense mechanisms of the body or mind. It may lead to a stage of adjustment or exhaustion, described by Hans Selye, an Austrian-Canadian endocrinologist.

General paralysis of the insane (Paresis) (GPI) A late manifestation of syphilis seen 20 years after the infection and characterized by alteration in higher function, and dementia. It is associated with euphoric grandiose state, agitated delirium, bilateral pyramidal signs, fits and widespread tremors. There is frontal and temporal lobe atrophy.

Generic *(jen-er'ik)* General; pertaining to a genus; distinctive.

Generic drugs Nonproprietary name of the drug describing its chemical structure.

Generic name The nonproprietary name assigned to a drug. Nonproprietary name of a medication.

Genesis *(jen'e-sis)* The origin of anything; the act of reproducing.

Genetic code Genetic information carried by specific DNA molecules that determine the specific amino acids and their arrangement in the polypeptides chain of each protein synthesized by the cell.

Genetic counseling The communication of information about disorders with a genetic component.

Genetic drift Tendency for variation in gene frequencies within a small population.

Genetic engineering (recombinant DNA technology) The manipulation of the genome of a living organism by insertion of genes or by genetic selection.

Genetics *(je-net'iks)* Biological science dealing with heredity and the laws governing it; the genetic makeup of a particular individual, family or group.

Genetics screening Undertaking investigations to detect presence of any inherited disorder.

Genic *(jen'ik)* Suffix meaning giving rise to; causing.

Genicular *(je-nik'u-ler)* Pertaining to the knee.

Geniculum *(js-nik'u-lam)* A small knee-shaped anatomical structure or abrupt bend.

Genioplasty Chin surgery to correct misalignment of chin, receding chin, or chin excess.

Genital *(jen'i-tal)* pertaining to reproductory organs or reproduction.

Genital herpes An infection with *Herpes simplex* acquired through sexual contact, characterized by vesicles on the genitals

Genital tract Organs that make up the male or female reproductive system.

Genital ulcers An open sore located on the genital area.

Genital warts Warts on the genitals and anus due to human papillomavirus.

Genitalia *(jen'i-tal'e-ah)* Reproductory organs.

Genogram *(je'no-gram)* A family assessment tool consisting of a family tree diagram depicting family dispersals, losses, roles of organizational patterns over three or more generations.

Genome *(je'nom)* A complete set of genes in the chromosomes that give instructions for growth, development and function of the organs.

Human genome It consists 3.2 billion base pairs. Arranged in 24 chromosomes. Humans are only 99% identical; and 0.1% makes them individual rather than identical clones.

Genome map Writing out of an entire chromosome, DNA sequence, or genome.

Genotype *(jen'o-tip)* The entire genetic constitution of an individual.

Gentamicin (*jen'tah-mi'cin*) Antibiotic elaborated by Micromonospora fungi, which is effective against gram-negative and gram-positive bacteria.

Gentian violet (crystal violet, methyl violet) A coal tar dye used as a stain in histology and also as an antibacterial and antifungal agent.

Genu Knee.

Genu recurvaturn Hyperextension at knee joint.

Genus (*je'nus*) Classification between family and species.

Genu valgum Knock knee.

Genu varum Bow legs.

Geophagia (*je-o-fa'ja*) Also known as geophagy. The habit of eating earth, soil or clay.

Geriatrics (*jer'e-at'riks*) The branch of medical science dealing with the problems of ageing and diseases of the elderly.

Germ (*jurm*) A microorganism; first rudiment of a developing part or organ.

Germ line Inherited material that comes from the ova or sperm and that is passed on to the offspring.

Germ theory Theory stating that certain diseases are the result of pathologic microorganisms in the body.

Germicide (*jer'mi-sid*) Agent that destroys the pathogenic microorganisms.

Germinal center The site in lymph nodes and lymphoid aggregates where normal lymphocyte transformation occurs.

German measles Rubella, an acute exanthematous viral infection noted in children. It may occur in pregnancy to result in various developmental defects. The infection from rubella virus, a single stranded RNA virus, after an incubation period of 2–3 weeks produces an evanescent rash on the face and neck spreading downwards, accompanied by fever, malaise, sore throat, palatal enanthema and rapidly extending maculopapular rash.

Germ cells (gonocyte) Gamete or their precursors.

Germ cells aplasia Absence of spermatocytes in the testes with infertility and high FSH.

Germ cells tumors Tumors arising from malignant degeneration of the germ cell epithelium, testicular tumors and benign cystic teratomas are examples.

Germinal epithelium The epithelial layer of the seminiferous tubules of the testicles.

Germinal vesicle The enlarged nucleus of the egg before completion of meiosis.

Germ layer Three primary cell layers (ectoderm, mesoderm, and endoderm) in the embryo from which the organs and tissues develop.

Gerontology (*je-ron-tol'o-je*) Scientific study of the ageing phenomenon as it affects cells and organisms.

Gerstmann's syndrome A rare neurological disorder consisting of a tetrad of symptoms including impairment in performing calculations (acalculia), discriminating their own fingers (finger agnosia), writing by hands (agraphia) and impairment if distinguishing left from right (left-right disorientation).

Gestaltism (*ge-stawl'tiz-am*) In psychology, concept based on a school of thought that looks at the human mind and behavior as a whole.

Gestation (*jes-ta'shun*) Period of development from fertilization of the ovum to the birth.

Ghon's focus Primary pulmonary tuberculosis, named after Anton Ghon, Czech pathologist.

Giant cell (*ji'ent*) A large tissue cell.

Giant cell carcinoma A highly malignant tumor occurring in the lung or thyroid.

Giant cell fibroblastoma A benign mesenchymal tumor occurring in children often located in the superficial tissues of the back and thigh.

Giant cell glioblastoma A firm well circumscribed tumor in the brain that is highly cellular, with hemorrhage and necrosis.

Giant cell hepatitis Giant cell transformation of the liver of the newborn as a reaction to increased conjugated hyperbilirubinemia of any etiology.

Giant cell myocarditis Focal granulomatous necrosis with multinucleated giant cells in the myocardium as a virallyinduced immune reaction.

Giant cell pneumonia A fulminant respiratory disease with dyspnea and tachycardia as a complication of measles.

Giant cell tumor A bony tumor in the weight bearing epiphysis of distal femur, proximal tibia and distal radius; a fibrous histiocytoma involving the flexor tendon sheath exhibiting presence of osteoclast like giant cells with hyalinization.

Giant-cell arteritis A large vessel vasculitis occurring predominantly in elderly people who present with severe headache.

Giardia (*je-ar'de-a*) A flagellate protozoal parasite, *Giardia lamblia*, described by a French biologist, Alfred Giard. It is a heart shaped single celled organism with two nucleus and four pairs of flagella. They attach to the intestinal mucosa and absorb nutrients.

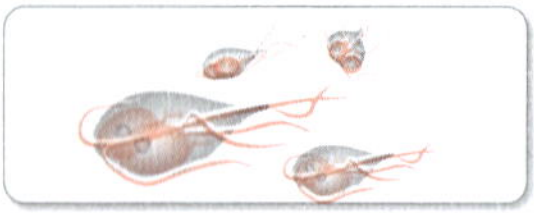

Giardia lamblia

Giardiasis (lambliasis) (*je"ahr-di'e-sis*) Infestation of the small intestine by *Giardia lamblia* giving rise to diarrhea and malabsorption. It is treated with metronidazole, tinidazole and furazolidone.

Gibbus (gibbosity) A hump; a deformity of spine.

Giemsa's stain (*gem'zas*) A stain with azure dyes used to stain the blood smear to demonstrate protozoan parasites, described by a German chemist, Gustav Giemsa.

GIT Gastrointestinal tract.

Gigantism (*ji'gan-tizm*) Increased size and stature of the body occurring before the closure of the growing ends of the bones due to hypersecretion of growth hormone.

Cerebral gigantism A rare genetic disorder caused by mutation in the NSD1 gene on chromosome 5, characterized by coarse, acromegaloid features with a large, dolichocephalic skull, antimongoloid slant of eyes and prominent jaw. Also known as sotos syndrome.

Pituitary gigantism Condition resulting from excessive secretion of GH (and therefore IGF1) before fusion of epiphyseal growth plates leading to tall stature, acral enlargement, facial changes, headaches, and excessive sweating.

Gilbert disease (*zhel-barz*) Benign hereditary hyperbilirubinemia and mild intermittent jaundice, described by a French physician, Nicolas Gilbert.

Gilchrist disease North American blastomycosis, named after Thomas Gilchrist, US dermatologist.

Gilles de la Tourette's syndrome Complexities with vocalizations, often with obscene utterances and rude gestures which may start in childhood and persist into adult life, which responds to dopaminergic receptor antagonists, named after Georges Gilles de la Tourette, a French physician.

Gingiva (*jin'ji-vah*) Gum, the part of the oral mucosa covering the tooth bearing border of the jaw.

Gingivectomy (*jin'ji-vek'to-me*) Surgical removal of diseased gingival tissue.

Gingivitis (*jin'ji-vi'tis*) Inflammation of the gums usually caused by poor dental hygiene.

Necrotizing ulcerative gingivitis A rapidly destructive, noncommunicable microbial disease of the gingiva in the context of an impaired host immune response.

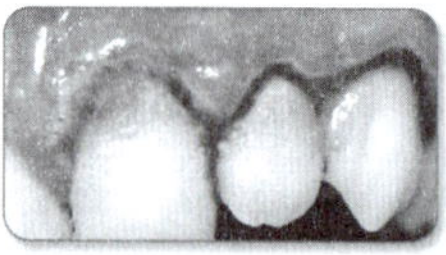

Necrotizing ulcerative gingivitis

Ginglymus (hinge joint) (*jin'gli-mas*) A joint in which movement is limited to one plane.

Girdle (*gur'del*) A zone or belt.

Pelvic girdle Portion of lower extremities composed of 2 hip (innominate bones) bones to which the lower limbs are attached.

Shoulder girdle Portion of upper extremity composed of two clavicles and two scapulae to which the upper limbs are attached.

Glabella (*glah-bel'a*) The area between the eyebrows above the nasion.

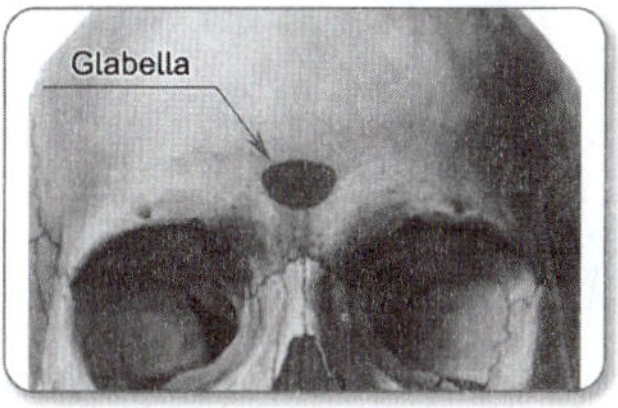

Glabella

Gladiolus (*glah-di'o-lus*) Body of the sternum.

Gland (*gland*) An aggregation of specialized cells concerned with secretion or elimination which is not related to their own metabolism; the two main types are the endocrine glands and the exocrine glands.

Apocrine gland A subtype of exocrine glands that releases its glandular apocrine secretions by the process of decapitation.

Bulbourethral gland Also called Cowper's Gland, either of two pea-shaped glands in the male, located beneath the prostate gland at the beginning of the internal portion of the penis.

Eccrine sweat gland Simple, coiled, tubular glands present throughout the body, most numerously on the soles of the feet.

Endocrine gland Consists of glands which release hormones internally.

Mammary gland An exocrine gland in humans and other mammals consists of disk of glandular tissue that produces milk to feed young offspring.

Parathyroid gland Small pea-sized endocrine glands that function to maintain the homeostasis of calcium and phosphorus in our bodies.

Pituitary gland Also called the master gland of the endocrine system because it controls the functions of many of the other endocrine glands.

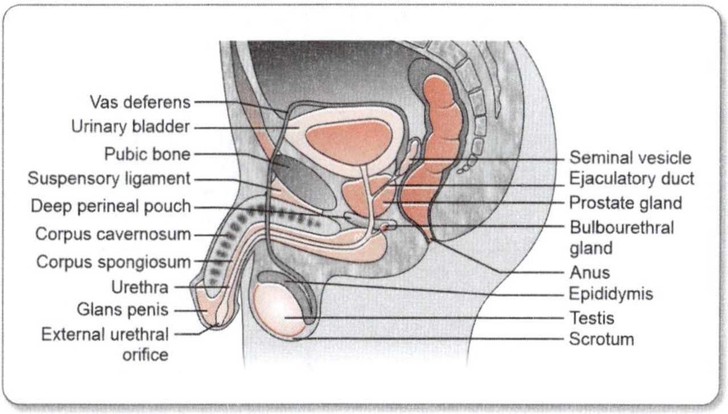

Bulbourethral gland (Male genitourinary tract)

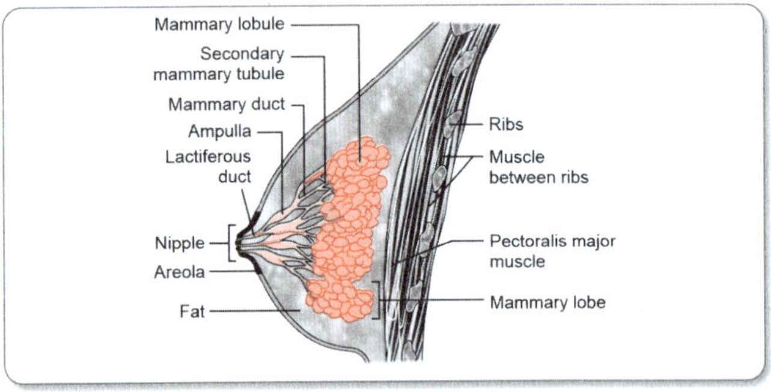

Mammary gland

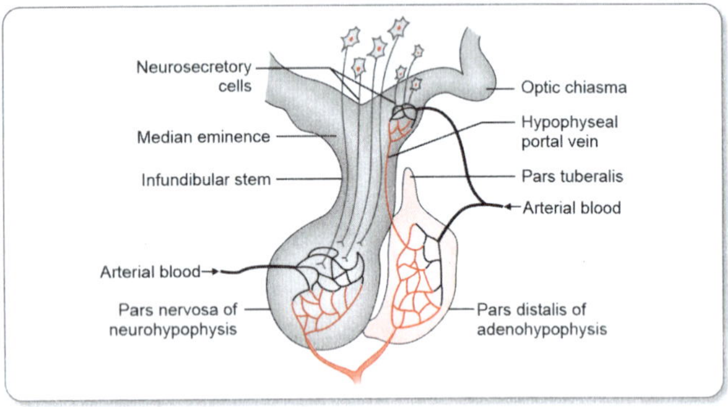

Pituitary gland

Salivary gland Exocrine glands that are positioned in the head, in and around the oral cavity and secrete their salivary contents into the mouth.

Sebaceous gland Small oil-producing gland present in the skin of mammals.

Glanders (equinia) (*glan'derz*) An infection caused by *Pseudomonas mallei*, it can be communicated to man from infected horses.

Glans (glans penis) (*glanz*) Conical, acorn-shaped structure.

Glans clitoris The small and highly sensitive cone-shaped tip of the clitoris.

Glans penis The head of the penis.

Glaucoma (*glaw-ko'mah*) Disease of the eye exhibiting raised intraocular pressure, causing internal damage and affecting the vision if untreated. It develops when the aqueous humor drainage is too slow to keep up with its production in anterior chamber.

Gleet (*gl'et*) A mucoid or purulent urethral discharge.

Gleason system A system that grades prostate cancer using numbers from 1 to 5 based on how much the cells in the cancerous tissue look like normal prostate tissue, named after Donald Gleason, a US pathologist.

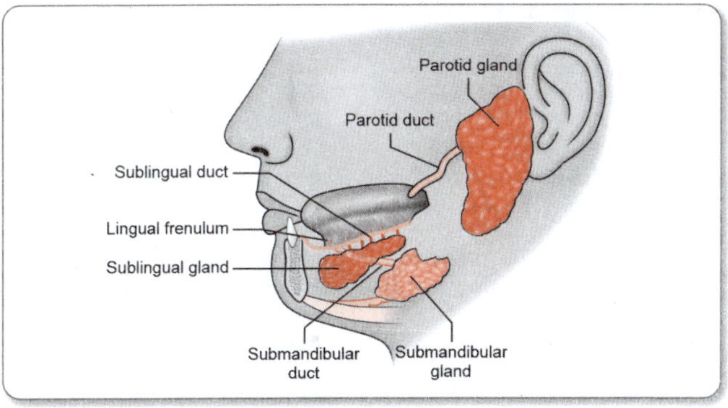

Salivary gland

Glenohumeral (*gle"no-hu'mer-al*) Related to glenoid of the scapula and the proximal humerus.

Glenoid cavity (glenoid fossa) A shallow depression with which the head of the humerus articulates.

Glia (neuroglia) (*gli'ah*) Neural cells having a connective tissue support, neuroglia.

Gliding joint A synovial joint in which articulation of contiguous bones allow one surface to move smoothly over an adjacent surface, as in wrist and ankle.

Glioblastoma (spongloblastoma) (*gli'o-bias-to'mah*) Malignant astrocytoma.

Glioma (*glio'mah*) Primary tumor of the brain with glial cells, that vary widely in its degree of malignancy and rate of growth.

Brainstem glioma Refer to all subtypes of astrocytomas that occur in the brainstem.

Nasal glioma A developmental abnormality of neurogenic origin with no malignant potential.

Optic glioma A slow growing brain tumor that arises in or around the optic nerve, which connects the eye to the brain.

Gliosome Lysosome in astrocyte.

Glipizide (*glipi-zid*) Short-acting oral hypoglycemic agent of sulphonyl urea group and is effective when given twice daily.

Globin (*glo'bin*) The protein of the hemoglobin.

Globulin (*glob'ulin*) A protein found in plasma, that play important role in the formation of antibodies.

Globulinuria The presence of globins in urine.

Globus (*glo'bus*) A spherical mass.

Globus hystericus An emotional disorder giving an uncomfortable sensation of having a lump in the throat.

Globus pallidus The smaller and more medial part of the lentiform nucleus of the brain.

Glomangioma (*glo-man"je-o'me*) Benign clusters of bluish-purple nodules that are often painful and sensitive to cold temperature and touch.

Glomerulonephritis (glomerular nephritis) (*glo-mer'u-lo-ne-fri-tis*) (GN) A group of diseases caused by immune mechanisms in which the glomeruli are primarily involved.

Acute glomerulonephritis Post-infections glomerulonephritis.

Chronic glomerulonephritis Terminal stage of many forms of glomerulonephritis. The kidneys are symmetrically contracted with smooth contour. Often there is hypertension.

Membranoproliferative glomerulonephritis Thickening of the glomerular basement membrane and proliferation of mesangial and endothelial cells.

Mesangial proliferative glomerulonephritis Mesangial widening and mesangial cellular proliferation similar to that seen in IgA nephropathy. It presents with features of nephrotic syndrome and runs a benign course.

Post infectious glomerulonephritis Acute nephritis developing 1–2 weeks after a history of acute respiratory infection or in association with infected scabies noted mostly in children with sudden onset of hematuria in the form of smoky urine, early morning puffiness of face, oliguria, and hypertension. There is endocapillary proliferative glomerulonephritis. Disease is self-limiting.

Rapidly progressive glomerulonephritis A clinical syndrome in which renal function deteriorates over a period of days or weeks in a patient with glomerulonephritis. There is crescent formation, hematuria, and azotemia. The condition may be due to antibodies to the glomerular basement membrane, or due to immune complexes or without any immunoglobulin deposition.

Glomerulus (*glo-mer'u-lus*) A tuft of convoluted mass of capillaries enclosed in Browman's capsule of the kidney. This is the site of filtration which is the first step in the formation of urine.

Glomus (*glo'mus*) A small body consisting of fine arterioles communicating directly with the venules, and a rich nerve supply, the aortic body and carotid body are examples.

Glossa (*glos'ah*) The tongue.

Glossectomy (*glos-sek'to-me*) Excision of a portion or whole of the tongue, as a treatment for cancer of tongue.

Glossina (*glo-si'na*) An African genus of dipteran flies, having features like long slender sharp proboscis and joint antennae bearing feathery appendages and that comprise the tsetse flies.

Glossitis (*glos-it'is*) Inflammation of the tongue.

Glossolalia (*glos'o-la'lea*) An expression of a revelatory message through unintelligible words.

Glossopharyngeal nerve Ninth cranial nerve.

Glossoplegia Paralysis of the tongue.

Glossopharyngeal (*glos'o-fer-in'ie-al*) Pertaining to the tongue and pharynx.

Glottis (*glot'is*) Larynx containing the vocal cords and the opening between them. It is the sound producing apparatus.

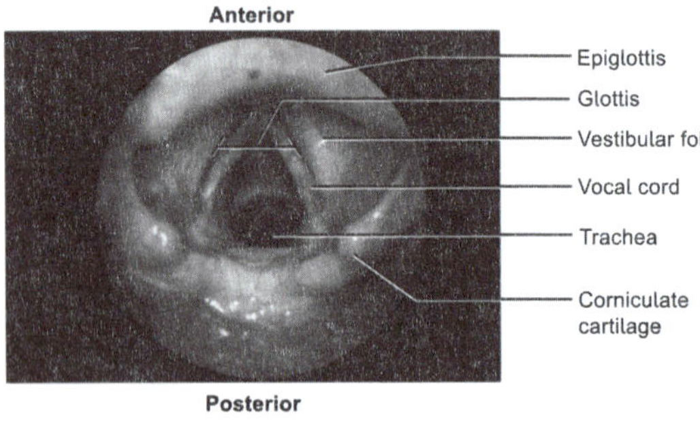

Glottis

Glossotrichia (*glos"so-trik'e-a*) Lengthening of papillae on the surface of the tongue, giving it a furry appearance.

Glottography (*glo-tog'ra-fe*) Measurement of the modulation of a sound by the vibration of the glottis.

Glucagon (*glu'ka-gon*) A polypeptide hormone secreted by the alpha cells of the islets of Langerhans, that stimulates the release of glucose into the blood stream.

Glucocerebrosidase (*glu'ko-se-re"bro-si'das*) A retaining β-glucosidase with acid pH optimum metabolizing the glycosphingolipid glucosylceramide to ceramide and glucose.

Glucocorticoid (*glu'ko-kor'ti-koid*) Corticoid hormone produced by the adrenal cortex that increases the gluconeogenesis, and suppresses inflammation.

Glucokinase (*glu'ko-ki'nas*) An enzyme found in the liver cells that in presence of ATP catalyzes the conversion of glucose to glucose-6-phosphate, which is the first step in glycolysis.

Glucometer (*gloo'ko-me-tur*) A battery-operated device used to measure blood glucose from a few drops of blood obtained from the finger.

Gluconeogenesis (*glu'ko-ne'o-jen'e-sis*) The synthesis of glucose from noncarbohydrate sources.

Glucoregulation Influenced by hormones, such as adrenaline and cortisol, that are sensitive to stressful or arousing cognitive tasks.

Glucosamine (*glu-ko'sah-min*) An amino derivative of glucose.

Glucose (dextrose) (*glu'kos*) A simple sugar, monosaccharide. It is the chief source of energy for living organisms.

Glucose tolerance test (GTT) A test of body's response to a dose of glucose after a period of fasting, used to diagnose diabetes mellitus.

Glucoside (*glu'ko-sid*) A glycoside that on hydrolysis yields glucose.

Glucuronic acid Carboxyl acid metabolite of glucose.

GLUT Glucose transport protein units, promote uptake of glucose by cells after insulin causes transfer of the GLUT from the Golgi apparatus to the cell membrane.

Glutamate (*glu'te-mat*) A neurotransmitter in the brain probably participating in memory.

Glutamic oxaloacetic transaminase (GOT) An enzyme that catalyzes the reversible transfer of an amino group, aspartic acid.

Glutamic pyruvic transaminase (GPT) An enzyme that catalyzes the reversible transfer of alanine.

Glutaminase (*glu-tam'i-nas*) An enzyme that catalyzes the breakdown of glutamine into glutamic acid and ammonia.

Glutamine (*glu'ta-min*) A nonessential amino acid.

Glutaric acid An alpha, omega-dicarboxylic acid that is a linear five-carbon dicarboxylic acid.

Glutaric acidemia Heterogeneous, genetic diseases that present with specific catabolic deficiencies of amino acid or fatty acid metabolism. It is of two types, type 1 and type 2.

Glutathione (*glu'ta-thi'on*) A tripeptide of glycine, cystine and glutamic acid.

Glutathione reductase Protect the red cells against damage due to oxidation.

Gluteal (*glu'te-al*) Relates to the buttocks.

Gluten (*glu'ten*) The insoluble protein derived from wheat.

Gluten free diet Elimination of gluten from diet avoiding products of wheat, oats, rye or barley.

Glyburide A sulfonylurea used in the treatment of noninsulin dependent diabetes mellitus.

Glyceride (*glis'er-id*) An ester of glycerol.

Glycerin (glycerol) (*glis'er-in*) Trihydroxypropane used as a solvent, a preservative and as an emollient in various skin diseases. It reduces intracranial and intraocular tensions.

Glycine (*gli'sen*) A nonessential simple amino acid.

Glycocholic acid A crystalline bile acid involved in the emulsification of fats, occurs as a sodium salt in the bile of mammals.

Glycogen (*gli'ko-jen*) Main carbohydrate reserve which is easily converted into glucose.

Glycogen storage diseases A group of familial enzyme defects affecting glycogen breakdown, usually with liver storage.

Glycogenesis (*gli'ko-jene-sis*) Formation of glycogen from glucose.

Glycogenolysis (*gli'ko-je-nol'i-sis*) Hydrolysis of glycogen to glucose.

Glycolipid (*gli-ko-lip'id*) A compound of fatty acid with a carbohydrate containing nitrogen found in myelin sheaths.

Glycolysis (*gli-kol'i-sis*) Nonmitochondrial conversion of glucose and ADP to lactate and ATP, major source of energy for voluntary and cardiac muscles.

Glycophilia (*gli"ko-fil'e-a*) A condition in which a small amount of glucose produces hyperglycemia.

Glycoprotein (*gli'ko-pro'ten*) A protein-carbohydrate compound.

Glycoside (*gli'co-si-d*) Any compound which on hydrolysis yields sugar and nonsugar residues.

Glycosialorrhea (*gli"ko-si'e-lo-re'a*) Excessive flow of saliva containing glucose.

Glycosuria The abnormal presence of glucose in the urine, which usually results from diabetes mellitus.

Glymidine Glycodiazine used for the treatment of noninsulin dependent (type-2) diabetes mellitus.

GMP Guanosine monophosphate.

Gnathic (*na-thi'c*) Relating to the jaw.

Gnathion (*nath'e-on*) The lowest point of the midline of the lower jaw.

Gnathostoma Spirurid nematodes characterized by the presence of a prominent cephalic bulb and body spines, and are typically associated with carnivorous mammal definitive hosts.

Gnotobiotic Relating to, living in or being a controlled environment containing one or a few kinds of organisms.

Goblet cell Mucus secreting cell in the bronchus, and intestinal tract.

Goiter (*goit'er*) Enlargement of the thyroid gland visible as a swelling on the neck.

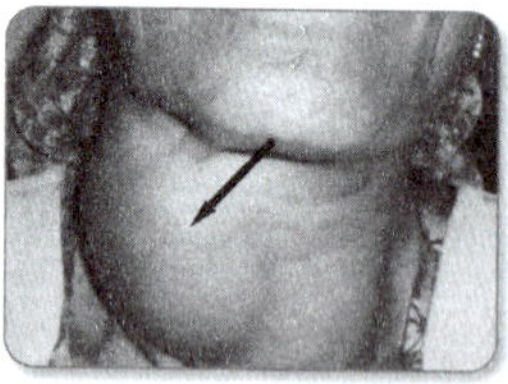

Goiter

Colloid goiter Late stage of diffuse hyperplastic goiter following reduction in TSH stimulation in which there are many inactive follicles filled with colloid.

Diffuse goiter Simple goiter due to puberty, pregnancy, iodine deficiency or due to colloid goiter.

Endemic goiter Occurrence of goiter in certain geographic areas where the iodine content of food and water is deficient.

Exophthalmic goiter Goiter with exophthalmos.

Nodular goiter Persistent fluctuating TSH stimulation may lead to formation of a solitary thyroid nodule.

Retrosternal goiter Goiter arising from the lower pole of the nodular goiter.

Simple goiter An euthyroid, nontoxic goiter which may be diffuse or nodular.

Toxic goiter Primary or secondary thyrotoxicosis. It may be diffuse or solitary and associated with excess production of the thyroid hormone.

Goldflam disease (*golt'flahm*) Myasthenia gravis, named after Samuel Goldflam, a Polish neurologist.

Golgi's apparatus A complex cellular organelle, described by an Italian anatomist Camillo Golgi.

Gomori's trichrome method A single step staining that combines the plasma stain (chronotrope 2R) and fiber stain (fast green FCF) in a phosphotungstic acid solution to which glacial acetic acid is added. (snap frozen human striated muscle are used as specimen).

Gomphosis (*gom-fo'sis*) The specialized fibrous joint that anchors the root of a tooth into its bony socket within the maxillary bone (upper jaw) or mandible bone (lower jaw) of the skull.

Gonad (*go'nad*) A sex gland, such as the testis and ovary that produces sperms or ova respectively.

Gonadotropin (gonadotropic hormone) (*go"na-do-tro'pin*) The hormones that stimulate the gonads, or sex glands, to carry out their reproductive or endocrine functions.

Goniometer (*go'ne-om'e-ter*) Instrument to measure the angles, used to quantitate joint movement.

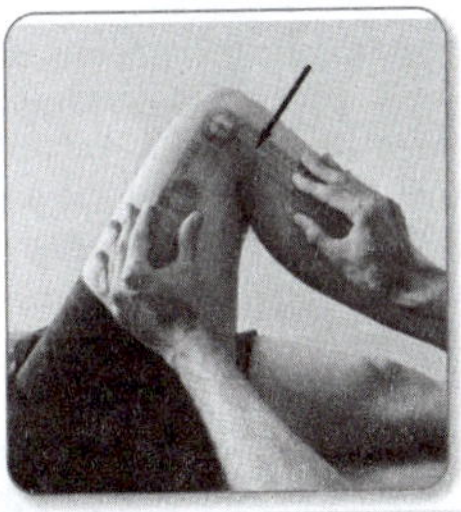

Goniometer used to measure range of motion of a knee joint

Gonion (*go'ne-on*) The point or apex of the angle of the lower jaw.

Goniopuncture A filtering operation, developed as a result of experiences with goniotomy, which seems of value in juvenile, and possibly congenital glaucoma.

Gonioscope (*glone-ah-skop*) An optical instrument for examining the angles of the anterior chamber of the eye.

Goniotomy (trabeculotomy) (*go'ne-ot'o-me*) An opening for glaucoma.

Gonococcus (*go'no-kok'us*) *Neisseria gonorrhea* species causing gonorrhea. It is gram-negative intracellular diplococcus.

Gonocyte Long-lived precursor germ cells responsible for the production of spermatogonial stem cells (SSCs).

Gonorrhea (*gon'o-re'ah*) A sexually transmitted disease predominantly affecting the lower genital tract, rectum and conjunctiva. The involvement of anterior urethra in male is associated with dysuria and purulent discharge. Involvement of lower cervical canal in women presents with vaginal discharge and dysuria. It is treated with penicillin.

Goodpasture syndrome An autoimmune disorder presenting with glomerulonephritis and pulmonary hemorrhage, described by an American pathologist, Earnest Goodpasture.

Gouge (*gouj*) A hollow chisel for cutting and removing bone.

Goundou (anakhre) A condition following an infection with yaws in which the nasal processes of the upper jaw bone thicken to form two large bony swellings, about 7 cm in diameter, on either side of the nose. The swellings not only obstruct the nostrils but also interfere with the field of vision.

Gout An acute inflammatory response to monosodium urate monohydrate crystals formed secondary to hyperuricemia.

Acute gout Urate gout presenting suddenly in the night involving the first metatarsophalangeal joint of the big toe. The joint and surrounding tissues are swollen, hot, red, shiny and extremely painful. It may provoke migratory attacks affecting other joints over subsequent days.

Chronic gout Tophaceous gout uncontrolled hyperuricemia of long duration with recurrent episodes of gout. Tophi consisting of chalky white urate crystals appear as firm, nodular swellings.

Intercritical gout First attack of gout may be followed by similar episodes within one year. There is increase in frequency of attacks and number of sites involved.

Graaffian follicle (*graf'e-an*) A small sac in the ovary that encloses an ovum, described by Dutch physician, Reijnier de Graaf.

Graft 1 (*graft*) Any healthy tissue or organ taken from one part of the body or from a donor and surgically implanted in another part of the body to repair or replace damaged tissue or organ.

Bypass graft A procedure used to treat coronary artery disease.

Graft versus host disease (GVHD) A rejection response that occurs following bone marrow transplant in the skin, gastrointestinal tract and liver when sensitized immunologically competent donor lymphocytes are transferred into an immunologically incompetent recipient tissues.

Gramicidin (*gram"i-si'din*) A heterogeneous mixture of six antibiotic peptides obtained from the soil bacterium *Bacillus brevis.*

Gram's stain (*gramz*) A procedure of staining bacteria with crystal violet and iodine, alcohol removes the stain from gram-negative but not from gram-positive organisms, described by a Danish physician, Hans Gram.

Grand mal (major epilepsy) (*gran-mal*) A major epilepsy exhibiting tonic-clonic seizures with loss of consciousness lasting up to 15 minutes.

Grand multiparity A woman who has had 5 or more viable pregnancies.

Granular cast A sign of many types of kidney diseases.

Granulation The process of creating granules by combining one or more powder particulates through compression activities and/or with a binding agent.

Granulocyte (*gran'u-lo-sit*) Any cell containing granules, usually refers to the white cells such as neutrophil, eosinophil and basophil.

Granuocytopenia A condition in which there is a lower-than-normal number of granulocytes (a type of white blood cell).

Granuloma (*gran"u-lo'ma*) A small nodular chronic inflammatory swelling.

Candidal granuloma Granuloma formed by candida infection.

Giant cell granuloma A benign reactive osseous proliferation that shares features with aneurysmal bone cyst.

Granuloma annulare Rounded skin lesion with raised edges.

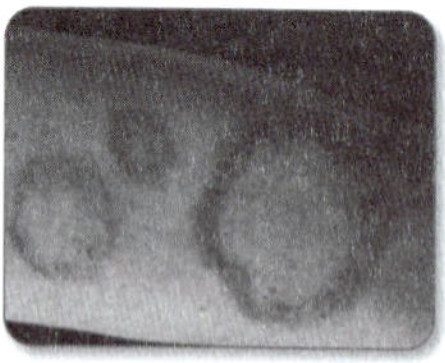

Granuloma annulare

Lethal granuloma A rare lethal granuloma characterized by necrosis of midface due to long standing inflammation.

Periapical granuloma Modified granuloma tissue adjacent to the root apex of a tooth due to chronic inflammation and infection.

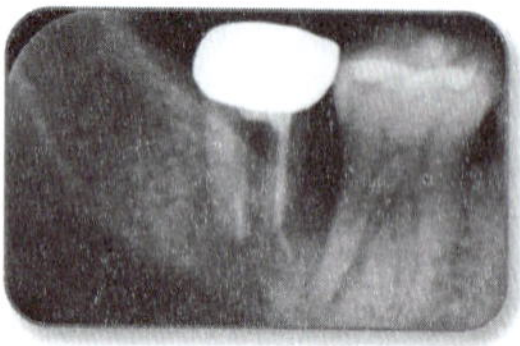

Periapical granuloma

Pyogenic granuloma An acquired benign proliferation of capillary blood vessels of the skin and oral cavity.

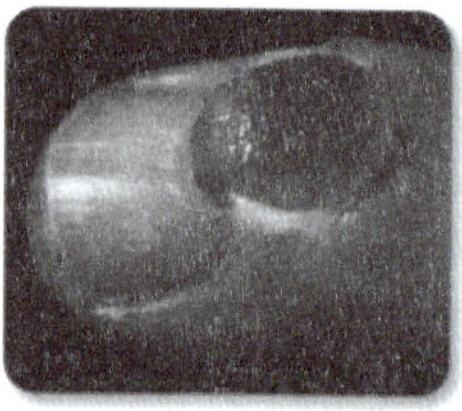

Pyogenic granuloma

Sarciud granuloma Seen in sarcoidosis.

Tuberculoid granuloma Granuloma due to tuberculosis.

Granuloma inguinale A sexually transmitted disease characterized by ulceration of the skin and subcutaneous tissue in the groin. It is caused by a small gram-negative, rod-shaped microorganism. *C. granulomatis.*

Granulomatosis *(gran"u-lo"ma-to'sis)* A chronic condition marked by the formation of numerous granulomas.

Granulopoiesis *(gran"u-lo-poi-e'sis)* The production of neutrophils, eosinophils, and basophils.

Graph- (grapho-) *(graf)* A nonlinear data structure consisting of vertices and edges.

Grattage *(grah-tahzh')* In order to stimulate healing, scraping away of granulations, in case of ulcer treatment.

Gravel Debris which is formed from a fragmented found in kidney stone.

Graves disease (exophthalmic goiter) Thyrotoxicosis associated with goiter and exophthalmos, described by an Irish physician, Robert Graves.

Gravid Pregnant.

Grawitz's tumor *(grah'vits-ez)* Renal cell carcinoma of the kidney, named after Paul Grawitz, a German pathologist.

Gray *(gra)* The international system (SI) unit of radiation dose, expressed as absorbed energy per unit mass of tissue. 1 Gy = 1 Joule/kilogram = 100 rad.

Gray baby syndrome A toxic condition seen in neonates especially premature infants following administration of chloramphenicol. The body mechanisms are not developed to detoxify and excrete the drug and present with ashen gray cyanosis, listlessness, and weakness.

Gray matter Gray area of the brain and spinal cord where the nerve fibers are not enclosed in a myelin sheath.

Green monkey disease Marburg disease.

Green stick fracture An incomplete fracture wherein the bone bends and exhibits the fracture only on the outer arc of the bend.

Grip *(grip)* Grasping or clasping.

Grippe *(F)* Influenza.

Griseofulvin *(gris"e-o-ful'vin)* An oral antibiotic used for the treatment of fungal infection.

Groin Junction between the abdomen and thigh.

Group practice Cooperative partnership of general practitioners.

Group therapy *psy* A form of psychosocial treatment where a small group of patients meet regularly to talk, interact, and discuss problems with each other and the therapist.

Growth factor Biologically active, naturally occurring substance capable of stimulating cell proliferation.

Growth hormone (hGH) A peptide hormone that stimulates growth, cell reproduction, cell regeneration in humans and other animals.

Grumous *(groo'mas)* Transformed from a liquid into a soft semisolid or solid mass.

Guaifenesin *(gwi-fen'a-sin)* The glyceryl ether of guaiacol $C_{10}H_{14}O_4$ that is used especially as an expectorant called also glyceryl guaiacolate.

Guanethidine *(gwahn-eth'i-den)* Antihypertensive agent which blocks release of noradrenaline from adrenergic nerve endings.

Guanfacine *(gwahn'fb-sen)* A class of medications belongs to centrally acting alpha2A-adrenergic receptor agonists used to treat high blood pressure (hypertension).

Guanine *(gwa-nen)* Purine base of nucleic acids that links with cytosine in double helix.

Guanosine *(gwan'o-sin)* The nucleoside formed from guanine and ribosome, and it is a major constituent of RNA and DNA.

Gubler's paralysis *(goob'lerz)* A brainstem lesion causing paralysis of the cranial nerves on one side and of the body on the opposite side, named after Adolphe Gubler, French physician.

Gubernaculum A card-like structure that unites two structures.

Guillain-Barré syndrome (GBS) *(ge-lan' ba-ra')* A neuropathy described by a French neurologists Georges Guillain and Jean Barre due to an immunologic injury presenting with sudden weakness of all four limbs in a previously healthy individual. The disease is symmetrical involving proximal and distal muscles, areflexia, sensory changes, postural hypotension, and cranial nerve paralysis involving bilateral facial and bulbar muscles. CSF shows albumin-ocytologic dissociation with increased protein with normal cells. Nerve conduction studies show demyelination. Those who survive recover remarkably, however, many fail to reach the previous level of activity.

Guillotine (*gil'o-ten*) A surgical instrument with a sliding blade.

Guillotine amputation A sharply defined loss of a portion or entire segments of extremities.

Guinea worm Dracunculus.

Gullet (*gul'at*) Comes from the Old French word 'golet' neck of a bottle; from the Latin 'gula', throat; esophagus.

Gum (*gum*) A plant extract that is sticky when moist but hard or drying; the fleshy tissue covering the alveolar processes of the jaws.

Gumboil (*gum'boil*) A dental abscess converted into a cyst with chronic drainage through a fistulous tract; parulis.

Gumma (*gum'e*) A soft gummy tumor noted in tertiary syphilis. It represents a hypersensitivity response to treponemal products. There is central caseating necrosis surrounded by epithelioid histiocytes and multinucleated giant cells.

Gumshield A protective device that is used to cover the teeth and gums; commonly used by boxers.

Gustation (*gus-ta'shun*) Sense of taste.

Gustatory (*gus'ta-tor'e*) Pertaining to the act or sense of taste.

Gustatory hallucination False perception of taste such as an unpleasant taste due to an uncinate seizure.

Gustatory organ Taste bud.

Gut (*gut*) Bowel, intestine.

Chromic gut Surgical cut which is treated with chromic salt to increase its resistance to absorption in tissue.

Postnatal gut A temporary extension of embryonic gut caudal to cloaca.

Surgical gut Catgut, an absorbable sterile suture is made from collagen.

Gut-associated lymphoid tissue (GALT) Presence of gastrointestinal immune system in the mucosa and submucosa of the gastrointestinal tract. It is prominent in the tonsils, Peyer's patches, and appendix.

Guthrie test (*guth're*) A screening test for phenylketonuria, to detect the presence of phenylalanine metabolites in the blood, named after Robert Guthrie, a US microbiologist.

Gutta A drop. pl. **guttae**.

Gutta percha *dent* An inert latex-like substance used for filling root canals.

Guttate Resembling a drop.

Gynecology (*gi'ne-kol-o-je*) A branch of medicine that deals with the diseases and routine physical care of the reproductive system of women.

Gynecomastia (*gi"ne-ko-mas'te-a, jin'e*) A condition of overdevelopment or enlargement of the breast tissue in men or boys.

Gypsum (*jip'sum*) A mineral containing crushed calcium sulphate hemihydrate which when calcinated becomes plaster of Paris.

Gyrus (*ji-rus*) One of the convolutions of the cerebral hemispheres of the brain. The gyri are separated by shallow grooves (sold) or deeper groves (fissures). pl. **gyri**.

H

Habituation (*he-bich'u-a-shun*) An adaptive response characterized by a decreased reactivity to a repeated stimulus.

Habitus (*hab'i-tes*) General physical appearance; body build.

Haemaphysalis (*he"ma-fis'a-lis*) A large genus of ticks of the family Ixodidae.

Haemophilus (*he-mof'il-us*) A small, nonmotile gram-negative bacterium that requires the growth factor (X or V or both), provided by blood. ***H. aegyptius*** causative agent of conjunctivitis. ***H. ducreyi*** causative agent of chancroid. ***H. influenzae*** causative agent of respiratory infections and meningitis. ***H. vaginalis*** bacterium causing vaginitis.

Hair (*har*) Any of the numerous fine, usually cylindrical, keratinous filaments growing from the skin of humans and animals; a pilus; a keratinized, thread-like outgrowth from the skin. A hair develops as a thin, flexible shaft of cornified cells from the hair follicle. It has a shaft and a root embedded in the follicle. The shaft consists of cuticle, cortex and medulla. The pigment found in the cortex is responsible for the color.

Anagen hair Actively growing hair.

Hair analysis Use of hair for detection of chronic heavy metal intoxication such as arsenic, lead and mercury.

Hair bulb Root of a strand of hair from which the color develops.

Hair cells Sensory receptors in the inner ear that transform sound vibrations into messages that travel to the brain.

Hair-on-end appearance A radiographic pattern seen as calcified spicules perpendicular to the bone surface seen in congenital hemolytic anemias such as sickle cell anemia, thalassemia, hereditary elliptosis and spherocytosis.

Hairpin vessels Minute blood vessels that are doubled upon themselves, seen at the metaphyseal-diaphyseal junction of normal bone.

Lanugo hair Fine hair of the fetus, usually shed at birth.

Telogen hair Nongrowing hair that is removed easily.

Terminal hair Coarse, deeply pigmented, stiff and thick hair seen in scalp, eyebrow, chest, axilla and pubic region. Androgens are responsible for such hair.

Vellous hair Fine, soft and downy hair of children and women.

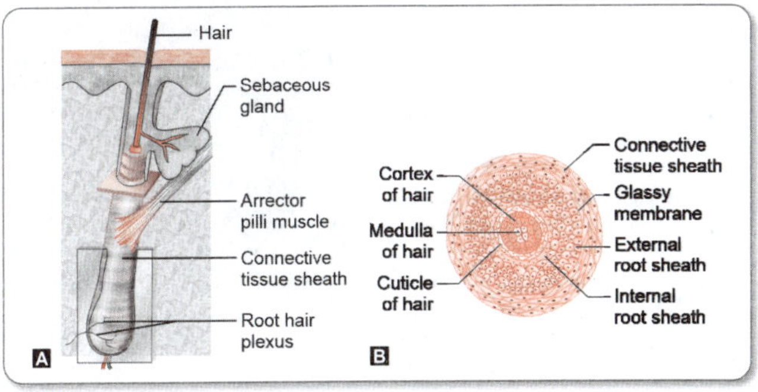

***A.** Hair in longitudinal section; **B.** Hair root—cross-section*

HAIR-AN syndrome Hyperandrogenism (HA), insulin resistance (IR) and acanthosis nigricans (AN).

Hairy cell leukemia A B cell leukemic lymphoproliferative disorder associated with splenomegaly, pancytopenia, recurrent infections and typical hairy cells in the blood and bone marrow. Interferon and purine analogs (deoxycoformycin chlorodeoxyadenosine) are useful in the management.

Hair follicle A cylindrical invagination of the epidermis in the corium layer of the skin and containing the root of a hair.

Halfway house A live-in treatment facility for individuals who have completed inpatient, or hospital-based psychiatric treatment, but who are not prepared to make a full transition to independent living.

Halitosis (*hal-i-to'sis*) Unpleasant breath due to oral infections and poor oral hygiene.

Hallberg effect Peaks and troughs in wave fields have opposite electrical signs.

Hallucination (*ha-loo-si-na'shun*) *psy* False sensory perceptions not associated with real external stimuli. Hallucination indicates a psychotic disturbance only when associated with impairment in reality testing.

Auditory hallucination False perception of sound, usually voices, often associated with chronic alcohol abuse; the sensory perceptions of hearing noises without an external stimulus.

Gustatory hallucination False perception of taste such as unpleasant taste due to an uncinate seizure.

Hypnagogic hallucination False sensory perception occurring while falling asleep.

Hypnopompic hallucination False sensory perception occurring while awakening from sleep.

Kinesthetic hallucination Movement of the body and a false perception of it.

Lilliputian hallucination False perception in which objects are seen as reduced in size.

Mood-congruent hallucination Hallucination whose content is consistent with either a depressed or manic mood.

Mood-incongruent hallucination Hallucination whose content is not consistent with either depressed or maniac mood.

Olfactory hallucination Referring to olfactory (relating to the sense of smell) perceptions in the absence of chemical stimuli, occur in nonclinical and clinical populations.

Somatic hallucination False sensation of things occurring in or to the body, most often visceral in origin.

Visual hallucination False perception involving sight, consisting of both formed images such as people and unformed images such as flashes of light.

Hallucinogen (*ha-loo'si-no-gen*) A drug that produces hallucinations.

Hallux (*hal'uks*) Pl. **halluces**. The big toe.

Hallux dolorosus Pain in the metatarsophalangeal joint of the big toe.

Hallux rigidus A painful deformity of big toe limiting movement at the metatarsophalangeal joint.

Hallux valgus Outward displacement of the big toe.

Hallux varus Inward displacement of the big toe.

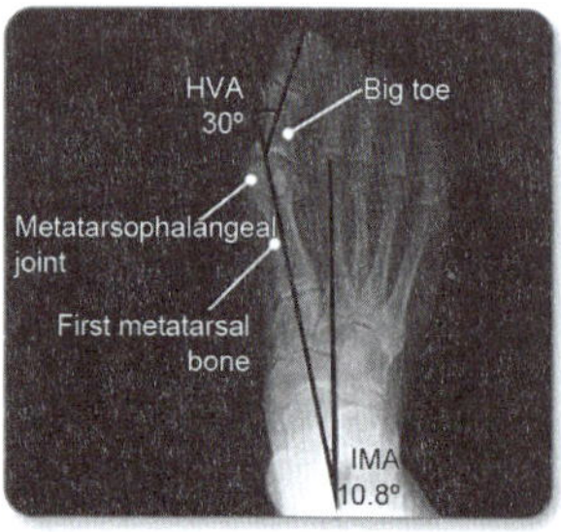

Hallux valgus showing intermetatarsal angle and lateral dislocation of sesamoids

Abbreviations: HVA, hallux valgus angle; IMA, inferior mesenteric artery

Halo The areola especially of the nipple; a ring surrounding macula; a circle of light surrounding a shining object.

Haloperidol (*ha-lo-per'i-dol*) A butyrophenone dopamine-blocking antipsychotic agent used for schizophrenia.

Haldol (Haloperidol): Treats schizophrenia and manages tics and vocal outbursts; antipsychotic medicine.

Halophilic Archaebacteria and eukarya which can thrive in salinity environment.

Halothane (*hal'o-than*) A fluorinated hydrocarbon used as a general anesthetic.

HALP Hyperalphalipoproteinemia; Hemoglobin, Albumin, Lymphocyte and Platelet (HALP score)—a score in patients with small cell lung cancer before first-line treatment with etoposide; hand-assisted laparoscopic proctocolectomy.

Hamartoma (*ham-ar-to'ma*) An error tumor consisting of components of mature tissues that are native to a site of origin. These components are arranged in an abnormal way as an island containing cartilage, fat, fibrous tissue, smooth muscle, nerve cells, epithelial tissue, and foci of calcification clefts.

Bile duct hamartoma Dilated cystic bile ducts, which are embryologic remnants that failed to involute during the period of embryogenesis.

Fibrous hamartoma Of infancy a rare, benign tumor of the subcutis and lower dermis, which usually occurs within the first 2 years of life.

Hepatic mesenchymal hamartoma A rare, benign, developmental tumor of the liver, with occasional risk of malignancy. Histologically, it appears as a disordered arrangement of the mesenchyme, bile ducts, and hepatic parenchyma.

Pulmonary hamartoma Benign malformation of the lung and it includes an abnormal mixture of tissue components such as cartilage, epithelium, fat or muscle which are common to the lung but the organ architecture is not preserved.

Sweat gland hamartoma A rare form of congenital tumorous malformation with proliferation of eccrine secretory coils and ducts, surrounding capillary angiomatous channels and occasionally other minor elements.

Hamate bone (unciform bone) The small medial bone at the ulnar side in the distal row of carpal bones.

Hamman's disease (*ham'anz*) Spontaneous mediastinal emphysema, named after Louis Hamman, US physician.

Hammer An instrument with a head attached transversely to the handle; hammer-shaped bone of the middle ear, malleus.

Hammer finger A flexion deformity of the distal interphalangeal joint of a finger caused by avulsion of the extensor tendon.

Percussion hammer A hammer with a rubber head used to elicit reflexes.

Hammer toe A joint involvement with flexion at the proximal interphalangeal joint with or without the distal interphalangeal joint and the metatarsophalangeal joint may he hyperextended.

Hamstring Any one of the three muscles on the posterior aspect of the thigh (semitendinosus, semimembranosus, and biceps femoris). These muscles flex the leg and adduct and extend the thigh; one of the tendons that forms the medial and lateral boundaries of the popliteal fossa.

Hamulus (*ham'u-lus*) Any hook-shaped structure.

Handicap Physical and mental disability that limits the performance.

Hand-Schuller-Christian disease (*hand-shil'erkris-chan*) Multifocal eosinophilic granuloma manifesting as histiocytic granulomas of the bone, exophthalmos, and diabetes insipidus. Seen in children, named after Alfred Hand Jr, US pediatrician, Arthur Schuller, Austrian neurologist and Henry Christian, US physician.

Hanot's cirrhosis *(a-noz)* Progressive biliary cirrhosis, named after Victor Hanot, French physician.

Hansen's bacillus *Mycobacterium leprae*, the causative agent of leprosy, discovered by Gerhard Hansen, Norwegian physician.

Haploid (monoploid) *(hap'loid)* Having half the normal number of chromosomes as in gametes, being 23 in humans.

Haplotype *(ha'plo-type)* A combination of related genes on the same chromosome, which are usually inherited together.

Happy puppet syndrome A puppet-like gait, fits of laughter and facial characteristics, *see* Angelman syndrome.

Haptene *(hap'ten)* A substance that normally does not act like an antigen, but that can be combined with carrier protein and then can initiate a specific antibody response.

Haptoglobin *(hap'to-glo'bin)* A mucoprotein to which hemoglobin released from lysed red cells into plasma is bound.

Harelip A congenital cleft in the upper lip usually due to failure of the median nasal and maxillary processes to unite.

Harrison's groove *(harr'i-sunz)* Horizontal depression on thoracic wall and it corresponds to the attachments of the diaphragm, noted at the xiphoid level in rickets described by Edwin Harrison, British physician.

Hartnup disease A rare hereditary disorder of renal and intestinal transport of tryptophan with clinical features resembling pellagra. The family name of the first reported case has been given to the disease; also called H disease.

Hashimoto's thyroiditis *(hash'i-mo'toz)* Autoimmune thyroiditis presenting with goitrous swelling of rubbery consistency. There is marked lymphocytic infiltration. Initially it may present with features of thyrotoxicosis, which over years may lead to hypothyroidism, named after Hakaru Hashimoto, Japanese surgeon.

Hashish *(hash'ish)* Extract of the hemp plant *Cannabis sativa* which is smoked or chewed for its euphoric effects.

Haustrum *(haws'trem)* The sac-like structure of the colon that in sequence gives the colon its segmented appearance.

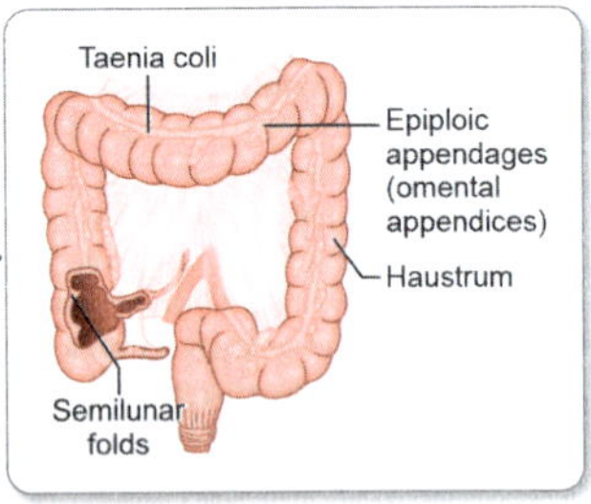

Haustra coli

Haversian canal Opening leading through the compact bone in a longitudinal direction and connecting with one another by transverse branches transmitting nutrient material, named after Clopton Havers, English anatomist and physician.

Haversian system A Haversian canal and its concentrically arranged lamellae, constituting the basic unit of the structure of compact bone.

Hay fever Allergic rhinitis, a type I hypersensitivity.

hCG Human chorionic gonadotropin; it is a hormone produced primarily by syncytiotrophoblastic cells of the placenta during pregnancy.

Head *(hed)* The part of the body containing the brain in the skull and organs of sight, hearing, smell and taste; the proximal end of a bone; the larger extremity of any structure or body.

Headache Cephalalgia, an acute or chronic diffuse pain in various parts of the head, not confined to the area of distribution of any nerve.

Cluster headache A migraine variant characterized by periodic, severe unilateral periorbital pain often accompanied by unilateral lacrimation and nasal congestion. The pain is brief and occurs at a particular time of the day.

Coital headache A sudden, often very severe headache at the climax of sexual intercourse in middle-aged men.

Exertional headache Brief headache during physical exertion.

Postlumbar puncture headache Headache developing on removal of CSF from lumbar puncture.

Spinal headache Frontal or occipital headache following spinal anesthesia.

Tension headache Dull or tight headache where the pain is constant and generalized. Emotional strain and anxiety are precipitating factors.

Health education A process that informs, motivates, and helps people to adopt and maintain healthy practices and lifestyles, advocates environmental changes and conducts professional training and research.

Hearing aid A sound-amplifying device used by the individuals with impaired hearing.

Heart (*hart*) cor. A hollow, muscular organ that maintains the circulation of the body by its pumping action. Two-thirds of its mass extends to the left of the midline. The wall of the heart consits of three layers outer epicardium, the middle myocardium made of cardiac muscle and inner endocardium. The pericardium envelops the heart. There are two upper thin-walled chambers right and left atria separated by the interatrial septum. They receive blood from the venae cavae and pulmonary veins, respectively. There are two lower, thick-walled chambers right and left ventricles separated by interventricular septum. The left ventricle pumps blood into the aorta and right ventricle pumps blood to the lungs through pulmonary artery. There are atrioventricular (mitral on left and tricuspid on right) and ventricular outflow (aortic and pulmonary) valves. The blood supply is by coronary arteries. The left main and right coronary arteries arise from the left and right coronary sinuses. The heart is innervated by both sympathetic and parasympathetic supply. The basic unit of contraction in the muscle is sarcomere.

Armored heart Calcium deposits in the pericardium.

Artificial heart A device that pumps blood like a normal left ventricle.

Athlete's heart Hypertrophy of the heart due to prolonged physical training.

Beri-beri heart Heart disease secondary to deficiency of thiamine.

Fatty heart Fatty degeneration of the heart; accumulation of fat in and around heart muscle.

Horizontal heart Rotation of electrical axis -30°.

Intermediate heart Direction of electrical axis to +30°.

Irritable heart Effort syndrome.

Left heart The left atrium and left ventricle that move blood into systemic circulation.

Right heart The right atrium and right ventricle that move the blood into the pulmonary circulation.

Semihorizontal heart Direction of the electrical axis at -0°.

Semivertical heart Direction of the electrical axis at +60°.

Univentricular heart Double-inlet ventricle in which one ventricular chamber receives flow from both tricuspid and mitral valves, single or common ventricle.

Vertical heart Electrical axis directed at +90°.

Water bottle heart Chest X-ray revealing markedly enlarged cardiac silhouette with a shape of water bottle in pericardial effusion.

Heart block A defect of conduction of impulse generated at SA node to the ventricles. It may be prolonged (first degree) leading to dropped beats (second degree) or with independent ventricular rhythm (complete).

Heartburn (pyrosis) Discomfort in the pit of the stomach or lower part of sternum due to acid reflux into esophagus.

Heart failure cell Hemosiderin-laden macrophages found in the alveoli and it indicates occurrence of repeated bleeding.

Heart lung machine An instrument that collects blood from both vena cavae, passes it through pump and oxygenator, and returns it to the femoral artery or ascending aorta. It temporarily takes over the function of the heart and lungs during heart surgery.

Heat exhaustion Caused by salt and water loss.

Heatstroke (sunstroke) Develops due to failure of body's thermoregulatory mechanism failure. It leads to widespread cellular damage.

Heat illness Represents a spectrum of disorders in which the thermoregulatory mechanisms of the body remain intact.

Hebephrenia (*he-be-fre'-ni-a*) Shallow inappropriate affect and silly regressive behavior and mannerisms.

Heberden's nodes Bony swellings close to distal interphalangeal joints due to osteoarthritis. Index finger is commonly affected, named after William Heberden, British physician.

Hebetude (*hebe'-tud*) Stupidity.

Hebetic Pertaining to youth.

Heel (*hel*) Calx.

Heel-to-knee test Coordination test for skilled movements. The heel has to be kept on the opposite knee and it should be drawn along the shin toward the ankle. The procedure is done on other side. In cerebellar disease, heel overshoots the knee and exhibits oscillation while it is moved down the leg. In sensory ataxia, heel is lifted high and falls off many times during its downward course.

Hegar's sign Early diagnosis of pregnancy between the sixth and tenth weeks, when the fundus and upper part of body of uterus are enlarged and lower uterine segment is soft and empty, cervix is soft and firm. Two fingers placed in the anterior vaginal fornix appear almost to meet the fingers of the other hand pressing backward and downward suprapubically, named after Alfred Hegar, German gynecologist.

Heimlich maneuver (*him'lik*) A first aid technique to dislodge an inhaled object in a choking person by administering rapid upward thrusts from below the sternum, named after HJ Heimlich, American physician.

Helcoplasty Act or process of repairing lesions by skin graft.

Helicotherapy Phototherapy.

Helix Pl. **halices**. A folded rim of cartilage forming the margin of auricle; a line in the shape of a coil.

Double helix Helical structure as surrounded by two strands of deoxyribonucleic acid, held together by hydrogen bonds, described by James Watson, US biochemist and Francis Crick, English biologist.

Helly's fluid A mixture of potassium dichromate, sodium sulfate, mercuric chloride, formaldehyde and distilled water used in preservation of bone marrow.

HELLP syndrome A syndrome noted in last trimester of pregnancy often with pregnancy-induced hypertension characterized by hemolysis, elevated liver enzymes, and low platelets.

Helminth A general term meaning worm. The helminths are parasitic invertebrates characterized by elongated, flat or round bodies like a fluke, tapeworm, or nematode.

Helminthiasis (*hel-min-thi'a-sis*) Helminths parasitizing humans. Helminths are largest of human parasites.

Helminthology The study of parasitic worms.

Heloma (*he-lo'ma*) Corn; collosity.

Hem- (hema-, hemo-, hemot(o)) (*he'm*) Combining word for blood.

Hemagglutination (*hem-a-glu-ti-na' shun*) The clumping of the red blood cells in presence of specific antibody or a microbial agent.

Hemagglutination inhibition reaction An immune reaction in which antigen-bearing erythrocytes are prevented from agglutinating.

Hemangioblastoma (Lindau's tumor) (*he-man'je-o-blasto'ma*) A slow growing well-circumscribed benign tumor consisting of proliferation of capillary vessel forming endothelial cells.

Hemangioma (*he-man'je-o'ma*) A developmental malformation of blood vessels in which there is intradermal or subdermal collection of dilated blood vessels. It is more common in the skin and subcutaneous tissues.

Capillary hemangioma Purple, or bright red lesion noted in childhood, pressure may cause disappearance of swelling or cause blanching.

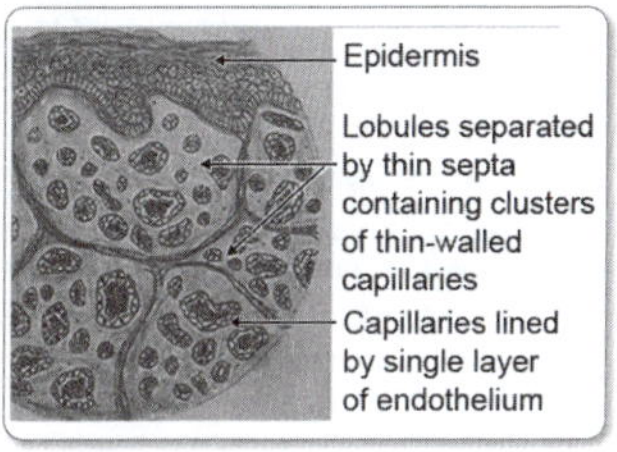

Capillary hemangioma

Cavernous hemangioma A congenital swelling containing multiple venous sinuses of varying caliber.

Plexiform hemangioma A diffuse pulsatile swelling of arteries and it feels like a bag of earthworms.

Senile hemangioma Red papule from weakened capillary wall.

Hemarthrosis (*hem'ar-thro'sis*) Bleeding into the joint usually from an injury which results in a swelling of the joint.

Hematemesis (*hem'at-em'e-sis*) The vomiting of blood. It occurs from upper gastrointestinal hemorrhage and it may be red with clots when bleeding is profuse, or black as coffee ground, when less severe.

Hematidrosis (hemathidrosis) (*he'mat-i-dro'sis*) Sweat containing blood or blood pigment.

Hematin (*he'ma-tin*) An iron-protoporphyrin containing ferric iron.

Hematinic (*hem'a-tin'ik*) Pertaining to blood; an agent that increases the level of hemoglobin and the number of red blood cells.

Hematocele (*hem'a-to-sel*) A collection of blood in a body cavity or potential space, commonly referred to a swelling of the membrane covering the testis.

Pelvic hematocele Collection of blood in pouch of Douglas.

Scrotal hematocele Collection of blood in scrotal sac.

Hematochezia (*hem'a-to-ke'zi-a*) The passage of blood in stools.

Hematocolpus (*hem'a-to-kol'pus*) Accumulation of menstrual blood in the vagina due to imperforate hymen or vaginal septum.

Hematocrit (*he-mat'o-krit*) The percentage volume of red blood cells in the blood; packed cell volume.

Hematocrit tube A narrow bore, thick-walled short glass tube of 11 cm length with calibrations to 100 mm and has a capacity to hold 1 mL of blood.

Hematocyst (*hem'o-to-cist*) Bleeding into a cyst; a hemorrhagic cyst.

Hematogenic, hematogenous (*hem'a-to-jen'ik, hem-a-toj'en-us*) Hemopoietic; anything produced from blood; spread through bloodstream.

Hematohidrosis (hemathidrosis, hematidrosis) (*he'mat-i-dro'sis*) Sweat containing blood or blood pigment.

Hematology (*hem'a-tol'o-jey*) The medical specialty concerned with the study of blood and blood forming tissues.

Hematoma (*he"me-to'ma*) An abnormal collection of blood outside of a blood vessel; a collection of blood inside the body, caused by bleeding from an injured vessel.

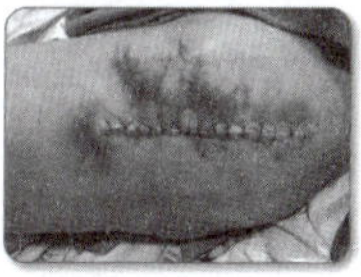

Postoperative hematoma

Muscle hematoma Occurs commonly in calf and psoas muscles in hemophilia.

Subdural hematoma Hematoma beneath the dura mater that produces neurologic symptoms by pressure on the brain.

Subungual hematoma A crimson, or gray-brown discoloration of nail plate, frequently of the big toe.

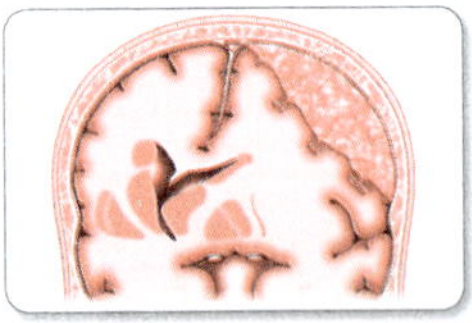

Subdural hematoma

Hematometra (*hem'a-to-me'tra*) Distension of uterus with blood either as an extension of hematocolpus or from obstruction of cervix.

Hematomyelia (*hem'a-to-mi-e'li-a*) Bleeding into the spinal cord.

Hematopoiesis (*hem'a-to-poi-e'sis*) Hemopoiesis

Extramedullary hematopoiesis The body's compensatory response to deficient erythropoiesis by the bone marrow or accelerated destruction of erythrocytes.

Hematoporphyrin (*hem'a-to-por'fi-rin*) Iron-free heme resulting from decomposition of hemoglobin.

Hematosalpinx (hemosalpinx) (*-sal'pinks*) Accumulation of blood in the fallopian tube, often associated with tubal pregnancy.

Hematoxylin (*he"me-tok'si-lin*) A natural dye from *Haematoxylum campechianum* used as the stain to examine tissues by light microscopy and it is used in conjunction with eosin, acting as a counterstain.

Hematuria (*hem'a-tu're-a*) Passage of blood in the urine.

Endemic hematuria Schistosomiasis.

Essential hematuria Hematuria whose cause is undetermined.

False hematuria Passage of red-colored urine following ingestion of food or drug containing pigment.

Microscopic hematuria Presence of red blood cells in urine recognized by microscopic examination.

Renal hematuria Hematuria resulting from extravasation of blood into the kidney where the urine is often smoky.

Urethral hematuria Bleeding into the urethra causing passage of bright red urine at the beginning of urination.

Vesical hematuria Bleeding into the urinary bladder causing hematuria.

Hemeralopia (*hem'er-a-lo'pe-a*) Day blindness.

Hemi- Combining word for half.

Hemiachromatopsia (*hem'e-a-kro'matop' se-a*) Color blindness in one half of the visual field.

Hemianopia (*hem'e-an'o-pe-a*) Blindness in one half of the visual field of one or both eyes.

Binasal hemianopia *see* Binasal hemianopia.

Bitemporal hemianopia *see* Bitemporal hemianopia.

Heteronymous hemianopia Blindness of both nasal or both temporal halves of the visual field.

Homonymous hemianopia Blindness affecting the nasal half of the visual field of one eye and the temporal half of the visual field of other eye.

Hemiballismus (*hem'e-bal-liz'mus*) A violent type of irregular, uncontrollable flinging movement affecting one half of the body.

Hemicolectomy Surgical removal of a part of colon.

Hemicrania (*hem'e-kra'ne-a*) Headache on one side of the scalp.

Hemimelia (*hem"e-me'le-a*) A developmental anomaly characterized by absence of all or part of the forearm of lower limb.

Hemin (*he'min*) Microscopic reddish-brown crystals, $C_{34}H_{32}N_4O_4FeCl$ formed when heating a sodium chloride crystal, a drop of glacial acetic acid, and some blood on a slide. These crystals are commonly employed to detect the presence of blood.

Hemiparesis (*hem'e-pa-re'sis*) Weakness affecting one side of the body.

Hemiplegia (hemiparesis) (*hem'e-ple'je-a*) Paralysis of one side of the body especially of the arm and leg. adj. **hemiplegic**.

Cerebral hemiplegia Hemiplegia due to a brain lesion.

Crossed hemiplegia Paralysis of one side of the face and opposite of the body.

Spastic hemiplegia Hemiplegia with spasticity of the affected muscles, accompanied by exaggerated deep reflexes.

Spinal hemiplegia Hemiplegia due to a lesion in the spinal cord.

Hemisacralization Fusion of 5th lumbar vertebra with left large transverse process which fuses with sacrum forming a psudoarticulation at that location.

Hemisphere (*hem'is-fer*) Half of a spherical structure or organ.

Cerebellar hemisphere Either of two lobes of the cerebellum situated lateral to the vermis.

Cerebral hemisphere One of the paired structures forming the bulk of the brain.

Dominant hemisphere That part of the cerebral hemisphere which is more concerned than the other in the integration of sensations and the control of voluntary functions.

Hemizygous Having only one copy of a given genetic locus.

Hemochromatosis (bronze diabetes, iron-storage disease) (*he'mo-kro'ma-to'sis*) A genetic disorder resulting in an excessive absorption and accumulation of iron in the liver, pancreas, and skin. There is bronzed skin, hepatomegaly, arthritis, congestive cardiac failure testicular atrophy and diabetes mellitus.

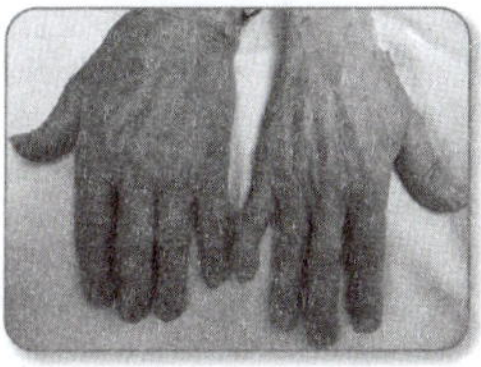

Hemochromatosis

Hemoconcentration Rise in the level of red blood cell count or hematocrit due to a fall in the plasma volume.

Hemocytometer (*he'mo-si-tom'et-er*) An instrument to count the blood cells.

Hemodialysis (*he'mo-di-al'i-sis*) A dialysis carried out in renal failure, in which blood is passed through a machine and purified before being returned to the body.

Hemodilution (*he'mo-di-lu'shun*) Fall in RBC count following bleeding and expansion of plasma volume.

Hemoglobin (*hem'o-glo'bin*) An iron-containing pigment in the red blood cells which carries o xygen to the tissues. Hemoglobin consists of four chains of globin, each surrounding a molecule of heme. There are four types of normal hemoglobin in man, the embryonic, fetal (HbF) and two adult types (HbA and HbA2).

Fetal hemoglobin The type of hemoglobin found in the normal fetus and it has the capacity to take up and give off oxygen at lower oxygen tensions.

Glycosylated hemoglobin HbA, or HbA1c that accounts for <4% of total hemoglobin in blood. Its estimation is helpful in assessing chronic glycemic control.

Hemoglobin C disease A benign hemoglobinopathy causing megaloblastic anemia in pregnancy and splenomegaly.

Hemoglobin H disease A condition due to failure of production of hemoglobin; a condition arising from heterozygosity for alpha thalassemia, noted in parts of Asia and around the Mediterranean.

Hemoglobin SC disease A mild variety of sickle cell anemia.

Mean corpuscular hemoglobin (MCH) The hemoglobin content of the average red cell.

Muscle hemoglobin Myoglobin.

Reduced hemoglobin Hemoglobin in the red cells following release of oxygen in the tissue.

Sickle cell hemoglobin Molecular abnormality characterized by presence of an abnormal hemoglobin HbS which is capable of altering its structure so that red cells assume a sickle shape.

Hemoglobinometer (*he'mo-glo'bi-nom'it-er*) A device used for determination of hemoglobin. Erythrocytes are lysed to get intracellular hemoglobin into solution and later its conversion into acid hematin. The resulting color is compared with permanent colored glass standard. The method is useful to measure only oxyhemoglobin.

Hemoglobinopathies (*he'mo-glo'bi-nop'a-thes*) Genetic disorders involving globin, the protein component of hemoglobin, divided into the thalassemia syndromes such as α and β thalassemia and variant hemoglobin such as sickle cell anemia.

Hemoglobinuria (*he'mo-glo'bi-nur'e-a*) The abnormal presence of hemoglobin in the urine.

Malarial hemoglobinuria Blackwater fever.

March hemoglobinuria Hemoglobinuria noted after prolonged or strenuous exercise.

Paroxysmal hemoglobinuria Intermittent attacks of hemoglobinuria due to increased fragility of red cells or presence of acute hemolysis.

Toxic hemoglobinuria Occurrence of hemoglobinuria from snake venom or toxic products of infection.

Hemogram (*he'mo-gram*) A detailed examination of the blood with special reference to the numbers, proportions and morphologic features of all formed elements.

Hemolysin (*he-mol'i-sin*) A toxic substance capable of causing lysis of red blood cells and liberation of their hemoglobin.

Hemolysis (*he-mol'i-sis*) The breakdown of red blood cells. It occurs as a normal process at the end of their life span, but occasionally occurs prematurely leading to anemia and jaundice.

Hemolytic (*he-mo-li'e-tik*) Referring to lysis of red cells.

Hemolytic disease of newborn A condition due to the incompatibility of fetal red cells with the maternal immune system.

Hemolytic jaundice Jaundice from increased destruction of red blood cells or their precursors in the marrow, causing increased bilirubin production. Jaundice is mild.

Hemolytic disease of the newborn A condition due to the incompatibility of fetal red cells with the maternal immune system.

Hemolytic uremia syndrome Condition occurring in children below two years with a prodrome of bloody diarrhea, hemolytic anemia and thrombocytopenia.

Hemopericardium (*he'mo-per'i-car'dium*) Blood in the pericardial sac.

Hemoperitoneum (*he'mo-per'i-to-ne'um*) Blood in the peritoneal cavity.

Hemophilia (*hem'o-fil'e-a*) An inherited coagulation defect characterized by a permanent tendency to hemorrhages due to a defect in the coagulation of blood.

Hemophilia A A sex-linked recessive condition with a deficiency of coagulation factor VIII, noted almost exclusively in males characterized by prolonged clotting time, hemarthroses, muscle hematoma and hemorrhage after trauma.

Hemophilia B Christmas disease condition clinically indistinguishable from hemophilia is due to hereditary deficiency of factor IX.

Hemophilia C Hemophilia due to a deficiency of factor XI.

Vascular hemophilia *see* Von Willebrand's disease.

Hemophthalmia (*he'mof-thal'mi-a*) An effusion of blood into the eye.

Hemopneumothorax (pneumobemothorax) (*he"mo-noo"mo- thor'aks*) Condition of having both air (pneumothorax) and blood (hemothorax) in the chest cavity.

A hemothorax, pneumothorax, or the combination of both can occur due to an injury to the lung or chest.

Hemopoiesis (*he'mo-poi-e'sis*) Formation and development of different types of blood cells and formed elements.

Hemopoietic (*he'mo-poi-et'ik*) Related to the blood; blood-forming organ.

Hemoptysis (*he-mop'ti-sis*) Coughing of blood or blood-stained sputum. It is bright red, and frothy coming from bronchial arteries.

Endemic hemoptysis Bouts of frank hemoptysis in lung due to infection by *Paragonimus westermani*.

Parasitic hemoptysis Hemoptysis due to fluke of genus *Paragonimus* causing cough, spitting up blood and slow deterioration.

Pseudohemoptysis Expectoration of red-colored sputum in *Serratia* infections.

Hemorrhage (bleeding) (*hem'o-rij*) Bleeding; an escape of blood from the blood vessels. It may be dark red and continuous (venous) or bright red and flowing in spurts (arterial). Capillary bleeding is red and occurs from tissues.

Hemorrhagic (*hem-o-raj'ik*) Relating to or characterized by hemorrhage.

Hemorrhagic pneumonia Hemorrhage into the alveoli.

Hemorrhoidectomy (*hem'o-royd-ek'to-me*) Excision of hemorrhoids.

Hemorrhoid (*hem'o-roid*) Pile; a mass of dilated, tortuous veins of the superior or inferior hemorrhoidal venous plexus at the anus.

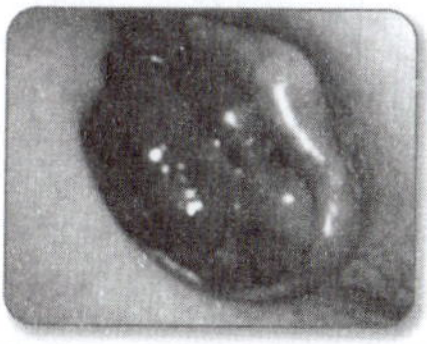

Hemorrhoid

Hemosalpinx (*he'mo-sal'pinks*) Hematosalpinx.

Hemosiderin (*he'mo-sid'er-in*) An insoluble iron-containing protein from hemoglobin following disintegration of red blood cells.

Hemosiderosis (*he'mo-sid'er-o'sis*) Abnormal accumulation of hemosiderin in tissues such as liver and spleen.

Idiopathic pulmonary hemosiderosis A condition characterized by intermittent intra-alveolar and intrabronchial hemorrhage form pulmonary capillaries presenting with recurrent hemoptysis and iron deficiency anemia.

Hemostasis (*he-mos'ta-sis*) The arrest of bleeding; the arrest of circulation in a part; stagnation of blood.

Hemostatic (styptic) (*he'mo-stat'ik*) Arresting bleeding; arresting the flow of blood within a blood vessel.

Hemothorax (*he'mo-thor'aks*) Blood in the pleural cavity.

Hemozoin Metabolic product of blood feeding parasites like malarial parasite. It is nonprotein component of hemoglobin.

Hendra virus An enveloped RNA virus closely related to Nipah virus causing respiratory infection, noted in Queensland, Australia.

Henipavirus (*hen'ipe-vi"res*) A genus of negative-strand RNA viruses in the family Paramyxoviridae, order Mononegavirales containing six established species, Two species have been identified to be zoonotic, causing disease in animals. These are the Hendra virus (HeV) and the Nipah virus (NiV).

Henle's loop The site of the majority of magnesium absorption from the kidneys.

Henry The practical unit of inductance in the meter-kilogram-second system, equivalent to the self-inductance of a circuit or the mutual inductance of two circuits, in which a change of one ampere per second produces an induced electromotive force of one volt.

Heparin (*hep'a-rin*) Naturally occurring glycosaminoglycan. It inhibits coagulation by enhancing the effect of antithrombin III in the inhibition of activated clotting factors IX, X, XI, XII and thrombin. Intravenous heparin is used for acute pulmonary embolism, acute myocardial infarction and deep vein thrombosis. It is also used while performing vascular procedures and inserting prosthetic heart valves. Bleeding is the most common complication. It has a short half-life.

Heparin sulfate A highly acidic linear polysaccharide with a very variable structure. It is ubiquitously expressed on cell surfaces and in the extracellular matrix and basement membrane of mammalian tissues.

Low-molecular-weight heparin (LMWH) Fragments of unfractionated heparin produced by either chemical or enzymatic depolymerization, used as parenteral anticoagulant for the prevention and treatment of thromboembolic diseases.

Unfractionated heparin (UFH) A crude product derived from the intestine of pigs, used as anticoagulant for acute thromboembolic disorders. It accelerates the inactivation of thrombin and FXa by antithrombin.

Hepatalgia Pain in or over the liver.

Hepatectomy Surgery to remove all or part of the liver.

Hepatic (*he-patik*) Pertaining to the liver.

Hepatic acinus Functional unit of the liver consisting of hepatocytes.

Hepatic amebiasis *see* Amebiasis.

Hepatic arterial disease Hepatic artery occlusion causing severe upper abdominal pain and high transaminase activity.

Hepatic decompensation Chronic liver failure when liver function can no longer maintain normal physiological conditions.

Hepatic failure Liver may fail in its function acutely presenting with mental changes progressing from confusion to stupor and coma or gradually leading to ascites, edema, hepatic encephalopathy jaundice, hypoalbuminemia and coagulation abnormality.

Hepatic lobule Division of liver into multiple smaller units comprising a central vein, radiating sinusoids separated from each other by hepatocyte plates and peripheral portal tracts.

Hepatic nodules Nodular regenerative hyperplasia giving rise to nodules in the liver.

Hepatic osteodystrophy Biliary cirrhosis associated with bone pain and fractures.

Hepatic duct The duct that carries bile out of the liver and it unites with the cystic duct to form the common bile duct.

Hepatic encephalopathy (portosystemic encephalopathy) A neuropsychiatric syndrome caused by liver disease. Liver failure and portosystemic shunting of blood are the underlying causes. It presents with change of intellect, personality, emotions and consciousness.

Hepatic flexure The bend of colon under liver where ascending colon becomes transverse colon.

Hepaticostomy The surgical procedure to create an incision or opening into a hepatic duct.

Hepatic vein Blood vessels that return low oxygen blood from liver, back to heart.

Hepatitis (*hep'a-ti'tis*) Inflammation of the liver which results in damage to hepatocytes with subsequent cell death.

Acute hepatitis Acute injury to the liver from viral infections (hepatitis A, B, C, D, E viral infections, EBV, CMV, herpes simplex) and drugs (rifampicin, isoniazid, chlorpromazine).

Alcoholic hepatitis Alcoholic liver disease presenting with jaundice, hepatomegaly, ascites, and encephalopathy. The toxic metabolites produced during conversion of acetaldehyde to acetate and immune reaction to liver cells are responsible for the condition.

Amoebic hepatitis Enlarged, tender liver, abscess in right lobe, fever and leukocytosis in patient with recent amebic colitis.

Anicteric hepatitis Viral hepatitis without jaundice.

Autoimmune hepatitis A chronic hepatitis occurring as an autoimmune disorder with presence of specific autoantibodies. It has an insidious onset with fatigue, anorexia, and jaundice.

Chronic hepatitis A disorder characterized by a mononuclear inflammatory cell infiltrate of the portal tracts, often due to hepatitis B.

Hepatitis A A self-limiting viral disease caused by hepatitis A virus, an RNA enterovirus. It spreads by fecal oral route in poor sanitation and rarely by blood. It has an incubation period of 2 weeks, presents with mild jaundice.

Hepatitis B This hepatitis is caused by HBV, a DNA virus and only hepadnavirus causing infection in humans. It is transmitted by parenteral route; other modes of spread are through saliva, sexual intercourse, and vertically from mother to child. Humans are the only source of infection. Individuals incubating or suffering from acute hepatitis are highly infectious. It causes a severe infection and chronic infection leads to chronic liver failure. These individuals are highly infectious when markers of continuing viral replication (HBeAg, HBV-DNA polymerase) are present.

Hepatitis C An RNA-containing flavivirus causing hepatitis. Humans appear to be sole source of infection and the spread is by inoculation with blood or blood products. Chronic infection with HCV may occur and is lifelong.

Hepatitis D An RNA defective virus which requires HBV for replication. It can infect individuals simultaneously with HBV and cause acute severe hepatitis and it can superinfect those who are already chronic carriers of HBV and lead to progressive chronic hepatitis and cirrhosis.

Hepatitis E Caused by HEV, an RNA virus, spreads by fecal-oral route and found in places with poor sanitation. It is responsible for large epidemics of water-borne hepatitis.

Interface hepatitis Hepatitis with invasion of inflammatory cell infiltrate into periportal parenchyma with loss of definition of the portal-peripheral interface, damage to the periportal hepatocytes and formation of hepatocyte 'rosettes'.

Toxic hepatitis Liver, main organ in which drugs are metabolized, may get impaired in its capacity to metabolize drugs and give rise to manifestations by hepatic damage.

Viral hepatitis This hepatitis is caused by specific hepatitis viruses and rarely from other viruses (cytomegalovirus, EBV, HSV, yellow fever virus).

Hepatization (*hep'a-ti-za'shun*) Transformation into a solid mass like the liver especially the consolidated lobe in pneumonia.

Hepatoblastoma (*hep'a-to-blas-to'ma*) A malignant hepatic tumor found in infants; the tumor is single, solid, well-circumscribed and contains immature histiocytes.

Hepatocellular (*hepa-to-cel'lu-lar*) Pertaining to or affecting liver cells.

Hepatocyte (*hep'a-tosit*) A liver cell.

Hepatolith (*hep'a-to-lith*) A calculus in the liver.

Hepatoma (*hep'a-to'ma*) Tumor of the liver; hepatocellular carcinoma.

Hepatomegaly (*hep'a-to-meg'a-le*) Enlargement of the liver. Liver is enlarged from infections (viral hepatitis, amebic hepatitis, malaria, kala-azar, hydatid disease, tuberculosis, infectious mononucleosis), congestion (congestive heart failure, portal hypertension), early stages of cirrhosis, toxic hepatitis, hematologic conditions (iron deficiency anemia, reticulosis, leukemia, multiple myeloma), metabolic (diabetes mellitus), amyloidosis, hepatoma and secondary deposits.

Hepatotoxic Damage to the liver caused by a medicine, chemical or herbal or dietary supplement.

Hereditary (*he-red'i-tar-e*) Capable of being passed from parent to offspring through genetic means.

Heredity (*he-red'it-e*) Genetic transmission of characters from parent to offspring.

Hernia (*her'ne-a*) Protrusion of a portion of an organ or tissue through a normal or abnormal opening in the wall of the cavity in which it lies. adj. **hernial**.

Abdominal hernia Hernia occurring through abdominal wall.

Barth's hernia Protrusion of a loop of intestine between a persistent vitelline duct and the abdominal wall.

Beclard's hernia Femoral hernia through the opening for saphenous vein.

Bochdalek hernia Congenital diaphragmatic hernia due to a defect in closure of pleuroperitoneal membrane.

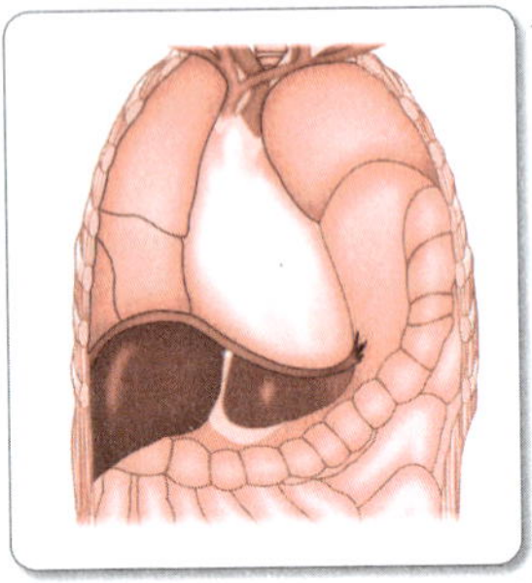

Bochdalek hernia

Cerebral hernia Protrusion of brain through the skull.

Complete hernia An indirect inguinal hernia in which the contents extend into the tunica vaginalis.

Congenital hernia Inguinal hernia that is present from birth. Most common congenital hernia is diaphragmatic hernia.

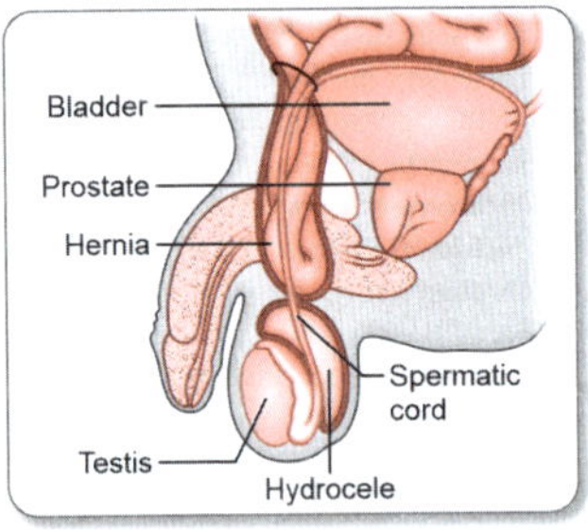

Congenital hernia

Crural hernia Femoral hernia.

Diaphragmatic hernia Protrusion of abdominal contents into the chest through the diaphragm.

Epigastric hernia A protrusion of extraperitoneal fat and occasionally a small peritoneal sac through the weakness in the linea alba between the xiphoid process and the umbilicus.

Fat hernia Protrusion of peritoneal fat through the abdominal wall.

Femoral hernia A protrusion of extraperitoneal fat, peritoneum and occasionally abdominal contents through the femoral canal.

Funicular hernia Inguinal hernia in which the proussus vagnialis is closed at its lower and just above the epididymes.

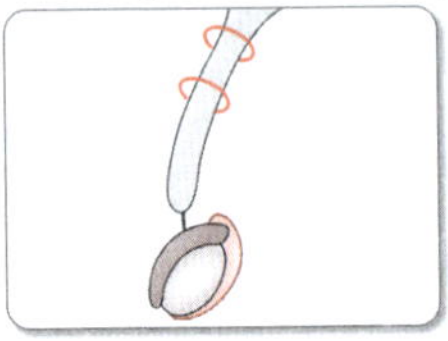

Funicular hernia

Gastroesophageal hernia Hiatus hernia in which distal end of the esophagus and part of the stomach protrude through the esophageal hiatus of the diaphragm.

Glissade hernia Sliding hernia. The posterior wall of the hernial sac is not formed by peritoneum alone, but also by viscus such as sigmoid colon and its mesentery on the left side and caecum on the right side and the contents of the sac may be intestine or omentum.

Incarcerated hernia Irreducible hernia.

Incisional hernia Hernia occurring through a surgical incision or scar indirect.

Infantile hernia Inguinal hernia seen in infants.

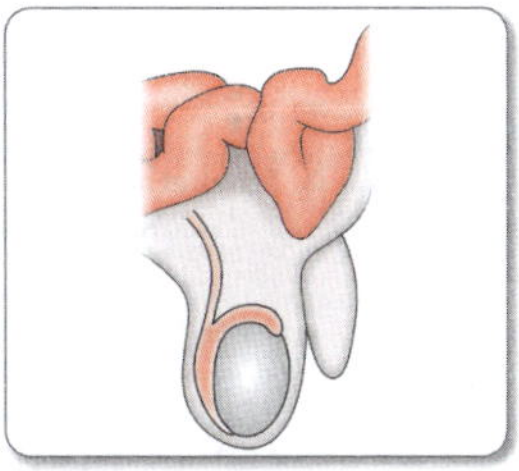

Infantile hernia

Inguinal hernia Most common of all forms of hernia; occurs through the inguinal canal. It may be direct or indirect. Direct inguinal hernia comes out through the Hasselbach's triangle, usually bilateral and incomplete that may be shaped spherical or globular. Common in old age.

Interstitial hernia Hernial sac lies between different layers of the abdominal wall which may be intraparietal, interparietal (intermuscular) or extraparietal.

Paraumbilical hernia Painless reducible swelling around the umbilicus liable to become irreducible.

Reducible hernia Hernia in which the contents of the hernial sac can be returned back by manipulation.

Sciatic hernia Protrusion of intestine through the great sacrosciatic foramen.

Scrotal hernia A complete inguinal hernia located in the scrotum.

Strangulated hernia An irreducible hernia which is constricted so as to compromise the blood supply.

Synovial hernia Protrusion of a fold of synovial membrane through the stratum fibrosum of a joint capsule.

Umbilical hernia Herniation of abdominal contents through the center of the abdominal scar.

Ventral hernia Hernia through the abdominal wall.

Vitreous hernia Prolapse of the vitreous into the anterior chamber.

Hernioplasty (*her'ne-o-plas'te*) Surgical correction of hernia.

Herniorrhaphy (*her'ne-or'a-fe*) Surgical repair of hernia, with suturing.

Heroin (diacetylmorphine) (*he'ro-in*) Diacetyl morphine.

Herpangina (*her'pan-ji-na*) An infectious febrile illness due to a coxsackievirus. The throat and posterior area of the mouth are covered with vesicles that rupture and ulcerate.

Herpes (*her'pez*) Any inflammatory disease characterized by small vesicles in clusters caused by herpesviruses. adj. **herpetic**.

Genital herpes Common sexually transmitted disease caused by herpes simplex virus (HSV) type 2. It is characterized by itchy or painful small grouped vesicles which break and produce ulcers in genital region with inguinal lymphadenopathy and fever.

Herpes encephalitis Inflammation of the brain caused by the spread of a herpes simplex virus.

Herpes febrilis Herpes simplex of the lips and nasal mucosa.

Herpes genitalis Genital herpes.

Herpes simplex Infection with the herpes simplex virus. It causes blister-like sores on the face, lips, mouth, or genitals.

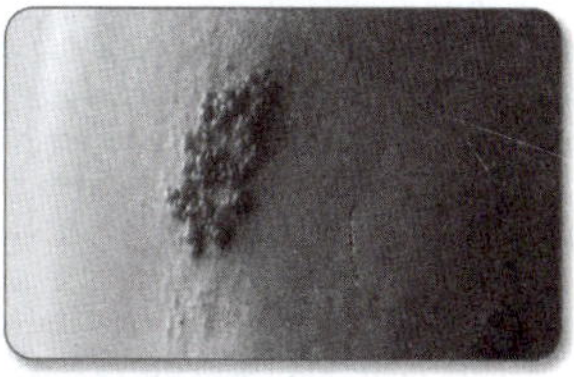

Herpes simplex

Herpesviridae A large family of DNA viruses, which includes HSV-1 and HSV-2, both of which can cause orolabial herpes and genital herpes.

Herpes whitlow Blistering of the skin on the fingers by herpes simplex viral infection.

Herpes zoster Shingles caused by varicella-zoster virus. It involves posterior root ganglia and presents with severe continuous pain in the distribution of the affected nerve root. The lesion after 3 or 4 days becomes red and vesicles appear which dry up and leave behind small scars. The condition may be followed by neuralgia.

Herpesvirus A group of viruses that includes herpes simplex virus, varicella-zoster virus, Epstein-Barr virus, and cytomegalovirus.

Hertz (*herts*) A unit of frequency equal to one cycle per second; Hz.

Heterochromatin (*het'er-o-kro'ma-tin*) Diversity of color in a part normally of one color; dark-appearing bands following Giemsa banding of chromosomes.

Heterochromia Condition characterized by a difference in the coloration of the iris (the colored part of the eye) between the two eyes or within the same eye. It occurs when there are variations in the concentration or distribution of melanin.

Binocular heterochromia An increase or decrease in pigmentation of one eye, with or without extraocular pigmentary defects.

Uniocular heterochromia A variegated or two-colored iris.

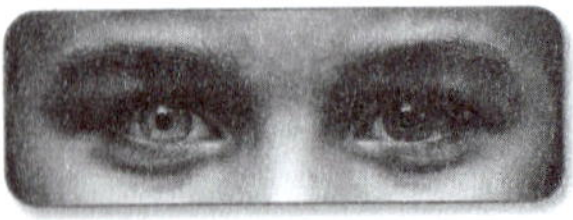

Heterochromia

Heterogametic The sex that produces two different kinds of gametes, which carry different sex chromosomes and therefore determines the sex of the offsping.

Heterogeneity The quality or state of being diverse in character or content.

Heterograft (xenograft) (*het'er-o-graft*) Xenograft, a graft transferred from an animal of one species to one of another species.

Heterophoria (*het'er-o-for'e-a*) A tendency for deviation of the eyes.

Heterophyes Genus of small digenetic trematode worms, belonging to the family Heterophyidae, is found to infest the small intestine, particularly in dogs, cats, and humans residing in Egypt and various regions of tropical Asia.

Heterophyiasis An infestation of the small intestine with parasitic fluke *Heterophyes*. Symptoms are abdominal pain and diarrhea.

Heteroplasty (*het'er-o-plas'te*) Tissue transplantation from one species to another heterotransplantation.

Heteropsia (*het'er-op'se-a*) Unequal vision in both eyes.

Heterosexuality (*het'er-o-sek'shu-al-ite*) Erotic attraction or sexual behavior between persons of the opposite sex.

Heterosis (*het"er-o'sis*) The tendency of a cross-bred individual to show qualities superior to those of both parents, also known as hybrid vigor.

Heterotopia (heterotopy) (*het'er-o-to'pe-a*) Ectopia; displacement of gray matter into deep cerebral white matter.

Heterotrophic (organotrophic) (*het"er-o-tro'fik*) Organism dependent on obtaining organic food from the environment because it is unable to synthesize organic material and eats other animals or plants, rather than making its own food.

Heterotropia (*het'er-o-tro'pe-a*) *see* Strabismus.

Band heterotropia Also known as double cortex syndrome, is a form of diffuse gray matter heterotopia affecting almost only women.

Periventricular nodular heterotropia The most common malformations of cortical development, and affected patients are frequently characterized by focal drug-resistant epilepsy.

Hexacanth The six hooked larva of a tapeworm.

Hexachlorophene Also known as Nabac, is an organochlorine compound that was once widely used as a disinfectant.

Hexachromia Ability to distinguish only 6 of the 7 colors of the spectrum. Most people can not distinguish indigo from blue or violet.

Hexobarbital (*hek'so-bar'bi-tal*) A short-acting barbiturate sedative and hypnotic.

Hexokinase (*hek'so-ki'nas*) An enzyme that catalyzes the transfer of a high energy phosphate group to a hexose.

Hexosamine (*hek'so-s'a-men*) The amine derivative of a hexose.

Hexose (*hek'sos*) A monosaccharide containing six carbon atoms in a molecule.

HGH or hGH Human growth hormone.

HHS Stands for Hyperosmolar Hyperglycemic State, is a serious complication of diabetes that happens when blood sugar levels are very high for a long period of time. Symptoms of HHS can include extreme thirst, frequent urination and confusion.

Hiatus (*hi-a'tus*) A gap, cleft or opening. adj. **hiatal**.

Hiatus hernia A condition in which part of the stomach pushes up through the diaphragm muscle.

Hib disease An infection caused by *Haemophilus influenzae* type B in children.

Hiccup (Hiccough) (*hik'up*) Spasms of the diaphragm usually due to irritation in the upper abdominal area.

Hickman line (*hik'man*) A type of catheter that is surgically implanted, whose one end leads into a large vein in the chest and the other end outside the chest.

Hidradenitis (Hidrosadenitis) (*hi'drad-e-nitis*) Inflammation of the sweat glands.

Neutrophilic eccrine hidradenitis A distinctive dermatosis occurring in patients with malignancy or undergoing chemotherapy.

Hidradenitis suppurativa Also called acne inversa, is a chronic inflammatory skin condition that affects apocrine gland-bearing skin in the axillae, groin, and under the breasts, characterized by persistent or recurrent boil-like nodules and abscesses that culminate in a purulent discharge, sinuses, and scarring.

Hidradenocarcinoma (*hi-drad'e-no-kar-cinoma*) Carcinoma of the sweat glands.

Hidrosis Sweating.

Hidrotic (*hi-drot'ik*) Pertaining to or characterized by or causing sweating.

High-resolution computed tomography (HRCT) A CT utilizing thin collimation and image reconstruction with high-spatial frequency algorithm.

Hilum (*hi'lum*) Pl. **hila**. A depression or a pit on an organ. It allows entry or exit to blood vessels and nerves. adj. **hilar**.

Hilum of lung Anatomic area situated between the lung laterally and the mediastinum medially, through which pass the bronchus, pulmonary vessels and is visible radiologically because of presence of surrounding aerated lung .

Hilum renale The entry and exit site for structures servicing the kidneys: vessels, nerves, lymphatics, and ureters.

Hindbrain (*hind'bran*) The most caudal part of the brain giving rise to cerebellum, pons and medulla oblongata.

Hindgut (*hind'gut*) The embryonic structure from which the colon is formed.

Hinge joint A joint in which the two bony surfaces fit tightly allowing flexion and extension as in knee or elbow joints.

Hip Coxa area of the body lateral to and including hip joint.

Snapping hip A condition in which hip is palpable or audible with snapping sensation, occurs during hip movement.

Hippocampal sclerosis A disorder characterized by hippocampal neuronal loss that causes medical temporal lobe epilepsy.

Hippocampus (*hip'o-kam-pus*) A curved elevation in the floor of the inferior horn of the lateral ventricle, and is thought to be involved in memory.

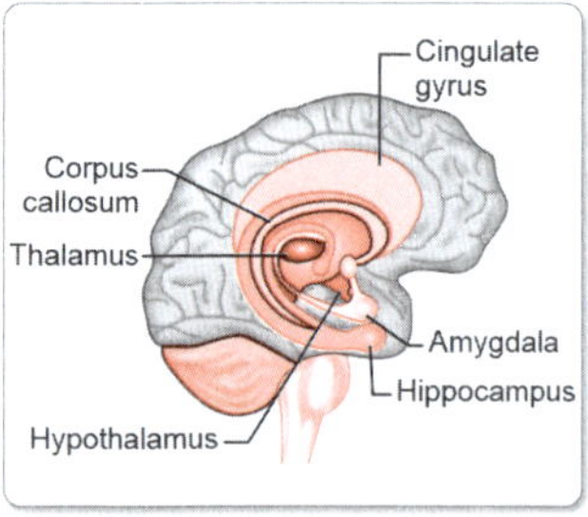

Hippocampus in limbic system

Hippocratic oath An oath demanded of physician about to enter upon the practice of his profession.

Hippus (*hip'us*) An abnormally exaggerated rhythmic contraction and dilatation of the pupil.

Hirschsprung's disease A condition that affects the large intestine and causes problems with passing stool.

Hirsutism (*hir'sut'izm*) Abnormal growth of hair, especially in women in a pattern that of a normal male due to an increased responsiveness of the hair follicles to the normal levels of androgenic hormones.

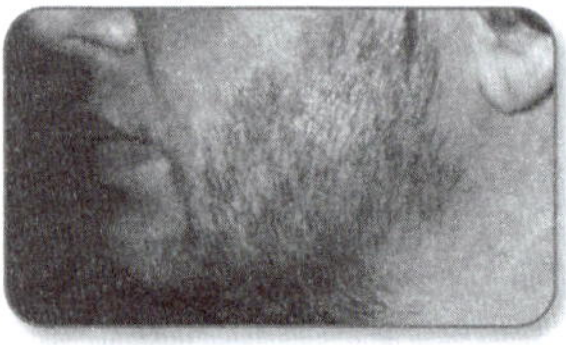

Hirsutism

Hirudin (*hi'rud'in*) The active principle of the buccal secretion of leeches. It prevents coagulation by acting as an antithrombin.

Hist- (histio-, histo-) Combining word for tissue.

Histamine (*his'ta-men*) A bioactive amine stored in mast cells and basophils. It may be secreted by monocytes, neural and endocrine cells. Histamine causes smooth muscle contraction, including bronchiolar and small vessel constriction, increased vascular permeability and secretion of nasal and bronchial glands. It is a powerful stimulant of gastric secretion.

Histaminergic (*his'ta-min-er'jic*) Referring to the effects of histamine at histamine receptors of target organ.

Histidine It is an essential amino acid. It is not made by the body, but is consumed in foods.

Histidinemia (*his'ti-din-e'mea*) An autosomal recessive condition characterized by a deficiency in histidase, the enzyme that converts histidine to urocanic acid in the liver and skin. Generally, asymptomatic. Rarely, it may have a neonatal onset with impaired speech, growth and mental retardation.

Histiocyte (*his'te-o-sit*) A resident macrophage. adj. **histiocytic**.

Histiocytoma (*his'te-o-si-to'ma*) A tumor-containing histiocytes.

Benign fibrous histiocytoma A mesenchymal tumor composed of fibroblasts and histiocytes arising in cutaneous and noncutaneous soft tissues.

Fibrous histiocytoma A benign soft tissue tumor that may present as a fibrous mass anywhere in the human body.

Generalized eruptive histiocytoma An unusual, benign disorder belonging to the group of non-Langerhans cell ('non-x') histiocytoses.

Malignant fibrous histiocytoma A neoplasm believed to originate from primitive mesenchymal cells; arising from soft tissue or bone, usually in the extremities or retroperitoneum.

Histiocytosis (*his'te-o-si-to'sis*) An uncommon condition of undetermined etiology presenting with involvement of flat bones and soft tissues like the lungs, skin, neurohypophysis, lymph nodes, liver and spleen, is characterized by granuloma formation with infiltration and proliferation of histiocytes.

Benign cephalic histiocytosis A rare self-limiting non-Langerhans histiocytosis that typically starts at the end of first year of life.

Histiocytosis X A group of disorders that includes fulminant Letterer-Siwe disease of early infancy, Hand-Schuller Christian disease of childhood, eosinophilic granuloma or Langerhans cell granulomatosis in young and middle-aged adults.

Langerhans cell histiocytosis A rare disorder that can damage tissue or cause lesions to form in one or more places in the body.

Malignant histiocytosis A progressive, neoplastic proliferation of atypical histiocytes and their precursors, which invade multiple organs.

Histochemistry (*his'to-kem'is-tre*) The study of chemistry of the cells and tissues.

Histocompatibility (*his'to-kom'pat'i-bil'it-e*) The state of being histocompatible.

Histocompatibility antigen One of the multiple antigens found in all nucleated cells in the body capable of identifying the cell as 'self' and it determines the compatibility of tissue for transformation.

Histogenesis (*his'to-jen'es-is*) The formation and development of tissues from the undifferentiated cells of the germ layers of the embryo.

Histogram (*his'to-gram*) A pictorial diagram of a frequency distribution and is represented by vertical bars or rectangles.

Histoid (*his'toid*) Resembling in structure one of the tissues in the body.

Histological grade A description of a tumor based on how abnormal the cancer cells and tissue look under a microscope and how quickly these cells are likely to grow and spread.

Histology (*his-tol'o-je*) The study of microscopic structure of organ tissues; the science dealing with the microscopic study of cells and tissues. adj. **histologic**.

Histone (*his'ton*) One of simple proteins that contains a high proportion of basic amino acids.

Histoplasma (*his'to-plas'ma*) A genus of fungi, *H. capsulatum* the causative agent of histoplasmosis. It exists in mycelial form in nature and in yeast phase in the human body temperature.

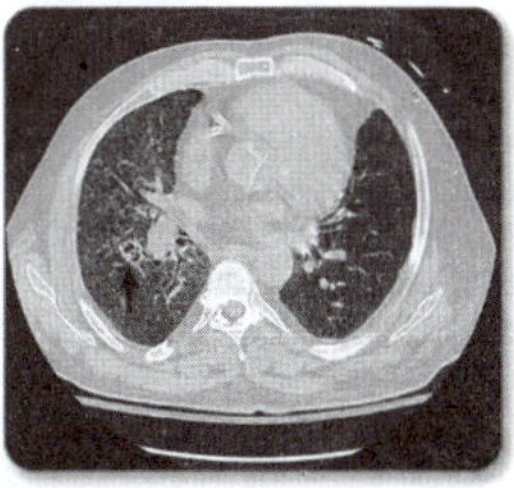

Histoplasma in lung

Histoplasmin Histoplasmin is a polyvalent mixture of antigens, only some of which are specific for *H. capsulatum*, skin test is used to check if you have been exposed to a fungus called *H. capsulatum*. The fungus causes an infection called histoplasmosis.

Histoplasmosis (*his'to-plaz-mo'sis*) The infection from *H. capsulatum* is acquired from the moist soil often contaminated by bird droppings in the river basins in temperate zones, especially in central United States. It presents as primary infection, or acute or chronic histoplasmosis.

Acute histoplasmosis Presents with cough, chest pain, fever, lassitude; multiple, soft pneumonic infiltrates in the lung leave behind multiple calcification.

Chronic histoplasmosis Associated with tissue necrosis and cavity formation. Amphotericin B is used in treatment.

Disseminated histoplasmosis Noted when histoplasmosis develops as an opportunistic infection.

Histotoxic (*his'to-tok'sik*) Any substance that is poisonous to the tissues.

HIV Human immunodeficiency virus.

HLA system Human leukocyte antigen system is important part of the immune system and is controlled by genes located on chromosome 6.

Hobnail liver A liver having many small knobby projections due to cirrhosis.

Hodgkin's disease A lymphoma of B cell origin. It may involve single lymph node region or extralymphatic site (stage 1), two or more lymph node regions or an extralymphatic site and lymph node regions on same side above or below diaphragm (stage 2), lymph nodes of both sides of diaphragm with or without localized extralymphatic involvement or involvement of spleen or both (stage 3), and diffuse involvement of one or more extralymphatic tissues (stage 4). Histologically, it is characterized by large malignant lymphoid cells. There is painless, rubbery lymphadenopathy or mediastinal masses. The spread is contiguous. Treatment includes radiotherapy, chemotherapy, or both, named after Thomas Hodgkin, British physician.

Holistic Pertains to the entire person, including the mind, body and spirit.

Holistic medicine Therapy that attempts to treat the patient as a whole person.

Holmes-Adie syndrome A rare neurological disorder affecting the pupil of the eye.

Holter monitor A device to record ECG tracing or a portable tape recorder while the patient carries normal activities, devised by Normann Holter, US biophysicist.

Holocrine (*hol'o-krin*) Secretion of the gland wherein the entire secretory cell containing secretory products is cast off as of sebaceous glands.

Homans' sign Calf pain on forced dorsiflexion of the ankle with knee extended in deep vein thrombosis, named after John Homans, US surgeon.

Homeopathy (*ho'me-op'a-the*) A system of therapeutics based on the theory that 'like cures like', founded by Samuel Hahnemann, German physician. He believed that administration of a large amount of a particular drug may cause symptoms of a disease and moderate dosage may reduce those symptoms.

Homeopathist A physician who practices homeopathy.

Homeostasis (*ho'me-o-sta'sis*) A relative constancy in the internal environment of the body maintained by a variety of active processes in the body.

Homeostasis (*ho'me-o-sta'sis*) A relative constancy in the internal environment of the body maintained by a variety of active processes in the body.

Homeothermy (*ho'me-o-ther'me*) Maintenance of a constant body temperature despite changes in the environmental temperature.

Homoeroticism Relating to or including sexual action between individuals of the same sex.

Homo The genus of primates, *H. sapiens* species of man.

Homogametic (*ho'mo-ga-met'ik*) A tissue made uniform in quality by grinding cells.

Homogenize (*ho'moj'in-iz*) To render homogeneous.

Homogentisic acid (*ho'mo-jen-tis'ik*) Alkapton; an intermediate in tyrosine metabolism.

Homograft (allograft) (*ho'mo-graft*) *see* Allograft, tissue or organ transplanted from one individual to another of same species.

Homolateral (*ho'mo-lateral*) Pertaining to the same side of the body; ipsilateral.

Homologous (*ho-mol'o-gus*) Corresponding or alike in certain characteristics.

Homoplastic (*ho'mo-plas'tik*) Similar in form and structure.

Homosexuality Sexual attraction to members of the same sex.

Homozygous (*ho"mo-zi-gos*) Possessing two identical forms of gene that controls a specific inherited trait.

Homunculus (*hom'an-cu-lus*) Little person.

Hook (*hook*) A curved instrument for traction or holding.

Hookworm (*hook'wurm*) A nematode parasite in the intestine and *Ancylostoma duodenale* (causing ancylostomiasis, Old World hookworm) and *Necator americanus* (New World hookworm) are two important species.

Hoover's sign (*hoo'verz*) Unilateral lag in motion of one side of the chest due to pleurisy or pleural effusion, elicited by comparing the displacement from the midline during a deep inspiration of the examiner's hands, each placed lightly over one hemithorax, with thumbs touching beneath the xiphoid process at the start of breath, named after Charles Hoover, US physician.

Hordeolum (*hor-de'o-lum*) Stye. Painful swelling from inflamed hair follicles at the margin of eyelid.

Hordeolum externa Inflammation of the sebaceous gland of an eyelash.

Hordeolum interna Acute purulent infection of meibomian gland.

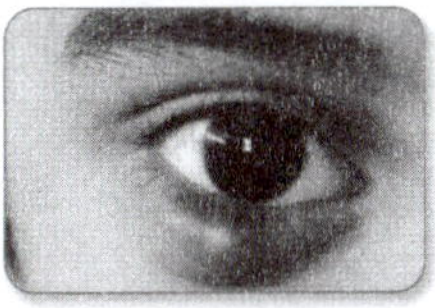

Hordeolum of right eye

Hormone (*hor'mon*) A chemical substance that is produced in the body by an organ or cells of an organ and released directly into the bloodstream. It has a specific regulatory action on the activity of a certain organ.

Adrenocortical hormones Hormones secreted by adrenal cortex. The major ones being glucocorticoids, mineralocorticoids, and androgens.

Adrenocorticotropic hormone ACTH corticotropin, hormone of anterior lobe of pituitary that stimulates the growth and functional activity of the adrenal cortex.

Androgenic hormone Masculinizing hormone.

Anterior pituitary hormone One of the several hormones secreted by the anterior lobe of the pituitary such as growth hormone, TSH, ACTH, FSH, ICSH, LH, prolactin and MSH.

Antidiuretic hormone ADH, a peptide hormone produced by the hypothalamus and stored in posterior pituitary. It increases reabsorption of water by kidneys; vasopressin.

Chorionic gonadotropic hormone Chorionic gonadotropin.

Corpus luteum hormone Progesterone secreted by corpus luteum.

Cortical hormone Adrenocortical hormone.

Corticotropin-releasing hormone (CRH) A neuropeptide from hypothalamus that stimulates the anterior pituitary to release ACTH.

Ectopic hormone Hormonal substances released from a neoplasm or cells outside the usual source of hormones.

Follicle-stimulating hormone (FSH) A gonadotropic hormone of anterior pituitary that stimulates growth and maturation of Graafian follicles in the ovary, and stimulates the epithelium of seminiferous tubules in the testis for spermatogenesis.

Follicle-stimulating hormone-releasing hormone (FSH-RH) A factor secreted by hypothalamus to promote release of FSH.

Gonadotropin-releasing hormone (GnRH) A hypothalamic hormone that stimulates anterior pituitary to release gonadotropins such as FSH and LH.

Growth hormone (GH) Somatotropin; a secretion of anterior pituitary that stimulates growth by directly influencing protein, carbohydrate and fat metabolism.

Growth hormone-releasing hormone (GHRH) A substance elaborated by hypothalamus. Stimulating the release of growth hormone from anterior pituitary.

Interstitial cell-stimulating hormone (ICSH) Luteinizing hormone.

Lactogenic hormone (LH) or prolactin hormone A gonadotropic hormone of the anterior pituitary that stimulates ripening of the follicles and secretion of progesterone by them, their rupture to release the ova and conversion of the ruptured follicle into the corpus luteum.

Luteinizing hormone-releasing hormone (LHRH) A hormone from the hypothalamus that stimulates anterior pituitary to release FSH and LH.

Luteotropic hormone (LTH) An anterior pituitary hormone that maintains the function of the corpus luteum.

Melanocyte-stimulating hormone (MSH) A peptide hormone secreted by the intermediate lobe of the pituitary that causes melanin formation and deposition in the body tissues and bring about darkening of skin.

Neurohypophysial hormones Posterior pituitary hormones.

Ovarian hormone One of the hormones secreted by the ovary, as an estrogen.

Parathyroid hormone A polypeptide hormone of the parathyroid gland which influences calcium and phosphorus metabolism.

Placental hormones Substances secreted by the placenta such as chorionic gonadotropin, relaxin and other substances.

Posterior pituitary hormones Substances such as vasopressin and oxytocin released from posterior pituitary.

Progestational hormone Progesterone.

Sex hormones Steroid hormones possessing estrogenic (female) or androgenic (male) activity.

Somatotropic hormone (STH) Somatotropin or growth hormone.

Steroid hormones Hormones possessing cyclopentanoperhydrophenanthrene ring in their molecules.

Thyroid hormones Thyroxine, triiodothyronine and calcitonin.

Thyroid-stimulating hormone (TSH) Thyrotropin.

Thyrotropin-releasing hormone (TRH) Hormone from the hypothalamus that stimulates anterior pituitary to release thyrotropin.

Hormone replacement therapy (HRT) Treatment with hormones to replace natural hormones when the body does not make in sufficient quantity.

Horn (*horn*) Cornu; a cutaneous outgrowth with a pointed projection; any horn-shaped structure.

Cutaneous horn A protrusion from the skin consisting of cornified material organized in the shape of a horn.

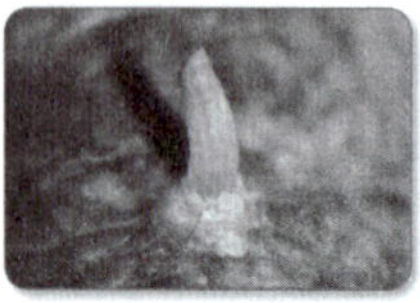

Cutaneous horn

Horn of pulp Extensions of pulp that protrude into the cusps of the tooth.

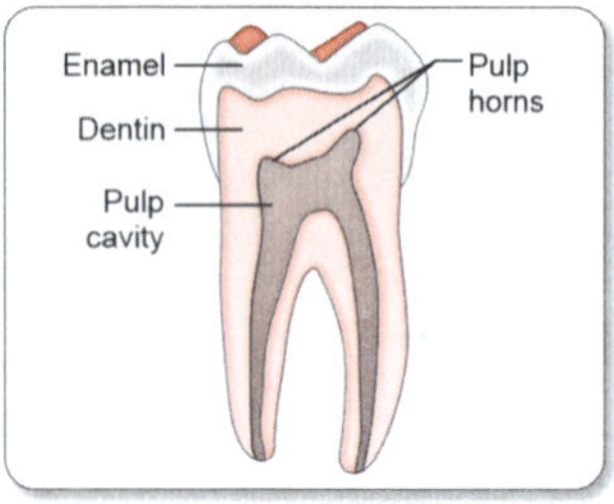

Horn of pulp

Sebaceous horn A hard outgrowth of the contents of a sebaceous cyst.

Horner's syndrome A syndrome characterized by ptosis, meiosis, enophthalmos and anhidrosis over one side of the face due to paralysis of the cervical sympathetic nerve trunk, named after Johann Horner, Swiss ophthalmologist.

Horseshoe kidney A condition in which the kidneys are fused together at the lower end or base.

Hospice (*hos'pis*) A hospital or a part of a hospital devoted for the care of dying patients.

Hospital (*hos'pit'l*) An institution for the care of the patients.

Base hospital The medical control hospital for a paramedic unit; a wind instrument that consists of a brass tube that is blown by means of a cup-shaped or funnel-shaped mouthpiece.

Flying hospital Air-borne fully equipped hospital established in 1996, a charitable humanitarian organization.

Teaching hospital Hospital in which undergraduate and postgraduate medical students receive clinical experience.

Housemaid's knee Swelling of prepatellar bursa situated over the lower half of the patella and in the upper half of the *ligamentum patellae.*

HTLV (Human T-cell lymphocytotropic virus) Human T-cell leukemia/lymphoma virus.

Human immunodeficiency virus (HIV) A Lentivirinae subfamily of retrovirus having an RNA genome. The viral enzyme reverse transcriptase has the property of transcribing a DNA copy of the RNA genome following viral penetration of the host cell. The DNA copy randomly integrates into host cell genome and it is used as a template to transcribe new RNA viral copies. HIV occurs in two types: HIVI and HIV2. HIV infects CD4+ helper T lymphocytes and causes attrition of the CD4 cell population resulting in gradual and increasing failure of immune function.

Human leukocyte antigens One of the important types of histocompatibility antigens studied to determine tissue compatibility between donors and recipients for transplants. These antigens are also associated with specific diseases.

Humectant (*hu-mek'tant*) A preparation intended to preserve moisture in the skin.

Humerus (*hu'mer-us*) *see* Table of Bones.

Humor (*hu'mer*) Pl. **humors**. One of the elemental body fluids such as blood, bile, and phlegm; a clear fluid with hyaline substance.

Aqueous humor The watery fluid that fills the anterior and posterior chambers of the eye.

Vitreous humor The fluid component of the vitreous.

Humoral Relating to a humor.

Huntington's chorea (Huntington's disease) An inherited disorder of CNS with onset in middle age exhibiting degeneration of cerebral cortex and basal ganglia. It is characterized by chorea, progressive dementia, named after George Huntington, US physician.

Hurler's syndrome A genetic disorder that causes severe mental retardation, named after Gertrud Hurler, German pediatrician.

Hutchinson-Gilford progeria syndrome A rare, sporadic autosomal dominant syndrome that involves premature aging, generally leading to death within approximately 13 years of age due to myocardial infarction or stroke.

Hyal- (hyalo-) Combining word for glassy; hyoid.

Hyaline (*hi-a-lin*) A glassy, homogeneous, translucent appearance.

Hyaline cartilage Smooth, semi- transparent cartilage.

Hyaline membrane disease Respiratory distress syndrome of the newborn characterized by loss of alveolar stability leading to progressive atelectasis of the affected lung presenting as respiratory distress at or shortly after birth.

Hyalitis (*hi'a-lit'is*) Inflammation of vitreous humor. The inflammatory changes extend into the vitreous from adjacent structures.

Hyaloid artery A branch of the ophthalmic artery, which is a branch of internal carotid artery.

Hyaloid canal (*hi'a-lo-id*) Remnant of a channel in the center of vitreous humor that carried an artery during the eyes' development in the fetus.

Hyaloid membrane A layer of collagen separating the vitreous humor from the rest of the eye.

Hyaluronic acid (*hi-a-lu'ro-nik*) A mucopolysaccharide forming a gelatinous substance in the tissue spaces and an intercellular cement substance throughout the body.

Hyaluronidases (*hi'a-lu-ron'i-das-us*) Any of the three enzymes (hyaluronoglucosaminidase, hyaluronoglucuronidase and hyaluronate lyase) that hydrolyzes hyaluronic acid.

Hybrid (*hibrid*) An animal or plant produced from two different species.

Hydatid (*hi'da-tid*) Hydatid cyst; any cyst like structure.

Hydatid cyst A cyst in the liver or lung containing the larva of *Echinococcus granulosus*.

Hydatids of Morgagni Benign, pedunculated, cystic structures arising from müllerian vestiges below the fallopian tube near the fimbria.

Sessile hydatid A cyst with watery contents that is produced by a tapeworm larva, esp. of the genus *Echinococcus*.

Hydatid disease (Hydatidosis, echinococciasis, echinococcosis) The manifestation of the liver and other organs with Echinococcus. Watery cysts full of tapeworm heads are formed which lodge in the organs to produce disease.

Hydatidiform mole (hydatid mole, vesicular mole) An intrauterine mass of grapelike enlarged chorionic villi. Such a degeneration from the proliferation of the trophoblast results in rapid growth of the uterus compared to the duration of gestation.

Hydatidosis (*hi-da-ti-do'sis*) Hydatid disease with presence of hydatid cysts.

Hydragogue Any purgative that causes evacuation of water from the bowels; producing a discharge of watery fluid; refers to cathartics that retain fluid in the intestine and help in the removal of edematous fluid.

Hydralazine (*hi-dral'a-zin*) A peripheral vasodilator used as an antihypertensive.

Hydramnios (hydramnion) Presence of excess amount of amniotic fluid in uterus during pregnancy.

Hydrargyria (*hi'drar-jir'e-a*) Mercury poisoning.

Hydrarthrosis (*hi-drar-thro'sis*) Collection of serous fluid in the joint cavity.

Hydremia An abnormally watery state of the blood.

Hydroa (hidroa) (*hi-dro'a*) Any bullous eruption.

Hydrocele (*hi'dro-sil*) It is a type of swelling in the scrotum, the pouch of skin that holds the testicles. This swelling happens when fluid collects in the thin sac that surrounds a testicle. Hydroceles are common in newborns.

Cervical hydrocele Hydrocele in the neck resulting from the accumulation of serous fluid in the persistent cervical duct or cleft.

Congenital hydrocele A hydrocele in the neck resulting from the accumulation of serous fluid in the persistent cervical duct or cleft.

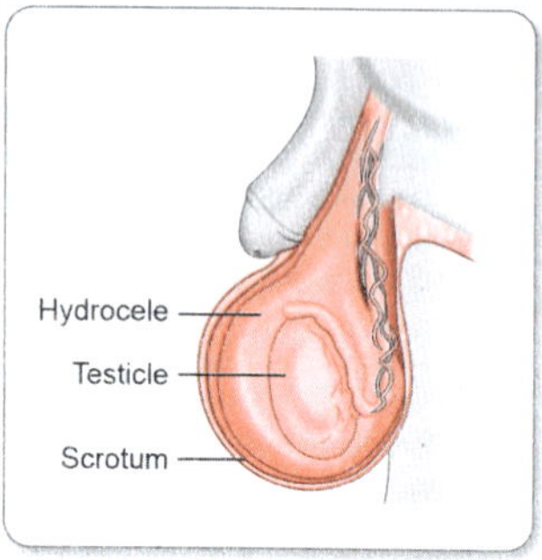

Hydrocele

Hydrocephalus (*hi'dro-sef'a-lus*) Distension of the cerebral ventricles by increased cerebrospinal fluid. It may be due to decreased absorption from congenital malformations, obliteration of aqueduct, hemorrhage, infection, neoplasms, and trauma. Rarely it can be due to an increased production of CSF.

The brain becomes edematous and the gyri flatten.

Hydrochloric acid (*hi'dro-klor'ik*) HCl; a strong acid that is a major component of gastric juice.

Hydrochlorothiazide (*hi'dro-klor'o-thi-a-zid*) An oral thiazide diuretic and antihypertensive.

Hydrocortisone (cortisol) (*hi'dro-kor'ti-son*) One of two main glucocorticoids secreted by adrenal cortex.

Hydrocyanic acid (prussic acid) (*hi'dro-si-an'ik*) Hydrogen cyanide, a colorless liquid poison.

Hydroflumethiazide (*hi'dro-flu'me-thi'a-zid*) A thiazide diuretic.

Hydrogenase (*hi'dro-jen-as*) An enzyme that catalyzes reduction by molecular hydrogen.

Hydrolase (*hi'dro-las*) Hydrolyzing enzyme that cleaves substrates by addition of H_2O.

Hydroma (*hi-dro'ma*) Hygroma.

Hydromeningocele (*hi'dro-me-ning'go-sel*) A sac formed by protrusion of the meninges containing cerebrospinal fluid.

Hydromyelia (*hi'dro-mi-el'e-a*) Fluid in the central canal of the spinal cord.

Hydromyelomeningocele (*hi'dro-mi'e-lo-mening'go-sel*) Projection of meningeal sac containing spinal cord tissue and cerebrospinal fluid through a spinal defect.

Hydronephrosis (*hi-dro'ne-fro'sis*) Dilatation of the pelvis and calices of one or both kidneys due to obstruction of the ureter to the flow of urine and leads to atrophy of renal parenchyma.

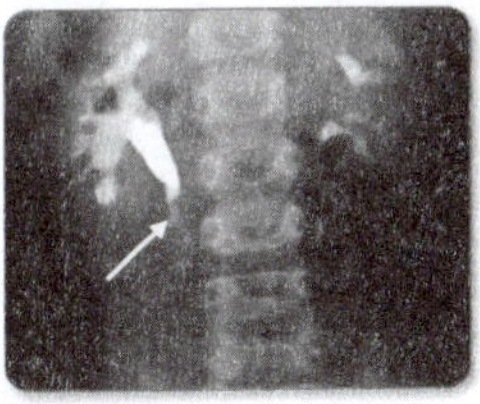

Hydronephrosis

Hydropericarditis (*hi-dro-per'i-kar-dit'is*) Collection of serous fluid in the pericardium.

Hydroperitoneum(*hi'dro-per'i-to-ne'um*) Ascites.

Hydrophobia (*hi'dro-fo'be-a*) Fear of water, *see* Rabies.

Hydrophthalmos (*hi'drof-thal'mos*) Distension of the eyeball due to accumulation of fluid within it as in infantile glaucoma.

Hydropneumopericardium A collection of fluid and gas in the pericardial sac.

Hydropneumoperitoneum (*hi'dro-nu-mo-per'it-o-ne'um*) A collection of fluid and gas in the peritoneal cavity.

Hydropneumothorax (pneumothydrothorax) (*hi'dro-thor'aks*) A collection of fluid and gas in the pleural cavity.

Hydrops fetalis Intrauterine death of fetus with edema and anemia due to severe Rhesus incompatibility.

Hydrosalpinx A condition where fluid accumulates in one or both fallopian tubes, creating a blockage.

Hydrotherapy (*hi'dr-o-tir'a-pi*) Use of water, ice, steam of hot and cold temperatures to maintain and restore health.

Hydrothorax (*hi'dro-thor'aks*) A collection of serous fluid in the pleural cavity.

Hydrotubation (*hi'dro-tu-ba'shun*) Injection of liquid medication or saline solution through the cervix into the uterine cavity and fallopian tubes for dilatation and medication of the tubes.

Hydroureter (*hi'dro-ur-et'er*) Distension of the ureter with urine or watery fluid due to obstruction.

Hydroxocobalamine Vitamin B_{12a} and is found in food, also used as a dietary supplement.

Hydroxychloroquine (*hi'drok'si-klor'o-kwin*) An antimalarial and anti-inflammatory preparation used in malaria and rheumatoid arthritis.

Hydroxyproline (*hi-drok'se-pro'len*) A hydroxylated proline found in high concentrations in collagen. It plays an important role in cross-linking collagen.

Hydroxysteroid It is a molecule derived from a steroid with a hydrogen replaced with a hydroxy group, the term often refers to steroids that are involved in the metabolism of hormones like cortisol, aldosterone, and sex hormones.

Hydroxyurea (*hi'drok'se-u-re'a*) An orally active cytotoxic agent used in refractory cases of chronic myeloid leukemia.

Hydroxyzine It is an antihistamine medication that is commonly used to treat various conditions, including allergies, anxiety, and certain skin conditions. It works by blocking the effects of histamine, a natural substance that the body releases during allergic reactions.

Hygiene (*hi'jen*) The science concerned with promotion and preservation of health.

Hygroma (hydroma) (*hi-gro'ma*) Cavernous lymphangioma especially of neck.

Hymen (*hi'men*) A thin, membranous ring surrounding the opening to vagina which gets torn during first sexual intercourse or by use of tampon.

Hymenolepis (*hi'me-nol'e-pis*) A genus of tapeworm *H. nana,* the dwarf tapeworm of 2.5 cm length capable completing its life cycle in a single host.

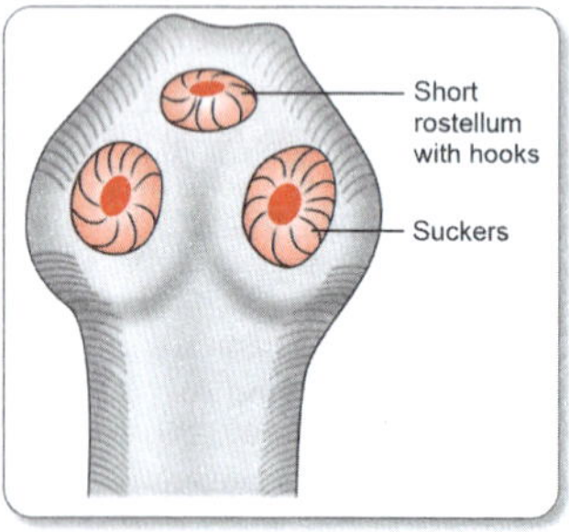

Hymenolepis nana—scolex

Hymenotomy Incision of the hymen at the entrance to the vagina.

Hyoglossus A muscle that serves to depress the tongue; originates on the hyoid bone.

Hyoscine (*hi'o-sin*) Scopolamine.

Hyoscyamine (*hi'o-si'a-men*) An anticholinergic alkaloid from Hyoscyamus and other solanaceous plants.

Hypalgesia (*hi'pal-je'ze-a*) Decreased pain sensation. adj. **hypalgesic**.

Hyper- Combining word meaning excessive or abnormally increased.

Hyperacusis (*hi'per-a-ku'sis*) Sounds heard with unusual loudness in paralysis of the stapedius muscle as it affects dampening influence on the stapes.

Hyperadrenalism (*hi'per-a-dren'a-lizm*) Cushing's syndrome.

Hyperalgesia (*hi'per-al-je'se-a*) Markedly increased pain sense. adj. **hyperalgesic**.

Hyperbaric (*hi'per-barik*) Referring to atmospheric pressure >1; solution more dense than the diluent or medium.

Hyperbaric oxygen Therapy exposing a person to oxygen at higher than normal atmosphere to increase oxygen supply in the tissues. It is indicated in decompression sickness, carbon monoxide poisoning, gas gangrene and arterial gas embolism.

Hyperbaric oxygen Therapy exposing a person to oxygen at higher than normal atmosphere to increase oxygen supply in the tissues. It is indicated in decompression sickness, carbon monoxide poisoning, gas gangrene and arterial gas embolism.

Hyperchromatism (*hi'per-kro'ma-tizm*) Excessive pigmentation; increased amount of chromatin in cell nuclei; increased staining capacity of the nuclei.

Hypercalcemia (*hi'per-kal-sem'e-a*) An abnormally high level of calcium in the blood.

Hypercalcuiria (hypercalcinuria) Excessive urinary calcium excretion, is the most common identifiable cause of calcium kidney stone disease. It may be secondary that is, a side effect of some other condition causing high levels of calcium in the bloodstream—or it may be idiopathic with normal blood calcium levels.

Hypercapnia (hypercarbia) (*hi'per-kap'ne-a*) An abnormally increased amount of carbon dioxide in the circulating blood.

Hyperchloremia (*hi'per-kap'ne-a*) An abnormally increased amount of carbon dioxide in the circulating blood.

Hyperchlorhydria (*hi'per-klor-hi'dre-a*) Presence of an increased amount of hydrochloric acid in the stomach.

Hypercholesterolemia (*hi'per-kol-es'ter-ol'e-me-a*) An abnormally high levels of cholesterol in the blood.

Famlial hypercholesterolemia An inherited condition that causes high levels of LDL (low-density lipoprotein) cholesterol beginning at birth, and heart attacks at an early age.

Autosomal dominant hypercholesterolemia Characterized by an isolated elevation of plasmatic low-density lipoprotein, which predisposes to premature coronary artery disease (CAD) and early death.

Polygenic hypercholesterolemia A familial condition where there is an elevation in serum cholesterol levels due to mutation in several small LDL raising alleles.

Hyperchromatism (*hi'per-kro'ma-tizm*) Excessive pigmentation; increased amount of chromatin in cell nuclei; increased staining capacity of the nuclei.

Hyperdactylism (polydacttlism) Presence of extra fingers or toes, also known as polydactyly.

Hyperdynamia (*hi'per-di-na'me-a*) Hyperkinesis exhibiting muscular restlessness. adj. **hyperdynamic**.

Hyperemesis Gravidarum: Extreme, persistent nausea and vomiting during pregnancy.

Hyperemia An excess of blood in the blood vessels in a specific part of the body.

Active hyperemia A normal and healthy response to an illness or physical activity.

Collateral hyperemia Increased blood flow through abundant collateral channels when the circulation through the main artery to a part is arrested.

Passive hyperemia Occurs most commonly in diseases of the heart and liver and in pregnancy.

Reactive hyperemia Increase in blood flow following arterial occlusion.

Hyperesthesia A neurological condition that causes a person extreme sensitivity to touch, pain, pressure, and thermal sensations. There is increased sensitivity of any of the sense organs, especially of the skin.

Acoustic hyperesthesia An excessive sensitivity of sound.

Muscular hyperesthesia Sensitivity to pain and tiredness.

Oneiric hyperesthesia the excessive perception of something, pertaining to dreams.

Optic hyperesthesia Sensitivity to light.

Tactile hyperesthesia Sensitivity to touch.

Hyperextension injury An injury caused by straightening of a joint beyond its normal limits.

Hyperglycemia (*hi'per-gli-se'mea*) An abnormally high level of glucose in the blood.

Hyperhidrosis (hyperhidrosis) (*hi'per-hi-dro'sis*) Increased sweating.

Hyperinsulinism (*hi'per-in'sul-in-izm*) An increased secretion of insulin by the islets of Langerhans resulting in hypoglycemia.

Hyperkalemia (*hi'per-kal-em'e-a*) Raised level of potassium ions in the circulating blood.

Hyperkinesia (*hi'per-ki'ne-zea*) Excessive activity or motor function.

Hyperkinetic syndrome A behavior disorder characterized by hyperactivity, short attention span, poor concentration, irritability, impulsiveness, variability.

Hyperlipemia (*hi'per-li-pe'me-a*) An excess amount of lipids in the blood.

Hyperkeratosis (*hi'per-ker'a-to'sis*) Hyperkeratinization; hypertrophy of the horny layers of epidermis especially of the palms and soles; hypertrophy of the cornea.

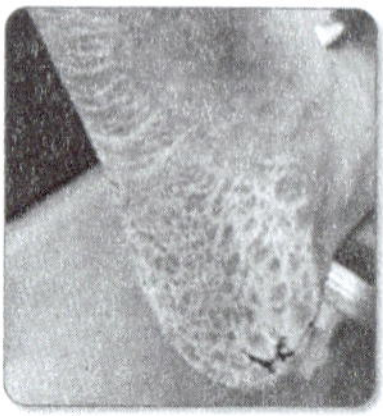

Hyperkeratosis showing in sole of right foot

Hyperlipoproteinemia (*hi'per-lip'o-pro'te-ne'me-a*) An increase in the level of lipoprotein in the blood.

Hypermotility (*hi'per-mo-til'it-e*) An abnormally increased motility.

Hypernatremia (*hi'per-na-tre'me-a*) Markedly increased plasma concentration of sodium ions.

Hypernephroma (Grawitz tumor, renal cell carcinoma) (*hi'per-ne-fro'ma*) Adenocarcinoma of the kidney presenting with painless, profuse, intermittent hematuria.

Hyperopia (farsightedness) (*hi'per-o'pe-a*) Hypermetropia; farsightedness.

Hyperosmia Refers to an increased sense of smell. It refers to a person's ability to perceive and distinguish odors at a more sensitive level than the average person's sense of smell. This can be temporary pain caused by things like pregnancy, medical conditions (such as migraines, sinus problems, epilepsy), or mental illness.

Hyperostosis (*hi'per-os'to'sis*) A proliferation of a bony matrix.

Diffuse idiopathic skeletal hyperostosis (DISH) A systemic condition characterized by characteristic ossification patterns that can occur in the spine and peripheral entheses.

Infantile cortical hyperostosis A largely self-limiting disorder which affects infants, causes bone changes, soft tissue swelling, and irritability.

Hyperparathyroidism (*hi'per-par'a-thi'roid-izm*) A condition associated with an autonomous secretion of parathyroid hormone by a single parathyroid adenoma (primary) or by hyperplasia secondary to chronic renal failure (secondary) or adenoma formation by continuous stimulation of parathyroid (tertiary).

Hyperpiesia Persistent and pathological high blood pressure for which no specific cause can be found.

Hyperpituitarism (*hi'per-pi-tu'i-ta-rizm*) Increased production of hormones of anterior pituitary, especially somatotropin and it leads to gigantism or acromegaly.

Hyperplasia (*hi'per-pla'zhea*) Overgrowth in numbers of tissue cells.

Gingival hyperplasia A simple overgrowth of gum tissue, specially the fibrous submucosa.

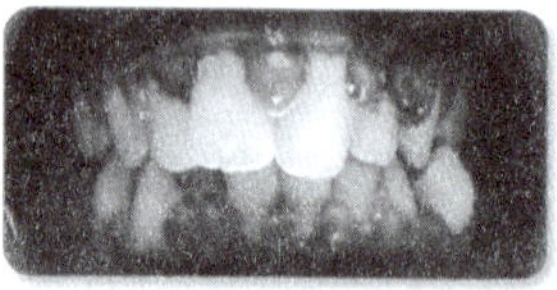

Gingival hyperplasia

Hyperpnea (*hi'perp-ne'a*) Deeper and more rapid breathing than normal.

Hyperpraxia (*hi'per-prak'se-a*) Excessively uneasy or restless.

Hyperpyrexia (*hi'per-pi-rek'se-a*) Extremely high fever with a temperature above 41°C.

Hyperresponsive (*hi'per-ri-spon-siv*) Characterized by an abnormal degree of responsiveness (as to a physical or emotional stimulus), e.g., airway hyperresponsiveness in bronchial asthma.

Hypersensitivity (*hi'per-sen'si-tiv'it-e*) Abnormal sensitivity to any stimulus exhibiting an excessive response; a state of altered reactivity in which body exhibits an exaggerated immune response to a foreign agent or allergen.

Hypersomnia (*hi'per-som'ne-a*) Excessive sleeping.

Hypersplenism (*hi'per-splen'izm*) Enlargement of spleen. The condition is associated with pancytopenia and hyperplasia of the marrow precursor cells. Splenectomy improves the condition.

Congestive hypersplenism Due to stasis of blood flow, mostly secondary to cirrhosis of the liver.

Hypersthenia (*hi'per-sthene'-a*) An excessive strength or tension of a part or all the body.

Hypertension (*hi'per-ten'shun*) Persistent high blood pressure. It is a quantitative deviation from the normal.

Accelerated hypertension Complicates hypertension of any etiology. There is accelerated microvascular damage with necrosis in the walls of small arteries and arterioles and intravascular thrombosis. The blood pressure is very high and there is rapidly progressive end-organ damage.

Borderline hypertension The arterial blood pressure being within normal range sometimes and in hypertensive range sometimes.

Essential hypertension Hypertension without any specific underlying cause.

Idiopathic intracranial hypertension Development of raised intracranial pressure without a space occupying lesion, ventricular dilatation, or impaired consciousness. Presents with headache, transient diplopia and visual abnormalities.

Malignant hypertension Accelerated hypertension.

Ocular hypertension Persistently elevated intraocular pressure in the absence of any other signs of glaucoma.

Portal hypertension Prolonged elevation of the portal venous pressure and is due to extrahepatic (sepsis) and intrahepatic parenchymal (cirrhosis) diseases. The clinical features are due to portal venous congestion and collateral vessel formation. Splenomegaly is constant.

Pregnancy-induced hypertension Hypertension complicating pregnancy with proteinuria and edema.

Primary hypertension Essential hypertension.

Pulmonary hypertension Markedly increased pressure in pulmonary circulation. There is marked narrowing of pulmonary vascular bed from anatomic or vasomotor mechanisms.

Renal hypertension Hypertension produced by renal diseases.

Renovascular hypertension Hypertension due to diminished blood flow to the kidney from renal artery stenosis.

Secondary hypertension Hypertension as a consequence of a specific disease or abnormality leading to sodium retention and/or peripheral vasoconstriction.

Venous hypertension Incompetent valves in deep leg veins resulting in retrograde blood flow to superficial system causing a rise in capillary hydrostatic pressure.

White-coat hypertension Recording of blood pressure by a doctor causing unrepresentative surge in blood pressure and it has been ascribed to anxiety.

Hyperthermia (hyperthermy) (*hi'per-therme'-a*) A body temperature of >42°C. It is characterized by vasodilatation, tachycardia, hypoxia, hyperkalemia, and cardiac failure.

Malignant hyperthermia A hypermetabolic myopathic syndrome that is chemically or stress induced, presenting by abrupt rise in temperature, vigorous muscular contractions, metabolic and respiratory acidosis, and ventricular arrhythmias, especially noted when inducing anesthesia.

Hyperthyroidism (*hi'per-thi'ro-id-izm*) A clinical syndrome resulting from exposure of the body tissues to excess circulating levels of free thyroid hormones. The condition is due to Graves disease, multinodular goiter or autonomously functioning solitary thyroid nodules. The condition develops insidiously and involves almost every system of the body. There is diffuse or nodular goiter, weight loss despite increased appetite, anorexia, palpitations, nervousness, irritability, muscle weakness, heat intolerance, fatigue, exophthalmos, lid retraction, amenorrhea, loss of libido and tremor.

Hypertonia (hypertonicity) (*hi'per-tone-a*) Increased tension of muscles or arteries.

Hypertonic (*hi'per-ton'ik*) Spastic; increased degree of tension; having an increased osmotic pressure than a reference solution.

Hypertrichosis (*hi'per-tri-ko'sis*) Excessive hair growth anywhere on the body in either males or females.

Hypertrophy (hypertrophia) (*hi-per'tro-fe*) An increase in the size of an organ that causes an increase in the size of its constituent cells.

Compensatory hypertrophy Hypertrophy results from an increased workload due to some physical defect, such as in an organ where one part is defective, or in one kidney when the other is absent or nonfunctional.

Facial hypertrophy Overgrowth of one side of the face.

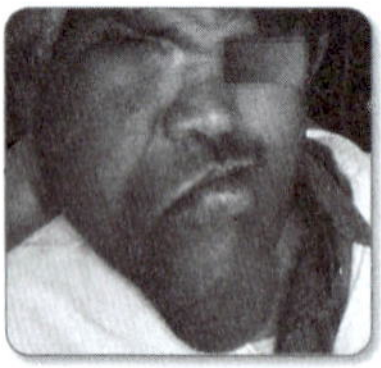

Facial hypertrophy

Physiologic hypertrophy Harmless, completely reversible increase in cardiac muscle mass that occurs in response to workload.

Ventricular hypertrophy Thickening of the walls of ventricles (lower chamber) of the heart.

Hypertropia (*hi'per-tro-pe-a*) Strabismus in which there is an upward deviation of the visual axis of an eye.

Hyperuricemia (lithemia) (*hi'per-u'ri-se'me-a*) Increased blood level of uric acid noted in renal failure, and disorder of purine metabolism such as gout.

Hyperuricemia (*hi'per-u'ri-se'me-a*) Increased blood level of uric acid noted in renal failure, and disorder of purine metabolism such as gout.

Hyperventilation (*hi'per-ven-til-a'shun*) Tachydyspnea noted in neurotics with anxiety attacks leading to respiratory alkalosis, tightness in the chest, dizziness, numbness of hands and feet, and tetany. Rebreathing air in a paper bag facilitates to increase CO_2.

Hypervitaminosis (*hi'per-vita-min-o'sis*) A condition caused by an excessive intake of vitamins especially vitamins A and D.

Hypervolemia (*hi'per-vol-em'e-a*) Plethora; an abnormally increased volume of blood.

Hyphedonia (*hip'he-do'ne-a*) An abnormally lessened degree of pleasure.

Hyphema (*hi-fe'ma*) Injury to the iris resulting in bleeding into the anterior chamber.

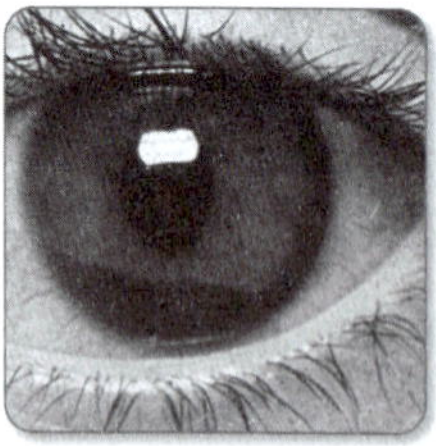

Hyphema

Hypnagogic Pertaining to, associated with, or happening during the phase of drowsiness that directly precedes falling asleep.

Hypnopompic Linked to the state of partial consciousness that comes before waking up.

Hypnosis (*hip-no'sis*) A state of suspended consciousness characterized by a heightened suggestibility.

Hypnotic (soporific) (*hip-not'ik*) Something, usually a drug, that induces sleep. Therapeutically it is a central nervous system depressant; relating to hypnotism; called also somniferous.

Hypnotism The act of putting someone into a mental state like sleep, in which their thoughts can be easily influenced by someone else; the process of inducing hypnosis.

Hypo- (*hi'po*) Less than normal; deficient, e.g., hypoglycemia.

Hypobaric (*hi'po-bar'ik*) Pertaining to pressure of ambient gases <1 atmosphere.

Hypobulia Lowered ability to make decisions or to act.

Hypocapnia (*hi'po-kap'ne-a*) Markedly decreased tension of carbon dioxide in the circulating blood.

Hypochloremia (*hi'po-klor-em'e-a*) Markedly decreased level of chloride ions in circulating blood.

Hypochlorhydria (*hi'po-klor-hi'dre-a*) Markedly decreased amount of hydrochloric acid in the stomach.

Hypochondria (*hi'po-kon'dre-a*) Exaggerated concern over one's health that is not based on real organic pathology, but rather on unrealistic interpretation of physical signs or sensations as abnormal; plural of hypochondrium.

Hypochondrium (*hi-po-kon'dre-um*) The area on either side of the abdomen covered by the costal cartilages, lateral to the epigastrium.

Hypoderma (*hi'po-derm'a*) The larvae belonging to genus of botflies causing cutaneous larva migrans.

Hypodermic (*hi'po-derm'ik*) Subcutaneous.

Hypodermic needle A hollow needle attached to a syringe that is used to inject medication under the skin, into a muscle or directly to blood vessel.

Hypodermoclysis (*hi'po-der-mok'li-sis*) Subcutaneous injection of a saline or other solution.

Hypodontia (*hi'po-don'shi-a*) Oligodontia; congenital absence of teeth.

Hypoesthesia (*hi'po-es-the'zea*) Markedly decreased sensitivity particularly to touch.

Hypofibrinogenemia (Fibrinogenopenia) (*hi'po-fi-brin'o-j'in-em'e-a*) Markedly decreased amount of fibrinogen in the circulating blood plasma.

Hypogammaglobulinemia (*hi'po-gam'a-glob'u-lin-em'e-a*) Decreased production of immunoglobulins which may be congenital with B cell defects or acquired as in chronic lymphocytic leukemia.

Hypogastrium (*hi'po-gas'tre-um*) Pubic region; the lower middle area of the abdomen below the umbilicus.

Hypogeusia (*hi'po-gu'ze-a*) A decrease in taste sensation.

Hypoglossal nerve The 12th paired cranial nerve which is under the tongue and has a purely somatic motor function.

Hypoglycemia (*hi'po-gli-sem'e-a*) A decrease in circulating glucose and occurs as a symptom.

Fasting hypoglycemia Caused by hypopituitarism, Addison's disease, adrenogenital syndrome, islet cell tumors, retroperitoneal sarcoma, hepatic disease, ectopic insulin production and glycogen storage disease.

Postprandial hypoglycemia Noted in postgastrectomy, oral hypoglycemic agents, insulin, alcohol, aspirin or idiopathic.

Hypogonadism (*hi'po-gon'ad-izm*) A clinical disorder characterized by decreased or absent phenotypic expression of a person's sexual genotype. It may be primary due to lack of end-organ response to FSH or LH produced normally by pituitary or secondary to defective hypothalamic or pituitary hormonal activity.

Hypohidrosis (hypoidrosis) (*hi'po-hi-dro'sis*) Decreased sweat production.

Acquired hypohidrosis Noted in Sjogren's syndrome, systemic sclerosis, psoriasis, pemphigus vulgaris, anticholinergics, hypothyroidism, diabetes insipidus, heat stroke, dehydration, peripheral neuropathies.

Inherited hypohidrosis Noted in ichthyosis, hereditary anhidrotic ectodermal dysplasia.

Hypoinsulinism Insuline deficiency either due to inadequate secretion of hormone by pancreas or inadequate treatment of diabetes mellitus.

Hypokalemia A lower than normal potassium level in your bloodstream.

Hypomania (*hi'po-mane-a*) Mild excitement with a moderate alteration in behavior.

Hypomenorrhea (*hi'po-meno-re-ah*) A decreased flow or a shortened duration of menstruation.

Hyponatremia (*hi'po-na-treme-a*) An abnormally low concentration of sodium ions in the circulating blood.

Dilutional hyponatremia Occurs due to the intake of water exceeds the kidney's ability to eliminate water.

Euvolemic hyponatremia Type of hyponatremia occurs when there is a normal total body of water and sodium.

Hypoparathyroidism (*hi'po-para-thi'roid-izm*) Parathyroid insufficiency due to diminution or absence of secretion of parathormones.

Pseudohypoparathyroidism Condition with normal or reduced parathormone secretion but lack of target tissue response to the hormone associated with congenital malformations.

Pseudo-pseudohypoparathyroidism Normal levels of PTH, calcium and phosphorus, with congenital abnormalities of pseudohypoparathyroidism.

Hypophoria (*hi'po-fore-a*) Downward deviation of the visual axis of one eye compared with the other eye.

Hypophysectomy (*hi-po-f'i-sek'to-me*) Surgical removal of the pituitary gland.

Hypophysis (*hi-po-f'i-sis*) Pea-sized conductor of endocrine orchestra presents in the sella turcica and is separated into an anterior lobe containing cells producing ACTH, FSH, GH (growth hormone or somatotropin), LH and TSH, intermediate lobe producing MSH and posterior lobe (neurohypophysis) which under the influence of hypothalamus produces antidiuretic hormone (vasopressin) and oxytocin.

Hypopiesis (*hi'po-pi-esis*) Hypotension.

Hypopituitarism (*hi'po-pi-tuit-ar-izm*) A condition due to diminished activity of the anterior lobe of the pituitary with inadequate secretion of one or more anterior pituitary hormones.

Hypoplasia (*hi'po-pla-zea*) Failure of an organ or tissue to develop fully.

Cartilage-hair hypoplasia A genetic disorder that affects the metaphyseal area of the long bone the wider part at the end causing lower extremity abnormalities.

Congenital adrenal hypoplasia A condition in which there is underdevelopment or hypotrophy of the adrenal cortex due to several clinical conditions.

Enamel hypoplasia A defect that causes a lesser quantity of enamel than normal.

Focal dermal hypoplasia A genetically inherited disorder that can affect the development of many different organ systems.

Renal hypoplasia A congenitally small kidney without dysplasia and can be bilateral or unilateral.

Hypoplastic left heart syndrome A congenital defect involving a rudimentary mitral valve and left ventricle, and with a hypoplastic aortic valve and ascending aorta.

Hypopnea (*hi'po-p'ne-a*) Significant decrease, not absence of airflow for at least 10 seconds.

Hypopraxia Abnormally decreased activity.

Hypoproteinemia Low levels of protein in the blood. Causes can be various health conditions.

Hypoprothrombinemia Disease characterized by a deficiency of blood clotting substance prothrobin, result is tendency to prolonged bleeding.

Hypopyon (*hi-po'pe-on*) Presence of pus in the anterior chamber of the eye, resulting from corneal ulceration and uveitis.

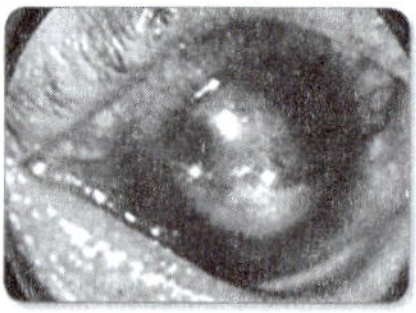

Hypopyon

Hyposensitive (*hi'po-sen'sit-iv*) Decreased ability to respond to stimuli.

Hyposensitization The state of being reduced in sensitivity especially to an allergen.

Hyposmia (*hi-poz'me-a*) Diminished sense of smell.

Hypospadias Condition in which the opening of the urethra is on the underside of the penis instead of at the tip; a developmental defect in which urethra opens on the undersurface of the penis.

Female hypospadias A rare genitourinary anomaly, often associated with other congenital malformations of the urinary tract.

Glandular hypospadias The most common form when opening is found near the head of the penis.

Hypostasis (*hi'pos'ta-sis*) Collection of fluid or blood in dependent parts.

Hyposthenia (*hi'pos-the'ne-a*) Weakness.

Hypotension (*hi'po-ten'shun*) An abnormally low blood pressure that reduces blood flow to the brain causing dizziness and fainting.

Hypotensive (*hi'po-ten'siv*) Characterized by low blood pressure; an agent causing a reduction in blood pressure.

Hypothalamus (*hi'po-thal'a-mus*) A portion of diencephalon of the brain forming the floor and part of the ventral wall of the third ventricle. It lies beneath the thalamus. It controls some metabolic activities, regulates body temperature and secretion of releasing and inhibiting hormones acting on pituitary gland. It integrates the activity of autonomic nervous system.

Hypothenar (*hi'po-the'na-r*) The fleshy mass at the ulnar side of the palm.

Hypothermia A dangerous fall in body temperature to below normal level (35°C or less), it causes drowsiness, and reduced breathing and heart rates and may lead to unconsciousness and death.

Accidental hypothermia An unintentional drop of core temperature below 35°C.

Induced hypothermia An intentional reduction of a patient's core temperature below 36°C.

Hypothymia (*hi'po-thi'me-a*) A state of depression; a diminished emotional response.

Hypothyroidism Reduced level of thyroid gland resulting in slow growth and mental development in children and metabolic changes in adults.

Hypotonia (*hi'po-to'ne-a*) A condition of diminished tone or tension; relaxation of arteries; diminished muscular tonicity.

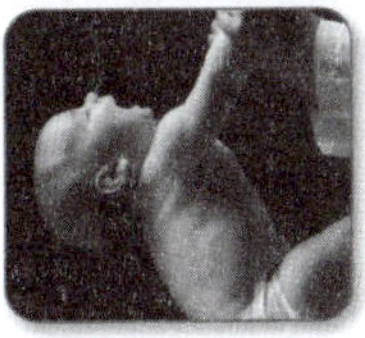

Hypotonia

Hypotonic (*hi'po-ton'ik*) Having a lesser concentration of solute than another solution hence exerting less osmotic pressure than that solution.

Hypotrichosis (*hi'po-tri-ko'sis*) A less than normal amount of hair on the scalp and/or body.

Hypotropia (*hi'po-tro'pe-a*) Downward deviation of the visual axis of one eye.

Hypoventilation (*hi'po-ven'ti-la'shun*) Reduced ventilation resulting in an increase in arterial carbon dioxide tension and decrease in arterial oxygen tension.

Hypovitaminosis A disorder caused by the deficiency of a vitamin.

Hypovolemia (oligemia) (*hi'po-vo-leme-a*) An abnormally low circulating blood volume.

Hypoxemia (*hi'pok-seme-a*) A decrease in PaO_2 below normal expected value. It may develop in presence of normal or lowered arterial carbon dioxide tension. An inadequate gas exchange due to ventilation-perfusion inequality, increased right-to-left intrapulmonary shunting of blood, impaired diffusion, and hypoventilation result in hypoxemia.

Hypoxia (*hi'pok'se-a*) An inadequate level of oxygen in the tissues, blood, or air.

Hypsarrhythmia (*hip'sa-rith'me-a*) The abnormal and characteristically chaotic electroencephalogram commonly found in patients with infantile spasms.

Hysterectomy (*his'ter-ek'to-me*) Surgical removal of the uterus.

Abdominal hysterectomy Excision of the uterus through the abdominal wall.

Cesarean hysterectomy Cesarean section followed by removal of the uterus.

Radical hysterectomy Removal of ovaries, fallopian tubes, lymph nodes and lymph channels with uterus and cervix.

Total hysterectomy Removal of uterus and cervix.

Hysteria (*his-ter'e-a*) The conversion of mental or emotional illness into physical symptoms such as blindness, paralysis.

Hysterical (*his-ter'ikal*) Relating to or suffering from hysteria.

Hysterical anesthesia Loss of sensory modalities resulting from emotional conflicts.

Hysterical dyspnea A frequent cause of dyspnea without any systemic cause, where dyspnea is evident at rest.

Hysterical fits Occur in emotionally charged situation in presence of onlookers and do not occur when patient is alone. Consciousness is not lost during fits. The movements are bizarre.

Hysterical neurosis A psychogenic loss or disorder of function manifested either as conversion reaction (sensory or motor) or as a dissociative reaction (psychic symptoms).

Hysterical personality Emotionally labile, dramatizing, defensive, and demanding, tendency to be untruthful.

Hysterical trans The twilight state or stupor. Patient gets detached from reality and may also be immobile and immersed in his own self.

Hysterosalpingography (*his'ter-o-sal'ping-gog'ra-fe*) An X-ray examination of the uterus and fallopian tubes used to investigate infertility.

Hysteroscope (uteroscope) (*his'ter-o-skop*) A viewing instrument for examination of the cervix and the interior of the uterus.

Hysterotomy (*his'ter-oto-me*) A miniature cesarean section, wherein the incision of uterus is made either transabdominally or vaginally to remove products of conception.

Hysterotrachelorrhaphy (*his'ter-o-tra-kel-or'a-fe*) Surgical repair of a lacerated cervix uteri.

HZV Herpes zoster virus.

Iasis Suffix indicating condition, especially pathologic.

Iatro A combining word for relating to a physician or to medicine.

Iatrogenic (*ia'trojen'ik*) Physician-produced.

Iatrogenic disease Any disease or disorder that has resulted in a patient from effects of treatment by a physician or a surgeon.

Ibuprofen A low-risk nonsteroidal anti-inflammatory drug.

Ichor (*i'kor*) Thin, fetid discharge from an ulcer or wound.

Ichthyosis (*ik'theo'sis*) Hypertrophy of horny layer characterized by thick, dry, scaly skin resembling fish skin. adj. **ichthyotic**.

Bullous ichthyosis A skin disorder characterized by epidermolytic hyperkeratosis with bullous lesions and hyperkeratosis in infants.

Ichthyosis congenita A severe variant of lamellar ichthyosis exhibiting thick sheet of hyperkeratosis.

Ichthyosis hystrix Ichthyosis characterized by bilateral symmetric epidermal naevus arranged in a geometrical pattern.

Ichthyosis vulgaris A skin disorder characterized by presence of brownish angulated scales over the body, especially on the front of the legs, inherited as an autosomal dominant character.

Ichthyosis vulgaris

Lamellar ichthyosis A rare autosomal recessive skin disorders characterized by hyperkeratosis or dry and scaly appearance.

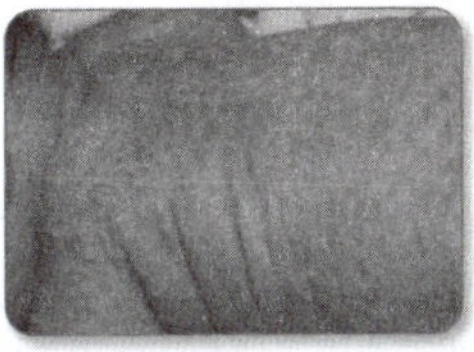

Lamellar ichthyosis

X-linked ichthyosis A skin disorder transmitted by recessive gene which manifests in males, though resembles autosomal dominant ichthyosis.

ICS Inhaled corticosteroids.

ICSH (Interstitial-cell stimulating bormone) Interstitial cell stimulating hormone, produced by the anterior lobe of pituitary gland.

Icterus (*ik'ter'us*) Jaundice.

Icterus gravis neonatorum Erythoblastosis fetalis is a hemolytic jaundice of the newborn baby with incompatibility between mother's serum and red blood cells of infant.

Icterus index Comparison of blood serum in intensity of color with that of potassium dichromate. Normally, it is 3–5. In presence of jaundice, the index shows a rise to 15 or more.

Icterus neonatorum Jaundice noted in infants between second and fifth days of life.

Ictus (*ik'tus*) A seizure, stroke sudden attack or a fit noted at birth.

Id *psy* Selfish and supremely egocentric.

ID Infections disease.

IDDM Insulin-dependent diabetes mellitus. *see* Diabetes mellitus.

Ideation (*i"de-a'shun*) The activity of forming ideas in the mind.

Identical twins One of a pair of twins of the same sex resembling one another closely who have developed from a single fertilized ovum.

Identification (*i'den-ti'fi-kashun*) For determination or establishment of individuality of a person-living or dead.

Ideomotor Not reflex but motivated by an idea.

Idiocy (*ide-o-se*) Severe mental retardation.

Idiogenetic (*i"de-o-ja-net'ik*) Originating ideas.

Idiopathic (*id"ie-o-path'ik*) Of undetermined origin.

Idiopathic CD4 lymphocytopenic syndrome A syndrome characterized by a low CD4 cell count that is unexplained by HIV infection or other medical conditions; ICL.

Idiopathic pulmonary fibrosis Appears as a fibrosing lesion in the alveolar walls.

Idiopathic scoliosis An abnormal condition characterized by a lateral curvature of the spine.

Idiosyncrasy (*id'e-o-sin'kra-se*) A habit or quality peculiar to any person; an abnormal susceptibility to some drug or protein peculiar to a person.

Idioventricular (*id'e-o-ven-trik'u-lar*) Relating to the cardiac ventricle alone when dissociated from the atrium.

Idoxuridine (IDU) (*i-doks-uri-den*) An analog of pyrimidine that inhibits viral DNA synthesis; used as topical antiviral agent to treat herpes.

Ifosfamide (*i-fos'fe-mid*) A cytotoxic alkylating agent of the nitrogen mustard group, a structural analog and similar in action to cyclophosphamide.

Ileal conduit An irreversible obstruction of the urinary tract, ureters may be anastomosed to an isolated loop of ilium opening on the abdominal wall.

Ileal pouch (perineal pouch) A reservior created by the surgeries after removing large intestine, usually due to coloretal disease.

Ileectomy Surgical removal of ileum or part of the ileum.

Ileitis (*il'ei'tis*) Inflammation of the ilium.

Regional ileitis A nonspecific, chronic, inflammatory, granulomatous lesion involving terminal ilium.

Ileocecal valve Sphincter that helps to close the ilium where it opens into the ascending colon.

Ileocolitis (*il'e-o-ko-li'tis*) Inflammation of ilium and colon.

Ileocolostomy (*il'e-o-ko-los'to-me*) Anastomosis between the ilium and colon.

Ileoproctostomy (Ileorectal anastomosis) A surgical operation in which the ileum is joined to the rectum; ilectomy.

Ileostomy (*il'e-os'to-me*) An operation to bring ilium through an incision in the abdominal wall and formed into an artificial outlet to allow discharge of feces into a bag attached to the skin.

Ileum (*il'e-um*) The longest and narrowest distal part of the small intestine connecting jejunum to the cecum.

Ileus (*il'e-us*) Impairment of the forward flow of the intestinal contents which is either paralytic secondary to electrolyte abnormalities, surgery, peritoneal irritation or mesenteric artery accidents or obstructive due to adhesive bands, foreign bodies, intussusception or tumors.

Paralytic ileus Ominous silence of abdomen without normal intermittent gushing and gurgling.

Iliacus A triangular muscle which passes from the pelvis through the groin on either side and together with the psoas, flexes the hip.

Ilium (*il'e-um*) The broad upper part of the hip bone; one of the bones of each half of the pelvis. It forms part of the acetabulum and provides attachment to several muscles.

Illusion (*il'lu-shun*) Misperceptions or misinterpretations of real external stimuli. adj. **illusory**.

Optical illusion A visual impression that is inaccurate.

Imagery (*im-ij-re*) Imagination; *psy* a technique in behavior therapy in which the patient is conditioned to substitute pleasant fantasies to counter the unpleasant feelings associated with anxiety.

Imago (*i-ma'go*) Sexually mature adult stage of an insect; a memory developed during childhood that has been clouded by imagination and idealism.

Image-guided biopsy A technique in which computer images are used to guide a biopsy needle to a lump that cannot be felt but has shown up on a mammogram; stereotactic biopsy.

Imbecility A state of mental retardation; feebleness of mind.

Imidazole (*im"id-azol*) A heterocyclic organic compound whose moleculecontainsafive-memberedhetero-aromatic ring of two non-adjacent nitrogen atoms, in which a carbon atom is placed between two nitrogen atoms.

Imipramine (*i-mip'ra-men*) A tricyclic anti-depressant drug.

Immersion foot A condition that can occur when your feet are cold and wet for a long time.

Immobilization Making part immovable.

Immune (*im-un'*) Resistant to a disease due to the development of antibodies.

Immune complexes Circulating aggregates of antibody antigen, whose deposition in the tissues such as blood vessel walls causes inflammation and tissue damage.

Immune deficiency Decreased effectiveness of the immune system. It is encountered in people who are malnourished, infected with HIV or undergoing chemotherapy for treatment of cancer.

Immune reaction Antigenic response to a specific antibody.

Immune reconstitution Improvement of the function of the immune system.

Immune response Reaction of the body to foreign substances.

Immune serum A serum containing naturally or artificially produced antibodies.

Immune system A collection of body cell substances and structures that works to protect the body from disease-causing organisms and from the development of cancer.

Immunity (*i-mu'-ni-te*) A state of resistance to a disease through the defense activities of the immune system; protection from a disease.

Active immunity Resistance to infection that is acquired as a result of previous infection with a disease-causing organism or following vaccination.

Adaptive immunity An immune system where distinct antigens generate specific responses and different lymphocytes recognize antigens. Reexposure to antigen induces more rapid and effective response.

Cell-mediated immunity (CMI) Antibacterial activity induced and expressed by T-Lymphocytes.

Humoral immunity Immunity mediated by antibody found in the plasma or lymph, synthesized by B lymphocytes.

Innate immunity Natural immunity where cellular and mediator events provide effective protection.

Passive immunity Injection of antibodies to provide temporary protection against a disease-causing organism.

Immunization (*im"u-ni-za'shen*) The process of inducting immunity as a preventive measure against specific infectious disease.

Immunization schedule (*see* **Table**).

Immunoassay (*im"u-no-as"a*) Laboratory methods to measure antibodies and antigens in a person's blood or tissue to diagnose infectious diseases.

Immunoelectrophoresis (*im"u-no-e-lek'-tro-fo-re-sis*) A method of electrophoresis and double diffusion to recognize the proteins based on their electrophoretic mobility and antigenic specificities.

Immunofluorescesnce (*im"u-no-flu"o-re's-ens*) Determination of the site of antigen or antibody in the tissue by fluorescence.

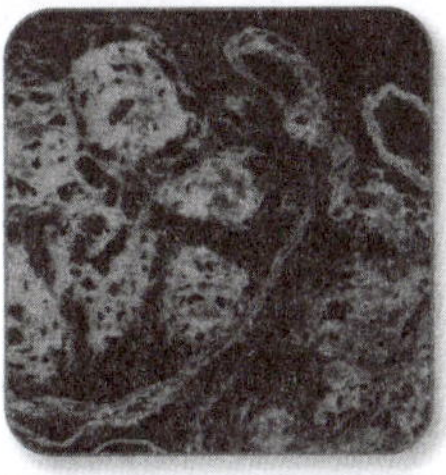

Immunofluorescence

Immunoglobulin (Ig) (*im"-u-no'-glob'u-lin*) A protein produced following exposure to an antigen possessing the activity of an antibody. They are the effector products of B cells in response to an antigen. There are five types of immunoglobulins - IgA, IgD, IgE, IgG and IgM (*see* **Table**).

Table: **Immunoglobulin**

IgA	Constitutes 20% of total immunoglobulins. Gut mucosa and lamina propria of the respiratory tract are major sites of IgA production. Secretory IgA provides local immunity.
IgD	Useful in the maturation and regulation of B-lymphocytes.
IgE	Produced in the lining of the respiratory and intestinal tracts, needed for immediate hypersensitivity reactions.
IgG	Constitutes 70% of total immunoglobulins and is distributed equally between the blood and extracellular fluid. It protects against immunoglobulin transported across the placenta and provides passively acquired immunity to the newborn. There are four subclasses of IgG, IgG1, IgG2, IgG3, and IgG4.
IgM	Earliest immunoglobulin to be synthesized by the fetus. An intravascular macromolecule stimulating complement activity.

Immunological tolerance The process by which immune cells are made unresponsive to self-antigens to prevent damage to healthy tissue.

Immunology (*im"u-nol'o-je*) The study of the molecular and cellular biology of antigen recognition and of immune reactions.

Immunosuppressive (*im"u-no-su-presh'un*) Prevention of activation of an excessive or inappropriate immune response by drugs such as corticosteroids cyclophosphamide, methotrexate or cyclosporine.

Immunosuppression (*im"u-no-su-presh'un*) Prevention of activation of an excessive or inappropriate immune response by drugs such as corticosteroids cyclophosphamide, methotrexate or cyclosporine.

Immunotherapy (*im"u-no'-ther'a-pe*) Passive immunization by preformed antibodies to build up a person's immunity to which he or she is allergic; use of body's immune system to counteract side effect of therapy especially cancer chemotherapy.

Immunotransfusion (*imu"no-trans-fu'zhan*) Reactions that occur when incompatible blood products are transfused into a patient's circulation, triggering a response from the patient's immune system.

Table: **Immunization schedule**

Vaccine	When to give	Dose	Route	Site
For pregnant women				
TT-1	Early in pregnancy	0.5 mL	Intramuscular	Upper arm
TT-2	4 weeks after TT-1	0.5 mL	Intramuscular	Upper arm
TT-booster	If received 2 TT doses in a pregnancy within last 3 years	0.5 mL	Intramuscular	Upper arm
For infants				

Contd...

Vaccine	When to give	Dose	Route	Site
BCG	At birth or as early as possible till 1 year of age	0.1 mL (0.05 mL till 1 month of age)	Intradermal	Left upper arm
Hepatitis	At birth or as early as possible within 24 hours	0.5 mL	Intramuscular	Anterolateral side of mid-thigh
OPV-0	At birth or as early as possible within 15 days	2 drops	Oral	Oral
OPV-1, 2 and 3	At 6 weeks, 10 weeks and 14 weeks	2 drops	Oral	Oral
DPT-1, 2 and 3	At 6 weeks, 10 weeks and 14 weeks	0.5 mL	Intramuscular	Anterolateral side of mid-thigh
HEP B-1, 2 and 3	At 6 weeks, 10 weeks and 14 weeks	0.5 mL	Intramuscular	Anterolateral side of mid-thigh
Measles	9 completed months–12 months	0.5 mL	Subcutaneous	Right upper arm
Vitamin–A (1st dose)	At 9 months with measles	1 mL (1 lakh IU)	Oral	Oral
For children				
DPT-booster	16–24 months	0.5 mL	Intramuscular	Anterolateral side of mid-thigh
Measles 2nd dose	16–24 months	0.5 mL	Subcutaneous	Right upper arm
OPV-booster	16–24 months	2 drops	Oral	Oral
Japanese encephalitis	16–24 months	0.5 mL	Subcutaneous	Left upper arm
Vitamin–A (2nd to 9th dose)	16 months then one dose every 6 months up to age of 5 years	2 mL (2 lakh IU)	Oral	Oral
DPT-booster	5–6 years	0.5 mL	Intramuscular	Upper arm
TT	10 years and 16 years	0.5 mL	Intramuscular	Upper arm

Impacted (*im-pak'ted*) Wedged in.

Impacted fracture A break in a bone in which the fragmented bony ends are forced into one another making it difficult to set.

Impacted tooth Tooth confined in its socket as to be incapable of normal eruption.

Impairment Any loss or abnormality of a structure of function.

Impalpable (*im-pal'pa-bl*) Not felt; not palpable; incapable of being perceived by touch.

Imperforate (*im-per'fo-rat*) not open.

Imperforate hymen A hymen without an opening.

Imperforate anus (proctatresia) Malformed opening at the anus which needs surgical correction.

Impetigo (*im-pe-ti'go*) A highly contagious skin infection showing confluent vesicles, pustules which rapture and exhibit bright yellow crusts.

Bockhart's impetigo Superficial folliculitis, infection at the opening of the hair follicles on legs and thighs presents with pustules, named after Max Bockhart, German physician.

Bullous impetigo Diffusely, scattered, tense bullae filled with clear fluid occurring in children.

Impetigo contagiosa A highly contagious form of impetigo affecting the most superficial layers of epidermis, occurs commonly on the face of children.

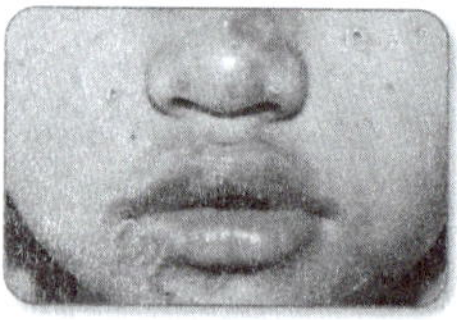

Bullous impetigo

Impetus (*im-pi-tus*) Driving energy, momentum, impulse, stimulus.

Implant (*im'plant*) To graft or to insert a natural or artificial material into a body surgically.

Implantation (*im'plan-ta'shun*) Process of grafting or insertion.

Implantation dermoid Painless, soft cyst in the pulps due to continued proliferation of fragment of epidermis that is driven beneath the dermis.

Impotence (*im'-po-ten's*) Inability to achieve or maintain a penile erection, adequate for the successful completion of intercourse, terminating in ejaculation.

Impression (*im'pre-shun*) *dent* A mold of the teeth, and the gums: a depression in a surface; an effect produced upon the mind; *dent* the imprint of all or part of the dental arch or teeth using appropriate dental materials.

Imprinting (*im-print'ing*) Differential effects of maternally and paternally derived DNA; a specialized form of learning occurring early in life and often influencing behavior later in life.

Impulse (*im'puls*) An act of driving outward with sudden force.

Cardiac impulse Heartbeat felt at the cardiac apex.

Excitatory impulse Impulse stimulating the activity.

Inhibitory impulse Impulse dampening the activity.

Nerve impulse An electrical change transmitted along the membrane of a nerve.

Proprioceptive impulse An afferent nerve impulse arising from stimuli originating in joints, muscles, tendons or other sensory endings.

Inarticulo mortis (*inahr-tik'u-lo mor'tis*) A Latin term used in law to describe the moment when someone is about to die. It is similar to the term in extremis.

Inbreeding A mating of closely related individuals.

Incarcerated hernia Herniation of a loop of intestine into a mesothelial sac that cannot return to its original position without surgery.

Incidence rate (inception rate) The incidence rate per 1000 persons in a population is the number of new cases that occur within a defined unit of time, divided by the persons exposed or at a risk during the same unit, multiplied by 1000.

Incineration (*in-sin'er-a'shun*) The act of burning.

Incision (*in-sizh'un*) A cut or a wound produced by a sharp instrument.

Incisor (*in-si'zor*) That which cuts.

Incisor teeth One of the four anterior teeth in each jaw at the front of the mouth used for cutting through food.

Incisure (*in-si'zher*) A deep indentation or notch in an edge or surface.

Inclusion body A particle of foreign (virus or lead) or metabolically inactive materials (Mellory body) within the cytoplasm or nucleus of a cell.

Incompatibility Quality of not being suitable for mixing.

Incompetence Insufficiency or inadequate ability to function.

Aortic incompetence Regurgitation of blood through the aortic valve.

Mitral incompetence Leaky mitral valve allowing regurgitation of blood from left ventricle to left atrium.

Pulmonary incompetence Inability of pulmonary valve to close permitting regurgitation of blood to right ventricle.

Tricuspid incompetence Leaky valve allowing blood to flow backward into right atrium.

Incontinence (*in-konti-nens*) Inability to control the passing of natural discharges or evacuations as urine or feces.

Fecal incontinence An involuntary passage of feces can develop following obstetric trauma, severe diarrhea or neurologic abnormalities.

Retention and overflow incontinence Incontinence.

Stress incontinence Laxity of pelvic floor musculature causing urine leak in women.

Urinary incontinence An involuntary loss of urine in large amounts, may be transient or persistent.

Incoordination (*in'ko-or'-di-na'shun*) Inability to produce a coordinated action; lack of coordination.

Incubation (*in'ku-ba'shun*) The process of incubating period; the period lapsing between entry of a pathogen and appearance of the clinical features; development of pathogens.

Incubation period (latent period) The time elapsed between exposure to a pathogenic organism and when signs and symptoms are first apparent.

Incubator An apparatus in which media inoculated with microorganisms are cultivated in appropriate temperature; enclosed crib where oxygen temperature and humidity are regulated to take care of prematurely born infants.

Incudectomy (*ing'ku-dek'to-me*) Surgical removal of all the parts of incus.

Incus (*in'kus*) The middle one of chain of small bones in the middle ear which conducts vibrations from the tympanic membrane to the inner ear; anvil.

Indapamide (*in-dap'a-mid*) A diuretic indicated for use as monotherapy or in combination with other blood pressure-lowering agents to treat hypertension.

Indian childhood cirrhosis A fatal familial disease of early childhood onset, first described in middle class Hindu families of rural India. It is characterized by fever, anorexia, hepatomegaly, fulminant cirrhosis and hepatic failure, excessive dietary copper intake appears to be the cause and discontinuation of use of copper cookware has reduced its incidence.

Indication (*in'dika-shun*) A sign or situation that indicates the proper treatment of a disease.

Indigestion (*in-di-jes'chen*) Common disorder producing nausea, belching, gas bloating, heart burn and abdominal cramps brought on by eating.

Indinavir (*in-din'a-vir*) An alpha-amino acid amide protease inhibitor used as a treatment therapy for Human immunodeficiency virus (HIV) infections.

Indole (*in'dol*) The product of bacterial decomposition of tryptophan. It is partially responsible for fecal odor.

Indolent (*in'do-lent*) Slow growing, causing little or no pain.

Indomethacin (*in'do-meth-a-sin*) An anti-inflammatory and antipyretic agent.

Indoxyl (*in-dok'sal*) A metabolite of dietary l-tryptophan that acts as a cardiotoxin and uremic toxin.

Induction (*in-duk'shun*) Initiation.

Induction chemotherapy During treatment for those presenting with an advance cancer.

Induction of labor Use of drugs to initiate the process of childbirth.

Induration (*in'du-ra'shun*) The process of hardening; the hardened area of a tissue.

Inebriant (*in-e'bre-ant*) An intoxicant.

Infant (*in'fent*) A young child; baby.

Infant mortality rate × 1000.

Infantile (*in'fan'til*) Pertaining to an infant.

Infantile glaucoma Buphthalmos, enlargement of the whole eye in infant.

Infantile paralysis Poliomyelitis

Infantile pyloric stenosis Presence of visible peristalsis from left to right where the infant vomits the water that is imbibed.

Infantile spasms A rare but serious type of epilepsy.

Infantilism (*in-fan'til-izm*) A condition wherein the characters of childhood persist into adult life.

Infant mortality rate (IMR) The number of deaths per 1000 love births of children under 1 year of age.

Infarct An area of necrosis due to a deficient blood supply.

Infarction The formation of an infarct.

Myocardial infarction An infarction in the cardiac muscle due to coronary occlusion.

Pulmonary infarction Infarction due to pulmonary embolism.

Infection (*in-fek'shun*) The invasion of the body by microorganisms that reproduce and multiply causing disease.

Acute infection An infection that occurs suddenly.

Airborne infection An infection caused by inhalation of microorganisms in the air.

Apical infection An infection located at the apex of a tooth.

Blood-borne infection An infection transmitted through contact with blood.

Chronic infection An infection having a prolonged course.

Cross infection The transfer of an infection from one patient to another in the hospital.

Droplet infection An infection acquired by inhalation of a microorganism in the air especially one added to the air by coughing or sneezing.

Endogenous infection Reactivation of a quiescent primary lesion as in tuberculosis.

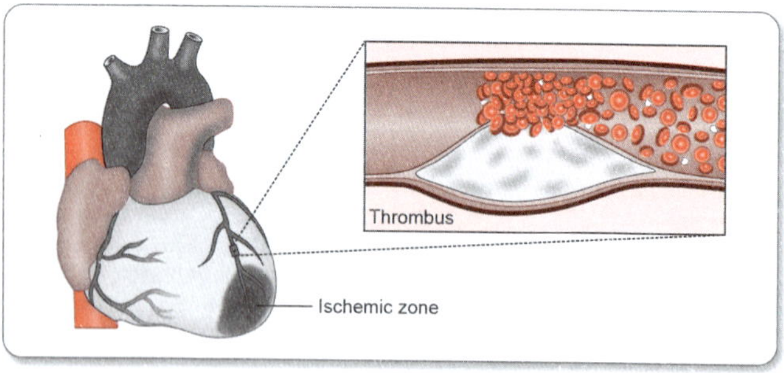

Myocardial infarction

Exogenous infection Infection acquired from outside from an active case.

Local infection Infection confined to the site of entry.

Nosocomial infection An infection acquired during hospitalization.

Opportunistic infection Any infection that results during immunocompromised conditions.

Pyogenic infection An infection resulting from pus-forming organism.

Secondary infection Infection made possible by a primary infection that lowers host's resistance.

Subacute infection An infection without presenting symptoms.

Systemic infection An infection in which the infecting agent is found throughout the body.

Infectious disease Any communicable disease.

Infectious mononucleosis Glandular fever caused by EB virus, characterized by exudative tonsillitis, petechial rashly madenopathy, splenomegaly.

Inferior alveolar nerve block (IANB): A technique of dental anesthesia, to numb the mandibular teeth, gingivae and lower lip.

Inferior liver margin sign A supine radiograph in pneumoperitoneum revealing collection of free gas under the inferior surface of the liver.

Infestation (*in-fes-ta'shen*) Presence of animal parasite such as lice or mites on the skin or hair or worms inside the body.

Infiltration (*in'fil-tra'shun*) Growth of tissue or cells which are not normal or in amounts in excess of the normal.

Cellular infiltration An infiltration of blood cells into tissues; invasion of malignant cells into adjacent tissues.

Fatty infiltration A deposit of fat in the tissues.

Inflammation (*in-flam-a'shun*) A bodily response to injury, infection or destruction characterized by heat, redness, pain, swelling and disturbed function referred to as *calor, rubor, dolor, tumor* and *functio laesa* respectively.

Influenza (*in'flu-en'za*) Flu; an acute infection of the respiratory tract by influenza virus A and B characterized by sudden onset of fever, headache, malaise, myalgias and arthralgias with dry cough and nasal discharge. Influenza C virus causes upper respiratory tract infection. The virus is transmitted in respiratory secretions. Treatment is symptomatic, amantadine and rimantadine can shorten illness if given early in cases of influenza A. Inactivated influenza vaccine offers protection against influenza A and B.

Infra Below.

Infracostal Below the ribs.

Infradiaphragmatic Below the diaphragm.

Inframammary Below the mammary gland.

Infranuclear Peripheral to a nucleus.

Infra patellar bursitis Painful swelling adjacent to insertion of the patellar tendon into tibial tubercle.

Infrascapular Beneath the shoulder blade.

Infraumbilical Below the umbilicus.

Infrared radiation (*in-fra-red'*) Electromagnetic radiation (EMR) with wavelengths longer than those of visible light and shorter than radio waves.

Infundibulum (*in'fun-dib'u-lum*) Structure having a funnel-shaped passage.

Infusion (*in-fu'zh'un*) The introduction of a fluid, drug or nutrient into a blood vessel or body cavity.

Infusion pump An apparatus designed to inject measured amounts of a drug over a period of time.

Ingress The act of entering.

Ingestion The act of taking any substance into the body through the mouth.

Ingravescent Gradually increasing in severity.

Inguinal (*ing'gwi-nal*) Pertaining to the groin.

Inguinal axillary veins Superficial venous communications between the axilla and femoral triangle.

Inguinal region The iliac region on either side of pubes.

Inguinal triangle Bounded by deep epigastric vessels, Poupart's ligament, and outer border of rectus sheath, described by Hesselbach, a German surgeon also called Hesselbach's triangle.

Inguinal canal A narrow passage in the lower part of the abdominal wall, extending from the internal (abdominal) ring to the external (subcutaneous) inguinal ring.

Inguinal hernia Protrusion of part of the intestines into the muscles of the groin.

Inguinal ligament (Poupart's ligament) A set of 2 bands that connect the oblique muscles of the abdomen to the pelvis, deep in the groin.

INH Isonicotinic acid hydrazide.

Inhalation (*in'ha-la'shun*) The act of drawing air or other substances into the lungs.

Inheritance (*in-her'i-tans*) The acquisition of characters from the parents to children through the influence of genes.

Inhibin (*in-hib'in*) A peptide hormone released by the testicular Sertoli cells that inhibits FSH, also produced by the ovarian granulosa cells in response to FSH.

Inhibition (*in'hi-bish'un*) Arrest a process.

Inhibitor A substance interfering with the process.

Innidiation The growth and multiplication of abnormal cells in another location to which they have been transported by means of lymph or blood stream, or both.

Inion (*in'e-on*) The most prominent point of the external occipital protuberance.

Initiation *mol* The first step in the synthesis of polypeptide chain. It requires the formation of a ribosome-mRNA-initiator tRNA complex.

Injection (*in-jek'shun*) The act of introduction of a drug, liquid or vaccine into the tissue or vasculature or an organ from a syringe through a needle.

Intralesional injection Injection of a large dose of a drug in a small volume of vehicle, directly in a place where it is required to act, example corticosteroids.

Intramuscular injection Injection into the muscles in the anterior thigh, deltoid or buttocks.

Intraosseous injection Injection of an anesthetic directly into the cancellous bone of the alveolar process adjacent to the tooth.

Intraperitoneal injection Injection into the peritoneal cavity.

Intrapleural injection Injection into the pleural cavity.

Intravenous injection Injection into a vein.

Subcutaneous injection Injection beneath the skin.

Inlay (*in'la*) *dent* A filling that is made outside of the tooth and then cemented into place.

Inlet A passage leading to a cavity.

Innate Genetically determined behavior patterns.

Innate releasing mechanism Sensory mechanism selectively responsive to specific external stimuli and responsible for triggering the stereotyped motor response.

Inner ear Labyrinth.

Innervation (*in'er-va'shun*) Nerve supply to an organ in a body.

Innominate artery Brachiocephalic artery.

Innominate bone Hip bone.

Innominate vein Brachiocephalic vein.

Inoculation (*in-ok'u-la'shun*) Introduction of infective agent, vaccine, serum into the tissues.

Inoculum (*in-ok'u-lum*) A substance introduced by inoculation.

Inodilator (*ino-di'la-tar, -di-la'tar*) An agent with both positive inotropic and vasodilator effects.

Inositol (*in-os'i-tol*) A member of vitamin B complex.

Inotropic (*in'o-trop'ik*) Affecting the force of muscular contractions.

Inotropic agent Agent that maintains tissue perfusion. These agents are sympathetic catecholamines such as dopamine and dobutamine.

Inpatient (*in'pa-shent*) A patient who is hospitalized.

Inquest A legal inquiry into the manner of a death.

Insanity (*in-san'i-te*) Mental derangement with unreliability of behavior with concomitant danger to himself and other.

Insect Organism belonging to class Insecta of the phylum Arthropoda, flies, mosquitoes, lice, fleas, ticks, spiders, bees, hornets and wasps are some examples.

Insecticide (*in-sek'ti-sid*) A preparation causing destruction of insects.

Insemination (*in-sem'in-a'shun*) Deposition of semen into the vagina or cervix.

Insertion The movable attachment of the distal end of the muscle; placement or implantation; *mol* the interposition of one or more nucleotides in a chain of DNA or RNA.

Insertion mutation A type of mutation involving the addition of genetic material.

Insight *psy* Ability of the patient to understand the true cause and meaning of a situation.

Impaired insight Diminished ability to understand the objective reality of situation.

Intellectual insight Understanding of the objective reality of a set of circumstances, without the ability to apply the understanding in any useful way to master the situation.

True insight Understanding of the objective reality of situation coupled with the motivation and emotional impetus to master the situation.

Insight psychotherapy *psy* Psychotherapy that aims to relieve emotional conflict by helping the patient understand the cause of a conflict.

In situ (*in si'tu*) (*L*) In place, confined to the site of origin.

Insomnia Inability in getting sleep or remaining asleep.

Inspiration (*in'spir-a'shun*) Inhalation, drawing air into the lungs.

Instillation (*in'stil-a'shun*) Administration of a liquid drop by drop.

Insufflation The act of blowing gas or powder into a body cavity.

Insula (*in'su-la*) Island; a triangular area of cerebral cortex lying in the floor of lateral fissure.

Insulin A protein hormone produced by the beta cells of the islets of Langerhans in the pancreas. It is essential to the body's use of glucose as an energy source. It lowers blood glucose by suppressing hepatic glucose production and stimulating peripheral uptake mainly in skeletal muscle and fat.

Insulinoma (*in'su-lin-o'ma*) A tumor of the beta cells of the islets of Langerhans that secretes excessive amounts of insulin. It causes a marked fall in the amount of glucose in the blood which can lead to collapse and coma.

Insulin pen A device with the size and shape of a pen to administer insulin. It is a syringe containing prefilled insulin cartridge with a very fine needle.

Insulin pump An implantable device that delivers insulin at low levels at a regulated rate.

Insulin-regulatable glucose transporter (IGRT) A protein expressed in muscle and fat that migrates from the cytoplasm to plasma membrane in response to insulin. It results in increased intracellular transport of glucose.

Insulin tolerance test A test of body's ability to utilize insulin. The blood glucose is measured periodically following administration of insulin. The blood glucose falls in 30 minutes and returns to normal after 90 minutes. The fall in glucose in patients with hypoglycemia is lower and is slower to return to normal.

Integration (*in'te-gra'shun*) Bringing together of various parts or functions so as to perform in harmony.

Integument (*in-teg'u-ment*) A covering, the skin.

Integumentum (*in-teg'u-men'tum*) A natural outer covering of an animal or a plant, such as skin, a seed coat, or a shell.

Intelligence quotient (IQ) Total score derived from a set of standarized tests or subsets designed to assess human intelligence.

Intelligence test An assessment that measures a range of cognitive abilities and provides a score as a measure of individual's intellectual abilities and potential.

Intensity modulated radiation therapy An advanced method of conformal radiation therapy in which the beams are aimed from several directions and the intensity of the beams is controlled by computers; IMRT.

Intention (*in-ten'shun*) A natural process of healing; purpose.

First intention Healing without granulation.

Second intention Healing by adhesion of two granulated surfaces.

Third intention Healing of an ulcer or cavity by filling with granulation tissue and cicatrization.

Intercartilaginous (*in'ter-kar"ti-laj'i-nus*) Between cartilaginous bone.

Intercalated (*in-ter'ka-lat"ed*) To interpolate; interpose.

Intercellular (*in"ter-sel'u-ler*) Between the cells.

Intercellular adhesion molecule-1 (ICAM-1) Production of a protein ligand induced by gamma-interferon required for neutrophils to migrate into inflamed tissue.

Intercostal muscles Muscle groups that are situated in between the ribs that create and move the chest wall.

Intercurrent (*in"ter-kur'ent*) Occurring during the course.

Interferon (*in-ter-fer'on*) Biologic substances elaborated by the viral infected host cells and they inhibit subsequent viral replication.

Interferon alpha and beta Produced by leukocytes and fibroblasts.

Interferon gamma Produced by T cells, NK cells and fibroblasts.

Interkinesis (*in'ter-ki-ne'sis*) Also known as interphase II, is a period of rest that cells of certain species experience between meiosis I and meiosis II.

Interleukins Protein substances that regulate immune responses. They are produced by several different cell types rapidly (*see* **Table**).

Intermittent (*inter-mit'ent*) Suspending activity at intervals.

Intermittent claudication An intermittent cramp-like pain occurring in the extremity during exercises and relieved by rest. It occurs due to accumulation of P substance in occlusive vascular diseases.

Intermittent limping A patient with endarteritis is unable to meet the demand of blood supply of the muscles on walking and the muscles go into cramp and patient limps intermittently.

Intermittent claudication An intermittent cramp-like pain occurring in the extremity during exercises and relieved by rest. It occurs due to accumulation of P substance in occlusive vascular diseases.

Intermittent fever Fever fluctuates between the normal body temperature and higher-than-normal levels through the day.

Intern (*in'tern*) A fresh medical graduate receiving training in the hospital by rotation in different disciplines over 12 months before being eligible to receive license to practice medicine.

International classification of disease ICD A system of disease classification which is regularly updated by WHO.

Interneuron (*in'ter-nur'on*) Neurons that are found exclusively in the central nervous system.

Interoceptor (*in'ter-o-sep'tar*) A sensory receptor that detects stimuli within the body, such as blood pressure and body position.

Interosseal Situated between the bones.

Interparietal bone (inca bone, incarial bone) A dermal bone situated between the parietal and supraoccipital.

Interpeduncular (*in'ter-pe-dunk'u-lar*) An unpaired CSF-filled subarachnoid cistern located between the cerebral peduncles.

Interphase (interkinesis) A stage of cell division during which there is replication of DNA; the area or zone where two phases of a substance (a gas and liquid) come in contact with each other.

Intersex (*in'ter-seks*) An individual exhibiting features of both sexes in varying degrees.

Interstice (*in-ter'stis*) An intervening space, especially a very small one.

Interstitial cells (e.g., Leydig cells) Any cell that lies in the spaces between the functional cells of a tissue.

Interstitial-cell-stimulating hormone Leutimizing hormone; A hormone made in the pituitary gland.

Interstitial cystitis A chronic condition causing bladder pressure, bladder pain and sometimes pelvic pain.

Interstitium (*in"ter-stishe-um*) A supporting or connective tissue or material that lies between the principal cells of an organ, or between structures in the body.

Intertrigo (*in'ter-tri-go*) Dermatitis occurring on opposed surfaces of the skin.

Acute intertrigo A painful deep fissure in a fold of skin with inflammatory changes in surrounding skin commonly the retroauricular fold or the interdigital areas.

Intertrigo hemorrhage Bleeding from internal organs presents with increasing pallor, increasing pulse-rate and there may be restlessness and air hunger.

Intertrochanteric (*in'ter-tro'kan-ter-ik*) Between the greater and lesser trochanter of the femur.

Interureteric (*in'ter-u're-ter'ik*) Related to interureteral.

Intestinal flora Bacteria and other organisms that live inside the intestines; these help in digestion and produce vitamins such as biotin and vitamin K.

Intestinal juice Clear to pale yellow, watery secretion composed of hormones, digestive enzymes, mucus, and neutralizing substances released from the glands and mucous-membrane lining of the small and large intestines.

Intestine (bowel, gut) (*in-tes'tin*) The largest portion of digestive system extending from the pyloric opening of the stomach to the anus; bowel; gut. It is divided into the small intestine and large intestine.

Large intestine Large intestine extends from the ileocecal junction to the anus and is of 1.5 m in length. The mucosa has no villi but contains mucous secreting glands. It absorbs water, minerals and vitamins and eliminates undigested material during defecation. It consists of cecum, vermiform appendix, ascending colon, transverse colon and descending colon, sigmoid colon, rectum, anal canal and anus.

Small intestine Small intestine consists of duodenum, jejunum and ilium. Duodenum receives chyme from the stomach through pyloric orifice and by common bile duct, bile from the liver and gall bladder and pancreatic juice from pancreas. Ilium opens into the cecum and ileocecal valve prevents regurgitation of intestinal contents. The wall of intestine contains circular folds of mucosa and submucosa containing villi and microvilli which provide surface area for absorption of products of digestion.

Intima (tunica intima) (*in'ti-ma*) An innermost layer of an artery containing continuous layer of endothelial cells.

Intolerance An inability to endure or an incapacity to bear pain; effects of a drug.

Intoxication The state of being intoxicated by a drug, or alcoholic beverage.

Water intoxication Excessive retention of water from excess ingestion of water, administration of hypotonic solutions, or oxytocin or increased secretion of ADH. It is characterized by abdominal cramps, dizziness, lethargy, convulsions and coma.

Intracellular (*in'tra-sel'u-lar*) Within the cell.

Intracranial (*in'tra-kre'ne-el*) Within the cranium or skull.

Intradermal (*in'tra-dermal*) Within the skin.

Intrafallopian (*in'tra-fa-lo'pe-an*) Withing fallopian tube.

Intramuscular Inside or into a muscle.

Intraocular Within the eyeball.

Intraoperative (*in'tra-op'er-a'tiv*) Occurring during operation.

Intraoperative radiation therapy Delivery of a single, high dose of external beam radiation to the tumor site; IORT.

Intrapartum (*in'tra-par-tum*) Occurrence during childbirth.

Intrathecal (*in'tra-the'kal*) Within the spinal canal.

Intrarenal resistive index A noninvasive ultrasound-based method to assess vascular resistance and elasticity used to assess the renal allograft function and the prediction of allograft and patient survival.

Intrauterine (*in'tra-u'ter-in*) Within the uterus.

Intrauterine contraceptive device (IUCD) A device with a small, flexible plastic frame. It often has copper wire of copper sleeves on it. It is inserted into a woman's uterus through her vagina. It has one or two strings or threads tied to them, which hang through the opening of the cervix into the vagina. It works chiefly by preventing sperm and ova from meeting. It is very effective and does not interfere with sex. Hormone-releasing IUDs release small amount of progesterone or levonorgestrel.

Intrauterine growth retardation A decreased rate of fetal growth may occur as a result of any condition that interfere with the blood supply to the placenta or general health and nutritional status of the mother.

Intravenous (*in-tra-ve'nus*) Inside a vein.

Intravenous pylogram (IVP) An imaging test used to look at the kidneys and ureters.

Intra vitam During life; while the subject is alive.

Intrinsic (*in-trin'sik*) Located in or originating from a tissue or organ.

Intrinsic asthma A variety of asthma where an extrinsic allergen cannot be identified as the cause, and asthmatic attacks are not mediated through IgE.

Intrinsic factor A vitamin B_{12} binding glycoprotein secreted by the gastric parietal cell.

Introitus (*in-tro'i-tus*) An opening or entrance into a canal or cavity as the vagina.

Introjection (*in"tro-jek-shun*) *psy* A defense mechanism whereby one deals with emotional conflicts by accepting blame beyond what is realistic.

Intromission (*in'tro-mish-un*) Insertion of one part into another, as insertion of the penis into the vagina.

Introversion (*in'tro-ver'shun*) The turning outside of an organ.

Introvert Individual having his interest toward himself.

Intubation (*intu-ba'shun*) The introduction of a tube into any hollow organ.

Intumescence (*in-too-mes'ens*) A swelling; the process of enlarging.

Intussusception (*in'tu-su-sep'shun*) One part of the intestine telescoping into the lumen of adjoining part. It is felt as a hard swelling as the wave of peristalsis begins often in the right hypochondrium. It may be associated with a red-current jelly exudate from the rectum.

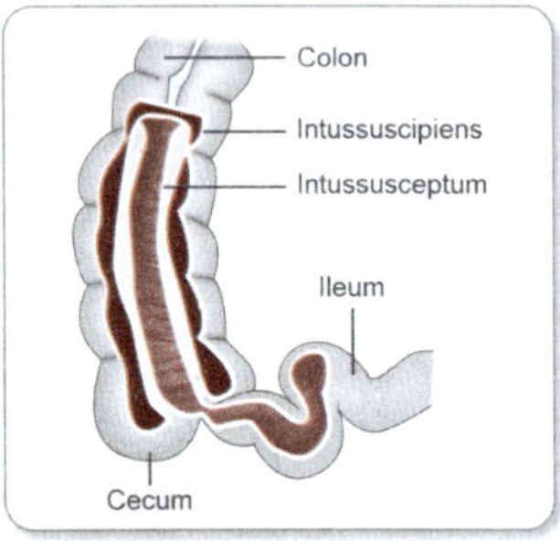

Enteric intussusception

Inulin A vegetable homopolysaccharide of D-fructose used to measure renal clearance.

Inunction (*in-ungk'shun*) The act of applying an ointment with friction.

Invagination The infolding of one part within another.

Invagination test A little finger when inserted into the inguinal canal if finds it empty in presence of a lump, the swelling cannot be inguinal hernia.

Invasion Attack, enter.

Inversion (*in-ver'shun*) A turning inside out; a chromosomal segment that has been broken off and reinserted in the same place, but with the genetic sequence in reverse order.

Invertebrate (*in-vur'te-brat*) Species of animals not possessing a backbone.

In vitro (*in-ve'tro*) (*L*) Within a test tube or in an artificial environment.

In vitro fertilization (IVF) A method of treating infertility. An ova is removed from a woman, and fertilized in the laboratory with sperm and reinserted into her uterus or a fallopian tube.

In vivo (Latin) Within the living, refers to tests, experiments and procedures that are done in or on a whole living organisms.

Involucrum (*in'vo-lu'kram*) A layer of new bone growth outside existing bone.

Involuntary muscle The muscles whose functioning cannot be controlled.

Involution (*in'vo-lu'shun*) Turning inward; a retrograde process; reduction in size.

Iodine (*i'o-din*) An essential micronutrient, mostly present in the thyroid gland in the form of thyroglobulin. It is essential to form thyroid hormone.

Iodipamide A contrast agent for cholecystography and intravenous cholangiography.

Iodism (*i'o-diz'm*) An abnormal local and systemic condition resulting from overdosage with, prolonged use of, or sensitivity to iodine or iodine compounds and marked by ptyalism, coryza, frontal headache, emaciation, and skin eruptions.

Iodoquinol (*i'odo-kwin'ol*) Belongs to the group of medicines called antiprotozoals. These medicines are used to treat infections caused by protozoa (tiny, one-celled animals). Iodoquinol is used most often in the treatment of an intestinal infection called amebiasis.

Ionophore (*i-on'o-for"*) A class of compounds that form complexes with specific ions and facilitate their transport across cell membranes.

Iontophoresis (*i-on'to-fo-re'sis*) The introduction of ions of soluble salts into the tissues by electric current; the process of electric current passing through a salt solution causing migration of positive ion to the negative pole and the negative ion to the positive pole.

Iopanoic acid A radiopaque dye used in cholecystography.

Iophendylate (*i'o-fen'di-lat*) A mixture of isomers used as contrast medium, mainly for brain and spinal cord visualization.

Ioxilan (*i-ok'si-lan*) A diagnostic contrast agent used in various medical imaging procedures, such as angiography, urography, and computed tomographic scans.

Ipecac (ipecacuanha) (*ip'e-kak*) the dried root of ipecacuanha, source of emetine.

Ipratropium (*ip"ra-tro'pe-um*) An anticholinergic drug used in the control of symptoms related to bronchospasm in chronic obstructive pulmonary disease (COPD).

Ipsilateral (homolateral) (*ip'si-lat'er-al*) Situated on the same side.

IQ Intelligence quotient, a measure of a person's intelligence. It is based on the results of special tests.

Iridauxesis Thickening of the iris.

Iridectasis (*ir'id-ek-ta'sis*) Dilatation of the iris or pupil.

Iridectomy Surgical removal of a part or all of the iris of the eye.

Iridencleisis (*ir'i-dan-kli'sis*) A surgical procedure especially for relief of glaucoma in which a small portion of the iris is implanted in a corneal incision to facilitate drainage of aqueous humor.

Iridocyclitis Inflammation of the iris and of the ciliary body.

Iridodialysis (*ir'i-do-di-ala-sis*) A condition in which the iris root is disinserted from the scleral spur.

Iridodonesis (*ir'id-o-do-ne'sis*) Abnormal tremulousness of the iris on movements of the eye.

Iridoplegia (*ir'id-o-ple'je-a*) Paralysis of the sphincter of the iris.

Iridotomy (*ir-i-dot'o-me*) Incision of the iris.

Iris (*i'ris*) The circular pigmented membrane suspended between the lens and the cornea with pupil at the center.

Iris lesions Ring-shaped papules with a central purpuric punctum and a peripheral rim of dusky erythema, as in erythema multiforme.

Iris bombe Bulging of iris forward by pressure of the aqueous humor.

Iritis (*i-ri'tis*) Inflammation of the iris which can impair vision. It is characterized by pain, photophobia, lacrimation and diminution of vision.

Iron (*i'ern*) A mineral essential for the production of hemoglobin and enzymes. Iron is used as a hematinic in the form of its salts and complexes such as ferrous sulphate, ferrous gluconate, ferrous fumarate and iron-dextran.

Iron deficiency anemia A microcytic hypochromic anemia caused by poor dietary intake, poor bioavailability of iron from cereal-based diets, increased requirements and blood loss.

Irradiation Treatment by ionizing radiation; spreading in all directions from a center.

Irreducible (*ir're-du'si-bl*) Not capable of being reduced as a fracture or hernia.

Irrigation Cleansing an area by flushing it with a stream of water or other fluid.

Bladder irrigation Washing out of bladder with water or other fluids, often normal saline.

Colonic irrigation Flushing of the colon with water.

Irritability Excitability; excessive response to a stimulus.

Irritable bowel syndrome (spastic colon, mucous colitis) (IBS) A functional bowel disorder in which abdominal pain is associated with defecation or a change in bowel habit.

Ischemia (*is-ke'me-a*) Deficiency of blood supply to an organ or tissue.

Myocardial Ischemia An imbalance between myocardial oxygen supply and demand leading to angina pectoris and if untreated to myocardial infarction.

Ischemic colitis Colicky abdominal pain with nausea, tenesmus, fever and bloody diarrhea resulting from atherosclerosis of the mesenteric arteries supplying the intestine.

Ischemic heart disease (*is'ke-mik*)Myocardial impairment due to imbalance between coronary blood flow and myocardial requirements. Atherosclerotic coronary artery disease forms the most common cause. Angina pectoris occurs when the vessel is critically narrowed so as to compromise the blood supply to the myocardium during period of stress. Unstable angina is noted when there is spasm over a fixed obstruction or when platelet aggregates occur or in presence of increased sympathetic flow resulting in increased myocardial oxygen consumption. Myocardial infarction occurs when a vessel gets totally occluded.

Ishiorectal abscess Hemochromatosis is an iron overload, in which body stores too much iron. It is often genetic.

Ischium (*is'ke-um*) The inferior dorsal part of the innominate (hip) bone.

Ischuria Retention or suppression of urine.

Island A structure detached from surrounding tissue or characterized by different structure.

Islet (*i'let*) A tiny isolated mass of one kind of tissue within another type.

Islets of Langerhans Groups of cells located inside the pancreas that secrete the hormone insulin and glucagon, named after Paul Langerhans, German pathologist.

Isoagglutination (*i'so-a-glu'ti-na'shun*) Agglutination of red blood cells as a result of the reaction between a isoagglutintin and specific antigen in or on the cells.

Isoagglutinin (Isobemagglutinin) (*iso'a-glu'ti-nin*) An isoantibody that causes agglutination of cells of genetically different members of the same species.

Isoantibody (*i-so-an'ti-bod'e*) Immune antibodies that are only produced following exposure to foreign red blood cell antigens.

Isoantigen (*i'so-an'ti-jen*) Formerly called alloantibodies, are antibodies produced by an individual against isoantigens produced by members of the same species.

Isodactylism A congenital defect in which all the fingers are the same length.

Isogamy (*i-sog'a-me*) A form of sexual reproduction that involves gametes of the same morphology.

Isograft Refers to tissue transplanted between genetically identical twins.

Isohemagglutinin Refers to the naturally occurring antibodies in the ABO blood group system.

Isoimmunization (*i'so-im'u-ni-za'shun*) The development of antibodies against the antigens of another individual of the same species. A condition that happens when a pregnant woman's blood protein is incompatible with the baby's causing her immune system to react and destroy the baby's blood cells.

Isolation The process of isolating; separation of a patient from other people to prevent him/her from infecting them or from being infected by them.

Isoleucine A crystalline, hydrophobic, essential amino acid $C_6H_{13}NO_2$ that is obtained in its levorotatory l-form by the hydrolysis of dietary protein and is isomeric with leucine.

Isomerase Any one of a class of enzymes that catalyze reactions involving a structural rearrangement of a molecule.

Isometric exercises (isometrics) Active exercise that strengthens the muscle by applying pressure against resistance.

Isometropia (*i'so-me-tro'pe-a*) The condition in which both eyes have equal refractive power.

Isthmectomy (*is-mek'tomi*) A surgical procedure that excises only the thyroid isthmus.

Isoniazid (isonicotinic acid hydrazide, INH) Isonicotinic acid hydrazide (INH); a powerful bactericidal agent acting on rapidly dividing extracellular tubercle bacilli, by interfering with the essential enzymes concerned in the terminal steps of the oxidative sequence of susceptible strains of tubercle bacilli.

Isopropamide A long acting quaternary antichalinergic drug, used in the treatment of peptic ulcer and other gastrointestinal disorders marked by hyperacidity and hypermotility.

Isoproterenol (Isoprenaline) (*i'so-pro'to-re-nol*) A beta- adrenergic agonist used as bronchodilator.

Isosorbide (*i'so-sor'bid*) A medication used to treat and prevent angina pectoris in patients with coronary heart disease.

Isosthenuria (*i'sos-then-u're-a*) The excretion of urine with the same osmolality as that of plasma despite variations in fluid intake.

Isotonic (*i'so-ton'ik*) A solution having same tonicity; maintenance of a constant amount of resistance during muscular contraction.

Isotope (*i'so-top*) A chemical element possessing the same number of protons and atomic number while differing in the number of neutrons and the atomic mass.

Isoxsuprine A beta-adrenergic agonist. It works by preventing the contractions of the smooth muscles in the uterus.

Isozyme (isoenzyme) (*i'so-zim*) A group of enzymes that catalyzes the same reaction but have different enzyme forms and catalytic efficiencies.

Isthmus (*is'mus*) A narrow connection between two larger parts.

Itch Pruritus; scabies.

Barber's itch Tinea barbae.

Dhobie itch Tinea cruris

Ground itch A local irritation; by penetration of the skin of the foot by hookworm larvae.

Swimmer's itch Dermatitis following swimming in water containing larval form of schistosomes.

Itch mite An extremely small, globular arthropod just visible to the naked eye. The female parasite, Sarcoptes scabei, is the example.

Itraconazole A triazole antifungal agent $C_{35}H_{38}Cl_2N_8O_4$ used orally especially to treat blastomycosis and histoplasmosis.

IUCD Intrauterine contraceptive device.

IUD (intrauterine device) Intrauterine device.

Ivermark's syndrome (*iver-mar-kz*)Histologic features of congenital hepatic fibrosis in addition to pancreatic cystic and dysplastic changes named after Bjorn Ivermark, Swedish Pathologist.

IVF *In vitro* fertilization.

IVP Intravenous pyelogram.

Ixodes (*iks-o'dez*) A genus of ticks of the family Ixodidae.

Ixodiasis (*ik'so-di'a-sis*) Disease caused by ticks of the superfamily Ixodidae.

Ixodidae (*iks-od'i-de*) A family of ticks which transmits disease in domestic animals and humans, such as Kyasanur forest disease, Rocky Mountain spotted fever, Lyme disease, ehrlichiosis and relapsing fever.

J

Jaccoud's fever Fever associated with slow and irregular pulse, noted in adults suffering from tuberculous meningitis, named after a French physician, Sigismond Jaccoud.

Jacksonian epilepsy *(jak-so'ne-an)* Named after John Hughlings Jackson, British neurologist characterized by unilateral clonic movements that begin in one group of muscles and spread gradually to adjacent group reflecting the march of the epileptic activity (e.g., mouth, thumb, great toe) through the motor cortex. The attacks may vary in duration from a few seconds to several hours.

Jacquemier'sign *(zhak-me-az)* Blue or purple color of vaginal mucosa sometimes noted after fourth week of pregnancy, described by Jean Jacquemier, a French obstetrician.

Jactitation *(jak'ti-ta-shun)* Rhythmic rolling, tossing from side to side seen in acute illness.

Jamaican neuropathy Tropical spastic paraparesis with sensory ataxia, optic atrophy and nerve deafness.

Jamais vu *(zham'-a-vu)* Psychomotor epilepsy with a mental reaction of false feeling of unfamiliarity with a real situation one has experienced.

Jarotzky's treatment *(yar-ot'skez)* Dietary therapy for peptic ulcer consisting of eggs, milk, bread and butter, formulated by Alexander Jarotzky, Moscow physician.

Jaundice *(jawn-dis)* Yellowish discoloration of the conjunctiva, sclera, mucosa under the tongue and skin due to deposition of bile pigments from hemolytic, hepatocellular or obstructive disorders of hepatobiliary system, and occurs as a symptom.

Acholuric jaundice Elevated unconjugated bilirubin that is not excreted by the kidney.

Induced jaundice Chemical compound and drugs causing liver damage due to either direct hepatotoxicity or by poison. Hypersensitivity may cause hepatic damage.

Leptospiral jaundice Jaundice present with leptospirosis.

Nonhemolytic jaundice Jaundice caused by an abnormality in the metabolism of bilirubin resulting in excessive accumulation of unconjugated bilirubin.

Physiologic jaundice Mild icterus neonatorum lasting the first few days of life.

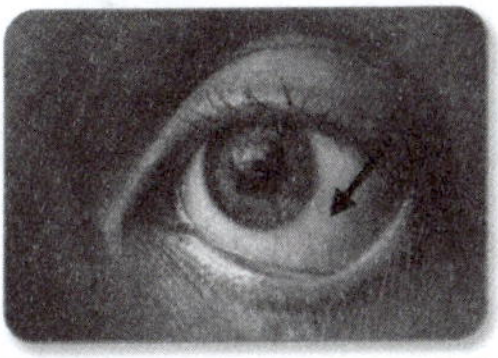

Jaundice

Jaw *(jaw)* Bony framework in the face bearing teeth, divided as upper and lower jaw (maxilla and mandible).

Cleft jaw An upper jaw (maxilla) which is relatively smaller than their lower jaw (mandible).

Dislocation of jaw Traumatic or spontaneous displacement of the mandible.

Hapsburg jaw A positional relationship of the mandible or maxilla to the skeletal base where either of the jaws protrudes beyond a predetermined imaginary line in the coronal plane of the skull.

Jaw drop Bilateral paralysis of the muscles of mastication resulting in failure to elevate the lower jaw.

Jaw jerk Reflex elicited by tapping chin with a rubber while mouth is half open and the jaw muscles relaxed.

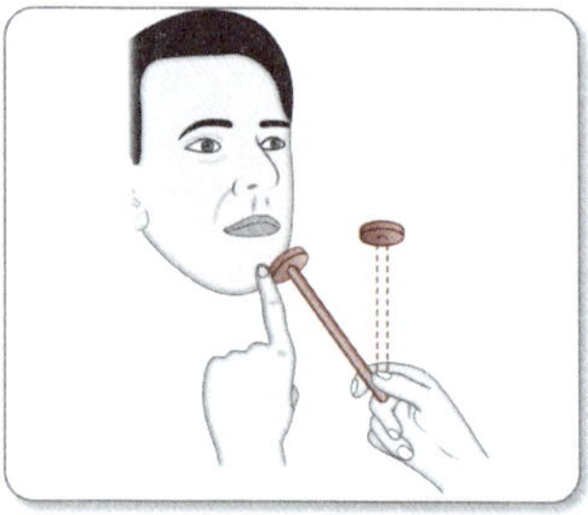

Jaw jerk

Jaw thrust A maneuver that manually displaces the jaw to establish an airway during resuscitation.

Jaw winking phenomenon Unilateral ptosis wherein lid is lifted following voluntary movements of the lower jaw due to faulty innervation of levator palpebrae; Marcus Gunn's syndrome.

Jaw wiring Surgical procedure where metal pins and wires are anchored into the jaw bones and surrounding tissue to prevent the jaw from moving; maxillomandibular fixation.

Pipe jaw A tool having two toothed jaws, one fixed and the other free to grip pipes and other tubular objects when the tool is turned in one direction only.

Jejunal ulcer A lesion in jejunum. It may develop after gastrojejunostomy.

Jejunectomy *(jeju-nek-to-me)* Excision of jejunum.

Jejunoileostomy An operation in which jejunum is joined to the ileum. Performed for intestinal disease like Crohn's disease.

Jejunostomy *(jeju-nos'to-me)* Formation of an artificial opening through the abdominal wall into the jejunum.

Jejunostomy feeding Administration of liquid foods through a hollow tube inserted into the jejunum through the abdominal wall.

Jejunotomy *(je'ju-no'to-me)* The surgical creation of a permanent opening between the jejunum and the surface of the abdominal wall.

Jejunum *(je-jun'um)* Empty; the middle portion of small intestine between duodenum and ileum. It is about 2.4 m long forming about two-fifths of the small intestine. adj. **jejunal**.

Jerk *(jurk)* A sudden reflex, involuntary muscular movement.

Biceps jerk A reflex contraction, of the biceps brachii on tapping the thumb of the evaluator, placed over the insertion of the tendon at the head of the radius in the cubital fossa.

Supinator jerk Flexion of the elbow and the finger flexion on striking the styloid process of the radius.

Tendon jerk The contraction of a muscle after tapping its tendon.

Triceps jerk An extension of forearm on tapping the stretched triceps tendon.

Jelly *(jel'e)* A translucent soft elastic material containing gelatin and pectin.

Cardiac jelly An acellular gelatinous matrix secreted by the myocardium which separates it from the endocardium in early heart development.

Contraceptive jelly A nongreasy jelly used in the vagina as a contraceptive agent.

Jiggers Infestation with jigger flea, *Tunga penetrans*.

Joint *(jo'ynt)* An articulation, a place of junction where two or more bones come in contact.

Ball and socket joint A joint in which the round end of one bone fits into the cavity of another enabling movement freely in almost all directions as in hip and shoulder joints.

Flail joint An unusually mobile joint.

Gliding joint Joints permitting a gliding motion as vertebral joints and finger joints.

Hinge joint Notably in elbows and knees, swing back and forth like doors on hinges.

Joint capsule Sac-like structure enclosing the ends of bone.

Joint cavity Articular space enclosed by the synovial membrane and articular cartilage.

Joint crepitus When a joint is moved with one hand while the other hand is laid, upon the joint fine crepitus may be appreciated in subacute and chronic affections of the joint and coarse crepitus in osteoarthritis.

Joint fracture A fracture of the articular surfaces of the bony structures of a joint.

Joint space Radiologic appearance produced by separation of bones by articular cartilages.

Saddle joint Each of the bones is concave in one direction, convex in the other and allow movement at right angles to each other, as in wrist and thumb.

Spheroidal joint A synovial joint in which a spheroidal surface of one joint (ball) moves within the concavity of (socket) the other bone.

Suture joint Inflexible joints in adult skull.

Synovial joint Union of the bony surfaces being surrounded by an articular capsule enclosing a cavity lined by synovial membrane.

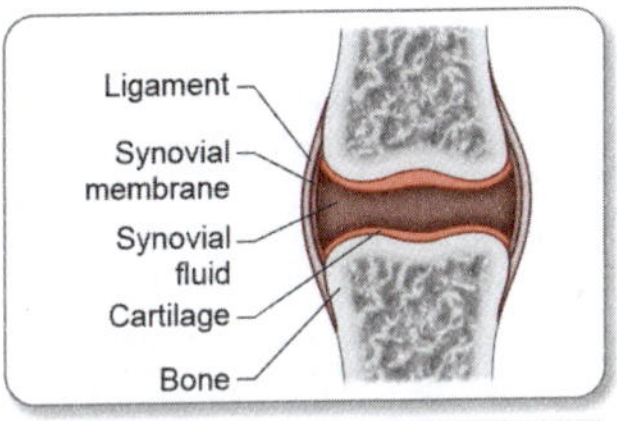

Synovial joint

Temporomandibular joint A bicondylar joint formed by the head of the mandible and the mandibular fossa, and the articular tubercle of the temporal bone.

Uniaxial joint One which permits movements in one axis only.

Jones' criteria *(jonz)* Major and minor manifestations of acute rheumatic fever, described by T.D. Jones, US physician. The major manifestations are polyarthritis, carditis, chorea, subcutaneous nodules and erythema marginatum. The minor manifestations include fever, arthralgia, previous rheumatic fever or known rheumatic heart disease, raised levels of ESR or C-reactive protein, protein, leukocytosis, first degree or second degree AV block. Presence of two major or one major and two minor criteria establishes the diagnosis of rheumatic fever.

Jones' test *(jonz)* Fluorescein instilled into conjunctiva reaches nasopharynx if lacrimal passage is patent.

Joubert's syndrome Nephronophthisis associated with mental retardation and ataxia.

Joule *(jool)* Unit of work or energy-named after English physicist, James Joule.

Jugular *(jug'u-lar)* Pertaining to neck.

Jugular foramen Opening formed by jugular notches of the temporal and occipital bones.

Jugular fossa Depression in petrosal part of the temporal bone.

Jugular ganglion Nodes of vagus and glossopharyngeal nerve in the jugular foramen.

Jugular venous pressure Vertical distance above sternal angle at which jugular veins collapse. It is measured from the sternal angle when the patient is propped up at 45° angle.

Jugular venous pulse Three positive (a,c,v) and two negative waves (x,y) in the neck veins. The oscillating top of the distended proximal portion of the internal jugular veins represents volumetric changes which faithfully reflect the right atrial pressure at all stages of the cardiac cycle.

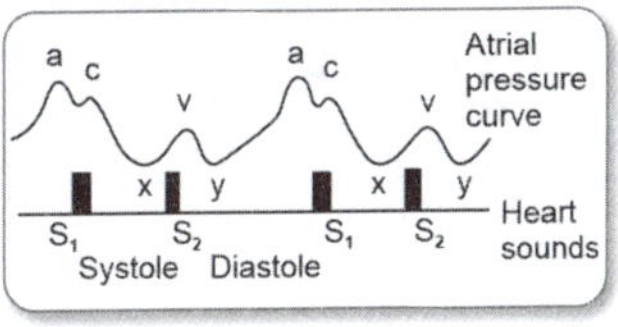

Jugular venous pulse

Jugular vein External, draining blood from exterior of the cranium and the deep parts of the face; and internal draining blood from the brain and superficial parts of the face and neck.

Junction *(junk-shun)* The place of meeting or coming together.

Dentinocemental junction The line of meeting of the dentin and cementum on the root of a tooth.

Dentino enamel junction The plane of meeting between dentin and enamel on the crown of a tooth.

Gap junction A narrow portion of the intercellular space containing channels linking adjacent cells and allowing passage of ions.

Gastroesophageal junction The site of transition from the stratified squamous epithelium of the esophagus to the simple columnar epithelium of the cardia of the stomach

Ileocecal junction The junction of the ileum and cecum, located in the right lower abdomen

Mucocutaneous junction The site of transition between skin and mucous membrane.

Myoneural junction Neouromuscular junction.

Neuromuscular junction The site of opposition between a nerve fiber and the motor end plate of the skeletal muscle which it innervates.

Sclerocorneal junction The line of union of the sclera and cornea.

Tight junction An intercellular junction at which adjacent plasma membranes are joined tightly together.

Juvenile *(ju'venil)* Young or immature.

Juvenile diabetes Insulin-dependent diabetes mellitus.

Juvenile polycystic kidney disease A recessively inherited disorder with multiple cysts in kidney with hepatic fibrosis and cysts which leads to renal and/or hepatic failure early.

Juvenile rheumatoid arthritis Arthritis developing in persons less than 16 years; juvenile chronic arthritis.

Juxta epiphyseal *(juks'ta ep-i-fiz-i-al)* Adjoining an epiphysis.

Juxta glomerular apparatus Granular cells in the wall of afferent arteriole before its entry into glomerulus, which secrete renin and possibly erythropoietin.

Juxta phrenic peak A triangular opacity with its base on the hemidiaphragm near the highest point of the dome, a radiographic sign of atelectasis.

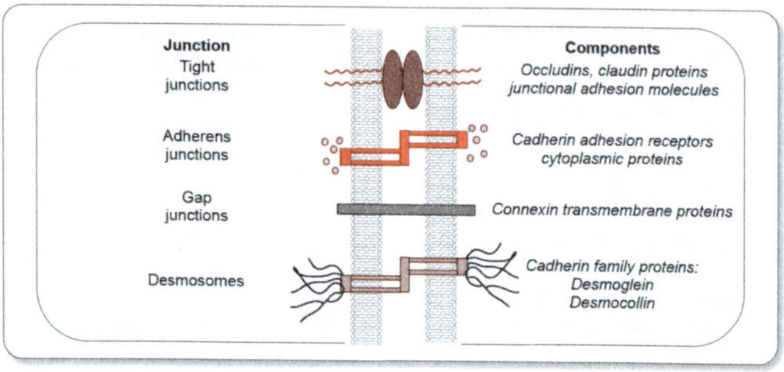

Various types of junctions

K

Kahn test (*kan*) A serologic precipitin test for syphilis, devised by American bacteriologist, Reuben Kahn; a three-dimensional projective test to assess psychosexual development, devised by American psychiatrist, Theodore Kahn.

Kala-azar (visceral leishmaniasis, dum-dum fever) (*ka'la-az'ar*) (*H*) Black disease, visceral leishmaniasis, an infections disease caused by *Leishmania donovani.* It is carried by sand flies (Phlebotomus). They multiply in the cells of reticuloendothelial system, and cause irregular fever, anemia and hepatosplenomegaly.

Kallmann's syndrome A condition characterized by absence of the sense of smell due to agenesis of the olfactory bulbs and by secondary hypogonadism; named after Franz Kallmann, American psychiatrist.

Kallidin (*kal'i-din*) A kinin liberated by the action of kallikrein or a plasma globulin; bradykinin.

Kallikrein (*kal'i-keri'n*) A group of enzymes that help in conversion of kininogen to a vasodilator substance, bradykinin.

Plasma kallikrein A trypsin-like serine protease whose activation results in the initiation and amplification of the plasma kallikrein/kinin system.

Tissue kallikrein A serine protease synthetized in renal tubular cells located upstream from the collecting duct where renal potassium balance is regulated.

Kanamycin (*kan'ah-mi-sin*) Antibiotic from *Streptomyces kanamyceticus* effective against aerobic, gram-negative bacteria and some gram-positive bacteria including mycobacteria.

Kaolin (*kao-'lin*) Hydrated aluminum silicate acting as an adsorbent.

Kaposi's sarcoma (*kap'o-se'*) A multifocal malignant neoplasm of reticuloendothelial cells involving skin.

Kary- (karyo-) Combining word for nucleus of a cell.

Karyokinesis (*kar'e-o-ki-nesis*) Division of the nucleus into two equal parts in the early stages of cell division, mitosis. adj. **karyokinetic**.

Karyolysis (*kar'e-ol'i-sis*) The dissolution of the nucleus of a cell, adj. **karyolytic**.

Karyoplasm (*kar'e-o-plasm*) Nucleoplasm, the substance of the nucleus of a cell.

Karyosome (*kar'e-o-som*) Condensed irregular clumps of chromatin dispersed in the chromatin network of a cell.

Karyotype (*kar-e-o-tip*) The chromosomal constitution of the cell nucleus.

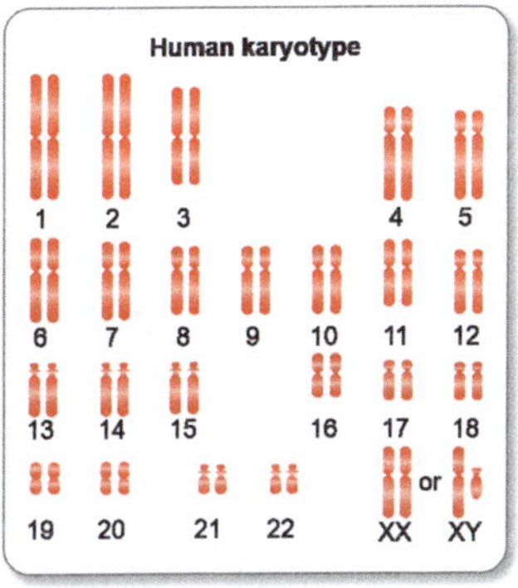

Karyotype

Kawasaki disease (mucocutaneous lymph node syndrome) Mucocutaneous lymph node syndrome of undetermined etiology affecting children under age 5 years. It presents with high fever, rash, conjunctivitis and cervical lymph node enlargement.

Kayser-fleischer ring (*ki'zer-fli'sher*) A gray-green to red-gold pigmented ring at the outer margin of cornea, described by German ophthalmologists **Bernhard Kayser** and ***Bruno Fleischer***. It is seen in Wilson's disease and pseudo-sclerosis.

Keloid (cheloid) (*ke'loyd*) A progressively enlarging firm, elevated scar with irregular margins at the site of a wound or burn of skin due to overgrowth of collagen. Its surgical removal is often followed by recurrence.

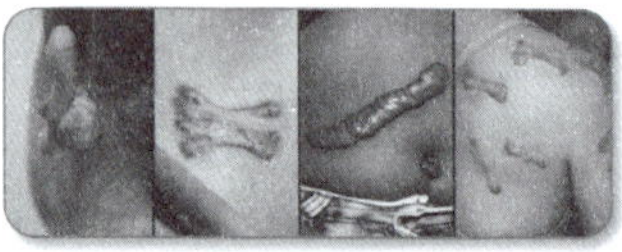

Keloid in various areas of body

Kelvin (*kel'vin*) The base SI unit of temperature, equal to 1/273.15 of the absolute temperature of the triple point of water.

Keratalgia (*ker'ah-tal'je-a*) Pain in the cornea.

Keratectasia (*ker'atek-ta'she-a*) Protrusion of a thin scarred cornea.

Keratectomy (*ker'ah-tek'to-me*) Excision of a portion of the cornea.

Photo refractive keratectomy A laser refractive procedure used to ablate the corneal stroma to correct refractive errors.

Keratin (*ker'a-tin*) A scleroprotein consisting of sulfur that is a major component of epidermis, hair, nails, horny tissues and the organic matrix of the enamel of the teeth.

Alpha keratin A fibrous structural protein, made up of amino acids. This protein is the primary component in hairs, horns, claws, nails and the epidermis layer of the skin.

Hard keratin A hard, waterproof protein found in the epidermis, hair, and nails, contains high level of cysteine (14%).

Soft keratin Keratin found in the epidermis of the skin as the flexible, tough stratum corneum in the form of flattened non-nucleated scales.

Keratinization (cornification) Process of development of/or conversion into keratin.

Keratitis (*ker'ah-tit'is*) Inflammation of the cornea.

Acanthamoeba keratitis Inflammation of cornea in which amoebae of the genus Acanthamoeba invade the clear portion of the cornea.

Catarrhal ulcerative keratitis Also known as phlyctenular corneal disease, noninfectious inflammatory processes of the peripheral cornea.

Fungal keratitis An inflammation of the cornea that is caused by a fungus.

Herpetic keratitis Inflammation of the cornea, caused by HSV.

Microbial keratitis Inflammation of the cornea, caused by bacteria.

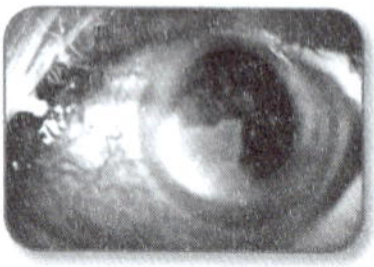

Microbial keratitis

Punctate keratitis Corneal inflammation of diverse causes characterized by scattered, fine, punctate corneal epithelial loss or damage.

Purulent keratitis Corneal inflammation resulting in pus formation.

Ulcerative keratitis Inflammation of cornea leading to corneal ulcer.

Vesicular keratitis Inflammation of cornea leading to developement of small, raised and clear vesicles.

Xerotic keratitis Softening, drying and ulceration of the cornea resulting from vitamin A deficiency.

Keratoacanthoma (molluscum sebaceum) (*ker'ah-to-ak'an-tho' ma*) Rapidly evolving tumor of the skin composed of keratinizing squamous cells originating from the pilosebaceous follicles. It may resolve spontaneously.

Eruptive keratoacanthoma Rare variant of keratoacanthoma (KA) that affects the skin and mucous membranes, is characterized by a sudden generalized eruption of severely pruritic, small folicular papules.

Keratocele (descemetocele) (*ker'ah-to-sel*) Hernia protrusion of Descemet's membrane of the cornea.

Keratoconjunctivitis (*ker'a-to-kon-junk'-ti-vi'tis*) Inflammation of the cornea and the conjunctiva.

Epidemic keratoconjunctivitis A viral conjunctivitis caused by a group of adenoviruses, EKC is highly contagious and has a tendency to occur in epidemics.

Flask keratoconjunctivitis Inflammation of the cornea and the conjunctiva leading to flask shaped ulcer.

Infectious keratoconjunctivitis Inflammation of the cornea and the conjunctiva caused by infection.

Keratoconjunctivitis sicca Dryness of cornea due to a deficiency of lacrimal secretion seen in Sjogren's syndrome, vitamin A deficiency and trachoma.

Keratoconus (*ker'o-toko'nos*) Conical protrusion of the central part of the cornea.

Keratoglobus (megalocornea) (*ker'ah-to-glo'bus*) Megalocornea. A rare, noninflammatory corneal ectasia characterized by diffuse protrusion and thinning of the cornea.

Keratoma (*ker'ah-to-mah*) A callus or callosity.

Keratomalacia (*ker'ah-to-ma-la'she-a*) Softening and necrosis of the cornea with absence of inflammation noted in vitamin A deficiency.

Keratome (*ker'a-tom*) A knife to incise cornea.

Keratometer (ophthalmometer) (*ker'a-tom'itar*) An instrument used for measurement of the curvature of the anterior surface of the cornea.

Keratoplasty (corneal graft) (*ker'ah-to-plas'te*) Corneal grafting.

Deep lamellar endothelial keratoplasty Refers to procedure in which Descemet's membrane and posterior corneal stroma is removed.

Descemet stripping endothelial keratoplasty Intended to transplant a healthy endothelial cell layer that will pump the fluid out of the cornea.

Optic keratoplasty A technique of performing full-thickness corneal transplantation where a diseased cornea is removed and replaced with a healthy and viable donor corneal button.

Refractive keratoplasty Surgery to reshape the cornea of the eye to correct vision problems such as myopia (nearsightedness) and hyperopia (farsightedness).

Tectonic keratoplasty A method in which a corneal button, preserved in glycerin is used as a seal over corneal perforation.

Keratoscope (Placido's disk) (*ker'a-to-skop'*) An instrument for determination of the symmetry of the curvature of cornea.

Keratosis (keratoma) (*ker'a-to-sis*) Horny growth.

Actinic keratosis A precancerous scaly spot found on sun-damaged skin, also known as solar keratosis.

Arsenic keratosis A precancerous dermatosis seen in patients with chronic arsenic toxicity.

Radiation keratosis A precancerous keratotic skin lesion that may arise on the skin many years after exposure to ionizing radiation.

Seborrheic keratosis Also known as seborrheic warts and basal cell papillomas, it is benign growth caused by a build-up of skin cells.

Stucco keratosis A type of benign, papular skin lesion that has a characteristic 'stuck on' appearance and commonly affects the distal limbs of elderly men.

Keratotomy (*ker'ah-tot'o-me*) Corneal incision.

Astigmatic keratotomy An outpatient surgical procedure to reduce or eliminate astigmatism.

Delimiting keratotomy Consists of an incision made completely through the cornea, tangential to the advancing border of the ulcer.

Radial keratotomy Involves multiple linear incisions in the anterior cornea that cause central cornea flattening and thereby reducing its focusing power.

Kerion (*ker'e-on*) An inflammatory condition that has produced a boggy swelling on the scalp, caused by a superficial fungal infection, *Trichophyton mentagrophytes* or *T. verrucosum*.

Kernicterus (*ker-nicter-us*) A grave form of *icterus neonatorum* presenting with severe neurologic symptoms with high levels of circulating bilirubin in newborn.

Kernig's sign (*ker'nigz*) Sign of meningitis, described by Russian physician, Vladimir Kernig, wherein there is an inability to extend the leg completely with thigh flexed upon the abdomen.

Ketoconazole A broad spectrum synthetic antifungal agent, used in the treatment of histoplasmosis, coccidioidomycosis and blastomycosis.

Ketogenesis (*ke'to-jen'e-sis*) The production of ketone bodies in the body.

Ketonemia (*ke'to'ne'mea*) A condition marked by an abnormal increase of ketone bodies in the circulating blood.

Ketonuria (acetonuria) (*ke'to-nu're-a*) Presence of ketone bodies in the urine; ketonuria.

Ketoprofen (*ke"to-pro'fen*) A nonsteroidal anti-inflammatory substance with analgesic and antipyretic properties.

Ketose (*ke'tos*) A sugar containing one ketone group per molecule in its cyclic form.

Ketosis (*ke-to'sis*) An abnormal accumulation of ketone bodies in the blood and tissues due to an inadequate utilization of carbohydrates.

Kidney (*kid'ne*) A pair of bean shaped organs in the lumbar region that filters the blood and excretes water, solute and waste products of metabolism.

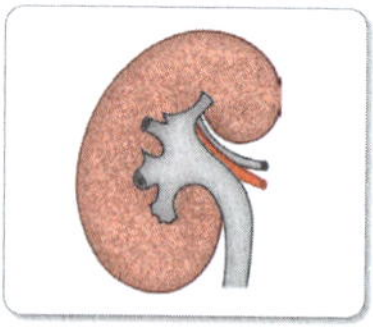

Kidney

Abdominal kidney An ectopic kidney situated above the iliac crest with its hilum at second lumbar vertebra.

Amyloid kidney Renal amyloidosis.

Artificial kidney A hemodialyzer; an extracorporeal machine through which blood circulates and gets rid of the substances that are normally excreted in the urine.

Cake kidney A bizarre shaped, irregularly lobed kidney.

Cement kidney Calcified contracted scarred kidney as in healed tuberculosis of the kidney.

Cicatricial kidney A shriveled, irregularly scarred kidney due to pyelonephritis.

Contracted kidney A scarred, granular, atrophic kidney.

Fatty kidney Kidney with fatty degeneration.

Flea-bitten kidney Kidney exhibiting petechiae on its surface.

Floating kidney Hypermobile kidney.

Fused kidney Fusion of renal anlagen resulting in a single anomalous kidney.

Goldblatt kidney Kidney with obstruction to its blood flow resulting in hypertension.

Horse-shoe kidney An anomalous kidney from fusion of the corresponding poles of renal analgen.

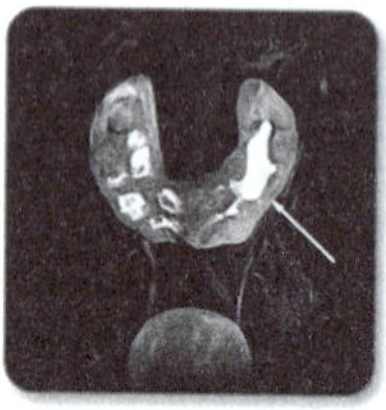

Horse-shoe kidney

Hypermobile kidney Freely mobile kidney.

Kidney machine Artificial kidney.

Kidney stone Renal calculus.

Lumbar kidney An ectopic kidney situated opposite sacral promontory in the iliac fossa.

Pelvic kidney Ectopic kidney situated opposite the sacrum and below the aortic bifurcation.

Polycystic kidney A genetic disease causing uncontrolled growth of cysts in the kidney eventually leading to kidney failure.

Primordial kidney An excretory structure or its rudiments developing in the embryo before the mesonephros; its duct is later used by the mesonephros, which arises caudal to it.

Sigmoid kidney A sigmoid kidney is an uncommon variant of the horseshoe kidney. Whereas the typical horseshoe kidney is fused only at the lower poles, in a sigmoid kidney both the upper and the lower poles are fused.

Sponge kidney A benign congenital abnormality, Anatomically it is characterized by cystic dilatation of the renal medullary collecting ducts..

Thoracic kidney The partial or complete protrusion of kidney above the level of diaphragm into the posterior mediastinum.

Waxy kidney A congenital condition characterized by the presence—seen best during urography—of spongy or porous appearing renal collecting tubules.

KID syndrome A triology of symptoms involving keratitis, ichthyosis and deafness.

Kilo- One thousand (10^3), a unit of measurement, K.

Kilocalorie (*kil'o-kal'o-re*) The amount of energy required to raise the temperature of 1 kilogram of water by 1°C; a unit of heat equal to 1000 calories (kcal).

Kin- (kine-) Movement.

Kinase (*ki'nas*) A phosphorylase subclass of transferase enzyme that catalyzes the transfer of a high energy phosphate from a donor molecule.

Kinematics (*kin'e-mat'iks*) The science concerned with movements of the parts of the body.

Kineplasty (*kin'e-plas'te*) Making use of the stump of an amputated extremity to produce motion of the prosthesis.

-kinesis (*ki-ne'sis*) Movement; stimulus-induced motion which responds to the intensity of the stimulus.

Kinesthesia (*kin'es-the'sea*) Appreciation of position, weight, tension and movement; sense of movement. adj. **kinesthetic**.

Kinesthesiometer A device to measure the angle of movement around a joint.

Kinetochore (*ki-ne'to-kor*) A specialized region of chromosome overlying the centromere, which is critical in mitosis.

Kinin (*ki'nin*) Vasoactive endogenous polypeptide inducing smooth muscle contraction.

Kiss of life Mouth to mouth resuscitation.

Klebsiella (*kleb'se-el'a*) A genus of gram-negative bacteria that appears as small, plump rods with rounded ends, named after German bacteriologist Theodore Klebs. It includes

K. pneumoniae Responsible for necrotizing pneumonia.

Klebs- Loeffler bacillus (*klebz'lef'ler*) *Corynebacterium diphtheriae*, named after German bacteriologists Theodor Klebs and Friedreich Loeffler.

Kleine-Levin syndrome A disorder occurring primarily in young males 3 or 4 times in a year marked by episodes of hypersomnia, hypersexual behavior and excessive eating.

Kleptomania (*klep'to-ma'ne-a*) An abnormal uncontrollable desire to steal things.

Klinefelter's syndrome (*klin'fel-ter*) A condition characterized by small testes, azoospermia, gynecomastia, excess elimination of urinary gonadotropins and subnormal intelligence.

Klippel-Trenaunay-Weber syndrome A macular vascular nexus in combination with bony and soft tissue hypertrophy and venous varicosities.

Klumpke's paralysis (*klump'kez*) Paralysis of intrinsic muscles of the hand which results in a claw hand. It is the result of an injury of the eighth cervical and first thoracic nerve roots as a result of forceful abduction of the shoulder mostly occurring during breech presentation with arms above the head.

Koch's bacillus (*koks*) *Mycobacterium tuberculosis*, named after Robert Koch, German bacteriologist.

Kobler's disease Inflammation of navicular bone of the foot.

Koilonychia (*koi'lo-nik'e-a*) Dystrophy of the nails which are abnormally thin and concave from side to side with edges turned up. Such spoon nails are seen in iron deficiency anemia.

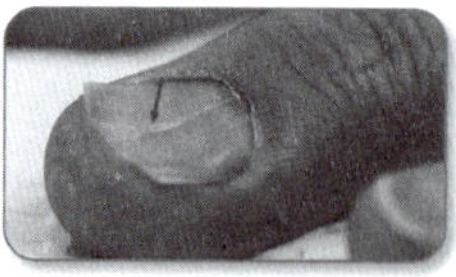

Koilonychia

Koplik's spots (*ko'plik*) Small bright red spots with a minute white speck in the center, on buccal and lingual mucosa, noted in measles before the appearance of rash, described by American pediatrician, Henry Koplik.

Koro Acute anxiety.

Korsakoff's syndrome (korsakoff's psychosis) Psychosis, described by Sergei Korsakoff, Russian neurologist. There is amnesia in chronic alcoholics due to deficiency of vitamin B1.

Kraurosis (*kraw-ro'sis*) A dried, shriveled condition.

Kraurosis vulvae Dryness, itching and atrophy of external genitalia in aged women.

K-ras gene One of the three proto-oncogenes.

Krebs cycle (citric acid cycle) (*krebz*) A sequence of enzymatic reaction involving metabolism of carbon chains of sugars, fatty acids and amino acids to yield carbon dioxide, carbon dioxide, water and high energy phosphate bonds, described by German-English biochemist Hans Krebs.

Krukenberg tumor (*kru'ken-bergz*) A neoplasm of the ovary developing as a metastasis of stomach cancer, named after Friedrich Krukenberg, German pathologist.

Krypton-81 m Radioactive gas used to evaluate regional ventilation .

Kupffer's cells (*kuf'er*) Large stellate or pyramidal intensely phagocytic reticuloendothelial cells lining the sinusoids of the liver, named after a German anatomist, Karl von Kupffer.

Kuru (trembling disease) (*ku'ru*) A fatal neurologic PRAM disease transmitted by subhuman primates in certain Melanesian tribes in New Guinea. It presents with cerebellar ataxia, tremors, dysarthria progressing to complete motor paralysis and death.

Kwashiorkor (*kwahshe-or'kor*) A protein-energy malnutrition seen in infants and young children after weaning from breast, characterized by edema, pigmentary changes in skin and hair, impaired growth and development and abdominal distension.

Kyasanur forest disease Monkey disease, an arbovirus disease, transmitted by soft wood tick, *Haemaphysalis spinigera*, maintained by monkeys in the forest areas of Shimoga, Udupi, Uttara Kannada, districts, Karnataka, India, characterized by fever, headache, muscular aches, back ache, orbital pain, prostration and occasionally hemorrhagic manifestations. The treatment is symptomatic.

Kymograph (*ki'mo-graf*) An instrument to record undulations of an artery.

Kyphos (*ki'fos*) The hump of the spine in kyphosis.

Kyphoscoliosis (*kifo-skole-o'sis*) Backward and lateral curvature of the spine.

Kyphosis (*ki'fo'sis*) An abnormally increased convex curvature of the thoracic spine, hunchback. adj. **kyphotic**.

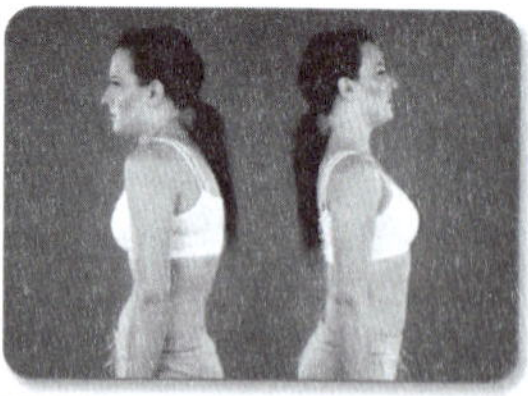

X-rays showing thoracic kyphosis (normal on right and kyphosis on left)

L

Labeling index The proportion of cells in a sample of tissue that are producing DNA. Ki-67 labeling index; a valuable tool that reflects tumor proliferation capability.

Labial (*la'be-al*) Pertaining to the lips.

Labial bar A connector installed labial or buccal to the dental arch.

Labial glands Small mucous or serous glands in the lips.

Labial notch A depression in the denture border.

Labio Combining word for lip.

Labiaplasty (cheiloplasty) (*lae'bea-pla'sti*) Surgical procedure in which labia minora are cut down to achieve reduction in size or better symmetry.

Labium (*la'be-um*) A lip with a fleshy border, pl. **labia.**

Labioclination (*la'be-o-kli-na'shan*) The outward tilting of incisor and canine teeth toward the lips.

Labor (*la'ber*) The physiological process of expulsion of the products of conception from the uterus *via* the cervix and vagina to the outside world.

Active labor Regular uterine contractions with increasing dilatation of the cervix and descent of the presenting part.

Complicated labor Labor occurring in association of an abnormality such as hemorrhage or inertia.

Dry labor Premature rupture of the membranes leading to drainage of most of the amniotic fluid and then occurrence of labor.

False labor Occurrence of uterine contractions which are not accompanied by effacement or dilatation of the cervix.

Induced labor Administration of oxytocin to stimulate uterine contractions.

Instrumental labor Application of forceps to complete the labor.

Missed labor Labor in which true labor pains stop as in dead fetus or extra uterine pregnancy.

Normal labor Progressive dilatation of the cervix with descent of presenting part.

Obstructed labor Obstruction to the fetal passage through the birth canal from fetal malposition, malpresentation and cephalopelvic disproportion.

Precipitate labor Labor of less than three hours in duration in a primigravida.

Preterm labor Premature labor wherein labor begins between 20 and 37 (i.e., <37 weeks) weeks of gestation.

Prolonged labor Abnormally slow progress of labor which may last 20 hours or more.

Spontaneous labor Labor taking place without any mechanical or operative interference.

Labioplasty (*la'be-o-plas'te*) Plastic operation on a lip.

Labrum (*la'burm*) An edge; rim; lip; lip-like structure.

Labyrinth (inner ear) (*lab-i-rinth*) Any group of interconnecting membranous cavities, cells or canals separated from the bony labyrinth by the perilymph both of which lie within the petrous portion of the temporal bone; internal ear comprises the semicircular canals, vestibule and cochlea.

Labyrinthitis (otitis Interna) (*lab-i-rin-thi'tis*) Inflammation of the three interconnecting fluid-filled chambers in the internal ear; otitis interna. The condition causes sudden vertigo typically precipitated or aggravated by movement, lasting minutes or hours. Nausea and vomiting are associated symptoms.

Lacerated (*las'er-at-ed*) Torn with a ragged edge.

Laceration (*las'er-a-shun*) A torn, jagged wound.

Laceratus (*la-ser'tus*) The muscular part of the arm.

Lacrimal apparatus A system of glands and ducts that produces tears and drains away from the inner corners of the eyes to the back of nose.

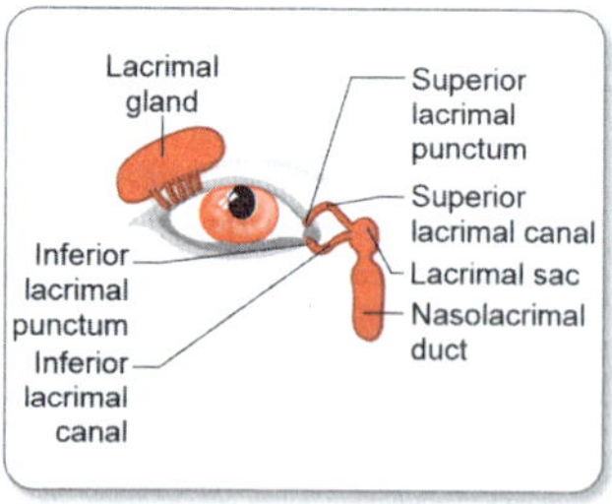

Lacrimal apparatus

Lacrimation (*lak'rim-a-shun*) The secretion and discharge of excessive amount of tears.

Lacrimator (*lak'rim-a-tor*) A substance irritating the eyes and producing tears.

Lactalbumin (*lak'tal-bu'min*) An albumin found in milk. It is found in higher concentration in human's milk than in cow's milk.

Lactase deficiency An inherited disorder with an inability to digest milk, sugar, lactose due to a deficiency of the enzyme, lactase on the intestinal brush borders.

Lactation (*lak-ta'shun*) The production and secretion of milk after childbirth; period of sucking.

Lactation suppression Suppression of milk production by high levels of estrogen in the blood.

Lacteal (*lak'te-al*) A lymphatic vessel carrying chyle from the intestine; pertaining to milk.

Lactic acid (*lak'tik*) A glycolytic product by the action of the lactic acid bacillus on milk or milk sugar; a weak acid produced during anaerobic exercise.

Lactic dehydrogenase LDH, an enzyme catalyzing the oxidation of lactate to pyruvate, also called lactate dehydrogenase. It is found in humans in several molecular forms called isoenzymes and any damage to the tissues is associated with release of an isoenzyme of LDH into the blood. Also known as lactate dehydrogenase.

Lactiferous (*lak'tif'er-us*) Producing milk.

Lactifuge (*lak'ti-fuj*) Causing the arrest of the secretion of milk.

Lactobacillus (*lak-to-ba-sil'us*) Gram-positive, nonmotile, rod-shaped bacteria capable of production of lactic acid from carbohydrates and cause souring of milk.

Lactobacillus acidophilus An organism capable of producing lactic acid by fermenting the sugars in the milk. It is found in milk and in the feces of bottle-fed infants.

Lactogenic hormone Prolacting—the hormone secreted by anterior lobe of pituitary.

Lactose intolerance A lactase deficiency causing an inability to digest lactose. The individual complains of bloating, nausea, diarrhea and abdominal cramps following intake of milk.

Lactosuria (*lak-to-su'rea*) Excretion of lactose in the urine which occur during pregnancy and lactation.

Lacuna (*la-ku'na*) A gap, space, pit or cavity, pl. **lacunae**, adj. **lacunar**.

Laetrile (*la'a-tril*) A partly man-made (synthetic) form of the natural substance amygdalin. Amygdalin is a plant substance found in raw nuts, bitter almonds, as well as apricot and cherry seeds. Plants like lima beans, clover and sorghum also contain amygdalin.

Lagena (*le-je'na*) An outpocketing of the saccule of birds, reptiles, and bony fishes corresponding to the cochlear duct of mammals.

Lagophthalmos (*lag'of-thal'mos*) An incomplete closure of the eyelids over the eyeball.

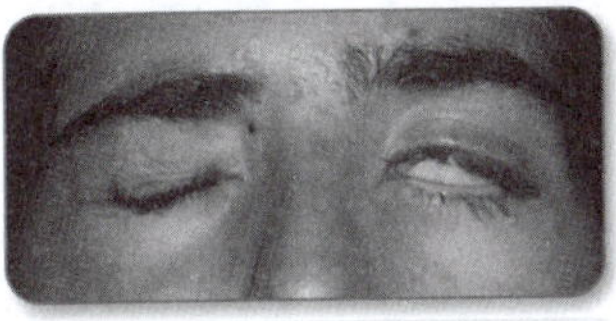

Lagophthalmos

Lallation (lalling) Infantile speech.

Laloplegia (*lal-o-ple'je-a*) Paralysis of the muscles concerned in the mechanism of speech.

Lamaze Method (*la-maz*) A method of preparation for uncomplicated vaginal delivery which includes relaxation, physical conditioning and breathing exercises, devised by Fernand Lamaze, a French obstetrician.

Lambda (*lam'da*) Junction of the sagittal and lambdoid sutures at the site of posterior fontanelle; a symbol for immunoglobulin light chain.

Lambda waves Sharp or sawtooth waves over the occipital areas in a normal *EEG*, and are evoked by visually scanning an object or a picture.

Lambdoid suture The junction of the occipital bone with the parietals.

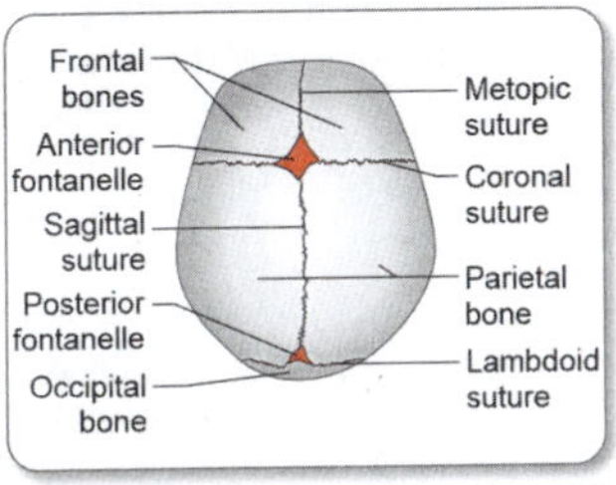

Lambdoid suture

Lambliasis (*lam-bli'a-sis*) Giardiasis.

Lamella (*la-mal'a*) A thin layer, thin plate or scale; disc of gelatin.

Lamina (*lam'i-na*) A thin, flat plate or layer or membrane, pl. **laminae**.

Lamina arcus vertebrae Two broad plates, extending dorsally and medially from the pedicles, fusing to complete the roof of the vertebral arch (*see figure*).

Rexed laminae A system identified in early 1950s by scientist Bror Rexed, consists of ten layers of gray matter (I–X), to label portions of the gray columns of the spinal cord.

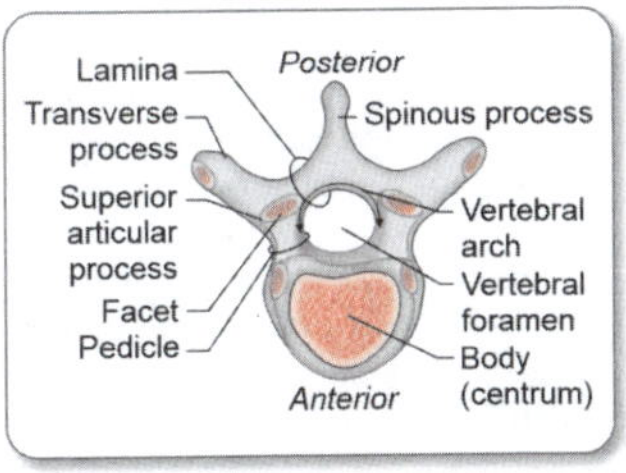

Thoracic vertebra—Lamina arcus vertebrae

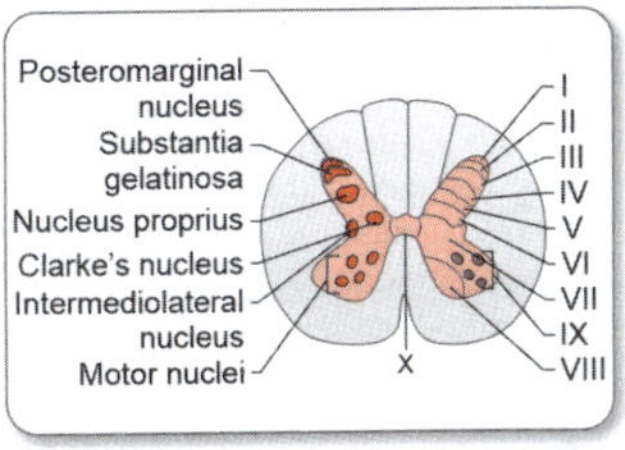

Rexed laminae in a cross-section of spinal cord

Laminectomy (rachiotomy) (*lam-i-nek'to-me*) Surgical removal of the entire lamina of a vertebra as a treatment of herniation of intervertebral disk.

Landsteiner's classification (*lan'sti-nerz*) A classification of blood in to A, B, AB and O groups based on the presence of antigens on the erythrocytes, named after Carl Landsteiner, physician, who worked in Vienna and New York.

Lanatoside (*lan-at'o-sid*) A glycoside obtained from the leaves of *Digitalis lanata*.

Lancet (*lan'set*) A surgical knife having a small, sharply pointed double edged blade.

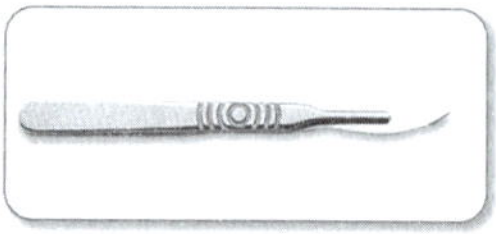

Lancet

Lancinating *(lan'si-nat'ting)* Sharply cutting or tearing.

Landry's paralysis Guillain-Barre syndrome, in which the body's immune system attacks part of the nervous system.

Lange's test *(lang'ez)* A test for diagnosis of neurosyphilis by the degree of gold precipitation of colloidal gold solution and cerebrospinal fluid named after Carl Lange, a German Physician.

Langerhans cell A macrophage that presents antigen to lymphocytes in the upper dermis which sends dendritic processes, named after Paul Langerhans, German pathologist.

Langhan's giant cell A giant cell composed of fused epithelioid cells. A large number of nuclei are arranged like garlands surrounding cytoplasm. These cells are diagnostic of tuberculosis when accompanied by caseation, described by T. Langhans, Swiss pathologist.

Lanugo *(la-nu'go)* Hair; fine, soft downy hair that covers a fetus and is shed before birth.

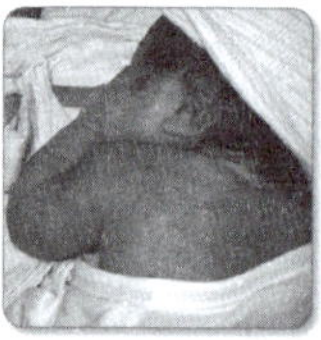

Lanugo

Laplace's law The well tension (T) is a function of the ventricular pressure (P) and the size of the chamber (radius = r), formulated by 18th century mathematician Laplace.

$$T = \frac{PT}{r}$$

Laparo Loin; abdomen.

Laparoscope (peritoneoscope) *(lap'a-ro-skop)* Peritoneoscope with a tiny camera at its tip to visualize internal organs in the abdominal cavity.

Laparoscopy (peritoneoscopy, abdominoscopy) *(lap-ar-os'ko-pe)* Examination of the interior of the abdominal cavity using a laparoscope. The laparoscope is inserted through a small incision in the abdomen and the image is displayed on TV screen.

Laparotomy *(lap-ar-ot'o-me)* Surgical incision to open up the abdomen.

Larva Immature form of an insect or a worm during the developmental stage, pl. **larvae**.

Cutaneous larva migrans An infectious syndrome caused by multiple types of hookworms.

Visceral larva migrans An infection caused by parasitic roundworms passed from animals to humans. It usually affects children.

Larva migrans An infestation with larvae that move through the skin or intestine.

Laryngectomy *(lar'in-jek'to-me)* Surgical removal of the larynx either partially or totally.

Laryngeal obstruction Obstruction to the entry of air from edema of glottis resulting in harsh respiration.

Laryngismus *(lar'in-jis'mus)* Spasm of the larynx.

Laryngitis *(lar-in-ji'tis)* Inflammation of the mucosa lining larynx that causes hoarseness.

Croupous laryngitis inflammation of the larynx, often with accompanying sore throat, hoarseness or loss of voice, and dry cough.

Syphilitic laryngitis A very frequent manifestation of secondary syphilis, the result of an extension downward of a syphilitic pharyngitis.

Tuberculous laryngitis The most common granulomatous disease of the larynx and has usually been considered to result from pulmonary tuberculosis (PT).

Laryngocele *(lar-in'go-sel)* A narrow necked pouch having connection with the larynx and the condition is suspected if a swelling of the neck appears when the patient blows his nose.

External laryngocele An abnormal cystic dilatation of the saccule of the outside part of larynx.

Internal laryngocele An abnormal cystic dilatation of the saccule of the inside part of larynx.

Laryngofissure Also known as median thyrotomy, a surgical procedure with vertically splitting the thyroid cartilage in the midline to gain access to the endolarynx. It provides good exposure to both anterior and posterior laryngeal structures with very minor morbidity.

Laryngology Also known as median thyrotomy, a surgical procedure with vertically splitting the thyroid cartilage in the midline to gain access to the endolarynx. It provides good exposure to both anterior and posterior laryngeal structures with very minor morbidity.

Laryngopharynx (*lar-in'go-far-inks*) The lower part of the pharynx, above the larynx.

Laryngoscope (*lar-in'go-far-inks*) The lower part of the pharynx, above the larynx.

Laryngoscopy (*lar'in-gos'ko-pe*) Visual examination of the larynx with a laryngoscope.

Laryngospasm An involuntary closure of the vocal cords and glottis in an attempt by the body to protect the airway.

Laryngotomy (Laryngofissure) (*lar-in-got'o-me*) Surgical incision of the larynx.

Laryngotracheobronchitis (*la-ring'go-tra'ke-o-brong-ki'tis*) Inflammation involving the larynx, trachea and bronchi.

Larynx (*lar'inks*) A musculocartilaginous structure concerned with voice production located between the pharynx and the trachea at the level of 3rd and 6th cervical vertebrae and comprises a number of articulated cartilages surrounding the upper end of the trachea and lined with ciliated mucous membrane; voice box containing vocal cords.

Laser (*la'zer*) Light amplification by stimulated emission of radiation; a device that transfers a narrow beam of visible light into an extremely intense monochromatic small beam of radiation with high energies which is able to cut and dissolve tissue.

LASIK Also known as laser-assisted in-situ keratomileusis, a laser-assisted surgical procedure for the correction of visual refractive errors.

Lassa fever A highly contagious fatal acute febrile disorder caused by an arena virus first reported in Lassa city in Nigeria. It is characterized by fever, headache, prostration and severe pharyngitis. There is lymphadenopathy, vomiting, diarrhea, a maculopapular rash and mucosal bleeding. Treatment is symptomatic.

Latent period The period between infection with virus or other microorganism and the onset of symptoms.

Lateral (*lat'er-al*) Pertaining to a side; away from the midline; situated on one side.

Lathyrism (*lath'ir-izm*) A spastic paraplegia developing from consumption of kesari dal, *Lathyrus sativus*. The disease affects men more frequently and more severely. It passes through non-stick, one-stick, two-stick and crawler stages. There is spasticity, a 'scissor type' of gait and weakness.

Laudanum (*law'dan-um*) A tincture containing opium.

Laughing gas An anesthetic gas, nitrous oxide.

Lavage (*la-vazh*) The washing out of a hollow cavity.

Bronchoalveolar lavage A procedure that is sometimes done during a bronchoscopy. It is also called bronchoalveolar washing.

Gastric lavage Washing out of the stomach using a stomach wash tube.

Peritoneal lavage An invasive emergency procedure used to detect hemoperitoneum and help determine the need for laparotomy following abdominal trauma.

Pleural lavage The washing of the thoracic cavity and is widely used in open chest trauma to minimize the incidence of inflammation, infection, and empyema.

Laxative (cathartic, purgative) *(lak'sa-tiv)* An agent that stimulates evacuation of soft, formed stools.

Bulk-forming laxative Not digested but absorb liquid in the intestines and swell to form a soft, bulky stool. The bowel is then stimulated normally by the presence of the bulky mass.

Lubricant laxative Such as mineral oil, taken by mouth encourage bowel movements by coating the bowel and the stool mass with a waterproof film. This keeps moisture in the stool. The stool remains soft and its passage is made easier.

Saline laxative Used for rapid emptying of the lower intestine and bowel.

LD50 Toxic unit that measures the lethal dose of a given substance.

Lead (*led*) Plumbum, a metal; the conductor connected to the electrocardiograph; insulates wires that connect a patient to a monitoring device.

Lead line A blue line consists of a series of gray-black dots situated about a mm from the free margin of the gums in patients who work with lead.

V leads Numbered from V1 to V6. They are positioned in specific positions on the rib cage. To position them accurately, it is important to be able to identify the "angle of Louis", or "sternal angle".

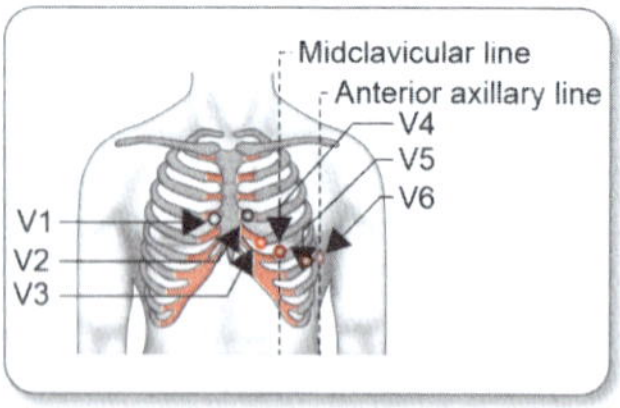

Positioning of V leads

Ledipasvir (*le-dip'as-veer*) A NS5A inhibitor direct acting antiviral medication used as part of combination therapy to treat chronic Hepatitis C, an infectious liver disease caused by infection with hepatitis C virus (HCV).

L-dopa Levodopa, 1-3,4 dihydroxyphenyl alanine useful in the treatment of Parkinsonism.

Lecithin (*les'ith-in*) A phospholipid. It is part of a cell membrane, also found in blood and egg yolk.

Lecithinase (*les'i-thin-as*) A phospholipase that catalyzes the decomposition of lecithin.

Leech (*letch*) A blood-sucking water worm. It is parasitic on humans and other animals. The worms are source of hirudin; an anticoagulant substance.

Legionella A genus of gram-negative rod-shaped bacteria.

Legionellosis Legionnaire's disease; a disease caused by *Legionella pneumophila*. It is a multisystem disorder affecting the lungs, kidney, alimentary tract and central nervous system. It presents with fever, chills, cough, dyspnea and prostration. There can be vomiting, abdominal pain, diarrhea, headache and mental confusion. It is treated with erythromycin. Rifampicin is added in severely ill-patients.

Leiomyoma (*li'o-mio'ma*) A benign tumor of smooth muscle containing a relatively small amount of fibrous tissue.

Uterine leiomyoma Uterine leiomyomata or fibroids are an extremely common benign neoplasm in women of reproductive age.

Leiomyosarcoma (*li'o-mi'o-sar-ko'ma*) a malignant tumor of smooth muscle.

Leiner's Disease (*li'nerz*) Exfoliative dermatitis, named after Karl Leiner, an Austrian pediatrician.

Leishman-Donovan bodies Small round or oval bodies found in the reticuloendothelial cells in a patient suffering from kala azar, described by an English army surgeon, William Leishman and Irish Physician Charles Donovan while working in Chennai, India.

Leishmania *(lesh-ma'ne-a)* A protozoan flagellate spread by bite of female sandfly responsible for leishmaniasis.

Leishmania donovani A species of intracellular parasites belonging to the genus *Leishmania*, a group of hemoflagellate kinetoplastids that cause the disease leishmaniasis.

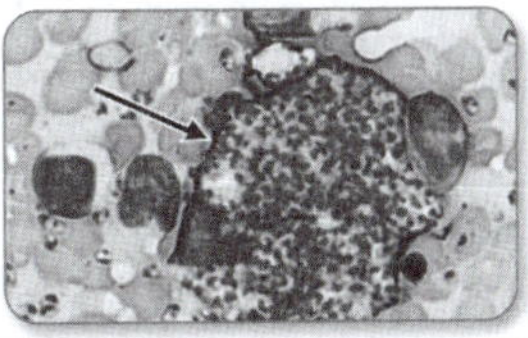

Leishmania donovani in stained preparation of bone marrow aspiration

Leishmaniasis *(lesh-ma-ni'-a-sis)* Infection from protozoa leishmania presenting in three different forms as visceral (kala-azar), cutaneous and mucocutaneous leishmaniasis.

Cutaneous leishmaniasis Single or multiple painless popular ulcerative lesions on the skin which leave an atrophic, depigmented scar after healing. Delhi boil or Bagdad sore is an example.

Mucocutaneous leishmaniasis Destructive lesions involving nasal and oropharyngeal region may occur following recovery from cutaneous ulcer.

Visceral leishmaniasis *see Kala-azar.*

Lema *(le'ma)* The dried secretion of the tarsal gland that collects in the inner canthus of the eye.

Lemniscus *(lem-nis'kus)* A band or bundle of sensory nerve fibers in the medulla and pons.

Lens *(lenz)* A transparent biconvex body lying in the internal compartment of the eye that adjust focus; a transparent refracting medium usually of glass which converges or scatters light rays.

Achromatic lens Lens that is designed to limit the effects of chromatic and spherical aberration.

Anastigmatic lens Photographic lens completely corrected for the three main optical aberrations: spherical aberration, coma, and astigmatism.

Biconcave lens Two inward curved surfaces. These lenses have a negative focal length.

Biconvex lens A simple lens which comprises two convex surfaces in spherical form, generally having the same kind of radius of curvature.

Contact lens Ocular prosthetic devices that can be worn to correct vision or for cosmetic or therapeutic.

Spherical lens A transparent material bound by two surfaces of which one or both surfaces are spherical, forms a lens.

Lenticonus *(len'ti-ko'nus)* A conical projection of the lens.

Lenticular Resembling a lens; having a shape of a lentil.

Lentigo *(len-ti'go)* A brown macule with a regular border on the skin due to excess deposition lipofuscin and is brought on by sun-exposure; a freckle.

Leontiasis *(le'on-ti-a-sis)* The lion-like appearance of the face in some cases of advanced lepromatous leprosy.

Lepidosis *(lep'i-do'sis)* Any scaly eruption.

Lepirudin A protein-based direct thrombin inhibitor used as an anticoagulant in patients with heparin-induced thrombocytopenia.

Leproma *(lep-ro'ma)* A granulomatous nodule caused by *Mycobacterium leprare.*

Lepromin *(lep'ro-min)* An extract of tissue infected with *Mycobacterium leprae* used in skin tests to determine tissue resistance in leprosy.

Leprosy (Hansen's disease) *(lep'ro-se)* Hansen's disease, a chronic granulomatous infectious disease caused by *Mycobacterium leprae*, the organisms were demonstrated by Hansen, a Norwegian physician.

Borderline leprosy Patients showing features closer to either lepromatous or tuberculoid leprosy. There can also be features lying midway between the two.

Indeterminate leprosy Early lesion of leprosy appearing as a hypopigmented macule.

Lepromatous leprosy Occurs in individuals with low resistance. It is a highly bacillary disseminated disease. The lesions are bilaterally symmetrical, ill-defined, hypopigmented macules or diffusely infiltrated plaques.

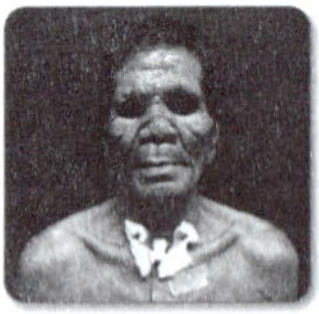

Lepromatous leprosy

Tuberculoid leprosy A high resistance form of the disease with individual exhibiting high degree of immunity. The lesions are well defined, anesthetic, and hidrotic and alopecia. The superficial nerves are thickened and tender.

Leptocyte (*lep'to-sit*) An unusually thin, flat red blood cell with a central rounded area of pigmentation like a *"bull's eye"* surrounded by a clear zone and a pigmented rim, often referred as 'target' or 'Mexican hat' cell.

Leptomeninges (*lep'to-men-in-jes*) Soft thin membranous covering of brain and spinal cord, the piamater and arachnoid mater.

Leptomeningitis (*lep'to-men-in-ji'tis*) Inflammation of the leptomeninges.

Leptophonia (*lep'to-fo'ne-a*) Feeble voice.

Leptospira (*lep-to-spi'ra*) A thin, spiral and hook-ended bacteria belonging to the family Treponemataceae. It has 240 serotypes and 23 serovars.

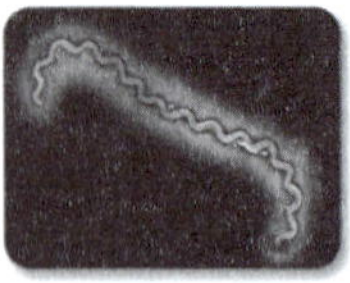

Leptospira

Leptospirosis (weii's disease) (*lep'to-spi-ro'sis*) Infection with species of *Leptospira interrogenes* that is acquired by domestic and wild animal hosts especially rodents. The illness is biphasic. Initially, there is frontal headache, muscular pains, fever and chills. Then, there is involvement of one organ system giving rise to any of the conditions such as hepatitis, nephritis, atypical pneumonia, influenza or gastroenteritis.

Leptotene (*lep'to-ten*) The early stage of prophase of cell division where the chromosomes become visible.

Lesbianism Sexual desire of women toward those of their own sex.

Lesion (*le'zhun*) A circumscribed area of pathologically altered tissue. Primary lesions are in the form of macules, papules, vesicles, pustules, blebs, bullae, chancres, tubercles, wheals and tumors. Secondary lesions are the result of primary lesions and consist of crusts, excoriations, fissures, scales, scars, pigmentations and ulcers.

Hill-Sachs Lesion A fracture in the long bone in the upper arm (humerus) that connects to the body at the shoulder.

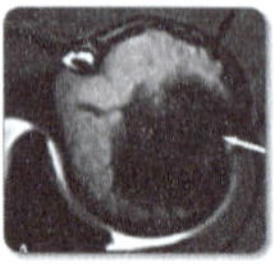

CT arthrography showing Hill-Sachs lesion of the articular surface of humerus head

Lethargy (*leth'ar-je*) Drowsiness; indifference.

Letterer-Siwe disease (*let'er-er-si'we*) A nonlipid reticuloendotheliosis of early childhood, described by German physician, Erich Letterer and Swedish physician, August Siwe.

Leukocytopoiesis Formation and development of the various types of white blood cells.

Leukonychia (*lu'ko-nik'e-a*) Partial or full discoloration of the nail plate on one or more fingernails or toenails.

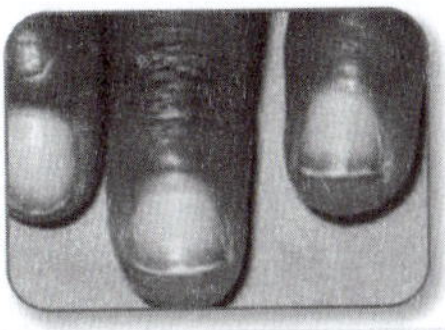

Leukonychia

Leukotaxis (*lu'ko-taks'is*) The quality or state of being leukotactic; the ability to attract WBCs.

Leukotome (*loo'ko-tom*) A needle used in leucotomy.

Leukotoxin The critical virulence factors of several gram-positive and gram-negative bacteria.

Leucovorin A folate analog used to treat the toxic effects of methotrexate and other folate antagonists, to treat megaloblastic anemia, and to provide palliative treatment of colorectal cancer.

Leuk- (leuko-, leuc-, leuco-) Combing word for white.

Leukemia (*loo-ke'me-a*) A form of cancer characterized by disorganized proliferation of abnormal leucocytes.

Acute leukemia Disorder of primitive stem cells which proliferate showing little or no differentiation. There are two main varieties, myeloid and lymphoid.

Chronic basophilic leukemia Resembles CGL. There is gross increase in basophils.

Chronic granulocytic leukemia (CGL), A malignant disease of myeloid stem cells noted in middle age and it passes through three stages—benign responsive; accelerated unresponsive and a terminal phase resembling acute leukemia. Majority show presence of Philadelphia chromosome.

Chronic lymphatic leukemia (CLL), A progressive proliferation of lymphocytes (usually B cells) with infiltration of the bone marrow causing a peripheral blood lymphocytosis, seen in elderly patients. Often, the condition is asymptomatic.

Chronic monocytic leukemia A blood picture of CGL with marked increase in the number of monocytes.

Hairy cell leukemia A variant of CGL rare and males are more frequently affected. There is presence of hairy cells having features of B lymphocytes and monocytes. The cytoplasm exhibits a number of villi giving a hairy appearance.

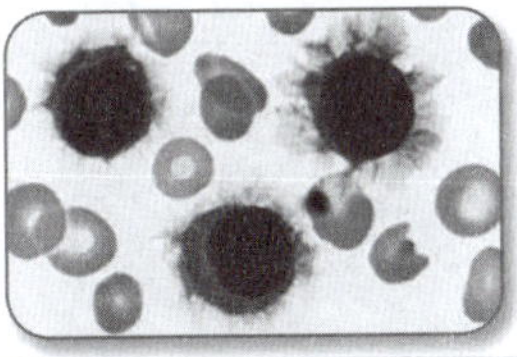

Hairy cell leukemia

Promyelocytic leukemia A rare variant of CLL, seen in males above 60 years of age, associated with gross splenomegaly and very high white cell count. Lymphadenopathy is rare.

Leukocidin (*lu'ko-ci-din*) A bacterial substance that destroys white blood cells.

Leukocyte (white blood cell) (*lu'ko-sit*) A white blood cell or corpuscle, WBC.

Leukocytosis (*lu'ko-si-to'sis*) An elevated white blood cell (WBC) count, typically above 11.0×10^9/L, on a peripheral blood smear collection.

Leukoderma (*lu-ko-der'ma*) A condition in which the skin pigment melanin is lost from areas of otherwise normal skin.

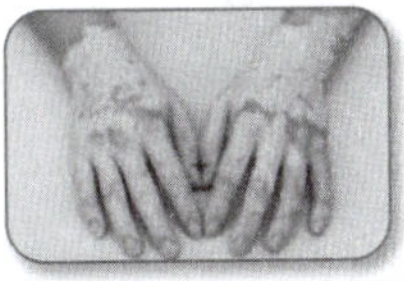

Leukoderma

Leukoma (*lu-ko'ma*) A scarring clouding of the cornea, which emerges because of its injury due to trauma, inflammatory or ulcerative process.

Leukopenia A condition where the body does not have enough disease-fighting leukocytes in the blood.

Leukoplakia (*lu'ko-pla'ke-a*) Raised white patch on the mucous membrane which has the potentiality to develop into cancer.

Hairy leukoplakia A condition triggered by the Epstein-Barr virus (EBV). It causes white hairy patches on the tongue.

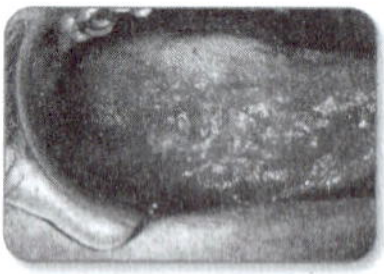

Hairy leukoplakia

Leukopoiesis (*lu'ko-poy-e'sis*) The process through which leukocytes are generated from hematopoietic stem cells of the bone marrow.

Leukorrhea (*lu'ko-re-a*) Flow of a whitish, yellowish, or greenish discharge from the vagina of the female that may be normal or that may be a sign of infection.

Leukotomy (*lu'kot'o-me*) The surgical operation of cutting some of the nerve fibers in the frontal lobes of the brain: formerly used for treating mental illness.

Levator (*le-va'tor*) A muscle or an instrument to raise a part.

Levator ani A broad muscle forming the floor of the pelvis.

Levator palpebrae superioris A muscle that elevates the upper eyelid.

Levamisole An anthelminthic drug that is commonly used for the treatment of parasitic, viral, and bacterial infections.

Levetiracetam (*le"ve-ti-ras'e-tam*) A novel antiepileptic drug used to treat partial, myoclonic, and tonic-clonic seizures.

Levodopa (L-dopa) Active from of dopa used in the treatment of Parkinsonism.

Levofloxacin (*le"vo-flok'se-sin*) A broad-spectrum, third-generation fluoroquinolone antibiotic used to treat bacterial infections.

Levothyroxine oral medication Used to treat hypothyroidism.

Levorphanol (*le-vor'fe-nol*) An opioid analgesic used to treat moderate to severe pain.

Levulinic acid An acid produced on addition of dilute hydrochloric acid on certain sugars.

Lewis blood group Antigen of red blood cells specified by Lewis that react with the antibodies designated anti Le after a patient in whose blood the antibodies were discovered, named after English propositus who first reported.

Leydig's cells Interstitial cells of the testis that secrete testosterone, named after a German anatomist, Franz Leydig.

LFP Liver function panel.

LFT Liver function tests, lung function tests.

LH Luteinizing hormone.

Lhermitte's sign (*lar'mits*) A sensation like an electric shock coursing down the spine when neck is flexed, described by Jacques Lhermittes, French neurologist. The etiology may be cervical spondylosis or multiple sclerosis.

Libido (*li-bi'do*) Sexual desire or drive.

Lice (*lis*) Plural of louse.

Lichen (*li'ken*) Discrete shiny, itchy popular skin lesions resembling lichens growing on rocks.

Lichen planus Pruritic purple polygonal papules.

Lichen sclerosus A chronic inflammatory skin disorder affecting the penile, vulval, and perianal areas.

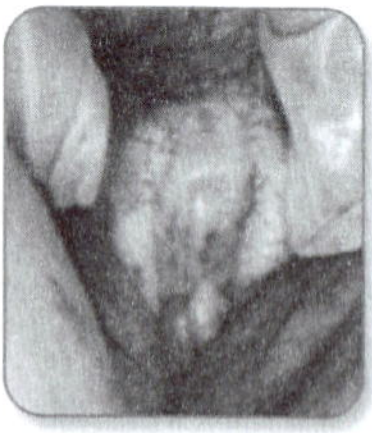

Lichen sclerosus

Lichen simplex chronicus A chronic itchy skin disorder characterized by well demarcated, erythematous patches, and plaques of thickened leathery skin.

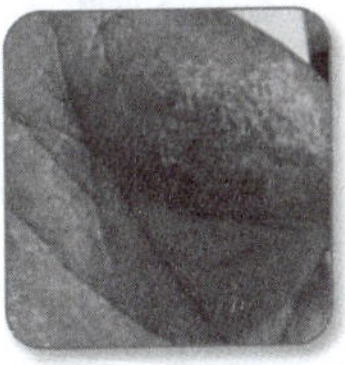

Lichen simplex chronicus

Nail lichen Lichen affecting nails.

Lichenification (*li-ken'i-fi-ka'shun*) Leathery induration and thickening of the skin.

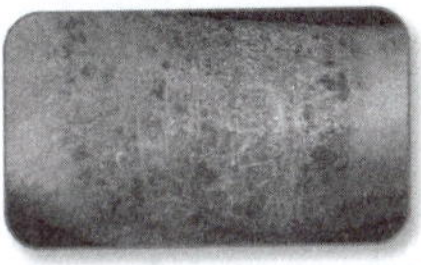

Lichenification

Lichenoid Resembling lichen.

Licorice Common name of *Glycyrrhiza glabra*, a flowering plant of the bean family *Fabaceae*, a herbaceous perennial legume from the root of which a sweet, aromatic flavoring is extracted, native to Western Asia, North Africa, and Southern Europe.

Lidocaine A local anesthetic used in a wide variety of superficial and invasive procedures.

Lieberkuhn glands (crypts of Lieberkunn) Tube-like glands found in the lining of the colon and rectum; these glands renew the lining of intestine and secrete mucus.

Lien (*li'en*) Spleen.

Lienitis Inflammed spleen.

Lientery A form of diarrhea in which the food is discharged undigested or only partly digested.

Life table A statistical record which reflects the course of mortality in a population.

Ligament (*lig'a-ment*) A tough slightly elastic band of fibrous tissue that binds together the bony ends in a joint.

Ligamentopexy (*lig'a-men'to-pek-si*) Fixation of the uterus by shortening the round ligament.

Ligature (*lig'a-chur*) Any material, such as a thread or wire used in surgery to tie off blood vessels to prevent bleeding around a structure.

Light chain disease Multiple myeloma producing only monoclonal light chain proteins.

Light reflex Reaction to light is dependent on the reflex arc with afferent fibers in the optic nerve, oculomotor nerve nuclei and efferent fibers in the oculomotor nerve.

Lightening An abrupt sensation of relief from the weight felt by the mother in the last weeks of pregnancy due to the descent of fetal head into pelvic cavity.

Lignocaine A local anesthetic of moderate potency and duration, but of good penetrating power and rapid onset of action; xylocaine.

Limbic system (*lim'bik*) A part of the brain which controls emotions and instincts.

Limbus (*lim'bus*) An edge or border of a part.

Limen (*li'men*) Entrance; threshold.

Liminal (*lim'i-nal*) Pertaining to a threshold.

Limping Walking with abnormal, jerky movements may arise from painful lesion, deformity, shortening or paralytic condition of the lower limb, trunk or abdomen.

Lincomycin (*lin"ko-mi'sin*) A lincosamide, narrow spectrum antibiotic with activity against gram-positive and cell wall-less bacteria including pathogenic species of *Streptococcus*, *Staphylococcus*, and Mycoplasma.

Linctus (*link'tus*) A confection a medical preparation taken by licking.

Lindane (gamma benzene bexachloride) (*lin'dan*) A neurotoxin ectoparasite that interferes with GABA neurotransmitter function by interacting with the GABA$_A$ receptor-chloride channel complex at the picrotoxin binding site. It ingested by humans, lindane affects the nervous system, liver, and kidneys, and may well be a carcinogen.

Linea (*line-a*) Line or strip distinguished from the adjacent tissues by its color or texture.

Linear accelerator (linac) Radiotherapy machine that emits photon or electron radiation megavolts redirected in many arcs for treating benign or malignant tumors throughout the body; linac.

Lingual (*ling'gual*) Relating to the tongue.

Lingual thyroid Ectopic thyroid as a round swelling at the back of the tongue which may produce dysphagia, dyspnea and hemorrhage.

Liniment An oily medicated liquid preparation for external application on the skin as a counterirritant or anodyne.

Linoleic acid An essential 18-carbon fatty acid with 2 unsaturated bonds obtained from vegetable oils.

Linolenic acid An essential 18-carbon fatty acid with 3 unsaturated bonds derived from either plants or animals.

Lint (*lint*) An absorbent surgical dressing material.

Liothyronine A medication used in thyroid hormone replacement therapy to treat hypothyroidism, to suppress TSH, and to help in the diagnosis of hyperthyroidism.

Lipase (steapsin) (*li'pas*) An enzyme secreted by pancreas that breaks down fat.

Lipase deficiency Decreased secretion of lipase by pancreas resulting in fats to pass through the intestine without being digested. It results in stools that are bulky, greasy and foul smelling.

Lipemia (*li-pe-mea*) A turbidity of the sample caused by accumulation of lipoprotein particles.

Lipid Group of fatty acids.

Lipidosis (lipoidosis) Disorder of metabolism that results in excessive accumulation of lipids in brain, liver, spleen or other parts of the body. It includes hereditary disorders such as Gaucher's disease, Tay Sachs disease and Niemann-pick disease. Usually, they occur as recessive disorders in Jews. It presents with dementia, epilepsy and blindness.

Lipoarthritis Inflammation of the periarticular fatty tissues of the knee.

Lipoblastomatosis Benign mesenchymal tumors of embryonal adipocytes, found primarily in young children.

Lipochondrodystrophy (*lip'o-kon-dro'dis' tro-fe*) A connective tissue disorder, Hurler's syndrome.

Lipochrome (*lip'o-krom*) A generic term for any natural, fat-soluble pigment including lipofuscin, carotenes and lycopenes.

Lipocoele (*lip'o'sel*) Presence of fatty tissue in a hernia sac.

Lipocrit An apparatus used to separate and analyze the amount of lipid in blood or other body fluid.

Lipodystrophy (*lip'o-dis'tro-fe*) Absence of subcutaneous fat associated with systemic abnormality.

Lipofuscin (*lip'ofus'sin*) A yellow to brown pigmented lipid degradation product after destruction of mitochondria or mitochondrial polyunsaturated lipid membrane; lysosomal digestion pigment accumulates with age in the muscle, heart, nerve cells and in lysosomes.

Lipogenesis (*lip'o-jen'e-sis*) Production of fat.

Lipogranuloma (*lip'o-gran-u-lo'ma*) A granulomatous condition in association with deposits of lipid substance in tissue.

Lipoic acid (*li'po'-ik*) Any of several microbial growth factors.

Lipoid (*lip'oyd*) Fat like.

Lipoid pneumonia A pneumonitis following inhalation of oil into the lungs. Liquid paraffin or nasal instillation of mineral oil may be inhaled by elderly people with neurologic disturbances. The malnourished young children may inhale milk or cod liver oil.

Lipolysis (*lip-ol'i-sis*) Hydrolysis of fat.

Lipoma (*li-po'ma*) A benign tumor of fatty tissue in the subcutaneous tissue, which is soft, mobile and slow growing.

Most lipomas fluctuate as fat is fluid at body temperature.

Lipomatosis (*li-po'ma-to'sis*) Abnormal deposits of in the tissue; adiposis.

Lipomyxoma A tumor composed partly of fatty and partly of mucous tissue.

Lipopolysaccharide (*lip'o-pol'e-sak'a–rid*) A compound formed by lipids and carbohydrates.

Lipotropin One of the two protein hormones produced by the pituitary gland that helps in releasing stored fat.

Liposarcoma (*li-po-sar-ko'ma*) A malignant condition consisting of lipoblasts or fatty tissue.

Liposome (*lip'o-som*) Synthetic spherical vesicle with a lipid bilayer. It functions as artificial membrane systems to deliver DNA, etc., into cell, and as a drug delivery system of toxic drugs.

Lipotropic Compound that helps catalyze the breakdown of fat during metabolism in the body.

Lipotropin One of the two protein hormones produced by the pituitary gland that helps in releasing stored fat.

Lippes loop (*li'pez*) An intrauterine contraceptive device, devised by Jacob Lippes, US obstetrician.

Lipping (*lip'ing*) Formation of a lip-like structure at the articular end of a bone.

Lipuria (*li-pu're-a*) Excretion of lipids in the urine.

Liquor (*lik'er*) Liquid.

Liquor folliculi Clear fluid containing cavities surrounding the ripening Graafian follicle.

Lissencephaly Smooth brain without gyri.

Listinopril An ACE inhibitor used to treat hypertension, heart failure and acute myocardial infarction.

Listeria A genus of gram-negative bacteria, named after Baron Lister, founder of modern antiseptic surgery, a Scottish surgeon.

Liter A metric unit of volume equal to one cubic decimeter.

Lithogogue Causing dislodgement or expulsion of a stone.

Lithiasis (*lith'i-a-sis*) Formation of calculi.

Lithium (Lithium carbonate) A soft, silvery-white, metal that heads group 1, the alkali metals group, of the periodic table of the elements, reacts less vigorously with water.

Lithogogue Causing dislodgement or expulsion of a stone.

Litholapaxy (lithotripsy) The procedure of removing bladder stones by crushing them and extracting them through a catheter.

Lithonephritis A condition in which the kidneys become inflamed due to the presence of calculi.

Lithonephrotomy Surgical removal of stone from the kidney.

Lithopedion A fetus that has died in the womb and has became calcified.

Lithotomy (*lith'ot'o-me*) Surgical removal of stone.

Lithotomy position The position assumed by the patient lying supine with the hips and knees flexed and the thighs abducted and rotated externally for vaginal examination.

Lithotripsy (*lith'o-trip'se*) The crushing of a calculus by concentrated ultrasonic shock waves. It is a nonsurgical, noninvasive method to dissolve renal and biliary tract calculi.

Lithotrite (*lith'o-trit*) An instrument used to crush a calculus.?

Lithuresis Passage of gravel in the urine.

Lithuria Presence of excessive amount of uric acid in the urine.

Little's disease Cerebral spastic paralysis or diplegia, described by William Little, a British physician.

Livedo (*li-e'do*) A discolored area on the skin due to passive congestion.

Liver (*liv'er*) The largest gland of the body lying in the right upper abdomen, containing a large number of minute lobules performing many functions essential to life.

Cirrhosis of liver A chronic generalized liver disease resulting from necrosis and regeneration of liver cells. It is characterized by liver cell dysfunction, increased hepatic fibrosis and nodular degeneration.

Liver abscess It may be pyogenic or amebic.

Liver cancer Primary, derived from hepatocytes known as hepatoma.

Liver fluke A flatworm which on infecting liver cause jaundice.

Liver tongue Blue-red tongue with engorged capillaries seen in advanced cirrhosis.

Livid (*liv'id*) Discolored.

Loa A genus of parasitic nematode responsible for loiasis

Lobe (*lob*) A well demarcated subdivision in any organ or gland.

Lobectomy (*lo-bek'to-me*) Surgical removal of a lobe.

Lobeline An alkaloid that has similarities to micotine or nicotine cholinergic receptors but is less patient.

Lobomycosis Rare, chronic, fungal infection of the skin and subcutaneous tissue.

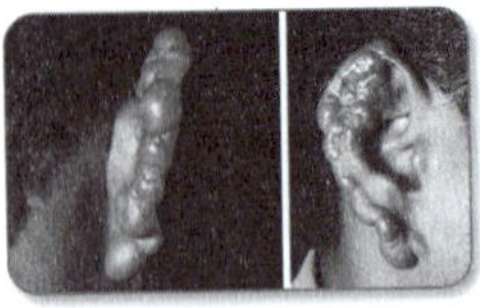

Lobomycosis for ear

Lobotomy (prefrontal leucotomy) (*lo'bo-tome*) A surgical procedure to treat psychiatric disorders where the nerves connecting the hypothalamus to the prefrontal cortex are severed by introducing surgical instruments into the frontal lobe of the brain.

Lobule (*lob'ul*) A small lobe or subdivision of a lobe; cartilage less and fleshy part of outer area of Ears.

Lochia (*lo'ke-a*) The vaginal discharge noted during the first three to four weeks following childbirth. It contains mucus, blood and tissue debris.

Lock jaw Painful spasm of the masseter muscles with stiffness of the jaw noted in tetanus.

Locomotor ataxia The inability to precisely control one's own body movements.

Loculus (*lok'u-lus*) A small space or cavity.

Locus (*lo'kus*) A site in the body or site of a gene on a chromosome.

Logopedics (*log'o-pe'di-ks*) The science concerned with the study and treatment of speech defects.

Loin (*loyn*) The part of the back on either side of the spine between the thorax and pelvis. Also known as lumbus.

Loop A turn or a curve.

Lomitapide A microsomal triglyceride transfer protein inhibitor used in homozygous familial hypercholesterolemia patients.

Loperamide An antidiarrheal medication, works by slowing down the contraction of the intestines thereby decreasing the speed at which the contents pass through it.

Lorazepam (*lor-az'e-pam*) A short-acting benzodiazepine mainly used in the treatment panic disorders, severe anxiety, and seizures.

Lordosis (*lor-do'sis*) Abnormal increase in the anterior curvature; saddle back.

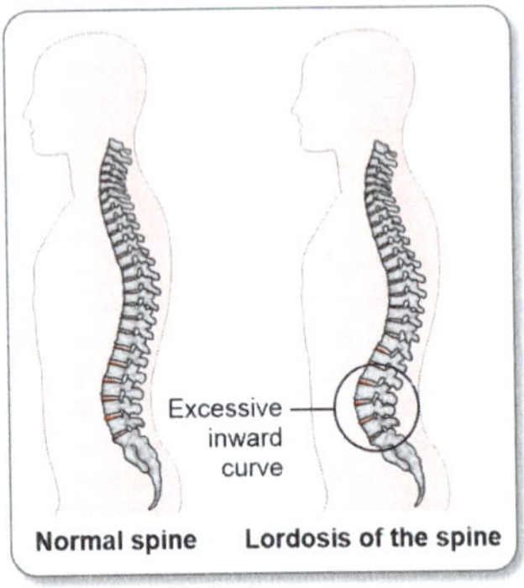

Illustration showing difference between normal spine and lumbar lordosis

Lorazepam (*lor-az'e-pam*) A short-acting benzodiazepine mainly used in the treatment panic disorders, severe anxiety, and seizures.

Losartan An angiotensin receptor blocker used to treat hypertension and diabetic nephropathy, and is used to reduce the risk of stroke.

Lotion (*lo'shun*) A liquid medicated suspension for external application to the body.

Loupe (*loop*) A convex lens to magnify light upon an object.

Louse An ectoparasitic insect infesting mammals. pl. **lice.**

Lovastatin An HMG-CoA reductase inhibitor belongs to class statin, used to lower LDL cholesterol and reduce the risk of cardiovascular disease and associated conditions, including myocardial infarction and stroke.

Lovset's maneuver Used to deliver the shoulders in a breech presentation, when the arms are extended.

Lozenge (*loz'enj*) A small disc-shaped body containing a drug.

LSD Lysergic acid diethylamide.

Lubb-dupp The lubb is the first heart sound associated with mitral and tricuspid valves closing, whereas Dupp is the second heart sound of the aortic and pulmonary valves closing soon after.

Ludwig's angina (*lud'vigz*) Diffuse purulent inflammation around the submaxillary glands due to streptococcal infection, named after Wilhelm von Ludwig, a German surgeon.

Lues Syphilis.

Lumbago (*lum-ba'go*) Pain in the lumbar region.

Lumbar (*lum'bar*) Pertaining to the loin.

Lumbar plexus An interlacing network of nerves located on either side of the spine in the low back.

Lumbar spine The part of the spine situated between the lowest pair of ribs and the top of pelvis; it consists of five lumbar vertebrae.

Lumbar puncture Insertion of a hollow needle into the lower part of the spinal canal to withdraw cerebrospinal fluid or to inject drugs, anesthetic agents or radiographic substances.

Lumbosacral Pertaining to the loin and groin.

Lumen (*lu'men*) Channel within a tubular structure.

Lumpectomy Segmental mastectomy.

Lunate bone Central bone in the wrist that is important for proper movement and support of the joint.

Lung Either of the organs of respiration situated on either side of the heart with in the side of the heart within the thoracic cavity. The right lung has three lobes (upper, middle and lower). The lungs have double arterial supply from pulmonary and bronchial arteries and double venous drainage. They provide a surface for transfer of gases through which blood gets rid of CO_2 and absorbs oxygen. The aim of the lungs is to achieve normal oxygenation (arterialization) of the mixed venous blood perfusing the pulmonary capillaries.

Lung aplasia A total absence of the lung and bronchi.

Budgerigar lung People exposed to droppings of Turkey pigeon are sensitized to avian serum proteins result in extrinsic allergic alveolitis.

Cheese worker's lung Exposure to mouldy cheese resulting in extrinsic allergic alveolitis.

Coffee worker's lung Coffee bean dust acting as a sensitizing agent to cause extrinsic allergic alveolitis.

Honeycomb lung An end result of many diverse interstitial lung diseases presenting radiologically with a pattern of coarse reticular interstitial areas of increased opacity with intervening cystic spaces, and pathologically cystic spaces with walls consisting of a variable amounts of fibrous tissue.

Lung scars Scars in the lung from a previous infection that acts as a weak point for action of environmental carcinogens.

Lung tumors *see* Bronchogenic carcinoma.

Lung volume Consists of four basic subdivisions as tidal volume, inspiratory reserve volume, expiratory reserve volume and residual volume. The former three are dynamic lung volumes. The lungs do not become totally airless at the end of each expiration and it can't be expelled (residual volume) (*see figure*).

Mushroom picker's lung Inhalation of mouldy mushroom compost dust resulting in extrinsic allergic alveolitis.

Pigeon fancier's lung People exposed to pigeon droppings are sensitized to avian serum proteins to result in extrinsic allergic alveolitis.

Lung abscess A localized collection of pus in the parenchyma of the lung as a result of tissue necrosis and suppuration from a pyogenic infection.

Lung agenesis A rare congenital abnormality exhibiting failure of development of the primitive lung bud.

Lung cancer Cancer of the lungs.

Lung collapse Shrinkage of lung volume either from the obstruction of a lobar bronchus or from presence of air or fluid in the pleural space.

Lung compliance A measure of the distensibility of lungs (C_L). It measures the ease with which the lung volume is changed and is expressed in liters/cm H_2O.

Lung rupture Expansion of the air in the lungs on ascent in divers, leading to its entry into the pleural space and the mediastinum.

Lunula (*lu'nu-la*) A small crescentic area.

Lupus (*lu'pus*) A chronic inflammation of connective tissue with skin lesions; wolf.

Lutein (*lu'tein*) A yellow pigment.

Luteinizing hormone (LH) Secretion of anterior pituitary and corpus luteum is formed by its influence. Ovulation requires a sudden surge of LH.

Lutetium Chemical element, a rare-earth metal of the lanthanide series of the periodic table, that is the densest and the highest-melting rare-earth element and the last member of the lanthanide series.

Lux A standard unit of measurement for illumination.

Luxation (*luks-a'shun*) Dislocation.

Lyase (*li-as*) Any member of an enzyme class that catalyzes the removal or addition of the elements of ammonia, carbon dioxide, or water at double bonds in different ways other than hydrolysis and oxidation.

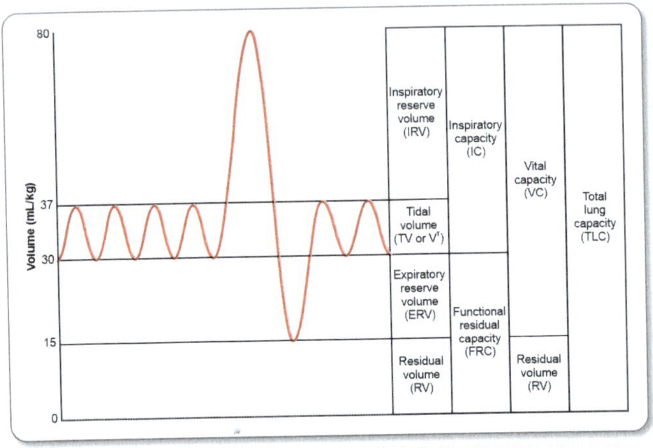

Lung volumes

Lycanthropy (*li-kan'thre-pe*) Mental disorder in which the patient believes that he is a wolf or some other nonhuman animal.

Lyme disease A multi-system disease by a bacterial (Borrelia burgdorferi) infection transmitted by tick bites initially described at old Lyme, Connecticut, USA.

Lymph (*limf*) A transparent, slightly yellowish fluid circulating in the lymphatics. It plays an important part in the immune system and in the absorption of fats from the intestine.

Lymph node A small gland that lies along the course of a vessel in the lymphatic system. It filters lymph and acts as a barrier to the spread of infection.

Lymphaden- (lymhadeno-) Lymph node.

Lymphadenectomy (*lim-fad'e-nek'to-me*) Excision of the lymph node.

Lymphadenitis (*lim-fad'en-i'tis*) Inflammation of one or more lymph nodes.

Lymphadenoma Rare benign tumor with nests and islands of bland epithelium composed in part of sebaceous elements, with lymphoid stroma. Also called sebaceous lymphadenoma if lymphoid stroma is prominent.

Lymphadenography (*lim-fad"e-nog're-fe*) A new method for the visualization of enlarged. Lymph nodes and lymphatic vessels.

Lymphagogue An agent that promotes lymph production or lymph flow.

Lymphangiectasis Superficial lymphatic dilatation caused by a wide range of scarring processes.

Lymphangiogram (*lim-fan'je-o-gram*) A roentgenogram of the lymphatic vessels.

Lymphangiography (*lim-fan'je-og'ra-fe*) Roentgenography of the lymphatic vessels following injection of contrast medium.

Lymphangioma (*lim-fan'je-o'ma*) A tumor composed of newly formed lymphatic vessels.

Lymphangiosarcoma A rare cancer which occurs in long-standing cases of primary or secondary lymphedema.

Lymphangitis (*lim'fan-ji'tis*) Inflammation of a lymphatic vessel or vessels.

Lymphatic (*lim-fat'ik*) Pertaining to lymph or lymph vessel.

Lymphatic system A part of immune system, consists of a large network of lymphatic vessels, lymph nodes, lymphoid organs, lymphatic tissue and lymph.

Lymphedema (*limf-e-de'ma*) Chronic edema of the extremities due to accumulation of interstitial fluid due to stasis of lymph.

Lymphapheresis Separation and removal of lymphocytes from the withdrawn blood, with the remainder of the blood retransfused into the donor. Also known as lymphocytopheresis.

Lymph node A small bean shaped structure that is part of the body's immune system.

Lymphoblast (*lim'fo-blast*) The immature precursor of the mature lymphocyte.

Lymphocyte (*lim-fo-sit*) A mononuclear leucocyte with a deeply staining nucleus containing dense chromatin and a pale-blue staining cytoplasm. It is divided into B and T lymphocytes responsible of humoral and cellular immunity respectively.

Lymphocytoblast A morphologically immature lymphocyte, once thought to represent an early stage in lymphocyte development but now known to be an activated lymphocyte that has been transformed in response to antigenic stimulation.

Lymphocytopenia A disorder in which enough WBC (lymphocytes) are not produced.

Lymphocytosis (*lim'fo-si-to-sis*) Increase in the number of normal lymphocytes in the blood.

Lymphogranuloma venereum An ulcerative disease of the genital area; it is sexually transmitted infection.

Lymphography (*lim-fog'ra-fe*) Roentgenography of the lymphatic vessels and lymph nodes following injection of contrast medium in a lymphatic vessel.

Lymphoid tissue A tissue rich in lymphocytes that is found in lymph nodes and in the spleen.

Lymphokine (*lim'fo-kin*) Mediator released by sensitized lymphocyte.

Lymphoma (*lim-fo'ma*) Any neoplastic condition of the lymphoid tissue. It consists of Hodgkin's disease, non-Hodgkin's lymphoma and T-cell lymphoma.

Lymphopenia (Lymphocytopenia) A disorder in which your blood doesn't have enough white blood cells called lymphocytes; also called lymphocytopenia.

Lymphopoiesis Production of new lymphocytes including B, T and NK cells.

Lymphorrhagia Escape of the lymph from injured lymphatic vessels.

Lymphosarcoma A malignant neoplastic disease of lymphoid tissue capable of arising in any lymphoid aggregate. It can be an acute or chronic and is almost invariably very radiosensitive.

Lymphuria Presence of lymph in the urine.

Lynestrenol Progestin containing medication, used for birth control and in the treatment of gynecological disorders.

Lysergic acid diethylamide (LSD) (LSD), Synthetic hallucinogen obtained from ergot alkaloids that produces mood elevations, sensory distortion and depersonalization and there can be panic attacks.

Lysin (*li'sin*) An antibody which can cause dissolution of cells.

Lysine (*li'sen*) An amino acid.

Lysis (*li'sis*) Dissolution by enzymes.

Lysogenic Harboring integration of the bacteriophage nucleic acid into the host bacterium's genome.

Lysophospholipid Small bioactive lipid molecules characterized by a single carbon chain and a polar head group.

Lyssavirus A genus of RNA viruses in the family Rhabdoviridae that infect neurons of mammals.

Lysosome (*li'so-som*) A minute membrane bound cytoplasmic organelle present in the cells that contains a variety of digestive enzymes.

Lysozyme (*li'so-zim*) A hydrolytic enzyme which hydrolyzes mucopolysaccharides and mucoproteins, found in tears, milk, saliva, serum and neutrophils and acts as an antibacterial enzyme.

M

μ mu, the 12th letter of Greek alphabet; symbol for the scientific prefix micro-, which indicates one millionth of a unit of measure; heavy chain of IgM.

μg A unit for measuring weight. There are one million micrograms in one gram.

μL Microliter, a measure of volume for a liquid, using the metric system. One microliter is equal to a millionth of a liter.

μm Micromole, a measure of the amount of a substance. The amount of a substance equal to a millionth of a mole.

MAC technique Monitored Anesthesia Care technique; Minimum alveolar concentration is often expressed as a percentage by volume, of a vapor in the alveoli of the lungs, needed to prevent movement (motor response) in 50% of subjects in response to surgical (pain) stimulus.

MacCallum's plaques Maplike thickening of the endocardium over myocardial lesion in acute rheumatic fever, named after William MacCallum, Canadian-US Pathologist.

Maceration (*mass-er-a'shun*) Process of softening a solid by steeping in a fluid; the chemical removal (dissolving) of muscles and other soft tissues in a specimen while leaving the sclerotized or chitinized parts that are needed for identification; in obstetrics, degenerative changes with discoloration and softening of tissues and eventual disintegration of a fetus retained in the uterus after its death.

Macro- (macro-) Large or long.

Macrocephaly (megalocephaly) (*mak-ro-sef'a-le*) Abnormally large and globular head, seen in hydrocephalus, acromegaly, osteitis deformans, or as a congenital condition.

Macroadenoma (*mak'ro-ad'e-no'ma*) A pituitary adenoma over 10 mm in diameter, large enough to be easily visualized by usual radiologic techniques; most are null-cell adenomas and are detected because they exert pressure on surrounding structures.

Macrobiotics (*ma'kro-bio-tiks*) Group of vegetarian diet with varying restrictions.

Macroblast (*mak'ro-blast"*) An abnormally large immature erythrocyte; a large young erythroblast with megaloblastic features.

Macrocheilia (*mak'ro-ki'le-a*) Abnormal size of the lips.

Macrocornea (*mak-ro-kor'ne-a*) Abnormal size of the cornea.

Macrocyte (megalocyte) Abnormally large erythrocyte with increased hemoglobin and decreased life span seen in hemolytic anemia, massive bleeding, hyperthyroidism and erythroblastosis fetalis.

Macrocythemia (*mak'ro-si'-the-mea*) A condition in which the erythrocytes are larger than normal, such as in macrocytic anemia and some types of liver disease; also called macrocytosis.

Macrocytosis (*mak'ro-si-to'sis*) Condition in which erythrocytes are larger than normal; macrocythemia.

Macrodactyly (*makro-dakte-le*) A condition of abnormally large fingers or toes.

Macrodontia (*mak'ro-gam'et*) A large immobile zygote formed by conjugation of female gamete with the microgamete (male). It is encountered in the plasmodium life cycle that occurs in human.

Macrogamete (*mak-ro-ga-met*) The larger of a pair of conjugating gametes, usually regarded as female, especially in protozoans.

Macrogametocyte (*mak'ro-ga-me'to-si't*) A large immobile reproductive cell developing from the merozoite of certain protozoa.

Macrogenitosomia (*mak'ro-jen'i-to-so'me-a*) Abnormal size of genitalia due to excess androgens.

Macroglia (*mak-rog'le-a*) Astrocyte.

Macroglobulin (*mak'ro-glob'u-lin*) Any large serum protein. Its level in the blood is increased in multiple myeloma, collagen disorders, cirrhosis of the liver and amyloidosis.

Macroglobulinemia (*mak'ro-glob'u-line'me-a*) Presence of macroglobulins in the blood, which causes increased viscosity of the blood, *see* Walden Strom macroglobulinemia.

Macroglossia (*mak'ro-glos'e-a*) Markedly enlarged tongue seen in acromegaly, cretinism, myxedema, primary amyloidosis, mongolism, hemangioma or lymphangioma.

Macrognathia (*mak-ro-na'the-a*) Abnormal size of the jaw.

Macrolide (*ma'kro-lid*) Antibiotic, any of a group of broad-spectrum antibiotics, e.g., erythromycin, clarithromycin, azithromycin and spiramycin which contain a lactone ring and inhibit protein synthesis in target bacteria.

Macromelia (*mak'ro-mel'e-a*) Excessive size of an organ or part especially limbs.

Macromyeloblast (*mak-ro-milo-blast*) An unusually large myeloblast.

Macronormoblast (*mak'ro-nor'mo-blast*) Same as macroblast.

Macrophage (clasmocyte) (*mak'ro-faj*) Cells of reticuloendothelial system possessing the ability to phagocytose bacteria and other foreign particles. They are monocytes comprising 3–5% of circulating leukocytes, tissue-bound macrophages located in the alveoli (dust cells), central nervous system (microglial cell), liver (Kupffer cells, lymph nodes), peritoneum and skin (Langerhans cells) and histiocytes found in connective tissues.

Alveolar macrophage Multipotent cells normally patrolling the interior of alveoli which recognize and destroy bacteria as the foreign organic particles.

Fixed macrophage A nonmotile macrophage.

Foamy macrophage Macrophages that stain positive with periodic acid-Schiff reagent and infiltrate small intestinal mucosa in Whipple's disease.

Free macrophage A wandering or amoeboid macrophage.

Macrophage activating factor MAF, a lymphokine that stimulates alteration in the appearance and activities of the macrophage cells so that they can kill some microbes.

Macrophage chemotactic factor Any cytokine that functions in tandem with macrophages mediating migration.

Macrophage migration inhibiting factor A substance that prevents the migration of macrophages in culture.

Macrophthalmia (*mak'rof-thal'me-a*) Abnormally large eyeball.

Macropsia (*mak-rop'se-a*) Condition wherein the objects look larger than they actually are.

Macroscopic (*mak-ro-skop'ik*) Large enough to be seen by the naked eye.

Macrosomia (*mak-ro-so'me-a*) Abnormally large body; an obstetric condition associated with other potentially life-threatening complications to both the mother and the fetus. It is the condition of having an abnormally large mouth, malunion of the maxillary and mandibular prominences, with extension of the oral orifice toward the ear. Can be unilateral or bilateral. Also known as macrosomatia.

Macula (*mak'u-la*) A small spot; a colored area.

Macula densa A specialized region in the distal renal tubule at which point specialised cells converge and macula densa is part of the juxtaglomerular apparatus.

Macula lutea Yellowish area of retina centered on *fovea centralis*.

Macula retinae A small area in the center of the retina where light is sharply focused to produce the detailed color vision needed for tasks such as reading and driving. When a full-thickness defect develops in the macula, the condition is referred to as macular hole.

Macula flava Located at the anterior and posterior ends of the bilateral vocal folds. Vocal fold ligaments run between the anterior and posterior maculae flavae. The maculae flavae seem to control the synthesis of fibrous components in the vocal ligament.

Macula sacculi Lies in a nearly vertical position. Its function is to detect vertical linear acceleration. It is a 2 mm by 3 mm patch of hair cells. Each hair cell of the macula contains 40–70 stereocilia and one true cilia, called a kinocilium.

Macula utriculi Present in a horizontal position and detects horizontal acceleration. The macula of utricle allows a person to perceive changes in longitudinal acceleration (in horizontal directions only).

Macule (macula) (*mak'ul*) Circumscribed area of variable size on the skin with an alteration in color and without any elevation as in leukoderma, mole, purpura, erythema, or leprosy.

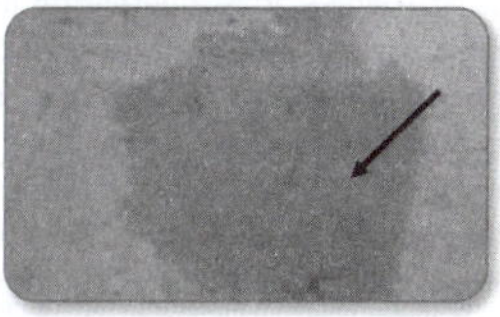

Macule

Maculopapular (*mak'u-lo-pap'u-lar*) An eruption consisting of both macules and papules.

Madarosis (*mad-a-ro'sis*) Loss of eyebrows or eyelashes.

Madura foot A chronic fungal disease of deep soft tissues and bones, most commonly of the limbs, named after the city Madurai, Tamil Nadu.

Madurella A fungus genus of Hyphomycetes, of uncertain position in the Sordariales, and sometimes classified as Mitosporic Ascomycota, is etiologic agent of eumycotic mycetoma.

Maduromycosis (*mad-u'ro-mi-ko'sis*) It is caused by two groups of organisms Eumycetes (*Madura mycetomatis, Madurella grisea)* and Actinomycetes (*Actinomadura madurae)*. They produce a chronic granuloma with a fibrous stroma and cyst-link space, which contain grains of colonies of matted organism. Those caused by Actinomycetes can be treated by rifampicin or streptomycin and dapsone or co-trimoxazole.

Mafenide A sulfonamide applied topically in the form of its acetate $C_7H_{10}N_2O_2S{\cdot}C_2H_4O_2$ as an antibacterial ointment especially in the treatment of burns.

Magenta tongue A deeply red-to-purple, smooth tongue seen in riboflavin deficiency.

Magnesium (*mag-neze'um)* A white mineral substance found in soft tissues, muscles, bones and body fluids. Magnesium is widely distributed in foods, especially whole grains, fruits and vegetables. It activates enzymes that catalyze reactions between phosphate ions and ATP. Its deficiency may be associated with tetany, weakness and mental depression.

Magnesium chloride Useful in treatment of electrolyte disturbances and in dialysis solution.

Magnesium citrate Used as a purgative.

Magnesium oxide White powder used as an antacid and laxative.

Magnesium carbonate A white odorless powder, on oral administration it neutralizes acid in the stomach.

Magnesium hydroxide Milk of magnesia used as a laxative and antacid.

Magnesium sulfate Epsom salt used as a cathartic, anticonvulsant and topically as an anti-inflammatory agent.

Magnesium trisilicate Used as an antacid.

Magnetic resonance imaging (MRI) the creation of images by the phenomenon of magnetic resonance which is a function of the distribution of hydrogen nuclei (protons) in the body. The MR image is a computerized interpretation of the physical interaction of unpaired protons with electromagnetic radiation in the presence of a magnetic field.

MAGPI operation Meatal Advancement and Glanduloplasty procedure is used for the repair of distal hypospasdias.

Maintenance dose The amount of dose required to keep a desired steady-state concentration in the tissues.

Mal A disorder or illness.

Grand mal Also known as tonic-clonic seizure, that produce bilateral, convulsive tonic and clonic muscle contractions.

Petit mal Also known as absence seizures, characterized by a brief altered state of consciousness and staring episodes.

Malabsorption (*mal'absorp'shun*) Impaired absorption of nutrients from gastrointestinal tract.

Congenital lactose malabsorption A disorder in which infants are unable to break down the lactose in breast milk or formula.

Congenital sucrose isomaltose Malabsorption A rare hereditary cause of chronic diarrhea in children. People with this condition lack the intestinal brush-border enzyme required for digestion of di- and oligosaccharides, including sucrose and isomaltose, leading to malabsorption.

Glucose-galactose Malabsorption A genetic condition in which a child's body cannot absorb the simple sugars glucose and galactose.

Malabsorption syndrome A complex of symptoms resulting from disorders in the intestinal absorption of nutrients characterized by abdominal distension, borborygmi, cramps, weight loss, undigested food in the stools, or bulky, pale and offensive stools, lethargy and malaise and deficiencies of specific vitamins, trace elements and minerals.

Malacia (*ma-la'she-a*) Abnormal softening of tissues or an organ.

Maladjustment (*mal'ad-just-ment*) A term used in psychology to refer to the inability to react successfully and satisfactorily to the demand of one's environment.

Malaise (*ma-laz*) Uneasiness; indisposition.

Malaria (ague, marsh fever, periodic fever, paludism) (*ma-la're-a*) A tropical disease caused by the presence of sporozoa plasmodium, species of protozoa and transmitted to humans by the bite of an infected female mosquito of the genus *Anopheles* that previously sucked the blood from a person with malaria. It mainly affects the hepatocytes and red blood cells and presents with fever and splenomegaly. Four species of plasmodium, *Plasmodium vivax, P falciparum, P. ovale* and *P. malariae* have man as their vertebrate host in their life cycle.

Acute malaria The most common presentation of malaria due to *P. vivax* and *P. falciparum.* It is characterized to cover the body with blankets (cold phase). There is uncontrollable shivering (rigors). It is followed by fever, headache, and flushing (hot phase). The fever remits in 3–8 hours with profuse sweating (wet phase). The paroxysm coincides with hemolysis.

Cerebral malaria Falciparum malaria in which brain is affected due to tendency of parasite to agglutinate in the capillaries and is manifested either by confusion or coma, usually without localizing signs.

Chronic malaria Persistent hepatic infection by *P. vivax* resulting in progressive splenomegaly.

Falciparum malaria Malaria caused by *P. falciparum.* It invades red cells of all ages and hemolysis is more severe. The condition is more dangerous than other forms of malaria. The fever has no particular pattern. Liver and spleen are enlarged and anemia develops rapidly.

Quartan malaria Malaria of short duration caused by *P. malariac* where sporulation occurs every 72 hours and bouts of fever every third day.

Quotidian malaria Malaria produced by *P. vivax* with classical bouts of fever on alternate days.

Tertian malaria Malaria in which sporulation occurs at 48 hours interval. Benign tertian malaria is caused by *P. vivax* and malignant tertian malaria by *P. falciparum*.

Vivax malaria Most common form of malaria produced by *P. vivax*. It is characterized by frequent recurrences.

Malformation (*mal-for-ma'shun*) Deformity; abnormal shape or structure.

Arnold-Chiari malformation A group of deformities of the posterior fossa and hindbrain, which includes the cerebellum, pons, and medulla oblongata. These deformities lead to problems ranging from cerebellar tonsillar herniation through the foramen magnum to the absence of the cerebellum, with or without other associated intracranial or extracranial defects such as hydrocephalus, encephalocele, syrinx, or spinal dysraphism.

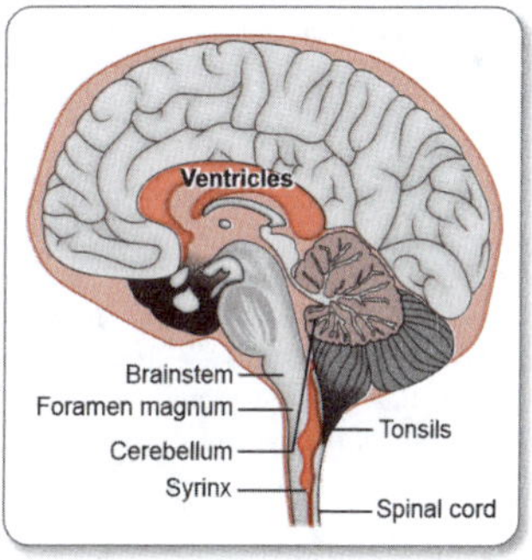

Arnold-Chiari malformation

Cavernous malformation Clusters of abnormal, tiny blood vessels and larger, stretched-out, thin-walled blood vessels filled with blood and located in the brain.

Capillary malformation A type of vascular anomaly, which is an anomaly or disorder of the vascular system, either in veins or arteries. Capillary malformation are commonly known as port wine stains. They look like a pink, red or purple patch of skin and occur in 1 in 300 newborns.

Chiari malformation Structural defects where the lower part of your brain presses on and through an opening in the base of the skull and cerebellum into the spinal canal.

Dandy-Walker malformation A posterior fossa anomaly characterized by agenesis or hypoplasia of the vermis and cystic enlargement of the fourth ventricle causing upward displacement of tentorium and torcula.

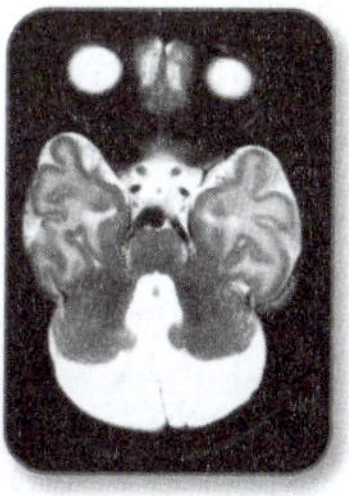

Dandy-Walker malformation

Vascular malformation An abnormal development of blood vessels. They might be found in the large arteries and veins, in smaller vessels called arterioles and venules, in microscopic capillaries, and/or in the lymphatic channels that carry lymphatic fluid and white blood cells outside of the arteries and veins.

Malignant (*ma-lig'nant*) Condition resisting treatment especially of cancerous growth; virulent.

Malignant hyperpyrexia A familial tendency to develop severe form of hyperpyrexia during the use of muscle relaxants or general anesthesia with succinylcholine or halothane.

Malignant hypertension A severe form of hypertension that progresses rapidly accompanied by widespread fibrinoid necrosis. It has a poor prognosis.

Malignant melanoma *see* Melanoma.

Malignant mimics Lesions that either grossly or microscopically mimic malignancy.

Malignant narcissism *psy* Personality disorder characterized by marked narcissistic and antisocial traits.

Malignant neoplasm A tumor that tends to invade and metastasize.

Malingering (*mal'in-ger'ing*) The act of intentionally feigning or exaggerating physical or physiological symptoms for personal gain.

Malleolus (*mal-e'o-lus*) Pl. **malleoli**. The bony protuberances on either side of the ankle joint.

External malleolus The prominent bone on the outer side of the ankle at the end of the fibula.

Internal malleolus The medial projection of bone from the distal tibia.

Lateral malleolus Protuberance in lower end of the fibula.

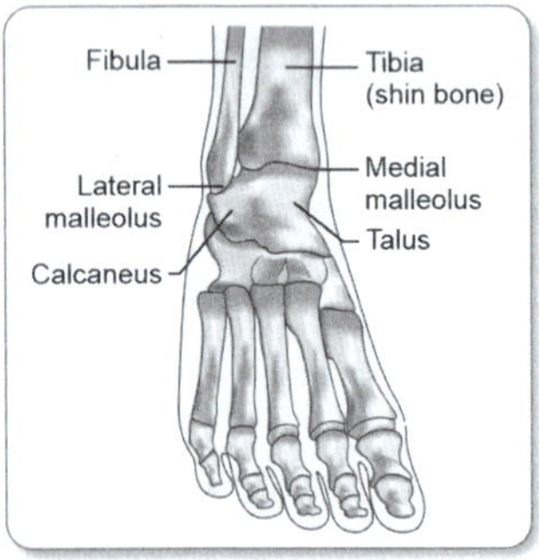

Lateral malleolus and medial malleolus joined with the talus in the ankle joint

Medial malleolus Protuberance in lower end of its tibia.

Malleus (*male-us*) Largest auditory ossicle in the middle ear that connects tympanum to incus.

Mallory-Weiss syndrome Tear of mucosa of the lower end of esophagus or gastroesophageal junction during severe vomiting especially in alcoholics, causing hemorrhage, named after Kenneth Mallory, US pathologist and Soma Weiss, US physician.

Malnutrition (*mal'nu-tri'shun*) Any disorder of nutrition caused by a deficiency of proper food substances. It may also be due to deficient breakdown, assimilation or utilization of the food.

Protein malnutrition A common childhood disorder which is primarily caused by deficiency of energy, protein, and micronutrients.

Protein energy/calorie malnutrition (PEM) An important worldwide cause of secondary immune deficiency. PEM may manifest as either marasmus, a wasting disease due to lack of protein and overall calories, or kwashiorkor, presented by generalized edema due to primary protein malnutrition.

Malocclusion (*mal'oklu'zhun*) Malposition and imperfect contact of the teeth in upper and lower jaw, causing a poor bite.

Malpighian body (*mal-pig'e-an*) Renal corpuscle consisting of a glomerulus enclosed in Bowman's capsule; periarticular lymphoid nodule in the spleen, named after Marcello Malpighi, Italian anatomist.

Malpighian layer Inner layer of epidermis that is a live cell segment consisting of basal cells and prickle cells.

Malposition (*mal-po-zi'shun*) Abnormal position of the parts of the body or of fetal presenting part in relation to the maternal pelvis.

Malpractice Professional misconduct or unreasonable lack of skill in the performance of a professional act.

Malpresentation (*mal'prez-an-ta'shun*) A faulty or abnormal fetal presentation.

Malt (*maw'lt*) Germinated grain, usually

barley, used in manufacture of beer.

Malt sugar Maltose.

Malta fever Brucellosis, named after Malta island.

Maltase (*mawl'tas*) An enzyme that converts maltose by hydrolysis to glucose.

Maltose (*mawltos*) A disaccharide formed from two units of glucose joined with an α(1→4) bond. In the isomer isomaltose, the two glucose molecules are joined with an α(1→6) bond. Maltose is the two-unit member of the amylose homologous series, the key structural motif of starch. When beta-amylase breaks down starch, it removes two glucose units at a time, producing maltose.

Malunion Union of fragments of fractured bone in a faulty position to affect function.

Mamillary bodies A pair of small round bodies, located on the under structure of the brain or diencephalon. They are associated with memory.

Mamma (*mam'a*) Pl. **Mammae** breast; modified cutaneous glandular structure on the anterior aspect of the thorax which secretes milk in females, for nourishment of the infants.

Mamma accessoria A milk-secreting gland located ectopic on the front of the chest and existing in addition to the two usual mammae.

Mamma areolata A condition of the breast in which there is bulging of the areola of the nipple.

Mamma masculine Masculine mammary glands which are rudimentary.

Mammary gland A milk secreting glandular structure situated in female on either side of the chest over the anterolateral area between the third and sixth ribs. Glandular tissue forms a radius of lobes containing alveoli, each lobe contains ducts for passage of milk from the alveoli to the nipple. The central part of the breast contains glandular tissue and the periphery consists of adipose tissue.

Mammography (*mam-og'ra-fe*) Radiography of the mammary gland.

Digital mammography Mammography system in which the X-ray film is replaced by solid-state detectors that convert X-rays into electrical signals. These detectors are similar to those found in digital cameras. The electrical signals are used to produce images of the breast that can be seen on a computer screen or printed on special film similar to conventional mammograms.

Mammoplasty Plastic reshaping of the breasts, performed to reduce or lift enlarged or sagging breasts; to enlarge small breasts or to reconstruct a breast with a plastic prosthesis, after removal of a tumor.

Mammothermography A diagnostic procedure in which thermography is used for examining the breast to detect abnormal growths.

Manchester operation An operation to support the uterus by shortening cervix and using the tissues around it to give support without removing the upper part of uterus.

Mancinism (*man'sin-izm*) State of being left handed.

Mandelic acid A urinary antiseptic.

Mandible (*man'di-b'l*) A large bone constituting lower jaw. It consists of a curved body and two perpendicular rami that join the body at almost right angles. The superior border contains sockets for 16 lower teeth.

Manganese (*man'ga-nez*) A metallic element, atomic number 25, found in many foods and tissues. Daily requirement is 2–3 mg. Its deficiency is rare.

Manganese poisoning Extrapyramidal manifestations may develop in workers exposed to manganese regularly.

Maneuver (*ma-nuvar*) Any skilled movement and procedure.

Allen maneuver With the elbow flexed at a right angle, the arm is extended horizontally and rotated externally at the shoulder, the head being rotated to the contralateral shoulder; obliteration of the radial pulse suggests scalenus anterior syndrome.

Barlow maneuver A dislocation maneuver used together with the Ortolani maneuver in diagnosing developmental dysplasia of the hip.

Heimlich maneuver A method of dislodging food or other material from the throat of a choking victim: the rescuer wraps their arms around the victim at the belt line and allows the victim's upper torso to hang forward; the rescuer makes a fist with one hand and grasps it with the other; with both hands placed against the victim's abdomen slightly above the navel and below the rib cage; then forcefully presses into the abdomen with a quick upward thrust. If the victim is sitting, the rescuer stands behind them and performs the same procedure. If the victim is prone, the rescuer turns him or her to lie on their back, kneels astride their torso, places both hands on their abdomen slightly above the navel, and presses forcefully with a sharp upward thrust. The maneuver may be repeated several times if necessary.

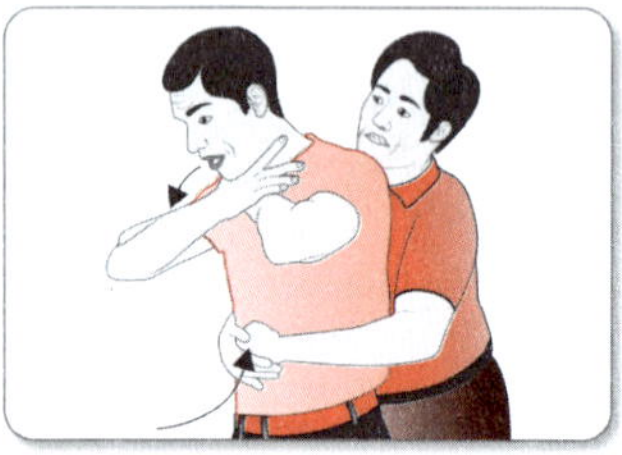

Heimlich maneuver

Leopold maneuvers Four maneuvers in palpating the abdomen for ascertaining the position and presentation of the fetus.

Valsalva maneuver Forcible exhalation effort against occluded nostrils and a closed mouth causes increased pressure in the eustachian tube and middle ear, so that the tympanic membrane moves outward; formerly used as a test of eustachian tube patency.

Mania (*ma'ne-a*) *psy* A hyperkinetic psychiatric reaction.

Mania episode A persistently elevated, expansive or irritable mood, increased energy, decreased sleep, distractibility, impaired judgment, grandiosity and flight of ideas.

Manic-depressive psychosis A mental condition that causes extreme mood swings that include emotional highs and lows.

Manikin (*man'i-kin*) A model of human body or its parts used to teach anatomy and nursing procedures.

Man-in-the-barrel syndrome A type of reverse paraplegia with severe weakness of upper extremity without weakness of lower extremity that may occur in comatose patients who survive an episode of severe hypotension.

Manipulation (*ma-nip'u-la'shun*) Any manual procedure; a joint mobilization technique; a method of realigning a fractured bone; influencing another person.

Mannitol (*man'i-tol*) Hexahydric alcohol obtained by reduction of fructose, used as an osmotic diuretic and to measure glomerular filtration.

Manometer (*man-om'et-er*) An instrument for determining liquid or gaseous pressure. The measurement is expressed in millimeters of either mercury or water, or in torn.

Manometry (*man-om-e-tre*) Measurement of pressure of gases or liquids by means of manometer.

Mantle A covering; cerebral cortex.

Mantoux test (*man-tu'*) An intradermal injection of 0.1 mL of purified protein derivative on flexor surface of forearm and measuring appearance of induration between 48 and 72 hours. An induration of 10 mm diameter is considered positive. It indicates person has been infected with *Mycobacterium tuberculosis*, named after Charles Mantoux, French physician.

Manubrium (*ma-nu'bre-um*) A handle-like structure.

Manubrium mallei Process of malleus that is attached to the middle layer of tympanic membrane, and tensor tympani muscle is attached to it.

Manubrium sterni The upper segment of the sternum articulating with the clavicle and the first two pairs of costal cartilages.

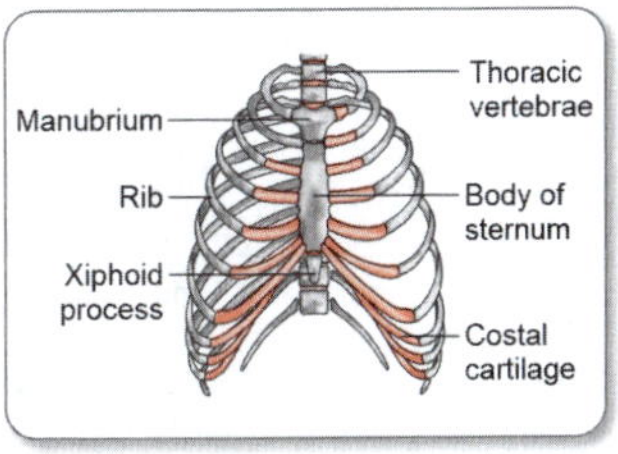

Manubrium sterni

MAO Monoamine oxidase; maximum acid output.

MAO inhibitor class of drugs that are used to treat depression and other neurological and psychiatric illnesses

Maple syrup urine disease MSUD branched chain ketoaciduria. A rare inborn error of metabolism due to decreased branched chain-ketoacid dehydrogenase complex activity resulting in accumulation of branched chain amino acids (valine, leucine and isoleucine). It has a neonatal onset, with dyspnea, spasticity, mental and growth retardation, feeding difficulties and convulsions. It is treated by excessive administration of thiamine.

Maprotiline (*ma-pro'ti-len*) is a tetracyclic antidepressant (TeCA) that is used in the treatment of depression, having pharmacological effects similar to those of the tricyclic antidepressants.

Marasmus (*mar-az'mus*) A state of severe malnutrition, due to decreased ingestion of protein and calories resulting from an inadequate diet, improper feeding habits or metabolic disturbances. It is characterized by failure to thrive, emaciation, weight loss, loss of skin turgor and subcutaneous atrophy. The children are listless, and wizened. There is muscular atrophy, hypotonia and hypothermia.

Marble bone disease Osteopetrosis, an autosomal recessive condition of early onset with failure to thrive, bone fragility and multiple fractures and bony over growth of cranial foramina resulting in proptosis, blindness, deafness and hydrocephalus, and osseous replacement of marrow spaces.

Marburg disease (green monkey disease) A viral hemorrhagic fever due to direct contact with infected monkey tissues. It presents with headache, fever, myalgia, rash and hemorrhage, first recognized in Marburg, Germany.

Marcus Gunn syndrome A congenital disorder in which the ptosis disappears on opening the mouth or on moving the jaw to one side; jaw winking phenomenon.

Marezine A drug used to treat and prevent nausea, vomiting and dizziness due to motion sickness or vertigo.

Marfan's syndrome (*mar-fahnz*) An autosomal dominant heritable disorder of connective tissue characterized by musculoskeletal, ocular and cardiovascular abnormalities. The affected persons are tall with long slender limbs; the lower segment (pubis to sole) length is greater than the upper segment (pubis to vertex) and arm span exceeds height. The muscles are underdeveloped and hypotonic. The fingers are long, tapering and spidery, there is upward bilateral dislocation of lens and diffuse dilatation of ascending aorta, described by Bernard-Jean Marfan, French physician.

Marijuana (marihuana) Refers to the dried leaves, flowers, stems, and seeds from the Cannabis sativa or Cannabis indica plant. The dried leaves, seed oil, and other parts of the cannabis plant are used for recreational and medicinal purposes.

Marrow (*mar'o*) The soft tissue filling the cavities of bones.

Marrow aspiration Procuring a specimen of bone marrow for examination using a special aspirating needle. It is obtained from the upper portion of the sternum or the iliac crest.

Red marrow Marrow found in spongy bones and is concerned with the production of different blood cells.

Spinal marrow The spinal cord.

Yellow marrow Marrow found in medullary cavities of the long bones. It is made up of fat cells and connective tissues.

MARS Molecular adsorbent recirculating system; a specific type of extracorporeal blood treatment which combines the removal of water and albumin-boar, toxins from patient's blood.

Marsupialization (*mar-su'pe-al-i-za'shun*) Process of conversion of a closed cavity into an open pouch by incising it and suturing the edges of the abdominal wound.

Massage systematic pressure Stroking and kneading of the body.

Cardiac massage Manual compression of the heart to restore heartbeat in cardiac arrest. It is done by applying intermittent pressure over the sternum (close cardiac massage) or through an incision in the chest well (open cardiac massage) to reinstate and maintain circulation carotid.

Sinus massage Firm rotatory pressure applied to one side of the neck over the carotid sinus to cause vagal stimulation to terminate tachycardia.

Masculinization (*mas'kul-in-i-za'shun*) The normal development of male sex characters at puberty; abnormal development of male secondary sex characters in the female and it may be due to testosterone producing tumors or intake of testosterone or anabolic steroids; virilization.

Masochism (*mas'o-kizm*) A perversion in which infliction of pain gives sexual gratification to the recipient, named after Leopold Masoch, Austrian novelist.

Masseter (*mas-se'ter*) *see* Table of muscles.

Mastalgia (*mast-al'je-a*) Pain in the breast.

Mast cell A type of cell that stains metachromatically due to its high proteoglycan content and electron dense granules and plays a role in the immune system and in allergic reactions. It releases mediators of inflammation in response to the presence of allergens.

Mast cell stabilizers Drugs that prevent the release of mediators of inflammation from the mast cells such as disodium cromoglycate and nedocromil sodium.

Mastectomy (*mas-tek'to-me*) Surgical removal of all or part of the breast as treatment of breast cancer.

Modified radical mastectomy Total mastectomy with removal of axillary lymph nodes, subcutaneous fat and involved skin but leaving the pectoral muscles intact.

Partial mastectomy Involves the surgical removal of cancerous breast tissue along with a rim of surrounding healthy tissue that will be used for further testing.

Radical mastectomy Removal of breast, skin, pectoral muscle, subcutaneous fat and axillary lymph nodes.

Simple mastectomy Removal of breast, nipple, areola and the involved overlying skin.

Skin-sparing mastectomy All of the breast skin, except the nipple and the areola, is preserved.

Total mastectomy Involves removal of the entire breast, including the breast tissue, areola and nipple.

Mastication (*mas'ti-ka'shun*) The process of chewing food. It helps in breaking of food and mixing with saliva in the mouth, adj. **masticatory**.

Mastitis (*mas-ti'tis*) Inflammation of the breast.

Chronic cystitis mastitis A condition rather than a disease. It is a common condition marked by benign (noncancerous) changes in breast tissue. These changes may include irregular lumps or cysts, breast discomfort, sensitive nipples, and itching.

Mastitis neonatorum An uncommon infection that usually occurs in term or near-term infants. It affects female infants twice as often as male infants.

Nocardial mastitis Mastitis due to nocardial infection.

Parenchymatous mastitis Inflammation of the parenchyma of the breast.

Puerperal mastitis An inflammatory condition of the breast that may occur in breastfeeding women during the puerperium.

Staphylococcal mastitis Mastitis due to staphylococcus infection.

Suppurative mastitis Inflammation (swelling) in the breast, which is usually caused by an infection.

Tuberculous mastitis A form of granulomatous mastitis secondary to Mycobacterium tuberculous infection of the breast.

Mastocytoma (*mas'to-si-to'ma*) Solitary in a child; purple granules characteristics of mast cells in dermis.

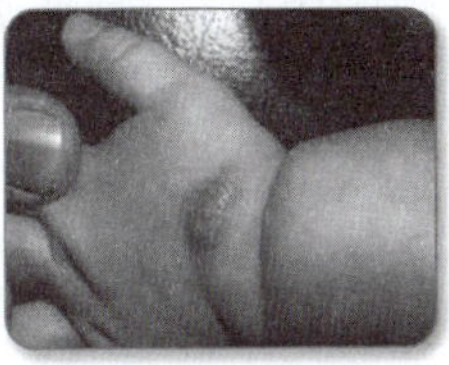

Mastocytoma

Mastoid (*mas'toyd*) Shaped like a breast; mastoid process of temporal bone; pertaining to the mastoid process, adj. **mastoidal.**

Mastoidectomy (*mas-to-id'ek-to-me*) Excision of mastoid air cells.

Bondy mastoidectomy A type of modified radical mastoidectomy in which the mastoid cavity is exteriorized without disturbing the intact ossicular chain and pars tensa.

Closed cavity mastoidectomy Excision of mastoid air cells, the lateral wall of the mastoid is removed and the posterosuperior wall of the external acoustic meatus is preserved. Also known as intact canal mastoidectomy.

Open cavity mastoidectomy Excision of mastoid air cells, the lateral wall of the mastoid is removed along with posterosuperior wall of the external acoustic meatus.

Radical mastoidectomy A canal wall down mastoidectomy in which the tympanic membrane and ossicles are not reconstructed, thus exteriorizing the middle ear and the mastoid.

Simple mastoidectomy A surgical procedure of the temporal bone that opens postauricular air cells by removing the thin bony partitions between them.

Mastoiditis (*mas-toyd-it'is*) Inflammation of the air cells of mastoid process.

Coalescent mastoiditis Acute otomastoiditis when mucoperiosteal disease extends to involve the bone.

Benzold mastoiditis A complication of acute otomastoiditis where the infection erodes through the cortex medial to the attachment of the sternocleidomastoid muscle, at the attachment site of the posterior belly of the digastric muscle, and extends into the infratemporal fossa.

Sclerosing mastoiditis Usually the result of repeated attacks of acute middle ear suppuration. within the mastoid cavity.

Silent mastoiditis An insidious progressive destruction of the mastoid process with or without otorrhea.

Mastoidotomy (*mas-toyd-ot'o-me*) Incision into the mastoid process.

Mastoid process A bony projection at the base of the temporal bones on each side of the skull.

Masturbation (*mas'ter-ba'shun*) Stimulation of genitals to induce orgasm by some means other than intercourse.

Mater (*ma'tur*) The trilaminal membranous covering of the brain and spinal cord.

Maternal mortality rate Maternal deaths at a place during a calendar year divided by the number of live births at the same place and year, multiplied with 1000 or 100,000.

Matrix (*ma'triks*) The basic substance from which a structure develops; the intercellular substance of a tissue; a mold for casting amalgams in dental restoration; a form for casting.

Amalgam matrix A mixture of 50% elemental mercury with a metallic alloy which mainly contains silver and tin. It is a type of band adaptable to the surface of the tooth it is restoring, enabling it to reproduce the tooth's anatomical contours.

Bone matrix The intercellular substance of bone.

Cartilage matrix Composed of collagens (primarily type II collagen with minor collagen types IX and XI) and proteoglycans.

Extracellular matrix Any substance produced by cells and excreted into the extracellular space within the tissue.

Functional matrix Helps physicians to organize patient information and guides them where to begin treatment.

Matrix unguis Nail bed.

Mitochondrial matrix The space within the inner membrane.

Nail matrix The origin of the nail plate.

Sarcoplasmic matrix A highly ordered structure consisting of an intricate network of tubules and cisternae specialized for regulating Ca^{2+} homeostasis in the context of muscle contraction.

Maturation (*mat'u-ra'shun*) The process of becoming mature or ripe as a graafian follicle; attainment of emotional and intellectual maturity; a process of cell division during which the number of chromosomes in the germ cells is reduced to one half; suppuration; attaining menarche; the completion of mineralization pattern.

Maturation index Squamous cell index to evaluate female estrogen status.

Maturational arrest Presence of immature nucleus in a relatively mature cytoplasm as in megaloblastic anemia due to a deficiency of vitamin B_{12} and/or folic acid; failure of testes to produce spermatozoa despite normal multiplication of earlier stages.

Maxilla (*mak-sil-ah*) The bone of the upper jaw, adj. **maxillary**.

Maxillodental (*mak-sil'o-den'tal*) Pertaining to the maxilla and the teeth it supports.

Maxillofacial (*mak-sil'o-fa'sheal*) Pertaining to the maxilla and face.

Maxillofacial syndrome Facial abnormalities due to improper ossification of the fetal cartilage in the facial area.

Maxillotomy (*mak'si-lot'o-me*) A surgical procedure of sectioning of the maxilla which permits movement of all or a part of the maxilla into the desired position.

Mayo's operation (*ma'oz*) Devised by William Mayo and Charles Mayo, US surgeons; excision of head of metatarsal bone for hallux valgus; excision of pyloric end of the stomach and construction of gastrojejunostomy; operation for radical cure of umbilical hernia; subcutaneous removal of varicose vein.

Mazindol A tricyclic compound with central nervous system stimulant properties similar to those of amphetamine. It releases and blocks reuptake of dopamine and noradrenaline, and the actions of these catecholamines, not serotonin, are responsible for its anorectic activity.

McBurney's point A point situated at the junction of lateral one third and medial two thirds of the right spinoumbilical line, denoting the site in appendicitis.

Mean (arithmetic mean) (*men*) *stat* An average, a numerical value intermediate between two extremes.

Measles (*me'zles*) A paramyxoma virus infection commonly noted in childhood. It spreads by droplet infection and begins as a catarrhal stage with fever, running nose, red watery eyes followed by cough, photophobia and Koplik's spots. After third day, a red macular or maculopapular rash develops. It is noted initially at the back of the ears and at the junction of the forehead and the hair. Within a short period, the whole skin is invaded by the rash, giving blotchy appearance. Fever settles when the rash begins to fade and desquamate. The condition may have complications such as post viral encephalitis, bronchopneumonia, corneal ulceration and weight loss. Live attenuated measles vaccine gives protection.

Black measles A severe form of measles with dark eruptions due to bleeding into the skin.

German measles Rubella.

Meatus (*me-a'tus*) An opening or passage. adj. **meatal.**

Acoustic meatus Either of two passages in the ear, external from external ear to tympanic membrane, and internal on the posterior surface of the petrous portion of temporal bone through which cochlear and vestibular nerves pass.

Meatus nasi One of the four portions of the nasal cavity (common, inferior, superior and middle) on either side of the septum.

Urinary meatus External opening of the urethra.

Mebendazole (*me-ben'da-zol*) A broad-spectrum anthelmintic used against trichuriasis, ascariasis, enterobiasis and hookworm infection.

Mecamylamine (*mek'a-mil'a-min*) A ganglion-blocking antihypertensive agent.

Mechanoreceptor (*mek'a-no-re-sep'tor*) A receptor that is excited by mechanical pressure.

Mechanotherapy (*mek'an-o-thera-pe*) Use of different mechanical apparatus to perform passive movements.

Mechlorethamine (*meklor-eth'a-men*) A vesicant and necrotizing irritant destructive to mucous membranes, mechlorethamine is an alkylating drug. It was formerly used as a war gas. The hydrochloride is used as an antineoplastic in Hodgkin's disease and lymphomas. It causes severe gastrointestinal and bone marrow damage.

Meckel's diverticulum (*mek'elz*) A blind pouch sometimes found in lower portions of ileum. It represents the persistent proximal end of the yolk stalk. It is a favored site for carcinoids, named after Johann Meckel the younger, German anatomist.

Meckel's syndrome An autosomal recessive disease with dysplasia and malformation of multiple organs characterized by occipital meningoencephalocele, microphelomia, lung hypoplasia, polycystic kidneys or renal hypodysplasia or dysplasia, bile duct dilatation, postaxial polydactyly and situs inversus.

Meclizine A histamine H_1 antagonist with antiemetic and antivertigo properties. It is used in the symptomatic treatment of motion sickness and control of vertigo associated with vestibular system diseases. It also exhibits anticholinergic, central nervous system depressant, and local anesthetic effects.

Meclofenamate (*mek'lo-fen'a-mat*) A nonsteroidal anti-inflammatory drug (NSAID) that is used to treat fever or mild to moderate pain in adults. Used in primary dysmenorrhea, heavy menstrual blood loss, rheumatoid arthritis, and osteoarthritis.

Meconium (*me-ko'ne-num*) The thick, sticky greenish black fecal material consisting of salts, amniotic fluid, mucus, bile and epithelial cells passed by newborn infant in the first 24 hours; opium

Meconium aspiration syndrome Breathing problems that a newborn baby may have when there are no other causes, and the baby has passed meconium into the amniotic fluid during labor or delivery.

Meconium ileus Ileus due to impacted meconium in the intestines, characteristic of cystic fibrosis.

Medial Pertaining to the middle; situated in or toward the midline.

Median (*me'de-an*) Middle; *stat* a number obtained by arranging the given series in order of magnitude and taking the middle number.

Median nerve *see* Table of nerves.

Median plane A vertical plane through the head and trunk dividing the body into right and left halves.

Mediastinitis (*me'de-as'ti-ni'tis*) Inflammation of the tissue of mediastinum.

Mediastinoscopy (*me'de-as'ti'nos'ko-pe*) Examination of the mediastinum by means of an endoscope through an incision in the neck.

Mediastinotomy (*me'de-as'ti-not'o-me*) Surgical incision of the mediastinum.

Mediastinum (*me'de-as-ti'num*) Pl. **mediastina**. A median septum between two parts of an organ; structure lying centrally within the chest spanning the region vertically from the thoracic inlet to the diaphragmatic hiatus, transversely between the parietal pleura, and coronally between the sternum and vertebral column. It contains all soft-tissue thoracic organs except the two lungs. It is divided empirically as anterior (posterior surface of sternum, the pericardium posteriorly and the visceral pleurae laterally), superiorly and extends from the pericardium anteriorly to the anterior surface posteriorly) and posterior (bounded by middle compartment anteriorly and the costophrenic angles laterally) compartments. adj. **mediastinal**.

Medical (*med'i-kal*) Pertaining to medical science; requiring treatment by medicines as distinct from surgical treatment.

Medical ethics Moral dilemmas affecting broad medical decisions.

Medical failure A patient not responding to a noninterventional method of treatment.

Medical grand rounds A medical education undertaken in a teaching hospital where the clinical case is presented and discussed.

Medical history A detailed record of present illness and past illness.

Medical informatics Application of information technology to various aspects of medical knowledge, practice and management.

Medical preparation A preparation of medical substance.

Medical record A written documentation of information regarding the patient's clinical history, physical findings, diagnostic tests and treatment.

Medical specialty Different branches of medical sciences providing specialized patient care.

Medical staff Licensed qualified medical persons.

Medical team A group of physicians and health care workers responsible for the patients' care while in hospital or in emergency.

Medical examiner A physician qualified and trained to undertake physical examination of person or to the task of investigation of the cause of death.

Medical Jurisprudence Application of the principles of law to the practice of medicine.

Medicare (*med'i-kar*) A program of health care covered by the health insurance for anyone aged 65 and older, and some people under 65 with certain disabilities or conditions.

Medicated (*med'i-kat"ad*) Impregnate with a medicinal substance.

Medication (*med'i-ka'shun*) The administration of remedies; impregnation with medicine; a medicament.

Medicine (*med'i-sin*) Any drug or remedy; the art and science of prevention of diseases, promotion of health and curing diseases; the study and treatment of diseases affecting internal organs; treatment of disease by medicines.

Adolescent medicine The branch of medicine dealing with the treatment of youth.

Aerospace medicine Branch of medicine concerned with the problems involved in aviation.

Alternative medicine The diagnosis and management of medical conditions by use of generally not accepted scientific disciplines such as Ayurveda, Homeopathy, Naturopathy, Holistic method, Siddha, Unani, Yoga, etc.

Clinical medicine Study and practice of medicine in the clinical setting at the bed side; the curriculum in a medical college after study of preclinical subjects.

Community medicine Medical science concerned with the population, with emphasis on preventive medicine

Complementary medicine Therapies which are not considered orthodox that can be used along with conventional medicine.

Emergency medicine The medical specialty dealing with acutely ill or injured who require immediate attention and treatment.

Empirical medicine Treatment born out of actual experience.

Environmental medicine Branch of medicine dealing with the effects of the environment on humans.

Essential medicine Those that satisfy the priority health care needs of the population. They are selected with due regard to public health relevance, evidence on efficacy and safety, and comparative cost.

Experimental medicine The study of diseases by experimentation upon animals or by clinical research.

Family medicine Medical specialty concerned with providing medical care to all members of the family.

Fetal medicine The medical specialty concerned with the study, development, care and treatment of the fetus.

Folk medicine Treatment of diseases by home remedy and measures based upon experience and knowledge passed from generation to generation.

Forensic medicine Medical jurisprudence.

Group medicine Practice of medicine by a group of physicians representing various specialties who are associated together in providing total care of the patient.

Holistic medicine Comprehensive health care of the patient affecting physical, mental, social and spiritual aspects.

Industrial medicine Specialty concerned with the diseases peculiar to the work environment.

Internal medicine Branch of medicine concerned with diagnosis and medical treatment of internal organs of the body.

Knidian medicine Anti-Hipppocratic School of Medicine at Knidos in Asia Minor which regarded disease as originating within the organism itself.

Legal medicine Forensic medicine.

Nuclear medicine The branch of medicine concerned with the use of radionuclides in the diagnosis and treatment of diseases.

Occupational medicine Industrial medicine.

Patent medicine A drug or remedy that is protected by patent and is available without a prescription.

Perinatal medicine The specialty concerned with care of the mother, fetus during pregnancy, labor and delivery.

Physical medicine Physiatry; treatment of diseases by mechanical devices or the physical agents such as heat, cold, light, electricity or manipulation.

Preclinical medicine The first year of training in a medical collage.

Preventive medicine Medical science concerned with the prevention of diseases and promotion of health.

Proprietary medicine A remedy where formula and mode of manufacture are the properties of the producer.

Psychosomatic medicine Branch of medicine that is concerned with mind-body interrelationship in diseases or abnormal states.

Rehabilitation medicine Branch of medicine concerned with the restoration of form and function following an injury or illness.

Socialized medicine The control of medical practice by a governmental agency.

Sports medicine The branch of medicine concerned with physiology, pathology and psychology as applied to the individuals who participate in sports and to the injuries sustained by athletes and sportsmen.

Tropical medicine Medical science dealing with the diseases occurring in tropics and subtropics especially diseases of parasitic origin.

Veterinary medicine The branch of medical science concerned with the diseases and health of animals.

Medicochirurgical (*med'i-ko-ki-rur'ji-kal*) Concerning both medicine and surgery.

Mediterranean fever A familial disease characterized by repetitive episodes of high fever, peritonitis, pleuritis and inflammatory arthritis, oral colchicine acts as a prophylactic and prevents the development of amyloidosis.

Medium (*med'e-um*) Pl. **media**. A means; anything through which an action is performed; substance used for cultivation of microorganisms; substance through which impulses are transmitted; the liquid holding a substance in solution or suspension.

Clearing medium A substance that makes histologic specimens transparent.

Contrast medium Radio-opaque substance such as barium used in radiography to permit visualization of internal organs.

Culture medium A liquid or solid matrix with nutrient substance on which microorganisms are cultivated, such as agar, broths or gelatin.

Differential medium Media that allow visualization of metabolic differences between groups or species of bacteria.

Dispersion medium A liquid in which colloid is dispersed.

Enriched medium A growth media that contains added growth factors such as blood, vitamins and yeast extracts.

Nutrient medium A medium to which nutrient substances have been added.

Refracting medium The transparent tissues and fluid through which light rays pass and get refracted and focused on retina.

Separating medium A substance applied to the surface of an impression or mold to prevent interaction of materials and to allow their separation after casting, in dentistry.

Transport medium A culture medium used to transport specimens for bacteriologic examination, as alkaline-peptone water to transport stool or vomitus in suspected cases of cholera.

Medroxyprogesterone (*med-rok'se-pro-jes'ter-on*) A long-acting progestational agent.

Medulla (*me-dul'a*) The marrow; innermost portion of an organ. adj. **medullary**.

Adrenal medulla Inner portion of the adrenal gland, that consists of cells displaying a chromaffin reaction and it secretes adrenaline and non-adrenaline.

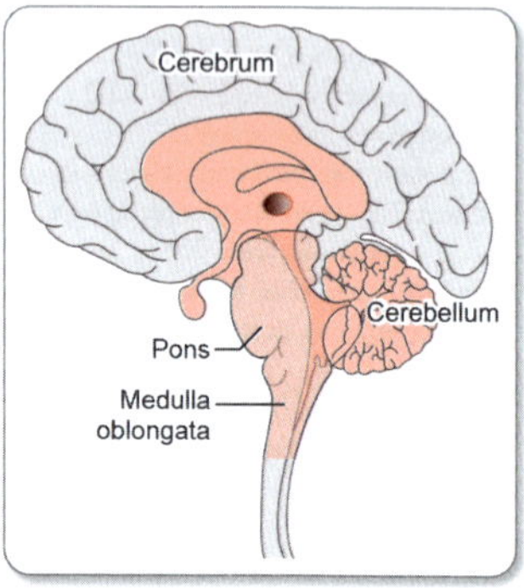

Medulla oblongata

Medulla of bone Bone marrow.

Medulla of hair shaft Central axis of some hairs

Medulla of kidneys Renal pyramid.

Medulla of ovary Central portion of

the ovary.

Medulla of thymus The central portion of each lobule of thymus containing reticular cells.

Medulla ossium Bone marrow. The tissue that fills the cavities of bone, having a stroma of reticular fibers and fat (yellow bone marrow) of developmental stages of erythrocytes, leukocytes and megakaryocytes (red bone marrow).

Medulla renis The renal pyramid composed chiefly of collecting ducts, loops of Henle and vasa recta.

Spinal medulla Spinal cord.

Medulla oblongata (Myelencephalon) The lowest sub division of brain stem, continuous with the pons above and the spinal cord below. It regulates all the vital functions such as heart rate, respiration, blood pressure, swallowing etc.

Medulloblastoma (*med-ul'o-blas-to'ma*) A tumor of childhood affecting the cerebellar vermis. A highly cellular tumor, presenting with a short history of headache, vomiting and truncal ataxia.

Mefenamic acid (*mef'a-nam'ik*) A nonsteroidal anti-inflammatory drug, with analgesic, anti-inflammatory, and antipyretic properties. It is an inhibitor of cyclooxygenase. Treats rheumatoid arthritis, osteoarthritis, dysmenorrhea, and mild to moderate pain, inflammation and fever.

Mefloquine An antimalarial agent acting on blood trophozoites and gametocytes. It acts more slowly than chloroquine or quinine. It is also used as a chemoprophylactic in chloroquine-resistant *P. falciparum* malaria.

Mega Combining word for large, oversize; indicates a unit of measurement of one million.

Megacolon (*meg'a-ko'lon*) Extreme dilatation of the colon and refractory constipation. It may be congenital or may develop later in life.

Acquired megacolon Colonic enlargement as a result of voluntary withholding of stool or chronic constipation and prolonged abuse of stimulant laxatives.

Congenital megacolon A congenital aganglionosis of large intestine, with failure of relaxation of internal anal sphincter. Constipation, abdominal distension and vomiting develop immediately after birth. *see* Hirschsprung's disease.

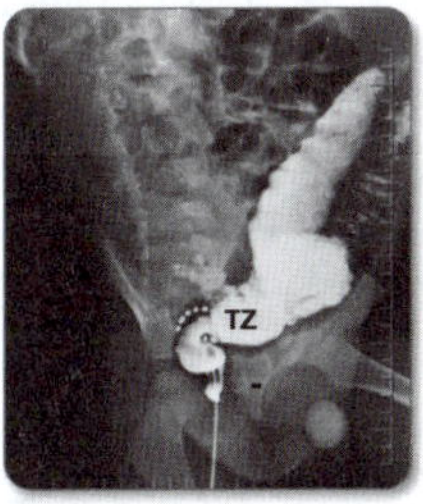

Congenital megacolon

Toxic megacolon Marked dilatation of the colon as a complication of ulcerative colitis.

Megakaryoblast (*meg-a-kar'i-o-blast*) Precursor of a megakaryocyte.

Megakaryocyte (*meg-a-kar'i-o-sit*) A large cell with a multilobed nucleus found in the bone marrow that gives rise to blood platelets.

Megal- (megalo-) Combining word for great or large.

Megaloblast (*meg'a-lo-blast*) An erythroid precursor with an enlarged nucleus related to vitamin B_{12} and/or folic acid deficiency which causes a change in the nuclear cytoplasm maturation.

Megalocephalic (*meg-a-lo-sef-al'ik*) Relating to or characterized by a large head.

Megalocephaly (*meg-a-lo-sef-a'le*) Megacephaly.

Megalocyte (*meg'a-lo-sit*) Markedly enlarged erythrocyte.

Megalomania (*meg'a-lo-ma'ne-a*) Overvaluation of one's importance.

Megaloureter (Megaureter) (*me'ga-lo-u-re'ter*) Markedly dilated ureter.

Megaly Combining word for an enlargement of specific organ or body part.

Megarectum A feces-filled dilated rectum resulting in constipation.

Megestrol (*mejes'trol*) Man-made version of the human hormone progesterone. It treats breast cancer and endometrial cancer by affecting female hormones involved in cancer growth, also used to treat loss of appetite, malnutrition, and severe weight loss in patients with AIDS.

Megaureter (*meg'-u-re'tar*) [mega- + ureter] Larger-than-normal (larger than 3/8-inch wide) ureters, diagnosed by ultrasound.

Meibomian cyst A red bump on eyelid. It forms when oil gland blocks.

Meibomian gland (tarsal glands) Row of large sebaceous glands within the upper lid discharging to lid margin.

Meiosis (reduction division) (*mi-o'sis*) Reduction cell division that produces ova or sperm, each of which contains half the genes of the original cell.

Meissner's plexus (submucous plexus) Autonomic nerve plexus found in the submucosa of the gut from the cardia downward that acts as a sensory side of peristaltic control.

Melancholia (*mel-an-ko'le-a*) *psy* Psychotic depression with an uninterested affect and lack of interest in activities that normally cause pleasure more common in women and is accompanied by helplessness, suicidal ideation or attempts.

Melanin (*mel'a-nin*) A complex polymer synthesized from DOPA and bound to a carrier protein by melanocytes. It gives skin, eyes and hair their color.

Melanism (melanosis) (*mel'a-niz'm*) Melanosis.

Melanocyte (Melanophore) (*mel'an-o-sit*) Melanin producing cell of neural crest origin found in basal layer of epidermis and hair matrix.

Melanocyte-stimulating hormone (MSH) A group of hormones produced by pituitary gland, hypothalamus and skin cells.

Melanocytoma of optic disk A deeply pigmented variant of melanocytic nevus that classically occurs in the optic disk, sometimes with contiguous involvement of the adjacent retina or choroid.

Melanoderma (*mel'an-o-der'ma*) Presence of an abnormally increased amount of melanin in the skin.

Melanoma (*mel'a-no'ma*) Tumor of melanocytes.

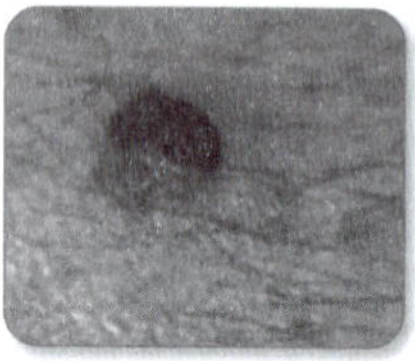

Melanoma

Acral melanoma Large macular lentiginous pigmented area on the palms and soles.

Lentigo maligna melanoma Slow-growing subtype of melanoma that often occurs on chronically sun-damaged skin, particularly the head and neck, in the elderly. Due to its clinical and histopathologic mimicry of benign lesions, it is often misdiagnosed for years or even decades, which can lead to increased morbidity and mortality.

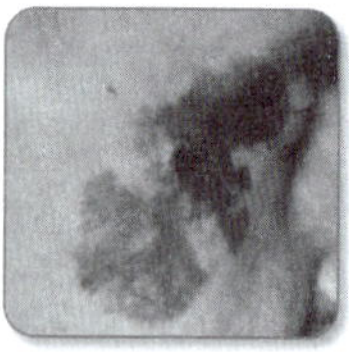

Lentigo maligna melanoma

Malignant melanoma A malignant tumor arising from melanocytes located in the epidermis, dermis or mucosal epithelium or from nevus cells.

The growth is asymmetrical with irregular border, color and elevation. It may spread to regional lymph nodes or produce distant disease.

Nodular melanoma Melanoma that develops on a pigmented nodule and has poor prognosis.

Melanonychia (*mel'a-no-nik'e-a*) Blackening of the nails by melanin pigmentation.

Melanophore (*mel'an-o-for*) A cell containing melanin pigment.

Melanoplakia (*mel'an-o-pla'ke-a*) The development of pigmented patches on the buccal mucosa and the tongue.

Melanosis (*mel'an-o'sis*) A condition with abnormal dark brown or brown-black pigmentation of tissues and organs; disorder from widespread metastases of melanoma.

Melanosis coli Segmental or global darkening of the colonic mucosa associated with chronic constipation due to prolonged use of laxatives containing anthraquinone.

Neurocutaneous melanosis A congenital disorder that includes melanocytic lesions of the skin and leptomeninges. Children with NM are at risk of developing malignant melanoma.

Oculocutaneous melanosis Also known as oculodermal melanocytosis, oculomucodermal melanocytosis, or congenital melanosis bulbi, is a benign mesodermal melanosis involving the distributions of the ophthalmic and maxillary trigeminal nerve with associated hyperpigmentation of the eye and its adnexa.

Riehl melanosis A noneczematous allergic contact dermatitis to fragrance, cosmetics, and sometimes occupational agents. It is specially marked by a reticulate gray-brown to black pigmentation involving the face and neck, interface dermatitis, and pigment incontinence.

Tar melanosis An occupational dermatosis that occurs among tar handlers after several years of exposure, characterized by a severe widespread itching that is soon followed by the appearance of reticular pigmentation, telangiectasis and a shiny appearance of the skin.

Transient neonatal pustular melanosis A normal and harmless skin condition that affects newborns. Infants with TNPM have skin bumps called pustules that are noticeable at birth. These pus-filled bumps rupture, causing white-encircled dark spots on the skin. These spots eventually fade.

Melanuria (*mel'an-ur'e-a*) Darkening of urine on standing due to the presence of melanin precursor, seen in extensive metastases from melanoma.

Melasma (*me-laz'ma*) chloasma; melanosis with sharply demarcated brown macules, usually symmetric on the face or neck, seen during pregnancy or at menopause or in those taking oral contraceptives.

Melatonin (*me-la'to-nin*) A hormone produced by the pineal gland in response to light.

MELD score The Model for End-stage Liver Disease determined by using the total serum bilirubin concentration, the international normalized ratio for the prothrombin time, and the serum creatinine concentration.

Melena (*me-le'na*) The passage of dark colored stools, generally due to upper gastrointestinal bleeding.

Melioidosis (*mel'e-oi-do'sis*) An infection caused by *Burkholderia pseudomallei,* a saprophyte found in soil and water. Infection is through abrasions characterized by fever, prostration, pneumonia, hepatosplenomegaly and multiple abscess. Ceftazidine and tetracyclines are useful.

Melituria Passage of any sugar such as glucose, fructose, maltose, or pentose in the urine.

Melomelus A fetus with a rudimentary limb attached to a normal limb.

Melphalan (*mel'fa-lan*) Alkylating cytotoxic agent used in myelomatosis.

Membrane (*mem'bran*) A thin layer or sheet of tissue that covers a part, lines a cavity or divides a cavity or connects two structures.

Basement membrane A sheet of amorphous extracellular material upon which the basal surfaces of epithelial cells rest; other cells associated with basement membranes are muscle cells, Schwann cells, fat cells, and capillaries. The membrane is interposed between the cellular elements and the underlying connective tissue. It comprises two layers, the basal lamina and the reticular lamina, and is composed of Type IV collagen (which is unique to basement membranes), laminin, fibronectin, and heparan sulfate proteoglycans.

Extraembryonic membranes Any of the membranes derived from embryonic tissue that lie outside the embryo, as the allantois, amnion, chorion and yolk sac.

Membrane bone Bone formed from fibrous tissue without intervention of cartilage.

Membrane potential Electrical potential due to the differences of ions on either side of a semipermeable membrane.

Membrane transport Active translocation of proteins from the site of production in the cell to the sites of storage or to the cell membrane for later release.

Placental membrane The semipermeable membrane that separates the fetal from the maternal blood in the placenta. In the human (hemochorial) placenta, it is composed of fetal vascular endothelium, connective tissue, cytotrophoblast, and syncytiotrophoblast, and it becomes thinner as pregnancy progresses. Sometimes inappropriately called the placental barrier; there are only a few substances that cannot pass through the membrane.

Serous membrane A connective tissue sheet lubricated with slippery serum.

Menarche (*me-nar'ke*) Onset or beginning of menstruation.

Mendel's Law Different forms of one character remain distinct without blending in crosses (of segregation); forms of any one character behave independently of those of any other character (of recombination), formulated by Gregor Mendel, Austrian monk and naturalist.

Mendelson's syndrome Acute lung injury from aspiration of acid gastric contents especially from general anesthesia, during labor, named after Curtis Mendelson, US obstetrician.

Meniere's disease (Meniere's syndrome) Labyrinthine vertigo. The condition is characterized by tinnitus, distorted hearing and paroxysmal attacks of vertigo, preceded by a sense of fullness in the ear, named after Prosper Meniere, French physician.

Meninges (*men-in-jez*) Membranes; the three membranes enclosing the brain and spinal cord, comprising the dura mater, the arachnoid and pia mater.

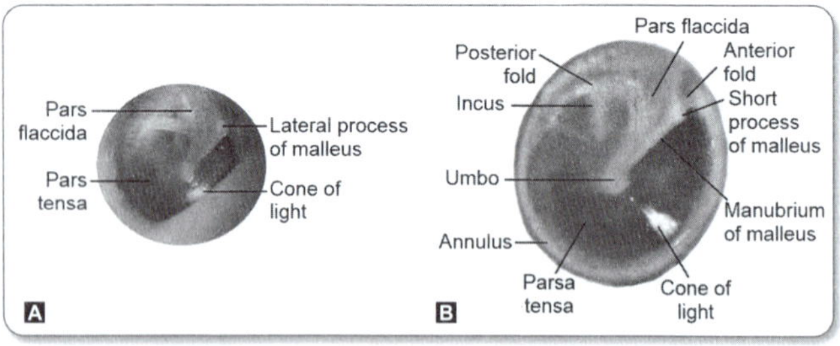

Membrana tympanica: ***A.*** *Otoscopic view;* ***B.*** *Diagrammatic view*

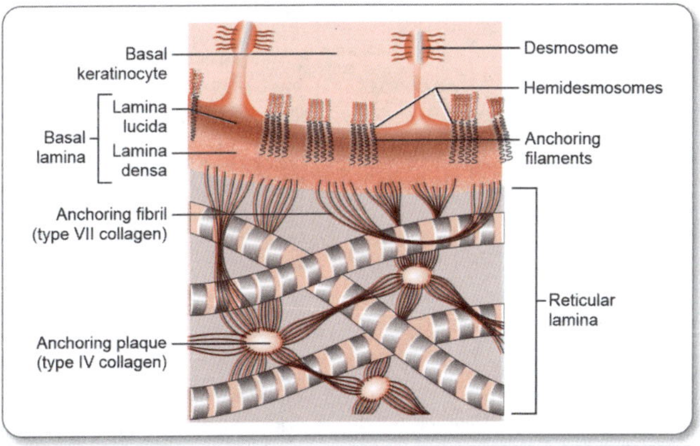

Basement membrane, comprising the lamina lucida and lamina densa, which together constitute the basal lamina, and the collagen-containing reticular lamina beneath, in a diagram of a section through epithelial tissue

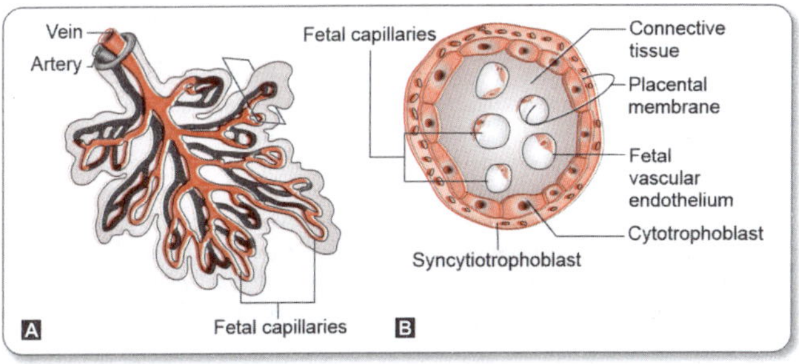

Placental membrane separating the blood in the fetal capillaries from the maternal blood in the intervillous space. ***A.*** *Chorionic villus containing the fetal vessels and surrounded by maternal blood in the intervillous space;* ***B.*** *Cross-section through a villus, showing the layers of the placental membrane separating the fetal blood from the maternal blood surrounding the villus.*

Meningioma (*me-nin'je-o'ma*) A fibroblastic tumor of the meninges seen in adults. It grows slowly and occurs most commonly in the cortical dura. It offers best prospects for complete removal by surgery.

Angioblastic meningioma A rare histological variant of meningioma. The clinical presentation was nonspecific and depended on the location of the tumor and was mainly due to the mass effect.

Chordoid meningioma An uncommon histopathological type of meningioma, frequently associated with Castleman's syndrome. Histologically, chordoid meningiomas are similar to chordomas. Because of their high proliferative index, they present aggressive biological behavior and high risk of

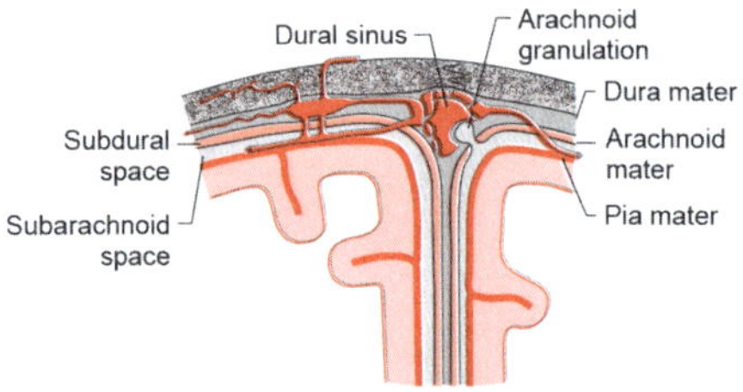

Cranial meninges

postoperative recurrence.

Cystic meningioma Meningiomas with intratumoral degenerative cyst formation as well as those with peritumoral arachnoid cysts or reactive intraparenchymal cysts.

Fibroblastic meningioma Characterized by spindle-shaped tumor cells, with narrow rod-shaped nuclei. These cells are embedded in abundant collagenous or reticulum background. Whorls are far less common than in meningothelial meningiomas, and psammoma bodies are only occasionally encountered.

Meningothelial meningioma A group of mostly benign, slow-growing neoplasms that most likely derive from the meningothelial cells of the arachnoid layer.

Orbital meningioma Typically benign tumors, most commonly originating from the dura of the sphenoid wing or the optic nerve sheath.

Papillary meningioma Rare meningeal tumors and are associated with aggressive clinical behavior as compared with other meningiomas. Because of their rare occurrence, they may pose a diagnostic dilemma to the unwary pathologist.

Psammomatous meningioma A histologic subtype of meningioma usually presented as a heavily calcified intracranial or spinal mass lesion.

Rhabdoid meningioma A rare and aggressive subtype of meningioma. Rhabdoid morphology is associated with a poor prognosis, regardless of tumor histogenesis. It resembles other types of rhabdoid tumors with a great tendency for recurrence.

Secretory meningioma A rare tumor, which has unique histopathological, immunohistochemical features and displays benign biological course.

Spinal meningioma A tumor that arises in the meninges, the thin membranes that cover and provide a protective wrapping for your brain and spinal cord.

Syncytial meningioma Characterized by sheets, whorls or syncytia of neoplastic cells which have round or oval centrally located nuclei with dispersed chromatin, smooth nuclear profiles and small indistinct nucleoli. They also sometimes demonstrate eosinophilic cytoplasmic invaginations (a.k.a. intranuclear pseudoinclusions). Lobules of the tumor are separated from each other with collagen sheets.

Tentorial meningioma A rare tumor located along the surface of the tentorium cerebella in the brain. These types of posterior fossa meningiomas can cause headaches, seizures, and difficulty walking.

Transitional meningioma Second most common subtype of benign meningioma that generally originates from the parasagittal region or sphenoid ridge of the brain.

Meningism (*men'in-jizm*) Meningitis-like symptoms without inflammation of the meninges.

Meningitis (*men'in-ji'tis*) Acute infection of meninges presenting with features of fever, headache, stiffness of neck and irritability.

Bacterial meningitis Develops secondary to a bacteremic illness or from direct spread from an adjacent focus of infection in the ear, sinus or skull fracture. *Neisseria meningitides, Haemophilus influenza* and *Streptococcus pneumoniae* are common causes. CSF is cloudy due to presence of neutrophils.

Fungal meningitis A recognized complication of HIV infection.

Tuberculous meningitis May develop after a primary infection in childhood or as part of military tuberculosis. SCF demonstrates a fine clot (cobweb) on standing, with a rise in protein and a marked fall in glucose. There is increased number of leukocytes.

Viral meningitis A benign and self-limiting illness. CSF headache is more severe than meningism. CSF shows excess leukocytes with normal proteins and glucose.

Meningocele (*me-ning'go-sel*) Protrusion of meninges through spina bifida.

Anterior meningocele A congenital defect seen in the anterior aspect of the spine. It is defined as a meningeal cyst that occurs in the presacral space secondary to agenesis of a portion of the anterior sacrum.

Cranial meningocele A rare central nervous system malformation characterized by herniation of meninges through a permanent defect in the skull. It is lined by arachnoid and contains cerebrospinal fluid, but no brain tissue.

Spinal meningocele A birth defect where there is a sac protruding from the spinal column.

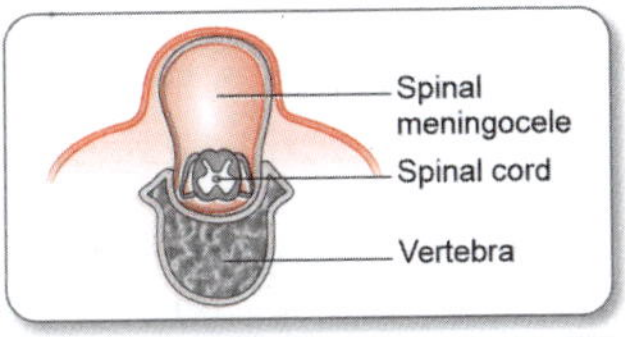

Cross-section of a spinal meningocele

Traumatic meningocele Occurs after injuries to the brachial or lumbosacral plexus.

Meningococcemia (*me-ning'gokok-seme'-a*) A disease caused by *Neisseria meningitidis* in the blood. It has a sudden onset with fever, chills, myalgia, headache, petechiae and severe prostration.

Meningococcus (*me-ning'go-kok'us*) Pl. **meningococci**. A bacterium of the genus *Neisseria meningitidis,* a non-motile, gram-negative diplococcus, often found in the nasopharynx of asymptomatic, cerebrospinal fever and meningitis.

Meningoencephalitis (*me-ning'go-en-sef'a-lit'is*) Inflammation of meninges and brain.

Amebic meningoencephalitis Inflammation of meninges and brain due to amebic infection.

Granulomatous meningoencephalitis Inflammation of meninges and brain due to granulomatous lesion.

Mumps meningoencephalitis Inflammation of meninges and brain due to mumps infection complication.

Primary amebic meningoencephalitis (PAM) A rare brain infection that is caused by Naegleria fowleri and is usually fatal.

Syphilitic meningoencephalitis Inflammation of meninges and brain due to untreated syphilis infection

Toxoplasmic meningoencephalitis Inflammation of meninges and brain due to toxoplasmic infection.

Meningoencephalocele (*me-ning'go-en-sef'a-lo-sel*) Protrusion of the meninges and brain through a congenital defect in the skull.

Meningomyelitis (*me-ning'go-mi'e-li'tis*) Inflammation of the spinal cord and meninges.

Meningomyelocele (*me-ning'go-mi'le-lo'sel*) Protrusion of the spinal cord or the cauda equina along with meninges through spina bifida. The cord and nerves appear as dark shadows in the brilliantly translucent swelling during transillumination test.

Meningovascular (*me-ningo-vas'ku-lar*) Pertaining to the blood vessels in the meninges or the meninges and blood vessels.

Meniscectomy Surgical removal of a meniscus, especially that of a knee.

Meniscus (*me-nis'kus*) Curved edge of liquid-solid line of contact; concavo-convex lens; a crescent-shaped structure as of cartilage of knee.

Meniscus sign *radiol* A semilunar radiolucency peripheral to a pulmonary mass lesion, seen in hydatid cyst, aspergilloma; a large semilunar hypodense zone in ulcerated gastric adenocarcinoma.

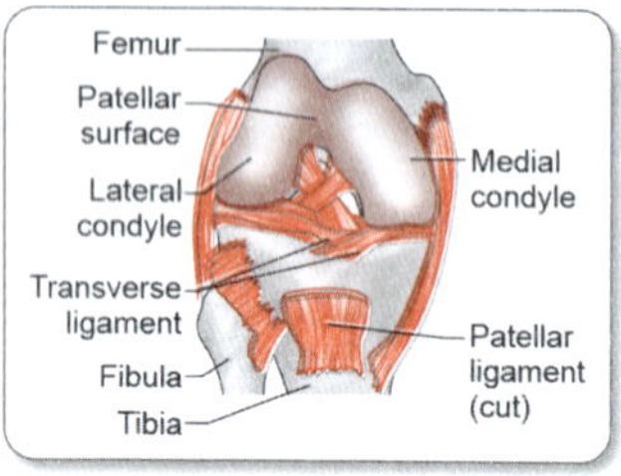

Articular menisci

Menopause (climacteric) (*men'o-pawz*) The cessation of menstrual activity which occurs between ages of 45 and 50, characterized by menstrual irregularity, hot flushes, irritability, increased weight, osteoporosis and atrophy of female tissues.

Menorrhagia (epimenorrhagia) (*men'or-a'jea*) Excessive or prolonged menstrual bleeding.

Menses (*men'sez*) The monthly flow of menstrual blood from the uterus.

Menstrual cycle A natural process which is complex and is controlled by female hormones, causing regular periods of bleeding. It has 4 phases-menstruation the follicular phase, ovulation and the luteal phase.

Menstruation (*men'stru-a'shun*) Cyclic endometrial shedding and discharge of bloody fluid from the uterus, and it occurs at approximately 4-week intervals.

Anovulatory menstruation Menstruation without the discharge of ovum.

Retained menstruation Hematocolpos.

Retrograde menstruation Backward flow of menstrual blood through the fallopian tubes.

Vicarious menstruation Periodic bleeding occurring from any surface other than uterine mucous membrane.

Mental (*ment'l*) Pertaining to the mind; pertaining to the chin.

Mental age *psy* The level of the mental ability of a person as determined by an intelligent test in relation to chronological age of an average person at this level.

Mental deficiency Lowered mental capacity.

Mental disorder Significant behavioral or psychological syndrome associated with distress or disability, not just an expected response to a particular event.

Mental retardation Impaired intellectual functioning and adaptive behavior.

Mental age *psy* The level of the mental ability of a person as determined by an intelligent test in relation to chronological age of an average person at this level.

Mental deficiency Lowered mental capacity.

Mental illness A wide range of conditions that affect mood, thinking and behavior.

Mental impairment A condition in which a part of the person's mind is damaged or is not working properly.

Mental retardation Impaired intellectual functioning and adaptive behavior.

Mentum (*men'tum*) chin.

Meperidine (*me-per'i-den*) A narcotic analgesic.

Mephenytoin (*me-fen'i-to'in*) An anticonvulsant agent.

Mepivacaine (*me-piv'a-kan*) A local anesthetic that is chemically related to bupivacaine but pharmacologically related to lidocaine. It is indicated for infiltration, nerve block, and epidural anesthesia. Mepivacaine is effective topically only in large doses and therefore, should not be used by this route.

Meprobamate (*me-pro'ba-mat*) An anxiolytic drug used for the short-term management of anxiety symptoms.

Meralgia paresthesia A sensory neuropathy resulting from compression of the lateral femoral cutaneous nerve at the level of inguinal ligament or in the fascia lata and it is characterized by pain and paresthesia involving lateral and occasionally anterior proximal thigh unilaterally.

Mercaptopurine (*mer'kap'to-pur'en*) A purine antimetabolite used in acute leukemia.

Mercurialism **(hydrargyria)** Chronic poisoning with mercury.

Mercury (*mer'kur-e*) A heavy, silver white metallic element, atomic no. 80, symbol Hg, fluid at ordinary temperatures used in barometers, thermometers, pesticides, dental fillings and pharmaceutical preparations.

Merocrine (eccrine) (*mer'o-krin*) A secretion in which the secreting cell remains intact while producing and discharging the secretory product.

Merozoite (*mer'o-zo-it*) A motile, pre- and extra-erythrocytic form of plasmodial parasites, resulting from the asexual division of plasmodia in the liver or erythrocytes which either infect other erythrocytes or spontaneously develop into sexual forms.

Mesaortitis Mesaortitisluica is form of cardiovascular syphilis that can present within the context of tertiary stage syphilis.

Mesarteritis Inflammation of the middle layer of an artery, often with inflammation of all layers of the artery wall. It is seen in syphilis, polyarteritis, temporal arteritis and Buerger's disease.

Mescaline (*mes'ka-len*) A psychedelic hallucinogen obtained from the small, spineless cactus Peyote (Lophophora williamsii), the San Pedro cactus, Peruvian torch cactus, and other mescaline-containing cacti. Its effects include an altered state of consciousness with altered thinking and changes in time and perception which are often described as happy, positive, enjoyable and 'illuminating'.

Mesencephalon (*mes'en-sef'a-lon*) The mid-brain.

Mesenchyme (*me'senz'kim*) Mesenchyma.

Mesentery (*mes'en-to're*) The peritoneal fold that encircles the small intestine and connects it to the posterior abdominal wall. adj. **mesenteric**.

Mesial (*me'ze-il*) Nearer the center of dental arch.

Mesiodens (*me'ze-o-dens*) A supernumerary tooth in the maxilla between the central incisor teeth.

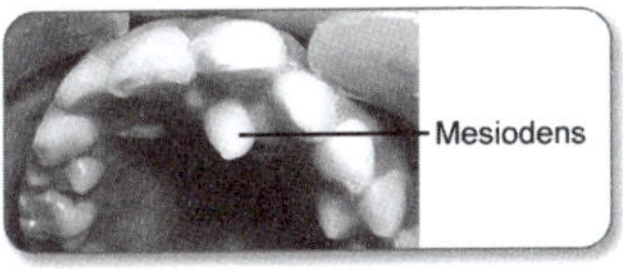

Mesiodens

Mesna (*mez'na*) Sodium 2-mercapto ethane sulfonate, a detoxifying medicine used to prevent hemorrhagic cystitis in patients receiving chemotherapy with either high-dose cyclophosphamide and ifosfamide.

Mesoappendix (*mes'o-a-pen'diks*) The peritoneal fold connecting the appendix to the ileum.

Mesocolon (*mes'o-ko'lon*) The peritoneal process attaching the colon to the posterior abdominal wall.

Ascending mesocolon The mesocolon that follow the course of ileocolic vessels and margin vessels along the mesocolic side of colon.

Descending mesocolon A section of the large intestine that passes downward.

Sigmoid mesocolon A fold of peritoneum that attaches the sigmoid colon to pelvic wall.

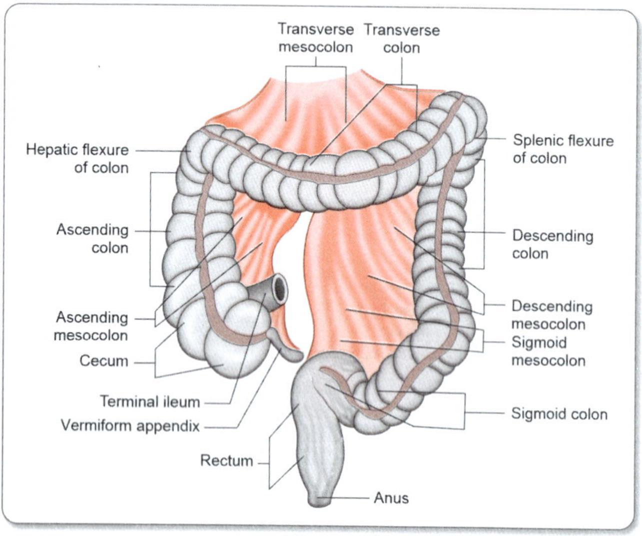

Mesocolon

Transverse mesocolon A broad, mesofold of peritoneum which connects the transverse colon to the posterior wall of abdomen.

Mesoderm (*meś'o-derm*) An embryonal tissue layer that gives rise to muscle, cartilage, bone and subcutaneous tissue, cardiovascular system, urogenital system except urinary bladder, serous membranes, spleen and adrenal glands.

Cardiogenic mesoderm The splanchnic mesoderm in the cardiogenic region where the heart develops; it gives rise to endocardial heart tubes that fuse to form the primordial cardiac tube, the heart primordium.

Extraembryonic mesoderm Tissue that supports the epithelium of the amnion and yolk sac and the chorionic villi, which arise from the trophoblastic tissues.

Head mesoderm A particular kind of tissue deriving from the paráxial mesoderm.

Peristomal mesoderm Mesoderm due to peristomal tissue.

Splanchnic mesoderm A layer continuous with mesoderm covering the yolk sac.

Mesometrium (*meso-me-tre-um*) The broad ligament of the uterus below the mesosalpinx.

Mesomorph (*mez'o-morf*) A body build characterized by predominance of tissues derived from mesoderm and the individual is stocky and muscular.

Mesonephros (wolffian body) (*mes'o-nef'ros*) The second stage in renal development which appears as an oblong mass along with the embryonal gonads and disappears with fetal maturation.

Mesophile (*mes'o-fil*) A microorganism with an optimum temperature between 25°C and 40°C, but growing between 10°C and 45°C.

Mesosalpinx (*meso'sal'pinks*) The part of the broad ligament covering the fallopian tube.

Mesosome (*mes'o-som*) An invagination of the bacterial cell membrane.

Mesotendineum (*mes'o-ten-din'e-um*) Synovial sheath of a tendon connecting the lining of tendon sheath to the fibrous sheath covering the tendon.

Mesothelioma (*mez'o-the'le-o-ma*) A neoplasm of serosal surfaces. Exposure to asbestos can lead to pleural, or latent period.

Peritoneal mesothelioma Presents as a diffuse abdominal mass due to omental infiltration and with ascites.

Pleural mesothelioma Diffuse malignant tumor spreading along pleural surface. It encases the lungs and invades tissues. There is accumulation of large amounts of hemorrhagic pleural fluid.

Malignant mesothelioma A cancer of the mesothelium that lines lungs, chest wall and abdomen.

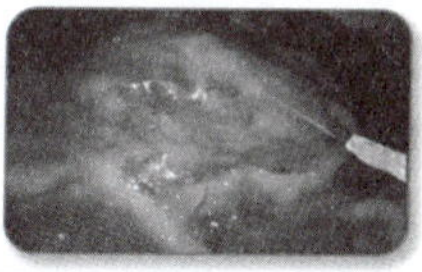

Malignant mesothelioma

Mesothelium (*mez'o-thel'e-um*) A single layer of flattened cells forming an epithelial lining of serous cavities.

Mesovarium (*mez'o-var'e-um*) A short peritoneal fold connecting the anterior border of the ovary with the posterior layer of the broad ligament of the uterus.

Mestranol (*mes'tra-nol*) Synthetic estrogen used in oral contraceptive.

Metabolism (*me-tabo-lizm*) The process of transforming food stuffs into tissue elements and into energy for use in the growth, repair and general function of the body.

Metabolism equivalent (MET) The amount of oxygen required per minute under quiet resting conditions, equal to 3.5 mL of oxygen consumed per kilogram of body weight per minute.

Metabolite (*met'a-lit*) Any product of metabolism.

Essential metabolite Steadily maintaining the mass flow to produce or consume the metabolites against any internal disturbances within the cell.

Metacarpal (*met'a-kar'pal*) Pertaining to the metacarpus; a bone of metacarpus.

Metacarpus (*met'a-kar'pus*) The part of the hand between the wrist and fingers. It is formed by five metacarpal bones that extend from the carpus to the phalanges.

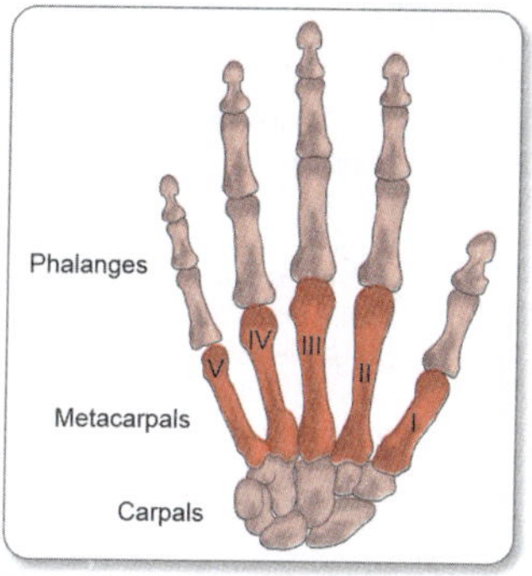

Metacarpus showing metacarpal bones, extending between carpus and phalanges and are numbered lateromedially

Metacentric (*met'a-sen'trik*) Location of centromere toward middle in a chromosome.

Metacercaria (*met'a-ser-ka're-a*) The encysted state in the life cycle of a trematode, which occurs in the intermediate host, a species of fresh water snail.

Metachromasia (metachromatism) (*met'a-kro-ma'zea*) The property of a tissue that enables it to stain differently from the colors used in the day.

Metagonimus (*met'a-gon'i-mus*) A genus of flukes that encyst on fish, and may infest man.

Metamorphopsia (*met'a-mor-fo'p-sea*) Distorted vision due to macular affections such as macular scar or edema.

Metamyelocyte (*met'a-mi'l-o-sit*) A maturing granulocyte between a myelocyte and a polymorphonuclear neutrophil, are confined to bone marrow. The nucleus chromatin.

Metanephros (*met'a-nef'ros*) The embryonic precursor of the adult kidney. It arises from mesonephric ducts.

Metaphase (*met'a-faz*) A stage in mitosis, wherein there is loss of nuclear membrane, with aggregation of chromosomes on equatorial plane and formation of nuclear spindle.

Metaphysis (*me-taf'i-sis*) The zone of growth between the epiphysis and diaphysis during development of a bone.

Metaplasia (*met'a-pla-zea*) The conversion of one type of adult cells into another, especially those of the epithelium.

Myeloid metaplasia A clinical and pathologic syndrome of varied cause which is characterized by the constant occurrence of extramedullary hematopoiesis in the spleen and almost always in the liver, splenomegaly and usually hepatomegaly, and an anemia with immature red and white cells in the peripheral blood.

Squamous metaplasia Refers to the transformation of mature, non-squamous epithelium into stratified squamous epithelium.

Metaproterenol (*met'a-pro-ter'e-nol*) Orciprenaline.

Metastasis (*me-tas'ta-sis*) Pl. **metastases**. Distal spread of a malignant cell either through blood or lymphatic vessel or along a serosal membrane. It develops a secondary focus of malignancy; transportation of microorganisms from one part of the body to another through the blood stream or lymph; the shifting of the manifestation of a disease from one part of the body to another.

Metachronus metastasis Metastasis developing after completion of the initial curative treatment. A positive resection margin is defined as the presence of tumor cells at, or within, 1 mm of the resection margin.

Retrograde metastasis Tumor spreading from the primary lesion down in the direction of the anal canal within the

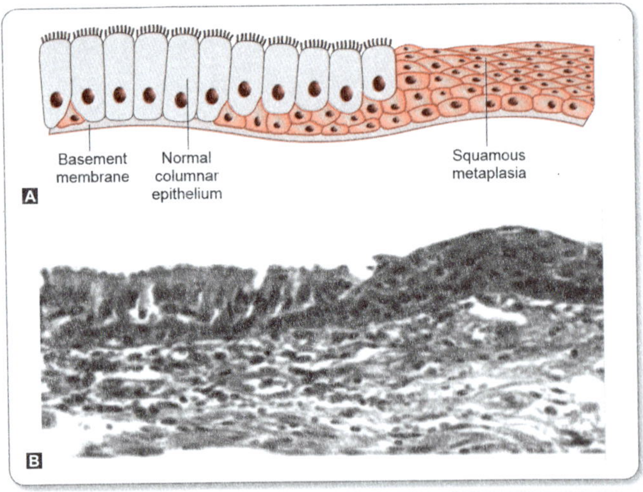

*Metaplasia of normal columnar (left) to squamous epithelium (right) in a bronchus, shown: **A.** Schematically and **B.** Histologically*

wall of the bowel or into immediately adjacent lymph nodes.

Synchronous metastasis The diagnosis of a distant metastasis or second carcinoma together with or within a three-month interval of the diagnosis of the primary colon cancer.

Metathesis (*me-tath'e-sis*) Transfer of a pathologic product from one place to another so as to decrease its effect.

Metatarsal (*met'a-tar'sil*) Pertaining to the metatarsus; a bone of metatarsus.

Metatarsal dome A rounded support under middle of forefoot to relieve metatarsalgia.

Metatarsalgia (*met'a-tar-sal'je-a*) Pain in the forefoot, symptom due to any abnormality of foot resulting in faulty distribution of weight.

Metatarsus (*met'a-tar'sus*) The part of the foot between the instep and the toes, consists of five metatarsal bones extending from the tarsus to the phalanges.

Metathalamus (*met'a-thal'a-mus*) The most caudal part of the thalamus composed of the medial and lateral geniculate bodies.

Metencephalon (*met'en-sef'a-lon*) The anterior of two major subdivisions of the rhombencephalon consisting of pons and cerebellum.

Meteorism (*met'e-o-rizm*) Tympanites.

Meter (*me'tar*) The base unit of length in the International System of Units that is equal to the distance traveled by light in a vacuum in $^1/_{299,792,458}$ second or to about 39.37 inches.

Metformin A biguanide oral hypoglycemic agent.

Methadone (*meth'a-don*) A synthetic, relatively long-acting oral opiate.

Methamphetamine A potent central nervous system stimulant that is mainly used as a recreational durg and less commonly as a second-line treatment for attention deficit hyperactivity disorder.

Methandriol Also known as methylandrostenedial, an androgen and anabolic steroid medication.

Methandrostenolone (*meth-an-dro'sten'o-lon*) An anabolic steroid possessing androgenic effects.

Methanol (*meth'a-nol*) A highly toxic polar alcohol used as an industrial solvent, often abused as an inebrient. It gets metabolized to formaldehyde and formate causing metabolic acidosis and damage to the optic nerve and blindness. Ethanol is used to reduce methanol metabolites and toxic effects.

Methapyrilene (*meth'a-pir'i-len*) An antihistaminic agent with sedative action.

Methaqualone Acts as a sedative, relieving anxiety and promoting sleep.

Methemalbumin (*met'he-mal-bu'min*) An albumin complex consisting of albumin and heme. The complex gives brown color to plasma and occurs in hemolytic and hemorrhagic disorders. Its presence in plasma is used to differentiate between hemorrhagic and edematous pancreatitis.

Methemoglobin (*met-he'mo-glo'bin*) A form of hemoglobin that has been oxidized, changing its heme iron configuration from the ferrous (Fe^{2+}) to the ferric (Fe^{3+}) state. Unlike normal hemoglobin, methemoglobin does not bind oxygen and as a result cannot deliver oxygen to the tissues.

Methenamine (hexamine) (*meth-en'a-men*) An anti- bacterial agent used in urinary tract infections.

Methenolone Androgen and anabolic steroid.

Methimazole (*methi-im'a-zol*) Antithyroid agent that inhibits synthesis of thyroid.

Methionine (*me-thi'o-nen*) A sulfur-containing essential amino acid.

Metixene An antiparkinson drug, a muscarinic antagonist and a histamine antagonist.

Methoserpidine Antihypertensive drug related to reserpine.

Methotrexate (*meth'o-trek-sat*) A folic acid antimetabolite used in choriocarcinoma and in combination with other agents for lymphoproliferative malignancy.

Methotrimeprazine Used in the management of psychosis, particularly those of schizophrenia and manic phases of bipolar disorder.

Methoxamine (*me-thok'sa-men*) An alpha adrenergic agonist used to treat hypotension.

Methoxyphenamine (*me-thok'si-fen'a-men*) Sympathomimetic bronchodilator.

Methyl alcohol (Methanol) CH_4O, solvent and antifreeze.

Methylcellulose (*meth'il-sel'u-los*) Hydrophilic colloid, used as bulk-making purgative and to adjust osmotic effects of lotions.

Methyclothiazide (*meth'i-klo-thi'a-zid*) [USP] A thiazide diuretic used for treatment of hypertension and edema; administered orally.

Methyldopa (*meth'il-do'pa*) A centrally acting antihypertensive, inhibits DOPA-decarboxylase.

Methylene blue (*meth'i-len*) A thiazine dye. Used as an indicator for the oxidation-reduction and as an agent to reduce methemoglobin. It is used in Wright-Giemsa stain and as a counter- stain.

Methylergonovine (*meth'il-er'go-no'vin*) [USP] An oxytocic used especially to prevent or combat postpartum or postabortion hemorrhage and atony; administered orally, intramuscularly, and intravenously.

Methylphenidate (*meth'il-fen'i-date*) An agent used to control attention deficit/hyperactivity disorder.

Methylprednisolone (*meth'il-pred-nis'o-lon*) A synthetic glucocorticosteroid.

Methyltestosterone (*meth'il-tes-tos'ter-on*) A methyl derivative of testosterone.

Methysergide (*meth'i-sur'jid*) Lysergic acid derivative, 5 HT antagonist used for prevention of migraine. Prolonged use is associated with retroperitoneal fibrosis.

Metoclopramide (*met'o-clo-pr'a-mide*) A prokinetic agent used as an antiemetic.

Metolazone (*me'tol'a-zon*) A thiazide diuretic.

Metoprolol (*met'o-pro'lol*) Adrenergic beta-blocker used in hypertension and arrhythmias.

Metr- (metro-) Combining word for uterus.

Metrectopia (*me'trek-to'pe-a*) Displacement of the uterus.

Metritis (*me-trit'is*) Inflammation of the uterus.

Metrocystosis (*me'tro-sis-to'sis*) Formation of cysts in uterus.

Metronidazole (*me'tro-ni'da-zol*) A nitroimidazole derivative having high activity against anaerobic bacteria and intestinal protozoa. It is effective against *Trichomonas vaginalis, Giardia lamblia* and *Entamoeba histolytica* and is active against infections caused by anaerobic bacteria, especially *B. fragilis*.

Metropathia Hemorrhagica (endometrial hyperplasia) Cystic glandular hyperplasia of endometrium resulting in abnormal, excessive uterine bleeding.

Metroptosis (*me'trop-to'sis*) Prolapse of the uterus.

Metrorrhagia (*me'tro-ra'je-a*) Irregular uterine bleeding superimposed on normal cycle.

MHC Major histocompatibility complex.

Mianserin Atypical antidepressant that is used primarily in the treatment of depression.

Miconazole (*mi-kon'a-zol*) Imidazole antifungal agent, topical for cutaneous candidiasis and intravenous for systemic candidiasis and intrathecal for cryptococcal meningitis.

Microadenoma (*mi'kro-ad'e-no'ma*) A pituitary adenoma of less than 1 cm in diameter.

Microaneurysm (*mi'kro-an'ur-izm*) Focal dilatation of capillaries occurring at arterio-capillary junctions, or at retinal capillaries.

Microangiopathy (*mi'kro-an'je-op'a-the*) Any defect of very small blood vessels, usually capillaries, common in diabetes mellitus.

Microbe (*mi'krob*) A microorganism including bacteria, spirochetes, rickettsiae and virus.

Microbiology (*mi'kro-bi-ol'o-je*) The science concerned with the study of microscopic and ultramicroscopic organisms.

Microblepharia (*mi'kro-ble-far'e-a*) A developmental abnormality wherein the eyelids have an abnormally small vertical dimension.

Microcephaly (*mi'kro-sefa-le*) Abnormally small brain.

Microhellia A congenital disorder where one's lips are unusually small.

Microcheiria (*mi'kro-ki're-a*) Abnormally small hands.

Microchimerism (*mik'ro-kemer-izm*) The intermingling of some cells from one person inside the body of another.

Micrococcus (*mi'kro-kok'us*) Pl. **micrococci.** A genus of bacteria belonging to the family of Micrococcaceae, that are gram-positive spherical cells. They occur in irregular masses, and are saprophytic or parasitic, such as *M. luteus.*

Microcyte (*mi'kro-sit*) A small non-nucleated red blood cell.

Hypochromic microcyte Smaller and paler microcyte.

Microcytotoxicity (*mi'kro-si'to-tok-sis-it-e*) Extremely minute quantities of substance damaging the cells.

Microcytosis Abnormally small size of red blood cells.

Microdactyly Abnormally small or short fingers.

Microdermabrasion (*mi'kro-der'ma-bra'zhun*) A cosmetic procedure for the skin that involves the mechanical abrasion and removal of all or part of the stratum corneum (as by a high pressure spray of granular crystals) and is used to rejuvenate the skin and to treat skin blemishes or imperfections.

Microdissection (*mi'kro-di-sek'shun*) Dissection of tissues under magnification.

Microdontia (*mi'kro-don'shi-a*) Markedly small dentition to the build of the body.

Microfilaria (*mi'kro-fi-la're-a*) Larvae of nematodes of the family Filarioidea. They are 170–320 microns long that migrate in blood or skin. The life cycle is completed when mosquitoes take up microfilariae while feeding on humans. Microfilariae appear in the blood at night and can be seen moving in a wet blood film.

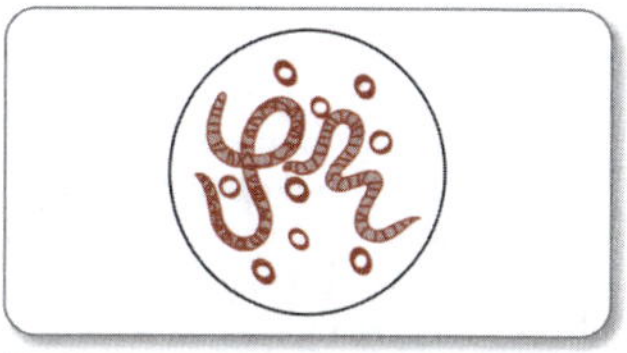

Microfilaria

Microgamete (*mi'kro-gam'et*) The smaller (male) of the two motile conjugating gametes in sexual cycle of plasmodium.

Microgametocyte (*mi'kro-ga-meto-sit*) The mother cell producing microgametes.

Microglia (*mi-krog'le-a*) Specialized form of macrophages in CNS.

Microglossia Abnormally small tongue.

Micrognathia (*mi'kro-nath'e-a*) Abnormally small jaws, especially mandible.

Microgram (*mi'kro-gram*) One millionth of a gram.

Micrograph (Photomicrograph) (*mi'kro-graf*) An instrument for magnifying and recording minute movements; photograph of an object or specimen as seen through a microscope; photograph taken through a light or electron microscope.

Microgyria (*mi'kro-ji're-a*) Shrinkage of convolutions from localized brain atrophy.

Microhematocrit A procedure for detemining the ratio of the volume of packed RBCs to the volume of whole blood by centrifuging a minute quantity of blood in a capillary tube coated with heparin.

Microinfarct (*mi'kro-in'farkt*) Very small infarct due to obstruction to the blood flow in arterioles or capillaries.

Micromanipulation (*mi'kro-ma-nip'u-la'shun*) Refers to the microscopic treatment of individual eggs, sperm, or embryos in an effort to improve fertilization and/or pregnancy rates. These techniques require specialized equipment and personnel.

Micromelia (*mi'kro-me'li-a*) Disproportionately small limbs.

Micrometastasis (*mi'kro-me-tas'ta-sis*) Metastasis in which the secondary deposits are too small to be detected.

Micrometer (*mi-krom'e-ter*) Thousandth of millimeter; a lens that is accurately marked for measuring microscopic forms.

Microorganism (microbe) (*mi'kro-or'ga-nizm*) A microscopic organism.

Microphakia (*mi'kro-fa'ke-a*) A congenital abnormality in which the lenses of the eye are small and spherical, often subjected to subluxation.

Microphotograph (*mi'kro-fot'o-graf*) A minute photograph of any object.

Micropipette (*mi'kro-pi-pet*) An extremely small pipette used to measure small quantities of liquids.

Micropsia (*mi'kro-p-se'a*) *psy* The visual perception that objects are smaller than they actually are.

Microradiography (*mi'kro-ra'de-og'ra-fe*) Technique of radiography of minute objects.

Microrefractometer (*mi'kro-re-frak-tom'it-er*) A refractometer used for the study of blood cells.

Microscope (*mi'kro-skop*) An instrument that gives an enlarged image of an object that is not visible to the naked eye.

Binocular microscope Microscope having two eye pieces.

Compound microscope Microscope having two or more lenses.

Dark field microscope A variant of light microscopy in which light is directed at an oblique angle and the specimen appears bright in a dark background, useful to observe spirochaetes.

Electron microscope A beam of electrons passes through the specimen providing a magnified image of an object on a fluorescent screen.

Fluorescent microscope A variant of light microscopy in which light is projected onto the specimen by halogen-quartz, mercury or xenon lamps and re-emitted at another wavelength.

Operative microscope Used in microsurgery.

Phase-contrast microscope Technique used to observe living cells.

Simple microscope Microscope consisting of a single magnifying lens.

Slit lamp microscope A low power light microscopy which has an attachment for examination of cornea.

Microscopic (*mi'kro-skop'ik*) Of extremely small size; visible only by the aid of the microscope; relating to a microscope or to microscopy.

Microsome (*mi'kro-som*) Smallest sized lipoprotein-rich cytoplasmic bodies, chiefly ribosomes.

Microsurgery (*mi'kro-surje-re*) Surgery utilizing operating microscope.

Microtome (*mi'kro-tom*) An instrument used to cut histological sections. The metal blades cut paraffin embedded tissues for high power microscopy and diamond blades cut plastic-embedded tissues for electron microscopy.

Microvillus (*mi'kro-vil'us*) Finger-like cell processes without showing complex structure of cilia. They are constructed of complex plasma membrane folds surrounding an actin microfilament core and form striated border of small intestinal mucosa to increase their cell surface area.

Microwave therapy A type of treatment in which body tissue is exposed to high temperatures to damage and kill cancer cells. Also called microwave thermotherapy.

Micturition (*mik'chur-a'shun*) Passing of urine.

Midbrain (mesencephon) (*mid'bran*) Upper segment of brain stem consisting of colliculi, tegmentum and cerebral peduncles.

Middle East Respiratory Syndrome A flulike respiratory infection that progresses to pneumonia caused by a corona virus with strong tropism for nonciliated bronchial epithelial cells; MERS.

Midgut (*mid'gut*) The central portion of the digestive tract, the small intestine; the portion of embryonic gut between the foregut and hindgut.

Midwifery (*mi'd-wif'ri*) Science dealing with care of women antepartum, intrapartum and postpartum.

Migraine (*mi'gran*) Paroxysmal headache, vomiting and focal usually visual, with malaise and irritability followed by a severe throbbing hemicranial headache, photophobia and vomiting. The etiology is unknown and there is a genetic predisposition with a great female preponderance.

Migraine equivalent A condition where the visual, sensory, motor or psychic disturbances are seen; characteristic of migraine is not followed by headache.

Migranous neuralgia A migraine variant with periodic unilateral periorbital pain, conjunctival injection, unilateral lacrimation and nasal congestion often in middle-aged male.

Miliaria (*mili'ar'e-a*) An eruption of minute vesicles and papules due to retention of sweat at the mouths of sweat follicles.

Miliaria rubra Prickly heat, papular lesions seen in persons exposed to hot environment especially in high humidity. They occur due to blockage of sweat glands by the prickle cell layer of epidermis.

Miliary (*mil'e-ar'e*) Like scattered millet seeds; characterized by lesions resembling millet seeds.

Miliary tuberculosis Presence of widespread lesions of tuberculosis occurring after a hematogenous dissemination of tubercle bacilli. It occurs in individuals who have inadequate cell-mediated immunity.

Milium (whitehead) (*mil'e-um*) Tiny keratin-filled cyst lying superficially within the skin, usually of face in the newborn.

Milk An opaque white liquid secreted by the mammary glands of female mammals serving for nourishment of their young; any whitish milky fluid; a pharmacopeial preparation containing a suspension of insoluble drugs in a water medium.

Milk teeth Temporary teeth of a young mammal (human) including four incisors, two canines and four molars in each jaw. These fall out during childhood and are replaced by the permanent teeth.

Millard-Gubler syndrome Paralysis of the lateral rectus with or without a lower motor neuron facial palsy and contralateral pyramidal tract signs due to a lesion in the pons, named after Auguste Millard and Adolphe Gubler, French physicians.

Miller-Fisher syndrome A variant of Guillain-Barre syndrome characterized by the acute onset of oculomotor dysfunction, ataxia, and loss of deep tendon reflexes with relative sparing of strength in the extensors and trunk, named after Charles Miller-Fisher, a Canadian Neurologist MFS.

Milliampere (*mil'e-am'per*) One thousandth of an ampere.

Milligram (*mili-gram*) (mg) One thousandth (10^{-3}) of a gram.

Milliliter (*mili-let'er*) (mL) One thousandth (10^{-3}) of a liter.

Millimeter (*mili-met'er*) (mm) One thousandth (10^{-3}) of a meter.

Milphosis (*mil'fo-sis*) The falling of eyelashes.

Milroy's edema Nonpitting edema due to congenital lymphatic deficiency, named after William Milroy, US physician.

Minamata disease Cerebral cortical atrophy due to methyl mercury poisoning, that occurred in Japan bay.

Mineralocorticoid (*min'er-al-o-kor'tikoid*) An adrenocortical hormone that influences sodium and potassium metabolism.

Minim (*min'im*) A unit of capacity such as liquid measure, equivalent of 0.0616 mL.

Minimal lesion nephropathy Common cause of nephrotic syndrome in children, which is immunologically mediated, follows infections and responds to immunosuppressants.

Minocycline (*mi-no-si'klen*) A semisynthetic antibiotic of tetracycline group.

Minoxidil (*mi-nok'si-dil*) A directly acting vasodilatory antihypertensive agent.

Miosis (myosis) (*mi-o'sis*) Contraction of the pupil; the period of decline of disease.

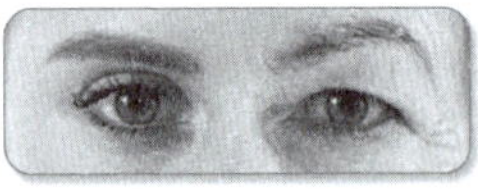

Miosis and eyelid ptosis of the left eye—Horner's syndrome

Miotic (*mi-ot'ik*) Pertaining to, characterized by or producing miosis; an agent producing miosis.

miRNA Micro RNA involved in regulation of gene expression through RNA interference.

Miracidium (*mi'ra-sid'e-um*) Free-swimming larva of schistosome, hatched in water to infect snails.

Mirtazapine (*mir"taz-a-pen*) An antidepressant compound unrelated to any of the classes of antidepressants; administered orally.

Miscarriage (*mis'kar-ij*) Loss of products of conception from the uterus before the fetus is viable.

Misopedia (*mis'o-pedea*) Hatred of children especially one's own.

Misoprostol (*mi-so-pros'tol*) A prostaglandin analog used to reduce the risk of NSAID related ulcers, manage miscarriages, prevent postpartum hemorrhage, and also for first trimester abortions.

Missed case A person suffering from a communicable disease in whom the symptoms and signs so minimal that either there is no request for medical assistance or the doctor fails to diagnose.

Mis-sense mutation The alteration of a single DNA nucleotide so resulting codon specifies different amino acids.

Mite (*mit*) A minute arthropod of the order Acarina that can act as a vector or intermediate host of pathogenic agents, or may cause dermatitis or tissue damage.

Mithramycin (*mith-ra-mi'sin*) A cytotoxic antibiotic from Streptomyces, used in teratoma and in hypercalcemia occurring in malignancy.

Mitobronitol A brominated analog of mannitol, is an anticancer agent, classified as an alkylating agent.

Mitochondria (*mi'to-kon'dre-a*) An organelle of the cell cytoplasm which is the main source of energy to the cell. It contains cytochrome enzymes. It has a smooth outercoat and an inner membrane arranged in the form of tubules or folds.

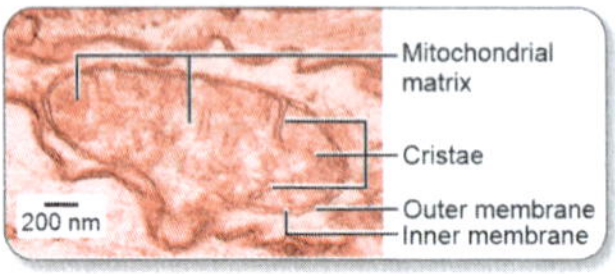

Electron micrograph of mitochondrion

Mitogen (*mi'to-jen*) A substance that induces mitosis especially in T cells.

Mitomycin (*mi'to-mi'sin*) An anti-tumor antibiotic from streptomyces.

Mitosis (*mi-to'sis*) Somatic cell division; process in which chromosomes duplicate and segregate during cell division.

Closed mitosis When the nuclear envelope persists.

Multipolar mitosis Aberrant mitotic figures, where the chromosomal material is pulled to more than two poles.

Open mitosis The segregation of chromosomes subsequent to nuclear envelope breakdown.

Pathologic mitosis Uncontrolled mitosis due to pathologic condition.

Mitotic Index The ratio between the number of population's cells undergoing mitosis to its total number of cells.

Mitoxantrone (*mi'to-zan'tron*) A chemotherapeutic agent used for the treatment of secondary progressive, progressive relapsing, or worsening relapsing-remitting multiple sclerosis.

Mitral (*mi'tral*) Relating to mitral or bicuspid valve; shaped like a bishop's miter.

Mitral stenosis Most common valvular lesion of rheumatic heart disease due to thickening of mitral cusps, fusion of valve commissures and shortening and fusion of chordae tendinae causing obstruction to the flow of blood across the mitral valve in diastole.

Mitral valvulotomy An operative procedure disrupting the fibrous union of the two cusps at either commissure.

Mitralization (*mi'tral-i-za'shun*) Straightening of the left border of the heart due to prominent left atrium and the pulmonary conus, an X-ray chest finding in mitral stenosis.

Mitral incompetence Occurs due to dilatation of the mitral annulus, shriveling of the cusps, alteration in the chordae, prolapse of the cusps, shortening of the cusps and rupture of chordae.

Mitral valve (bicuspid valve) (MVP) Barlow's syndrome, floppy valve syndrome, an abnormal displacement of one or both mitral leaflets into the left atrial cavity during systole. Presents with chest pain and a mid-systolic click.

Mitsuda reaction A skin test to detect delayed hypersensitivity in leprosy, subcutaneous injection of lepromin (Dharmendra antigen) giving a second reaction with induration 3–4 weeks after injection, named after Kensuke Mitsuda, Japanese physician.

Mittelschmerz (*mit'al-shmartz*) Pain associated with ovulation, usually occurring in the middle of the menstrual cycle.

Mixed connective tissue disease (MCTD) has signs and symptoms of a combination of disorders-primary lupus, scleroderma and polymyositis.

MLC (MLR) Medicolegal case.

MLD Minimum lethal dose.

mm Hg Millimeters of mercury, to measure blood pressure.

Mobitz type I block *ECG* Second degree heart block where PR interval increases progressively till a QRS is totally missed. Clinically the pulse exhibits a regular irregularity.

Mobitz type II block *ECG* Second degree heart block that is a very serious arrhythmia, it is mostly due to a block in His-Purkinje system. The PR interval of conducted beats is fixed; but some of the P waves fail to be conducted to the ventricles and are not followed by QRS. The P waves outnumber the QRS complexes.

Modafinil (*mo-dafi-nil"*) A central nervous system stimulant medication used to treat sleepiness due to narcolepsy, shift work sleep disorder, and obstructive sleep apnea.

Modality (*mo-dal'i-te*) Method of procedure; any form of therapeutic intervention; different forms of sensation.

Mode (*mod*) *stat* In a set of measurements the value which appears the most.

Modiolus (*mo-di'o-lus*) Conical bony axis of cochlea.

MODY Maturity-onset diabetes of the young, an autosomal dominant variant of NIDDM, and the responsible gene is located on the long arm of chromosome 20.

Molar tooth A tooth having a crown with four to five cusps on the grinding surface, attached to lower jaw with a bifid root and upper jaw with three conical roots. They are three in permanent dentition situated on either side behind premolars. Their number is two in deciduous dentition and are situated on either side behind the canines.

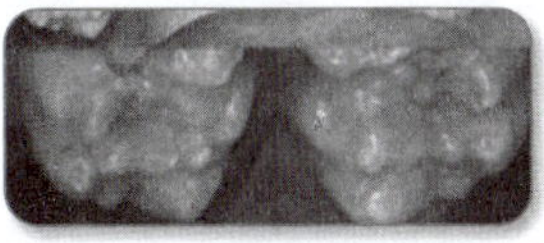

Mulberry molars in congenital syphilis

Molarity (*mo-lar'it-e*) The amount of substance of a solution that is expressed in moles of solute per liter of solution (mol/L).

Mold (*mold*) Fungi which produce spores.

Molding (*mold'ing*) Changes that the fetal skull undergoes to accommodate itself into the birth canal.

Molecular biology Study of biology at the molecular level, involving DNA, RNA and proteins.

Molluscum (*mo-lus'kum*) Any of small round superficial skin lumps.

Molluscum bodies Intracytoplasmic inclusion bodies seen within the epithelial cells of molluscum contagiosum.

Molluscum contagiosum A viral disease caused by a DNA pox virus, the largest virus affecting the human beings. The virus gets implanted on the skin by contact with other infected persons. It presents with pearly white or pink smooth surfaced papules of 2–10 mm size over any part of the body in diffusely scattered clusters.

Molluscum fibrosum Soft pink skin nodule of neurofibromatosis.

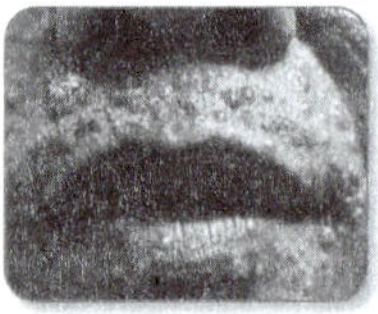

Molluscum contagiosum infection

Mongolism (*mong'go-lizm*) Down's syndrome; trisomy 21.

Monilia (*mo-nil'e-a*) Candida.

Moniliasis Candidiasis a yeast infection, caused by candida albicans.

Monoamine Oxidase (MAO) (MAO) Enzyme that converts methylamine groups to aldehydes.

Monoarthritis Inflammation of one joint rather than multiple joints.

Monoblast (*mon'o-blast*) An immature cell that develops into a monocyte.

Monochromat (*mon"o-kro'mat*) A person who has monochromatic vision; also called achromat.

Monoclonal antibody A highly specific antibody formed by fusing an immortal cell from mouse myeloma to a cell producing an antibody against a desired antigen.

Monocular (*mon-ok'ul-ar*) Relating to or having only one eye; having only one eye piece, as in microscope.

Monocyte (*mon'o-sit*) Large mononuclear leukocyte of blood.

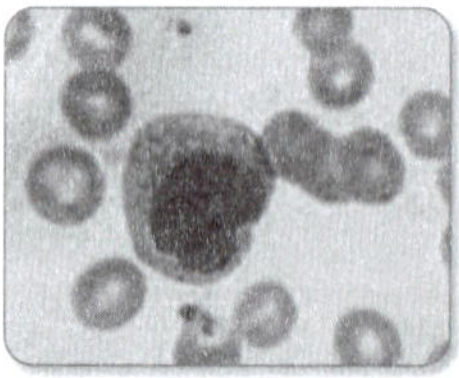

Monocyte

Monocytosis Increase in the number of monocytes in the blood seen in chronic infections, monocytic leukemia and Crohn's disease.

Monodactylism The congenital absence of all but digit on each hand and foot.

Monoiodotyrosine (*mon'o-i-o'-do-ti'ro-sen*) An amino acid intermediate in the synthesis of thyroxine and triiodothyronine.

Monomania (*mon'o-ma'ne-a*) Preoccupation with a single object.

Mononeuritis (*mon'o-nu-ri'tis*) Inflammation of a single nerve.

Mononucleosis (*mon'o-nu'kle-o'sis*) Presence of increased number of mononuclear leukocytes in the peripheral blood, especially forms that are not normal.

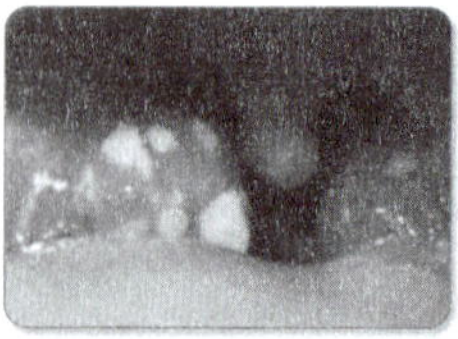

Severe pharyngotonsillitis caused by infectious mononucleosis

Infectious mononucleosis Glandular fever; an acute infectious disease caused by Epstein-Barr virus that occurs in young adults. The virus infects and replicates primarily in B lymphocytes. It presents with malaise, tiredness, headache, anorexia and fever. There is lymphadenopathy, splenomegaly, exudative tonsillitis and rash.

Monophobia A fear of dread of oneself being alone, isolated abandoned and ignored.

Monophyletic (*mon'o-fi-letik*) Having a single source of origin.

Monoplegia (*mon'o-ple'jea*) Paralysis of only one limb. adj. **monoplegic**.

Monorchism The state of having only one testicle within the scrotum.

Monosaccharide (*mon'o-sak'a-rid*) A simple sugar that cannot be further hydrolyzed.

Monosomy (*mon'o-so'me*) Presence of one chromosome only of a pair.

Monozygotic twins Genetically, identical twins formed by the division into two at an early stage in the development of an embryo derived from a single fertilized ovum.

Mons A prominence.

Mons pubis, Mons veneris The prominence caused by a pad of fatty tissue over the symphysis pubis in female.

Moraxella (*mo-rak'sel'a*) A genus of gram-negative coccobacillus that are parasitic on the mucous membrane of man and animals; *M. lacunata* causes conjunctivitis.

Morbid (*mor'bid*) Diseased or pathologic; *psy* abnormal or deviant.

Morbidity (*mor'bid'it-e*) Prevalence of the disease in a community; a diseased state.

Morbilli (*mor-bil'i*) Measles.

Morbilliform (*mor-bil'i-form*) Measles-like; resembling the eruptions of measles.

Morbus (*mor'bus*) Disease.

Mordant (*mord'ant*) A substance that fixes a stain or dye.

Moribund (*mor'i-bund*) In a dying state.

Morning sickness Pregnancy-related nausea, often accompanied by vomiting on getting up in the morning, noted in the first 2–12 weeks of gestation.

Moron (*mor'on*) Mentally subnormal.

Morphea (*mor'fe'a*) Localized scleroderma.

Deep morphea A variant of morphea (localized scleroderma) in which inflammation and sclerosis are found in the deep dermis, panniculus, fascia or superficial muscle.

Generalized morphea A form of scleroderma that involves isolated patches of hardened skin on the face, hands and feet, or anywhere else on the body, with no internal organ involvement.

Guttate morphea lesions Multiple and primarily involve the neck and the upper portion of the trunk. The lesions are small (<10 mm in diameter) and superficial, with less induration and a sharply demarcated border. The sclerotic lesions of guttate morphea are typically whitish in color.

Morphine (*mor'fen*) An opium alkaloid with powerful analgesic properties.

Morphology (*mor-fol'o-je*) The study of the structure of animals or plants.

Morqio-Brailsford disease A type of mucopolysaccharidoses; a rare disease with features of short stature, atlantoaxial instability with risk of cord damage, odontoid hypoplasia, spine deformities and restrictive lung disease.

Mortality (mortality rate) (*mor-tal'it-e*) The state of being mortal; death rate.

Early neonatal mortality Number of child deaths <7 days of life expressed as per 1,000 live births in the reference year.

Fetal mortality The number of fetal deaths per 1,000 live births per year.

Infant mortality The number of deaths of children less than one year per 1,000 live births per year.

Late neonatal mortality Number of child deaths of 7 days to 28 completed days of life expressed as per 1,000 live births in the reference year.

Maternal mortality The number of deaths of women during child bearing per 100,000 births.

Neonatal mortality The number of deaths of infants less than 28 days per 1,000 live births per year.

Perinatal mortality Number of deaths of fetuses weighing at least 500 g plus the number of early neonatal deaths, per 1,000 total births.

Post neonatal mortality Number of child deaths of 29 days to less than 1 year of age expressed as per 1,000 live births in the reference year.

Under-5 mortality Probability of dying between birth and exactly five years of age expressed per 1,000 live births.

Mortification (*mort'i-fi-ka'shun*) Gangrene; necrosis.

Morula (*mor'ula*) Earliest embryo as a solid clump of cells from first division occurring in fallopian tube.

Mosaicism (*mos'ay-sis'm*) A genetic condition resulting from a mutation crossing over, or nondisjunction of chromosomes during cell division causing a variation in the number of chromosomes in the cells.

Mosquito (*mus-keto*) A blood sucking dipterous insect of the family Culicidae which includes *Aedes*, *Anopheles*, *Culex* and *Haemagogus* and they act as vectors of many diseases including malaria, filariasis, dengue, viral encephalitis and yellow fever.

Motion sickness (travel sickness) A clinical manifestation occurring in response to real or apparent motion to which a person is not adapted and presents with nausea, pallor, sweating and vomiting.

Motor (*mot'er*) Producing motion; nerve structure by which impulses are generated and transmitted.

Motor neuron disease A group of chronic neurologic disorders that selectively affect with varying combination of the anterior horn cells of the spinal cord and lower brainstem.

MOTT Mycobacteria other than tuberculosis; also referred to as nontuberculous mycobacteria (NTM)—Mycobacteria other than *M. tuberculosis* and *M. bovis*, or atypical mycobacteria.

Mountain sickness Sudden exposure to altitude above 2,500 m may lead to hyperventilation, tachycardia, palpitation and headache resulting from lowered oxygen tension. In susceptible individuals untoward symptoms follow after 6 to 7 hours of ascent, in pulmonary (cough, dyspnea, giddiness, irritability, insomnia, convulsions) or hypoxic (muscle cramps, anorexia) forms.

Moxibustion (*mok'si-bu'stan*) A form of therapy that uses burning of mugwort leaves (a herb).

Moxisylyte A vasodilator that is used in urology for the erectile dysfunction. It is an α1–adrenergic antagonist.

MSH Melanocyte-stimulating hormone.

Mucilage (*myoo'se-lij*) A watery solution of gummy substance used as a vehicle or demulcent.

Mucin (*mu-sin*) A secretion containing mucopolysaccharides, such as that from mucous glands and it is also found in the ground and it is also found in the ground substance of connective tissue. adj. **mucinoid**.

Mucocele (*mu'ko-sel*) A benign, mucus-containing cystic lesion of the minor salivary gland. This type of lesion is most commonly referred to as mucocele. The more common is a mucus extravasation cyst; the other is a mucus retention cyst.

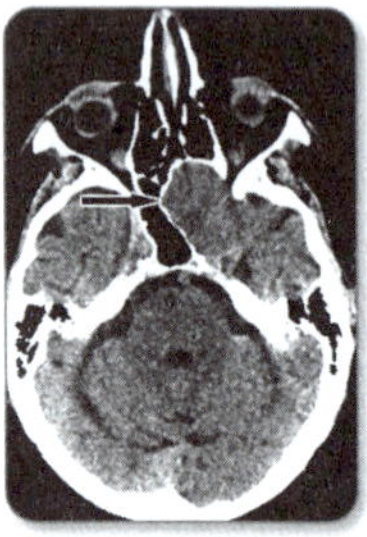

Mucocele

Mucolytic (*mu'ko-lit'ik*) Ability of reducing the viscosity of mucus; an agent that reduces the viscosity of mucus.

Mucopolysaccharide (*mu'ko-pol'i-sak'a-rid*) A group of polysaccharides containing hexosamine, including glycosaminoglycans and neutral polysaccharides; glycosaminoglycan.

Mucoprotein (*mu'ko-pro'ten*) A protein-polysaccharide complex.

Tamm-Horsfall mucoprotein A matrix of urinary casts derived from the ascending loop of Henle named, after Igor Tamm, Russian born US virologist and Frank Horsfall, US physician.

Mucopurulent (*mu'ko-pu'ru-lent*) Containing both mucus and pus.

Mucopus (*mu'ko-pus*) Mucus blended with pus.

Mucor (*mu'kor*) A genus of fungi found in dead or decaying matter, belong to the family of Mucoraceae and may cause mucormycosis.

Mucormycosis (*mu'kor-mi-ko'sis*) Infection with certain species of *Mucor*, *Rhizopus* and *Absidia*, common saprophytic fungi which can cause an opportunistic infection in the lung.

Mucosa (*mu-ko'sa*) Mucous membrane.

Mucoviscidosis (*mu'ko-vis'i-do-sis*) Cystic fibrosis.

Mucus (*mu'kus*) A clear viscid fluid that is produced by mucous membrane. It consists of mucopolysaccharides, enzymes, IgA and other proteins, desquamated epithelial cells and in organic salts.

MUGA scan (Multiple-gated arteriography) Uses a radioactive material that targets the heart, along with a gamma camera and a computer. It creates images of the blood flowing through the heart.

Mullerian duct Paramesonephric ducts from which in female the fallopian tubes, uterus and part of vagina develop; and in male appendix, testis and prostatic utricle, named after Johannes Muller, German physician.

Multifactorial diseases Diseases which result from an intervention of environmental factors with multiple genes at different loci.

Multifocal motor neuropathy A rare but treatable acquired motor neuropathy that may simulate motor neuron disease.

Multigravida (*mul'ti-grav'i-da*) A pregnant woman who has been pregnant one or more times previously.

Multipara (*mul-tip'a-ra*) A woman who has given birth at least two times to viable fetuses, whether alive or dead.

Multiple sclerosis (disseminated sclerosis) (MS) Disorder of CNS white matter with preservation of axons compared with loss of myelin. It presents with multiplicity of lesions with sclerotic appearance that are scattered throughout CNS. Relapses and remissions are common. It presents with muscle weakness, ocular disturbance, gait ataxia, paresthesia, dysarthria and mental disturbances.

Mummification (*mum'i-fi-ka'shun*) Dry gangrene; drying and shriveling of a body as a dead and retained fetus.

Mumps An inflammatory disease caused by a paramyxovirus infection leading to acute painful inflammation of the parotid and occasionally other salivary glands. Orchitis, oophoritis, pancreatitis, meningitis and encephalitis may occur as complications.

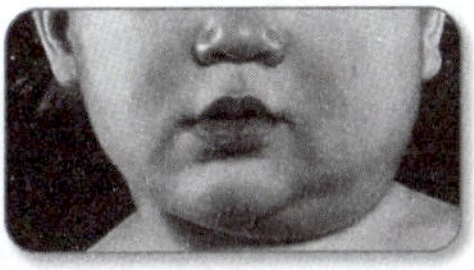

Mumps of left side

Munchausen syndrome (*mun-chou'zen*) Repeated feigning of major disorders to obtain hospital admissions, name derived from Baron Karl Munchausen, a fictional literary character; a subtype of factitious disorder.

Murmur (bruit) (*mur'mur*) Vibrations heard due to a turbulent blood flow with an increase in its velocity at or near a valve or of an abnormal communication within the heart. They are audible on auscultation of the heart, or blood vessels.

Aortic diastolic murmur Failure of cusps of aortic valves coming in apposition during the diastole resulting in a high pitched soft blowing murmur.

Aortic systolic murmur An ejection systolic murmur heard in aortic stenosis, dilatation of the ascending aorta, and in hyperkinetic states.

Apical diastolic murmur A diastolic filling murmur at the apex.

Austin-Flint murmur A diastolic rumble at the apex in severe aortic incompetence.

Cardiac murmur A murmur produced within the heart.

Cardiopulmonary murmur An innocent murmur synchronous with the heartbeat, that disappears when the breath is held.

Carey Coombs murmur A short lived diastolic murmur at the apex in mitral valvulitis due to acute rheumatic fever.

Continuous murmur Murmur heard continuously during systole and diastole due to continuous flow of blood through an abnormal communication from a region of high pressure to low pressure with a large pressure gradient between the two regions.

Crescendo murmur A murmur increasing in its intensity due to atrial systole facilitating increased blood flow across the stenotic valve from left atrium to the left ventricle.

Diastolic murmur A murmur heard during diastole.

Duroziez murmur Systolic and diastolic murmur audible on compression of femoral artery in aortic incompetence.

Ejection murmur Murmur produced by the forward flow of blood across the right or left ventricular outflow tract. Murmur is midsystolic, medium pitched with intensity ascending and descending in a diamond-shaped configuration.

Flint murmur Austin-Flint murmur.

Flow murmur Increased velocity and volume of blood flow across a normal mitral valve producing short mid-diastolic rumble at the apex.

Gibson's murmur A machinery murmur audible over left second and third intercostal space near the sternum in patent ductus arteriosus.

Graham Steell's murmur An early diastolic murmur in the second left intercostal space next to sternum heard in pulmonary incompetence.

Hemic murmur Faint systolic murmur over the pulmonary area and to a lesser extent over the apex in severe anemia.

Innocent murmur Functional murmur.

Late systolic murmur Heard at the apex in mild mitral incompetence due to an unusual distortion of the mitral valve leaflet, chordae tendinae or papillary muscles.

Machinery murmur Gibson's murmur.

Mitral diastolic murmur Narrowing of the orifice of the mitral valve causing a low pitched, rumbling mid-diastolic murmur.

Mitral systolic murmur A soft blowing pansystolic murmur at the apex, that is conducted toward the axilla due mitral valve incompetence.

Obstructive murmur A murmur produced as a result of a forward flow of blood across a stenosed region.

Organic murmur Murmur when arises from the damaged heart.

Pansystolic murmur A murmur begins with the first heart sound and continues through to the second heart sound. The intensity of the murmur is uniform.

Presystolic murmur Atrial systolic ejection murmur.

Pulmonary diastolic murmur Graham Steell's murmur.

Pulmonary systolic murmur An early to midsystolic murmur of FDA or tricuspid stenosis audible at the apex due to transmission of the murmur.

Tricuspid regurgitant murmur A pansystolic murmur heard over tricuspid area that tends to get louder on inspiration.

Tricuspid stenotic murmur A low pitched presystolic scratchy murmur audible near the lower end of sternum and it has a crescendo-decrescendo character.

Muscarinic receptors Cholinergic receptors mostly of parasympathetic nervous system stimulated by muscarine.

Muscle (*mus'l*) Tissue composed of contractile cells or fibers that cause movement of an organ or part of the body. They are classified as skeletal, cardiac or smooth muscles.

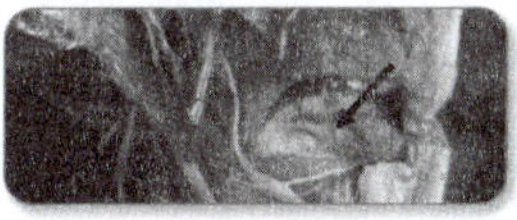

Genioglossus muscle (arrow showing)

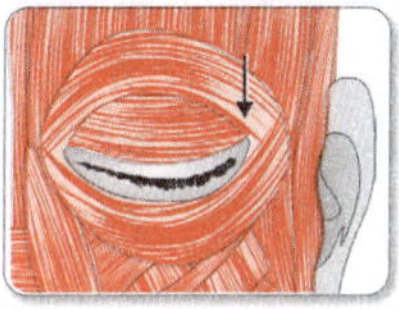

Orbicularis oculi muscle (arrow showing)

Muscle relaxant A drug to reduce muscle tone.

Muscle spindle Small voluntary muscle fibers covered by sensory nerve endings.

Muscular cirrhosis of the lung Pulmonary muscular hyperplasia, a variant of diffuse fibrosing alveolitis presenting with honeycombing radiologically.

Muscular dystrophy A group of muscular diseases that cause progressive weakness and loss of muscle mass.

Muscularis (*mus'ku-la'ris*) Relating to muscle coat of a hollow organ or tubular structure.

Muscularis mucosa Unstriated muscular tissue layer of mucous membrane.

Musculocutaneous (*mus'ku-lo-kut'e-neus*) Pertaining to or comprising the skeleton and the muscles, as musculoskeletal system.

Musculophrenic (*mus'ku-lo-fren'ik*) Belonging to or supplying both the diaphragm and the adjoining muscles.

Musculotendinous (*mus'ku-lo-ten'di-nus*) Belonging to or composed of muscle and tendon.

Mutagen (*mu'ta-jen*) An agent that causes genetic mutations.

Mutant (*mut'nt*) An organism that has undergone genetic mutation; produced by mutation.

Mutation (*mu-te'shun*) An alteration in genetic material. It could be a single base change (point mutation) or more extensive losses of DNA (deletion).

Nonsense mutation A single DNA base change resulting in a premature stop codon, there is gene mutation that ends the gene rather than continuing with the sequence of base pairs.

Point mutation Genetic change involving a single base pair.

Mutism (*mut'izm*) Inability to speak.

Akinetic mutism A situation of being immobile or silent with loss of emotional feeling due to lesions of the upper brain stem.

Elective mutism Inability to speak due to hysteria.

Mutualism (*mu'chu-al-iz-m*) An interaction between individuals of different species that results in positive (beneficial) effects on per capita reproduction and/or survival of the interacting populations.

My- (myo-) Combining word for muscle.

Myalgia (*mi-al'je-a*) Pain in a muscle.

Myasthenia gravis A defect at neuromuscular junction, wherein the antibodies against acetylcholine receptors do not permit acetylcholine to combine with the receptors, thus blocking the chemical transmission. The thymus gland acts as a source of antigen directing humoral and cellular immune responses. There is easy fatigability of muscles, worsened on exertion and the disability is relieved by rest. Diplopia, ptosis, ophthalmoplegia, dysphagia and dysphonia occur due to involvement of muscles supplied by cranial nerves.

Myatonia (*mi-at'o-nea*) Defective muscle tone.

Myatrophy (*mi-at'ro-fe*) Atrophy of a muscle.

Mycelium (*mi-se'le-um*) Mass of interlaced hyphae (fungus) or of filamentous bacteria (actinomycetes).

Mycetoma (*mi-se-to'ma*) A chronic granulomatous inflammation caused by several species of fungi or actinomycetes.

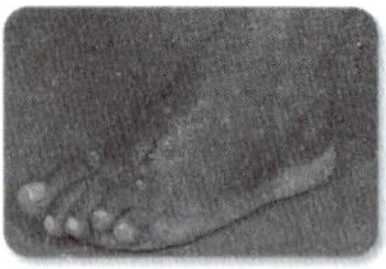

Mycetoma

Mycobacterium (*mi'ko-bak-ter'e-um*) A genus of aerobic nonmotile, gram-positive acid-fast bacteria, belonging to the family Mycobacteriaceae. It consists of parasitic and saprophytic species. pl. **mycobacteria**. *M. avium*, complex causes a chronic pulmonary disease resembling tuberculosis. *M. balnei* (formerly known as *M. marinum*) causes swimming pool granuloma.

Mycobacterium bovis Causative agent of tuberculosis in cattle, transmitted to man through milk.

Mycobacterium kansasii A photochromogen produces a chronic pulmonary disease resembling tuberculosis.

Mycobacterium leprae An obligate parasitic species which causes leprosy.

Mycobacterium marinum A species causing swimming pool granuloma.

Mycobacterium scrofulaceum A scotochromogen causes cervical lymphadenitis exclusively in children.

Mycobacterium tuberculosis The tubercle bacillus, the cause of tuberculosis in man, most commonly of the lungs.

Nontuberculous mycobacterium (NTM) Ubiquitously distributed in the environment and can cause disease similar to tuberculosis, also celled atypical mycobacteria, anonymous mycobacteria, or mycobacteria other than *M. tuberculosis.*

Mycology (*mi-kol'o-je*) The science concerned with the study of fungi.

Mycoplasma (*mi'ko-plaz'ma*) An incomplete intracellular and extracellular infectious particle that causes pneumonia and genitourinary infection.

Mycoplasma agalactiae A species of bacteria in the genus Mycoplasma. This genus of bacteria lacks a cell wall around their cell membrane, a small fastidious bacterium which has no cell wall and a very small genome. It is resistant to penicillin, the etiologic agent associated with the specific disease entity contagious mastitis.

Mycoplasma hominis A species of bacteria in the genus Mycoplasma. M. hominis has the ability to penetrate the interior of human cells. a potential underestimated pathogen causing both genitourinary and extragenital infections including neonatal infections.

Mycoplasma pneumoniae A very small bacterium in the class Mollicutes. It is a human pathogen that causes the disease mycoplasma pneumonia, a form of atypical bacterial pneumonia related to cold agglutinin disease. M. pneumoniae is characterized by the absence of a peptidoglycan cell wall and resulting resistance to many antibacterial agents. The persistence of M. pneumoniae infections even after treatment is associated with its ability to mimic host cell surface composition.

Mycosis (*mi-ko'sis*) Fungal infection.

Deep mycosis fungal infection involving subcutaneous tissue and organs.

Subcutaneous mycosis Subcutaneous fungal infection such as sporotrichosis, chromomycosis, phycomycosis and rhinosporidiosis.

Superficial mycosis Fungal infection limited to the dead keratinized tissue of the skin wherein the cellular response of the host is minimal and it includes superficial mycoses and dermatophytosis.

Systemic mycosis Fungal infection affecting various systems of the body.

Mycosis fungoides Cutaneous T cell lymphoma.

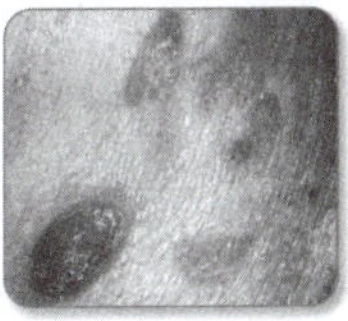

Mycosis fungoides

Mydriasis (*mi'dri-a'sis*) Dilatation of pupil.

Mydriatic (*mi'dre-at'ik*) Mydriasis; drug causing dilatation of pupil.

Myectomy (*mi-ek'to-me*) Excision of a muscle.

Myel- (myelo-) Combining word for marrow, spinal cord.

Myelencephalon (*mi'il-en-sef'a-lon*) Medulla oblongata.

Myelin (*mi'e-lin*) A complex lipid material of axon sheath. It is rich in cerebrosides and phosphatidyl ethanolamine.

Myelinated (medullated) nerve fiber (*mi'a-li-nat''ad*) Having a myelin sheath.

Myelinated (*mi'a-li-nat''ad*) Having a myelin sheath.

Myelinization (*mi'e-lin'i-za'shun*) Formation of a myelin sheath around a nerve fiber.

Myelitis (*mi'e-li'tis*) Inflammatory lesions of the spinal cord encompassing which may be infective or noninfective.

Acute necrotic myelitis A necrotizing myelitis affecting the white matter of the cord, characterized by acute onset paraplegia or quadriplegia with sensory deficit and sphincter paralysis.

Ascending myelitis Symptoms of spinal syndrome ascending progressively.

Transverse myelitis Transverse and complete spinal syndrome with flaccid paralysis, sensory loss below the lesion, presence of a zone of increased sensation between the area of sensory loss and the area of normal sensation, and involvement of bladder.

Myeloblast (*mi'e-lo-blast*) Earliest recognizable granulocyte precursor. It has basophilic cytoplasm without granules.

Myelocele (*mi'e-lo-cel*) Protrusion of the spinal cord through a defect in the vertebral column.

Myelocyte (*mi'e-lo-sit*) Granulocyte precursor in the bone marrow. It has a round nucleus with numerous granules in the cytoplasm.

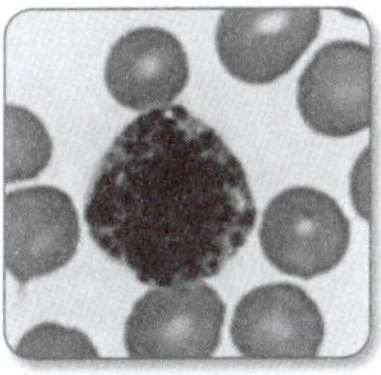

Neutrophilic myelocyte

Myelofibrosis (*mi'e-lo-fi-bro'sis*) Replacement of bone marrow by fibrous tissue. There is extramedullary hemopoiesis with massive splenomegaly.

Myelography (*mi'e-log'ra-fe*) X-ray to demonstrate spinal subarachnoid space, taken after introduction of contrast agent into the theca and positioning the patient to allow the dye to pass up or down.

Myeloid (*mi'e-loid*) Pertaining to or derived from bone marrow; spinal cord; pertaining to certain features of myelocytic forms in the bone marrow.

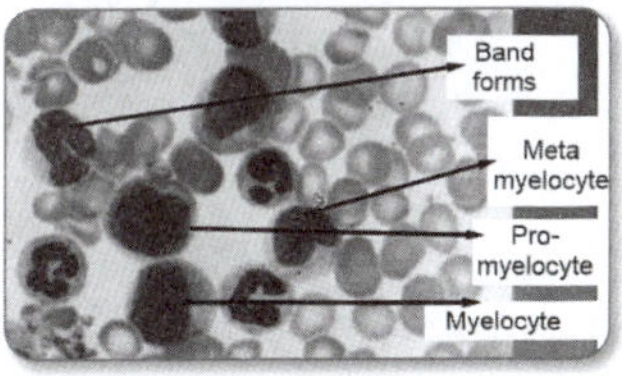

Myeloid leukemia

Myeloid metaplasia Spleen and liver with a leukoerythroblastic blood picture.

Myeloid leukemia A disorder of unrestrained and excessive proliferation of hematopoietic tissue showing full range of granulocyte precursors from myeloblasts to mature neutrophils in the peripheral blood. It is associated with extramedullary hemopoiesis with active marrow tissue.

Myeloma (multiple myeloma, myelomatosis) (*mi'e-lo-ma*) A tumor composed of cells derived from hemopoietic tissue of bone marrow.

Multiple myeloma A malignant proliferation of plasma cells. The plasma cells produce an immunoglobulin of a single heavy and light chain. The malignant plasma cells are present in the bone marrow and a small number in the peripheral blood. It causes bone erosion, pathological fracture, renal damage, increased blood viscosity and impaired immune function.

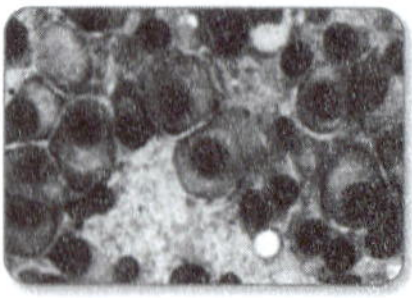

Multiple myeloma in bone marrow with large plasma cells

Myelomatosis (*mi'e-lo-ma-to'sis*) Multiple myeloma.

Myelomeningocele (*mi'e-lo-me-ning'go-sel*) Hernia protrusion of the spinal cord and its meninges through a defect in the vertebral column.

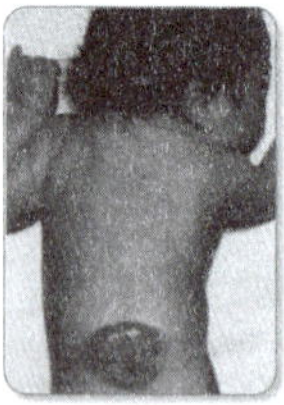

Myelomeningocele

Myelosuppression (*mi'e-lo-su-presh'un*) Bone marrow suppression.

Myenteron (*mi-en'ter-on*) The muscular coat of the intestine.

Myiasis Invasion of tissues or body cavities by the maggots (larvae) of dipterous flies.

Mylohyoid (*mi'elo-hi'oid*) Belonging to molar teeth and the hyoid bone.

Myoblast (*mi'o-blast*) A primitive muscle cell.

Myocardial infarction Myocardial damage, due to the formation of occlusive thrombus at the site of rupture of an atheromatous plaque in a coronary artery. It presents with pain, breathlessness, anxiety, nausea, vomiting, collapse or syncope.

Myocarditis (*mi'o-kar-di'tis*) An acute inflammatory condition that may complicate a wide variety of infections, mostly from viruses. It may present with inappropriate tachycardia or fulminant heart failure. Some forms may lead to chronic low grade myocarditis or dilated cardiomyopathy.

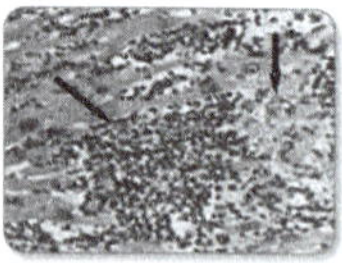

Infectious myocarditis

Bacterial myocarditis Myocarditis due to bacterial infection.

Giant cell myocarditis A rare, rapidly progressive, and frequently fatal myocardial disease in young and middle-aged adults. The disease due to T-cell lymphocyte-mediated inflammation of the myocardial mucles.

Hypersensitivity myocarditis An inflammatory disease of the myocardium usually related to a drug allergy.

Idiopathic myocarditis Rare, malignant, autoimmune myocarditis which is histopathologically characterized by multinucleated giant cells, myocyte necrosis, and infiltration of inflammatory lymphocytes.

Parenchymatous myocarditis Myocarditis in the parenchymal cell.

Protozoal myocarditis An inflammatory disease of the myocardium usually related to protozoal infection.

Rheumatic myocarditis A condition in which the heart valves have been permanently damaged by rheumatic fever.

Tuberculous myocarditis An inflammatory disease of the myocardium related to secondary infection of tuberculosis.

Viral myocarditis An inflammatory disease of the myocardium usually related to viral infection.

Myocardium (*mi'o-kar'de-um*) The middle and thickest layer of the heart wall composed of cardiac muscle.

Myoclonus (*mi-ok'lo-nus*) A brief involuntary random muscle contraction occurring either with rest, in response to sensory stimuli, or with voluntary movements.

Myocyte (*mi'o-sit*) A muscle cell.

Myodystonia (*mi'o-dis-to'ne-a*) A disorder of muscular tone characterized by slow relaxation interrupted by a succession of slight contractions following an electrical stimulation of a muscle.

Myoepithelium (*mi'o-ep'i-the'le-um*) Contractile cells forming outer layer of secretory epithelium, as of breast, salivary and sweat glands.

Myofibril (*mi'o-fi'bril*) One of the slender, longitudinal fibrils occurring in a skeletal or cardiac muscle fiber.

Myogenic (*mi'o-jen'ik*) The development of muscle tissue, especially its embryonic development.

Myoglobin (*mi'o-glo'bin*) Hemoglobin in the muscle having one heme per globin unit instead of four.

Myoglobinuria Metabolic abnormality in which the muscle becomes starved for energy, leading to release of myoglobin into the circulation; causing brown discoloration of the urine and increases the risk of acute renal failure.

Myograph (*mi'o-graf*) An instrument by which tracings are made of muscle contraction.

Myokymia (*mi'o-ki-me-a*) Irregular twitching of muscle fibers.

Myology (*mi-ol'o-je*) The branch of science concerned with the study of the muscles and their parts.

Myoma (*mi-o-ma*) A benign tumor of muscle tissue.

Myomectomy (*mi'o-mek-to-me*) Surgical removal of a myoma, specifically of a uterine myoma.

Myometritis (*mi'o-me-trit'is*) Inflammation of the muscular wall of the uterus.

Myometrium (*mi'o-me'tre-um*) The muscular wall of the uterus .

Myoneural junction A functional unit consisting of highly specialised structures neuromuscular junction.

Myopathy (*mi-op-a-the*) Any abnormality of the muscular tissue especially involving the skeletal muscle.

Carcinomatous myopathy Eaton-Lambert syndrome.

Centronuclear myopathy Slowly progressive generalized muscle weakness and atrophy beginning in childhood. The nuclei of most muscle fibers are found near the center of the fiber.

Congenital myopathy An inherited disorder, central core disease with its gene being located on chromosome 19, associated with structural changes in muscle fibers, floppy at birth or early childhood, generally nonprogressive, weakness more prominent in proximal muscles.

Distal myopathy Myopathy affecting predominantly distal portions of the limbs, has an autosomal dominant inheritance.

Myotubular myopathy Centronuclear myopathy.

Nemaline myopathy Myopathy with dystrophic facial features and skeletal deformities, deteriorates rapidly.

Ocular myopathy Begins in early childhood with bilateral symmetrical ptosis and progressive external ophthalmoplegia.

Proximal myotonic myopathy Autosomal dominant condition with proximal muscle weakness, cataract and myotonia.

Thyrotoxic myopathy Generalized muscle weakness with predilection to girdle muscles in thyrotoxicosis.

Myopia (nearsightedness) (*mi-o'pe-a*) Short sight in which parallel rays entering the eye focus in front of the retina. adj. **myopic**.

Curvature myopia Myopia due to excessive corneal curvature.

Index myopia Myopia doe to abnormal refractivity of the media of the eye.

Malignant myopia Progressive myopia leading to retinal detachment and blindness.

Progressive myopia Myopia increasing during adult life.

Myoplasm (*mi-o-plazm*) The contractile part of muscle cell.

Myoplasty (*mi'o-plas'te*) Plastic surgery of muscle tissue.

Myosarcoma (*mi-o-sar-ko'ma*) A malignant tumor derived from muscle tissue.

Myosin (*mi'o-sin*) Fibrous protein of skeletal and heart muscle.

Myositis (*mi'o-sit'is*) Inflammation of a muscle.

Inclusion body myositis A progressive inflammatory myopathy affecting muscles of pelvis and lower limbs.

Multiple myositis Polymyositis.

Myositis epidemic Pleurodynia.

Myositis fibrosa Induration of a muscle through an interstitial growth of fibrous tissue.

Myositis ossificans Myositis accompanied by calcium deposits in the muscle.

Myositis purulenta Suppurative myositis with abscesses.

Traumatic myositis Myositis due to injury.

Trichinous myositis Myositis due to the presence of *Trichinella spiralis*.

Myotatic reflex Muscle contraction in response to stretching a muscle.

Myotome (*mi'o-tom*) A knife used for cutting muscles; that part of an embryonic somite that gives rise to striated muscle; all muscles derived from one somite and innervated from a single spinal segment.

Myotomy (*mi-ot'o-me*) The cutting or dissection of a muscle or of muscular tissue.

Myotonia (*mi'o-to-ne-a*) Delayed relaxation after contraction.

Myotonia congenita An inherited condition beginning in early childhood characterized by difficulty in getting up and walking, difficulty in relaxing a grip, and generalized muscular hypertrophy. There is reduced chloride membrane conductance and reduced number of chloride channels.

Myotonic An inability to relax muscles at will.

Myotonus (*mi-ot'o-nus*) A tonic spasm of muscle.

Myringa (*mi-ring'ga*) The tympanic membrane.

Myringitis (*mir'in-jit'is*) Inflammation of tympanic membrane.

Bullous myringitis An infectious condition characterized by bullae or vesicles on tympanic membrane.

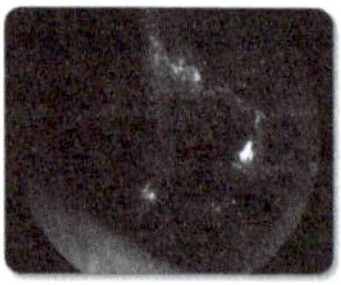

Bullous myringitis

Myringoplasty (tympanoplasty) Replacement of eardrum with temporal fascia.

Myringotomy (tympanotomy) (*mir'in-got'o-me*) Tympanectomy.

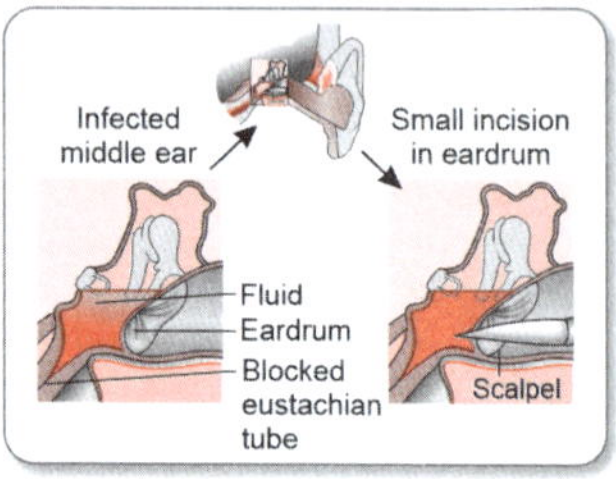

Myringotomy

Myxedema (*mik'se-de'ma*) Primary hypothyroidism in juveniles and adults, it has an insidious onset, slowing of activities, lethargy, somnolence, constipation, gain in weight, increased sensitivity to cold, accumulation of fluid and adipose tissue, lusterless thick, dry skin with scanty hair, husky voice, and nonpitting edema.

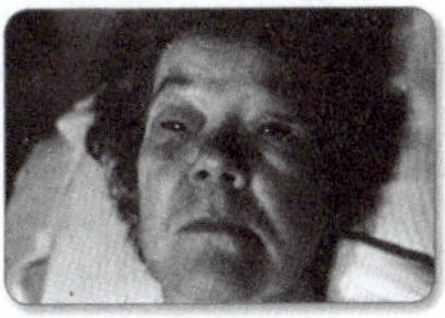

Myxedema in adult hypothyroidism

Myxedema coma Untreated cases of myxedema leading to somnolence, stupor and coma.

Myxedema madness Psychiatric disturbance in myxedema.

Pretibial myxedema Localized myxedematous deposits in front of the leg in hyperthyroidism.

Myxofibroma (*mik'so-fi-bro'ma*) A benign fibrous connective tissue tumor which contains primitive mesenchymal tissues.

Myxoma (*mik'so'ma*) A slow growing soft, lobulated tumor occurring in subcutaneous tissue, spinal cord, urinary bladder, bones and heart.

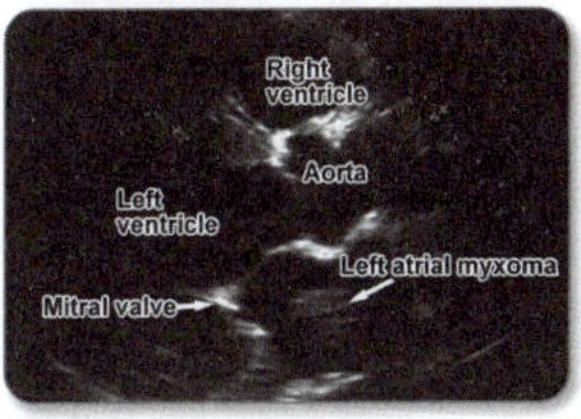

Left atrial myxoma

Myxosarcoma (*mik'so-sar-ko'ma*) A sarcoma containing tissue having resemblance to primitive mesenchymal tissue.

Myxovirus (*mik'so-virus*) RNA viruses having affinity to mucous surfaces. Includes influenza viruses A, B and C and parainfluenza and respiratory syncytial virus that cause the respiratory infections.

N

Nabothian cyst (*nabo'the'-en*) A cyst formed in a nabothian gland of uterine cervix. It appears pearly white and firm has no adverse effects.

Nabothian gland One of many small, mucus-secreting glands of uterine cervix, named after Martin Naboth, German physician.

NAD (nicotinamide adenine dinucleotide) No appreciable disease; nothing abnormal detected.

Nadolol (*nad'e-lol*) A β-adrenergic blocking agent, used in treatment of hypertension and angina pectoris.

NADP Nicotinamide adenine dinucleotide phosphate.

Naegleria Free-living soil amoebae that may produce primary amoebic meningoencephalitis. The organisms are carried in the nose and the throat of asymptomatic carriers.

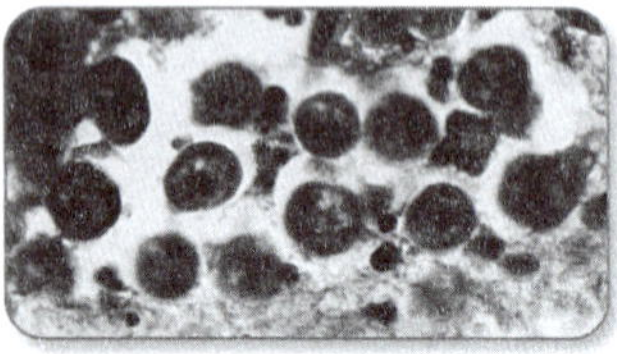

Naegleria fowleri in brain tissue

Naegele's obliquity The sagittal suture nearer the promontory than the symphysis when the vertex engages in the pelvic brim; anterior asynclitism.

Naga sore Tropical skin ulcer.

Nail (*nal*) An epidermal plate with keratin covering the sensitive tips of the fingers and toes; a slender metallic rod used in operation to fasten pieces of broken bone. pl. **nails**.

Brittle nail Weakening of nail edges with splitting and softening often due to effects of solvents, detergents and soaps.

Hippocratic nail The coarse curved nail of a clubbed finger; *see* Clubbed digits.

Ingrown nail Growth of the nail edge into the soft tissue, a result of improper pairing of the nails or pressure on a nail edge from improperly fitted footwear.

Nail bed The portion of the tip of a finger or toe covered by the root and body of the nail.

Nail biting A neurotic condition wherein the edges of the nails are bitten.

Nail fold A fold of skin supporting the nail at its base.

Nail groove A shallow depression between the nail bed and the nail wall.

Nail patella syndrome An autosomal dominant disease involving structures of mesodermal and ectodermal origin and presenting with defective nails of thumb and great toe, flexion contraction of multiple joints, defective or absent patellae, lordosis, renal abnormalities, exostosis of ileum and pigmentary anomalies of iris, cataract, microcornea and ptosis; hereditary osteo-onychodysplasia.

Nail plate The hard portion of the dorsum of the fingers and thumb.

Smith-Petersen nail A three-fanged nail to fix the fractures of the neck of the femur devised by Marius Smith Petersen, US orthopedic surgeon.

Spoon nail Koilonychias, a nail with depressed center and elevated lateral edges seen in iron deficiency anemia.

Terry nail's Apparent leukonychia in which the white discoloration affects the entire nail except for 1–2 mm at the distal margin; it is frequently seen in cirrhosis, congestive heart failure, and certain other conditions.

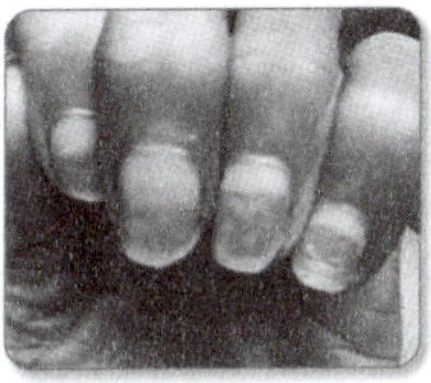

Terry nails

Nalidixic acid (*nal-i-diks'ik*) A quinolone preparation active against bacterial urinary tract infections.

Nalorphine (*nal'or-fen*) A morphine antagonist.

Nandrolone (*nan'dro-lon*) An anabolic androgenic steroid.

Nano- Division by 10^9, dwarf.

Nanometer (nm) (*nan'o-me"ter*) One billionth (10^{-9}) of a meter.

Naphazoline (*naf-az'o-len*) A vasoconstrictor used as a topical nasal decongestant and as a mydriatic.

Naprapathy (*nap'ra-pathe*) Treatment of disease by manipulation of joints, muscles and ligaments, and nutritional therapy.

Naproxen (*ne-prok'sen*) A nonsteroid anti-inflammatory drug.

Narcissism (*nar'si-sizm*) Self-love, which may include sexual attraction toward self.

Primary narcissism The earliest type of narcissism, in which the infant's libido is directed toward his or her own body and its satisfaction rather than toward the environment or objects.

Secondary narcissism The isolation may be necessary to carry out the self-soothing grandiose fantasies as well as the focus on love for the self.

Narco Illegal drugs.

Narcolepsy (*nar'ko-lep'se*) A sudden collapse into sleep at irregular intervals during daytime whose cause is undetermined.

Narcosis (*nar-ko'sis*) Depression of neuronal excitability causing stupor/ or sleep.

Basal narcosis Preliminary unconsciousness induced in a patient by administration of an opioid drug prior to administration of a general anesthetic by inhalation.

Carbon dioxide narcosis A clinical picture of lethargy, drowsiness, flapping tremors, altered consciousness due to sudden increase in arterial carbon dioxide tension.

Nitrogen narcosis Also known as depth intoxication or rapture of the deep, is a change in consciousness and neuromuscular function caused by breathing compressed inert gas.

Narcotic (*nar-kot'ik*) A substance capable of inducing stupor and insensibility.

Narcotic addict A person who has become dependent on narcotics.

Narcotic analgesics Pain killing drugs used in the treatment of pain. They diminish perception of pain by combining with pain receptors on brain cells and block transmission of pain signals.

Narcotic antagonist A drug used in the treatment of narcotic-induced respiratory depression, such as nalorphine and naloxone.

Narcotic poisoning Poisoning by narcotics which causes depression, decreased heart rate and respiration, sleep and coma.

Nares (*na'rez*) (sing, na'ris) The external orifices of the nose; called also nostrils.

Nasal bone Either of two small bones forming the arch of the nose.

Nasal cavity One of a pair of cavities that open on the face through the pear-shaped anterior nasal aperture and communicate with the pharynx.

Nasal concha turbinate bone Bony plates located on the lateral wall of the nasal cavity.

Nasion (*na'ze-on*) A point on the skull which corresponds to middle of the nasofrontal suture; the depression at the root of the nose.

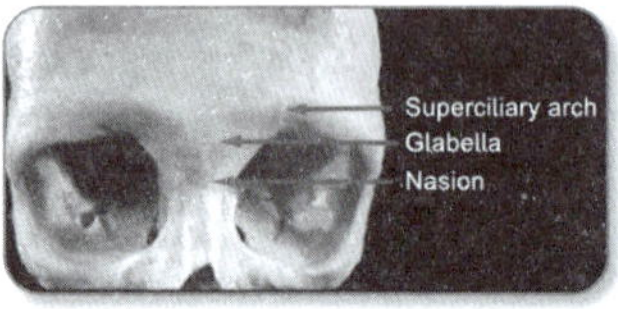

Nasion

Nasogastric tube A narrow plastic or rubber tube that is passed through the nose down esophagus and into the stomach to introduce fluids into or remove secretions from the stomach.

Nasolacrimal (*na'zo-lak'ri-mal*) Relating to the nasal cavity and lacrimal apparatus.

Nasolacrimal groove A groove on the nasal surface of the upper jaw, which is the site of the nasolacrimal duct.

Nasolacrimal reflex Reflex secretion of tears produced by stimulation of nasal mucosa by irritating substances.

Nasolacrimal duct A channel that carries tears from the lacrimal sac to the nasal cavity.

Nasopharynx (rhinopharynx) (*na'zo-far'inks*) The part of the pharynx above the soft palate which opens above into the nasal cavity; back of the throat.

Nasopharyngolaryngoscopy (*na"zo-fe-ring"go-le-ring'go-skope*) Instrumentation to get the view of the larynx and laryngopharynx and to demonstrate the lesions.

Natalizumab (*nat"a-liz'u-mab*) A monoclonal anti-integrin antibody which binds to the alpha 4 subunit of integrins to prevent migration of immune cells, and is used to treat Crohn's disease or multiple sclerosis.

Nates (*na'tez*) The buttocks; breech.

Natriuresis (*na'tre-u-re'sis*) Increased urinary elimination of sodium.

Pressure natriuresis refers to the phenomenon whereby increasing renal perfusion pressure (due in part to systemic hypertension) enhances sodium excretion.

Natriuretic (*na'tre-u-ret'ik*) Agent increasing urinary elimination of sodium.

Natural Killer cell (NK cell) NK cells, large granular lymphocytes with a high cytoplasmic: nuclear ratio and an intrinsic non-antibody mediated ability to kill various cells.

Naturopathy (*na'chur-op'a-the*) A system of healing that espouses the philosophy that disease is the result of violation of natural laws of living.

Nausea (*naw'ze-a*) An unpleasant sensation of impending desire to vomit. It is usually associated with salivation, inhibition of gastric peristalsis and rise in the tone of the duodenum and proximal jejunum.

Navel (*na'vel*) Umbilicus; a small depression in the middle of abdomen.

Navicular bone Scaphoid bones in the carpus and tarsus.

Nearsightedness (*ner'sit"id-nis*) Myopia.

Nearthrosis (*ne'ar-thro'sis*) A new joint following total joint replacement; an abnormal articulation developing after a nonunited fracture.

Nebula (*neb'u-la*) A faint corneal opacity; cloudiness in urine.

Nebulizer (*neb'u-liz'er*) A device which makes liquid medication into an extremely fine mist or aerosol, which is administered through a face mask.

Ultrasonic nebulizer An aerosol produced by vibrating ultrasonic transducer under water.

Necator (*ne-ka'tor*) Hookworm; cold murderer

Necator americanus A new world nematode that resembles Ankylostoma duodenale, but shorter and slender.

Necatoriasis (*ne-ka'tor-i-asis*) Hookworm disease caused by *Necator americanus*.

Necro- (*nek"ro*) A combining word for death.

Necrobiosis (*nek-ro-bi-o'sis*) Gradual degeneration of cells or tissues.

Necrobiosis lipoidica Reddish-yellow shiny plaques on shins, with atrophy and telangiectasia, often associated with diabetes mellitus.

Necrology (*ne-karol'o-je*) Study of the causes of death; mortality statistics.

Necromania/necrophilism An irresistible sexual attraction to dead bodies.

Necropsy (*nek'rop-se*) Autopsy.

Necrosis (mortification) (*ne-kro'sis*) Death of cells, tissue or organ within living body.

Anemic necrosis Necrosis following deficient blood supply.

Aseptic necrosis Occurring without infection.

Caseous necrosis Necrosis with cheesy material.

Central necrosis Necrosis occurring only in the central part.

Coagulation necrosis Occurrence of coagulation in necrotic area due to lack of blood supply.

Colliquative necrosis Necrosis caused by liquefaction of tissues.

Fat necrosis Necrosis in fatty tissue.

Fibrinoid necrosis Not a true necrosis, but a homogeneous, granular eosinophilic material seen in necrotizing vasculitis.

Liquefactive necrosis Necrosis that occurs during abscess formation caused by enzymatic degradation.

Necrosis of renal papillae Damage to one or both kidneys caused by overexposure to pain medicines, occurs with analgesic nephropathy.

Pathergic necrosis Dissolution of tissue without apparent cause as in Wegener's granulomatosis.

Putrefactive necrosis Necrosis by bacterial decomposition.

Subcutaneous fat necrosis of newborn A rare, self-limited panniculitis that typically occurs in full-term or post-term newborn infants within the first few weeks of life.

Necrospermia (*nek"ro-spur'me-a*) A condition in which the spermatozoa of the semen are either motionless or dead.

Necrotomy (*ne-krot'o-me*) Dissection of a dead body; sequestrectomy.

Necrotizing (*nek'roti-zing*) Causing the death of tissues.

Necrotizing enterocolitis A disease of premature infants affecting the terminal ileum characterized by abdominal distension, vomiting, gangrene, sepsis and perforation, less common in breast-fed children.

Necrotizing vasculitis An inflammatory condition of blood vessels characterized by necrosis, fibrosis and proliferation of the inner layer of the vessel wall.

Needle (*ne'del*) A slender, sharply pointed instrument used for suturing, ligaturing or puncturing.

Needle aspiration Removal of material from a clinically or radiologically identified mass by aspirating it through a hollow needle attached to a syringe.

Needle biopsy Removal of a piece of tissue for examination by cutting it with a wide-bore hollow needle.

Needle holder A surgical forceps to hold and pass a suturing needle through tissue.

Needle-stick injury Accidental puncture by the needle.

Negative (*neg'a-tiv*) Numerical value less than zero; an absence or not present.

Negative feedback A decrease in function in response to a stimulus.

Negative pressure Less than ambient atmospheric pressure.

Negativism (*neg'a-tiv-izm*) Performing opposite of what is asked.

Neisseria (*nis-se're-a*) Gram-negative cocci occurring in pairs with the adjacent sides flattened, named after Albert Neisser, Polish dermatologist.

Neisseria gonorrhoeae Gonococcus gram-negative, nonmotile, diplococcus which appear as flattened pairs within the cytoplasm of neutrophils.

Neisseria meningitidis Meningococcus nonmotile, gram-negative diplococcus frequently found in the nasopharynx.

Nelfinavir (*nel-fin'a-vir*) Belongs to the class of drugs known as protease inhibitors; it is an antiretroviral medication used in the treatment of HIV/AIDS.

Nelson's syndrome Bilateral adrenalectomy may be followed after a few years by enlargement of the pituitary, pressure effects on optic chiasma and raised intracranial pressure and increased pigmentation, named after Donald Nelson, US physician.

Nematode (roundworm) (*nem'ah-tod*) Parasitic worms such as intestinal and filarial round worms.

Nembutal A barbiturate that acts as a depressant or sedative also used for short-term to treat insomnia.

Neo- A prefix meaning 'new'.

Neoadjuvant chemotherapy A type of cancer treatment where chemotherapy drugs are administered before surgical extraction of the tumor.

Neocerebellum (*ne'o-ser'e-bel'um*) The large lateral portion of the cerebellar hemisphere; little brain.

Neogenesis (*ne'o-jen'e-sis*) Regeneration, as of tissue.

Neologism (*ne-ol'e-jiz"am*) A new word or expression or a new meaing for an existing word; *psy* a meaningless word used by a psychoic person.

Neomycin (*ne'o-mi'sin*) Aminoglycoside antibiotic used topically and for gut sterilization.

Neonatal death The death of a live-born infant during the first 28 days after birth.

Neonatal screening Screening an infant shortly after birth for conditions that are treatable but not clinically evident in the newborn period.

Neonate (*ne'o-nat*) A neonatal infant; a newborn child from birth up to four weeks of age.

Neopallium (*ne'o-pale-am*) Neocortex.

Neoplasia (*ne'o-pla'ze-a*) The pathologic process resulting in the formation and growth of a neoplasm.

Neoplasm (*ne'o-plazm*) A tumor; an abnormal growth serving no function.

Benign neoplasm A localized growth that does not spread by metastases or infiltration.

Gestational trophoblastic neoplasm A group of neoplastic disorders develop from placenta having H. mole, *choriocarcinoma* and *chorioadenoma.*

Intraductal papillary mucinous neoplasm Grossly visible noninvasive mucinous epithelial neoplasm arising from main pancreatic duct or branch ducts, usually >5 mm, composed of various cell types with various cytologic and architectural atypia.

Malignant neoplasm Tumor that infiltrates and spreads by metastasis.

Multiple endocrine neoplasm (MEN) A group of autosomal dominant disorders characterize by hyperplasia and hyperfunctions of two or more components of endocrine system.

Neostigmine (*ne'o-stig'min*) A cholinergic agent to improve muscle function in myasthenia gravis.

Nephelometer (*nef'a-lom'e-ter*) An instrument dedicated to the measurement of the turbidity or cloudiness of a sample. Turbidity is usually caused by the presence of insoluble particles suspended in a liquid or gas.

Nephron (*nef'ron*) The microscopic functional unit of the kidney consisting of the renal corpuscle (a glomerulus enclosed within Bowman's capsule) and the tubule (proximal convoluted tubule, loop of Henle and distal convoluted tubule) that filter waste products from the blood and regulate the excretion of salts and water in the urine. Each kidney has one million nephrons.

Nephralgia (*ne'fral'je-a*) Renal pain.

Nephrectomy (*ne-frek'to-me*) Surgical removal of the kidney.

Nephritis (Bright's disease) (*ne-fri'tis*) Inflammation of the kidneys.

Acute nephritis A group of symptoms that occur with some disorders that cause swelling and inflammation of the glomeruli in the kidney, or glomerulonephritis.

Hemorrhagic nephritis A disease of serious prognosis, for it not infrequently leaves behind it a more or less severely damaged kidney in which all the glomeruli present evidences of a diffuse injury.

Heymann nephritis Experimental autoimmune disease of rats characterized by immune-complex (IC) depositions on the epithelial side of the glomerular basement membrane (GBM) and by proteinuria.

Masugi nephritis Also known as Nephrotoxic serum nephritis (NTS), is induced in rats by administration of antiserum to rat renal structural proteins.

Suppurative nephritis The inflammation produces numerous small, yellow nodules, well delineated and surrounded by a red rim and usually more frequent in the cortex than in the medulla. The lesions may progress to form abscesses or secondary ischemic infarcts.

Nephroblastoma (Wilms' tumor) (*nef'ro-blas-to'ma*) Wilms tumor, rapidly growing tumor of the kidney that occurs in children.

Nephrocalcinosis (*nef'ro-kal'si-no'sis*) Diffusely scattered calcification in the kidneys.

Nephrogenic cord Bilateral condensations of the intermediate mesoderm. The cords extend from the cervical segments of the embryo. Nephogenic cords are located on the posterior wall of the embryo, which is where the kidneys are located.

Nephrolithiasis (*nef'ro-li-thi'a-sis*) The presence of calculi in the kidneys or the urinary passages. It is characterized by the combination of renal colic with hematuria, presence of stones in the urine or radiologic visualization of the stone.

Nephrolithotomy (*nef'ro-li-thot'o-me*) Incision into the kidney to remove a stone.

Nephrology (*ne-frolo'-je*) The branch of medical science concerned with renal disorders.

Nephron (*nef'ron*) The microscopic functional unit of the kidney consisting of the renal corpuscle (a glomerulus enclosed within Bowman's capsule) and the tubule (proximal convoluted tubule, loop of Henle and distal convoluted tubule) that filter waste products from the blood and regulate the excretion of salts and water in the urine. Each kidney has one million nephrons.

Nephropexy (*nef'ro-pek'se*) Surgical fixation of a floating kidney.

Nephroptosis (*nef'rop-to'sis*) Prolapse of the kidney.

Nephropyelography (*nef'ro-pi"e-log' ra-fe*) Radiography of the kidney and renal pelvis.

Nephrosclerosis (*nef'ro-skle'ro-sis*) Scarred contracted kidney, commonly seen in arteriosclerotic kidneys.

Benign nephrosclerosis Refers to renal damage resulting from essential hypertension, usually defined as a diastolic blood pressure in excess of 90 mm Hg.

Malignant nephrosclerosis Hardening of the walls of the small arteries and arterioles (small arteries that convey blood from arteries to the even smaller capillaries) of the kidney.

Nephroscope (*nef'ro-skop*) Instrument used to remove stones measuring one-third of an inch (1 cm) or larger.

Nephrosis (*ne-fro'sis*) Nephrotic syndrome wherein there is a non-inflammatory derangement of glomerular function characterized by an increased glomerular leak with loss of albumin.

Nephrostomy (*ne-fros'to-me*) Introduction of a small tube into the kidney to drain urine to the abdominal surface bypassing the ureter; the procedure done to facilitate healing of the ureter after surgery.

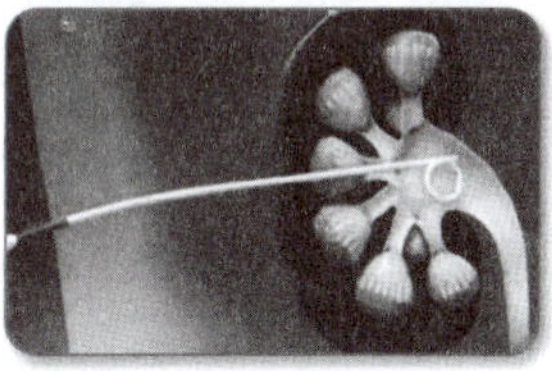

Nephrostomy

Nephrotic syndrome (*ne-frot'ik*) A condition characterized by hypoalbuminemia, hyperlipidemia, edema and hypercoagulability resulting from increased glomerular permeability to protein leading to massive proteinuria (3.5 g in 24 hours).

Nephrotomography (*nefro-to-mogra-fe*) A combination of rapid intravenous nephrography and body-section radiography. The procedure has been found to be of considerable value in the differentiation of renal cysts from neoplasms.

Nephrotomy (*ne-frot'o-me*) Surgical incision of the kidney.

Nephroureterectomy (ureteronephrectomy) (*nef'ro-u're-ter-ek'to-me*) Surgical removal of a kidney and its ureter.

Nerve (*nerv*) A whitish cord consisting of fibers held together by a connective tissue that transmits electrochemical messages back and forth between the brain and spinal cord and other parts of the body (*see* **Table**).

Afferent nerve A nerve that conducts sensory impulses from receptors to the central nervous system.

Efferent nerve A nerve that conducts motor impulses from CNS to the effector organs and tissues.

Mixed nerve Nerve containing both sensory and motor fibers.

Nerve compression Pressure on a nerve to cause its damage and muscle weakness.

Nerve conduction studies Noninvasive method to assess a nerve's ability to carry an impulse. It provides information on latency periods and conduction velocities.

Nerve entrapment A nerve entrapment is caused when a peripheral nerve loses mobility, flexibility or becomes compressed by surrounding tissues.

Nerve excitability The readiness of a nerve cell to respond to a stimulus.

Nerve plexus An interwoven network of nerves such as brachial or lumbar plexus.

Nerve sheath Coverings for nerve fiber.

Nerve block Injection of a narcotic into or around a nerve to produce loss of sensation in a part of the body supplied by that nerve.

Nerve cell The basic unit of the nervous system that detects sensory information

Table: Nerves

Abducent nerve	**Sixth cranial nerve** arises from the nucleus situated in the floor of the fourth ventricle at the level of pons, and emerges between the porns and medulla, runs through cavernous sinus and enters orbit to supply lateral rectus, has a very long intracranial course, making it vulnerable to the effects of pressure.
Accessory nerve	**Eleventh cranial nerve** has two roots— cranial and spinal arising from a nucleus in the floor of fourth ventricle along glossopharyngeal and vagus nerves and the upper portion of the spinal cord. The cranial branch emerging from the medulla joins the vagus nerve contributing sensory innervation to the palate, pharynx and larynx. The spinal accessory supplies upper part of the trapezius and sternomastoid muscle.
Alveolar—inferior	Branch from mandibular nerve, supplies teeth and gums of lower jaw, akin of chin and lower lip, motor to mylohyoid arid anterior belly of digastric, branches are inferior dental, mental, gingival and muscular.

Contd...

Alveloar—superior	Originates from maxillary nerve by anterior, middle and posterior branches, supplies upper jaw, teeth and maxillary sinus.
Anococcygeal	Originates from coccygeal plexus, supplies sacrococcygeal joint, coccyx and skin over coccyx.
Auditory nerve	**Eighth cranial nerve. Vestibulocochlear nerve** has two divisions—cochlear concerned with hearing and vestibular with equilibrium. The auditory fibers arise from the cochlear (spiral) ganglion having receptors in spiral organ of cochlea terminate in the dorsal and ventral nuclei situated in the pons. The vestibular fibers arising from vestibular ganglion having receptors in the semicircular canals, ventricle and saccule, terminate in a group of nuclei in the pons and medulla. The secondary auditory tracts after partial decussation end in the inferior colliculi and the medial geniculate bodies. The fibers arising from them pass through internal capsule to the cortical center for hearing in the first and second temporosphenoid convulsions of the brain. The vestibular fibers are connected with the cerebellum.
Auricular—great	Origin from cervical plexus, supplies parotid gland, mastoid process and pinna.
Auriculotemporal	Branch of mandibular nerve, supplies parotid gland, skin of temporal region and tympanic membrane, external acoustic meatus and pinna.
Axillary	C5, 6 from posterior cord of brachial plexus, muscular and cutaneous branches supply deltoid and teres minor muscle and skin over back of arm.
Buccal	Sensory branch from mandibular nerve, supplies skin and mucous membrane of cheek, gum, molar and premolar teeth.
Cardiac—superior, middle and inferior cervical	Originates from superior cervical, middle cervical and cervicothoracic ganglion, carries sympathetic supply and pain afferents from heart.
Cardiac—thoracic	Originates from thoracic 2 to 5 sympathetic ganglia supplies heart through plexus formation.
Carotid—external and internal	Origin from superior cervical ganglion, supplies cranial blood vessels and glands *via* plexuses.
Cervical	Origin from cervical segments of spinal cord. 8 pairs, upper cervical branches from cervical plexus, lower branches contribute in the formation of brachial plexus.
Cervical—transverse	Origin from cervical plexus, supplies skin of side and front of neck by its superior and inferior branches.

Contd...

Ciliary—long	Branch of mucociliary nerve of ophthalmic division of trigeminal nerve, supplies dilator pupillae and cornea.
Ciliary—short	Originates from ciliary ganglion by 10–12 branches, carries sympathetic, parasympathetic and sensory fibers to smooth muscles and eye ball coverings.
Cranial nerve	There are 12 pairs of cranial nerves and they are classified into three categories depending on their function as sensory, motor and mixed. **Motor nerve** oculomotor, trochlear, abducent, and hypoglossal **mixed nerve** trigeminal, facial, glossopharyngeal, vagus and spinal accessory **sensory nerve** olfactory, optic and auditory. The cranial nerves have been numbered serially by Roman numerals.
Cutaneous nerve of arm	Superior lateral, inferior lateral, medial and posterior branches from axillary, radial and medial cord of brachial plexus supplying skin on the medial, lateral and posterior aspects of arm.
Cutaneous nerves of forearm	Lateral, medial and posterior branches of musculocutaneous nerve, medial cord of brachial plexus and radial nerve respectively supply corresponding areas of forearm for general sensation.
Cutaneous nerves of calf	Lateral and medial branches of common fibular and tibial nerve supplies lateral and posterior aspects of leg.
Cutaneous nerves of thigh	Lateral—arises from lumbar plexus. Supplies front and lateral sides of thigh and calf.
Cutaneous nerves of thigh	Posterior—arises from sacral plexus. Supplies skin of buttock, genitalia and back of thigh and calf.
Dorsal nerve of clitoris	A branch from pudendal nerve, supplies deep transverse muscle of perineum, sphincter urethrae muscle, skin, prepuce and glans of clitoris.
Dorsal nerve of penis	A branch from pudendal nerve, supplies deep transverse muscle of perineum, sphincter urethrae muscle, skin, prepuce and glans of penis.
Dorsal scapular	Branch of brachial plexus, motor supply of rhomboid and levator scapulae muscle.
Ethmoidal nerve	Anterior and posterior—branches from nasociliary of ophthalmic nerve supply upper part of nasal septum, nasal cavity, ethmoidal and sphenoidal air sinuses, skin of the nose.
Facial nerve	**Seventh cranial nerve.** The motor fibers take their origin from the nucleus situated in the lower part of the pons lateral to that of the abducent nerve, and emerge at pontomedullary junction.

Contd...

	It enters the internal auditory meatus along auditory nerve and reach geniculate ganglion. The nerve pursues its course in the facial canal close to middle ear emerges through the stylomastoid foramen and divides into many branches to supply all the muscles of facial expression except locator palpebrae. It gives branch to platysma and stapedius muscle. The secretomotor fibers in the greater superficial petrosal nerve supply lacrimal, submandibular, and sublingual salivary glands. The taste sensation from the anterior two thirds of the tongue is carried by the lingual nerve and the taste fibers leave and go in the chorda tympani which join the facial nerve and reach geniculate ganglion. The axons from the ganglia pass along the facial nerve (nervous intermedius) and reach medulla and terminate in the tractus solitarius. Sensations from the skin of external auditory meatus and part of pinna are also carried by sensory part of the facial nerve.
Femoral	Originates from lumbar plexus, supplies skin of the thigh and leg, hip and knee joints and muscles of front of thigh by its muscular, articular and cutaneous branches.
Frontal	Branch of ophthalmic division of trigeminal nerve, divides into supratrochlear and supraorbital nerve for sensory innervation of forehead and scalp.
Genitofemoral	Origin from lumbar plexus, divides into genital and femoral branches to supply cremaster muscle and skin of scrotum or labium majus and thigh.
Glossopharyngeal nerve	**Ninth cranial nerve.** Takes its origin in an elongated nucleus in the medulla in the floor of fourth ventricle and emerges by several roots along the lateral aspect of the medulla and leave the skull through the jugular foramen along accessory nerve. The nerve innervates stylopharyngeus muscle and middle constrictor of the pharynx. The sensory fibers carry sensation from the upper part of the pharynx and taste as well as somatic sensations from the posterior third of tongue, through tympanic, pharyngeal, tonsillar and lingual branches.
Gluteal—inferior	Origin from sacral plexus, supplies gluteus maximus muscle.
Gluteal—superior	Origin from sacral plexus, supplies gluteus medius, gluteus minimus, tensor fascia lata and hip joint.
Iliohypogastric	Origin from lumbar plexus (L_1) supplies skin above pelvis and lateral side of buttock by its lateral and anterior branches, may supply pyramidalis muscle also.
Ilioinguinal	Origin from lumbar plexus (L_1) passes through inguinal canal to supply skin of scrotum, labia-majora and thigh by its anterior scrotal or labial branches.

Contd...

Infraorbital	Continuation of maxillary division of trigeminal, branches are middle and anterior superior alveolar, inferior palpebral, internal and external nasal and labial to supply upper incisor, premolars, skin and conjunctiva of lower eye lid, nose, part of septum, skin of upper lip and mucous membrane of mouth.
Infratrochlear	Branch of nasociliary from ophthalmic, supplies skin of root of nose, lower eye lid, conjunctiva and lacrimal duct.
Intercostobra-chial	Formed by second and third intercostal nerves, supplies skin on posterior and medial aspects of arm.
Intermedius of facial	Parasympathetic and special sensory root of facial supplying lacrimal, palatine, submandibular and sublingual glands and anterior 2/3rd of tongue through greater petrosal and chorda tympani branches.
Interosseous of forearm—anterior	Branch of median nerve, supplies flexor pollicis longus, flexor digitorum profundus, pronator quadratus muscles and wrist and intercarpal joints.
Interosseous of forearm—posterior	Branch of radial nerve, supplies abductor pollicis longus, extensors of thumb and index finger, wrist and intercarpal joints.
Interosseous of leg	Branch of tibial nerve, supplies interosseous membrane and inferior tibiofibular joint.
Lacrimal	Branch of ophthalmic division of trigeminal, supplies lacrimal gland, conjunctiva and skin of upper eye lid.
Laryngeal—external	Motor branch of superior laryngeal nerve to supply cricothyroid and inferior constrictor muscle.
Laryngeal—internal	Sensory branch of superior laryngeal nerve to supply mucosa of epiglottis, base of tongue and larynx.
Laryngeal—recurrent	Branch of vagus nerve, supplies intrinsic muscles of larynx by its inferior branch and mucosa of trachea and esophagus, contributes in the formation of cardiac plexus.
Laryngeal—superior	Origin from inferior ganglion of vagus, supplies cricothyroid muscle, inferior constrictor, mucous PI membrane of posterior part of tongue and larynx by its external and internal branches.
Lingual	Sensory branch of mandibular nerve, supplies anterior 2/3 of tongue and adjacent areas of mouth and gums.
Lumbar	Origin from lumbar segments of spinal cord, 5 pairs, ventral branches of these nerves contribute in the formation of lumbosacral plexus.
Mandibular	*see* Trigeminal nerve.
Masseteric	Branch of mandibular nerve, supplies masseter muscle.

Contd...

Maxillary	*see* Trigeminal nerve.
Median	Origin from lateral and medial cord of brachial plexus (C_6–T_1) supplies skin of hand, flexor muscles of front of forearm, short muscles of the thumb and elbow joint.
Mental	Continuation of inferior alveolar nerve, supplies skin of chin and lower lip.
Musculocutaneous	Origin from lateral cord of brachial plexus (C_5–C_7), supplies coracobrachialis, biceps brachialis, skin of forearm and elbow joint.
Nasociliary	Branch of ophthalmic division of trigeminal nerve, supplies ethmoidal air sinuses by ethmoidal branches, and skin of upper eyelid by infratrochlear branch gives long ciliary branch to supply sclera of eyeball and a communicating branch to ciliary ganglion.
Nasopalatine	Parasympathetic and sensory branch from pterygopalatine ganglion, supplies mucosa and glands of nasal septum and anterior part of hard palate.
Obturator	Origin from lumbar plexus (L_3–L_4), supplies adductor muscles, gracilis, skin of medial side of thigh and hip joint.
Obturator—accessory	Origin from lumbar (L_3 and L_4), supplies pectineus muscle and hip joint.
Obturator—internal	Origin from ventral branches of L_5-S_2, supplies gemellus superior and obturator internus muscle.
Occipital—greater	Origin from dorsal branch of cervical second, supplies semispinalis capitis and skin of head posteriorly.
Occipital—lesser	Origin from cervical plexus, sensory supply to skin of medial surface of pinna and adjacent area of head.
Occipital—third	Arises from dorsal branch of cervical third, supplies skin of back of neck and head.
Oculomotor nerve	Third cranial nerve. Takes origin from a series of nuclei in the mid-brain. The nuclei in the front (Edinger-Westphal nucleus) supply parasympathetic innervation to the ciliary muscles, and iris and nuclei behind are concerned with innervation to the extraocular muscles. The nerve passing through cavernous enters the orbit, divides into superior, medial and inferior rectus, inferior oblique and levator palpebrae.
Ophthalmic	*see* Trigeminal nerve.
Olfactory nerve	First cranial nerve, nerve of smell, arises from the sensory cells in the olfactory epithelium located in the upper part of the nasal fossa, consists of 15–20 bundles, passes through cribriform plate of ethmoid, ends in olfactory bulb. The fibers forming the olfactory tract emerge from the olfactory bulb and reach the uncus of hippocampal gyms (olfactory area) in the cerebral cortex.

Contd...

Optic nerve	**Second cranial nerve**, nerve of vision. The fibers originate in the retina and pass behind as optic nerve. The nerves of both sides meet at optic chiasma. There is partial decussation and the fibers from the temporal half of the same side and nasal half of the retina of the opposite side emerge as optic tract and terminate in the internal geniculate body. The optic radiation arising from the lateral geniculate body passes through the posterior limb of the internal capsule on either side to reach visual cortex in occipital lobe.
Palatine—greater	Origin from pterygopalatine ganglion, supplies palate.
Palatine—lesser	Origin from pterygopalatine ganglion, supplies soft palate and tonsil.
Perineal	Branch of pudendal nerve, supplies bulbospongiosus, ischiocavernosus, bulb of penis, sphincter ani externus, levator ani, superficial transverse perinei and skin of scrotum and labia majora.
Petrosal—deep	Sympathetic nerve from internal carotid plexus, forms nerve of pterygoid canal with greater petrosal to supply lacrimal, nasal and palatine glands through branches from pterygopalatine ganglion.
Petrosal—greater	Branch from geniculate ganglia, joins deep petrosal to form nerve of pterygoid canal, parasympathetic and sensory supply to lacrimal, nasal, palatine, glands and nasopharynx through branches from pterygopalatine ganglion.
Petrosal—lesser	Origin from tympanic plexus, carrying fibers of glossopharyngeal nerve supply parotid gland through auriculotemporal nerve, having parasympathetic post-ganglionic fibers in otic ganglion.
Phrenic	Origin from cervical plexus (C4–C5), supplies diaphragm, pleura, pericardiurn, peritoneum and a communicating branch to sympathetic plexus.
Phrenic—accessory	Separate origin and course from cervical fifth, enters the thorax and joins phrenic nerve.
Plantar—lateral	Origin as terminal branch of tibial nerve, passing through layers of sole muscles, supplies intrinsic muscles of sole and gives cutaneous branches to skin of lateral half of sole and fourth and fifth toes.
Plantar—medial	Origin as larger terminal branch of tibial nerve, supplies intrinsic muscles of the sole of the medial side and cutaneous supply to skin of medial half of sole and first to fourth toe.
Nerve of pterygoid canal	Formed by union of deep petrosal and greater petrosal nerve carrying sympathetic and parasympathetic fibers, joins pterygopalatine ganglion.

Contd...

Pudendal	Origin from sacral plexus (S_2–S_4), supplies muscles, skin and erectile tissue of perineum by its branch inferior rectal, and perineal and dorsal nerve of penis and clitoris.
Radial	Origin from posterior cord of brachial plexus, supplies extensor muscles at the back of the arm and forearm, joints and skin of back of arm, forearm and hand.
Rectal—inferior	Origin as a branch of pudendal nerve, supplies sphincter ani exterior muscle, lower part of anal canal and skin around anus.
Sacral	Five pairs of sacral nerves arising from sacral segments of spinal cord, contributes in the formation of sacral plexus (S1–S4).
Saphenous	Termination of femoral nerve, supplies skin on medial side of leg and foot, forms subsartorial plexus and supplies knee joint.
Sciatic	Origin from sacral plexus (L4–S3), divides into common peroneal and tibial nerve.
Splanchnic	• Greater—origin from thoracic sympathetic chain and ganglia (T5–T10), ends in celiac ganglion. • Lesser—from sympathetic chain or thoracic ganglion (T9–T10), joins celiac plexus and communicates with renal and superior mesenteric plexuses. • Lowest—from last ganglion of sympathetic trunk, joins aorticorenal and other plexus. Lumbar from lumbar ganglia, joins celiac, mesenteric and superior hypogastric plexus. Pelvic origin from sacral plexus (S3–S4), joins inferior hypogastric plexus and supplies pelvic viscera. • Sacral—from sacral part of sympathetic chain, supplies pelvic viscera and blood vessels.
Subcostal	Ventral branch of spinal nerve T12, supplies transversalis, oblique, rectus abdominis and skin of lower abdomen and lateral part of gluteal region.
Suboccipital	Origin as dorsal branch of C1 supplies muscles of suboccipital triangle and semispinalis capitis.
Subscapular	Origin from posterior cord of brachial plexus (C5), two nerves—upper and lower—supply subscapularis and teres major muscles.
Supraclavicular	Medial, intermediate and lateral, originate from cervical plexus (C3–C4), supplies skin of shoulder, pectoral and deltoid region.
Supraorbital	Terminal branch of frontal nerve, supplies skin of upper eyelid, forehead, scalp and mucosa of frontal sinus.
Suprascapular	Origin from upper trunk of brachial plexus, supplies supraspinatus, infraspinatus muscles and also to shoulder joint and acromioclavicular joint.
Supratrochlear	Terminal branch of frontal nerve, supplies skin of forehead and upper eyelid.

Contd...

Sural	Formed by union of medial sural and a communicating branch from common peroneal, supplies skin of the back of leg, lateral side of foot and heel.
Temporal—deep	Branch of mandibular supplies temporal muscle.
Thoracic—long	Origin from ventral branches of T5–T7 of brachial plexus, supplies serratus anterior muscle.
Thoracodorsal	Origin from posterior cord of brachial plexus (C7–C8), supplies latissimus dorsi muscle.
Tibial	Continuation of sciatic nerve in lower pan of thigh, supplies semimembranosus, semitendinosus, biceps abductor magnus and muscles of calf and sole and toes. Also supplies joints and skin of back of leg, sole and toes.
Trigeminal nerve	**Fifth cranial nerve.** Has a long sensory nucleus extending from the pons to the upper cervical portion of the spinal cord and a small motor nucleus in the pons near the floor of the fourth ventricle. The sensory part has three divisions—ophthalmic, maxillary and mandibular—which carry the sensations from the face, teeth, mouth and nasal cavity and its motor part is related to mandibular division and it innervates the muscles of mastication (pterygoids, masseter, temporalis, tensor tympani and tensor palati). Mandibular branch carries sensations from the lower part of the face, the lower lip, ear, tongue and lower teeth. Maxillary branch carries sensations from the cheek, upper lip, lower eyelid and its conjunctiva, side of the nose, mucous membrane of the nose, upper teeth, upper part of the pharynx and tonsils. Ophthalmic branch carries sensations from the upper eyelid and its medial part of the conjunctiva, nose up to the tip, forehead and anterior part of the scalp. The sensations carried through the sensory divisions reach the Gasserian (trigeminal) ganglion. The sensory root originating from the ganglion terminates in the brain stem. 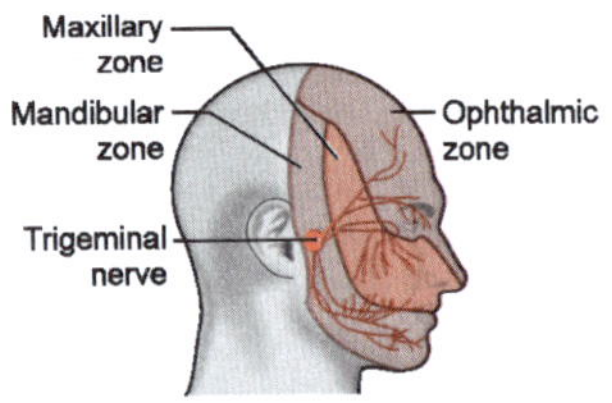 *Distribution of trigeminal nerve*

Contd...

Trochlear nerve	**Fourth cranial nerve.** Arises in the midbrain caudal to the nucleus of oculomotor nerve. The nerve fibers decussate unlike other cranial nerves before it emerges near the roof of the fourth ventricle. It supplies superior oblique muscle of the eyeball.
Tympanic	Origin from inferior ganglion of glossopharyngeal contributes in the formation of tympanic plexus, supplies mucous membrane of tympanic cavity, auditory tube and mastoid air cells.
Ulnar	Origin from medial cord of brachial plexus (C8–T1) supplies flexor muscles on the front of arm and short muscles of the hand. Also carries sensory fibers from skin of the joint and medial part of hand and 11/2 fingers on medial side.
Vagus	**Tenth cranial nerve** arises from the nucleus in medulla in the floor of fourth ventricle and emerges by several rootlets from the lateral side of the medulla and passes through jugular foramen, continues in the neck, thorax and abdomen. It carries sensations from the pharynx and larynx. Motor fibers innervate muscles of the soft palate, pharynx and larynx. The parasympathetic branches supply to the thoracic and abdominal viscera. Branches are superior and recurrent laryngeal, meningeal, auricular, pharyngeal, cardiac and other visceral plexus.
Vestibular	Part of VIIIth cranial nerve, fibers arise from vestibular ganglion, receptors in semicircular canals, ventricle and saccule of internal ear concerned with sense of equilibration.
Vestibulocochlear	*see* Auditory nerve.
Vidian	Formed by union of deep petrosal and greater petrosal nerve, carries sympathetic and parasympathetic fibers to nasal mucous membrane.
Zygomatic	Origin as a branch from maxillary nerve, communicates with lacrimal nerve, sensory for skin of temple and adjacent part of face.

and transmits it from one part of the body to another.

Nerve ending The termination of a nerve fiber in a peripheral structure.

Nerve fiber Axon of a neuron which may be myelinated or unmyelinated.

Nerve gases Also called nerve agents are organic chemicals which disrupt the mechanisms by which nerves transfer messages to organs.

Nerve impulse The electrochemical process involved in neural transmission.

Nervous system The extensive, intricate network of structures that activates, coordinates and controls the functions of the body. It consists of central nervous system comprising the brain and the spinal cord, and the peripheral nervous system.

Nesbit's operation A procedure to correct curvature of the penis during erection; only indicated if the penis is too bent to permit penetration and the disease has stabilized.

Nettle rash An urticarial eruption following stinging nettle, a common weed.

Neural (*nu'ral*) Relating to nerve cells or its processes.

Neural crest The dorsal region of the embryonic nervous system that gives rise to the sensory and autonomic nervous systems and melanocytes.

Neural tube Tube in the back of an embryo that develops into the spinal cord and brain.

Neural tube defects Failure of normal development of the spinal cord or brain in an embryo resulting in birth defects such as spina bifida and anencephaly.

Neuralgia (*nu-ral'je-a*) Severe pain in the course or distribution of a nerve due to irritation or damage to a nerve.

Glossopharyngeal neuralgia Recurrent, paroxysmal intense pain originating in the tonsillar fossa and may radiate to the ear on the same side.

Occipital neuralgia Paroxysmal pain in the occipital, suboccipital and posterior parietal areas on one side due to spontaneous irritation of the greater occipital nerve.

Postherpetic neuralgia Severe burning pain may occur following herpes zoster and persist for a long time.

Post-traumatic neuralgia Occurrence of persistent pain and sensory changes following trauma to a peripheral nerve.

Temporomandibular neuralgia Recurrent unilateral, severe pain originating in one temporomandibular joint and spreading either into the face or into the temporal muscle.

Trigeminal neuralgia Recurrent paroxysmal, brief episodes of intense pain over one side of the face confined to one of the three divisions of trigeminal nerve.

Neural plate A key developmental structure that serves as the basis for the nervous system. It is shaped by the intrinsic movements of the epidermal and neural plate regions.

Neural spine Backward extending spinous process, which serves to attach muscles and ligaments.

Neurapraxia (*nur"a-prak'se-a*) The mildest form of traumatic peripheral nerve injury. It is characterized by focal segmental demyelination at the site of injury without disruption of axon continuity and its surrounding connective tissues. This condition results in blockage of nerve conduction and transient weakness or paresthesia.

Neurasthenia (*nu'ras-the'ne-a*) Fatigue accompanying depression; nervous debility.

Neurectasis Surgical procedure for stretching a peripheral nerve.

Neurectomy (*nu-rek'to-me*) Excision of a segment of a nerve.

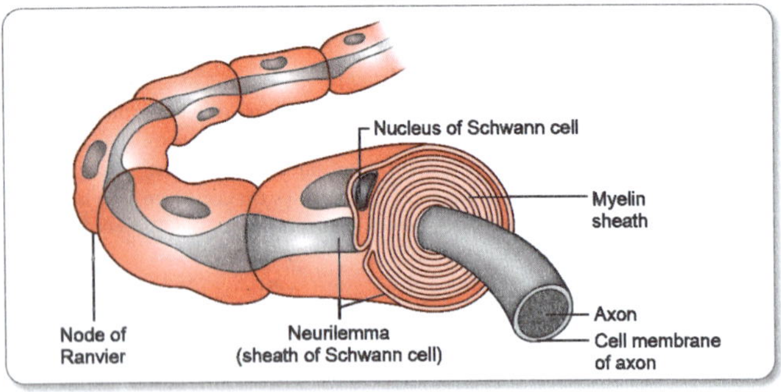

Neurilemma with enclosing axon in a peripheral nerve

Neurilemma (neurolemma) (*nu'ri-lem'ma*) Sheath of Schwann, the external sheath of a nerve fiber.

Neurilemmoma (*nu'ri-lem-mo-ma*) Schwannoma, benign encapsulated tumor from cells structurally identical to Schwann cells, neurinoma; a benign tumor that can arise from any nerve in the body, but tends to favor certain nerves located in the head and neck, as well as nerves that are involved in flexing the upper and lower extremities.

Neurinoma (*nu'ri-no'ma*) A tumor of the nerve sheath.

Neuritis (*nu-ri'tis*) Inflammation of a nerve.

Neuroanatomy (*nu'ro-a-nat'o-me*) The anatomy of the nervous system.

Neurobiotaxis The growth of a nerve fiber toward the tissue it will innervate, during embryological development.

Neuroblast (*nu'ro-blast*) An embryonic nerve cell that develops into a neuron.

Neuroblastoma (*nu'ro-blas-to'ma*) A malignant tumor with neuroblasts that usually originates in the adrenal medulla. It may also originate in any part of the sympathetic nervous system.

Neurocranium (*nu'ro-kra'ne-um*) The part of the skull enclosing the brain.

Cartilaginous neurocranium The **cartilaginous** part, or chondrocranium, which forms bones of the base of the skull.

Membranous neurocranium Consists of neural crest cells and paraxial mesoderm which form the main portion of the roof and lateral sides of the neurocranium.

Neurodermatitis (neurodermatosis) (*nu-ro-der'ma-ti'tis*) A chronic indurated and thickened skin lesion often associated with emotional stress.

Neuroendocrine tumors Growth with malignant potential that secretes one or more hormones with neuroendocrine properties. They are derived from embryonic neural crest cells, also called APUD tumors carcinoids, insulinoma, VIPoma, somatostatinoma, glucagonoma and Zollinger-Ellison syndrome are some examples.

Neuroepithelioma (*nu'ro-epi-the'le-o'ma*) Retinoblastoma.

Neuroepithelium (*nu'ro-epi-the'le-um*) Epithelial cells receptive to external stimuli.

Neuroepithelium cristae ampullaris Epithelial cells with hair cells and supporting cells covered by neuroepithelium.

Neurofibril (*nu'ro-fi-bril*) Filamentous structures in the nerve cell.

Neurofibroma (neurilemmoma, neurinoma, neuroma, schwanmoma) (*nu'ro-fi-bro'ma*) Schwannoma, a benign, nonencapsulated soft tumor due to proliferation of Schwann cells; neurilemmoma. It presents with single or multiple nodules of variable size which are freely mobile.

Cutaneous/dermal neurofibroma A neoplasm of peripheral nerve Schwann cells that present as a soft nodule in the dermis of the skin.

Plexiform neurofibroma An irregular, thick and noncircumscribed tumor of peripheral nerve sheath which can involve multiple nerve fascicles.

Solitary neurofibroma A common nerve sheath tumor. It presents as a skin-colored, soft-to-firm papule or nodule with a smooth surface.

Neurofibromatosis (von recklinghausen's disease) (*nu'ro-fi-bro-ma-to'sis*) Multiple subcutaneous slow growing soft fibrous swellings that grow from nerves.

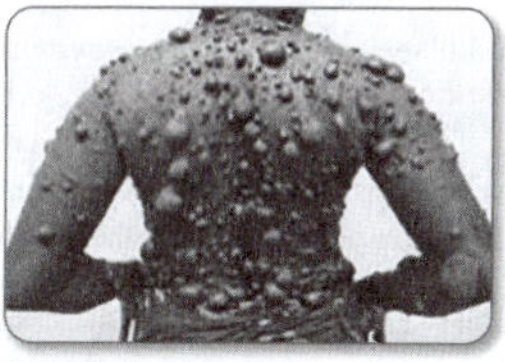

Neurofibromatosis

Generalized neurofibromatosis Von Recklinghausen's disease, presence of multiple nodules all over the body with pale brown pigmentation of the skin.

Plexiform neurofibromatosis Multiple fibromyxomatous masses hanging down loosely on folds of skin and subcutaneous tissue, usually on the face affecting the branches of trigeminal nerve.

Neurogenesis (*nu'ro-jen'e-sis*) Formation of nervous tissue.

Neurogenic (*nu'ro-jen'ik*) Originating in or caused by nervous system.

Flaccid neurogenic bladder Interference with voluntary and reflex control of urinary bladder from segmental lesions at S_2 to S_4 level. There is loss of the sensation of bladder fullness causing 'overflow' incontinence.

Neurogenic abdominal pain Burning pain limited to the distribution of peripheral nerve.

Neurogenic arthropathy Painless disorganization of joint.

Neurogenic bladder Loss of bladder control due to spinal lesion. It is accompanied by urgency, increased frequency, decreased functional capacity, and spastic contractions and poor voluntary control.

Neurogenic claudication Symptoms of dysfunction of cauda equina appear on walking or prolonged standing and subside by rest.

Neurogenic fracture A fracture associated with the destruction of nerve supply to a specific bone.

Neurogenic shock A form of shock resulting from peripheral vasodilation spastic.

Neuroglia (*nu-rog'le-a*) Non-neuronal cellular elements of nervous system.

Neurohormone (*nu'ro-hor-mo'n*) A chemical messenger formed by neurosecretory cell such as acetylcholine, dopamine, epinephrine, norepinephrine and serotonin.

Neurohormone (*nu'ro-hor-mo'n*) A chemical messenger formed by neurosecretory cell such as acetylcholine, dopamine, epinephrine, norepinephrine and serotonin.

Neurohypophysis (*nu'ro-hi-pof'i-sis*) Posterior lobe of pituitary, that is the source of antidiuretic hormone (ADH) and oxytocin.

Neurology (*nu-rol'o-je*) The branch of medical science concerned with the nervous system and its disorders.

Clinical neurology The branch of medicine that deals with the nervous system and its disorders.

Interverntional neurology An advanced, minimally-invasive surgical treatment for complex brain and spinal cord vascular diseases that is performed from inside the blood vessels. Also known as endovascular neurosurgery.

Vascular neurology focuses on the treatment of vascular issues that involve the central nervous system, including stroke, brain hemorrhages and other kinds of brain bleeds.

Neuroma (*nu-ro'ma*) A combing word for a benign tumor of nerve tissue.

Neuromuscular junction (myoneural junction) A functional unit consisting at highly specialized structures at the nerve terminal and at the muscle end plate as well as the gap between them across which electrochemical communication occurs.

Neuromyelitis optica (Devic's disease) A central system disorder that causes inflammation in nerves of the eye and the spinal cord.

Neuron (nerve cell) (*nu'ron*) Nerve cell, the basic of the nervous system consisting of nerve cell body, the axon and the dendrites.

Bipolar neuron A neuron having one axon and one dendrite.

Motor neuron Neuron that transmits nerve impulses from the brain and the spinal cord to the muscles and the glandular tissue.

Multipolar neuron Neuron possessing one axon and several dendrites, most neurons in the brain and the spinal cord are examples.

Sensory neuron Neuron that transmits nerve impulses toward the spinal cord and the brain.

Unipolar neuron Embryonic structure whose dendrites and axons are fused into a single fiber, which after a short distance gets separated into two processes.

Neuronopathy (*nuro-nopa'-the*) Refers to the conditions that result when nerves that carry messages to and from the brain and spinal cord from and to the rest of the body are damaged or diseased.

Neuroplasty (*nur'o-plas'te*) A procedure to remove pressure caused by excessive scar tissue in the epidural space.

Neuropathic bladder Lack of bladder control due to a brain, spinal cord or nerve problem.

Neuropathy (*nu-ropa'-the*) Any disorder affecting any of the peripheral nerves.

Congenital neuropathy Hereditary sensory radicular neuropathy or hypertrophic interstitial neuropathy.

Entrapment neuropathy Compression of a peripheral nerve against bone or tendon. In early stages, there is numbness and paresthesia and later a fixed sensory loss and muscle atrophy.

Giant axonal neuropathy An autosomal recessive neuropathy of childhood due to mutation in the GAN gene (locus: 16q24.1), which encodes gigaxonin, a protein involved in the ubiquitin-proteasome system targeting damaged proteins for destruction. There are central and peripheral nervous system symptoms and enlarged axons made up of masses of tightly woven neurofilaments.

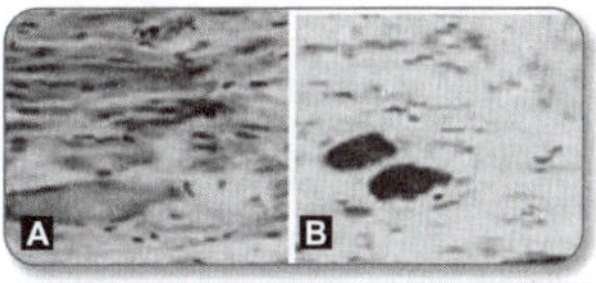

*Giant axonal neuropathy. **A.** Eosinophilic enlarged axons, surrounded by rings of Schwann cells; **B.** Neurofilaments in axonal spheroids*

Peripheral neuropathy Non-acute traumatic degeneration of the nerves of the limbs. It includes rapid onset post-infective polyneuritis, slow onset hereditary sensorimotor neuropathy, subacute or chronic distal neuropathy and mononeuropathies.

Toxic neuropathy Tobacco, or alcohol-related amblyopia.

Neurophysiology (*nu'ro-fiz'e-ol'o-je*) Physiology of the nervous system.

Neuropil (*nur'o-pil*) Any area in the nervous system composed of mostly unmyelinated axons, dendrites and glial cell processes that form a synaptically dense region containing a relatively low number of cell bodies.

Neuroretinitis (*nur"o-ret"i-ni'tis*) Inflammation of the optic nerve and retina.

Neurosecretion (*nu'ro-se-kre'shun*) The release of a chemical substance at the axon terminal.

Neurosis (*nu-ro'sis*) An emotional nervous disorder.

Neurosurgery (*nu'ro-sur'jer-e*) Surgery of the nervous system.

Neurosyphilis (*nu'ro-sif'i-lis*) Syphilitic involvement of the nervous system characterized by tabes dorsalis, and general paralysis of insane.

Asymptomatic neurosyphilis Neurosyphilis is present, but the individual reports no symptoms.

Meningovascular neurosyphilis Characterized by endarteritis of blood vessels anywhere in the CNS causing thrombosis and infarction and, unlike other causes of stroke, prodromal symptoms characterized by vertigo, insomnia and emotional lability that occur for months as prodromal symptoms.

Neurotomy (*nu-rot'o-me*) Surgical division of a nerve; interruption of a nerve through surgical cutting or production of artificial lesions.

Neurotoxic (*nu'ro-tok'sik*) Poisonous to the nervous system.

Neurotransmitter (*nu'ro-tran's-mi-ter*) Any chemical mediator released by a presynaptic cell, that is capable of transmitting an electrical impulse.

Neurotrophic A group of proteins that play a critical role in the growth, survival and maintenance of neurons.

Neurotropic (*nu'ro-trop'ik*) Having affinity for nervous system.

Neurotropic factors Proteins that stimulate growth of nerve cells during normal development of fetus and after injury.

Neutropenia (*nu-tro-pe'ne-a*) An abnormal decrease in the number of neutrophils in the circulating blood.

Cyclical neutropenia Rare disorder showing periodic reduction in neutrophils at 3–4-week intervals.

Idiopathic benign neutropenia Fall in neutrophil count due to migration of neutrophils from circulating pool to the marginating pool. It is not associated with an increased tendency for infections.

Severe neutropenia Marked neutropenia as a toxic reaction to several drugs or as a part of pancytopenia.

Neutrophil (polymorph) (*nu'tro-fil*) A mature granulocytic white blood cell whose granules exhibit no special affinity to acid or basic dyes. It is responsible for the body's protection against infection.

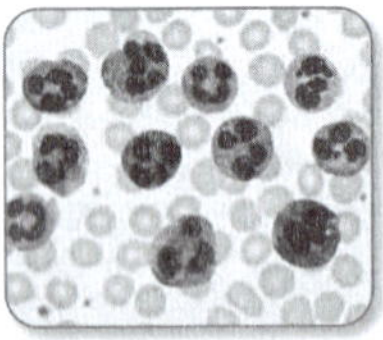

Polymorphonuclear neutrophil

Neutrophil leukocytosis Increase in neutrophil count, occurs in many bacterial infections, inflammations, tissue necrosis, myeloproliferative disorders, acute hemorrhage and acute hemolysis.

Nevus (*nevas*) A benign (not cancer) growth on the skin that is formed by a cluster of melanocytes (cells that make a substance called melanin).

Cellular blue nevus A usually congenital type of large blue nevus found in the dermis or subcutaneous tissue around the buttocks or sacrococcygeal region. It consists of deeply pigmented, dendritic, spindle-shaped melanocytes alternating with cellular islands of spindle cells with pale cytoplasm. Occasionally one may undergo malignant transformation to melanoma.

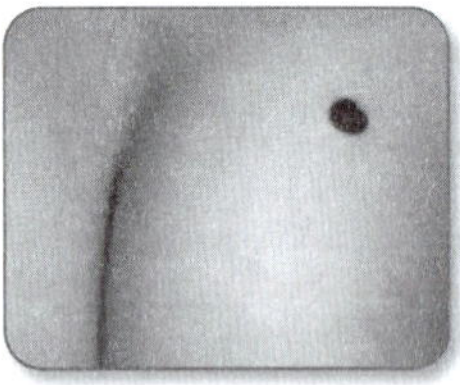

Cellular blue nevus

Giant congenital pigmented nevus A melanocytic lesion present at birth that will reach a diameter ≥20 cm in adulthood.

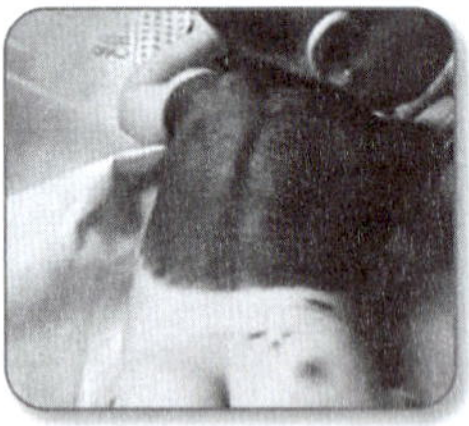

Giant congenital pigmented nevus

Pigmented nevus Any nevus containing melanin, such as a Becker nevus, melanocytic nevus, or nevus spilus. Also called nevus pigmentosus; melanocytic nevus.

New Drug application (NDA) is an application through which drug manufacturers or its agents requests permission from US FDA for a license to market a drug for one or more specified indications.

Newton (*nu'tan*) The newton (symbol: N) is the unit of force in the International System of Units (SI). It is defined as 1 kg m/s^2, the force which gives a mass of 1 kg an acceleration of 1 m/sec. Named after Isaac Newton in recognition of his work on classical mechanics, specifically Newton's Second Law of Motion.

Nexus (*nek'sus*) Junction; connection between two cells.

Niacin (*ni'a-sin*) Nicotinic acid and nicotinamide possessing equal biological potency, a part of Vitamin B complex.

Niacinamide (*ni-a-sin-am'id*) Nicotinamide, biologically active form of nicotinic acid.

Niche (*nick*) A recess in a wall; an ulcerated or eroded region.

Nicholson's method To overcome abdominal rigidity, the base of the palm of the left hand is placed upon the lower part of the sternum and increasing pressure is exerted. Eventually the examiner is leaning quite heavily on the chest with the result the patient breaths abdominally. While the patient draws his breath, the abdominal muscles show a decrease in their tonicity, where upon the right hand palpates the abdomen, named after Neville Nicholson, English surgeon.

Nicotine (*nik'o-ten*) A poisonous volatile alkaloid from tobacco.

Nicotinamide (*nik"o-tin'a-mid*) INN for niacinamide.

Nicotinamide adenine dinucleotide phosphate (NADP) A coenzyme composed of nicotinamide mononucleotide (NMN) coupled by pyrophosphate linkage to the 5/-phosphate of adenosine 2/,5/-bisphosphate. It serves as an electron carrier in numerous reactions, being alternately oxidized (NADP+) and reduced (NADPH). Formerly called also triphosphopyridine nucleotide (TPN).

Nicotinamide mononucleotide (NMN) A nucleotide containing covalently linked nicotinamide and ribose 5-phosphate. It is a constituent of NAD and NADP.

Nicotinamide adenine dinucleotide (NAD) A coenzyme composed of nicotinamide mononucleotide (NMN) coupled to adenosine monophosphate (AMP) by pyrophosphate linkage. It is found widely in nature and is involved in numerous enzymatic reactions in which it serves as an electron carrier by being alternately oxidized (NAD+) and reduced (NADH).

Nictitation (*nik"ti-ta'shan*) A reflex that closes and opens the eyes rapidly.

Nidation (*ni-da'shun*) Embedding.

Nidus (*ni'dus*) Central point; point of lodgment; focus of infection.

Nifedipine (*ni-fed'i-pen*) A calcium channel blocker.

Nifuratel Drug used in gynecology. It is a local antiprotozoal and antifungal agent that may be given orally.

Night blindness Decreased ability to see in dim light due to defective rod function with delayed dark adaptation and perceptual threshold. It is noted in deficiency of vitamin A, retinitis pigmentosa, late stages of glaucoma, cataract, optic atrophy and in retinal degeneration.

Night stick fracture An undisplaced fracture of the ulnar shaft caused by a direct blow.

Night terror Sleep disorder, occurring mainly in children, in which an individual awakens suddenly in an agitated, almost terrified state.

Ninhydrin test A chemical test used to identify ammonia, primary/secondary amines or amino acids.

Nipple (mamilla, papilla) (*nip'l*) Papilla; the protuberance at the top of breast through which lactiferous ducts discharge. It contains erectile tissue and is surrounded by pigmented areola.

Nipple discharge Serous and/or serosanguinous discharge from the breasts in peri- and post-menopausal women.

Nipple shield A device to protect the nipples of a lactating woman.

Retracted nipple A nipple whose tip lies below the level of surrounding skin.

Nissl granules (*nisl*) Coarse RNA aggregations in cytoplasm of nerve cells which are the site of protein synthesis, named after Franz Nissl, German neurologist.

Nit An empty egg shell of louse attached to hair or clothing.

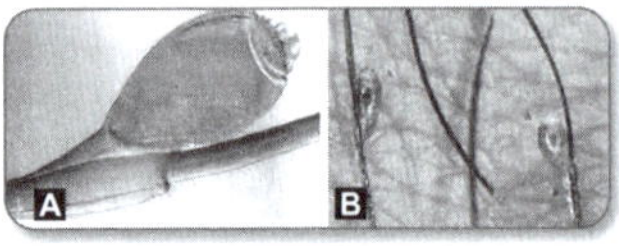

Nits of Pthirus pubis: ***A.*** *Microscopic appearance;* ***B.*** *On hair*

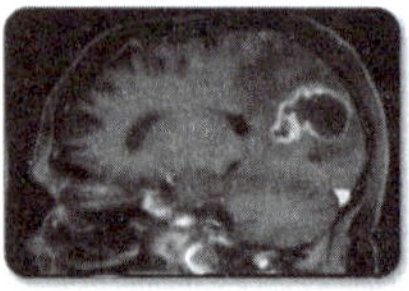

Nocardiosis—multiple gadolinium MRI scan

Nitric acid HNO_3, a colorless, corrossive liquid.

Nitrofurantoin (*ni'tro-fu-ran'to-in*) A urinary antiseptic.

Nitroglycerin (glyceryl trinitrate) (*ni-tro'glis'erin*) Glycerol trinitrate. An organic nitrate used as a short-acting vasodilator agent for the treatment of anginal pain.

Nitrous oxide (*ni'trus*) N_2O, laughing gas, first general anesthetic.

Nizatidine (*ni-za'ti-den*) A histamine H_2 receptor antagonist that inhibits stomach acid production, and is commonly used in the treatment of peptic ulcer disease and gastroesophageal reflux disease.

NMR Nuclear magnetic resonance.

Nocardia (*no'kar-de-a*) A genus of aerobic nonmotile actinomycetes, of which *N. asteroids* and *N. brasiliensis* are pathogenic, named after Edmund-Nocard, French veterinary pathologist. *Nocardia madurae* organism causes Madura foot.

Nocardiosis (*no-kahr"de-o'sis*) An infectious disease caused by Nocardia that classically manifests as an opportunistic infection in immunocompromised hosts. Pulmonary nocardiosis and disseminated forms of the infection are opportunistic diseases occurring mainly in patients deficient in T cell-mediated immunity. Patients with the greatest susceptibility to this include those with solid organ transplant, hematopoietic stem cell transplant recipients, human immunodeficiency virus (HIV) infected patients, patients taking corticosteroids chronically, or patients with ongoing malignant processes.

Nociceptive (*no'se-sep'tiv*) Capable of appreciation or transmission of pain.

Nociceptive reflex A reflex caused by a painful stimulus.

Nociceptive stimulus A painful stimulus.

Nociperception (*no"si-par-sep'shan*) Nociception.

Noctambulation To walk about at night.

Nocturia (*nok-tu're-a*) Increased urination at night disturbing a person's sleep. It can be an early symptom in diabetes mellitus, chronic renal insufficiency or early congestive heart failure.

Node (*nod*) A small circumscribed mass of tissue.

Nodes of Ranvier Constrictions occurring on myelinated nerve fibers at regular interval of about 1 mm; at these sites the myelin sheath is absent and the axon is enclosed only by Schwann cell processes.

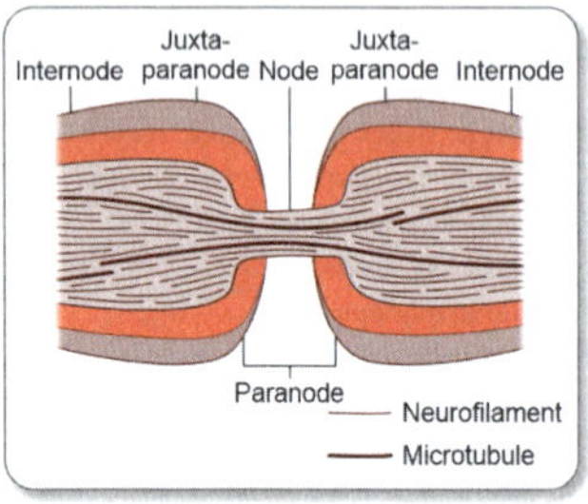

Node of Ranvier (diagrammatic)

Nodule (*nod'ul*) a small, rounded mass of tissue of variable size and shape.

Apple jelly nodules Minute translucent nodules of a distinctive yellow to reddish brown color, visible on diascopic examination of the lesions of lupus vulgaris.

Aschoff nodules Aschoff bodies.

Babes nodules Collections of microglial cells around neurons in the central nervous system, seen in rabies and other types of viral encephalitis; called also Babes nodes or tubercles.

Bohn nodules Inclusion cysts found in the mouths of newborns along the buccal and lingual aspects of the dental ridges and on the palate away from the raphe; they are considered to be remnants of mucous gland tissue trapped during fetal development. Called also Bohn pearls.

Brenner nodules Nodular masses of tumor in the cyst wall in cases of Brenner tumor.

Busacca nodules An accumulation of epithelioid cells and lymphocytes occurring in chronic inflammation of the iris, usually on its anterior surface around the region of the ciliary zone.

Cirrhotic nodule A regenerative nodule surrounded by fibrous septa.

Coal nodule A palpable lesion of the lung seen in coal workers' pneumoconiosis, containing coal dust, dust-filled macrophages, and collagen fibers; develops from a coal macule.

Cold nodule A thyroid nodule that is less detectable than surrounding tissues on a radionuclide scan because of low uptake of the tracer; up to one in four may be malignant.

Cortical nodules Nodules of closely packed lymphocytes in the cortical portion of a lymph gland.

Dalen-Fuchs nodules Small hemispherical mounds principally composed of epithelioid cells and cells of the retinal epithelium, seen in sympathetic ophthalmia and certain other disorders.

Koeppe nodules White to gray nodules observed at the pupillary border in chronic inflammation of the iris, and consisting of accumulations of epithelioid cells and lymphocytes.

Lisch nodules Hamartomas of the iris, occurring in neurofibromatosis.

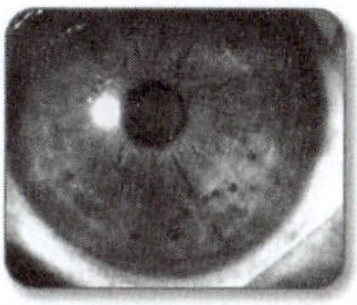

Lisch nodules

Nodules of Arantius Noduli valvularum semilunarium valvae aortae.

Nodule of cerebellum Nodulus vermis.

Teacher/Singer's nodules Vocal cord nodules.

Thyroid nodules Pathological nodules in the thyroid gland, often filled with colloid; some are indicative of adenoma or carcinoma.

Noma (*no'ma*) A gangrenous stomatitis; cancrum oris. An acute necrotizing polymicrobial and ulcerating infection of the orofacial tissues seen in malnourished children, which rapidly erodes deep tissues exposing bone and teeth.

Nondisjunction (*non'dis-junk'shun*) Failure of chromosome to separate during cell division resulting in passage of both chromosomes to the same daughter cell and result in serious genetic disorder.

Nonsecretor (*non"se-kre'ter*) An individual with A or B type blood whose saliva and other body secretions do not contain the A or B blood group antigens.

Norclozapine (*nor"-cloz'uh-peen*) A major active metabolite of the atypical antipsychotic drug clozapine. Unlike clozapine, it possesses intrinsic activity at the D2/D3 receptors, and acts as a weak partial agonist at these sites. Used in treatment of schizophrenia and schizo affective disorders.

Norepinephrine (noradrenaline) (*nor"ep-i-nefrin)* Also called noradrenaline or noradrenalin, is an organic chemical in the catecholamine family that functions in the brain and body as both a hormone and neurotransmitter; functions as a peripheral vasoconstrictor by acting on alpha-adrenergic receptors. It is also an inotropic stimulator of the heart and dilator of coronary arteries as a result of its activity at the beta-adrenergic receptors.

Norethandrolone (*nor'eth-an'dro-lon*) Anabolic steroid.

Norethindrone (*nor-eth'in-dron*) A progestational agent having some anabolic, estrogenic, and androgenic properties; used as an oral contraceptive, alone or in combination with an estrogen component.

Norfloxacin (*nor-flok'sesin*) A quinolone antibacterial agent used in the treatment of infections of urinary tract.

Normoblast (*nor'mo-blast*) A nucleated red blood cell and its presence suggests hemolysis; erythroblast.

Normocyte (*nor'mo-sit*) Normal mature red cell having a diameter of 7 microns.

Normotensive (*nor"mo-ten'siv*) Characterized by normal tone, tension, or pressure, as by normal blood pressure.

Nortriptyline (*nor-trip'ti-len*) An antidepressant that falls under the pharmacological category of tricyclics (secondary amine), more commonly known as TCAs. Used for treating nerve pain, depression and bedwetting in children (nocturnal enuresis).

Nose (*noz*) Nasus, a central projection of the face which acts as an organ of smell and the opening to the nasal cavities that warms, moistens and filters inhaled air as it moves into respiratory tract.

Saddle nose Depressed bridge of nose due to erosion of nasal bones seen in congenital syphilis and leprosy.

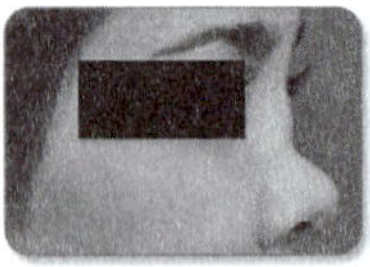

Saddle nose

Nose bleed Bleeding from nose due to injury, hypertension, foreign body or fracture.

Nosocomial infection An infection acquired in a hospital by pathogens that were not in incubation period when the person concerned was admitted for treatment.

Nosology (*no-sol'o-je*) Scientific classification of diseases.

Nosopsyllus (*nos"o-silus*) A genus of fleas. N fasciatus, the rat flea of North America and Europe, is a vector of murine typhus and probably of plague.

Nostril (*nos'tril*) One of the external orifices of the nose.

Notch (*Noch*) Incisure; an indentation or a depression in a bone or organ.

Notifiable disease A group of communicable diseases which are considered to be serious menaces to public health. Once a communicable disease is detected, it should be notified immediately to the local health authorities to permit immediate action to control the spread of the disease.

Notochord (*no'toko-rd*) The axial fibrocellular structure around which the vertebral primordia develop.

Novacin (*no'va-kan*) Brand name of aminoglycoside antibiotic, prescribed for serious bacterial infections of throat, lung, sinus, kidney, urinary tract, skin and soft tissues. It inhibits the production of bacterial proteins, which causes bacterial cell death.

NSAID Nonsteroidal anti-inflammatory drug.

Nucha (*nu'ka*) The back of the neck.

Nuclear magnetic resonance (NMR) Noninvasive, imaging technique without use of ionizing radiation.

Nuclear medicine An area of medicine that uses radioisotopes for the diagnosis and treatment of disease.

Nuclease (*nu'kle-as*) Any enzyme catalyzing the hydrolysis of nucleic acids, consists of DNAase (DNase) and RNAase (RNase) enzymes.

Nucleic acid (*nu'kle'ik*) Polymer of nucleotide, DNA or RNA which possess a complex chemical structure consisting of pentoses (sugars), phosphoric acid and purines and pyrimidines (nitrogenous bases).

Nucleolus (*nu'kle'o-lus*) A small round mass within the cell nucleus concerned with the production of nucleoprotein. pl. **nucleoli**.

Nucleoplasm (Karyoplasm) (*nu'kle-o-plaz"m*) A type of protoplasm that is composed of thick fluid and constitutes chromatin fibers made up of DNA and usually found in the nucleus of the eukaryotic cells. This fluid contains primarily water, dissolved ions, and a complex mixture of molecules.

Nucleoprotein (*nu'kle-o-pro'te-in*) A complex of protein and nucleic acid.

Nucleoside (*nu'kle-o-sid*) A compound of sugar (ribose or deoxyribose) with a purine or pyrimidine base.

Nucleoside analog Chemical that interferes with the replication of viruses.

Nucleoside base Chemical that forms the building blocks of DNA or RNA and their sequence gives the picture of genetic code.

Nucleotide (*nu'kle-o-tid*) The basic unit of nucleic acids DNA/RNA, which is made up of a purine or pyrimidine base (A adenine, T thymine, U uracil, G guanine or C cytosine), a pentose sugar (ribose or deoxyribose) and a phosphate group.

Nucleotide analog A chemical substance that resembles a nucleotide.

Nucleus (*nu'kle-us*) Oval mass containing chromatin and nucleoli which acts as the central unit of a living cell. pl. **nuclei**.

Nucleus caudatus (Caudata nucleus) An elongated, arched gray mass closely related to the lateral ventricle throughout its entire extent and consisting of a head, body, and tail. The caudate nucleus and putamen form a functional unit (the neostriatum) of the corpus striatum.

Nucleus cuneatus (Cuneate nucleus) A nucleus in the medulla oblongata at the rostral end of the fasciculus cuneatus, in which the fibers of this fasciculus synapse; the cells project to the thalamus via the medial lemniscus.

Nucleus lentiformis (Lentiform nucleus) The part of the corpus striatum somewhat resembling a biconvex lens, divided into an external, larger, lateral part (putamen) and an internal, smaller, medial part (globus pallidus). The glo-

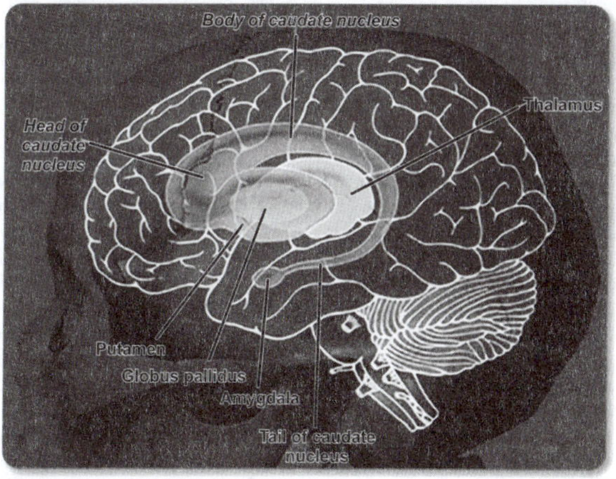

Caudate nucleus

bus in turn is divided into lateral and medial segments by the internal medullary lamina; the medial segment may be subdivided into lateral and medial parts by the accessory medullary lamina. Also known as lenticular n.

Nucleus pulposus A semifluid mass of fine white and elastic fibers that form the central portion of an intervertebral disk; it has been regarded as the persistent remains of the embryonic notochord.

Nucleus ruber (Red nucleus) A distinctive oval nucleus (pink in fresh specimens because of an iron-containing pigment in many of the cells) centrally placed in the upper mesencephalic reticular formation; it receives fibers from the cerebellar nuclei cerebral cortex and projects fibers to the cerebellum, brainstem, and spinal cord.

Nude mouse A researcher's tool for transplant research, specially created by mutation. It does not possess a thymus gland and lacks immune system and body hair.

Null cell (*nul cel*) A lymphocyte that develops in the bone marrow and lacks the characteristic surface markers of the T and B lymphocytes; examples of null cells are natural killer or NK cells.

Null hypothesis A type of statistical hypothesis that proposes that no statistical significance exists in a set of given observations.

Nullipara (*nu-lli'pa-ra*) A woman who has never borne a child.?

Nurse (*ners*) A person involved in the care of the sick persons; a woman taking care of an infant or young child; to suckle a child.

Nursemaid's elbow Subluxation of the head of the radius.

Nurse midwife (*nurs-mid'wif*) A registered nurse with additional training as a midwife who delivers infants and provides prenatal and postpartum care, newborn care, and some routine care (such as gynecological exams) of women.

Nurse midwifery (*nurs-mid'wi-fbr-e*) The independent management of care of essentially normal newborns and women, (antepartum, intrapartum, postpartum), and/or gynecologically, occurring within a health care system which provides for medical consultation, collaborative management, or referral, and is in accord with the functions, standards, and qualifications as defined by the American College of Nurse-Midwives.

Registered nurse A person who has passed general nursing and midwifery examination after training in a recognized school of nursing and has been granted a license to practice nursing profession.

Wet nurse A woman who breast-feeds a baby that is not her own.

Nutraceutical (*nu-tre-su'ti-kal*) A chemical substance considered a nutrient and used for prevention or treatment of disease.

Nutrient (*nu'tre-ent*) Food material that is used by the body to sustain life and health and the examples are carbohydrates, fats, proteins, vitamins and minerals.

Nutrient enema Introduction of saline or glucose into the body via the rectum.

Nutrient medium Culture medium that provides the essential nutrients required for growth of microorganism, usually carbohydrates and proteins.

Nutrition (*nu-tri'shun*) Food material that is metabolized by the body facilitating the building of tissue and liberation of energy.

Enteral nutrition Introduction of nutrients, through a nasogastric tube.

Nux vomica (*nuks vom'i-ka*) Vomiting nut, tree producing strychnine.

Nyctalopia (*nik'ta-lo'pe-ah*) Night blindness encountered in Vitamin A deficiency, retinitis pigmentosa and chorioretinitis.

Nyctophilia Abnormal liking or love for darkness.

Nyctophobia (*nik'to-fo'be-a*) Abnormal fear of darkness.

Nyctophobia (*nik'to-fo'be-a*) Abnormal fear of darkness.

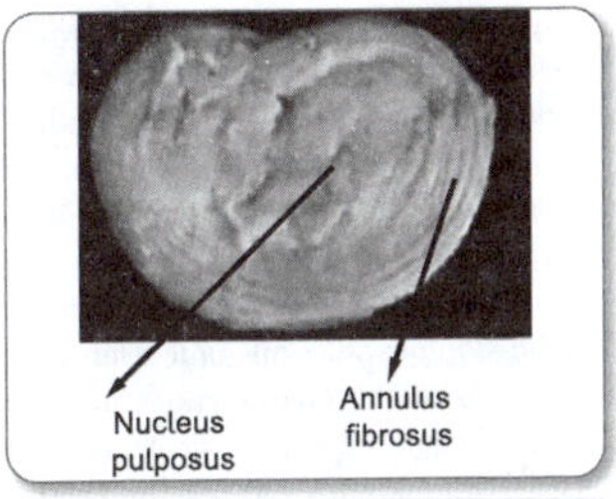

Intervertebral disk showing nucleus pulposus and annulus fibrosus

Nymph *(nimf)* A stage between larva and adult in the life cycle of certain arthropods.

Nymphomania *(nim'fo-ma'ne-a)* Abnormally excessive sexual desire in women.

Nystagmus *(nis-tag'mus)* Involuntary, often rhythmic oscillation of the eyeballs. The movements may be up-and-down, side-to-side or rotary. The speed of the movements may be the same in both directions, or quicker in one direction than another; in the latter case the quicker movements indicate the direction of the nystagmus. Nystagmus may be due to disorders of the vestibular system, lesions affecting the central pathways concerned in ocular movements or to weakness of ocular muscles.

Ataxic nystagmus Nystagmus in abducting eye than in adducting eye during lateral gaze noted in multiple sclerosis involving medial longitudinal fasciculus.

Cerebellar nystagmus Nystagmus in lateral lobe lesions with the fast component toward the side of lesion.

Downbeat nystagmus Nystagmus with fast phase downwards in a lesion at lower medulla.

Gaze-evoked nystagmus Nystagmus in the direction of gaze.

Horizontal nystagmus Nystagmus at extremes of gaze, often it has no pathologic significance.

Jerking nystagmus Nystagmus of constant direction irrespective of direction of gaze and suggests labyrinthine or cerebellar lesion.

Miner's nystagmus Nystagmus of retinal origin noted in miners who work in dim light.

Optokinetic nystagmus A normal reflex phenomenon involving occipital cortex and frontal eye fields. Nystagmus has a slow phase in the direction of movement of the rotating object and a quick corrective phase in opposite direction.

Pendular nystagmus Nystagmus of visual origin and often rotary on central fixation of the eyes. It has a smooth equal oscillation in either direction.

Positional nystagmus Nystagmus associated with benign epidemic vertigo and with posterior fossa tumors, may be induced only by certain movements of the head.

Rebound nystagmus Nystagmus that reverses direction as the eccentric gaze position is held, noted in cerebellar atrophy.

Rotary nystagmus Oscillatory movements of the eyeballs affecting more than one place.

See-saw nystagmus A rare variety in which one eye moves upward while the other moves downward, occurs in lesion of suprasellar region.

Vestibular nystagmus Occurs following damage to inner ear, eighth cranial nerve or its central connections. It is greater on looking away from the side of destructive lesion and the fast component is always directed away from the side of lesion.

Vertical nystagmus Nystagmus that locates the lesion to brain stem.

Upbeat nystagmus Nystagmus with fast components upwards due to lesions at level of superior colliculus.

Nystatin *(nis'ta-tin)* Polyene antifungal agent for candida.

O

Ω Symbol for ohm, SI unit for electrical resistance.

ω Omega, the 24th and last letter of the Greek alphabet.

Oat cell carcinoma A histologic subtype of small cell carcinoma of the lung.

Obesity (*o-be'si-te*) An excessive accumulation of fat in the body resulting in an increase in body weight >20% or more over the maximum desirable weight for his/her weight.

Endogenous obesity Obesity caused by a metabolic abnormality.

Exogenous obesity Obesity due to excessive intake of food.

Hypothalamic obesity Obesity due to a dysfunction of hypothalamus especially the appetite-regulating center.

Obesity hypoventilation syndrome Alveolar hypoventilation during wakefulness and most of them have severe obstructive sleep apnea.

Obex (*o'beks*) Posterior limit of the fourth ventricle marking the beginning of the central canal.

Objective (*ob-jek-tiv*) Lens in a microscope near the object that is being examined aim;

Objective lens Nearest lens to the object being observed under the microscope.

Objective sign A clinical observation that can be seen, heard, measured or recorded.

Objective symptom A symptom that is accompanied by signs.

Oil immersion objective A microscope objective with the space between the objective lens and specimen is filled with oil.

Obligate (*ob'li-gat*) Compulsory, ability to survive in a particular environment.

Obligate aerobe An organism that cannot grow in the absence of oxygen.

Obligate anaerobe An organism that cannot grow in the presence of oxygen such as *Clostridia* organisms.

Obligate parasite An organism that depends entirely on its host for survival.

Obsession (*ob-sesh'un*) *psy* A mental state with an irresistible thought or feeling that cannot be eliminated from consciousness by logical effort which is associated with anxiety.

Obstetric (*obstet'rik*) Relating to childbirth and the processes associated with it; pertaining to obstetrics and midwifery.

Obstipation (*osti-pa'shun*) Severe constipation.

Obstructive (*ob-struk'-tev*) Causing obstruction.

Obstructive sleep apnea Disturbed sleep and respiration due to obstruction to the extrathoracic upper airway at the level of oropharynx. It is sucked in and closed when the patient breaths during sleep.

Obtund (*ob-tund'*) To dull or blunt the level of alertness or consciousness.

Obturator (*obtu-rat'or*) A disk or plate used in closing an opening or a cavity.

Obturator block Obturator nerve is blocked by an anesthetic as it lies in the obturator canal for operations involving the knee joint and medial aspects of the thigh.

Obturator externus The flat triangular muscle covering the outer surface of the anterior wall of the pelvis.

Obturator internus A muscle that covers a large part of the inferior aspect of the lesser pelvis, where it surrounds the obturator foramen.

Obturator membrane A tough fibrous membrane covering the obturator foramen on either side of the pelvis.

Obturator nerve Nerve to adductors of the lower limb and it arises from 3rd and 4th lumbar plexus.

Obturator neuralgia Paroxysmal stabbing pain in the distribution of the great auricular or occipital nerves. The affected nerve may be tender on palpation.

Obturator sign A unilateral increase on the bulk of obturator muscle seen as a soft tissue bulge on inner pelvis with medial displacement of the normal fat line, radiologically it is a feature of infective arthritis.

Obturator test On flexing the right thigh and internally rotating the hip joint, the obturator internus is flexed. An inflamed obtusion appendix in its contact causes pain in the hypogastrium.

Obturator foramen A membrane between the rami of hip bone.

Obturator muscle Two muscles on either side of the pelvis that rotate the thighs outward.

Obtusion *(ob-tu'zhun)* Blunting of sensibility.

Occipital bone Bone in the back of the skull between the parietal and temporal bones.

Occiput (*ok'si-put*) The back portion of the skull. adj. **occipital.**

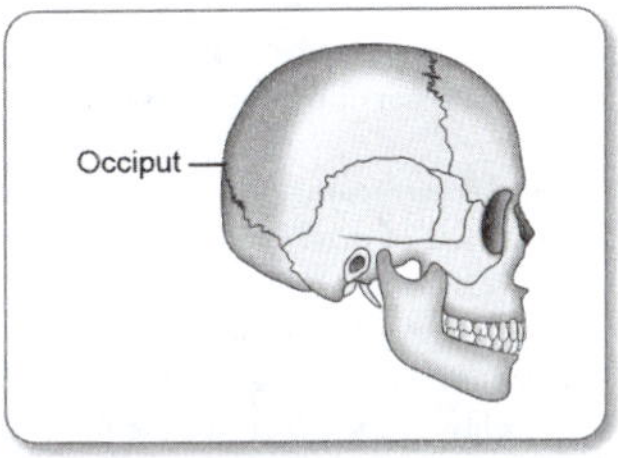

Occiput

Occlusal *(o-kloo'z'l)* pertaining to a closure of an opening such as contact between the teeth of upper and lower jaws.

Occlusal adjustment The grinding of the occluding surfaces of teeth to improve the relation between opposing surface of teeth.

Occlusal contouring The modification by grinding of irregularities of occlusal tooth forms.

Occlusal form The shape of the occluding surfaces of a tooth or teeth.

Occlusal plane A plane passing through the occlusal surfaces of the teeth.

Occlusal rest A support which is part of a removable partial denture.

Occlusal surface The surface of teeth in one arch that makes contact with the corresponding surface of the teeth in the opposite arch.

Occlusal trauma Injury to a tooth and surrounding structures caused by malocclusion stresses.

Occlusal rim The wax occlusal extension of a denture base used to establish jaw and tooth relationships during the construction of a complete or partial denture, also known as bite block or bite rim.

Occlusion (*o-kloo'zhun*) The act of closure; blockage of any channel or opening in the body.

Abnormal occlusion Malocclusion.

Balanced occlusion A type of occlusion in which teeth work harmoniously.

Coronary occlusion Partial or complete occlusion of a coronary artery of heart.

Occlusion rim An artificial dental structure with occluding surfaces attached to temporary or permanent denture bases.

Protrusive occlusion Anteropulsion.

Retrusive occlusion Distoclusion.

Venous occlusion Obstruction of vein.

Occult (*ok-ult*) Concealed, obscure, den.

Occult blood The presence of blood in body fluids or in feces that cannot be seen by the naked eye but can be detected by chemical tests.

Occult cancer A malignancy of unknown origin that first manifests itself as metastasis and it reflects poor prognosis.

Occult fracture Fracture that cannot be found by examination initially but may be evident in radiograph taken subsequently.

Occult hydrocephalus Normal pressure hydrocephalus wherein the ventricles are dilated without an increase in the intracranial pressure. It is associated with progressive dementia, ataxia and urinary incontinence in elderly persons.

Occult infection A bacterial infection in an obscure site presenting with polymorphonuclear leukocytosis and fever of unknown origin.

Occult pneumothorax Pneumothorax seen only on the CT scan.

Occult primary malignancy A histologically proven metastatic malignant tumor with no identifiable primary on routine investigations.

Occupational disease A disease caused by particular job usually resulting from prolonged exposure to harmful substances in the work place.

Occupational mortality A death that occurs while a person is at work or doing work related tasks.

Occupational therapy Utilization of work, self care and play as therapeutic measures to increase the function, to enhance competence and to prevent disability.

Ochronosis (*o'kro-n-o'sis*) An inborn error of protein metabolism causing pigmentation of the body tissues by the deposition of alkapton bodies. There is dusky discoloration of the sclerae and ears, arthritis and darkening of urine on standing due to the presence of homogentisic acid. There is lack of homogentisic acid oxidase in the liver and kidney resulting in accumulation of homogentisic acid.

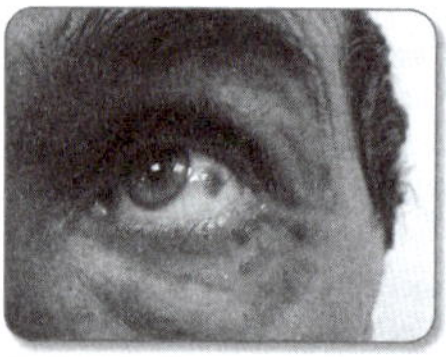

Ochronosis in left eye

Oct- (octa-, octi-, octo-) Combining word for the number eight or series of eight.

Ocular (*ok'u-lar*) Relating to the eye and its structure; pl. **oculi**; eyepiece of a microscope.

Ocular bobbing Sudden, brisk, downward diving eve movements seen in pontine or cerebellar hemorrhage.

Ocular cysticercosis Cysticercosis of the eye may present as retinitis, uveitis, conjunctivitis or choroidal atrophy.

Ocular dysmetria A visual disorder wherein the eyes are unable to fix the gaze on an object or follow a moving object properly.

Ocular fundi Examination with ophthalmoscope the optic disk, arteries, veins, hemorrhages and exudates.

Ocular herpes A herpes virus infection of the eye.

Ocular hypertelorism Markedly widened bridge of the nose and increased distance in between the eyes.

Ocular hypoteleorism Marked narrowing of the bridge of the nose and decreased distance between the eyes.

Ocular larva migrans The larva of toxocara may affect eye producing a posterior chorioretinitis or an intraretinal granuloma.

Ocular movements Horizontal, vertical, diagonal or rotatory movements of the eye.

Ocular myopathy Slowly progressive weakness of ocular muscles exhibiting decreased movements of the eye and ptosis. It may be unilateral or bilateral.

Ocular tension Pressure in the eyeball roughly assessed by palpating the eyeball or accurately by tonometer.

Oculist (*ok'u-list*) Ophthalmologist.

Oculo- (*ok'ulo*) Referable to the eye.

Oculogyric crisis (OGC) A rare, acute dystonic ration involving the extraocularmuscles.

Oculomotor (*ok'u-lo-mot'or*) Relating to the movements of the eye.

Oculomotor nucleus A nucleus of a third cranial nerve in the midbrain.

Oculomotor palsy The eye is deviated downward and outward. There will be paresis, pupils are dilated and fixed. There is an inability to move the eyeball inward and upward.

Oculomotor nerve Third cranial nerve arising in the midbrain. It supplies the medial, superior and inferior recti, inferior oblique, levator palpebrum superioris, ciliary muscle and sphincter muscles of the iris.

Oculonasal (*ok'u-lo-na'zal*) Pertaining to the eye and the nose.

Odaxesmus (*o'dak-sez'mus*) The biting of the tongue, lip or cheek during an epileptic attack.

Oddi's sphincter (*od'ez*) Muscular sphincter at the opening of the common bile duct and pancreatic duct into the duodenum, described by Italian physician, Ruggero Oddi.

O'Donoghue's knee triad Rupture of medial collateral ligament, damage to medial meniscus and rupture of anterior cruciate ligament, described by O'Donoghue, US orthopedic surgeon.

Odontoblast (*o-don'to-blast*) Cell concerned with deposition of dentin and with formation of dentin and with formation of the outer surface of the dental pulp.

Odontoid process Tooth-like projection from the upper surface of the body of second cervical vertebra (axis) which serves as a pivot for the rotation of the first cervical vertebra (atlas) allowing the head to turn.

Odontology (*o'don-tol'o-je*) Dentistry.

Odontoma (*o'don-to'ma*) Benign tumor of tooth.

Ameloblastic odontoma A benign, slow growing, expansile epithelial odontogenic tumor with odontogenic mesenchyme. nonaggressive benign tumor contains enamel, dentin, cementum, and pulp either arranged in an orderly manner resembling a rudimentary tooth.

Complex composite odontoma As a mixed structure of disorganized tissue mass.

Composite odontoma A malformation in which all the dental tissues are presented in a more orderly pattern so that the lesion consists of many tooth-like structures.

Coronary odontoma A tumor involving the teeth or the tissue that surrounds or produces teeth.

Dilated odontoma Lesion appears as a roughly spherical mass that does not resemble a tooth but in a way appears tooth-like on radiographs due to somewhat similar radiodensity.

Odontoma adamantium Immature precursor of complex odontoma.

Odontorrhagia (*o-don'to-ra'je-a*) Hemorrhage from a tooth socket following extraction.

Odynia Pain.

Odynophagia (*o-din'o-fa'jea*) Painful swallowing of food characteristic of monilial and herpes esophagitis.

Oedipus complex (*ed'i-pus*) Sexual feelings of a son toward his mother. Oedipus of Greek mythology, killed his father unknowingly and married his mother.

Oesophagostomum (*e-sof'a-gos'to-mum*) A genus of nematodes of the family Strongylidae, a nodular parasitic worm in the intestines of various animals; the larvae often encyst in the intestinal wall, while the adults are mostly free in the lumen.

Okra sign Radiologically the upper duodenal bulb may appear mildly twisted and filled with air, whose cross-sectional view may appear like a transected okra *Hibiscus esculentus.*

Ointment (*oint'ment*) A semisolid medicinal preparation for external application to the body.

Benzoic and salicylic acid ointment A combination medicine used to treat skin irritation and inflammation caused by burns, insect bites, fungal infections, or eczema.

Hydrophilic ointment As a moisturizer to treat or prevent dry, rough, scaly, itchy skin and minor skin irritations.

Lubricating ophthalmic ointment Keeps the eye moist, helps to protect the eye from injury and infection, and decreases symptoms of dry eyes such as burning, itching, and feeling as if something is in the eye.

Polyethylene ointment Alleviates Psoriasis-like inflammation.

Rose water ointment Contains cetyl esters, wax, white wax, mineral oil, sodium borate, and purified water, for irrigation USP is indicated for use as an irrigating fluid or pharmaceutic aid.

Oleandomycin (*o'le-an'do-mi'sin*) An antimicrobial macrolide.

Olecranon process The proximal articular portion of the ulna is olecranon. Along with the coronoid process, it forms the greater sigmoid notch which articulates with the humerus to provide flexion and extension of the elbow.

Oleic acid (*o-leik*) An organic acid prepared from animal fats and vegetable oils and it is used as an emulsifying agent.

Oleo- Referable to oil.

Oleothorax (*o-le-o-tho'raks*) The therapeutic injection of oil into the pleural cavity.

Oleum Oil; pl. **olea**.

Olfactory (*ol'fak-ter-e*) Relating to the sense of smell.

Olfactory bulb The area of forebrain where the olfactory nerves terminate and olfactory tracts arise.

Olfactory spectogram Test to determine the quality and quantity of sense of smell with seven primary odors—camphoraceous, ethereal, floral, musky, minty, pungent and putrid.

Olig- (oligo-) A combining word for, scanty, little.

Oligemia (*ol'i-geme-a*) Deficiency in the volume of the blood; an increased radiographic lucency.

Oligoarthritis Joint stiffness and swelling that most often affects large joints, such as knees, elbows and ankles, diagnosed in the age group of <16 years.

Oligodactyly (*ol'i-go-dak'ti-le*) Congenital absence of one or more fingers or toes.

Oligodendrocyte (*ol'i-go-den'dro-sit*) A cell of the oligodendroglia. Its dendritic projections coil around axons of neural cells.

Oligodendroglioma (*ol'i-go-den'dro-glio-ma*) A slow-growing neoplasm found on cerebral hemispheres, particularly the frontal lobes consisting of oligodendrocytes.

Oligodipsia (*ol'i-go-dip'se-a*) Hypodipsia.

Oligodontia (*ol'i-go-don'she-a*) Presence of less than normal number of teeth.

Oligohydramnios (*ol'i-go-hi-dram'ne-os*) The presence of abnormally small amount of amniotic fluid in the uterus during pregnancy. It can result in miscarriage, fetal deformities or fetal death; oligoamnios.

Oligomenorrhea (*ol'i-go-men'o-re'a*) Markedly decreased menstrual flow.

Oligophrenia Less than normal mental development. It is of 2 types; First, the associated with damage to the CNS; 2nd is associated with damage to the endocrine system.

Oligospermia (*ol'i-go-sperme-a*) Decrease in the number of spermatozoa in the semen. It forms a major cause of sterility.

Oliguria (*ol'i-gu're-a*) Scanty urine. Amount of urine voided is <500 mL in every 24 hours, and is noted in peripheral circulatory failure, acute nephritis, dehydration and cardiac failure.

o.m. (*L. omni mane*) Every morning.

-oma A suffix meaning tumor, neoplasm.

Omentectomy (*o'men'tek'to-me*) Excision of all or part of the omentum.

Omentopexy (*o-men'to-pek'se*) Fixing the omentum to some other tissue, and is performed to establish collateral circulation.

Omentum (epiploon) (*o'men'tum*) A fold of peritoneum extending from the stomach to adjacent abdominal organs.

Greater omentum An extension of the peritoneum covering the transverse colon and the coils of the small intestine. It is attached along the greater curvature of the stomach and the first part of the duodenum.

Lesser omentum A peritoneal extension from the peritoneal layers covering the stomach and the first part of the duodenum which extends from the portal fissure of the liver to the diaphragm where the layers separate to enclose the end of the esophagus.

Ommaya reservoir A small, plastic device that is implanted in patient's brain. It allows the doctor to deliver medicine directly to the fluid around brain and spinal cord. It also allows the CSF sample to be taken for test.

Omphal- (omphalo-) Umbilicus.

Omphalitis (*om'fa-lit'is*) Inflammation of the umbilicus due to infection of the umbilical stump following its septic cutting and improper hygiene.

Omphalocele (*om'fa-lo-sel*) Protrusion of a part of the intestine at birth through a defect in the abdominal wall at the umbilicus.

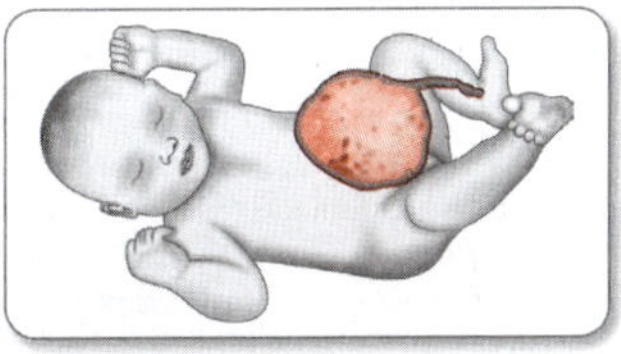

Omphalocele

Omphalus (*om'fa-lus*) The umbilicus.

Onchocerca (*ong'ko-ser'ka*) A filariform nematode whose adult, *Onchocerca volvulus* lives in subcutaneous tissues.

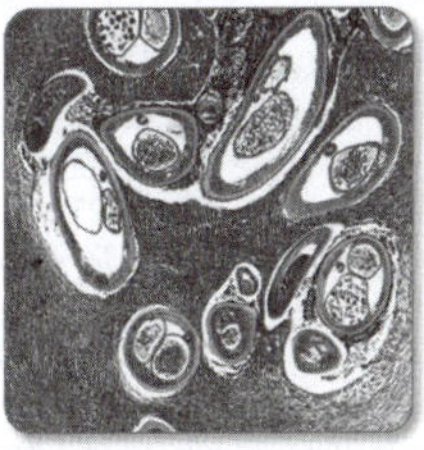

Onchocerca volvulus

Onchocerca dermopathy Skin changes in *Onchocerca* may be in the form of lizard skin (shiny), leopard skin (spotted) and elephant skin (thickened).

Onchocerciasis (*ongko-ser-ki'a-sis*) Infection by nematodes of genus *Onchocerca*. It presents with an itchy and erythematous rash, cutaneous lymphedema with leathery thickening of the skin and impaired visual acuity. It is treated with diethyl carbamazine or ivermectin; river blindness.

Onco- Relating to a tumor.

Oncofeal antigen Proteins, occurring in both tumorous and fetal tissues. These proteins are typically present only during fetal development but are found in adults with certain kinds of cancer.

Oncogene (*ong-ko-jen*) Dominantly acting altered genes that are capable of inducing malignant transformation, such 'cancer genes' are derived from oncogenic RNA viruses and from normal genes.

Oncogenesis (*ong'ko-jene-sis*) The production of tumors. adj. **oncogenetic**.

Oncogenic (*ong'ko-jenik*) Giving rise to tumors (either benign or malignant) or causing tumor formation; said especially of tumor-inducing viruses.

Oncogenic virus Any DNA virus (human papillomavirus) or RNA virus (retrovirus) that has the ability to cause malignant transformation of cells.

Oncolysis (*ong-kol'i-sis*) Destruction of tumor cells.

Oncometer An instrument for measuring variations in size or volume of the internal organs of the body.

Oncosphere (hexacanth) (*ong'-ko-sfer*) Larva of tapeworm which exists in the tissues of vertebrates and invertebrates.

Oncotic (*ong-kotik*) Pertaining to, caused by, or marked by swelling.

Oncotic pressure The osmotic pressure of a colloid in solution.

Oneir- (oneiro-) Combining word for dream.

Oneirism (*o-ni'rizm*) A waking dream state.

Onomatomania (*on'o-mat'o-ma'ne-a*) A mental derangement regarding words or names.

Onomatopoeic (*on'o-ma-to-poik*) Related to the use of words whose sounds suggest their sense.

Ontogeny (*on-toj'i-ne*) Development of the individual organism. adj. **ontogenic**.

Onychauxis (*oni-kawk'sis*) Thickening of the nails.

Onychia (*o-nik'e-a*) Inflammation of the matrix of the nails, resulting in loss of the nail.

Onychogryphosis (*oni-ko-gri-fo'sis*) Ram's horn nails; a disorder of nail plate growth that is characterized by an opaque, yellow-brown thickening of the nail plate with associated gross hyperkeratosis, elongation, and increased curvature.

Onycholysis (*oni-kol'i-sis*) Separation of a nail from nail bed.

Onychomadesis (*on'i-ko-ma-de'sis*) Proximal separation of the nail plate from the nail matrix due to a temporary cessation of nail growth. It can occur in children of all ages including neonates.

Onychomycosis (*on'i-ko-mi-ko'sis*) Fungal infection of the nail; tinea unguium.

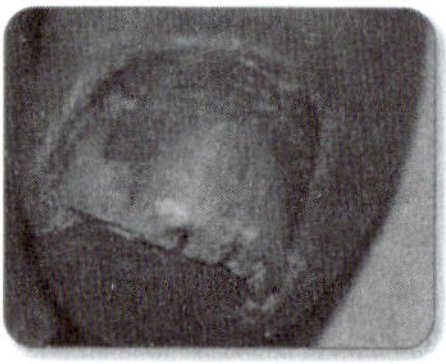

Onychomycosis

Onychosis (*oni-ko'sis*) Disease of the nail.

O'nyong'nyong disease (*o'ni-ang-ni-ang*) A mosquito-borne dengue-like alpha virus infection seen in Uganda, characterized by weakening of the joints and generalized lymphadenopathy.

Oo- A prefix meaning 'of or pertaining to an egg or ovum'.

Oocyst (*o'o-sist*) The encysted zygote in the wall of a mosquito's stomach.

Oocyte (*o'o-sit*) A developing egg cell.

Oogenesis (*o'o-jen'e-sis*) The process of formation of the female gametes or ova.

Oogonium (*o'o-go'ne-am*) An immature female reproductive cell that gives rise to primary oocytes by mitosis.

Ookinete (*o'o-ki-net'*) The fertilized form of the malarial parasite in the body of the mosquito.

Oophorectomy (ovariectomy) (*o-of'o-rek'to-me*) The surgical removal of the one or both ovaries; ovariectomy.

Oophorohysterectomy (*o-of'o-ro-his'ter-ek'to-me*) Surgical removal of the uterus and ovaries.

Oophoritis (ovaritis) (*o-of'o-rit'is*) Inflammation of the ovary.

Oophoropexy (*o-ofo-ro-pek"se*) The operation of elevating and fixing an ovary to the abdominal wall.

Oophoroplasty (*o-of'o-ro-plaste*) Plastic surgery of the ovary.

Oophorosalpingitis (*o-of'o-rosal'pin-je'itis*) An inflammation of both the ovary and fallopian tube.

Operant (*op'er-ant*) Any response that recurs at a given rate without any specific external stimulus.

Operating microscope (*op'er-a-ting*) A binocular microscope used in delicate surgery especially surgery of the eye or ear.

Operculum (*o-per'ku-lum*) A lid or covering.

Cartilaginous operculum A lid or covering consist of cartilage.

Dental operculum Any gum tissue that covers or partially covers the biting surface of a tooth.

Frontal operculum The part of the frontal lobe that overlies the rostrodorsal portion of the insula in primates.

Frontoparietal operculum Covers the upper part of the insular lobe from the front to the back.

Occipital operculum Part of the occipital lobe.

Parietal operculum Part of the parietal lobe.

Temporal operculum Contains Heschl's gyrus which serves as the primary auditory complex.

Trophoblastic operculum A bony plate that covers and protects the gills of most bony fishes.

Operon (*opĕr-on*) *Mol* A segment of chromosome consisting of an operator gene and closely linked structural gene possessing related function; two or more prokaryote genes that are transcribed into a single mRNA.

OPG Stands for Orthopantomogram, which is a type of X-ray scan that provides a panoramic view of the jaw and teeth.

Ophthalmectomy (*of'thal-mek'to-me*) Enucleation of the eyeball.

Ophthalmia (*of-thal'me-a*) Severe inflammation of the eye.

Ophthalmia neonatorum Purulent infection of the eyes of the infant from gonococcus or *Chlamydia*.

Ophthalmic (*of-thal'mik*) Relating to the eye.

Ophthalmic nerve The first division of the trigeminal nerve supplying the eyeball, forehead, scalp, lacrimal gland and dura mater.

Ophthalmitis (*of'thal-mi'tis*) Inflammation of the eye.

Ophthalmodynamometry (*of'thal'mo-di'na-momĕ-tre*) Determination of the retinal artery pressure.

Ophthalmologist (*of'thal-molŏ-jist*) Specialist trained in the diagnosis and management of diseases of the eye.

Ophthalmology (*of'thal'molŏ-je*) Science dealing with the eye and its disorders.

Ophthalmomalacia (*of'thalmo-ma-lăshe-a*) Abnormal softness of the eye.

Ophthalmometer (*of'thal-momĕ-ter*) Instrument to measure refractive powers.

Ophthalmometry (*of'thal-momĕ-tre*) Determination of the refractive powers and defects of the eye.

Ophthalmomyotomy (*of-thal'mo-mi-otŏ-me*) Surgical division of the muscles of the eye.

Ophthalmoplasty (*of-thal'mo-plas'te*) Plastic surgery of the eye or of its appendages.

Ophthalmoplegia (*of'thal'mo-pleje-a*) Partial or total paralysis of the muscles that move the eyes.

Exophthalic ophthalmoplegia Protrusion of the eyeballs due to increased water content of orbital tissues incidental to thyroid disorders, usually hyperthyroidism.

Nuclear ophthalmoplegia An ocular movement disorder that presents as an inability to perform conjugate lateral gaze and ophthalmoplegia due to damage to the interneuron between two nuclei of cranial nerves (CN) VI and CN III (internuclear).

Orbital ophthalmoplegia Ophthalmoplegia due to a lesion within the orbit.

Progressive ophthalmoplegia A disorder characterized by slowly progressive paralysis of the extraocular muscles.

Supranuclear ophthalmoplegia Unable to move their eyes at will in all directions, especially looking upward.

Total ophthalmoplegia Loss of function of all eye muscles, both internal and external.

Ophthalmorrhexis (*of-thal'mo-rek'sis*) Rupture of the eyeball.

Ophthalmoscope (*of'thal'mo-skop*) An illuminated viewing instrument to examine the retina.

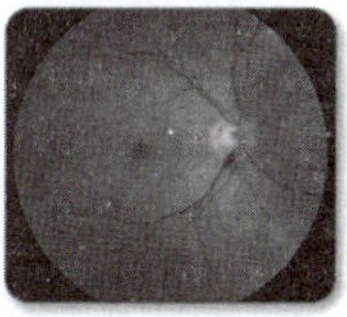

Normal fundal view by ophthalmoscope

Ophthalmotomy (*ofthal-moto-me*) The operation of incising the eyeball.

Ophthalmotonometry A diagnostic test that measures the intraocular pressure inside the eyes. It helps to assess the risk of glaucoma.

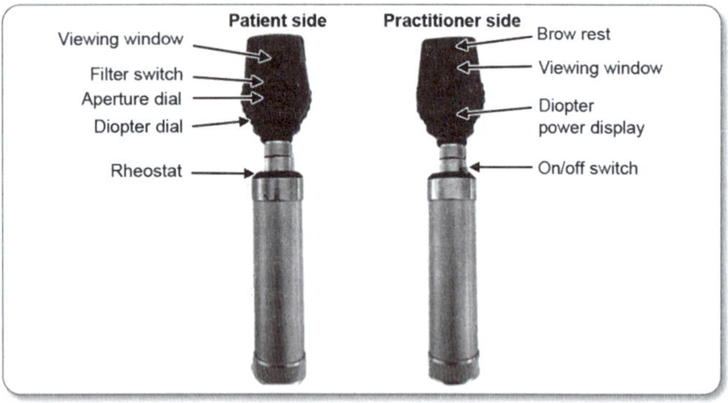

Ophthalmoscope

Opiate (*ope-at*) Any natural or synthetic (fentanyl) semisynthetic (morphine) alkaloid narcotic possessing opium-like activity.

Opiate poisoning Toxic effects of the potent narcotic causing depression of brain centers and coma.

Opiate receptor Any of a group of cells in the brain that bind to opiate drugs.

Opisthorchiasis (*o'pis-thor-ki'a-sis*) Infection with *Opisthorchis viverrini* (Southeast Asian liver fluke) or *O. felineus* (cat liver fluke), which is acquired by eating infected raw or undercooked fish that contains infectious metacercariae (encysted stage).

Opisthorchis (*o'pis-thor'kis*) A genus of trematodes, characterized by having the testes near the posterior end of the body.

Opisthotonos (*o'pis-thoto-nos*) A spasm wherein the head and the heels are bent back making the body like a bow noted in extreme cases of tetanus.

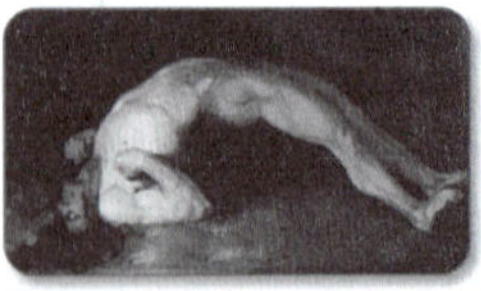

Opisthotonos

Opium (*o'pe-um*) Exudate from capsules of *Papaver somniferum*. Morphine, heroin and codeine are extracted from opium.

Crude opium One of the oldest recreational and medicinal drugs in the world, extracted from the unripe pods of the poppy flower, opium serves as the raw material for production of numerous drugs, both legal like morphine, codeine, hydromorphone, oxycodone, hydrocodone, etc., and illegal like heroin.

Denarcotized opium Powdered opium treated with purified petroleum benzine that removes certain nauseating and odorous constituents.

Opponens (*o-po'nens*) Opposing.

Opponens pollicis muscle In the thumb tested by touching the top of the little finger with the point of the thumb.

Opportunistic infections (*op'or-tu-nis'tik*) Infections caused by organisms which rarely produce disease in a healthy person but frequently cause disease in persons whose immune system is weakened by a disease such as AIDS or as a result of immunosuppressive therapy.

Opsonic index A numerical measure of potency of a given individual's serum to opsonize foreign material or bacteria, ready for phagocytosis.

Opsonin (*op-so'nin*) A substance that binds to red cells, bacteria or other exogenous agents enhancing their susceptibility to phagocytosis.

Opsonization (*op'so-ni-za'shun*) Rendering of bacteria and other cells subject to phagocytosis.

Optic (*op'tik*) Pertaining to the eyes or to sight.

Optic chiasma (optic commissure) Optic nerves of both sides meet at this point lying in close contact with pituitary gland and there is decussation of fibers from the inner half of each retina.

Optic density A number describing the blackening of an X-ray film in any specified location.

Optic disk Pink, oval or circular prominent structure of retina whose margins are sharp with a small central depression.

Optic disk drusen Condensations of hyaline-like material within the substance of the optic nerve head.

Optic fundus Fundus of the eye.

Optic glioma A slow-growing tumor on the optic nerve or in the chiasma. It consists of glial cells and presents with loss of vision, strabismus, exophthalmos and ocular paralysis.

Optic radiation Axons of nerve cells of lateral geniculate body carrying visual information.

Optic righting A basic neuromuscular reaction enabling a person to change body position that involves a reflex that automatically orients the head to a new optical or visual fixation point, depending on the body position change.

Optic stalk One of a pair of slender embryonic structures that becomes the optic nerve.

Optic tract Nerve fibers running backward and laterally around each cerebral peduncle from the optic chiasma to the lateral geniculate body.

Optic atrophy Optic disk is paler than normal and may even be white.

Optic cup The optic disc has a center portion called the 'cup' which is normally quite small in comparison to the entire optic disc.

Optical coherence tomography (OCT) An imaging technology using an infrared light to obtain cross-sectional images of tissues.

Optic foramen An aperture in the root of the lesser wing of the sphenoidal bone transmitting the optic nerve.

Optician (*op-tish'an*) Person who fits and supplies spectacles or contact lenses.

Optic nerve Second cranial nerve that transmits information about visual images received from the retina to the lateral geniculate body. It also acts as an afferent pathway for the pupillary reflexes.

Optic neuritis Inflammatory demyelinating or vascular disease affecting optic nerve leading to loss of vision.

Opticociliary (*op'ti-ko-sile-ar-e*) Pertaining to the optic and ciliary nerves.

Optometer (refractometer) (*op-tom'e-ter*) Instrument measuring the power and range of vision.

Optometrist (*op-tom'e-trist*) A person trained to test the eyes and prescribe spectacles and other visual aids.

Oral (*or'al*) Pertaining to the mouth.

Oral allergy syndrome Contact with certain fresh fruit juices results in urticaria and angioedema of the lips and oropharynx.

Oral cancer A malignant neoplasm on the lip or in the mouth.

Oral glucose tolerance test Test to determine the ability to metabolize sugar. Performed in the morning after 3 days of unrestricted diet and physical activity, but the patient should be fasting at least 10 hours before and a loading dose of glucose of 75 g (adults) or 1.75 g/kg (children) given.

Oral hygiene Maintenance of the tissues and structures of the mouth clean by brushing the teeth, massaging the gums.

Oral hypoglycemic agents They are sulfonylureas (tolbutamide, chlorpropamide, glypizide, glibenclamide, glyclazide and glimepiride), biguanides (phenformin, metformin), guargum and acarbose.

Oral poliovirus vaccine An attenuated live poliovirus vaccine that confers immunity to poliomyelitis prepared by Albert Sabin, US virologist.

Oral rehydration therapy (ORT) Administration of 3.5 g sodium chloride, 2.5 g sodium bicarbonate, 1.5 g potassium chloride and 20 g of glucose dissolved in one liter of water orally at frequent intervals to correct dehydration caused by diarrhea.

Oral surgery Surgery concerned with operations in and around the mouth.

Oral temperature Recording of body temperature with the centigrade clinical thermometer. Orally, before its use, the thermometer should be washed with water and the mercury column brought down by shaking it. The thermometer should be kept beneath the tongue and the mouth closed. It must be allowed to stay for 1–2 minutes. The normal temperature is 37°C (98.6°F) with average from 36.6°C to 37.2°C (98°–99°F).

Oral ulceration Ulceration in oral mucosa, which may occur as aphthous ulcers or in association with systemic disorders.

Oral white patches White lesions in the oral mucosa either due to *Candida* infection or are rarely seen in SLE.

Oral cavity The cavity of the mouth including the tongue and teeth.

Oral contraceptive Used as effective spacing method of contraception and they prevent release of the ovum from the ovary. Combined pill consisting of 30–35 mcg of a synthetic estrogen with 0.5–1.0 mg progesterone taken orally for 21 consecutive days beginning on the fifth day of the menstrual cycle, followed by a break of 7 days during which period menstruation occurs. Mini pill consists of progesterone only and it is given throughout the cycle. Morning after pill or postcoital pill contains very high doses of estrogen and is used in an unprotected intercourse.

Orbicularis Muscles in the face supplied by facial nerve.

Orbicularis oculi Muscle of the eye which helps in closing the eye tightly.

Orbicularis oris Muscle of lips that helps to purse the lips.

Orbit (*or'bit*) Socket in the skull containing the eyeball, protective pads of fat, blood vessels, muscles and nerves; also called eye socket or orbita.

Orbitotomy (*or'bi-tot'o-me*) The operation of incising or opening into the orbit through the orbital margin.

Orchialgia (*or-ke-al'je-a*) Pain in the testis.

Orchiectomy (*or'ke-ek'to-me*) Surgical removal of one or both testes.

Orchiopexy (*or'ke-o-pek'se*) Surgical fixation of an undescended testis into the scrotum.

Orchiotomy (*o"ke-ot'o-me*) An incision into a testis, such as for drainage; called also orchidotomy.

Orchitis (*or-kit'is*) Inflammation of one or both testes characterized by swelling and pain. Treatment includes support and elevation of the scrotum, cold packs and analgesics.

Mumps orchitis Pain and swelling of the testicle (orchitis), seen as complication of mumps infection.

Orf Also known as ecthyma contagiosum, contagious pustular dermatitis, infectious labial dermatitis, scabby mouth, or sore mouth, is a viral disease seen in sheep. Also referred as sheep pox.

Organ (*or'gan*) Any part of the body perforating a specific function.

Organ bank A repository for a long-term storage of certain tissues destined for transplantation.

Organ donation Permission given by a person or from relatives after the death of a person for surgical removal of one or more organs for use in transplant surgery.

Organ of Corti The true organ of hearing named after Alfonso Corti, Italian anatomist. It is a spiral structure within the cochlea containing hair cells that are stimulated by sound vibrations.

Organ recital Giving a list of complaints from multiple organs and organ systems by a hypochondriac.

Organ transplantation Transfer of an organ (kidney, heart, liver) between members of the same species.

Organelle (*or'gan-el'ae*) Specialized structure within a cell which is separated from the rest of the cell by a membrane composed of lipids and proteins, where chemical and metabolic functions take place.

Organic (*or-gan'ik*) Pertaining to an organ.

Organic amnestic syndrome A marked impairment of memory occurring in clear consciousness. It is associated with impairment of short-term memory. It may be noted in severe thiamine deficiency secondary to chronic alcohol abuse.

Organic brain syndrome Cerebral degeneration in the form of cortical atrophy.

Organic delusional disorder A mental state dominated by delusions which are very often persecutory.

Organic disease Disorder accompanied by demonstrable changes in the body structure.

Organic mental disorders Disorders characterized by progressive deterioration of the mental processes. They develop from brain dysfunction or brain damage.

Organism (*or'gan-izm*) Any living individual either animal or plant. It is an organized system of parts that ordinarily work together in a unified manner.

Organ of Jacobson (vomeronasal organ) An organ of chemoreception that is part of olfactory system of amphibians, reptiles and mammals, although not found in all tetrapods. It occurs as a patch of sensory cells within the nasal chamber that detects heavy moisture-borne odor particles.

Organotrophic (*or'ga-no-tro'fik*) Heterotrophic.

Orgasm (*or'gazm*) Peak of sexual excitement, experienced as an intensely pleasurable sensation.

Oriental sore (Baghdad boil, Delhi boil, Aleppo boil) Cutaneous leishmaniasis caused by *Leishmania tropica*.

Orientation (*or'en-ta-shun*) Determination of one's position with respect to space and time.

Origin (*or'i-jin*) The point of beginning.

Ornithine (*or'ni-then*) An amino acid formed on hydrolysis of arginine by arginase.

Ornithosis (*or'ni-tho'sis*) An acute generalized, infectious disease of birds transmitted to man and is caused by *Chlamydia psittaci*, psittacosis, parrot fever. Illness is like influenza and effective treatment is tetracycline or erythromycin.

Oro- A combining word for related to mouth.

Oroantral fistula An epithelialized pathological unnatural communication between the oral cavity and the maxillary sinus.

Orphan (*or'fen*) Destitute; a child whose parents have died or are not known.

Orphan disease An illness due to its rarity has received less attention.

Orphan drugs Drugs used to treat rare diseases but are not profitable to the manufacturer.

Orphan virus A virus that has been isolated and identified although it has not been associated with any particular disease.

Oropharynx (*or'o-far'inks*) The region of pharynx lying between the soft palate and epiglottis.

Oroya fever Also known as carrion's disease is a bacterial infection caused by the bartonella bacilliformis bacteria.

Orphenadrine (*or-fen'e-dren*) An anticholinergic drug of the ethanolamine antihistamine class; it is closely related to diphenhydramine. It is a muscle relaxant that is used to treat muscle pain and to help with motor control in Parkinson's disease.

Ortho- Combining word for straight, regular, upright.

Orthochromatic (*or'tho-kro-mat'ik*) Having normal color or staining normally.

Orthodiagraph A fluoroscopic device used in making orthodiagrams.

Orthodonic appliance A dental device that is fabricated specifically for treatment of a dental condition.

Orthodontics (*or'tho-don'tiks*) Branch of dentistry referring to corrective dental work for irregularities of teeth; orthodontia.

Orthopantomogram (OPG) A common-radiograph used to indentify the hard tissues of the oral cavity and surrounding skeletal structures.

Orthopedics (*ortho-pe diks*) The branch of surgery concerned with the disease of the skeletal system.

Orthopercussion (*ortho-per-kush'un*) Percussion wherein the terminal phalanx of the pleximeter finger is held perpendicular to the chest wall.

Orthophoria (*or"tho-fo're-a*) A normal condition of balance of the ocular muscles of the two eyes in which their lines of vision meet at the object toward which they are directed.

Orthopneic position (*or'thop'ne-ik*) A posture that enables to breath comfortably. The patient sits and bends forward with the arms supported on a table.

Orthopnoea (*or'tho-p-ne'a*) Dyspnea in the recumbent, but not in the upright position. It is usually relieved by two or three pillows under the head and neck. It is a hallmark of pulmonary congestion that stiffens the lungs.

Orthopraxis (*or"tho-prak'sis*) Correct practice or the belief that right action is as important as religious faith.

Orthoptics The science of correcting defects in binocular vision that have resulted from defects in optic musculature.

Orthostatic (*ortho-sta-tik*) Caused by standing erect.

Orthostatic hypotension Blood pressure falling when the individual assumes the standing posture; postural hypotension.

Orthostatic proteinuria A benign condition where apparently healthy persons excrete small amounts of protein in relation to assuming erect posture.

Os Any orifice of the body, bone; mouth, opening.

Os hamatum hamate bone The medial bone in the distal row of carpal bones; called also fourth carpal or unciform bone.

Os sutura'le pi; os'sa sutura'lia sutural bone Any of the small irregular bones in the sutures between the bones of the skull, most frequently in the course of the lambdoid suture and often at the fontanelles (ossa fonticulorum); called also epactal bone and Wormian bone.

Oscilloscope (*a-silo-skop*) A laboratory instrument commonly used to display and analyze the waveform of electronic signals on fluorescent screen of a cathode ray tube. In effect, the device draws a graph of the instantaneous signal voltage as a function of time.

Osculum (*os'ku-lum*) Minute opening.

Osmolagnia (*oz-mo-lag'ne-a*) Sexual excitation produced by odor.

Osmolal gap (*os'mo-lal-gap*) An osmometer measurement indicating a serum osmolality that is >10 Osm/L greater than the calculated osmolality. It suggests the presence of an osmotically active substance that is not accounted for by the calculated osmolality. Ethanol produces an increase in measured osmolality over the calculated osmolality.

Osmoreceptor (*oz'mo-re-sep'tor*) A sensory receptor stimulated by changes in the osmotic pressure or by sensation of odors.

Osmosis (*oz-mo'sis*) The passage of a solvent from a less concentrated solution to a concentrated one through a semi-permeable membrane.

Osseous (*os'e-us*) Bony

Osseous labyrinth The bony portion of the internal ear. It consists of three cavities: vestibule, semicircular canals, and cochlea. It contains perilymph in which a membranous labyrinth is suspended.

Ossicle (*os'i-kl*) A small bone.

Ossicle of Bertin A shell-shaped structure; Bertin bone.

Wormian ossicle Supernumerary bones of the skull that form as a result of extra ossification centers during development in utero.

Ossification (osteogenedis) (*os'i-fi-ka'shun*) The process of formation of bone; conversion of cartilage into bone.

Intracartilaginous ossification Preceded by cartilage as in the bones of the limb.

Intramembranous ossification Preceded by membrane as in the formation of the roof and sides of the skull.

Ostectomy (*os-tek'to-me*) The excision of a bone.

Osteitis (*oste-itis*) Inflammation of a bone; ostitis.

Acute osteitis A bacterial infection of the bone and surrounding soft tissues, that occurs within 8 weeks of trauma or an operation.

Alveolar osteitis Inflammation of the alveolar bone.

Caseous osteitis Tuberculous caries in bone.

Chronic nonsuppurative osteitis A chronic bone disease and may be associated with a reparative periosteum entity called proliferative periostitis (PP).

Chronic osteitis A rare autoinflammatory disorder characterized by the presence of sterile bone lesions.

Cortical osteitis Inflammation of bony structures, in particular the cortex.

Garre's osteitis A type of chronic osteomyelitis also called periostitis ossificans and Garré's sclerosing osteomyelitis.

Gummatous osteitis Inflammation of a bone as a consequence of infection or trauma or degeneration.

Osteitis deformans A chronic bone disorder characterized by excessive breakdown and regrowth in the affected bone; *see* Paget's disease.

Osteitis fibrosa cystica *see* Hyperparathyroidism. There is replacement of normal bone by cysts and fibrous tissue; a disorder involving the bone which is resulted from excessive production of parathyroid hormone (PTH) due to parathyroid gland hyperactivity; osteitis fibrosa osteoplastica.

Sclerosing osteitis An inflammatory condition believed to be a local bony reaction to a low-grade inflammatory stimulus or to bacteria of low virulence.

Osteo A prefix meaning 'of or relating to a bone'.

Osteoarthritis (osteoarthrosis) (*os'te-o-ar-thri'tis*) Degenerative joint disease characterized by both degeneration of articular cartilage and simultaneous proliferation of new bone, cartilage and connective tissue. The joints most frequently involved are those of the spine, hip, knees and hands.

Facet osteoarthritis Happens when the cartilage that covers the ends of the joints, wears out and becomes thin.

Interphalangeal osteoarthritis Arthritis of the fingers.

Osteoarthritis deformans A chronic, proliferative, noninfectious inflammation, which gradually leads to progressive mutilation of the joint.

Osteoarthropathy (*os'te-o-ar-throp'a-the*) Any disease of the joints and bones.

Familial osteoarthropathy A rare disorder that is considered to be a form of avascular necrosis of the proximal interphalangeal joints of the fingers and toes.

Hypertrophic osteoarthropathy A syndrome characterized by a combination of clinical findings of severe disabling arthralgia and arthritis, digital clubbing, and periostosis of tubular bones, with or without synovial effusion; swelling around the wrists and ankles from periosteal thickening.

Hypertrophic pulmonary osteoarthropathy A condition that affects some people with lung cancer. It most often causes inflammation of bones and joints in the wrists and ankles. Another common symptom is clubbing of the fingers.

Idiopathic hypertrophic osteoarthropathy A condition occurring predominantly in males at the age of puberty or adolescence and characterized by the osteo-arthropathic syndrome—clubbing of the digits, enlargement of bones and joints, and thickening of the skin of the face—in the absence of any demonstrable primary disease.

Osteoarthrosis (*os'te-o-ar-thro'sis*) Non-inflammatory joint involvement.

Osteoarthrotomy (*os"te-o-ahr-throt'a-me*) Surgical removal of the articulating end of a bone.

Osteoblast (*os'te-o-blast*) Cell arising from a fibroblast concerned with building new bone.

Osteochondritis (*os'te-o-kon-dri'tis*) Inflammation of bone and cartilage.

Osteochondritis ischiopubica A rare cause of pain in the pediatric pelvis due to late closure in synchondrosis ischiopubic, whose main symptom is an asymmetric pain that can cause a limitation in movement or limp.

Osteochondritis juvenalis Inflammation of a growing area of bone in a child or adolescent. It causes local pain and distortion of a joint.

Osteochondritis necroticans Necrosis and destruction in the cartilage of the sesamoid bone of the great toe.

Osteochondritis dissecans A disorder following an injury, releasing small fragments of cartilage or bone into the joint space especially of the knee and elbow.

Osteochondroma (*oste-o-kon-dro'ma*) A benign tumor of bone originating from the growing epiphyseal cartilage. It grows outward from the bone like a mushroom and is capped by cartilage.

Osteochondrosis (*oste-o-kon-dro'sis*) A disease of ossification center in children which exhibits degeneration followed by regeneration.

Osteochondrosis deformans tibiae A deformity of abrupt angulation into varus below the knee and inward rotation of the tibia.

Osteoclasis (osteoclasia, osteoclasty) (*os'te-o-kla'sis*) Forcible bending or incomplete breaking of a bone to correct deformities of the long bones.

Osteoclast (*os'te-o-klast*) Cell concerned with the absorption and removal of bone; an instrument useful in the surgical fractures of bone.

Osteoclastoma (*os'-te-o-klas-to'ma*) Giant cell tumor of bone. Though benign, it tends to recur after removal, noted in young adults. It presents with pain at the site of the tumor and a gradually increasing local swelling. There is destruction of the bone with expansion of the cortex.

Osteocyte (*os'-te-o-sit*) An osteoblast within the bony matrix.

Osteodystrophy (*os'-te-o-dis'tro-fe*) Defective bone formation.

Albright hereditary osteodystrophy A hereditary condition due to inactivating GNAS1 gene mutation.

Renal osteodystrophy A bone disease that occurs in adults and children with chronic kidney disease.

Osteogenesis (*os'-te-o-jen'e-sis*) Formation of bone.

Osteogenesis imperfecta (fragilitas ossium) A genetic disorder in which bones are abnormally soft and easily broken. It is associated with blue sclerae, deafness, scoliosis, thin hyperextensible skin, visceral herniation, ligamentous laxity and easy bruising; fragilitas ossium; brittle bone disease.

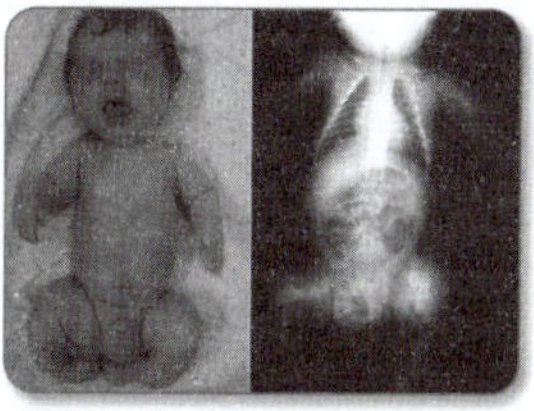

Osteogenesis imperfecta

Osteology (*os'-te-ol'o-je*) The scientific study of the bone.

Osteolysis (*os'-te-ol'i-sis*) Degeneration and dissolution of bone, resulting from disease, infection or lack of a blood supply.

Osteoma (*os-te-o'ma*) A bony tumor, that may occur on any bone. It may be composed of hard compact bone (ivory osteoma) or of spongy bone (cancellous osteoma).

Osteoma myelofibrosis A chronic progressive condition characterized by panmyelosis and variable marrow fibrosis, massive splenomegaly secondary to extramedullary hematopoiesis.

Osteomalacia (*os'-te-o-mal-a-she-a*) Softening, weakening and demineralization of adult bones due to vitamin D deficiency, phosphate depletion or chronic metabolic acidosis. It presents with bone pain and tenderness. There can be proximal myopathy. Radiologically the bones appear less dense than normal and the long bones may show areas of decalcification treated by vitamin D_2.

Hepatic osteomalacia A frequent condition in patients with chronic liver disease, particularly in cholestatic diseases. Hepatic osteodystrophy is mainly due to osteoporosis, which is clinically relevant especially in patients with advanced liver disease and after liver transplantation.

Oncogenic osteomalacia A paraneoplastic syndrome of renal phosphate wasting caused by a bone or soft tissue tumor.

Puerperal osteomalacia A type resulting from exhaustion of skeletal stores of calcium and phosphorus by repeated pregnancies and lactation.

Senile osteomalacia A multifactorial skeletal disease, characterized by a reduction in bone mass and deterioration of the microarchitectural structure of bone tissue, with a resulting increase of bone fragility and of fracture risk.

Osteomyelitis (*os'-te-o-mi-el-i'tis*) Inflammation of bone and bone marrow due to a pyogenic infection.

Acute hematogenous osteomyelitis An infection that usually affects the growing skeleton, involving primarily the most vascularized regions of the bone.

Acute osteomyelitis Infection of the bone with pyogenic organisms—usually the *Staphylococcus aureus*. A minor injury to bone renders it vulnerable to infection by organisms circulating in the blood. Occurs in children, has rapid onset with pain over the affected bone and fever.

Chronic osteomyelitis Occurs as a sequel to acute osteomyelitis. It is common in long bones. The bone is thickened and denser than normal with presence of sequestra. Often a sinus track leads to skin surface. In addition to rest and antibiotics, the fragments of infected dead bone have to be removed.

Conchiolin osteomyelitis A condition seen in workers in mother-of-pearl, probably due to the inhaled dust being deposited in the bone marrow.

Diffuse sclerosing osteomyelitis A rare inflammatory disease of bone, which affects the mandible and other long bones.

Focal sclerosing osteomyelitis A periapical lesion that involves reactive osteogenesis evoked by chronic inflammation of the dental pulp.

Garre's osteomyelitis A rare chronic inflammatory disease resulting in thickening of cortices with loss of medullary canal without any signs of active infection.

Sclerosing nonsuppurative osteomyelitis It is also known as Garré's sclerosing osteomyelitis, chronic osteomyelitis with proliferative periostitis, ossifying periostitis, or nonsuppurative chronic sclerosing osteomyelitis.

Typhoid osteomyelitis Caused due to *Salmonella typhi* infection, the lesion is usually single and well-localized and runs a chronic course.

Vertebral osteomyelitis A type of osteomyelitis that affects the vertebrae. It is a rare bone infection concentrated in the vertebral column.

Osteopathy (*os'-te-op-a-the*) Any disease of a bone; a system of medicine relying on manipulation of various body parts to regain a state of wellness; a form of manipulation of the spinal and other joints based on realignment.

Hunger osteopathy A nonspecific term for any diet-related bone disease, which may include the osteomalacia of rickets, anorexia nervosa (or starvation-related osteopenia) and/or osteoporosis, as well as other conditions.

Hypertrophic osteopathy An unusual disorder involving bilaterally symmetrical proliferation of fibrous tissue and periosteal bone in the appendicular and, less frequently, the axial skeleton, involving the metaphyseal and diaphyseal regions of several bones of all limbs.

Osteopetrosis (Albers-Schonberg disease, marble-bone disease) (*os-te-o-pe-tro'sis*) A rare genetic disorder showing abnormally hard, dense bone due to a faulty bone resorption. There is increased liability of fracture and anemia.

Osteophyte (*os'-te-o-fit*) An overgrowth of a bone at the edge of a joint, seen in osteoarthritis.

Osteoporosis (*os-te-o-por-o'sis*) A systemic skeletal disease characterized by low bone mass and microarchitectural deterioration with a consequent increase in bone fragility and susceptibility to fracture.

Juvenile osteoporosis A skeletal disorder characterized by thinning of the bones (osteoporosis) that begins in childhood. Osteoporosis is caused by a shortage of calcium and other minerals in bones.

Osteoporosis of disuse A state of bone loss due to local skeletal unloading or systemic immobilization.

Postmenopausal osteoporosis Generalized skeletal disorder in which because of decreased bone density or deteriorating bone quality, there is increased risk of fracture.

Senile osteoporosis Bone loss that results from aging; diffuse osteoporosis of unknown cause affecting elderly, especially women. There is reduction of total bone mass and compression fracture of vertebrae may be noted.

Osteosarcoma (*os'-te-o-sar-ko'ma*) *see* Osteogenic sarcoma.

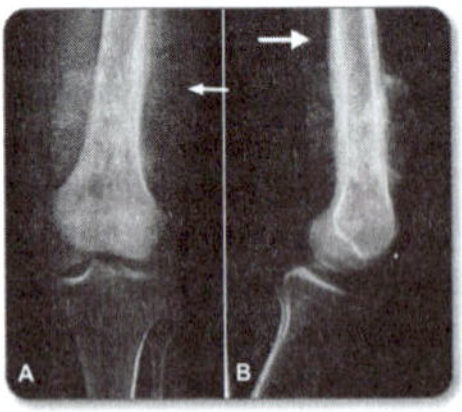

Osteosarcoma: ***A.*** *PA view;* ***B.*** *Lateral view*

Chondroblastic osteosarcoma A histological entity characterized by predominant presence of chondroid matrix, which tends to exhibit a high degree of hyaline cartilage and is intimately associated with the nonchondroid element (osteoid or bone matrix).

Extraosseus osteosarcoma A malignant neoplasm that produces osteoid, bone, and chondroid material without direct attachment to bone or periosteum.

Gnathic osteosarcoma A subtype of osteosarcoma that primarily affects the mandible (horizontal ramus) and maxilla (alveolar ridge, sinus floor, and palate).

Intracranial osteosarcoma A highly malignant neoplasm of bone and can occur anywhere in the body, but is most commonly found in the long bones.

Telangiectatic osteosarcoma Typically a purely lytic lesion with a permeative destructive growth pattern.

Osteosclerosis (*os-te-o-skle-ro'sis*) Hardening or an abnormal density of bone.

Osteotome (*os-te-o-tom*) A chisel-like knife useful to cut the bone.

Osteotomy (*os-te-ot'o-me*) The surgical cutting of a bone to correct a deformity or to change its length or to improve the joint stability.

Ostium (*os-te-um*) Opening between cavities or an opening into a tube.

Ostium abdominale tubae uterinae A small opening or orifice, as in a body organ or passage.

Ostium anatomicum internum uteri (*L*) Anatomical internal os of uterus.

Ostium aortae Opening of the right coronary artery is in the right aortic sinus and that of the left coronary artery is in the left aortic sinus, just above the aortic valve ring.

Ostium appendicis vermiformis The opening of the vermiform appendix into the lumen of the cecum.

Ostium atrioventriculare dextrum (*L*) An atrioventricular opening that leads from the right atrium into the right ventricle of the heart.

Ostium cardiacum The orifice between the esophagus and the stomach: called also cardiac orifice.

Ostium secundum An opening in the upper portion of the membrane dividing the embryonic heart into right and left sides, appearing later than the ostium primum.

Ostwald coefficient The amount of gas which dissolves in a unit volume of solvent, measured under the conditions of temperature and pressure at which solution takes place, described by Wilhelm Ostwald, Russian-German physical chemist.

Otalgia (*os-tal'je-a*) Earache.

Otitis (*o-ti'tis*) Inflammation of the ear.

Otitis externa An inflammation or infection of the external auditory canal (EAC), the auricle, or both.

Otitis externa acute bacterial An inflammation or infection of the external auditory canal (EAC), the auricle, or both due to *Pseudomonas aeruginosa* and *Staphylococcus aureus* infection.

Otitis externa circumscribed An abscess-forming infection of a hair follicle (i.e., a furuncle) in the cartilaginous part of the external auditory canal, mostly due to *Staphylococcus aureus*.

Otitis externa fungi An inflammation or infection of the external auditory canal (EAC), the auricle, or both because of fungal infection.

Otitis externa malignant An infection that affects the external auditory canal and temporal bone. The causative organism is usually *Pseudomonas aeruginosa*, and the disease commonly manifests in elderly patients with diabetes.

Otitis externa necrotizing A severe infection of the ear canal with frequent bone erosion and local complications.

Otitis interna Inflammation of the inner ear often resulting from an infection that inflames one or both of the labyrinthine compartments.

Otitis media Inflammation of the middle ear. It may be acute, noted in children, characterized by severe pain, fever and varying degree of deafness. The tympanic membrane is bulging, reddish and sometimes pulsatile. It may resolve or lead to perforation. Chronic otitis media presents with continuous discharge of pus and deafness. There is a hole in the tympanic membrane.

Otitis media adhesive A condition in which the tympanic membrane is depressed and adheres to the fibrous scar tissue caused by chronic inflammation in the inner wall of the middle ear cavity, resulting in the loss of aeration in the tympanic cavity.

Otitis media atelectasis A condition of retraction and atrophy of the tympanic membrane in chronic otitis media with effusion.

Otitis media catarrhal Otitis media with catarrhal stage.

Otitis media mucoid Mucus accumulation in the middle ear cavity.

Otitis media purulent An acute, suppurative infectious process marked by the presence of infected middle ear fluid and inflammation of the mucosa lining the middle ear space.

Otitis media serous Also called serous otitis media or "glue ear," is defined as the presence of middle ear fluid without signs of acute infection.

Otitis media suppurative An initial episode of acute otitis media and is characterized by a persistent discharge from the middle ear through a tympanic perforation.

Otocranium (*o"to-kra-neum*) The area of the petrous part of the temporal bone surrounding the osseous labyrinth.

Otocyst (*o'to-sist*) The auditory vesicle of the embryo, the primordium of the internal ear or the auditory sac of certain animals.

Otolaryngology (*o'to-lar'in-gol-o-je*) Branch of medical science dealing with the diseases of the ear, nose and throat.

Otolith (Otoconium) (*o'to-lith*) A calcareous mass in the inner ear.

Otology (*o-tol' o-je*) Branch of medical science dealing with the ear.

Otomycosis (*o'to-mi-ko'sis*) Fungal infection of the external ear and ear canal.

Otoplasty (*o'to-plas-te*) A reconstructive surgery of the cartilage in the ears.

Otorhinolaryngology (*o'to-ri-no-lar-in-gol-o-je*) Branch of medicine dealing with the disease of ear, nose, pharynx and larynx.

Otorrhagia Presence of blood coming from the ear canal. Cause can be minor injury to more serious underlying conditions.

Otorrhea (*oto-rea*) A discharge from the ear. It may be serous, purulent or sanguineous.

Otosclerosis (*o'to-skle-ro'sis*) An inherited disorder exhibiting irregular ossification in the bony labyrinth of inner ear especially of the stapes, causing tinnitus and later deafness. Stapedectomy is necessary to restore hearing.

Otoscope (auriscope) (*o'to-sk-op*) An instrument consisting of a light, magnifying lens and a device for insufflation, used to examine the external ear and tympanic membrane.

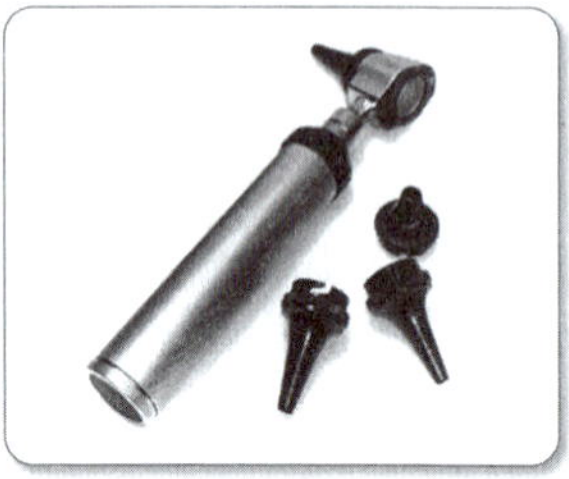

Otoscope set

Ouch-ouch disease A form of renal osteodystrophy with marked bony pain, described in Japanese women due to accumulation of cadmium in bone from eating fish contaminated by industrial pollutants.

Ouabain (*wa-ba'in*) A rapid and short-acting digitalis preparation.

Outbreeding (*out-breding*) The breeding of genetically unrelated species; also known as crossbreeding.

Outpatient (*out'pa-shunt*) A patient who gets the diagnosis and treatment in a clinic or hospital without getting admitted.

Oval window An oval-shaped aperture in the wall of the middle ear leading to the inner ear.

Ovarian (*o-va're-an*) Concerned with ovary.

Ovarian cycle A sex cycle having a follicular phase and a luteal phase with ovulation intervening.

Ovarian hyperstimulation syndrome Ovarian enlargement, ascites, pleural effusion, hypovolemia, hemoconcentration and oliguria. It is a serious complication of ovulation induction with human chorionic gonadotropin and occasionally clomiphene.

Ovarian pregnancy Ectopic gestation on ovary.

Ovarian tumor A malignant tumor of the ovary that is diagnosed only in advanced stage as a palpable abdominal or pelvic mass accompanied by irregular or excessive menses or postmenopausal bleeding. It spreads over the surface of peritoneum. It requires total abdominal hysterectomy and bilateral salpingo-oophorectomy with omentectomy.

Ovarian cyst A globular sac filled with fluid or semisolid material that develops in or on the ovary.

Ovariectomy (*o'va-re-ek'to-me*) Surgical removal of an ovary.

Ovariotomy (*o-var"e-ot'o-me*) Oophorectomy or removal of an ovarian tumor.

Abdominal ovariotomy Ovariotomy performed through the abdominal wall.

Vaginal ovariotomy Ovariotomy performed through the vagina.

Ovaritis (*o'va-ri'tis*) Oophoritis.

Ovary (*o'va-re*) Female gonad found on each side of the lower abdomen besides the uterus in a fold of the broad ligament.

Polycystic ovaries Ovaries become enlarged and contain many fluid-filled sacs (follicles) that surround the eggs.

Overbite (*o'ver-bit*) Vertical overlapping of lower teeth by upper teeth.

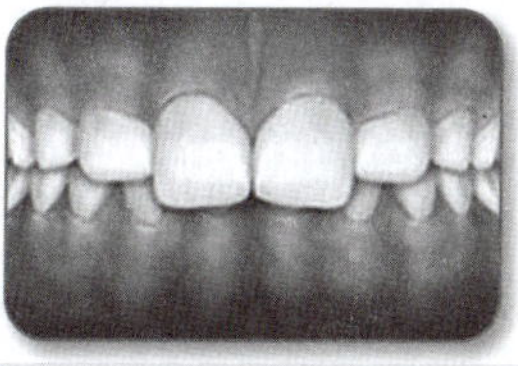

Overbite

Overcompensation (*o'var-kom"pen-sa'shan*) Excessive reaction to a feeling of inferiority, guilt, or inadequacy leading to an exaggerated attempt to overcome the feeling due to psychological or physical deficiency.

Overjet A horizontal projection of upper teeth beyond lower teeth.

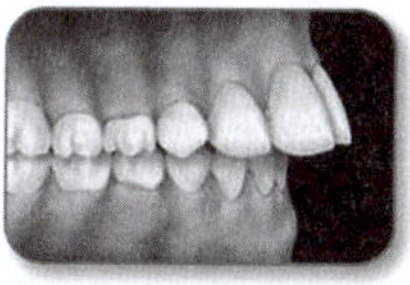

Overjet

Oviduct (*o'vi-dukt*) Fallopian tube.

Ovulation (*ov'u-la'shun*) The discharge of a ovum from the Graafian follicle of the ovary in a cyclic fashion. It usually occurs on the fourteenth day after the first day of the last menstrual period.

Ovum (egg cell) (*o'vum*) The female reproductive cell; an egg cell. pl. **ova**.

Oxacillin (*ok'sasil'in*) A penicillinase-resistant penicillin antibiotic. Used in the treatment of severe infections caused by penicillinase-producing staphylococci.

Oxalosis (*ok"sa-lo-sis*) Generalized deposition of calcium oxalate in renal and extrarenal tissues, as may occur in primary hyperoxaluria.

Oxaluria (*ok"sal-u're-a*) Hyperoxaluria.

Oxazepam (*ok-saz'e-pam*) A short-to-intermediate-acting benzodiazepine. Oxazepam is used for the treatment of anxiety and insomnia and in the control of symptoms of alcohol withdrawal syndrome.

Oxidase (*ok'si-das*) An enzyme that catalyzes the reduction of molecular oxygen.

Oxidoreductase (*ok"si-do-re-duk'tas*) Any member of a class of enzymes, commonly known as dehydrogenases or oxidases, that catalyze the removal of hydrogen atoms and electrons from the compounds on which they act.

Oximeter (*ok-simė-ter*) A photoelectric device useful in determination of oxygen saturation of blood. Light at certain wavelengths is shone on the blood and the amount of light reflected or transmitted is measured.

Ear oximeter A tool for wearable, unobtrusive monitoring of core blood oxygen saturation.

Finger oximeter Small beams of light pass through the blood in your finger, measuring the amount of oxygen.

Oxtriphylline (*oks-trefil'en*) A xanthine derivative, useful as a bronchodilator.

Oxycephaly (turricephaly) (*ok'se-sef'a-le*) A malformed skull developing from premature closure of the corona and sagittal sutures. There is an accelerated upward growth of the head giving it a long, narrow pointed appearance.

Oxygen (*ok'si-jen*) A colorless, odorless, tasteless gas that is essential for life. It is used in the cell mitochondria and energy is produced through citric acid cycle in the form of adenosine triphosphate.

Heavy oxygen An isotope of oxygen having a mass number greater than 16, especially oxygen of mass 18.

Oxygen capacity The maximum amount of oxygen that can be made to combine chemically with hemoglobin. 1 gram of hemoglobin can bind a maximum of 1.34 mL of oxygen.

Oxygen concentrator A device that separates oxygen from the air.

Oxygen consumption Utilization of oxygen per minute by the metabolizing tissues.

Oxygen content Amount of total oxygen present in the blood.

Oxygen cost of breathing The rate at which the respiratory muscles consume oxygen as they ventilate the lungs.

Oxygen debt The differences, with time between the oxygen demand and the actual oxygen consumption per minute.

Oxygen delivery Amount of oxygen delivered to the tissues and it depends on the total oxygen content of the blood and cardiac output.

Oxygen delivery devices Devices to deliver oxygen such a cannulae, prongs and masks.

Oxygen dissociation curve A sigmoid curve that describes the relationship between hemoglobin oxygen saturation and tension.

Oxygen free radicals Active sources of oxygen produced in the body by normal activity and by external agents that damage cells highly reactive, toxic molecules that appear when electrons are added to oxygen in the presence of hydrogen ions.

Oxygen hood A device placed over the head of neonatal patients to deliver high concentrations of oxygen.

Oxygen mask Mask to deliver oxygen at high concentration. It may be simple without any valve or reservoir, partial rebreathing with a unidirectional valve on either side and air-entrainment type to provide a constant fraction of inspired oxygen regulated by Venturi design.

Oxygen ratio Estimated by dividing PaO_2 in mm Hg by inspired oxygen concentration (FiO_2) in percent (PaO_2/FiO_2). Normally it is 4.

Oxygen saturation The proportion of hemoglobin (Hb) combining with oxygen. It reflects the degree of oxygenation of the blood.

Oxygen tension Partial pressure of oxygen in the arterial blood and it is 80 to 100 mm Hg at sea level.

Oxygen toxicity Occurrence of toxic features when the concentration of inhaled oxygen is high, and it causes damage to the pulmonary capillaries and alveolar epithelium.

Oxygen-15 An isotope used in positron emission tomography (PET); used in simple chemical forms to study oxygen metabolism, blood flow and blood volume in man, using the technique of PET.

Oxygenator (*ok'si-je-na'tor*) A mechanical device that oxygenates venous blood outside.

Bubble oxygenator Uses bubbles that are introduced directly into the blood.

Disk oxygenator A device for oxygenating blood during extracorporeal circulation.

Film oxygenator A device, encased in a container of oxygen, that makes possible reduction of a thin film of blood to facilitate the exchange of gases.

Intravascular oxygenator A new alternative method for augmenting blood gas transfer in patients with acute respiratory failure.

Membrane oxygenator A device used to add oxygen to, and remove carbon dioxide from the blood.

Rotating oxygenator Of a design differing from other rotating oxygenators in that the large surface area necessary for filming blood at high.

Screen oxygenator Consisted of five vertical stainless steel mesh screens suspended in a chamber through which oxygen flowed.

Oxygen deficit The sum of minute differences between the measured oxygen uptake and the oxygen uptake during steady state work at the same rate.

Oxygen tent A canopy that encloses the head and neck of a patient under high oxygen tension.

Oxyhemoglobin (*ok'se-hemo-glo'bin*) Oxygenated hemoglobin; oxygen combined with hemoglobin; HbO_2. Each gram of hemoglobin can bind 1.39 mL of oxygen.

Oxymesterone Also known as methandrostenediolone; it is an orally active anabolic androgenic steroid.

Oxyntic (*ok-sin'tik*) Secreting acid.

Oxypertine An antipsychotic drug that's used to treat schizophrenia, mania, disturbed behavior, and severe anxiety.

Oxyphencyclimine A synthetic drug used to treat peptic ulcers and gastrointestinal spasms.

Oxytetracycline Bacteriostatic antibiotic that inhibits growth of a wide range of gram-positive and gram-negative bacteria.

Oxytocic (*ok-se-to'sik*) Characterized by, or promoting oxytocia; an agent that hastens evacuation of the uterus by stimulating contractions of the myometrium.

Oxytocin (*ok'se-to-sin*) A hypothalamic polypeptide hormone released into the pituitary gland that induces and stimulates the contraction of the uterus during labor and stimulates the flow of milk for breastfeeding.

Oxyuriasis (*ok'se-u-ri'as-is*) Infection with *Enterobius vermicularis*.

Oxyuris (*ok'se-ur'is*) A genus of nematodes; also called pinworms.

Ozena (*o-ze'na*) Primary atrophic rhinitis or seen in late stage of rhinoscleroma with a thick mucopurulent discharge, mucosal crusting, and fetor, often associated with the presence of *Klebsiella pneumoniae* subsp. *ozaenae*.

Ozonator (*ozo-na'tur*) An apparatus for generating ozone and diffusing it in the atmosphere of a room.

Ozone (*o'zon*) O_3, a form of oxygen present in upper atmosphere that protects Earth from the harmful effects of ultraviolet radiation of the sun.

Ozostomia (*o'zo-sto'me-a*) Foul-smelling breath; halitosis.

P

P24 antigen The core antigen of the human immunodeficiency virus type 1, (HIV-1), which is held responsible for AIDS.

Pacchionian corpuscles (*pak-e-o'ni-an*) Prominent arachnoid villi, named after Antonio Pacchioni, Italian anatomist.

Pacemaker (*pas'ma-ker*) Any rhythmic center that establishes a pace of activity; an electronic device used to stimulate or regulate the heart beat.

Pacemaker syndrome A complication of implanted pacemakers, characterized by vertigo, syncope, dyspnea, weakness, postural hypotension, decreased effort tolerance and palpable hepatic and jugular pulsations, and it is due to alternating atrioventricular asynchrony.

Wandering pacemaker A disturbance of the normal cardiac rhythm in which the site that controls the pacemaker shifts from beat to beat usually between the sinus and AV nodes.

Pachy Combining word for 'thick'.

Pachydactyly (*pak'e-dak'ti-le*) Enlargement of the fingers or toes.

Pachyderma (*pak'e-der'-ma*) Abnormal thickening of the skin.

Pachyglossia (*pak'e-glos'e-a*) Abnormally thick tongue.

Pachygyria (*pak'e-ji're-a*) A congenital malformation of the cerebral hemisphere due to abnormal cell migration resulting in unusually thick convolution of the cerebral cortex.

Pachymeningitis (*pak'e-men'in-jit'is*) Inflammation of the dura mater.

Pachymeninx (*pak'e-me'ninks*) Pl. **pachymeninges**. The dura mater.

Pachyonychia (*pak'e-o-nik'e-a*) Abnormal thickening of the finger nails or toe nails.

Pachysalpingitis (*pak'e-salpin-jitis*) Chronic inflammation of fallopian tube with thickening.

Pachytene (*pak'i-ten*) The stage of prophase in meiosis in which the pairing of homologous chromosomes is complete. They may twine about each other and undergo longitudinal cleavage to become a set of four intertwined chromatids.

Pacinian corpuscles (*pa-sin'e-an*) Large encapsulated touch receptors especially of skin, named after Filippo Pacini, Italian anatomist.

Pack (*pak*) To wrap the body in a sheet, or blanket; to fill up a cavity with cotton or gauge.

Packed cell volume (PCV) The percentage of volume of red blood cells in the blood determined by using Wintrobe hematocrit tube. Normal PCV is 45%.

Pad A cushion of soft material used to apply or relieve pressure on a part or organ; a fatty mass.

Pad sign Padded-out appearance of duodenal loop in carcinoma of head of pancreas on barium meal.

Paget's disease A weeping eczematoid erosive lesion of the nipple that is associated with underlying intraductal breast carcinoma.

Painful arc syndrome A disorder in which the arm cannot be raised between 45° and 160° laterally.

Paint (*pant*) A solution of medicaments for application to the skin.

Palate (*pal'at*) Roof of the mouth, the partition separating the nasal and oral cavities.

Bony palate The concave bony plate formed by maxilla and palatine bones and it forms the anterior portion of the palate.

Cleft palate Congenital fissure in the midline of the palate which is often associated with cleft lips.

Gothic palate An excessively high arched palate.

Hard palate Bony palate.

Pendulous palate Uvula.

Soft palate Posterior muscular portion of the palate that separates the mouth and pharynx.

Palatine (*pal'a-tin*) Relating to palate; palate bones.

Palatoplasty (*pal'a-to-plas'te*) Surgical reconstruction of the palate.

Palatopharyngoplasty A surgical procedure for the soft palate and pharynx to eliminate redundant mucosa.

Palatorrhaphy (*pal-a-tora-fe*) Surgical repair of a cleft palate.

Paleocerebellum (*pale-o-sere-bel'um*) Medial part of the cerebellum comprising vermis and adjacent medial zone of cerebellar hemisphere having spinocerebellar fibers and is concerned with equilibrium and movements of locomotion.

Paleopathology (*pa'le-o-pa-thol-o-je*) A branch of pathology related to ancient diseases as evidenced in bones, mummies and archeological artifacts.

Paleostriatum (*pa'le-o-stri-at'um*) The globus pallidus.

Paleothalamus (*pa'le-o-thal'a-mus*) The medial portion of the thalamus.

Palilalia A language disorder characterized by the involuntary repitition of syllabled, words or phrases.

Palindromia (*pal'in-dro'me-a*) Intermittent recurring episodes.

Palingraphia Mirror writing.

Paliphrasia A form of stammering with repitition of phases while speaking.

Palliative (*pal'e-a'tiv*) Giving relief; a drug giving relief.

Palliative care Improvement of the quality of life when treatment to cure disease and prolong life is no longer a realistic objective.

Palliative surgery Therapeutic procedure undertaken to reduce the severity of symptoms and improve the quality of life in presence of advanced stage of malignancy.

Palliative therapy Any treatment of a terminally ill patient to alleviate pain and suffering without undertaking any aggressive procedures.

Pallidectomy (*pal'i-dek'to-me*) Surgical removal of the globus pallidus.

Pallidum (Paleostriatum) (*pali-dum*) Dense collection of gray matter deep in each cerebral hemisphere that make basal ganglia.

Pallium (*pal'e-um*) The cerebral cortex.

Pallor (*pal'er*) Paleness as of skin and mucous membrane.

Palmitic acid (*pa-mit'ik*) A 16-carbon saturated fatty acid found in most oils and fats.

Palpation (*pal-pa'shun*) The act of feeling with the hand, one of the cardinal methods of physical examination.

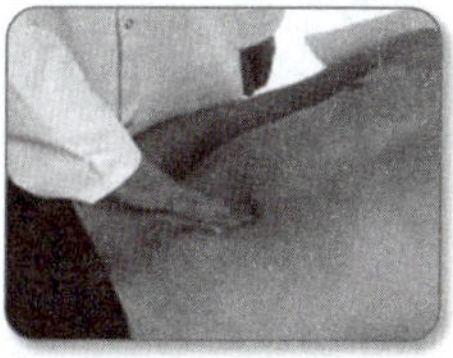

Palpation of liver

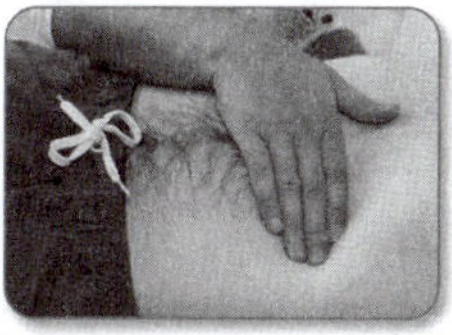

Palpation of spleen

Palsy (*pawl'ze*) Paralysis.

Birth palsy Obstetric paralysis, from an injury received at birth or due to anoxic injury of the fetal brain *in utero.*

Bulbar palsy Progressive muscular paralysis occurring due to degeneration of the nuclei of lower cranial nerves.

Facial palsy Bell's palsy.

Pressure palsy Temporary paralysis due to pressure on nerve trunk.

Shaking palsy Paralysis agitans.

Pamidronate (*pam''i-dro'nat*) A bisphosphonate, treats high calcium levels in the blood caused by cancer. It may also be used with chemotherapy to treat weakened bones caused by cancer. It can also be used to treat Paget's disease of the bone.

PAN- (pant(o)-) Polyarteritis nodosa.

Panagraphy (*pan-a'gra-fe*) View of all teeth in one jaw with X-ray source in mouth and film in cassette wrapped round jaw.

Panacea (*pan-a-se'a*) Cure all, remedy, single solution for multiple problems; a remedy claimed to be curative to all ills.

Pancarditis (*pan'kar-dit'is*) Diffuse inflammation of all tissues of the heart as in rheumatic fever.

Pancreas (*pan'kre-as*) A lobulated gland functioning as an exocrine and endocrine organ, devoid of capsule, extending from the concavity of the duodenum to the spleen in a horizontal position in front of first and second lumbar vertebrae. It is divided into head attached to the duodenum, body and tail reaching the spleen. The exocrine portion consists of acini which secrete pancreatic juice that drains into main pancreatic duct. It joins the common bile duct and empties into the duodenum. The islets of Langerhans distributed throughout the gland have alpha, beta and delta cells secreting glucagon, insulin and somatostatin respectively and function as an endocrine gland.

Pancreas divisum Birth defect in which parts of the pancreas do not join together.

Pancreatectomy (*pan'kre-a-tek-to-me*) Excision of the pancreas.

Pancreatic juice Liquid secreted by (20v-800mL/day) by pancreas having enzymes.

Pancreatin (*pan'kre-a-tin*) Enzymes containing amylase, protease, and lipase obtained from hog or ox and used to facilitate digestion.

Pancreatitis (*pan'kre-a-ti'tis*) Inflammation of the pancreas.

Acute pancreatitis Pancreatitis due to interstitial inflammation, edema, necrosis and hemorrhage. There is premature release of proteases which digest the pancreas and surrounding tissue and the condition is characterized by severe constant upper abdominal pain, nausea, vomiting and marked epigastric tenderness.

Chronic pancreatitis A chronic inflammatory disease characterized by fibrosis and destruction of exocrine pancreatic tissue, resulting from alcohol abuse in majority of cases.

Pancreatogram Used to diagnose and treat problems of biliary system. It is done by Endoscopic Retrograde Cholangio Pancreatography (ERCP). It uses a type of X-ray.

Pancreatotomy (*pan"kre-a-tot'o-me*) Incision of the pancreas.

Pancreozymin (*pan'kre-o-zi'min*) A duodenal hormone that stimulates the pancreas for production of amylase.

Pancytopenia (*pan'sit-o-pe'ne-a*) Hypoplasia or aplasia of bone marrow resulting in deficiency of all types of blood cells.

Pandemic (*pan-dem'ik*) A widespread epidemic disease affecting a large number of people at the same time and in many geographic regions.

Pandy's test (*pan'dez*) Presence of globulin in CSF tested by addition of 70% phenol which produces turbidity, named after Pandy Kalman, Hungarian psychiatrist.

Panencephalitis (*pan'en-sef'a-lit'is*) Encephalitis producing lesions of both the gray and white matter of the brain.

Panhysterectomy (*pa'n-his-ter-ek'to-me*) Surgical removal of the entire uterus including the cervix uteri.

Panmixis Random mating of individuals within a population. The breeding individuals show no tendency to choose partners with particular traits.

Panniculitis (*pan-nik'u-li'tis*) Inflammation of subcutaneous fat in the anterior wall of the abdomen.

Panniculus (*pa-nik'u-lus*) A layer of membrane, such as subcutaneous fat layer.

Pannus (*pan'us*) Fibrovascular proliferative response occurring in the cornea and conjunctiva due to *Chlamydia trachomatis*; a nonspecific immune response in the form of a reticulated membrane of granulation tissue in chronic proliferodestructive phase of rheumatoid arthritis.

Panophthalmitis (*pan'of-thal-mit'is*) Inflammation of all parts of the eye.

Panstrongylus (*pan-stron'ji-lus*) A genus Panstrongylus, belongs to the subfamily Triatominae. It is found in South America, a blood-sucking sylvatic insect noted as a putative vector of minor importance in the transmission of *Trypanosoma cruzi* to humans; this is a parasite, which causes Chagas disease. The insect is described as sylvatic; subsisting primarily in humid forests, and is also known to inhabit vertebrate nesting places such as those of the armadillo (dasypus novemcinctus or dasypus), and is also involved in enzootic transmission of *T. cruzi* to those species.

Pant- (panto-) To gasp for breath; to breathe rapidly and shallowly.

Pantoprazole (*pan-to'pra-zol*) A proton pump inhibitor used to treat erosive esophagitis, gastric acid hypersecretion, and to promote healing of tissue damage caused by gastric acid.

Pantothenic acid A member of vitamin B complex, widespread in food that helps in the release of energy in the cells.

Pantropic (*pan-tro'pik*) Found throughout the tropical regions.

Papain (*pa-pa'in*) A proteolytic enzyme from *Carica papaya* which catalyzes the hydrolysis of proteins and polypeptides to amino acids.

Papanicolaou test (Pap test) Pap smear, a cytologic sampling from the uterine cervix that serves to detect and squamous cell carcinoma of the cervix, described by George Papanicolaou, Greek-US physician.

Papaverine (*pa-pav'er-in*) Isoquinoline alkaloid found in opium, a smooth muscle relaxant.

Papilla (*pa-pil'ah*) Pl. **papillae**. A small nipple-shaped projection. adj. **papillary**.

Circumvallate papilla Large papillae found near the base on the dorsal surface of the tongue arranged in a V-shape.

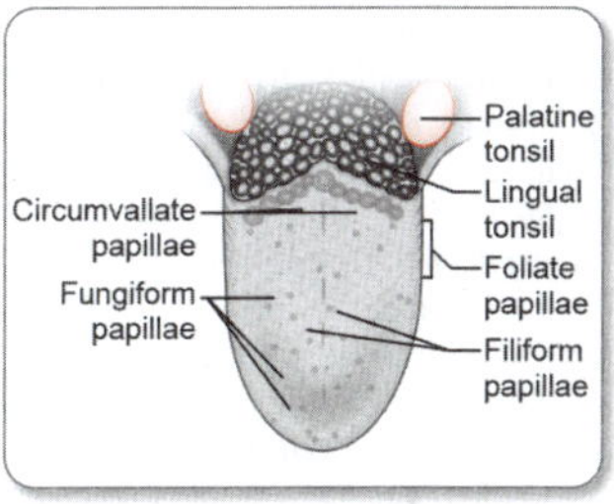

Circumvallate papillae

Conical papilla Numerous projections on the dorsum of the tongue.

Dental papilla A mesenchymal tissue giving rise to dentine and dental tissue.

Duodenal papilla The point of opening of the common bile duct into the duodenum.

Filiform papilla Elongated conical projection on the dorsum of the tongue.

Foliate papilla Numerous projections arranged in several folds in the lateral margins of the tongue.

Fungiform papilla Numerous minute flat papillae on the dorsum of the tongue resembling a fungus.

Gingival papilla Gingival tissue between the adjacent teeth.

Hair papilla A conical projection containing capillaries at the bottom of hair follicles.

Incisive papilla A slight projection of mucosa on the anterior portion of raphe of the palate.

Interdental papilla The gingiva that fills the space between adjacent teeth.

Lacrimal papilla A slight projection from the margin of each eyelid near the medial commissure, in the center of which there is opening of the lacrimal duct.

Lingual papilla Any of the tiny projections such as conical, filiform, fungiform and vallate papillae covering the anterior two-thirds of the tongue.

Optic papilla Optic disc.

Papilla basilaris Organ of corti.

Papilla mamma Nipple, teat.

Parotid papilla The projection at the opening of the parotid duct into the mouth opposite second upper molar tooth.

Papilla pili Hair papilla.

Renal papilla The apex of a renal pyramid which projects into a minor calyx.

Tactile papilla A dermal papilla containing a tactile cell or corpuscle.

Urethral papilla A slight projection in the vestibule of the vagina marking the urethral orifice.

Papilledema (*pap"il-e-de'ma*) Edematous swelling of optic disc due to raised intracranial tension.

Papillitis (*pap'i-lits*) Inflammation of a papilla; a type of optic neuritis affecting the optic disc.

Papilloma (*pap'il-o'ma*) A benign epithelial tumor; epithelial tumor of skin or mucous membrane consisting of villous outgrowths such as warts, polyps or condylomas.

Papillomatosis (*pap'il-o'ma-to'sis*) Development of multiple papillomas.

Papilloretinitis (*pap'il-o-ret'i-ni'tis*) Inflammation of the optic disc and retina.

Papillotomy (*pap'il-ot'o-me*) Incision of a papilla.

Papovavirus (*pa-po'va-vi'rus*) Any virus of the family papovaviridae.

Pappataci fever A vector borne arboviral (sand fly fever virus) infection. After 2–6 days of incubation period, it causes fever and headache.

Papule (*pap'ul*) A small, circumscribed, solid, elevated lesion of the skin. adj. **papular**.

Papulo- (*pap"u-lo-ne-krot'ik*) A chronic, recurrent, symmetrical eruption of necrotizing papules that ulcerate, crust, and heal after a few weeks with varioliform scarring.

Papulosquamous disorders Skin lesions characterized by well-demarcated, red or purple popules and plaques with scales such as psoriasis.

Para- (*par'ah*) A woman who has produced viable young regardless of whether the child was alive at birth used with Roman numerals to designate such pregnancies as para 0 (none-nullipara), para 1 (one-primipara), para 2 (two-secondipara), para 3 (three-tripara), para 4 (four-quadripara) etc. A multiple birth is considered a single parous experience.

Para-aminobenzoic acid (*para-a-mi'no-ben-zoik*) PABA, a folic acid precursor.

Para-aminosalicylic acid (PAS) Substance cleared entirely from plasma while passing through the kidney.

Paracentesis (*par'a-sen-te'sis*) A procedure in which a body cavity is punctured from outside with a needle or trocar to remove fluid for therapeutic and diagnostic purpose.

Paracholia Disordered bile secretion.

Paracoccidioides (*par'a-kok-sid'e-oidez*) A dimorphic fungus and one of the two species that cause paracoccidioidomycosis (the other being Paracoccidioides lutzii). The fungus has been affiliated with the family Ajellomycetaceae (division Ascomycota) although a sexual state or teleomorph has not yet been found.

Paracrine (*par'a-krin*) Action of hormones on cells close to secreting cells.

Paracusis (*par'a-ku'sis*) Any perversion of hearing.

Paradidymis (*par'a-did'i-mis*) A small vestigial structure in the spermatic cord.

Paradox (*par'a-doks*) Contradiction.

Paradoxical Different from normal expectation.

Paradoxical embolism Emboli that occur when thrombotic material passes through right-to-left cardiac shunts.

Paradoxical hypoxia Administration of oxygen may lead to temporary deterioration of consciousness.

Paradoxical pulse A decrease of greater than 10 mm in the systolic blood pressure upon inspiration.

Paraffin *par'a-fin)* A hydrocarbon wax used for embedding histological specimens; a light mineral oil as liquid paraffin.

Paraffin section A stained section of tissue mounted on a glass slide and examined by light microscopy.

Paraffinoma *(par-a-fi-no'ma)* A granuloma produced by prolonged exposure to paraffin.

Paraldehyde *(par-al'de-hid)* Hypnotic and anticonvulsant possessing a peculiar smell.

Paraganglion *(par'a-gang'gle-on)* Pl. **paraganglia**. A collection of chromaffin cells derived from neural ectoderm. They are found outside the adrenal medulla near the sympathetic ganglia.

Parageusia (parageusis) *(par'a-gu'ze-a)* Perversion of the taste sensation.

Paragonimiasis (endemic hemoptysis) *(par'a-gon'i-mi-a-sis)* Infestation with flukes belonging to the genus *Paragonimus. P. westermani* cysts in the lung present with hemoptysis and clubbing. Liver and brain may be affected. Praziquantel is used in the treatment.

Paragonimus *(par'a-gon-i-mus)* A genus of trematode parasite *P. westermani*, most common fluke that lives in the lungs, whose ova are expectorated or eliminated in feces. Miracidia emerge in water from these eggs and are taken by fresh-water snail. The larvae emerging from snail encyst in freshwater crabs as Metacercariae which when eaten, raw or undercooked, can infect man.

Paragranuloma *(par'a-gran'u-lo'ma)* A benign form of Hodgkin's disease affecting lymph nodes.

Paralysis *(pa-ral'i-sis)* Loss of power of motor system concerned with voluntary movement in a muscle due to a lesion of neural or muscular mechanism.

Bulbar paralysis Progressive bulbar palsy.

Compressive paralysis Paralysis caused by pressure on a nerve.

Decubitus paralysis Paralysis due to pressure on a nerve due to lying in one position for a long period.

Hysterical paralysis Loss of movement without any organic cause.

Infantile paralysis Poliomyelitis.

Vasomotor paralysis Paralysis of vasomotor centers.

Paralytic ileus A situation in which the peristalsis of the intestine slows down or stop, noted following abdominal surgery, electrolyte abnormalities (hypokalemia) or peritonitis.

Paramedian incision A vertical incision 1–2.5 cm away from midline of abdomen with lateral retraction of rectus muscle.

Paramethadione Oxidizing anticonvulsant that acts on the CNS to reduce the number of seizures.

Parametritis (pelvic cellulitis) *(par'a-me-tri'tis)* Inflammation of the parametrium.

Parametrium *(par'a-me'tre-um)* Loose connective tissue in broad ligament beside cervix and fornices.

Paramimia *(par'a-mim'e-a)* The use of wrong or improper gestures in speaking.

Paramnesia *(par'am-ne'ze-a)* Recall of events that have not taken place.

Paramyoclonus *(par-a-mi-ok'lo-nus)* Myoclonus in a widely different group of muscles.

Paramyotonia congenita A rare non-progressive genetic disorder that affects the skeletal muscles.

Paranasal sinuses *(par'a-na'zal)* Around or near the nose.

Paraneoplastic syndrome Comorbid conditions due to remote or biologic effects of malignancy, which may be the first sign of a neoplasm or its recurrence.

Paranoia (*par'a-noi-a*) A disorder characterized by the false belief that people or events are in some way related to oneself.

Paranoid Unrealistic distrust of others that they are trying to harm or are saying bad things about you.

Paraparesis (*par'a-pa-re'sis*) Partial paralysis of the lower limbs.

Paraphasia (*par'a-fa'ze-a*) Production of incoherent speech.

Paraphimosis A true urologic emergency that occurs in uncircumsized males when the foreskin becomes trapped behind the corona of the glans penis.

Paraphrenia A chronic psychotic disorder characterized by a strong delusional component with preservation of thought and personality.

Paraplegia (*par'a-ple-jea*) A term used to describe the inability to voluntarily move the lower parts of the body.

Paraprotein (*par'a-pro'ten*) Various proteins found in large amounts in blood or urine in disease and not normal constituent.

Parapsoriasis (*par'a-sor-i'a-sis*) A chronic maculopapular scaly erythroderma appearing in persistent and often enlarging plaque.

Parapsychology The study of alleged psychic phenomena and other paranormal claims such as near-death experiences.

Paraquat (*par'a-kwaht*) A powerful herbicide, fatal poisoning can occur by its accidental ingestion. It acts like a corrosive poison and causes hepatic and renal damage. Lung involvement leads to inexorable pulmonary fibrosis.

Parasite (*par'a-sit*) Organisms that live in or on other organisms; some of which cause disease in people.

External parasite A parasite that lives on the skin such as lice, fleas, ticks or mites.

Facultative parasite An organism capable of living independently of its host at times.

Incidental parasite A parasite that normally lives on another than its present host.

Internal parasite A parasite such as a protozoon or worm that lives within the body of the host.

Malarial parasite Any one of the species of plasmodium that can cause malaria

Obligate parasite A parasite that is entirely dependent or the host.

Specific parasite A parasite needing a specific host to complete its life cycle.

Parasitology (*par'a-si-tol'o-je*) The scientific study of parasites and parasitism.

Parasomnia (*par'a-somne-a*) A sleep disorder that involves unusual and undesirable physical events or experiences that disrupt sleep.

Parasternal (*par'a-stur'nal*) Situated close to the sternum.

Parasuicide (*par'a-su'i-sid*) An apparent attempt at suicide by self-poisoning or self-mutilation.

Paraympathetic nervous system Responsible for the body's rest and digestion response when the body is relaxed, feeding or resting.

Parasympatholytic A substance or activity that reduces the activity of the parasympathetic nervous system.

Parasympathomimetic (*par'a-tho-mi-met'ik*) Producing effects resembling those resulting from stimulation of parasympathetic nervous system; relating to an agent producing features resembling that caused by stimulation of the parasympathetic nervous system.

Paratendinitis (*para-ten'di'-ni'tis*) Damage to the tendon sheath, diagnosed by eliciting tenderness around the full circumference of the tendon.

Paratenon (*par'a-ten'on*) Connective tissue immediately surrounding tendon.

Parathion (*par'a-thi'on*) An acetyl-cholinesterase-inhibiting organophosphate insecticide.

Parathormone (*par'a-thor'mon*) Parathyroid hormone.

Parathyroidectomy Surgery to remove the parathyroid tumors.

Parathyroid glands (*par'a-thi'roid*) Situated beside thyroid gland; one of the four small endocrine glands on the back of or at lower edge of thyroid gland or embedded within its substance. They secrete parathyroid hormone that regulates calcium and phosphorus metabolism.

Parathyroid hormone (Parathormone) A hormone released by parathyroid glands to control calcium levels in the blood.

Pareidolia (*par'i-do'hlea*) The tendency for perception to impose a meaningful interpretation on a nebulous stimulus, usually visual, so that one sees an object, pattern, or meaning where there is none.

Parenchyma (*pa-reng'ki-ma*) The essential part of an organ consisting of functional elements as distinguished from its framework.

Parenteral (*pa-ren'ter-al*) Administration of drugs, nutrients or other substances by any other route other than the digestive tract.

Paresis (*pa-re'sis*) Partial paralysis.

Paresthesia (*par'es-the'ze-a*) A tingling in the skin; a 'pins and needles' sensation.

Paries (*par'e-ez*) A wall.

Parietal (*par-ri'e-t'l*) Pertaining to the walls of a cavity; pertaining to or located near the parietal bone.

Parietal cell Large eosinophilic cell of a gland concerned with production of hydrochloric acid.

Parietal layer Serosal lining of the external surface of the cavity.

Parietal lobe Part of each cerebral hemisphere that is involved in pain and touch sensations, speech and control of spatial orientation.

Parietal bone A cranial bone forming part of the side and top of the head.

Parietal cells Large eosinophilic cell of a gland concerned with production of hydrochloric acid.

Parietal lobe Part of each cerebral hemisphere that is involved in pain and touch sensations, speech and control of spatial orientation.

Parity (*par'it-e*) The condition of having given birth to an offspring alive or dead. Multiple births are considered a single pars; equality or similarity.

Parkinsonism (*par'kin-son-izm*) A degenerative disease affecting the basal ganglia presenting with slowness of movement (bradykinesia), increased tone (rigidity), tremor and loss of postural reflexes.

Secondary parkinsonism Develops from definable causes, such as drugs (phenothiazines, reserpine, lithium), toxins (manganese, 1-meth l 4-phenyl y tetrahydropyridine), carbon monoxide, encephalitis lethargica, atherosclerosis, Wilson's disease or head injury (punch-drunk syndrome).

Paromomycin (*par'o-mo-mi'sin*) An aminoglycoside antibiotic useful in treating amebiasis.

Paronychia (*par'o-nik'e-a*) An infection of the nail fold especially of the lateral, and it becomes red, swollen, tender and very painful. It involves a single nail at a time.

Chronic paronychia Asymptomatic erythematous swelling of the posterior nail fold of one or more fingers.

Paroophoron (*par'o-ofo-ron*) A group of rudimentary tubules in the broad ligament between the epoophoron and the uterus that constitutes a remnant of the lower part of the mesonephros in the female corresponding to the paradidymis of the male.

Parosmia A disorder in which the odors of certain things are distorted.

Parotid gland The largest pair of salivary glands which are present on either side of the face, just below and in front of the ear.

Parotitis (*par'o-tit'is*) Inflammation of the parotid gland.

Parous Having given birth to one or more viable children.

Paroxysm (*par'ok-sizm*) A sudden attack or worsening or recurrence of symptoms or of a disease or a spasm or seizure.

Parrot disease Psittacosis, associated with birds that can result in a flue-like illness or serious pneumonia in many people. Parrots are carries of the chlamydia psittaci, the causative agent.

Pars A part or portion of a structure.

Partial seizure A localized abnormal electrical discharge in the brain that affects isolated body or mental functions.

Partial thromboplastin time Activated partial thromboplastin time (aPTT) one stage coagulation test that is sensitive to deficiencies of antihemophilic factors.

Parturition (*par'tu-ri'shun*) Childbirth.

PAS Pars aminosalicylic acid; periodic acid-Schiff (stain).

Pascal (*pas-kal*) Pressure expressed in newtons per square meter, named after Blaise Pascal, French scientist.

Paschen bodies Particles or inclusion bodies that occur in the cells of skin rashes in patients with cowpox or smallpox.

Past pointing Misjudging the distances in cerebellar lesions, resulting in missing the target.

Paste A soft semisolid that flows slowly.

Pasteurella (*pas'tu-rel'a*) A genus of gram-negative bacteria belonging to the family Pasteurellaceae, and it includes *P. multocida*, named after Louis Pasteur French chemist and bacteriologist.

Pasteurization (*pas'cher-i-za'shun*) The process of heating of milk or other liquids for about 30 minutes at 60°C which kills the bacteria and prevents the spread of milk-borne pathogens.

Patch test Application of allergens to the skin of the back to detect type IV hypersensitivity used in the diagnosis and as a test for safety of drugs.

Patella (*pa-tel'a*) The knee cap, *see* Table of bones. adj. **patellar**.

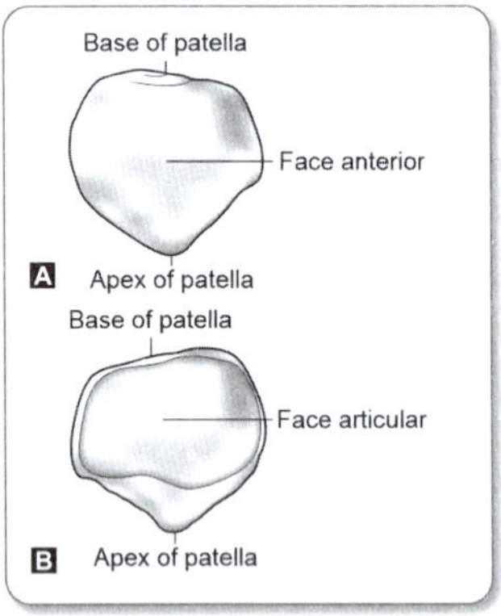

*Patella: **A.** Anterior view; **B.** Posterior view*

Patellar reflex A stretch reflex produced by the extension of the knee joint upon the ipsilateral stimulation of the patellar tendon. This tests the L2, L3 and L4 segments of the spinal cord.

Patent ductus arteriosus (PDA) During fetal life, the blood from the pulmonary artery passes through the ductus arteriosus into the aorta, that closes after birth. It may remain persistent producing a continuous murmur and enlarged pulmonary artery. Later there can be reversed shunt.

Pathogen (*path'o-jen*) Any disease producing agent or microorganism. adj. **pathogenic**.

Pathogenesis (*path'o-jen'e-sis*) The process by which a disease originates and develops.

Pathognomonic (*path'og-no-mon'ik*) Characteristic of a disease.

Pathological Related to pathology.

Pathology (*pa-thol'o-je*) Branch of medical science dealing with the structural and functional changes that result from disease processes.

Cellular pathology Interpretation of diseases on the basis of cellular alterations.

Clinical pathology Use of laboratory methods as pertains to diagnosis of the disease.

Comparative pathology The disease of animals especially in relation to human pathology.

Oral pathology Morbid anatomic or functional change due to disease of oral and paraoral structures.

Speech pathology Function and organic speech defects and disorders.

Surgical pathology Examination of tissues removed from living patients for the purpose of diagnosis.

Pauciarthritis The number of joints with pauciarthritis juvenile rheumatoid arthritis (PJRA) affects, the large joints which is four or less.

Pavementation (Paveminting) Sticking of WBCs to the linings of the capillaries when inflammation occurs.

Peau d' orange (*po-dor-anj*) Multiple dimples seen in the skin resembling an orange, due to lymphatic edema.

Pecten (*pek'ten*) A structure possessing comb-like processes or projections.

Pectoral Relating to the chest.

Pectoral girdle A set of bones in the appendicular skeleton connecting the arm on either side.

Pectoral muscles Each of the 4 large paired muscles that cover the front of the ribcage and serve to draw the fore-limbs towards the chest.

Pectoriloquy (*pek-to-ril'o-kwi*) An increased vocal resonance with transmission of voice sounds through the pulmonary structures.

Spoken pectoriloquy Spoken words are clearly audible as if speaking right into the listener's ears.

Whispering pectoriloquy Distinctly audible syllables of the whispering sounds, heard over an area of consolidation, or over a big cavity communicating with a patent bronchus.

Pectus (*pek'tus*) Chest, thorax or the breast.

Pectus carinatum Pigeon chest.

Pectus excavatum Funnel chest.

Pederasty (*ped'er-as'te*) Anal intercourse, especially when practiced on boys.

Pediatric (*pe'de-at'rik*) Relating to pediatrics.

Pediatric advanced life support (PALS) The treatment measures including the basic and advanced life support required to stabilize critically ill child.

Pedicle (*ped'ik'l*) A foot-like structure; a stalk by which a tumor attaches to the normal tissue; a stalk through which a skin flap in plastic surgery receives its blood supply.

Pediculicide (*pe-dik'ul-i-sid*) Destroying the lice; an agent that destroys lice.

Pediculosis (*pe-dik'u-lo'sis*) An infestation caused by lice.

Pediculosis capitis Infestation by head louse, *Pediculus humanus capitis*, affecting scalp hair, transmitted by close contact. The lice are brown in color and live on the scalp and lay eggs (nits), which stick to hairs. It causes severe itching.

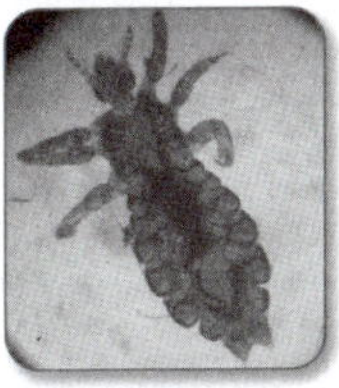

Pediculosis capitis

Pediculosis corporis Caused by body louse *P. humanus corporis*. It is white in color and lives in seams of the clothes, causes itching and severe excoriations, transmitted by close contact in individuals with poor hygiene.

Pediculosis pubis Caused by *Pthirus pubis*, infests hairs in the pubic region, moustache, beard, axillae and eye lashes and causes intense itching often transmitted by sexual contact.

Pedodontics (*pe-do-don'tiks*) The branch of dentistry dealing with dental care and treatment of children.

Pedophilia (*pe-do-fil'e-a*) Abnormal fondness for children by an adult for sexual purpose; *psy* a sexual perversion to have sexual relations with children.

Peduncle (*pe-dung'k'l*) Pedicle; band of connecting nerve fibers.

Mamillary peduncle A band of fibers connecting the tegmentum of the midbrain to the mamillary body.

Olfactory peduncle The long stalk of the olfactory bulb.

Pineal peduncle A band from either side of pineal gland extending to the fornix.

Thalamic peduncle One of the four radiations extending from the thalamus to the cerebral cortex.

Pellagra (*pe-lag'-ra*) A syndrome due to niacin deficiency in individuals with high intake of maize (deficient in tryptophan) or *jowar* (high leucine content) characterized by dermatitis on exposed parts of the body, diarrhea and mental changes.

Pellicle (*pel'ik'l*) A thin piece of skin; a thin film on the surface of liquids.

Pelvic girdle (hip girdle) A ring like bony structure, located in the lower part of the trunk. It connects the axial skeleton to the lower limbs.

Pelvic inflammatory diseases (PID) An infection of one or more of the female upper reproductive organs, including uterus, fallopian tubes and ovaries.

Pelvimetry (*pel-vim'e-tre*) Measurement of the diameters of the pelvis.

Pelvis (*pel'vis*) Pl. **pelves**. The basin-shaped bony structure at the base of the spine consisting of the ilium (hip bone), the sacrum and coccyx; a cup-shaped cavity as the pelvis of the kidney.

Android pelvis A masculine pelvis.

Anthropometric pelvis A female pelvis with a long anteroposterior diameter and a narrow transverse diameter.

Assimilation pelvis A deformity in which transverse processes of the last lumbar vertebra are fused with the sacrum or the last sacral with the first coccygeal body; pelvis with pelvic bone laterally compressed.

Beaked pelvis Osteomalacic pelvis.

Brachypellic pelvis Pelvis with transverse diameter exceeding the anteroposterior diameter.

Champagne glass pelvis Pelvic radiograph exhibiting flattening of the iliac wings with pelvic inlet resembling a champagne bottle, noted in achondroplasia.

Contracted pelvis Pelvis with less than normal measurements in all dimensions.

Cordate pelvis Sacrum projecting forward between the ilia, making the brim of pelvis heart shaped.

Dolichopellic pelvis An elongated pelvis with the anteroposterior diameter being greater than the transverse diameter.

Flat pelvis A pelvis in which the anteroposterior diameter is uniformly contracted.

Funnel-shaped pelvis Pelvis with normal inlet but a greatly narrowed outlet.

Gynecoid pelvis Normal female pelvis, a rounded oval pelvis with rounded anterior and posterior segments.

Infantile pelvis Generally contracted pelvis with oval shape with slender bones.

Kyphotic pelvis Backward curvature of lumbar spine making pelvis.

Masculine pelvis minor True pelvis, the cavity of pelvis below the brim.

Mesatipellic pelvis A pelvis with equal anteroposterior and transverse diameters.

Osteomalacic pelvis Beaked pelvis, pelvic aperture with the shape of a heart of clover leaf and pubic bones beak-shaped, a deformity due to osteomalacia.

Pelvis justo major An unusually large gynecoid pelvis with all dimensions increased.

Pelvis justo minor A small gynecoid pelvis with all its diameters smaller than normal.

Pelvis major False pelvis, the expanded portion of pelvis above brim.

Platypellic pelvis A flat oval pelvis in which the transverse diameter is longer than the anteroposterior diameter.

Rachitic pelvis A contracted and deformed pelvis.

Renal pelvis Flat, funnel-shaped expansion of the upper end of the ureter receiving the calices of the kidney.

Split pelvis Absence of symphysis pubis with separated pelvic bones.

Spondylolisthetic pelvis Pelvic brim being occluded by a dislocation forward of body of the lower lumbar vertebra.

True pelvis Pelvis minor.

Pemphigoid (*pem'fi-goid*) Occurrence of tense large blisters associated with an erythematous discoloration of skin.

Bullous pemphigoid Large tense and unilocular blisters in and around axilla and limbs.

Pemphigoid gestationis Blistering condition affecting periumbilical region and limbs, in young pregnant females.

Pemphigus (*pem'fi-gus*) An autoimmune disease caused by reaction of IgG with a protein (glycocalyx) found on the surface of the epidermal cells. It leads to activation of some proteases, which cause separation of epidermal cells from one another (acantholysis) and formation of intraepidermal bullae.

Pemphigus erythematosus Lesions surrounded by erythema and found on the butterfly area of the face.

Pemphigus vegetans Lesions are vegetating growths in the skin folds such as axillae and groins. Bullae are less in number.

Pemphigus vulgaris An autoimmune disorder with appearance of crops of intraepidermal bullae in the mouth, face, neck and trunk. Pressure on bullae enlarges them due to splitting of the skin. Bullae contain clear or purulent fluid which on healing leave behind pigmentation and scarring.

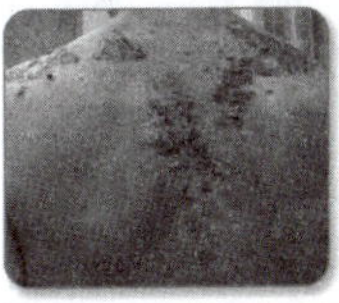

Pemphigus vulgaris

Penetrance (*pene'-trans*) The frequency with which a mutant gene produces its characteristic effect in those possessing it; the extent to which something enters an object or part.

Penia Combining word for deficiency.

Penicillamine (*pen'i-sil'a-men*) A hydrolytic degradation product of penicillin used to facilitate urinary excretion of heavy metals such as copper, mercury, zinc or lead.

Penicillinase (*pen'i-sil'i-nas*) A β-lactamase which can cleave the β-lactam ring and inactivate penicillin. The plasmids which code for the enzyme are transmissible between bacteria.

Penicillin V (*pen'i-sil'in*) Antibiotic with a basic structure of a four-membered β- lactam ring produced by the molds, *Pencillium notatum* and *P. chrysogenum*. It is bactericidal killing bacteria by interfering with their cell wall synthesis. It acts on both gram-positive and certain gram-negative organisms. Penicillinase is capable of inactivating the penicillin. Hypersensitivity forms the most important reaction.

Penicillium (*pen'i-sil'e-um*) A genus of fungi belonging to class Ascomycetes or the order Aspergillales yielding many antibiotic substances.

Penile (*pe'nil*) Pertaining to the penis.

Penile prosthesis Two artificial cylinders that fill with fluid to allow the penis to become hard for an erection.

Penis (*pe'nis*) The male organ of copulation and urination. It is suspended from the front and sides of pubic arch and is composed of erectile tissues arranged in three columns. There are two lateral columns, called corpora cavernosa and a median column corpus spongiosum containing urethra. Glans penis is a cone-shaped head of the penis containing urethral orifice, and is covered by the foreskin (prepuce). Sexual excitement causes hyperemia facilitating filling of corpora cavernosa and erection. It becomes flaccid on subsidence of hyperemia.

Pentaerythritol (*pen'ta-e-rith'ri-tol*) An organic nitrate used in the treatment of angina pectoris.

Pentagastrin (*pen'ta-gas'trin*) A synthetic gastrin used to test the ability of the stomach to secrete hydrochloric acid.

Pentazocine (*pen-taz'o-sen*) A synthetic narcotic analgesic.

Pentobarbital (*pen'to-bar'bi-tal*) A hypnotic barbiturate.

Pentosan (*pen'to-san*) A sulfated pentosyl polysaccharide used to treat bladder pain and discomfort due to interstitial cystitis.

Pentostatin (*pen'to-stat'in*) An adenosine deaminase inhibitor used to treat hairy cell leukemia.

Pentosuria (*pen'to-su're-a*) The excretion of one or more pentoses in the urine.

Pentoxifylline A xanthine derivative used as a drug to treat muscle pain in people with peripheral artery disease.

Peotillomania (*pe'o-til'o-ma-ne-a*) A nervous habit of constant pulling of the penis.

Pepsin (*pep'sin*) The principal enzyme secreted in the stomach that helps in digestion of protein. It is formed from pepsinogen by the chief cells of gastric glands and reduces proteins to smaller molecules such as proteoses and pentoses.

Pepsinogen (*pep-sin'o-jen*) A proenzyme secreted by the chief cells of the gastric mucosa.

Peptic (*pep'tik*) Relating to gastric digestion; pertaining to pepsin.

Peptic ulcer An ulcer in the lower esophagus, stomach or duodenum. Chronic peptic ulcer presents with pain in the epigastrium, clock like regularity of pain in relation to intake of food - on eating (gastric) and on empty stomach (duodenal).

Peptidase (*pepti-das*) An enzyme capable of hydrolyzing one of the peptide links of a peptide to produce an amino acid.

Peptide (*pep'tid*) Compound of two or more amino acids wherein—carboxyl group of one is united with the –amino group of the other.

Peptone (*pep'ton*) Intermediate polypeptide products formed in partial hydrolysis of proteins.

Peptonuria A high protein level in urine.

Perception (*per-sep'shun*) Process of transferring physical stimulation into psychological information; mental process by which sensory stimuli are brought to awareness.

Percussion (*per-kush'un*) A technique to produce sound waves by tapping the surface with the finger and it varies in its quality depending on the density of the underlying tissues.

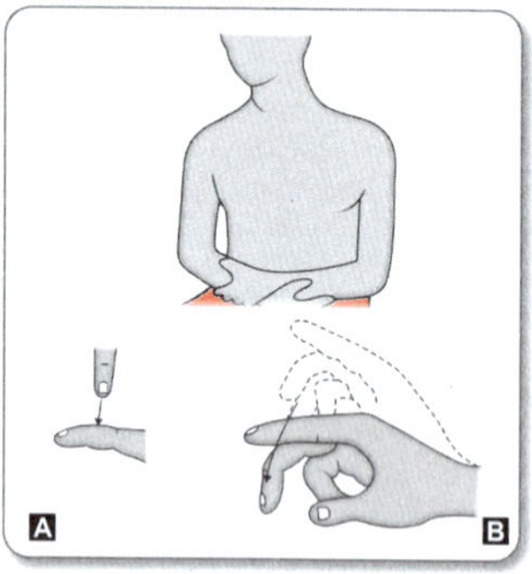

Percussion-position of pleximeter finger and plexor finger

Auscultatory percussion Auscultation of the sounds produced by percussion.

Direct percussion Percussion wherein the finger strikes directly over the bony region without the intervention of any other finger as on clavicle.

Immediate percussion Direct percussion.

Mediate percussion A type of percussion, done by using the middle finger of one hand as a plexor and of the middle finger of other hand applied firmly on the surface as pleximeter.

Percutaneous (*per'ku-ta'ne-us*) Performed in through the skin.

Percutaneous transluminal coronary angioplasty (PTCA) An interventional procedure consisting of balloon expansion of one or more stenosed coronary arteries.

Percutaneous nephrolithotomy A procedure used to remove kidney stones from the body when they cannot pass on their own.

Perfusion (*per-fu'zhun*) The passage of blood or other fluid through a vascular bed of an organ or tissue; pouring of a fluid; supply of nutrients to an organ by injecting into an artery.

Periadenitis (*per'e-ad'e-ni'tis*) Inflammation of tissues around a gland.

Perianal hematoma External hemorrhoid of anal area.

Periapical (*per'e-a'pi-kal*) Surrounding the apex of the root of a tooth.

Periarteritis nodosa A serious inflammatory blood vessels disease.

Periathritis A type of arthritis that occurs due to inflammation of tissues around a joint.

Peribronchiolitis (*per'i-bronk'-e-o-lit'is*) Inflammation of tissues around the bronchioles.

Pericardial (*per"e-karde-el*) Related to pericardium.

Pericardiectomy (*per'e-kar-de-ek'to-me*) Surgical removal of a portion of the pericardium.

Pericardiocentesis (*per'e-kar-de-o-sen-te'sis*) Paracentesis of the pericardium.

Pericardiolysis (*per'e-kar'de-ol'i-sis*) The operative separation of adhesions between the visceral and parietal pericardium.

Pericardiorrhaphy (*per'e-kar'de-or'a-fe*) Suture of the pericardium.

Pericardiostomy (*per'e-kar'de-os'to-me*) Creation of an opening into the pericardium.

Pericardiotomy (*per'e-kar'de-ot'o-me*) Incision of the pericardium.

Pericarditis (*per'e-kar-di'tis*) Inflammation of the pericardium due to various reasons such as infections, immunological reactions, trauma etc.

Acute fibrinous pericarditis Pericarditis with a fibrinous exudate.

Adhesive pericarditis Fibrinous pericarditis leading to varying degrees of adhesion formation between the two layers of the pericardium or between the pericardium and the heart or the neighboring structures.

Constrictive pericarditis Progressive thickening, fibrosis and calcification of the pericardium.

Fibrinous pericarditis Acute pericarditis with fibrinous exudate.

Hemorrhagic pericarditis Hemorrhagic effusion in the pericardium often due to malignant disease.

Purulent pericarditis Purulent collection of fluid in pericardium as a complication of septicemia or by direct spread of an intrathoracic infection.

Serous pericarditis A large effusion of turbid, straw colored fluid in the pericardium.

Pericardium A protective fluid filled sac that surrounds heart.

Perichondritis An inflammation of the skin and tissue surrounding the cartilage of the outer ear.

Perichondrium (*per'e-kon'dre-um*) A membrane of fibrous connective tissue around cartilage.

Pericoronitis *dent* Irritation or inflammation of the gum produced by the crown of an incompletely erupted tooth.

Pericranium (*per'e-kra'ne-um*) The periosteum of the skull. adj. **pericranial**.

Pericystitis Inflammation of the cellular tissues around the urinary bladder.

Pericyte (*per'i-sit*) An elongated contractile cell found in close association to the outside of capillary wall.

Periderm (*per'i-durm*) A thin layer of flat cells covering the epidermis in the fetus, that disappears before birth.

Perifolliculitis (*per'i-fo-lik'ul-itis*) Inflammation surrounding the hair follicles.

Perihepatitis (*per'e-hep'a-titis*) Inflammation of the peritoneal covering of the liver.

Perikaryon (*per'e-kar'e-on*) The cytoplasm around a nucleus; the cell body of a nerve cell as distinguished from its axon and dendrites; an odontoblast excluding the dentinal fiber.

Perilymph (*pe'ri-limf*) Fluid found within the space between membranous and bony labyrinths of the ear.

Perimeter Boundary of an area; instrument for perimetry.

Perimetritis Inflammation of the membrane on the outer surface of the uterus.

Perimetrium (*per'i-me'tre-um*) The serous membrane covering the uterus.

Perimysium (*per'i-mis'e-um*) The fibrous sheath surrounding each of the primary bundles of skeletal muscle fibers.

Perimysium (*per'i-mis'e-um*) The fibrous sheath surrounding each of the primary bundles of skeletal muscle fibers.

Perinatal (*per'i-nat'l*) Relating to the period just before, during or just after birth. It pertains to the period beginning after 28th week of pregnancy to one to four weeks after birth.

Perinatal mortality rate The number of still births plus neonatal deaths per 1000 total births.

Perineal pouch A potential space between the deep fascia of the pelvic floor (superiorly) and the perineal membrane (inferiorly). It contains part of urethra, external urethral sphincter and vagina in the female.

Perineopalsty A surgical procedure to repair the perineum and external organs of vagina.

Perineorrhaphy (*per'i-ne-or'a-fe*) Suture of the perineum.

Perinephric abscess Perinephric abscess

Perinephritis (*per'e-ne-frit'is*) The inflammation of perinephric tissue.

Perineum (*per'e-ne'um*) The tissue between the external genitalia and the anus that extends internally up to the muscles at the base of the pelvis and the surrounding bony structures; superficial area corresponding to the inferior outlet of pelvis.

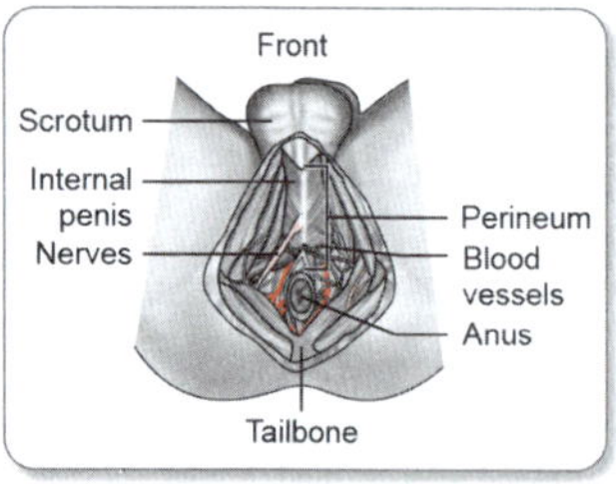

Male perineum

Perineurium (*per'e-nur'e-um*) Fibrous sheath of separate fascicles in a peripheral nerve.

Periodic acid– Schiff (PAS) reaction Tissue section is treated with Schiff's reagent which gives red or magenta color if glycoprotein, certain polysaccharides or fatty acids are present.

Periodic fever 3 or more episodes of unexplained fever in a 6-month period, occurring at least 7 days apart.

Periodontal abscess A localized accumulation of pus within the gingival wall of a peridontal pocket.

Periodontal pocket Presence of an abnormal depth of the gingival sulcus near the point at which the gingival tissue contacts the tooth.

Periodontitis (*per'e-don-ti'tis*) A disease of the tissues that surround and support the teeth, characterized by inflammation of gingivae, degeneration and resorption of dental periosteum, alveolar bone and cementum. There is loosening of teeth and recession of gingivae.

Periodontium (*per'e-don'she-um*) The tissues that surround and support the teeth. They are gingivae, cementum, periodontal membrane and alveolar bone.

Periodontology A specialty of dentistry that studies supporting structures, diseases and conditions of teeth.

Periosteum (*per'e-oste-um*) The thick, fibrous membrane that covers the bones except the articular cartilage. It consists of two layers—an inner osteogenic layer forming new bone tissue and an outer connective tissue layer containing blood vessels and nerves.

Periostitis (*per'e-os-titis*) Painful inflammation of the periosteum, resulting from injury or infection.

Peripartum cardiomyopathy A type of heart muscle disease that develops during or immediately after pregnancy.

Peripheral nervous system All the nerves that fan out from the central nervous system to the rest of the body.

Periphlebitis (*per'i-fle-bit'is*) Inflammation of tissues around a vein or of the outer coat of vein.

Perisalpingitis (*per'i-sal'pin-jitis*) Inflammation of tissues around the fallopian tube.

Perisplenitis (*per'i-sple-nit'is*) Inflammation of the peritoneal covering of the spleen.

Perisplenitis (*per'i-sple-nit'is*) Inflammation of the peritoneal covering of the spleen.

Peristalsis (*per'i-stal'sis*) Involuntary, wave- like alternate contraction and relaxation occurring in tubular structures, especially alimentary canal by which the contents are propelled onward.

Mass peristalsis Forced peristaltic movements of short duration seen in large intestine which allows the movement of its contents from one part to another.

Reversed peristalsis Peristalsis in a direction the reverse of normal, which forces the contents backward.

Peristaphyline (*per'i-staf'i-lin*) Around the uvula.

Peritendineum (*per'i-ten-din'e-um*) One of the fibrous sheaths covering tendons and extending between the fibers composing the tendon.

Peritendinitis (*per'i-ten'di-ni'tis*) Inflammation of the sheath of a tendon.

Peritenonitis (*per'i-ten'o-ni'tis*) *see* Peritendinitis.

Peritoneocentesis (*per'i-to-ne'o-sen-te-sis*) Paracentesis of the abdominal cavity.

Peritomy (*pe-rit'o-me*) Excision of a ring of conjunctiva around the cornea; circumcision.

Peritoneoscope (*per'i-to'ne-o-skop*) A long, slender telescope with a light at one end and an eye piece at the other. It facilitates inspection of the peritoneal cavity through a small incision in the abdominal wall.

Peritoneum (*per'i-to-ne'um*) The serous membrane lining the wall of the abdominal cavity (parietal p) and pelvic cavities and reflecting over the viscera contained therein (visceral p) and it forms two sacs, the peritoneal (greater) sac and the omental bursa (lesser sac) connected by the foramen epiploicum.

Peritonitis (*per'i-to-nitis*) Inflammation of the peritoneum.

Peritonsillar abscess An area of pus filled tissue at the back of the mouth, next to one of the tonsils.

Peritrichous (*pe-rit'ri-kus*) Microorganism having cilia or flagella around the entire surface.

Perityphlitis (*per'i-tif-li'tis*) Inflammation of the peritoneum around the cecum.

Periureteral (*per'i-u-re'ter-al*) Around a ureter.

Periureteritis (*per'i-u-re'ter-i'tis*) Inflammation of tissues around the ureter.

Perivasculitis (*per'i-vas'ku-li'tis*) Inflammation of the tissues surrounding a blood vessel.

Perle (*perl*) (*Fr*) A soft capsule containing medicine.

Perleche (*per-lesh*) (*Fr*) An inflammation with exudation, epithelial desquamation and fissuring at the corners of the mouth, especially in children.

Pernicious (*per-nish'us*) Fatal; harmful.

Pernicious anemia Anemia due to intrinsic factor deficiency.

Pernicious trend *psy* Abnormal departure from usual ideas and social interests.

Pernio (*per'ne-o*) *see* Chilblain.

Perniosis Chillblains; itchy, swollen, painful lumps or patches on the skin.

Peroneal (*per'o-ne'al*) Pertaining to the muscle fibula.

Peroneal atrophy Progressive peroneal muscle atrophy.

Peroneal nerve palsy Entrapment neuropathy causing foot drop, dorsiflexion and eversion of foot.

Peroneus Any of several muscles on the outer side of the leg, which assists in extending the foot and turning it outward.

Peroxidase (*per-ok'si-das*) Iron-porphyrin enzyme facilitating the transfer of oxygen from peroxide to a tissue requiring oxygen.

Peroxisome (*pe-roks'i-som*) Membrane-bound vesicles containing enzymes such as perioxidase, catalase and d-amino oxidase, concentrated in liver and kidney cells.

Perphenazine (*per-fen'a-zen*) A tranquilizer used as an antipsychotic and as an antiemetic.

Perseveration (*per-sev"er-a'shen*) Persisting response to a prior stimulus after a new stimulus has been presented, often associated with organic brain disease.

Personality (*pers'on-al'i-te*) The characteristics, attitude, intellectual qualities, emotional dispositions and behavior of an individual which sets him/her apart from others. It refers chiefly to the mental aspects than the physique.

Personality disorder *psy* Persistent and pervasive patterns of inner experience and behavior that deviate markedly from the expectations of the individual's culture and cause significant distress or impaired functioning.

Perspiration (*per'spi-ra'shun*) Sweating; the secretion of the sweat glands of the skin; sweat, a weak solution of sodium chloride.

Insensible perspiration Evaporation of water vapor from the body without producing any moisture on the skin.

Sensible perspiration Perspiration producing moisture on the skin.

Perthes' disease A rare childhood condition in which bone in the femur head part of ball and socket hip joint dies from lack of blood supply osteonecrosis. When the blood supply returns to the femur head, the bone improves its strength.

Perversion (*per-ver'ihun*) Deviation from the normal course.

Pes The foot; any foot-like process, pl. **pedes**.

Pes anserinus The three main branches of the facial nerve; the tendinous expansions of the sartorius, gracilis and semitendinosus muscles.

Pes cavus Marked concavity of the sole of the foot.

Pes contortus Talipes equinovarus.

Pes equinovalgus A deformity in which heel is elevated and turned outward.

Pes equinovarus A deformity in which heel is turned inward and foot is plantar flexed.

Pes equinus A deformity in which heel does not touch the ground while walking.

Pes hippocampi The lower part of hippocampus major.

Pes planus Flat foot.

Pes valgus Talipes valgus.

Pes varus Talipes varus.

Pes cavus Marked concavity of the sole of the foot.

Pes planus Flat foot.

Pessary Vaginal suppository.

Pesticide (*pes'ti-sid*) Any chemical agent used to kill pests. They are in the form of fumigants, fungicides, herbicides or insecticides.

Petechia (*pe-te'ke-a*) Pinpoint non-blanching spots that measure less than 2 mm in size and affect the skin and mucous membranes.

Petit mal A mild form of epilepsy, characterized by brief spells of unconsciouness without loss of posture.

Petri dish A container with two flattened clear glass or plastic plates allowing examination of bacterial culture, devised by R J Petri, assistant to Robert Koch in Berlin.

Petrissage (malaxation) (*pe'tre-sahzh*) Kneading of tissues in massage.

Petrositis (*pe'tro-sit'is*) Inflammation of the petrous portion of the temporal bone.

Petrous bone Stone-like hard densest bone, such as temporal bone's petrous part between the sphenoid and occipital bones.

-pexy Combining word for surgical fixation.

Peyer's patches Submucosal lymphoid aggregates of ileal mucosa, named after Johann Peyer, Swiss physician.

Peyronie's disease Fibromatous contracture of penis due to hardening of the corpora cavernosa of the penis, named after Francois Peyronie, French surgeon.

pH Potential of hydrogen. It is the symbol for the logarithm of the reciprocal of the H ion concentration. It is expressed in molarity. A solution with a pH 7.4 is neutral, above 7.4 it is alkaline and below 7.4 it is acidic.

PHA Phytohemagglutinin

Phacoemulsification (*fak'o-i-mul'si-fi-ka'shun*) A method of fragmentation, emulsification and aspiration of a cataract by using a low-frequency ultrasonic vibrations.

Phacomatosis (*fa'ko-ma-to'sis*) A group of hereditary diseases characterized by hamartomas in the tissues of ectodermal origin.

Phacometachoresis (*fa'ko-met'a-kor-e'sis*) Displacement of the lens of the eye.

Phage Combining word for one that eats or destroys.

Phagedena (*faf'a-de'nb*) Rapidly spreading, destructive ulceration of soft tissue.

Phagia Combining word for eating; swallowing(*fag'o-sit*) A cell of the immune system that can surround, engulf and digest microorganisms, foreign particles and cellular debris.

Phagocyte (*fag'o-sit*) A cell of the immune system that can surround, engulf and digest microorganisms, foreign particles and cellular debris.

Phagocytosis (*fag'o-si-to'sis*) The process of engulfing of microorganisms, necrotic tissue or other foreign bodies by phagocytes and their digestion.

Phalangeal cells Elongated supporting cells of the organ of Corti with bases that rest on the basilar membrane adjacent to the pillar cells.

Phalangectomy (*fal'an-jek-to-me*) Excision of a phalanx.

Phalanges The bones that make up the fingers (hand) and toes (foot). There are 56 phalanges in the human body.

Phalangitis (*fal'an-jit'is*) Inflammation of one or more phalanges.

Phalanx (*fa'lang-ks*) One of the bones of the fingers or toes, two for the thumb or big toe, and three each for other digits, are referred to as proximal, middle and distal, beginning from the metacarpus; one of a set of plates made up of inner and outer phalangeal cells forming the reticular membrane of organ of Corti.

Phalloplasty (*falo-plas'te*) The construction or reconstruction of a penis.

Phallus (*fal'us*) Penis. adj. **phallic**.

Phanero- (*fan'er-o'sis*) The process of becoming apparent.

Phaneromania An irresistible desire to pick at superficial body parts such as nail-biting.

Phantom (*fant'um*) Model of organs or of the body.

Phantom bone disease Disappearing bone disease characterized by extensive bone resorption.

Phantom breast Sensation that a surgically removed breast is still present.

Phantom limb The perception that a limb is present after it has been amputated.

Phantom tumor A well circumscribed accumulation of fluid in the interlobar spaces seen on chest radiographs which may occur in congestive heart failure.

Phantom tumor A well circumscribed accumulation of fluid in the interlobar spaces seen on chest radiographs which may occur in congestive heart failure.

Pharmaceutical (*far'ma-sut'ikal*) Relating to pharmacy or drugs.

Pharmacist (*farma-sist*) A person qualified in pharmacy who is licensed to prepare and dispense drugs.

Pharmacodynamics (*farma-ko-di-nam'iks*) The study of the effects of a given concentration of drug at its site of action.

Pharmacognosy (*far'ma-kog'no-se*) A branch of pharmacology concerned with the natural drugs and their characteristics and source.

Pharmacokinetics (*far'ma-ko-ki-net'iks*) Movement and concentrations of drugs in relevant tissues as function of time.

Pharmacology (*far'ma-kol'o-je*) The science concerned with the study of drugs, their structure, absorption, distribution, biotransformation, effects and side effects.

Molecular pharmacology Pharmacology that considers molecules as the fundamental functional units. It explains the pharmacological effects of biologically active compounds at the molecular level.

Pharmacomania An obsession or addiction to taking drugs.

Pharmacopoeia (*far'ma-ko-pe-a*) A standard text giving a detailed description of drugs, their actions, indications, dosage, methods of preparation and side effects.

Pharmacy (*far'ma-se*) The branch of health sciences concerned with the preparation, dispensing and utilization of drugs; a place where drugs are prepared and dispensed; a drug store.

Pharyng- (pharyngo-) Combining word for pharynx.

Pharyngeal (*fa-rin'je-al*) Pertaining to the pharynx.

Pharyngeal arches Series of primitive structures appearing in the fourth and fifth week of the embryo which give rise to major structures of the head and neck.

Pharyngeal bursa A midline recess over nasopharyngeal tonsil; a groove in embryonic pharyngeal wall representing pharyngeal cleft.

Pharyngeal clefts Primitive structures seen in the five-week embryo, one of which (first) gives rise to external auditory canal.

Pharyngeal pouches Embryonic structures occurring as outpouchings along the lateral wall of the pharyngeal cleft.

Pharyngeal A midline recess over nasopharyngeal tonsil; a groove in embryonic pharyngeal wall representing pharyngeal cleft.

Pharyngectomy (*far'in-jek'to-me*) Excision of part of the pharynx.

Pharyngismus (*far'in-jiz'mus*) Spasm of the pharyngeal muscles.

Pharyngitis (*far'in-jit'is*) Inflammation of the pharynx.

Pharyngocele (*fa-ring'go-sel*) A herniation or a diverticulum of the pharynx.

Pharyngoplegia (*fa-ring"go-ple'je-a*) Paralysis of the muscles of the pharynx.

Pharyngoscope (*fa'ring'go-skop*) An instrument for direct visual examination of the pharynx.

Phenacemide Ureal anticonvulsant used to control severe epilepsy.

Phenacetin (*fe-nas'e-tin*) An analgesic and antipyretic.

Phenazopyridine (*fen'a-zo-per-'i-den)* An azo dye, is a urinary analgesic used as an adjuvant medicine in the outpatient setting to treat patients with urinary tract infections (UTIs) and related conditions.

Phenelzine (*fen'al-zen*) A hallucinogen formerly used as a veterinary anesthetic, and briefly as a general anesthetic for humans. Phencyclidine is similar to ketamine in structure and in many of its effects. Like ketamine, it can produce a dissociative state. It exerts its pharmacological action through inhibition of NMDA receptors (receptors, N-methyl-D-aspartate). As a drug of abuse, it is known as PCP and Angel Dust.

Pheniramine (*fen'ir'a-men*) An antihistamine.

Phenmetrazine (*fen-met'ra-zen*) A sympathomimetic amine, which is similar to an amphetamine, used as adjunct therapy for the short-term management of exogenous obesity.

Phenobarbital (*fe'no-bar'bi-tal*) A long-acting barbiturate used as a sedative and hypnotic.

Phenol (carbolic acid) (*fe'nol*) Phenyl alcohol; phenic or carbolic acid, used as an antiseptic and disinfectant. It can be ingested in 3–4% solution to cause neurolysis.

Phenolphthalein (*fe'nol-thal'en*) Bright red crystalline powder used as an indicator in tissue culture media, and by parenteral injection as a test for renal function. It is also a laxative.

Phenothiazine (*fe'no-thi'a-zin*) The parent compound for synthesis of a variety of antipsychotic agents such as chlorpromazine, mepazine and prochlorperazine.

Phenotype (*fe'no-tip*) All the observable characteristics of an organism as determined by the genetic and environmental factors.

Phenoxybenzamine (*fe-nok'se-ben'za-men*) An alpha—adrenergic receptor blocking agent and is used to treat hypertension.

Phensuximide (*fen-suk'si-mid*) An anticonvulsant used in petit mal epilepsy.

Phentermine (*fen'tar-men*) A sympathomimetic anorectic agent used as a short-term adjunct therapy that is included in a regimen of weight reduction in cases of exogenous obesity.

Phentolamine (*fen-tol'a-men*) A potent alpha-adrenergic blocking agent useful in treatment of hypertension due to pheochromocytoma.

Phenylbutazone (*fen'il-buta-zon*) An analgesic, anti-inflammatory and antipyretic agent used in treatment of rheumatoid arthritis.

Phenylephrine (*fen'il-efren*) An adrenergic compound used to produce nasal decongestion.

Phenylketonuria (*fen'il-ke-to-nu'rea*) A genetic disorder in which the body is not capable of oxidizing the amino acid phenylalanine to tyrosine and it leads to severe mental retardation. Dietary restriction of phenylalanine is vital in the treatment.

Phenylpropanolamine (*fen'il-pro'pa-nol'a-men*) A sympathomimetic nasal decongestant.

Phenytoin (*fen'i-to-in*) An anticonvulsant and antiarrhythmic agent.

Pheochromocytoma (*fe'o-kro'mo-si-to-ma*) A benign tumor of adrenal medulla that secretes the hormones adrenaline and noradrenaline, leading to intermittent, life-threatening increase in blood pressure.

Pheochromocytoma triad Headaches, sweating and tachycardia in a patient with hypertension.

Phimosis (*fi-mo'sis*) Tightness of foreskin preventing it from being drawn back over the head of the penis.

Phleb- (phlebo-) Combining word for vein.

Phlebectomy (*fle-bek'to-me*) Excision of a segment of a vein.

Phlebitis (*fle'-bit'is*) Inflammation of a vein, which often leads to development of a blood clot.

Phlebography (*fle-bog'ra-fe*) The recording of the venous pulse; the radiography of a vein filled with contrast media.

Phlebolithiasis (*fleb'o-li-thi'a-sis*) Development of calcareous deposit in the venous wall.

Phlebosclerosis (venosclerosis) (*fleb'o-sk-le-ro'sis*) Fibrous thickening of the walls of a vein.

PHlebothrombosis (*fleb'o-throm-bo'sis*) A condition in which a blood clot forms in a vein without any inflammation.

Phlebotomus (*fle-bot'o-mus*) A genus of blood sucking sand flies which transmit diseases such as kala azar, cutaneous leishmaniasis and phlebotomus fever.

Phlebotomy (venesection) (*fle-bot'o-me*) Venesection; incision of a vein to withdraw blood.

Phlegm (*flem*) Sputum; viscid mucus, especially from respiratory tract; one of the four humors of the body.

Phlegmon (*fleg'mon*) A localized area of acute inflammation of the soft tissues.

Phlyctena (*flik-te'na*) A small vesicle following first degree burns.

Phobia (*fo'be-a*) A persistent, irrational fear of a particular object, person, place or situation.

Phocomelia (*fo'ko-me'le-a*) A congenital skeletal limb deformity due to the idiopathic absence of the radial elements of a limb bud.

Phon Combining word for sound, speech, voice.

Phonasthenia (*fo'nas-the'ne-a*) Weakness of voice.

Phonation (*fo-na'shun*) The production of sounds by means of vocal cords.

Phonocardiography (*fo'no-kar'de-og' ra-fe*) Recording of heart sounds with a phonocardiograph.

Phonocatheter (*fo'no-kath'e-ter*) A device that appears like a conventional catheter, with a microphone at the tip; used in recording the sounds of the heart and great vessels.

Phonomyography (*fo-no-mi-og'ra-fe*) Recording of the sounds produced by muscle contraction.

Phonosurgery A surgical procedure done on the vocal cords and adjacent tissues to improve the timbre, tone and quality of the voice.

Phosgene (*fos'gen*) Carbon chloride $COCl_2$ a highly poisonous gas, used in chemical warfare.

Phosphagen (*fos'fa-jen*) An energy storing compound that is chiefly found in muscles and nervous tissues in animals.

Phosphatase (*fos-fa-tas*) Any of a group of enzymes that catalyze the hydrolysis of phosphonic acid esters.

Acid phosphatase A phosphatase acting at an optimum pH of 5.4 and is present in prostate gland.

Alkaline phosphatase A phosphatase acting at an optimum pH of 8.6. It is present in teeth, developing bone, plasma, kidney and intestine. The level is very high in infancy which gradually decreases later.

Phosphatemia (*fosfa-te'me-a*) The occurrence of phosphate in the blood especially in excessive amounts.

Phosphatidylcholine (*fos'fa-tid'l-ko'len*) A chemical contained in eggs, soybeans, mustard, sunflower, and other foods. It is found naturally in the body in all cells. Phosphatidylcholine is also a source of choline in the body. It is used for ulcerative colitis. There is some scientific research that supports this use.

Phosphaturia (phosphuria) (*fos'fa-tur'e-a*) Excessive excretion of phosphates in the urine.

Phosphocreatine (PC) A cardioprotective agent indicated for use in cardiac surgery.

Phosphofructokinase A kinase enzyme that phosphorylates fructose 6-phosphate in glycolysis.

Phospholipid (*fos'fo-lip'id*) A lipid containing phosphorus. It includes lecithin and sphingomyelin. The lipid portion of cell membranes is essentially made up of phospholipids.

Phosphonecrosis (*fos'fo-ne-kro'sis*) The destruction of tissues caused by excessive amounts of phosphorus in the system. The organs likely to suffer are the liver, kidneys, muscles, bones, and the cardiovascular system.

Phosphorus (*fos'for-us*) A nonmetallic chemical, symbol P, atomic no. 15. It occurs as phosphate in all living cells and forms major component of mineral phase of bone. It is actively involved in metabolic process.

Phosphorylase (*fos-for'i-las*) A transferase, as involved in transfer of an inorganic phosphate group to some organic acceptor; any of the group of enzymes that catalyze phosphorolysis.

Photalgia (*fo-tal'je-a*) Pain caused by light as in eye.

Photocoagulation (*fo'to-ko-ag'ul-a'shun*) Destruction of tissue by heating effect of intensely focused light.

Photodermatitis (*fo'to-der'ma-tit'is*) Dermatitis caused by exposure to ultraviolet light.

Photomicrograph (*fo'to-mi'kro-graf*) An enlarged photograph of an object viewed with a microscope.

Photophobia (*fo"to-fo'be-a*) Abnormal intolerance to visual perception of light.

Photophthalmia Inflammation of the eye.

Photopic The normal adaptation of the eye to light; day vision.

Photopsia A visual disturbance that happens when one sees light without looking at a light.

Photoretinitis (*fo'to-ret'in-it'is*) Decreased visual acuity from a macular burn due to excessive exposure to sunlight or other intense light.

Photosensitivity Abnormal reaction to exposure to sunlight, usually in the form of rash. It can result from some disorders or from ingestion of particular drugs.

Photosynthesis (*fo'to-sin'the-sis*) The process by which plants are able to produce carbohydrates by combining carbon dioxide and water in the chlorophyll tissue under the influence of light.

PHototaxis (*fo'to-tak'sis*) Reaction of living protoplasm to the stimulus of light.

Photuria Excretion of phosphorescent urine, which glows in the dark, due to the presence of certain phosphorus containing compounds derived from phosphates.

Phren- (phreno-) Combining word for diaphragm; phrenic nerve; mind.

Phrenic avulsion Phrenic nerve injury which may present diaphragmatic dysfunction, unilateral diaphragmatic paralysis or bilateral diaphragmatic paralysis.

Phrenicectomy (*fren'i-sek'to-me*) Resection of a part of phrenic nerve.

Phreniclasia (*fren'i-kla'ze-a*) Phrenic nerve crush with a clamp causing paralysis of the diaphragm.

Phrenic (*fren'ik*) Pertaining to the diaphragm or mind.

Phrenic nerve A nerve that runs from the spinal cord to the diaphragm. It causes the diaphragm to contract and reflex which helps to control breathing.

Phreniclasia (*fren'i-kla'ze-a*) Phrenic nerve crush with a clamp causing paralysis of the diaphragm.

Phrenology (*fre'nol-o-gi*) A pseudo-scientific practice of determining a person's mental characteristics and personality by studying the shape and contours of the skull; this practice has ben wholly discredited by scientific research.

Phthiriasis (*thi-ri'a-sis*) Infestation with Phthirus pubis.

Phthisis (*thesis*) A wasting disease of the body; tuberculosis.

Phthisis bulbi Degeneration of the ocular globe accompanied by retinal necrosis, atrophy, thickening of sclera, and loss of function.

Phycomycosis (*-mi-ko'sis*) An acute fungal disease caused by phycomycetes.

Phylogenesis The biological process by which development of an organism is studied.

Physical (*fiz'ik-l*) Relating to the body.

Physical dependence Need to continue using a drug to maintain normal body function and to avoid withdrawal illness; addiction.

Physical examination Examination of the body by inspection, palpation, percussion and auscultation.

Physical fitness The ability to undertake daily tasks without undue fatigue.

Physical therapy Treatment using physical methods such as exercise or agents such as heat, light or water.

Physician (*fi-zish'un*) A person who has successfully completed the prescribed medical curriculum in a medical institution recognized by the medical council and who has obtained the license from the medical council to practice medicine; a person who practices medicine as distinct from surgery.

Physiological solution (*fizè-o-loji-kal*) Pertaining to normal physiology.

Physiology (*fizè-olò-je*) The science concerned with the normal functions of the living organism and its components including the physical and chemical processes involved.

Physiotherapy (*fizè-o-thèra-pe*) Physical therapy; the prevention and treatment of disease or injury with physical methods such as exercise and machines.

Physostigmine (*fi'so-stig'men*) A cholinergic alkaloid inactivating cholinesterase, thus prolonging the action of acetylcholine.

Phytohemagglutinin (PHA) (*fi'to-hemà-glut'in-in*) A phytomitogen from plants that agglutinates red blood cells.

Phytonadione (*fi-tòna-diòn*) A vitamin K1 medication used to treat and manage vitamin K deficiency, which is a significant risk factor for intracranial hemorrhage and other bleeds.

Phytophotodermatitis (*fi'to-fo'to-der' ma-ti'tis*) A cutaneous phototoxic inflammatory eruption resulting from contact with light-sensitizing botanical substances, also known as furanocoumarins, and long-wave ultraviolet A (UV-A, 320-380 nm) radiation.

Phytotoxin (*fi'to-tok'sin*) Any toxin of plant origin.

Pia (pia mater) (*pi'a*) Pia mater.

Piaglia (*pi'a-glia*) Related to pia mater and glial cells.

Pica (*pi'ka*) A perverted appetite with craving for unnatural articles as food.

Pick's disease A form of presenile dementia affecting frontal and temporal lobes, and characterized by personality change, named after Arnold Pick, Czeck physician.

Picornavirus (*pi-kor'na-vi'rus*) An extremely small nonenveloped virus having a core of single stained RNA. It includes polioviruses, coxsackie viruses and echoviruses.

Picric acid (trinitrophenol) Trinitrophenol used in application in burns, eczema and pruritus.

Piedra (*pe-àdra*) A fungal disease of the beard and moustache in which the fungi form sheath-like nodular masses.

Pigeon toes When feet point inward instead of forward Pigeon toes are common in young children.

Pigment (*pig'mint*) Any coloring matter of the body; a stain used in histologic work; a medicinal preparation for external use, applied to the skin like a paint. adj. **pigmentary**.

Bile pigment A complex, highly colored substance such as bilirubin, biliverdin and their derivatives such as urobilinogen, urobilin, which imparts brown color to intestinal contents and feces.

Blood pigment A pigment in red blood cell (hemoglobin) and a derivative of it (hematin, methemoglobin, hemosiderin).

Respiratory pigments The oxygen carrying pigments such as hemoglobin, myoglobin or cytochromes participating in the oxidative processes of the body.

Retinal pigment Visual pigment.

Skin pigment Melanin and carotene.

Urinary pigment Urochrome and sometimes urobilin.

Uveal pigment Melanin in the choroid layer of the eye, ciliary processes and the posterior surface of the iris.

Visual pigment The photopigment of retinal cones (photopsins) and rods (scotopsins) that absorb light and initiate the phenomenon of vision.

Wear and tear pigment Accumulation of lipofuscin in aging cells.

Pigmentation (*pig'men-tàshun*) Coloration of skin or tissues due to deposition of pigment.

Piles Hemorrhoids; swollen veins in the anus and lower rectum.

Pili (fimbriae) (*pili*) A hair-like appendage found on the surface of many bacteria and archaea. They function to attach the cells to surfaces.

Pill (*pil*) A little ball of medicine; oral contraceptive agent.

Pep pill Stimulating drugs used to keep the person from falling asleep.

Pillar (*pi'lar*) A column of stone, wood or metal that is used for supporting part of a building.

Pilocarpine (*pi'lo-kar'pen*) A cholinergic alkaloid from leaves of pilocarpus, used as an ophthalmic miotic agent in glaucoma.

Piloerection (*pi'lo-e-rek'shun*) Erection of the hair.

Pilomotor nerves (*pi'lo-mo'ter*) Referring to the arrector muscles, whose contraction results in goose flesh and piloerection.

Pilonidal sinus (*pi'lo-nid'al*) Referring to a growth of hair in deeper layer of skin or in a dermoid cyst.

Pilosebaceous Of or relating to hair follicle and its sebaceous gland.

Pilus (*pi'lus*) A hair; one of the minute filamentous appendages of certain bacteria.

Pimecrolimus (*pim"e-kro-li'mus*) A calcineurin inhibitor that is used to treat atopic dermatitis (eczema).

Pimozide (*pi'mo-zid*) An antipsychotic used to manage debilitating motor and phonic tics in patients with Tourette's Disorder.

Pimple (*pim'pl*) A papule or a small pustule.

Pincement One of the techniques used in massage, in which pinches of the patient's flesh are taken between finger, thumb and twisted or rolled before release. This is said to improve tone of skin.

Pineal gland A cone-shaped gland located in the roof of the third ventricle.

Pinguecula (*ping-gwe'ku-la*) A yellowish raised growth on the conjunctiva typically adjacent to the border where the colored part of the eye meets the white part of the eye. It usually appears on the side closer to the nose, is present in both eyes and relatively permanent; also called pinguicula.

Pink eye Acute contagious conjunctivitis by *Haemophilus aegyptius* or *H. ducreyi*.

Pinna (auricle) (*pin'a*) Pl. **pinnae**; the auricle or projected part of the external ear composed of elastic cartilage and covered by skin, that collects and directs sound waves into the external auditory meatus; a feather or wing.

Pinna nasi A protruding cartilaginous extension on each nostril.

Pinocytosis (*pi'no-si-to'sis*) The process by which cells ingest liquid to form small vesicles.

Pinta Pinta (*pen'ta*) A nonvenereal disease caused by the spirochaete, *Treponema carateum*, transmitted by direct mucocutaneous inoculation.

Pinworm (threadworm) *Enterobius vermicularis*, causing Enterobiasis.

Piperazine (*pi'per-a-zen*) Anthelmintic used in the treatment of round worm and thread worm infestation.

Piriformis syndrome An entrapment neuropathy of sciatic nerve characterized by pain in the hip and buttock that radiates up into the lower back and down the leg.

Piroxicam (*pir-ok'si-kam*) An analgesic and anti-inflammatory agent.

Pisiform bone A small bone found in the proximal row of the wrist (carpus). It is situated where the ulna joins the wrist, within the tendon of the flexor carpiulnaris muscle.

Pit A tiny hollow; a shallow depression on pressure in edema; a small depression in the enamel surface of a tooth.

Pithiatism (*pithe'a-ti'zm*) A disorder created by suggestion and curable by persuasion; hysteria.

Pithing (*pith'ing*) Destruction of CNS piercing brain or spinal cord.

Pitting The formation of a small depression, usually by scarring; a splenic function removing intracytoplasmic inclusions such as siderotic granules or Howell-Jolly bodies; remaining indented for some time after removal of firm finger pressure, as in edema.

Pituicyte (*pi-tu'i-sit*) Supporting cell of posterior pituitary gland.

Pituitary gland (hypophysis) Master of endocrine orchestra, a pea-sized structure lying in the sella turcica of the sphenoid bone and attached to the hypothalamus by the infundibulum. The pituitary gland has two anatomically and functionally separate portions. The anterior pituitary is derived from an outgrowth of ectoderm (Rathke's pouch) in the roof of the mouth and contains many glandular epithelial cells. The secretions regulate a wide range of bodily activities. The hormones are human growth hormone (hGH) prolactin, adrenocorticotropic hormone (ACTH), thyroid-stimulating hormone (TSH), follicle-stimulating hormone (FSH), luteinizing hormone (LH) and melanocyte-stimulating hormone (MSH). The posterior pituitary arises as an outgrowth of neurohypophyseal bud. Though it does not synthesize hormones, it is concerned with storage and release of oxytocin and antidiuretic hormone (ADH). In addition, there is an atrophied intermediate lobe (*Pars intermedia*).

Pituitary dwarfism A condition caused by hyposecretion of human growth hormone during growth years.

Pituitary tumor Mostly benign adenomas, may be hormonally silent or hormonally active.

Pityriasis (*pit'i-ri'a-sis*) A non-inflammatory skin disorder with scale formation.

Pityriasis alba A condition characterized by ill defined, hypopigmented macules, located on the cheeks, noted before puberty, probably because of lack of sebaceous secretion; pityriasis simplex.

Pityriasis capitis Dandruff.

Pityriasis rosea A condition characterized by sudden eruption of asymptomatic, oval or circular erythematous, scaly lesions where margins are more prominent and pink and are found on the upper trunk and arms. A herald patch appears two to three days before appearance of eruptions.

Pityriasis rubra pilaris A follicular keratotic condition characterized by skin colored follicular papules on the extremities and trunk.

Pityriasis versicolor Tinea versicolor, a fungal infection caused by *Pityrosporum orbiculare* (Malassezia furfur) which affects the stratum corneum in the form of discrete hypo- or hyperpigmented macules with overlying scales over the trunk, arms and face.

Pityrosporum (*pit'i-ros'po-ram*) A condition where the yeast, pityrosporum, gets down into the hair follicles and multiplies, setting up an itchy, acne-like eruption.

Pivot joint A conical surface of one bone articulates with a ring formed partly by another bone and partly by a ligament, as in the joint between the atlas and axis, and between the proximal ends of radius and ulna.

Placebo (*pla-se'bo*) A substance having no pharmacological effect but given merely to satisfy a patient who considers it to be a medicine; a substance having no pharmacological effect but administered as a control in testing experimentally or clinically the efficacy of a biologically active preparation.

Placebo effect A positive or negative response to a drug resulting from a person's expectations rather than from any real chemical effects.

Placenta (*pla-sen'ta*) A special structure through which the exchange of materials between fetal and maternal circulation occurs.

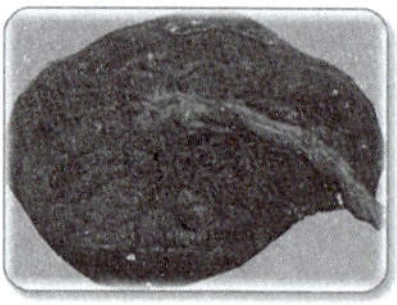

Placenta

Placenta accreta Firm attachment of placenta to the uterine wall preventing its separation at labor.

Placenta previa Implantation of placenta in lower uterine segments.

Placentography (*pla'sen-tog'ra-fe*) Radiographic examination of the placenta.

Placode (*plak'od*) A plate-like thickening of the epithelium, usually the ectoderm.

Plagiocephaly (*pla-je-o-sef'a-le*) Oblique skull showing bulge anteriorly on one side and posteriorly on other side.

Plague (*plag*) A communicable disease caused by *Yersinia pestis* acquired by humans from rats or by droplet infection.

Bubonic plague Condition acquired by bite of infected fleas (xenopsylla) carrying disease from dying rats. It has a sudden onset with high fever, dry skin, headache and swelling at the site of the affected lymph node (bubo). The condition may lead to toxemia and death.

Domestic plague Plague spread by rodents living with man.

Pneumonic plague Spread of plague between humans by droplets containing *Y. pestis*. It is characterized by cough and dyspnea, expectoration of highly frothy blood-stained sputum.

Septicemic plague Patients with plague exhibiting severe toxemia, hypotension and mental confusion.

Sylvatic plague Plague afflicting mainly rodents and independent of human population.

Plane (*plan*) A flat, relatively smooth surface; a specified level, as the plane of anesthesia; between the tissue layers; anatomical planes of body are imaginary flat surfaces used as reference points to divide the body into sections for anatomical study.

Plane wart A variety of viral papilloma of the skin exhibiting several small round flat plaques on the face and back of hands.

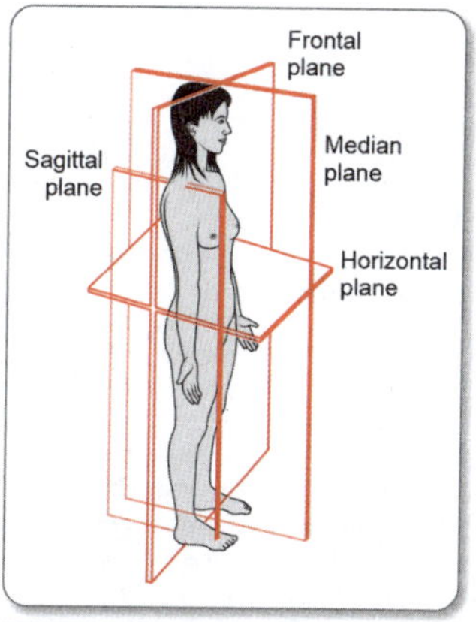

Anatomical planes of body

Planoconcave (*pla'no-kon'kav*) Pertaining to a lens that is plane on one side and concave on the other.

Planoconvex (*pla'no-kon'veks*) Pertaining to a lens that is plane on one side and convex on the other.

Plantar (*plan'tar*) Pertaining to the sole of the foot.

Equivocal plantar response Stroking of the outer side of the sole of the foot may elicit only dorsiflexion of big toe without any fanning of the toes or without dorsiflexion of the big toe; it is noted in early pyramidal disease or in its minimal involvement.

Extensor plantar response Extension of big toe at the metatarsophalangeal joint due to the contraction of the extensor hallucis longus, and extension and spread of the other toes like a fan when the outer side of the sole of the foot is stroked. It indicates involving the corticospinal tract.

Plantar fasciitis Tenderness under the heel from plantar fibromatosis or tear of plantar fascia.

Plantar flexion Bending of the foot in the direction of the sole.

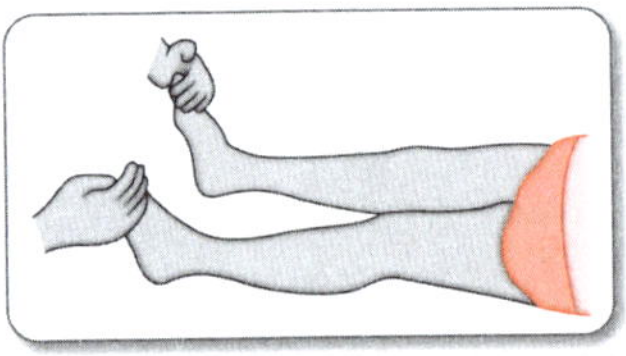

Plantar flexion

Plantar response/reflex There is flexion of the great toe at the metatarsophalangeal joint and flexion and abduction of other toes when the outer side of the sole of the foot is stroked lightly.

Plantar wart A hard, horny, rough surfaced area on the sole of the foot caused by papovavirus.

Plantar arch Formed from the continuation of the lateral planter artery and the anastomoses between the deep branch of dorsalis pedis artery. It supplies sole of the foot.

Plantigrade Foot posture in which the entire sole of the foot is placed on the ground.

Plaque (*plak*) A cholesterol-containing mass in the tunica media of arteries; a mass of bacterial cells, polysaccharide and other debris that adheres to the teeth; areas of demyelination in disseminated sclerosis.

Plasia Combining word for formation; growth; proliferation.

Plasm- (plasma-) (*plazm*) Plasma.

Plasma (blood plasma) (*plaz'ma*) The extracellular fluid found in blood vessels and lymphatics.

Plasma cell Plasmacyte with abundant RNA in cytoplasm.

Plasma exchange therapy Removal of plasma from the body and replacement with normal plasma.

Plasma thromboplastin Antecedent clotting factor XI that activates Christmas factor.

Plasma thromboplastin component Christmas factor IX.

Plasmacytoma (*plaz'ma-si-to'ma*) A tumor composed of plasma cells.

Plasmalogen (*plaz-mal'o-jen*) A class of glycerophospholipids which contain a vinyl-ether and an ester bond at the sn-1 and sn-2 positions, respectively, in the glycerol backbone.

Plasmapheresis (*plaz'ma-fer-e'sis*) A procedure in which blood is removed from the body, its components are separated, disease causing components such as toxins, metabolic products and antibodies are removed, and the remainder is returned to the body.

Plasmin (fibrinolysin) (*plaz'min*) Fibrinolytic enzyme derived from plasma plasminogen blood.

Plasminogen (*plaz'min'o-jen*) The substance that when activated forms plasmin.

Plasmodium (*plaz-mo'de-um*) Pl. **plasmodia**. A genus of protozoa belonging to subphylum sporozoa. It includes the malarial parasite.

Plasmodium falciparum The causative agent of malignant tertian malaria.

Plasmodium malariae The causative agent of quartan malaria.

Plasmodium ovale The causative agent of benign tertian malaria.

Plasmodium vivax The causative agent of benign tertian malaria.

Plasmolysis (*plaz'mol'i-sis*) Shrinkage of cytoplasm of the cell due to loss of water.

Plaster A solid material which can be spread when heated and which becomes adhesive at the body temperature; a topical preparation used to apply drugs to the surface to obtain their systemic effects.

Adhesive plaster A plaster made of a strong cloth that has a coating of an adhesive substance on one side. It is used to keep the edges of a wound in apposition, and to protect raw surfaces.

Dental plaster A semisolid paste that hardens to a model material.

Plaster cast A rigid dressing made of gauze impregnated with plaster of Paris used in immobilization of bone fractures.

Plaster lung Extensive pulmonary consolidation seen in *Klebsiella pneumoniae* infection.

Plaster of Paris Exsiccated calcium sulfate (gypsum cement) which when mixed with water forms a paste that sets rapidly. It is used for casts.

Plaster of Paris Exsiccated calcium sulfate (gypsum cement) which when mixed with water forms a paste that sets rapidly. It is used for casts.

Plastic surgery Surgery aimed at restoring the lost functions and in some instances improving personal appearance.

Plastron The sternum and attached cartilages.

Platelet (thrombocyte) (*plat'let*) A round or oval disc of 2–4 mm in diameter, found in the blood and their number varies from 1,50,000–4,00,000/mm^3. They are fragments of megakaryocytes. They play an important role in blood coagulation, hemostasis and formation of thrombus.

Platelet activating factor (PAF) A phospholipid synthesized by leukocytes, macrophages and endothelial cells that produces platelet aggregation, neutrophil release of enzymes and amines, and increased vascular permeability.

Platelet plug Aggregation platelets at a damaged blood vessel to prevent loss of blood.

Platelet-derived growth factor (PDGF) Molecules released from platelets, which help to heal wounds and to repair damage to blood vessel walls. They also help blood vessels grow.

Platy A combining word for broad.

Platyhelminth (*plat'e-hel-minth*) Flat worm.

Platysma (*pla-tizma mi-oy-dez*) A broad thin plate-like muscle that extends from fascia of both sides of neck to the jaw and muscles around the mouth.

Pledget (*plej'et*) A small compress of gauze or absorbent cotton that is used to absorb fluid or as a protective; a small spherical mass of cotton used with forceps for topical application of medicinal substances.

Pleiotropy (*pli'o-tro'pe*) Different effects of a gene on apparently unrelated characteristics such as the phenotype, organ systems or functions.

Pleocytosis (*ple'o-si-to'sis*) Increase in the number of cells, especially in CSF.

Pleomastia A condition of having more than two mammary glands or nipples.

Pleomorphism (*ple-o-mor'fizm*) The occurrence of more than one form in a life cycle; the property of crystallizing into two or more different forms.

Pleoptics (*ple-op'tiks*) Ocular exercises to stimulate and train an amblyopic eye.

Plerocercoid Larval tapeworm of *Diphyllobothrium latum* found in fish, which develops into adult when eaten by men.

Plessimeter (Pleximeter) (*ple-sim'e-ter*) Pleximeter.

Plessor (plexor) (*ples'or*) Plexor.

Plethora (*pleth'o-ra*) Excess amount of fluid; appearance of having more blood.

Plethysmography (*pleth'iz-mogra-fe*) A technique that measures the changes in the volume of an organ, limb or the body.

Impedance plethysmography Measurement of changes in limb volume with each arterial pulse and during occlusion of the cuff of the venous return from a limb to determine the acute venous obstruction or vascular insufficiency in an extremity.

Whole body plethysmography Measurement of thoracic gas volume and airway resistance.

Pleur- (pleuro-) Combining word for pleura; rib; side.

Pleura (*plu'ra*) The serous membrane that covers the lungs and lines the chest wall and the diaphragm; pl. **pleurae**.

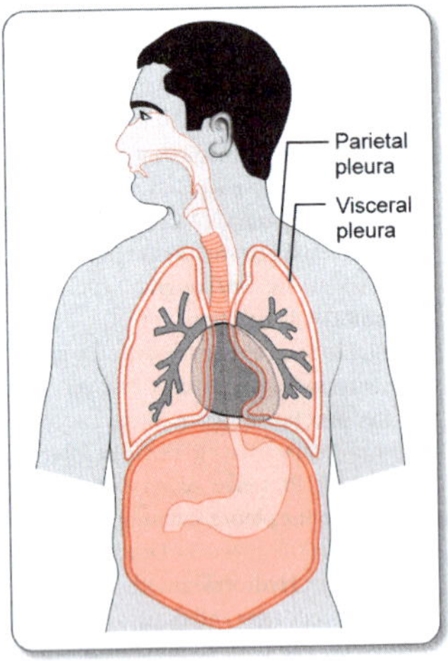

Pleura

Parietal pleura The membrane lining the inner surface of chest wall, cervical tissues, mediastinum and diaphragm.

Visceral pleura The membrane encasing the lung including the interlobar fissures.

Pleuracentesis A minimally invasive procedure that removes fluid from the pleural space.

Pleural cavity Small potential space between the visceral and parietal pleurae.

Pleurectomy (*plu-rek'to-me*) Surgical removal of part of the pleura.

Pleurisy (*plu'ris-e*) Inflammation of the pleura.

Pleurocele (*plu'ro-sel*) Hernia of the lungs and pleura; collection of serous fluid in the pleural cavity.

Pleurodesis (*plu'ro-de'sis*) Production of adhesions between the parietal and visceral pleura.

Chemical pleurodesis Instillation of chemical irritants such as quinacrine, tetracycline, cyclophosphamide or iodized talc into the pleural space to produce pleural irritation, fibrosis and adhesion.

Pleurodynia (*plu'ro-din'e-a*) Sharp pain in the intercostal muscles.

Epidemic pleurodynia *see* Bornholm disease.

Pleurohepatitis (*plu'ro-hep'a-ti'tis*) Inflammation of the pleura and the liver.

Pleurolysis (pneumolysis) (*plu-rol'i-sis*) Loosening of parietal pleura from intrathoracic fascia.

Pleuropneumonia (*plu'ro-nu-mo'ne-a*) Pleurisy in association with pneumonia.

Pleuropneumonia-like organisms (PPLO) (*plu'ro-nu-mo'ne-a*) Pleurisy in association with pneumonia.

Pleurotomy (*plu-rot'o-me*) Incision of the pleura.

Pleximeter (*plek-sim'e-ter*) A finger or a device held over the surface of the body for receiving the blow of a finger or the percussion hammer, in mediate percussion.

Plexor (*pleks'or*) A hammer or a finger for striking on the pleximeter in percussion.

Plexogenic (*plek'so-jen'ik*) Giving rise to weblike or plexiform structures.

Plexus (*pleks'us*) A network of nerves or of blood vessels or lymphatics.

Plica (*pli'ka*) A fold; pl. **plicae**.

Plicamycin (*pli"ka-mi'sin*) An antineoplastic antibiotic produced by Streptomyces plicatus. It has been used in the treatment of testicular cancer, Paget's disease of bone, and, rarely, the management of hypercalcemia.

Plication (*pli-ka-shun*) The stitching of folds or tucks in the wall of organ to decrease its size.

Plombage (*plom-bazh*) A method of causing collapse of the diseased lung by stripping parietal pleura from the chest wall and packing the space by small plastic balls.

Plumbism (*plum'bizm*) Poisoning from lead.

Plummer-Vinson syndrome (*plum'er-vin'sun*) An iron deficiency anemia associated with dysphagia and koilonychia, named after Henry Plummer, US physician and Porter Vinson, US surgeon.

Pluripotent (*plu-rip'o-tent*) An embryonic cell capable of developing into different kinds of cells; capable of different actions.

Pneumatization (*nu'ma-ti-za'shun*) The formation of air-filled cells or cavities, usually in bone such as paranasal sinuses and mastoid process of temporal bone.

Pneumolithiasis (*nu'mo-lith-i'as-is*) Formation of concretions in the lung.

Pneumomassage (*nu'mo-ma-saz*) Massage of tympanum with air to facilitate movement of the ossicles of the inner ear.

Pneumatocele (*nu-mat'o-sel*) A small, thin-walled structures consisting of single or multiple air-filled cysts secondary to alveolar and bronchiolar necrosis.

Pneumaturia (*nu'mat-u're-a*) Passage of gas or air from the urethra during or after urination, as a result of infected urine or intestinal fistula.

Pneumo Combining word for air, lung.

Pneumocephalus (pneumocele) (*nu'mo-ce'fa-lus*) Presence of air in the ventricles of the brain.

Pneumococcus (*nu'mo-kok'us*) An oval-shaped, encapsulated, gram-positive organism occupying in pairs (diplococcus) and having a lancet-shaped ends. There are more than 80 serologic types of pneumococci and cause pneumonia, otitis media, bronchitis, and meningitis.

Pneumoconiosis (*nu'mo-ko'ne-o'sis*) Occupational pulmonary diseases caused by prolonged inhalation of dusts which accumulate in lungs causing tissue reactions, in the form of fibrosis, pneumonia, bronchiolitis, extrinsic allergic alveolitis and asthma.

Pneumocystis (*nu'mo-sis'tis-ka-ri'ne-i*) A round or elongated organism of 2–4 microns length that causes an opportunistic infection in an immunocompromised host. AIDS patients develop pneumonia from its infection. The infection is limited to the lungs.

Pneumoencephalography (*nu'mo-en-sef'a-log'ra-fe*) Radiography of the subarachnoid space and the ventricles following removal of CSF and injection of air or oxygen *via* lumbar puncture.

Pneumography (*nu'mo-grafe*) An anatomical description of the lungs; graphic recording of respiratory movements; radiography of a part or organ after injection of air.

Pneumohemothorax (*nu'mo-hem'o-tho'raks*) Presence of gas or air and blood in the pleural cavity.

Pneumohydrothorax (*nu'mo-hi'dro-tho'raks*) Hydropneumothorax; presence of air or gas and fluid in the pleural cavity.

Pneumolysis The separation of an adherent lung from the pleura, to permit collapse of the lung.

Pneumonectomy (*nu'mon-ek'to-me*) Excision of all or part of the lung.

Pneumonia (*nu-mo'ne-a*) Consolidation of a part or the whole of the lung from an acute inflammatory exudate into the alveolar spaces.

Acute eosinophilic pneumonia Acute respiratory failure with marked eosinophilia.

Aspiration pneumonia Pneumonia resulting from aspiration of foreign material, usually food particles or vomit into the bronchi.

Atypical pneumonia Pneumonia caused by virus or mycoplasma.

Bacterial pneumonia Bacterial infection of the alveoli.

Bronchial pneumonia Acute inflammation of the walls of the smaller bronchial tubes varying amounts of pulmonary consolidation due to spread of the inflammation into peribronchiolar alveoli and the alveolar ducts.

Chlamydial pneumonia Pneumonia produced by *Chlamydia pneumoniae*.

Chronic eosinophilic pneumonia Insidious condition with dyspnea, non-productive cough, eosinophilia and radiologic peripheral homogeneous density.

Community acquired pneumonia Pneumonia developing from infection acquired from patients or convalescent carriers through droplets.

Desquamative interstitial pneumonia Diffuse proliferation of alveolar lining cells which desquamate into the air sacs that produce a gradual onset of dyspnea and dry cough.

Double pneumonia Lobar pneumonia affecting both lungs.

Gram-negative pneumonia Infection from aerobic gram-negative organisms in situations of poor resistance and altered defense mechanisms.

Hypostatic pneumonia Pneumonia that usually results from the collection of fluid in the dorsal region of the lungs, occurs especially in those (elderly or bedridden patients) confined to a supine position for extended periods.

Influenzal pneumonia Pneumonia due to *Haemophilus influenzae;* pneumonia complicating influenza.

Klebsiella pneumonia Infection from *Klebsiella pneumoniae* with a necrotizing pneumonia.

Legionella pneumonia Infection by *Legionella pneumophila.*

Lipoid pneumonia Diffuse pneumonia or fibrotic granuloma from inhalation of oil into the lung.

Lungs lobar pneumonia Pneumonia involving one or more lobes of the lung, usually caused by *Streptococcus pneumoniae.*

Mycoplasmal pneumonia Pneumonia caused by *Mycoplasma pneumoniae.*

Nonbacterial pneumonia Pneumonia involving interstitium of the lungs.

Nosocomial pneumonia Pneumonia developing after hospitalization, the infection was not incubating at the time of admission.

Pneumococcal pneumonia The most common bacterial pneumonia caused by *Streptococcus pneumoniae* characterized by chills, fever, chest pain, cough and rusty sputum.

Pneumocystic carinii pneumonia Pulmonary infection from *Pneumocystis carinii* in immunocompromised patients especially those with AIDS.

Radiation pneumonia An inflammatory condition of the lung caused by thoracic irradiation.

Rickettsial pneumonia Infection from *Coxiella burnetii* developing in persons with history of contact with cattle or sheep.

Staphylococcal pneumonia Pneumonia in infants and children by *Staphylococcus aureus.*

Streptococcal pneumonia Pneumonia occurring as a complication of viral infections (*Streptococcus pyogenes*) or following secondary invasion during lowered resistance (*Streptococcus viridans*).

Tuberculous pneumonia Pneumonia caused by *M. tuberculosis* with rapid and widespread inflammatory exudate.

Varicella pneumonia Involvement of lungs during the course of chickenpox that may leave behind multiple calcification.

Viral pneumonia Occurrence of pneumonia as a primary viral infection in infants (respiratory syncytial virus and para influenza virus) and in elderly, debilitated individuals (adenovirus and influenza virus).

Pnemonitis Lung inflammation causing difficulty in breathing and is often accompanied by a cough.

Pneumopericardium (*nu'mo-per-i-kar'de-um*) Presence of air or gas in the pericardial cavity.

Pneumoperitoneum (*nu'mo-per-i-to-ne'um*) Air or gas in the peritoneal cavity, as in laparoscopic procedure.

Pneumoradiography (*nu'mo-ra-de-og'ra-fe*) Radiography of a part following injection of air or oxygen.

Pneumothorax (*nu-mo-tho'raks*) Presence of air in the pleural space where air (gas) can enter either from the lung parenchyma and airways; (internal) or from outside (external).

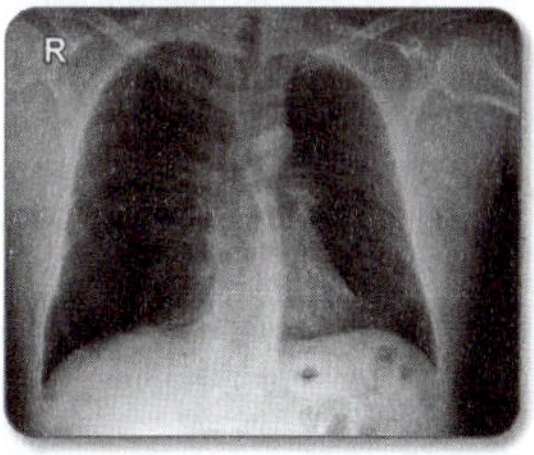

Pneumothorax

Artificial pneumothorax Deliberate introduction of air into the pleural space.

Catamenial pneumothorax Pneumothorax during menstruation.

Closed pneumothorax Pneumothorax with the opening sealed by deposition of fibrin and the pleural pressure is negative.

Noisy pneumothorax A shallow left sided pneumothorax producing a crunching or clicking sounds near the apex of the cardia.

Open pneumothorax Pneumothorax with communication between the lung and the pleural space that remains patent, allowing free movement of air in and out of pleural cavity during respiration.

Shallow pneumothorax Pneumothorax with at least 300–500 mL of air in the pleural cavity.

Simple pneumothorax Closed pneumothorax.

Spontaneous pneumothorax Spontaneous occurrence of pneumothorax developing secondary to an underlying pulmonary lesion or from congenital weakness of the pleura.

Tension pneumothorax A flap of opening acting as a check valve allowing entry of air into pleural cavity during inspiration. There is progressive increase in size of pneumothorax with positive intrapleural pressure and shift of mediastinum to the opposite side.

Traumatic pneumothorax Pneumothorax that develops following injuries over the chest or rib fractures.

Valvular pneumothorax Tension pneumothorax.

Pock (*pok*) A pustule of eruptive fever, or small pox.

Pocket (*pok'et*) A sac-like cavity.

Pocket dosimeter *radiol* A small ionizing chamber worn by persons exposed to ionizing radiation.

Pod- Combining word for foot.

Podocyte (*pod'o-sit*) Epithelial cell with many foot plates, that form the inner layer of Bowman's capsule of renal glomerulus which have spaces for the passage of glomerular filtrate.

Podagra (*po-dag'ra*) Joint pain in the big toe especially in gout.

Podalic (*po-dal'ik*) Pertaining to the feet; of or in the direction of feet especially the use of feet inversion during labor.

Poikiloblast (*poy'ki-lo-blast"*) An abnormally shaped erythroblast; a large crystal of a metamorphic rock with a texture marked by the inclusion of small idioblasts.

Poikilocyte An irregularly shaped red blood cell.

Poikilocytosis (*poy'kil-o-si-to'sis*) A pear-shaped erythrocyte, seen in myelofibrosis.

Poikiloderma (*poy'ki-lo-derma*) A mottled appearance of the skin due to hyperpigmentation followed by atrophy.

Poikilothermia The inability to regulate core body temperature.

Point (*poynt*) A spot or small area; the sharp end of any object; to approach the surface as in an abscess about to rupture; a position of space, time or degree.

McBurney's point The point on the lower right quadrant of the abdomen at which tenderness is maximal in cases of acute appendicitis.

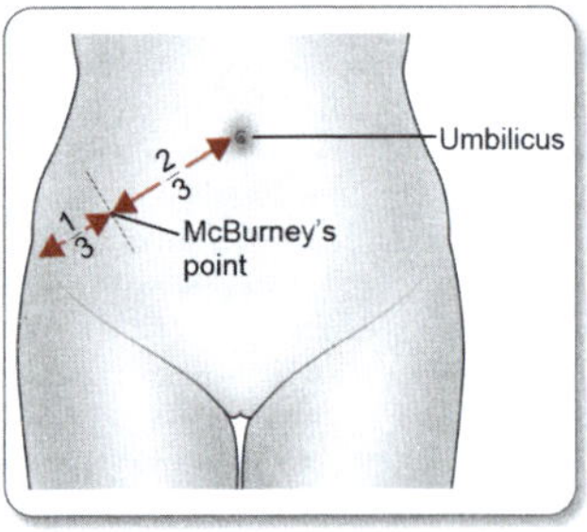

McBurney's point

Point mutation A change in one of the nucleotides on the double-stranded DNA molecule.

Point prevalence Prevalence of a disease at a specific point in time.

Pointillage (*pwan'te-yazh*) Massage with finger tips.

Poiseuille's law (*pwa-zu'yez*) A formula stating rate of flow of liquid through small vessels is directly proportional to pressure and fourth power of radius of the tube and inversely proportional to the viscosity of the fluid and length of the tube, described by Jean Poiseuille, French physiologist.

Poison (*poi'zn*) A chemical substance that usually kills, injures or impairs an organism.

Polar body One of the two small bodies containing chromosomes discarded from ovum during meiotic division.

Pole (*pol*) One of two points at the extremities of the axis of any organ or body.

Polioencephalitis (*po'le-o-en-sef'ah-litis*) All inflammation of the gray matter of the brain.

Polioencephalomyelitis (*pol'e-o-en-sef'al-o-mi'el-i'tis*) Inflammation of the gray matter of the brain and spinal cord.

Poliomyelitis (infantile paralysis, polio) (*pol'e-o-mi'el-i-tis*) An acute disease caused by one of three polioviruses. The virus infects the gray matter of the spinal cord, brain stem and cortex and has a particular propensity to damage anterior horn cells. After an incubation period of 1–2 weeks, it presents as a febrile illness or as an aseptic meningitis or encephalitis from which many patients recover. In some weakness may develop in one muscle group and can lead to widespread paresis, and cause residual disability. In early stages bed rest is necessary as exercise may worsen the paralysis or precipitate it. Residual disability needs physiotherapy and orthopedic measures. The condition is prevented by immunization with oral polio vaccine.

Poliosis (*pol'e-o'sis*) Gray or whiteness of hair.

Poliovirus (*po'le-o-vi'rus*) The causative agent of poliomyelitis. It consists of three serotypes named type I, II and III and belong to the enterovirus group. Infection occurs through the nasopharynx. Widespread use of oral vaccines through Pulse Polio Program is expected to eliminate the infection.

Pollex (*pol'eks*) The thumb.

Pollex valgus Deviation of the thumb toward the ulnar side.

Pollex varus Deviation of the thumb toward the radial side.

Pollinosis (*pol'in-o'sis*) A hypersensitivity reaction to pollen; hay fever.

Polyarteritis nodosa (periarteritis nodosa) (*pol'e-ar'ter-i-tis*) A systemic necrotizing arteritis that affects muscular arteries throughout the body especially in the kidneys, heart, gastrointestinal tract and peripheral nervous system. The clinical features include fever, myalgia, weight loss, rashes, gangrene, mononeuritis multiplex, hematuria, loin pain, acute and chronic renal failure, abdominal pain and hypertension.

Polyarthritis (*pol-e-ar-thri'tis*) Inflammation of several joints.

Polyadenitis (*pol'e-ad'e-ni'tis*) Inflammation of several lymph nodes, especially cervical lymph nodes.

Polyadenomatosis (*pol'e-ad'e-no-ma-to'sis*) Adenoma of several glands particularly endocrine glands.

Polyblennia (*pol'e-ble'ne-a*) Secretion of an abnormal amount of mucus.

Polychromasia (Polychromatophilia) (*pol'e-kro-ma'se-a*) Staining readily with acid, basic and neutral dyes.

Polycoria (*pol'e-ko're-a*) Presence of two or more pupils in one iris.

Polycystic disease of the kidneys (*pol'e-sis'tik*) Having many cysts.

Polycystic kidney Cystic disease of the kidney that may be juvenile with a recessive inheritance or adult with dominant inheritance. It may present with abdominal lump, hematuria, hypertension, and chronic renal failure.

Polycystic liver Gradual cystic dilation of intralobular bile ducts (Meyenburg complexes) that fail to involute in embryonic development of the liver.

Polycystic ovary Multiple cysts present in ovary.

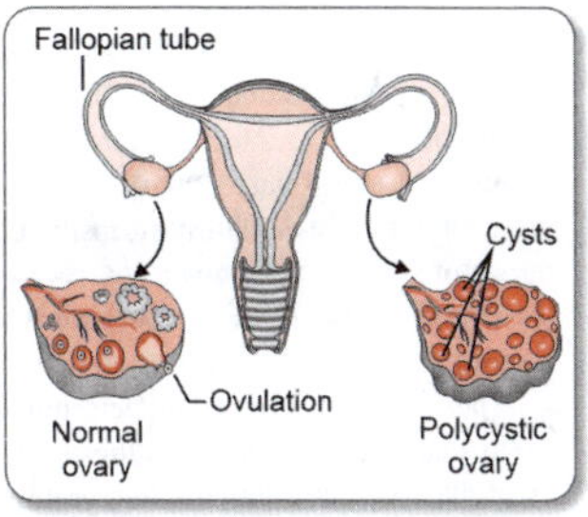

Polycystic ovary

Polycystic ovary disease (PCOD) Endocrinopathy characterized by oligomenorrhea, androgen excess and a high prevalence of glucose intolerance and type 2 diabetes mellitus.

Polycystic ovary syndrome Endocrinopathy characterized by oligomenorrhea, androgen excess and a high prevalence of glucose intolerance and type 2 diabetes mellitus.

Polycythemia (*pol'e-si-the'me-a*) An increase in the number of red blood cells.

Polycythemia rubra vera A malignant myeloproliferative disorder with predominant expansion of mature erythroid cell population. It presents with splenomegaly, pruritus, hyperviscosity and gastrointestinal bleeding.

Secondary polycythemia Increased red cell mass due to a raised level of erythropoietin.

Polydactylism (*pol'e-dak'ti-lizm*) Polydactyly.

Polydipsia (*pol'e-dap'se-a*) Frequent drinking from excessive thirst.

Polygene (*pol'e-jen*) One of a group of genes acting together to bring about quantitative changes of a particular character.

Polymastia (pleomastia) (*pol'e-mas'te-a*) Presence of supernumerary breasts.

Polymer (*pol'i-mer*) A substance formed by a combination of simple molecules (monomers).

Polymerase (*pol-im'er-as*) An enzyme that catalyzes polymerization.

Polymorph (polymorphonuclear leukocyte) (*pol'i-morf*) A polymorphonuclear leukocyte.

Polymorphism (*pol"e-mor'fiz-em*) A part of the DNA sequence that can occur in two forms; occurrence in more than one form.

Polymyalgia rheumatic A condition of undetermined etiology, seen in elderly characterized by sudden pain and severe stiffness of proximal muscles and periarticular tissues.

Polymyositis (*pol'e-mi'o-si'tis*) An inflammatory muscle disease presenting with progressive painful, proximal upper and lower limb weakness, dysphagia and respiratory muscle weakness. There is arthralgia, malaise and fever.

Polymyxin B (*pol'e-miks'in*) Polypeptide antibiotic from *Bacillus aerosporus*, active against many gram-negative bacteria.

Polyneuritis (*pol'e-nu'ri'tis*) Inflammation of several peripheral nerves simultaneously.

Polyneuropathy (*pol'i-nu-rop'a-the*) Neuropathy of several peripheral nerves simultaneously.

Acute inflammatory polyneuropathy Guillain-Barre syndrome, an acute demyelinating predominantly motor polyradiculoneuropathy.

Polynucleotide (*pole-nu'kle-o-tid*) A linear polymer whose molecule is composed of many nucleotide units, constituting a section of a nucleic acid molecule.

Polyopia (*pol"e-o'pe-a*) The visual perception of multiple images even after removal of an object from the visual field.

Polyorchidism (*pol'e-or'ki-dism*) Presence of one or more supernumerary testes.

Polyp (Polypus) A growth with a pedicle protruding from a mucous membrane commonly found in structures which are vascular such as nose, uterus, colon and rectum. They bleed easily and may become malignant.

Polypectomy (*pol'i-pek'to-me*) Excision of a polyp.

Polypeptide (*pol'e-pep'tid*) A peptide formed by the union of a large number of amino acids.

Polyphagia (*pol'e-fa-jea*) Excessive eating.

Polypharmacy (*pol'e-far-ma'se*) Treatment with multiple drugs.

Polyploid (*pol'e-ploi'de*) The heritable condition of possessing more than two complete sets of chromosomes.

Polypoid (*pol'e-poid*) Resembling a polyp.

Polyposis (*pol'e-po'sis*) Multiple polyps.

Familial adenomatous polyposis An autosomal dominant disorder from germ line cell mutation of the APC gene on chromosome S, and develop in the colon, stomach and duodenum.

Juvenile polyposis Mucus filled hamartomatous polyps found in the colon and rectum.

Polypus (*pol'e-pus*) Pl. **polypi**. A polyp.

Polyradiculitis (polyradiculopatny) (*pol'e-ra-dicu-li'tis*) Inflammation of the roots of the nerves.

Polyriosome (polysome) A group of ribosomes bound to an mRNA molecule like beads on a thread.

Polysaccharide (*pol'e-sak'a-rid*) A carbohydrate which on hydrolysis yields many molecules of monosaccharides.

Polyserositis (*pol'e-ser'o-sit'is*) Fibrotic thickening of serosa of multiple sacs with effusion.

Polysome (*pol'e-som*) Aggregate of ribosome around a messenger RNA molecule.

Polyspermia (*pol'e-sper'me-a*) An abnormally profuse secretion of seminal fluid; polyspermy.

Polyspermy (Polyspermia) (*pol'e-sper'me*) Fertilization of an ovum by many spermatozoa.

Polythelia (*pol'e-thel'e-a*) Presence of supernumerary nipples on the breast or elsewhere.

Polyuria (*pol'e-ur'e-a*) Passage of excess amount of urine noted in excess fluid intake, hyperglycemia and diabetes insipidus.

Pompholyx (*pom'fo-liks*) Intense pruritus of the palmoplantar surfaces, with crops of vesicles and bullae, and it can be provoked by heat, stress and nickel ingestion.

Pons (*ponz*) The portion of the brain stem that forms a 'bridge' between the medulla and the midbrain, anterior to the cerebellum. It contains fiber tracts connecting the medulla and cerebellum with the upper portions of the brain. The abducens, facial and cochlear division of the eight nerves take their origin in pons; any bridge-like structure connecting parts of the same structure or organ.

Pons varolii (pons) A component of the brainstem that forms a bridge between the midbrain and medulla oblongta.

Popliteal (*pop'lit'e-al*) Relating to the area behind the knee.

Popliteal cyst Cyst communicating with knee, but fluid is prevented from returning to the joint by valve-like mechanism; Baker's cyst.

Porcelain The puffy, pale facies in adults with myxoedema due to accumulation of glycosaminoglycans.

Pore (*por*) A small opening of the secretory duct of the sweat gland; a minute opening on an epithelial surface.

Alveolar pores Opening between adjacent pulmonary alveoli.

Gustatory pores External opening of taste buds.

Nuclear pore A small octagonal opening where the inner and outer membranes of the nuclear envelopes are continuous.

Pores of Kohn Alveolar pores, named after Hans Kohn, German pathologist.

Slit pores Small slit-like spaces between the interdigitating pedicles of podocytes of the renal glomerulus.

Porencephaly (*por'en-sefa-le*) Presence of abnormal cavity (*ies*) in the brain filled with CSF.

Porphin (*por'fin*) A tetrapyrrole nucleus forming the basis of porphyrins.

Porphobilinogen (*por'fo-bi'lin-o-jin*) An intermediate product in heme synthesis. It is found in the urine in large quantities in cases of acute porphyria.

Porphyria (*por-fir'e-as*) A heterogeneous group of disorders due to inherited or acquired abnormalities of enzymes involved in the biosynthesis of heme resulting in excess production, accumulation and excretion of intermediate compounds, the porphyrins, and/or its precursors—delta aminolevulinic acid and porphobilinogen.

Acute intermittent porphyrias Hereditary hepatic porphyria with an increased production of 8-aminolevulinic acid. It is associated with abdominal colic, intermittent hypertension, psychosis and neuropathy. There is increased urinary excretion of 8- aminolevulinic acid and porphobilinogen.

Congenital erythropoietic porphyrias Increased formation of porphyrin by erythroid cells in the bone marrow leading to severe porphyrinuria. There is an increased cutaneous photosensitivity.

Porphyrias cutanea tarda A condition noted in middle aged, often in males with bullous skin eruptions on exposure to sunlight, which heal by scarring. It develops in those with liver dysfunction in whom alcohol acts as a precipitating agent.

Hepatic porphyrias Acute intermittent porphyria.

Symptomatic porphyrias Cutaneous hepatic porphyria.

Variegate porphyrias Increased production of protoporphyrin exhibiting clinical features of acute porphyria with those of cutaneous porphyria.

Porphyrin (*por'fi-rins*) Pigments consisting of four pyrroles joined in a ring of porphyrin structure and are categorized as uro-, copro- or protoporphyrin depending on their structure. Both uro and coproporphyrins can be eliminated in the urine. An increased production of protoporphyrin is associated with its excretion in the urine.

Porphyrinuria (*por'fi-ri-nu're-a*) An increased elimination of uro and coproporphyrins; and an increased elimination of protoporphyrin in the urine turn reddish-brown on standing.

Porro's operation (*por'oz*) Cesarean section followed by removal of uterus, fallopian tubes and ovaries, named after Edoardo Porro, Italian obstetrician.

Porta (*por'ta*) Pl. **portae**. Hilum; the point of entry of the blood vessels and nerves to an organ.

Porta hepatis A transverse fissure on the visceral surface of the liver where portal vein and hepatic artery enter as the hepatic duct leaves.

Porta lienis The hilus of the spleen.

Porta pulmonis Pulmonary hilus for entry and exit of bronchi, vessels and nerves.

Porta renis The hilus of the kidney.

Portacaval (*por'ta-ka'val*) A specific type of circulatory anastomosis that occurs between the veins of the portal circulation and the vena cava.

Portacaval shunt A surgical procedure that diverts blood away from the portal venous system into the inferior vena cava, reducing portal hypertension.

Portal (*por'tal*) Relating to any porta; the point of entry into the body of a pathogenic microorganism; the point of exit of the infectious agent from a carrier.

Portal cirrhosis Diffuse process of fibrosis that converts the liver into structurally abnormal nodules.

Portal pyemia Suppurative infection of portal veins especially within the liver.

Portal hypertension Obstruction to the portal vein or its radicals leading to development of back pressure and rise in the pressure and its radicals. There is splenomegaly and development of collaterals between the radicals of the portal vein and systemic veins as varices.

Port-wine nevus Nevus flammeus; a congenital neurovascular malformation that appears as deep redpurple macular lesions.

Port wine urine Transparent red urine found in myoglobinuria.

Positron emission tomography (PET) Scanning, a noninvasive imaging modality that uses radionuclides to detect biochemical and pathological abnormalities in living tissues, such as cerebral cortex.

Posology (*po-sol'o-je*) The science of dosage of remedies.

Postcentral (*post-sen'tral*) Behind a center; behind the fissure of Rolando.

Postcibal (*post-si'bal*) After food.

Postcoital contraception A medication or device that is used to prevent pregnancy after sexual intercourse.

Postcoital test Examination of cervical mucus for motile sperms.

Posterior (*pos-te're-ur*) Toward the back or dorsal; situated behind; toward the caudal end.

Postero- (*pos'ter-o*) Combining word for posterior; situated behind; toward the back.

Postganglionic (*post'gan-gle-on'ik*) Distal to the ganglia.

Posthitis (*pos-thi'tis*) Inflammation of the prepuce.

Posthumous birth (*pos-thu-mus*) Occurring after death; born after the death of the father; cesarean delivery after death of the mother.

Postmortem Medical examination of the body after death to know about the cause of death; autopsy.

Postoperative Following operation.

Postoperative care Care undertaken after a surgical operation.

Postpartum (*post-par'tum*) After childbirth.

Postprandial (*post-pran'de-al*) Postcibal; after taking food.

Postprandial syndrome Symptoms suggestive of, but not actually due to hypoglycemia occurring 1–2 hours after the food.

Postural muscles (antigravity muscles) (*pos'tu-ral*) Relating to the posture.

Postural drainage Drainage of secretions from the bronchi or abscess cavity in the lung by positioning the patient in such a way so that gravity will allow drainage from the involved segment or lobe.

Postsphygmic (*post-sfig'mik*) After a pulse wave.

Poststenotic (*post'ste-not'ik*) Distal to a stenosed or a constricted area, especially of an artery.

Postsynaptic (*post'si-nap'tik*) Distal to a synapse.

Post-traumatic Following or related to trauma.

Potassium (*pot'tas'e-um*) An alkaline metallic element, atomic no. 19; symbol K (kalium).

Pott's disease Caries spine, named after Sir Percivall Pott, British surgeon.

Pouch (*powch*) A pocket; cul-de-sac.

Poultice (fomentation) (*pol'tis*) A soft, moist, hot mass of mustard, linseed or soap and oil between layers of gauze or linen applied to the skin to create moist local heat or counter irritation.

Poupart's ligament (*pu-parz*) Inguinal ligament, named after Francis Poupart, French anatomist.

Pox (*poks*) Any infectious disease with pustular skin eruption.

Poxvirus Large, brick-shaped viruses with double-stranded DNA, causing small pox, vaccinia and molluscum contagiosum.

PPLO Pleuro pneumonia like organisms, e.g., Mycoplasma.

Practolol Beta-adrenergic blocking agent used in resistant ventricular arrhythmias.

Prader-Willi syndrome A genetic mutation disorder characterized by obesity, hypogonadism and mental retardation due to lack of paternal contribution to the chromosome 15 region, named after Andrea Prader and Heinrich Willi, Swiss Pediatricians.

Pralidoxime A cholinesterase reactivator used in the treatment of organophosphorous insecticide poisoning.

Prazosin Alpha-blocking vasodilator used as an antihypertensive agent.

Pre- Prefix indicating before, in front of.

Preagonal (*pre-ag'o-nal*) Immediately preceding death.

Precocious puberty Appearance of secondary sexual characteristics before age of 8 years in the girls and age of 9 years in boys.

Precancerous (*pre-kan'ser-us*) Pertaining to any lesion that is considered a precancer.

Precipitin (*pre-sip'i-tin*) An antibody that interacts with an antigen forming a precipitate that sediments out of solution.

Precipitinogen (*pre-sip'i-tin'o-jen*) An antigen that stimulates the production of specific precipitin following injection into the animal body.

Precision A measurement of the reproducibility of a test or assay.

Precocity (*pre-kos'i-te*) Unusually, early or rapid development of physical or mental traits.

Precordium (*pre-kor'de-um*) The region of the thorax immediately in front of or over the heart.

Precuneus (*pre-ku'ne-us*) A division of the medial surface of a cerebral hemisphere between the cuneus and paracentral lobule.

Predisposition (*pre'dis-pozi'shun*) A tendency or susceptibility to a disease.

Prednisolone (*pred-nis'o-lon*) Synthetic glucocorticoid with minimum mineral activity.

Prednisolone (*pred-nis'o-lon*) Synthetic glucocorticoid with minimum mineral activity.

Prednisone (*pred'ni-son*) Synthetic glucocorticoid that is converted to prednisolone in the body.

Preeclampsia (pregnancy- induced hypertension) (*pre'e-klamp'se-a*) A triad of edema, proteinuria and hypertension during pregnancy and it may be progressive, presenting increased risk to the fetus and mother.

Prefrontal (*pre-fron'tal*) Situated in the anterior part of the frontal lobe or region.

Prefrontal leukotomy Extensive division of white matter of frontal lobes to reduce tension in schizophrenia.

Preganglionic (*pre'gang-le-on'ik*) Situated proximal to or preceding a ganglion.

Pregnancy (*preg'nan-se*) Gestation; the state of a woman after conception until the birth of the baby.

Abdominal pregnancy Implantation and development of the ovum in the peritoneal cavity.

Ampullary pregnancy Tubal pregnancy in the ampulla of the fallopian tube.

Bigeminal pregnancy Pregnancy with twins in utero.

Cervical pregnancy Implantation of the ovum in cervical canal.

Cornual pregnancy Development of impregnated ovum in one of the cornua of the uterus.

Ectopic pregnancy Development of an impregnated ovum outside the cavity of the uterus.

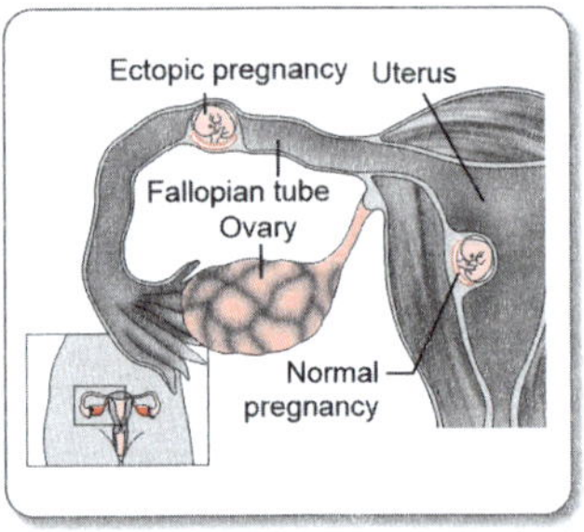

Ectopic pregnancy

False pregnancy Pseudocyesis.

Heterotopic pregnancy Combined intrauterine and extrauterine pregnancies high.

Risk pregnancy Pregnancy with coexisting diseases causing a greater risk to the health of the mother, embryo or both.

Hydatid pregnancy Pregnancy leading to the development of hydatidiform mole.

Intraligamentary pregnancy Ectopic pregnancy within the broad ligament.

Intramural pregnancy Development of the fertilized ovum in the uterine portion of the fallopian tube.

Membranous pregnancy Embryo lying in direct contact with the uterine wall.

Molar pregnancy Ovum developing into a mole instead of an embryo.

Multiple pregnancy Presence of two or more fetuses simultaneously in the uterus.

Ovarian pregnancy Development of a fertilized ovum in an ovarian follicle.

Postdate pregnancy Pregnancy that extends beyond 42 weeks of gestation.

Tubal pregnancy Development of embryo in the fallopian tube.

Tuboabdominal pregnancy Development of an ectopic pregnancy partly in the tube and partly in the abdominal cavity.

Tubo-ovarian pregnancy Development of the fertilized ovum at the fimbriated end of the fallopian tube and involving ovary.

Uteroabdominal pregnancy Twin pregnancy with one embryo developing in the uterus and other in the abdominal cavity.

Pregnancy-induced hypertension (PIH) Gestational hypertension high blood pressure that occurs in the latter half of pregnancy but does not affect kidneys or release protein in urine.

Pregnanediol (*preg'nan-di'ol*) Product of progesterone excreted in urine, the amount is markedly increased in late pregnancy.

Pregnenolone (*preg-nen'o-lon*) A steroid that serves as an intermediate in the biosynthesis of numerous hormones including progesterone.

Premature beat Happens when the heart beats earlier than it should. This briefly interrupts the heart's rhythm.

Premature birth Born before 37th week of pregnancy, but mature enough to survive. Premature babies may have serious health problems.

Premature ejaculation Occurs in men when semen ejaculates sooner than wanted during sex.

Premedication (*pre'med-i-ka'shun*) Drugs administered in preparation for anesthesia.

Premenstrual (*pre-men'stru-al*) Relating to the period before menstruation.

Premenstrual dysphoric disorder Occurrence of depressed mood, anxiety, marked affective lability and decreased interest in activities before menstruation.

Premenstrual tension syndrome Premenstrual dysphoric disorder.

Premenstruum (*pre-men'stroo-um*) The period preceding menstruation.

Premolar (*pre-mo'ler*) Anterior to a molar tooth; a bicuspid tooth.

Premyelocyte (*pre-mi'el-o-sit*) Promyelocyte, precursor of myelocyte.

Prenatal (*pre-na'tl*) Antenatal; preceding birth.

Prenatal care Care of the woman during pregnancy.

Prenatal surgery Intrauterine surgical procedures.

Prenatal diagnosis (antenatal diagnosis) Diagnosis of a disease or malformation while the fetus in utero.

Preoperative Before undertaking surgery.

Preoperative care Care of the patient before operative procedure.

Prepubertal (*pre-pu'ber-tal*) Before puberty.

Prepuce (foreskin) (*pre'pus*) Foreskin; the free fold of skin that covers the glans penis.

Preputial glands (*pre-pu'shal*) Relating to prepuce.

Preputial gland Modified sebaceous gland on the inner surface of prepuce secreting smegma.

Preputial sinus Space between foreskin and glans.

Prepyramidal fissure Situated in the middle lobe of cerebellum, in front of the pyramid.

Presbyopia (*prez-be-o'pe-a*) Age-related loss of range of visual accommodation.

Prescription (*pre-skrip'shun*) A written direction for the preparation and administration of any medication; a medicinal preparation compounded according to directions. It consists of subscription (to take, with symbol R_x), transcription (ingredients), subscription (direction regarding preparation) and signature (direction on the manner of taking and signature of the prescribing physician).

Presenility (*pre'se-nill-ti*) Premature old age.

Presentation (*pre-zen-ta'shun*) Lie, axis of the fetus; the position of the fetus presenting itself to the examining finger of obstetrician; the relationship of the long axis of the fetus to that of the mother.

Antigen presentation Presentation of antigen at the surface of macrophages to lymphocytes for induction of an immune response.

Breech presentation Presentation of the fetal buttocks in labor. It may be complete (thighs of the fetus flexed on the abdomen and legs flexed upon the thighs), frank (legs extended against the trunk and feet lying against the face) or incomplete (prolapse of the feet or knees into maternal vagina).

Brow presentation Presentation of fetal brow or face in labor.

Cephalic presentation Presentation of any part of the fetal head during labor.

Compound presentation Prolapse, of an extremity of the fetus alongside the head in cephalic presentation or alongside the breech at the commencement of the labor.

Face presentation Presentation of the fetal face during labor.

Footling presentation Presentation of the fetal feet during labor.

Funic presentation Presentation of umbilical cord in labor.

Longitudinal presentation Presentation in which the long axis of the fetus is parallel to the long axis of the mother.

Oblique presentation Presentation in which the long axis of the fetus is oblique to that of the mother.

Pelvic presentation Breech presentation.

Placental presentation Placenta previa.

Shoulder presentation Presentation of the fetal shoulder during labor.

Vertex presentation Presentation of the upper and back portion of fetal head in labor.

Pressor (*pres'or*) Exciting to vasomotor activity; producing increased blood pressure.

Pressure point A location used for exertion of pressure to control bleeding.

Pressure sore A bed sore; a decubital ulcer appearing on dependent sites usually on lumbosacral region, most common in bedridden elderly persons.

Presymptomatic (*pre'sim-po-mat'ik*) The state of health before the manifestations of a disease.

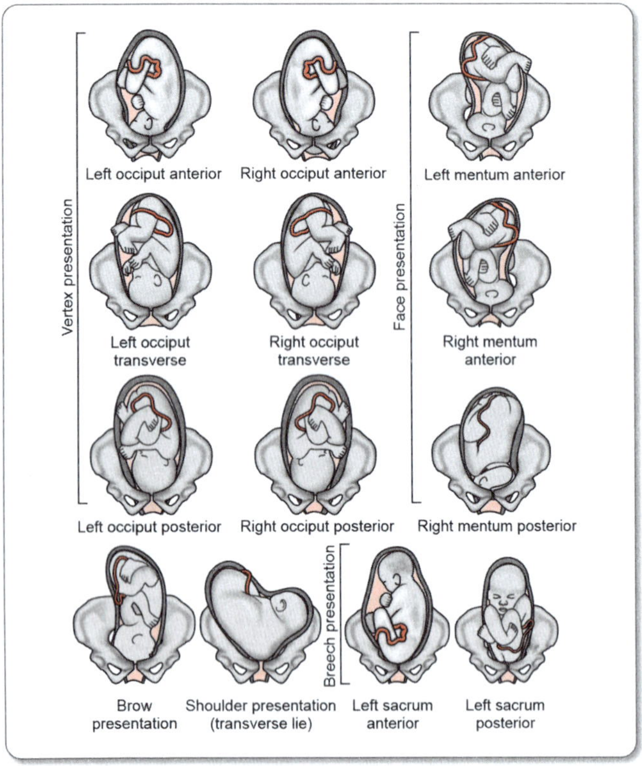

Presentation of fetus

Presystole (*pre-sis'to-le*) Late diastole; relating to the period immediately before systole.

Prevalence rate The total number of cases of a disease existing in a population divided by the total population.

Preventive dentistry Branch of dentistry concerned with avoiding tooth decay ad gum diseases.

Preventive medicine Organized activities of the community to prevent occurrence as well as progression of disease and disability and timely application of all means to promote health of individuals and of the community as a whole.

Priapism (*pri'a-pizm*) Prolonged and unusually painful penile erection occurring in the absence of sexual excitement or desire.

Priapitis (*pri-a-pi'tis*) Inflammation of the penis.

Prickle cells Type of epidermal cell also known as spinons cells. These produce keratin and appear prickly.

Prickly heat (heat rash) Miliaria; papular itching eruption of the skin due to blockage of sweat ducts.

Prilocaine (*pril'o-kan*) A local anesthetic used in dental procedures.

Primaquine (*prim'a-kwin*) 8 Aminoquinoline, antimalarial agent, active against exoerythrocytic parasites, used in eradication of parasites.

Primary care Least specialized level of medical care rendered by a primary physician; an integral part of the whole health system that ensures greater community participation, and acts as the first point of contact for health and social needs.

Prime (*prim*) First in order of time, rank of importance; full health and strength; an initial treatment that is carried out before administering a large dose of the same or different medicine.

Primidone (*prim'i-don*) An antiepileptic agent.

Primigravida (*pri-mi-grav'i-da*) A woman who is pregnant for the first time.

Elderly primigravida A woman who is 35 years of age or above becoming pregnant for the first time.

Primipara (*pri-mip'ara*) A woman who has given birth for the first time to an infant or infants.

Primitive streak (*pri'mi-tiv*) Structures in the earliest stage of development.

Primordial (*pri-mor'de-al*) Relating to primordium; primitive.

Proantithrombin (*pro'an-ti-throm'bin*) A substance found in the blood which gets converted into antithrombin by heparin.

Proarrhythmia A situation likely to lead for development of an arrhythmia; increased occurrence of existing arrhythmias, a serious reaction to antiarrhythmic medications in some people.

Probability *stat* Proportion of positive results to be expected if trial were repeated any number of times.

Proband The affected individual from which a pedigree is constructed.

Probang (*pro'bang*) A flexible thin rod with a sponge attached to the end useful for application of medicine and to determine the site of stricture.

Probe (*prob*) A single stranded segment of DNA/RNA which is labeled with a radioactive substance or chemical and it will bind to its complementary single-stranded target sequence; a slender rod with a blunt bulbous tip; used for exploring an open body part.

Probenecid Uricosuric agent used in gout; concomitant use with benzyl penicillin, raises the blood levels of penicillin by delaying its excretion by the kidney.

Probucol Anticholesterolemic agent, increasing excretion of bile.

Procainamide A cardiac depressant used in arrhythmias especially originating in the ventricle.

Procaine hydrochloride (*pro'kan*) Short-acting local anesthetic.

Procaine penicillin G Long-acting procaine benzyl penicillin.

Procarbazine A chemotherapeutic agent used for the treatment by Hodgkin's lymphoma and brain cancers.

Procerus muscle A muscle arising from the skin over the nose. It is connected to the forehead. It draws the eyebrows down.

Process (*pros'es*) A prominence or projection as from a bone; a method of action; progress, as of a disease.

Prochlorperazine A phenothiazine drug used in the treatment of nausea and vomiting.

Procidentia (*pro'si-den'she-a*) A prolapse of any organ or part as in uterus.

Proct- (procto-) Combining word for anus, rectum.

Proctalgia (proctodynia) (*prok-tal'je-a*) Pain in the anus or in the rectum.

Proctalgia Brief attacks of severe pain in rectal region.

Proctectasia (*prok'tek-ta'se-a*) Dilatation of anus or rectum.

Proctectomy (*prok-tek'to-mi*) Surgical resection of the rectum.

Proctenclisis (*prok'ten-kli'sis*) Stricture of anus or rectum.

Proctitis (*prok-ti'tis*) Inflammation of the mucous membrane of the rectum.

Proctocele (rectocele) (*prok'to-sel*) Prolapse or herniation of the rectum.

Proctocolectomy (*prok'to-ko-lek'to-me*) Surgical resection of the rectum and part or all of the colon.

Proctocolitis (*prok'to-ko-li'tis*) Inflammation of the rectum and colon.

Proctocolpoplasty (*prok'to-kol'po-plas'te*) Surgical closure of a rectovaginal fistula.

Proctodeum (*prok'to-de'um*) Anal pit; an ectodermally lined depression at the terminal portion of embryonic hindgut from which anal and urogenital external orifices are developed.

Proctodynia (*prok'to-din'e-a*) Pain in the rectum or anus.

Proctology (*prok'tol'o-je*) A surgical specialty concerned with the diseases of colon, rectum and anus.

Proctoparalysis (*prok'to-par-al'i-sis*) Paralysis of the anal sphincter leading to incontinence of feces.

Proctorrhaphy (*prok-tor'a-fe*) Suturing of a rectum or anus.

Proctoscope (*prok'to-skop*) A speculum for inspection of the rectum.

Proctosigmoiditis (*prok'to-sig'moyd-i-tis*) Inflammation of rectum and sigmoid colon.

Proctotomy (*prok'tot'o-me*) An incision into the rectum, as for the division of a stricture.

Procyclidine Anticholinergic agent used in the treatment of Parkinsonism.

Prodromal (*pro-dro'mal*) Pertaining to the early stage of a disease.

Prodrome (*pro'dro-m*) An early or premonitory symptom of a disease; running ahead of a symptom or group of symptoms that appears shortly before an acute attack of illness.

Proenzyme (zymogen) (*pro-en'zim*) Inactive precursor of an enzyme, requiring some change to make it active; zymogen.

Proerythroblast (*pro'e-rith'ro-blast*) Earliest recognizable cell of red cell series.

Profundus (*pro-fun'dus*) Deep.

Progeria (*pro-je're-a*) A condition characterized by markedly premature ageing of childhood onset, in which the morbid conditions encountered in elderly are noted during puberty and death from old age occurs by 20.

Progesterone (*pro-jes'te-rn*) Steroid hormone of secretory phase of menstrual cycle.

Progestogen (*pro-jes'to-jen*) A hormonal substance that produces effects similar to those due to progesterone.

Proglottis (*pro-glot'tis*) Related to proglottid; pl. **proglottids**.

Prognathism (*prog'na-thizm*) The condition of being prognathic.

Prognosis (*prog-no'sis*) To forecast the outcome of the disease.

Proinsulin Precursor of insulin consisting of A and B chains linked by C-peptide.

Projection The act of throwing forward.; a prominence; the referring of sensation to the object producing it; localization of visual impressions; the act of extending; an unconscious defense mechanism.

Projective test *psy* A type of psychological test that assesses a person's thinking patterns, observational ability, feelings and attitudes.

Prolactin (lactogenic hormone, luteotrophic hormone, luteotropin) (*pro-lak'tin*) Anterior pituitary hormone concerned with maintenance of lactation.

Prolapse (*pro-laps*) Abnormal descent of a structure, usually within or into cavity due to laxity of its attachments.

Prolapse of cord Appearance of umbilical cord in vagina before birth of child.

Prolapsed intervertebral disk (PID) When the outer fibers of the intervertebral disc are injured and soft material nucleus kulposus enclosure ruptures.

Proline (*pro-len*) Amino acid derived from glutamic acid.

PROM Premature rupture of membranes, leading to leakage of amniotic fluid prior to the onset of labor.

Promazine (*pro'ma-zen*) Antipsychotic and antiemetic agent.

Promegakaryocyte (*pro-meg'a-kar'e-o-sit*) A precursor of a megakaryocyte.

Promethazine (*pro-meth'a-zen*) Antihistamine agent.

Prominence (*prom'i-nens*) A projection or protrusion.

Promontory (*prom'on-tor'e*) Bulge above the oval window in the middle ear, marking the basal turn of cochlea; upper anterior edge of first sacral segment.

Promyelocyte (Premyelocyte) (*pro-mi'e-lo-sit*) Early precursor of granulocytes.

Pronation (*pro-na'shun*) The act of assuming or of being placed in a prone position.

Pronator A muscle which turns a part into prone position.

Pronator syndrome Entrapment of median nerve at the elbow with pain in the wrist, paresthesia of the hand and tenderness of proximal thenar muscles.

Prone (*pron*) Lying face downward; denoting a hand with the palm or a foot with sole turned downward.

Pronephros (*pro-nef'ros*) The primordial kidney consisting of a series of tortuous tubules emptying into the cloaca by a primary nephric duct.

Pronucleus (*pro-nu'kle-us*) The nuclear material of the sperm or of the ovum after fertilization of the ovum; each carries a haploid number of chromosomes.

Propantheline (*pro-pan'the-len*) An anticholinergic agent.

Properdin (*pro-perd'in*) A globulin fraction of serum that participates in the alternate pathway to activate the terminal components of complement.

Prophase (*pro'faz*) The first phase of mitosis or meiosis that consists of increase in thickness of chromosomes, division of centriole and migration of the two daughter centrioles toward either pole of the cell.

Prophylactic (*pro-fi-lak'tik*) Preventing disease; an agent that helps in the prevention of infection or disease.

Prophylaxis (*pro-fi-lak'sis*) The prevention of the disease.

Propositus (proband) (*pro-poz'i-tus*) Proband; a premise.

Propoxyphene (*pro-pok'se-fen*) An analgesic agent.

Propranolol A beta-adrenergic blocking agent used in the treatment of angina pectoris, cardiac arrhythmia and hypertension.

Proprietary name The patented name of the drug under which a manufacturer markets the product.

Proprioceptor (*pro'pre-o-sep'tor*) One of a variety of sensory receptor that responds to stimuli originating within the body, as to pressure, position or stretch.

Proptometer (*prop-tom'e-ter*) An instrument for measuring the extent of exophthalmos.

Proptosis (*prop-to'sis*) A forward displacement of any organ, as in exophthalmos.

Propylthiouracil (*pro'pil-thi'o-u'rah-sil*) An inhibitor of thyroid biosynthesis.

Prorenin (*pro're-nin*) A protein that constitutes a precursor for renin, the hormone that activates the renin angiotensin system, which serves to raise blood pressure.

Prosencephalon (*pros'en-sef'a-lon*) The embryonic forebrain which undergoes division into diencephalon and telencephalon.

Prostaglandin (*pros'ta-glan'din*) (PG) Oxidative metabolic product of arachidonic acid by cyclooxygenase enzymes. The important examples are PGE_2, PGF_{2a}, PGD_2, PGI_2 (prostacyclin). Prostaglandins have a variety of biological effects and act as local intracellular or intercellular modulators of biochemical activity of the tissues in which they are formed.

Prostaglandin synthase (*pros'ta-glan'din sin'thas*) An enzyme involved in eicosanoid and glutathione metabolism, a member of MAPEG family. It generates prostaglandin E (PGE) from prostaglandin H2.

Prostatectomy (*pros'ta-tek'to-me*) Surgical removal of part or all of the prostate.

Prostate gland (*pros'tat*) A gland having a median lobe and two lateral lobes surrounding the neck of the bladder and urethra in the male. It is partly muscular and partly glandular. The secretion from the gland drains into the prostatic portion of the urethra. The secretion is thin opalescent fluid forming part of the semen.

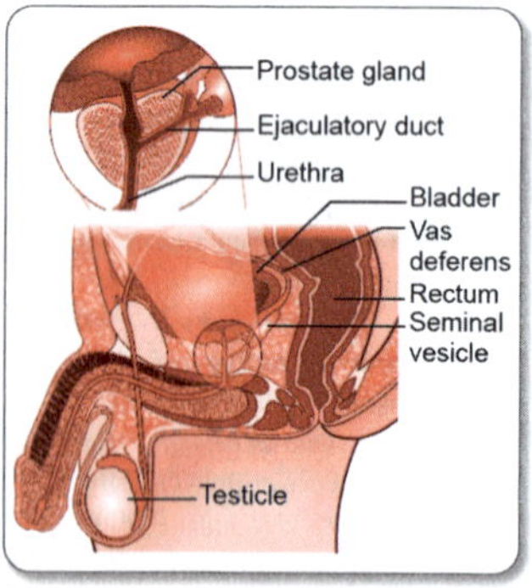

Male reproductive system showing prostate gland

Prostatitis (*pros'ta-ti'tis*) Inflammation of the prostate.

Prostatolithotomy (*pros'tat'o-li'thot'o-me*) Incision of prostate for removal of a calculus.

Prostatorrhea (*pros'ta-to-re'a*) An abnormal discharge from prostate gland.

Prosthesis (pl. Prostheses) (*pros'the-sis*) Device that replaces organ or part of the body such as a limb, tooth, eye or heart valve and performs some of its function; pl. **prostheses**.

Prosthetic (*pros'thet'ik*) Relating to a prosthesis.

Prosthetic anemia Mild form of hemolytic anemia in patients with artificial heart valves.

Protamine (*pro'ta-min*) A heparin antagonist.

Protamine zinc insulin A long-acting insulin.

Protanopia (*pro-tan-o'pe-a*) A form of color blindness where a person is not capable of distinguishing shades of red color.

Protease (*pro'te-as*) An enzyme acting as a catalyst in the breakdown of protein.

Protease inhibitor Anti-HIV drugs such as amprenavir, atazanavir, indinavir, lopinavir, nelfinavir, ritonavir, and saquinavir.

Protein (*pro'ten*) Any of a group of complex nitrogenous compounds containing carbon, hydrogen, oxygen, nitrogen and sulphur. They serve as enzymes, hormones, immunoglobulins and are involved in oxygen transport, electron transport and muscle contraction.

Protein-activated receptor A thrombin receptor on platelets; PAR-1.

Protein C A potent anticoagulant which inactivates coagulation factors V and VIII.

Protein energy malnutrition (PEM) A variety of interrelated clinical syndromes that occur as a result of lack of protein and calories in proper proportions. Occurs most frequently in infants and young children and presents with loss of subcutaneous fat and muscle wasting (marasmus) or with edema, hepatomegaly, skin and hair changes (kwashiorkor).

Protein kinase (*pro'ten ki'nas*) An enzyme that transfers a phosphoryl group (-PO32-) from ATP to the side chain of a serine, threonine, or tyrosine residue in a protein.

Protein losing enteropathy A condition exhibiting an increased transmucosal efflux of plasma proteins from the intestinal lumen due to increased permeability.

Protein sparing Addition of carbohydrates and fats to a low-protein diet to minimize protein catabolism.

Protein tyrosine kinase (*pro'tenti'ro-sen ki'nas*) A group comprising the protein kinases that catalyze the phosphorylation of tyrosine residues in specific proteins.

Proteinuria (*pro'te-n-u're-a*) Excretion of protein in the urine.

Proteolysis (*pro'te-ol'i-sis*) Hydrolysis of protein.

Proteolytic (*pro'te-o'lit'ik*) Relating to or causing proteolysis.

Proteose (*pro'te-os*) A mixture of intermediate products of proteolysis between protein and peptone.

Proteus (*pro'te-us*) A genus of gram-negative motile bacilli found in fecal matter and decaying material. It includes *P. mirabilis* and *P. vulgaris*.

Proteus syndrome A somatic mosaicism characterized by patchy or segmental overgrowth and hyperplasia of skin, connective tissue, and other tissues along with susceptibility to the development of tumors.

Prothipendyl A neurotropic agent indicated in the treatment of restlessness and agitation in patients with psychiatric conditions.

Prothrombin A plasma protein precursor of thrombin. It is synthesized in the liver if there is adequate amount of vitamin.

K prothrombin time The time taken for clotting following addition of thromboplastin and calcium to decalcified plasma.

Protionamide An antitubercular thiomide-derivative used in the treatment of multi drug resistant (MOR) tuberculosis and leprosy.

Protodiastole (*pro'to-di-as'to-le*) Earliest phase of ventricular diastole immediately following second heart sound.

Proto-oncogene Normal genes involved in cellular proliferation.

Protopathic (*pro'to-path'ik*) Pertaining to the somatins of pain and temperature.

Protoplasm (*pro'to-plasm*) The living substance of a cell consisting of water, mineral and organic compounds.

Protoplast (*pro'to-plast*) The protoplasm of a cell without its containing membrane; the original.

Protoporphyrin (*pro'to-por'fi-rin*) A porphyrin that combines with iron and protein to produce hemoglobin, myoglobin and catalase.

Protozoa Simplest organisms of animal kingdom consisting of unicellular organisms. They possess a flexible membrane and ability to move. Common examples are Plasmodium, Entamoeba, Giardia, and Leishmania.

Protozoan (*pro'ta-zo'an*) A member of protozoa; relating to protozoa.

Protozoology A branch of zoology that is concerned with the study of protozoa.

Protriptyline (*pro-trip'ti-len*) A tricyclic antidepressant of the dibenzocycloheptadiene class.

Protrusion (*pro-troo'zhun*) The state of being thrust forward or projected; a forward position of the mandible.

Protuberance (*pro-tu'ber-ans*) A prominence, eminence or projection.

Provitamin (*pro-vi'ta-min*) An inactive substance that can be converted in the body to a corresponding active vitamin.

Proximal (*prok'sim-al*) Nearest to a center or median line.

Prurigo *pro-ri'go*) Any of the several constantly recurring, discrete pale, deep seated, intensely itchy papules on the extensor surface of the limbs, followed by crusting and lichenification. adj. **pruriginous**.

Pruritus (*proo-ritus*) Severe itching, adj. **pruritic**.

Pruritus ani Intense itching around the anus.

Pruritus vulvae Intense itching of female external genitalia.

Prussic acid A poison that occurs naturally in plant foods such as apricot or apricot kernels, bitter almonds and flaxseed.

Psammoma (*sam-o'ma*) A neoplasm containing psammoma bodies, that occurs in meninges, choroid plexus, pineal body and ovaries.

Psammoma bodies Round laminated calcified masses due to degenerated papillary clusters of cellular debris in benign prostatic hypertrophy.

Psellism (*sel'izm*) Defective pronunciation, stuttering or stammering.

Pseudoarthrosis (nearthrosis) (*soo'dar-thro'sis*) A new false joint arising at the site of ununited fracture.

Pseudobulbar palsy Multifocal infarction in the brain resulting in dysarthria, dysphonia, dysphagia, bilateral facial weakness and lack of emotional expression or exhibit inappropriate responses to environmental cues.

Pseudoagglutinaton Misleading appearance of clumping which occurs during an antigen antibody reaction in a lab as a result of incorrect temperature or acidity of the solution used.

Pseudoclaudication (*soo"do-klaw'di-ka'shun*) Patients with lumbar spondylosis exhibiting unilateral or bilateral pain, paresthesia and weakness in the lower limbs exaggerated by walking and relieved by rest.

Pseudocholinesterase (*soo"do-ko'lin-es'ter'as*) An enzyme found in the liver and plasma that hydrolyses succinylcholine and acetylcholine.

Pseudocoxalgia (*soo"do-kok-saljea*) The radiographic changes outside the femoral head.

Pseudocrisis (*soo"do-kri'sis*) A temporary fall in the body temperature to be followed by a rise.

Pseudocroup (*soo"do-kroop*), Laryngismus stridulus.

Pseudocryptorchidism A testicle drawn into the inguinal canal by cold temperature, fear or genital manipulation.

Pseudocyesis (phantom pregnancy) False pregnancy women with pseudocyesis have pregnancy symptoms, but test will confirm there is no pregnancy.

Pseudocyst (*soo"do-sist*) A dilated space that is not lined by epithelium or mesothelium, seen in acute pancreatitis.

Pseudogout (*soo"do-gowt*) An arthropathy in elderly females characterized by deposition of calcium pyrophosphate dihydrate crystals in large joints.

Pseudobermaphroditism A condition in which the individual has single chromosome (sex) and gonadal sex but may show combined features of both sexes in the external genitalia, causing doubt as to true sex.

Pseudohypertrophy (*soo"do-hi-per'tro-fe*) Increase in the size of an organ or structure due to hypertrophy or hyperplasia of the supporting structure and not of parenchyma.

Pseudohypoparathyroidism (*soo"do-hi'po-par'a-thiroi-dizm*) A situation of a congenital androgen resistance to parathormone with features of round face, short neck and short metacarpals and short metatarsals. There is hypocalcemia and hyperphosphatemia.

Pseudologia fantastica Pathological lying about matters big or small, regardless of the situation. It is a psychiatric disorder and is a symptom of personality disorder.

Pseudomembrane (*soo"do-mem'bran*) A thin, adherent, gray-white exudate in the oropharynx, whose removal cause, bleeding. It is composed of necrotic debris and neutrophils.

Pseudomonas (*soo"do-mo'nas*) A genus of small, motile gram-negative bacilli with polar flagella. They exist as saprophytes, but can be sometimes pathogenic such as *P. aeruginosa, P. pseudomallei.*

Pseudomutuality A relationship between two persons in which conflict of views or opinions is solved by simply ignoring it.

Pseudomyxoma A condition with poorly circumscribed gelatinous masses containing mucin secreting cells that may arise from the ovary.

Pseudoneuritis (*soo"do-nu-ri'tis*) Pseudopapilledema.

Pseudophakia An artificial or fake lens (intraocular lens) that is implanted in eye to replace the clouded lens removed during cataract surgery.

Pseudoplegia Paralysis of the limbs not associated with organic abnormalities. It may be a symptom of conversion disorder.

Pseudopodium (*soo"do-po'de-um*) A temporary protruding process of an amoeba or of a leucocyte.

Pseudopolyposis (*soo"do-pol'i-po'sis*) Markers of episodes of severe inflammation.

Pseudopseudohypoparathyroidism Persons exhibiting skeletal features of pseudohypoparathyroidism without metabolic abnormalities.

Pseudosyndactyly (*soo"do-sin-dak'ti-le*) A mitten hand deformity of hands and feet in dystrophic epidermolysis bullosa.

Pseudotumor cerebri Benign intracranial hypertension.

Psiolosis A chronic disorder that occurs in tropical and non-tropical forms and in both children and adults. It is characterized by foul-smelling diarrhea and emaciation.

Psittacosis (*sit'a-ko'sis*) An acute systemic infection due to *Chalantydia psittaci* transmitted by infected parrots, parakeets and fowls. ***C psittaci*** is gram negative intracellular bacteria and produces clinical manifestations varying from a flu-like illness to severe fatal pneumonia.

Psoas (psoas major) (*so'as*) One of the two muscles of the loins..

Psoas sign Loss of the sharp delineation of the psoas muscle border on a plain erect abdominal film, indicative of the presence of intra abdominal or retroperitoneal condition.

Psoriasis (*so-ri'a-sis*) A chronic disorder characterized by well defined, scaly, erythematous plaques on the extensor surfaces of the extremities like elbows and knees, trunk, back and scalp. It may be localized or generalized and is considered an autoimmune disease.

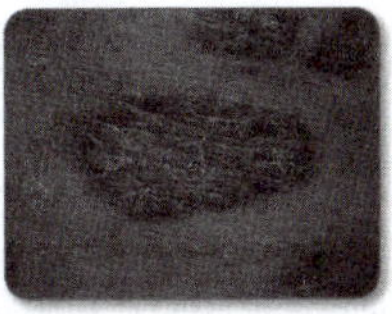

Psoriasis

Exfoliative psoriasis Sudden widespread involvement of psoriasis after abrupt discontinuation of treatment associated with itching and burning.

Guttate psoriasis Sudden crops of erythematous shiny papules on the trunk and proximal part of extremities in children and young adult.

Pustular psoriasis Tiny, superficial, sterile pustules appearing either on the surface of psoriatic lesions or on previously unaffected skin.

Psoriasis vulgaris Erythematous, scaly, well-defined plaques on extremities, trunk and scalp and nail involvement is common.

Psoriatic arthritis Seronegative polyarthritis affecting distal interphalangeal joints of the fingers and toes in Association with psoriatic lesions of the skin and nails.

Psyche (*si'ke*) The human soul, mind or spirit.

Psychedelic (*sy'ke-de'lik*) Relating to or denoting drugs that produce hallucinations.

Psychiatrist (*si-ki'a-trist*) A specialist in psychiatry.

Psychiatry (*si-ki'a-tre*) Medical specialty concerned with mental disorders or diseases, and problems of emotional character.

Psychic (*si'-kik*) Pertaining to the mind; a person sensitive to nonphysical forces.

Psychoanalysis (*si'ko-a-nal'i-sis*) A division of psychiatry concerned with exploration of patient's personality.

Psychodrama (*si'ko-dra"ma*) A structured form of therapy in which a person dramatizes a personal problem or conflict, usually in front of a group of other therapy participants.

Psychogenic (*si-ko-jen'ik*) Psychogenetic.

Psychokinesis (*si'ko-ki-ne'sis*) Impulsive behavior; influence of mind upon a physical matter.

Psychologist (*si-kol'o-jist*) A person, not a physician, who has been trained in the study of human behavior and psychology.

Psychology (*si-kol'o-je*) The study of behavior and of functions and processes of the mind, and its relation to the social and physical environment of an individual or a group of individuals; a profession dealing with understanding of, prevention of and finding a solution to individual or social problems.

Psychometrics A field of study within psychology concerned with the theory and technique of measurement.

Psychomotor (*si'ko-mo'tor*) Pertaining to or causing voluntary movements associated with mental processes.

Psychomotor epilepsy Complex partial seizures, characterized by a clouding of consiousness and by strange repititions movements called automatism.

Psychoneurosis (*si'ko-nu-ro'sis*) An emotional or behavioral disorder arising from unresolved unconscious conflicts.

Psychopath (*si'ko-path*) A person exhibiting an antisocial behavior.

Psychopathology (*si'ko-path-ol'o-je*) The study of the etiology, processes, and features of mental disorders; the behavioral manifestation of any mental disorder.

Psychopharmacology (*si-ko-far'ma-kol'o-je*) The scientific study of the effect of drugs on behavior and normal and abnormal mental functions.

Psychophysology The study of the relatioship between physiological and psychological phenomena.

Psychosexual development Freud's stages. Children's pleasure-seeking urges are focused on a different area (erogenous zone) of the body, at each of the five stages of development—oral, anal, phalic, latency and genital.

Psychosis (*si-ko'sis*) Any mental disorder of organic or emotional origin exhibiting a gross impairment in reality testing. The person fails to evaluate the correctness of his or her perceptions and thoughts and makes incorrect references about the reality even when it is contrary.

Psychosomatic (*si'ko-so-mat'ik*) Bodily diseases stimulated, or caused by mental factors; the expression of emotional conflict through physical symptoms; of or pertaining to psychosomatic medicine.

Psychosurgery (*si-ko-sur'jer-e*) Operative treatment designed to correct psychological diseases.

Psychotherapy (*si-ko-ther'a-pe*) Treatment aimed at helping the patient to solve his psychiatric and emotional problems.

Pscychoticism A personality type that is prone to take risks, might engage in anti-social activities, impulsiveness, or non-conformist behavior.

Psychrophilic (*si-kro-fil'ik*) Preferring cold, refers to the bacteria thriving at low temperatures.

Psychotropic drug Drug altering emotional and behavioral response.

Pterion (*te're-on*) Point of suture of frontal, parietal, temporal and sphenoid bones.

Pteroylglutamic acid (*ter"o-il-gloo-tam' ik*) Folic acid.

Pterygium (*ter-ij'e-um*) A thick triangular tissue that extends medially from the nasal border of the cornea to the inner canthus of the eye.

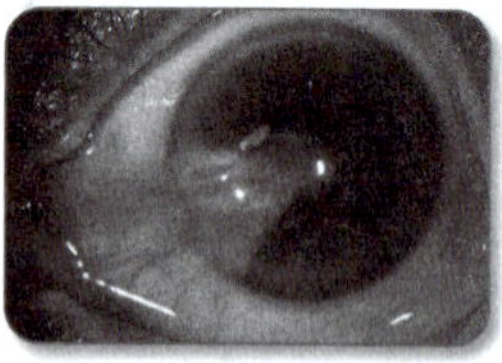

Pterygium

Pterygoid process Each of a pair of a projections from the sphenoid bone in the skull.

Ptomaine (*to'man*) A nitrogenous substance produced by putrefactive bacteria acting on proteins and amino acids.

Ptosis (*to'sis*) Drooping of an organ or part such as upper eyelid or visceral organs.

Ptyalin (*ti'a-lin*) An enzyme found in the saliva that hydrolyzes starch and glycogen.

Ptyalism (Sialorrhea) (*ti'a-lizm*) Excessive salivary secretion.

Ptyalography (*ti-al-og'ra-fe*) Sialography.

Ptyalolith A calculus in the salivary gland or duct.

Puberty (*pu'ber-te*) Transformation of child into an voting adult at which the individual becomes capable of reproduction.

Precocious puberty Development of pubertal changes at an unusually early age.

Pubes (*pu'bez*) The anterior part of the innominate bone; the pubic region; the pubic hair.

Pubiotomy (*pu-be-ot'o-me*) Incision across pubis undertaken to enlarge the pelvic passage to facilitate the delivery of fetus in malformed pelvis.

Pubis (*pu'bis*) Pl. **pubes.** Pubic bone.

Public health The science and art of preventing disease, prolonging life and promoting health through organized community efforts.

Pudendum (*pu-den'dam*) The external genital organs of a human being and especially of a woman.

Pudendum femininum Vulva.

Pudendum muliebre Female external genitals.

PUFA Polyunsaturated fatty acids.

Puerperal (*pu-er'per-al*) Concerning the puerperium.

Puerperal eclampsia Eclampsia during puerperium.

Puerperal fever Septicemia following childbirth.

Puerperal infection A postpartum infection, is a bacterial infection of the genital tract that develops after childbirth, miscarriage, or induced abortion.

Puerperal pyrexia (*pu-er'per-al*) Concerning the puerperium.

Puerperium (*pu'er-pe're-um*) The period from the termination of labor to complete involution of the uterus, lasting approximately 6 weeks.

Pulex (*pu'leks*) A genus of fleas that is the type genus of the family Pulicidae and includes the most common flea that regularly attacks human beings.

Pulicide (*pu'li-sid*) An agent that destroys fleas.

Pulmo- (pulmono(ʊ)-) A combining word for lung.

Pulmonary (*pul'mo-ne-re*) Pertaining to the lungs or respiratory system.

Pulmonary agenesis A congenital anomaly exhibiting failure of development of the primitive lung bud.

Pulmonary alveolar proteinosis Non-inflammatory progressive pulmonary disease presenting with dyspnea due to intra-alveolar extracellular deposition of granular lipoproteinaceous material.

Pulmonary angiitis Tissue reactions characterized by focal destructive and infiltrative vascular disease in the lung.

Pulmonary atresia Atretic pulmonary valve with hypoplastic pulmonary artery.

Pulmonary congestion An excessive accumulation of fluid in the lungs, usually associated with either an inflammation or congestive heart failure.

Pulmonary hemosiderosis Recurrent hemoptysis and iron deficiency due to intrapulmonary hemorrhage.

Pulmonary metastases Metastatic spread of malignancy to the lung from carcinomatous conditions in different parts of the body.

Pulmonary stenosis Narrowing of pulmonary valve orifice.

Pulmonary thromboembolism A condition associated with the obstruction of pulmonary artery by a thrombus arising from an extrapulmonary source.

Pulmonary circulation A vast network of arteries, veins and lymphatics that function to exchange blood and other tissue fluids between the heart, the lungs and back.

Pulmonary embolism Pulmonary thromboembolism.

Pulmonary hypertension Marked narrowing of pulmonary vascular bed from anatomic or vasomotor mechanisms, either singly or together, result in an increased vascular resistance to the blood flow through the lungs and pulmonary hypertension.

Pulp Soft part of an organ; soft part of a fruit; a mass of partially digested, food; the soft vascular part of the center of tooth; *dent* soft innermost layer of a tooth containing blood vessels and nerves.

Pulp chamber Area within the natural crown of the tooth occupied by dental pulp.

Pulpitis (*pul-pi'tis*) Inflammation of the pulp of a tooth.

Pulse A wave of expansion felt due to systolic ejection of the left ventricle in already filled arteries.

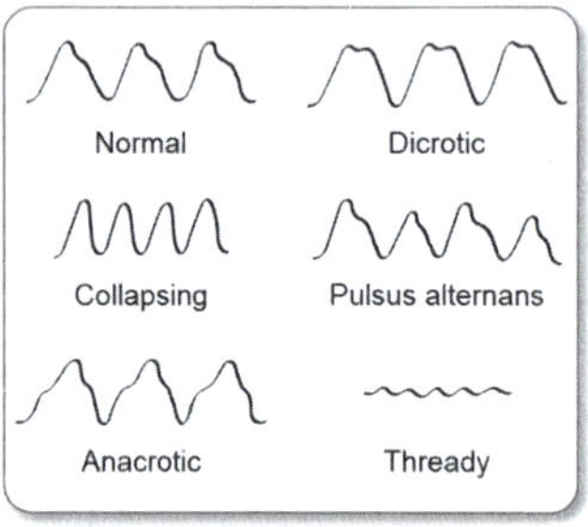

Pulse

Anacrotic pulse A prominent initial tidal wave than the main wave.

Capillary pulse Pulsations noted in the regions adjoining the poorly vascular and richly vascular areas of the capillary systems, commonly in the nailbed.

Carotid pulse Pulsations noted in the carotid artery.

Collapsing pulse Pulse showing a rapid upstroke due to markedly increased stroke volume and a fall due to regurgitation of blood back into the left ventricle during diastole and to decreased systemic vascular resistance, seen in aortic incompetence and hyperdynamic circulatory states.

Dicrotic pulse A double arterial pulse due to an exaggerated dicrotic wave in the early diastole.

Plateau pulse A sustained peak with a slow upstroke and a downstroke as in aortic stenosis.

Pulse deficit Radial pulse being less than ventricular rate as in atrial fibrillation.

Pulse pressure The difference between the systolic and diastolic pressures, normally a value of about 40 mm Hg.

Radial pulse Normal pulse felt in the radial artery at the wrist.

Thready pulse Rapid pulse with low volume and low force as in shock.

Unequal pulse A pulse in which beats vary in force.

Venous pulse Pulsations in the jugular vein exhibiting a wavy pattern with three distinct positive waves during each cardiac cycle and are better seen than felt.

Waterhammer pulse Collapsing pulse appreciated when the arm of the patient is raised above the level of the head.

Pulsus paradoxus An exaggerated inspiratory fall in blood pressure during quiet breathing and there is a decrease in the pulse amplitude or disappearance of pulse during quiet breathing.

Pulvinar (*pul-vi-nar*) A part of thalamus comprising a portion of the posterior nucleus.

Punch-drunk syndrome An instrument to make a small circular hole in a material or tissue.

Punch biopsy Removal of a living tissue for microscopic examination by a punch, as in bone marrow aspirates.

Punctum (*punk'tum*) Pl. **puncta**. Point.

Puncture (*punk'chur*) A hole made by a sharp pointed instrument; to make a hole by a pointed instrument.

Pupil The contractile circular opening in the center of the iris of the eye. It lies behind the anterior chamber of the eye and the cornea and in front of the lens. It contracts when exposed to strong light and when focused on a near object and dilates in the dark and when focused on a distant object.

Pupillary reflex (light reflex) (*pu-piler-e*) Pertaining to the pupil.

Purgation (*pur-ga'shun*) Cleaning; evacuation of the bowel by a purgative.

Purgative (*pur'ga-tiv*) Cleansing; an agent stimulating the bowel movements.

Purine (*pu'ren*) Any one of a large group of nitrogenous compounds. They are end products in the digestion of certain proteins in the diet, and some are synthesized in the body.

Purine base Any of the purine derivates such as xanthine and uric acid.

Purkinje cells (*pur-kin'je*) Large neuron of the cerebellar cortex, named after Johannes Purkinje, Polish physiologist.

Purkinje fibers Myocardial fibers that are a continuation of the bundle branches and extend into the ventricular walls.

Purpura (*pur'pu-ra*) A disorder characterized by bleeding into the skin often associated with bleeding from mucous membranes. It is caused by thrombocytopenia or thrombocytopathy or primary disorders affecting the blood vessels. The bleeding is circumscribed showing a clearcut margin with the surface and not blanching on application of pressure.

Anaphylactoid purpura An immune complex-mediated disease associated with vasculitis involving small blood vessels.

Drug-induced purpura Vascular purpura following exposure to drugs such as penicillin, sulphonamides, aspirin and sedatives.

Henoch-Schonlein purpura Anaphylactoid purpura.

Immune thrombocytopenic purpura Condition exhibiting antibodies directed against platelet components. There are purpuric spots and ecchymoses over limbs, chest and back. There is marked reduction in the number of platelets.

Purpura fulminans (*pur'pu-ra-ful'minanz*) A life threatening cutaneous hemorrhage and necrosis caused by disseminated intravascular coagulation and dermal vascular thrombosis.

Senile purpura Chronic disorder in elderly with purpura and ecchymoses on the extensor surfaces of the forearms.

Symptomatic purpura Purpura occurring in infections.

Vascular purpura Nonthrombocytopenic purpura, with bruising and spontaneous bleeding from small vessels due to abnormality in the capillaries.

Purulent (*pur'u-lent*) Suppurative; forming or containing pus.

Pus A pale yellow or green creamy liquid consisting of dead leukocytes that occurs at the site of bacterial infection.

Pustule (*pus'tul*) A small circumscribed elevation of the skin containing purulent fluid.

Putamen (*pu-ta'men*) A part of the lentiform nucleus situated lateral to the globus pallidus.

Putrefaction (*pu'tre-fak'shun*) Decomposition of animal matter.

Putrescine A toxic diamine formed by putrefaction from the decarboxylation of arginine and ornithine. Putrescine is a solid. This compound belongs to the polyamines.

Pyarthrosis (*pi-ar-thro'sis*) Pus in a joint cavity.

Pyelitis (*pi'e-li'tis*) Inflammation of the pelvis of the kidney and its calices.

Pyelocystitis (*pi'e-lo-sis-ti'tis*) Inflammation of the renal pelvis and the bladder.

Pyelogram (*pi'e-lo-gram*) Radiograph of the renal pelves and ureters following intravenous injection of a radioopaque substance.

Pyelography (urography) (*pi'e-log'ra-fe*) Radiography, of the renal pelves and ureters following injection of a radio-opaque contrast substance.

Pyelolithotomy (*pi'e-lo-li-thot'o-me*) The surgical removal of calculus from the pelvis of a kidney.

Pyelonephritis (*pi-e-lo-ne-fri'tis*) Inflammation of the kidney and renal pelvis.

Pyeloplasty (*pi'e-lo-plas'te*) Surgical repair of the pelvis of the kidney.

Pyelotomy (*pi'e-lot'o-me*) Incision of the

Pyemia (*pi-e'me-a*) A diseased state in which pyogenic bacteria are circulating in the blood, characterized by the development of abscesses in various organs.

Pyemotes (*pi"e-mo'tez*) A genus of mites that are usually ectoparasites of insects but that include one which causes grain itch in humans when transferred to the skin.

Pyknolepsy Petit mal epilepsy; characterized by a brief altered state of consciousness and absence of seizures.

Pyknosis (*pik-no'sis*) Reduction in the size of the cell or its nucleus, usually associated with hyperchromatosis.

Pylephlebitis (portal pyemia) (*pi'le-flebi'tis*) Inflammation of the portal vein.

Pylethrombosis Formation of a blood clot in a vein that is not inflamed. Physical inactivity can lead to the condition.

Pylorectomy (*pi'lo-rek'to-me*) Operative removal of the pylorus.

Pyloric (*pi-lor'ik*) Pertaining to the distal portion of the stomach.

Pyloric sphincter A thick, circular muscle in the distal end of the stomach that controls the passage of food into the small intestine.

Pyloric stenosis An uncommon condition in infants that blocks food from entering the small intestine.

Pyloromyotomy (Ramstedt's operation) (*pi-lor'o-mi-ot'o-me*) Incision and suture of the pyloric sphincter.

Pyloroplasty (*pi-lor'o-plas'te*) A surgical procedure to widen the muscular outlet from the stomach.

Pylorospasm (*pi-lor'o-spazm*) Spasmodic contraction of the pyloric orifice.

Pylorus (*pi-lor'us*) The inferior region of the stomach that connects to the duodenum. It has two parts, the pyloric antrum which connects to the body of the stomach and the pyloric canal which leads into the duodenum. Pylorus has a sphincter at the site of its communication with the duodenum.

Pyocele (*pi'o-sel*) A hydrocele where the fluid has become purulent due to secondary infection. It is an acutely tender swelling with positive fluctuation but negative transillumination test.

Pyocolpos A rare complication of hydrocolpos, which in turn is the accumulation of secretions within the vagina and failure to exteriorize, secondary to mostly an imperforate hymen.

Pyocyanin A blue-green pigment secreted by P. aeruginosa.

Pyoderma (*pi'o-derma*) Any purulent skin disease, such as impetigo.

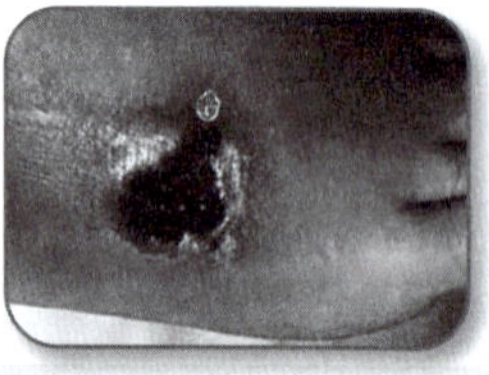

Pyoderma gangrenosum

Pyogenic (*pi'o-jen'ik*) Producing pus.

Pyogenic microorganism A microorganism producing pus.

Pyometra (*pi'o-me'tra*) Accumulation of pus in the uterine cavity.

Pyometritis (*pio'-me-tri'tis*) Purulent inflammation of the uterus.

Pyomyositis (*pi'o-mi'o-si'tis*) A bacterial infection of the skeletal muscles which results in a pus-filled abscess.

Pyonephrosis (*pi'o-nef-ro'sis*) Accumulation of pus in the renal pelvis.

Pyopneumothorax (*pi'o-nu'mo-tho'raks*) The collection of pus and gas in the pleural cavity.

Pyorrhea (*pi'o-re-a*) Discharge of pus.

Pyosalpingitis Inflammation of a fallopian tube, with the formation of pus.

Pyosalpingo-oophoritis (*pi'o-sal-pin'go-o'of-o-ri'tis*) Inflammation of the ovary and fallopian tube with collection of pus.

Pyosalpinx (*pi'o-sal'pinks*) Collection of pus in the fallopian tube.

Pyosis Formation or discharge of pus; suppuration.

Pyothorax (*pi'o-tho'raks*) Empyema thoracis.

Pyramid (*pir'a-mid*) A mass of tissue rising to an apex as in cerebellum and kidneys.

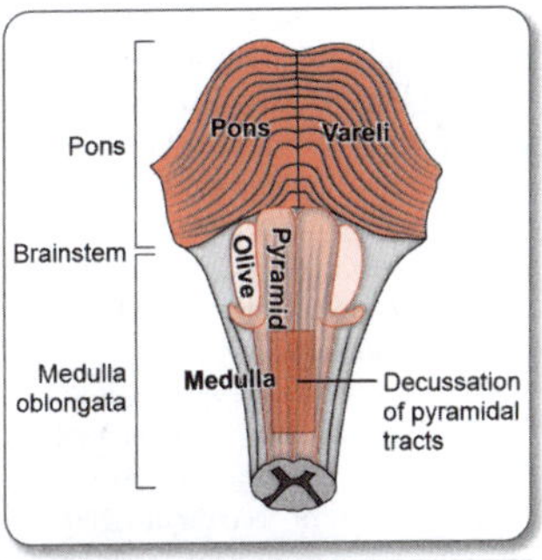

Pyramid of medulla oblongata

Pyramidal cell (*pi-ram'i-dal*) In the shape of a pyramid.

Pyrazinamide (*pi'ra-zin'a-mid*) A bactericidal antituberculosis drug that has action more marked on intracellular bacilli and in an acid medium. It has a potent sterilizing action on slowly multiplying bacilli inside the macrophages.

Pyret (pyreto-) (*pi're-to-li-sis*) Delirious state induced by high fever.

Pyrexia (*pi-rek-se'a*) Fever.

Pyridoxal phosphate (*pir'i-dok'sal*) The active form of vitamin B_{12}; a coenzyme in a variety of enzymatic reactions.

Pyridoxine (*pir'i-dok'sen*) A water soluble vitamin, part of the B complex group derived from pyridine. It functions as coenzyme for the synthesis and break-down of amino acids, the conversion of tryptophan to niacin, the breakdown of glycogen to glucose-1 phosphate and the formation of heme in hemoglobin.

Pyrilamine A first generation antihistamine, targeting the H1 receptor. It has mild hypnotic properties and some local anesthetic action and is used for allergies (including skin eruptions) both parenterally and locally. It is a common ingredient of cold remedies.

Pyrimidine (*pi-rim'i-den*) An organic compound of heterocyclic nitrogen found in nucleic acids and in antiviral drugs.

Pyrogen (*pi'ro-jen*) An agent inducing fever.

Pyromania (*pi'ro-ma'ne-a*) An impulse control disorder with an uncontrollable urge to set fires; deliberate and purposeful fire setting on more than one occasion.

Pyrosis (*pi-ro'sis*) Heart burn.

Pyruvic acid (pyruvate) (*pi-roo'vik*) An end product of glycolysis in the anaerobic metabolism of glucose.

Pyrvinium (*pir-vin'e-um*) A cyanine dye derived drug used in the treatment of threadworm infestation.

Pyuria (*pi-u're-a*) Discharge of pus in the urine and is a sign of urinary tract infection.

Q

Q fever Query or Queensland fever. An acute zoonotic rickettsial infection caused by *Coxiella burnetti*. It follows an occupational contact with livestock and presents with influenza-like picture.

QRST complex *ECG* The Q, R, S and T waves of an electrocardiogram. The T wave following the QRS complex, reflects ventricular repolarization.

QT interval *ECG* Duration of ventricular systole is measured in the electrocardiogram from the beginning of the Q wave to the end of T wave and it varies with the heartbeat. It represents repolarization of the heart.

QT syndrome *ECG* A combination of prolonged QT interval and *torsades de pointes*.

Quadrantanopia (*kwahd'rant-a-no'pea*) Hemianopia in one fourth of the visual field, bounded by a vertical and a horizontal radius. Also known as tetartanopia and quadrant hemianopia.

Quadrantectomy (*kwahd'ran-tak'to-me*) Partial surgical removal of a quadrant of breast.

Quadrate lobe A small lobe of liver located on the visceral surface, lying in contact with pylorus and duodenum.

Quadratus (*kwahd'ratus*) Four-sided.

Quadriceps (*kwod'ri-seps*) Having four heads.

Quadriceps femoris Powerful anterior thigh muscle with four heads (rectus femoris, vastus lateralis, vastus medialis and vastus intermedius) that extend the knee joint.

Quadriceps reflex Extension of the leg following contraction of quadriceps muscle from patellar tap.

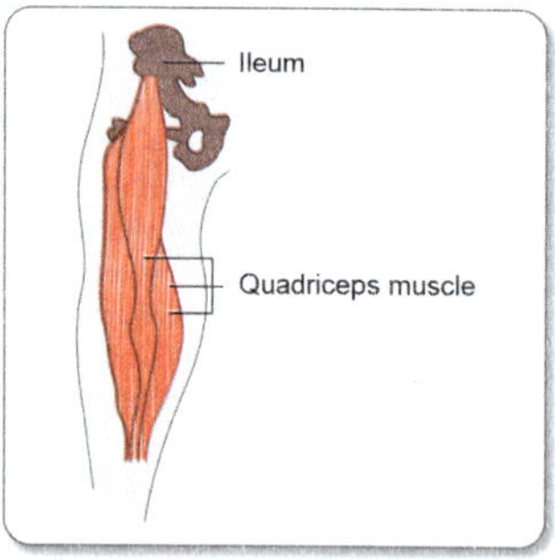

Quadriceps

Quadriplegia (tetraplegia) (*kwod'ri-ple'je-a*) Paralysis of all four limbs; tetraplegia.

Flaccid quadriplegia Can occur in brainstem lesions with neuronal shock, polyneuropathy, due to Guillain-Barré syndrome, diphtheria, or porphyria, myasthenic crisis, periodic dyskalemic paralysis and polymyositis.

Spastic quadriplegia Can occur in high cervical cord lesions such as cervical spondylosis, craniovertebral anomalies, or in cortical lesions such as cerebral palsy or decerebrate rigidity.

Quarantine (*kwor'an-ten*) Isolation or detention of a person who has been exposed to a communicable disease, which is imposed for the maximal incubation period with the purpose of preventing its further dissemination.

Quartan fever The fever caused by *Plasmodium malariae* in which fever spikes appear every third day.

Queckenstedt's test (*kwek'en-stets*) Absence of variation in pressure of the cerebrospinal fluid when the jugular veins are compressed. It indicates a block in the vertebral canal.

Quellung reaction A swelling of the capsule of the bacteria on exposure to specific antisera.

Quickening (*kwik'en-ing*) A subjective feeling caused by the fetal movement within the uterus, usually noted early in the fifth month of pregnancy as 'fluttering of a bird' by the mother.

Quiescent (*kwies'ent*) Quiet, being at rest, still inactive.

Quinacrine (*kwin'ah-krin*) An alkaloid used in the suppressive treatment of malaria, and in the treatment of tapeworm infestation and giardiasis; mepacrine.

Quinestradol Oral estrogen whose action is confirmed to the lower genital tract.

Quinestrol (*kwin-es'trol*) A long-acting estrogen.

Quinidine (*kwin'i-din*) An alkaloid isomeric with quinine, used to regulate heart rhythm in cardiac arrhythmias. It suppresses excitability and slows conduction in atrial or ventricular muscle.

Quinine (*kwi'nin*) An alkaloid obtained from cinchona bark. Its hydrochloride and sulfate preparations are used in treatment of chloroquine resistant malaria.

Quinism A chronic encephalopathy due to intoxication by mefloquine quinacrine or chloroquine. It is associated with dysfunction of brain and brainstem.

Quinsy (*kwin'ze*) Painful abscess of tonsils; suppurative tonsillitis with peritonsillar abscess.

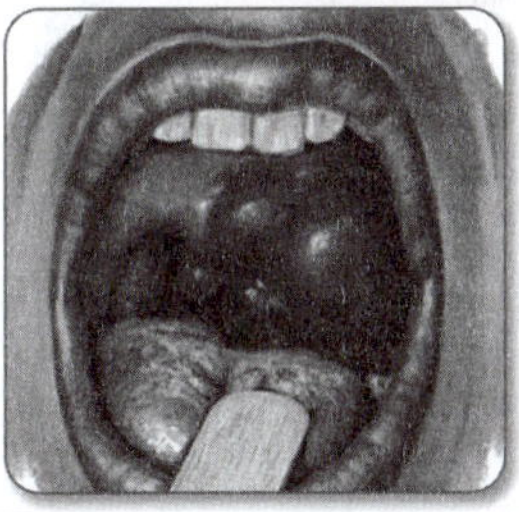

Quinsy

Quotidian fever A malarial fever with daily occurrence.

Q wave *ECG* A small negative deflection preceding R wave electrocardiogram which is caused from left to right of the interventricular system.

R

RAAS Renin angiotensinogen-angiotensin system.

Rabeprazole (*ra-bep'ra-zol*) Proton pump inhibitor (PPI), works by reducing the amount of acid in the stomach which helps in relief of acid related indigestion and heartburn.

Rabies (hydrophobia) (*ra-bez*) Hydrophobia, a highly fatal infection caused by a bullet-shaped neurotropic rhabdovirus transmitted by the bite of carnivorous animals. The incubation period, varies from 4 to 8 weeks or longer. The patient becomes increasingly anxious and develops characteristic fear of water, hydrophobia. There is cranial nerve lesions and hyperpyrexia. Death occurs within a week of the onset of symptoms. Postexposure prophylaxis is by administration of human diploid cell strain vaccine; 1.0 mL given intramuscularly on days 0, 3, 7, 14, and 28.

Raccoon sign Periorbital ecchymosis and it may be a feature of basilar skull fracture; black eyes.

Racemose (*ras'e-mos*) Branching with nodular ends, resembling a bunch of grapes.

Racemose aneurysm Marked dilatation of lengthened and tortuous blood vessels.

Racephedrine (*ra-sefa-dren*) Synthetic or man-made racemic ephedrine used in the form of its hydrochloride.

Rachiotomy (*ra-ki-oto'mi*) Laminectomy.

Rachis (*ra'kis*) The spinal column.

Rachischisis (*ra-kis'ki-sis*) Refers to cases of neural tube defect involving at least the cervical spine region and extending for varying degrees down the spinal column.

Rachitic (*ra-kit'ik*) Rickety; pertaining to rickets.

Rachitic dwarf A person whose retarded growth is caused by rickets.

Rachitic rosary Bulbous widening of the costochondral junction due to softened epiphysis, seen in vitamin D-deficient rickets, childhood hypophosphatemia and in adenosine deaminase deficiency.

Rad A unit to measure the dose absorbed from ionizing radiation.

Radial (*ra'di-al*) Lateral aspect of the upper limb; relating to the radius.

Radial bursa Tendon sheath of flexor pollicis in palm and thumb.

Radial immunodiffusion A method for quantifying serum proteins, complement proteins and immunoglobulins.

Radial keratotomy Tiny shallow incisions made on the cornea to make it bulge slightly to correct for near sightedness.

Radial nerve palsy Weakness of extension of wrist and fingers due to paralysis of wrist and finger extensors and supinator. The condition is often precipitated by sleeping in abnormal posture.

Radial pulse The pulse of the radial artery felt at the wrist over the radius.

Radial artery An artery in the forearm, beginning at the bifurcation of the brachial artery giving branches to the forearm, wrist and hand.

Radial nerve The largest branch of the brachial plexus. The nerve supplies the skin of the arm and forearm and, in the arm triceps, brachialis, brachioradialis, extensor carpi longus *et* brevis and anconeus and in the forearm the extensor group of muscles including supinator.

Radial reflex Reflex elicited by tapping over the distal radius with the response being flexion of the forearm.

Radiation (*ra-de-a'shun*) Sending energy in the form of X-rays, radio waves, visible light, ultraviolet light and gamma rays.

Radiation burn A burn resulting from exposure to radiant energy (sunlight, X-ray or nuclear emissions).

Radiation cataract A cataract developing after an excessive exposure of the eye to X-rays or other type of radiation.

Radiation dermatitis Inflammation of the skin caused by exposure to ionizing radiation.

Radiation fibrosis Development of fibrosis in all patients with radiation pneumonitis 6–12 months after radiotherapy.

Radiation pneumonitis Radiation injury of the lung developing 2–6 months following radiation therapy.

Radiation sickness Acute radiation injury presenting with anorexia, nausea, vomiting, fatigue, leukopenia and thrombocytopenia.

Radical (*rad'i-kal*) A group of atoms acting as a single unit, which do not change while passing from one com-pound to another; oriented toward the root.

Radical dissection The surgical excision of tissue in an extensive area surrounding the operative site. It is undertaken in malignancy to decrease the chance of recurrence.

Radical mastectomy Excision of entire breast, axillary lymph nodes, pectoral muscles and all fat, fascia and adjacent tissues in cancer of the breast.

Radical treatment Vigorous treatment that aims at the complete cure of the disease rather than mere relief.

Radiation sickness Acute radiation injury presenting with anorexia, nausea, vomiting, fatigue, leukopenia and thrombocytopenia.

Radiculitis (*ra-dik-u-li-tis*) Inflammation of a spinal nerve root present within the dura, accompanied by pain and hyperesthesia.

Radioactivity (*ra'de-o-ak-tiv'i-te*) The property of emission of rays (alpha, beta, gamma) as a consequence of its nuclear degeneration.

Induced radioactivity Radioactivity produced by bombarding an element with high velocity particles.

Radiograph (*ra'de-o-graf*) Roentgenogram wherein a shadow image is produced on a sensitized film by radiography.

Bite-wing radiograph A radiograph used to detect decay between teeth and changes in bone caused by periodontal disease.

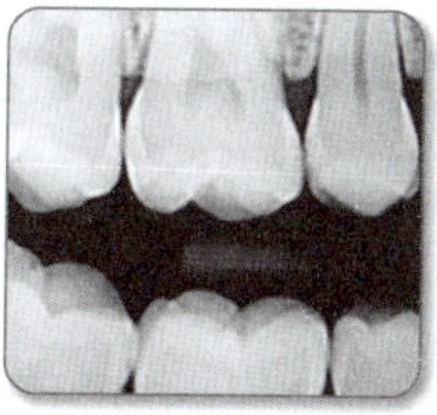

Bite-wing radiograph

Cephalometric radiograph A radiograph of skull with head fixed in cephalostat.

Lateral skull radiograph A nonangled lateral radiograph of skull.

Radiography (*rade-og'ra-fi*) Roentgenography; production of images upon a photographic plate of film of any region of the body by passing X-rays.

Digital radiography A type of radiography that uses sensitive X-ray plates to directly capture data during patient examination.

Electron radiography A type of radiography in which a latent electrons image is produced on clear mash by passing X-ray through a gas with high atomic number.

Spot-film radiography A type of radiograph which forms localized instantaneous radiographic exposures during fluoroscopy.

Radioimmunoassay (*ra'de-o-im'u-no-as'sa*) RIA, an immunologic procedure utilizing a radioisotope substance to measure the amount of specific antibodies or antigens present in the test fluid.

Radioisotope (*ra-de-o-i'so-top*) An unstable isotope that decays to a stable state by emitting radiation.

Radiologist (*ra'de-o-lojist*) Roentgenologist, a specialist in radiography.

Radiology (*ra'de-olo-ji*) Roentgenology, a branch of science concerned with radiant energy.

Radionecrosis Necrosis occurring after excessive exposure to radiation.

Radionuclide (*rade-o-noo'klid*) An isotope exhibiting radioactivity.

Radionuclide imaging Examination of different parts of the body especially the heart using thallium 201.

Radionuclide scanning To produce a three-dimensional image by a camera that rotates around the person being examined; SPECT.

Radiopaque (*ra-de-o-pak*) Relatively impenetrable to radiation and such substances are used to make organs to stand out more clearly on X-ray images.

Radiopaque dye A chemical substance that does not permit the passage of X-rays.

Radioscopy (*ra"de-os'ko-pe*) Examination of the inner structure of opaque objects using X-rays or other penetrating radiation.

Radiosensitive (*ra'de-o-sen'sitiv*) Affected by radiation.

Radiosensitizer Any substance that makes tumor cells easier to kill with radiation therapy.

Radiotherapy (*ra'de-o-ther'epe*) The medical specialty concerned with use of radiant energy from a cobalt source in the treatment of disease; exposure of a defined area of the body to a source of ionizing radiation under carefully controlled conditions.

Radium (*ra'de-um*) A radioactive metallic element, symbol Ra, atomic no. 88.

Radium insertion An introduction of metallic radium into body cavity, such as uterus or cervix to treat cancer.

Radium therapy The use of radium and its radioactive emissions to treat malignant condition.

Radius (*radi-us*) The lateral short bone of the forearm lying parallel to the ulna.

Radix Root.

Radon A radioactive gas resulting from the decay of uranium. Symbol Rn, atomic no. 86.

Radon seed A small sealed tube containing radon for insertion into body tissues in the treatment of malignancies.

Rai staging system Five-stage to determine survival of untreated patients with chronic lymphocytic leukemia.

Rale (*rahl*) Crepitation; crackles heard as, a moist adventitious sounds on auscultation of the chest.

Ramelteon A melatonin receptor agonist used to treat insomnia.

Ramsay Hunt's syndrome Herpes zoster infection of the geniculate ganglion, characterized by rash over the palate and over external ear, severe ear pain, neuron facial palsy, named after James Ramsay Hunt, US neurologist.

Ramstedt's procedure Used in the treatment of infantile pyloric stenosis; pyloromyotomy.

Ramus (*ra'mus*) A branch. pl. **rami**.

Ranitidine (*ranit'iden*) A histamine H_2 receptor antagonist indicated in the treatment of peptic ulcers and gastric hyper-secretory states.

Ranula (*ran'u-la*) Sublingual cyst. A mucocele in the floor of the mouth caused by obstruction of the ducts of sublingual salivary glands.

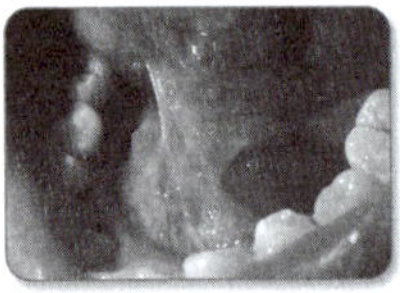

Ranula

Raphe (*ra'fe*) A line of union of two contiguous bilaterally symmetrical structures.

Abdominal raphe A fibrous white streak running vertically along the median line from the umbilicus to the pubis.

Raphe of tongue A fibrous wall forming a line of union between the right and left sides of the tongue.

Ras genes A family of oncogenes and proto-oncogenes first identified in a rat sarcoma, which encode oncoproteins or proto-oncoproteins.

Rash A cutaneous eruption.

Butterfly rash A red or purplish facial rash with a "butterfly" pattern.

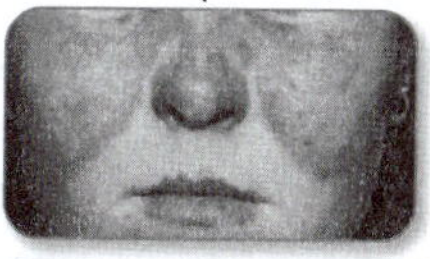

Butterfly rash

Heliotrope rash A reddish purple rash on or around the eyelids.

Pleomorphic rash All stages of rash are present at one point of time.

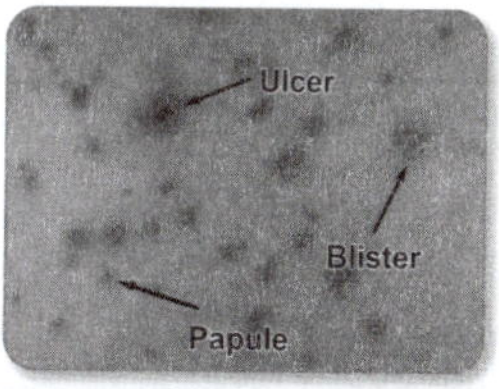

Pleomorphic rash

Rasp A coarse file used in surgery - also known as raspatory and xyster; a harsh, grating noise.

Raspatory A surgical instrument for abrading.

RAST Radio allergosorbent test.

Rat-bite fever (sodoku) Febrile illness following rat-bite carrying *spirillum minus* or *Streptobacillus moniliformis.* It is characterized by fever, headache, malaise, nausea, vomiting and rash. There is a swelling at the site of the wound and regional lymphadenopathy. It responds to penicillin.

Rathke's pouch (*rat'kez*) A depression that forms the roof of the mouth of an embryo. The walls of the diverticulum develop into the anterior lobe of the pituitary gland, described by Martin Rathke, German anatomist.

Raxibacumab A human IgG1λ monoclonal antibody used in conjunction with an antibacterial regimen to treat patients with inhalational anthrax caused by *Bacillus anthracis* and for prophylaxis of inhalational anthrax when appropriate.

Raynaud's disease (*ra-noz*) A disorder wherein exposure to cold causes sudden contraction of small arteries supplying the fingers and toes, named after Maurice Raynaud, French physician.

RBBB Right bundle branch block.

RCA Right coronary artery, Regulator of complement activation.

Reaction A response in opposition to a stimulus, substance or treatment.

Allergic reaction Hypersensitivity reaction to a particular allergen; symptoms can vary greatly in intensity.

Allograft reaction A response by host T lymphocytes reacting to transplantation antigens that are carried on allogeneic lymphoreticular cells.

Arthus reaction A form of type III allergy reactions producing an antigen-antibody immune complex.

Delayed hypersensitivity reaction An immunologic reaction that is mediated primarily by T cells and monocytes and presents hours to days after the antigen crosses into the skin.

Fight or flight reaction Alarm reaction.

Graft versus host reaction A systemic disorder that occurs when the graft's immune cells recognize the host as foreign and attack the recipient's body cells.

Immediate hypersensitivity reaction Occur within 24 hours of exposure to the antigen or allergen.

Reaction formation (*re-ak'shun for-ma'shun*) A defense mechanism in which people express the opposite of their true feelings, sometimes to an exaggerated extent.

Reactive (*re-ak'tiv*) To be ready to react or respond to something else.

Regain (*re'a-gan*) Alternatively known as homocytotropic antibody or Prausnitz-Küstner antibody, refers to a specific type of antibody present in the bloodstream and skin of individuals with allergic hypersensitivity. It is also detected in minor quantities in the blood of individuals who are normally sensitive. Majority belongs to the immunoglobulin E (IgE) category.

Reamer (*rem'ar*) A specialized surgical tool employed in a range of medical procedures, notably in orthopedic and dental surgeries. Its purpose is to carefully enlarge and contour an opening or hollow space within bone or tissue.

Rebound tenderness Deep pressure is exerted over the site of pain on the abdomen. The hand is removed suddenly and the patient experiences sharp pain indicating inflammation of the parietal peritoneum.

Receptor (*re-sep'tor*) A nerve cell responding to a specific stimulus by producing nerve impulses or an area on the surface of a cell to which a chemical substance binds to have its effect.

Adrenergic receptor Membrane-bound proteins that mediate the peripheral and central actions of norepinephrine and epinephrine (*see* **Table**).

Receptor defect A defect in a receptor that prevents the chemical that normally binds to it from having its effect.

Receptor site A location on a cell surface where certain molecules attach to interact with cellular components.

Recess (*re'ses*) A small hollow cavity.

Pyriform recess A pear-shaped inlet in the wall of laryngeal pharynx.

Tubotympanic recess The dorsal portion of the embryonic first endodermal pharyngeal pouch; it develops into the middle ear cavity.

Recessive (*re-ses'iv*) Receding; suppressed; pertaining to gene whose effect is masked or hidden in presence of a dominant gene at the same locus.

Recipient (*ris'i-pe-ant*) The person who receives a blood transfusion, or tissue graft or organ.

RECIST Response evaluation criteria in solid tumors.

Reconstructive surgery Surgical procedure attempting to restore a tissue close to its original structure.

Recombinant DNA A DNA molecule in which rearrangement of the genes has been artificially induced by enzymes.

Recrudescence (*re-kru-des'ens*) A recurrence of morbid process or its symptom following a period of improvement.

Recruitment (*re-kroot'mant*) The process of actively seeking out, finding and hiring candidates for a specific position or job.

Recreational drug Any substance with pharmacologic effects that is taken voluntarily for personal pleasure.

Rectal (*rek'tal*) Relating to the rectum.

Rectal abscess An abscess in the perianal region.

Rectal alimentation Administration of nourishment in a concentrated form by instillation through rectum.

Rectal reflex Defecation response to the presence of an accumulation of feces in the rectum; defecation reflex.

Rectal temperature Temperature measured in the rectum, which is generally 0.3°–0.4°C or 0.5°–0.75°F higher than mouth temperature.

Rectectomy (*rek-tek'to-me*) Resection of the rectum.

Rectocele (*rek't-o-sel*) A protrusion of the rectum and the posterior wall of the vagina into the vagina.

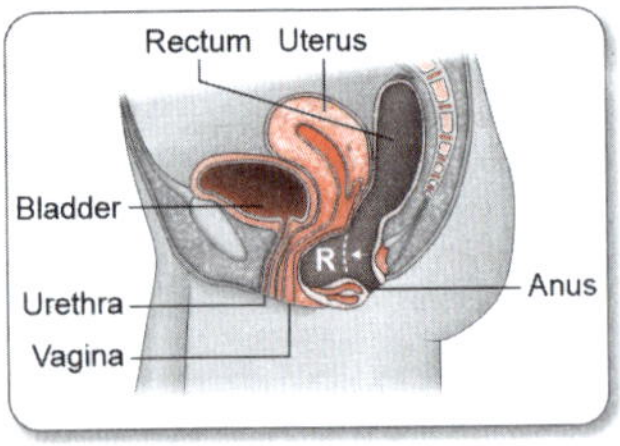

Rectocele (R)

Rectosigmoid (*rek-to-sig'moyd*) Pertaining to rectum and sigmoid colon.

Table: Adrenergic receptors

Receptor Type	Tissue Distribution	Mechanism of Action	Physiological Effects	Agonist	Antagonist
α_1	Vascular smooth muscles, Visceral smooth muscles	Gq-protein coupled activates Phospholipase C, IP3+DAG	Smooth muscle contractions, Gluconeogenesis, Vasoconstriction	Norepinephrine, Phenylephrine, Methoxamine	Doxazosin, Phentolamine, Prazosin
α_2	Presynaptic terminals, Pancreas, Platelets, Ciliary epithelium, Salivary glands	Gi-protein coupled inhibits Adenyl cyclase	Inhibits release of Neurotransmitter	Clonidine, Monoxidine	Yohimbine, Idazoxan, Tolazoline
β_1	Heart, Kidney, some presynaptic terminals	Gs-protein coupled activates Adenyl cyclase +PKA	Increase heart rate and Renin secretion	Isoproterenol, Norepinephrine, Dobutamine	Propranolol, Metoprolol, Atenolol
β_2	Visceral smooth muscles, Bronchioles, Liver, Skeletal muscles	Gs-protein coupled activates Adenyl cyclase +PKA, Ca-channels	Vasodilation, Bronchodilation, inhibits insulin secretion	Isoproterenol, Salbutamol, salmeterol, albuterol, Formoterol, Terbutaline, Levalbuterol	Propranolol, ICI-118, 551, Nadolol, Butoxamine
β_3	Adipose Tissue	Gs-protein coupled activates Adenyl cyclase +PKA	Increase lipolysis	Isoproterenol, Amibegron, Solabegron	SRS9230A

Rectum (*rek'tum*) The end part of the alimentary tract extending from the sigmoid colon to the anal canal where feces collect before being eliminated. It is about 12 cm long.

Rectus A straight abdominal muscle.

Recurrent (*re-kur'ent*) Reappearance of symptoms or lesion after an interval; turning back on oneself.

Recurrent bandage A bandage that is wrapped several times around itself as in head or an amputated stump.

Reduction (*re-duk'shun*) Repositioning; restoration; gain one or more electrons by a compound; addition of a hydrogen to substance; removal of oxygen from a substance; the correction of a fracture, hernia or luxation.

Reduction diet A diet that is low in calories, used for reduction of body weight.

Reduction of fracture The technique of manipulating or surgically realigning displaced broken bony ends.

Reduction division The first cell devision in meiosis, by which germ cells are formed.

Reed-Sternberg cell A large, multinucleated reticuloendothelial cell found in Hodgkin's disease, named after Dorothy Reed, US pathologist and Karl Sternberg, Austrian pathologist.

Referred pain (synalgia) Pain felt at a site different from the location of the injured or diseased part of the body.

Reference range A set of values for an analysate being measured in a patient which is regarded as encompassing the usual maximum or minimum for the given analysate.

Referral Referring a patient for second opinion or treatment to a specialist.

Referred pain Pain felt at a site different from the location of the injured or diseased part of the body.

Reflex (*re'fleks*) An involuntary motor response in response to a stimulus.

Abdominal reflex Reflex elicited by scratching the abdominal wall with a blunt point when the patient is recumbent and relaxed. There is contraction of abdominal muscles with drawing of the *linea alba* and the umbilicus toward the stimulus. The reflex is lost in upper motor neuron lesions, acute abdominal conditions and in abdominal distension.

Anal reflex Scratching the skin around the anus results in immediate contraction of the voluntary anal sphincter.

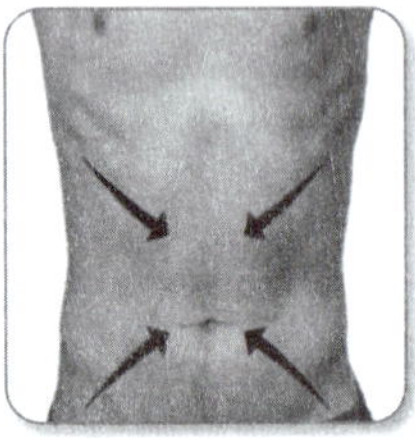

Abdominal reflex

Ciliospinal reflex Normally, when the skin of the neck is pinched due to reflex excitation of the pupil dilating fibers in cervical sympathetic. It is lost in the lesions of the sympathetic tract and pathway in the spinal cord. The loss of reflex is useful to assess the depth of coma and to diagnose brain death.

Cremasteric reflex It is elicited by stroking the inner parts of the upper thigh in male patients. There is drawing of the testicle upward due to contraction of *dortos* muscle. It is not elicited in pyramidal tract lesion and in conditions associated with hydrocele, or orchitis and in elderly men.

Deep reflex Muscle or monosynaptic stretch reflex, a single sharp tap with a soft rubber hammer on the tendon of a slightly stretched muscle results in a brief contraction of the muscle.

Glabellar reflex There is blinking when the middle of the forehead above the level of the nose is tapped with the finger. Normally it stops quickly on continuing tapping, but it continues to occur rhythmically in senile dementia and Parkinsonism.

Gonda's reflex Extension of big toe with slight dorsiflexion of the foot occur on squeezing the calf in gross lesions of corticospinal tract.

Grading of reflex Tendon reflexes are graded on their briskness as 0 (absent), 1 (normal), 2 (brisk), 3 (very brisk) and 4 (clonus).

Grasp reflex Grasping of the examiner's finger when it is drawn across the patient's palm between the thumb and index fingers in lesions of contralateral frontal lobe, reflex is normally present in infancy.

Moro reflex An involuntary protective motor response against abrupt disruption of body balance or extremely sudden stimulation.

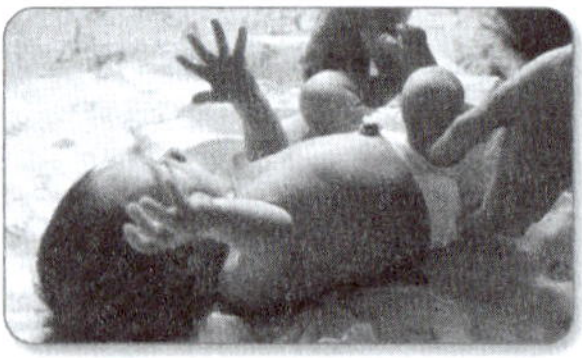

Moro reflex

Myotonic reflex Delayed return of contract muscle to the resting phase as in myxedema.

Organic reflex Act of swallowing, micturition and defecation are a reflex phenomenon and depend on movement of striated and unstriated muscles.

Palatal reflex Reflex contraction and elevation of soft palate and uvula on touching posterior wall of the pharynx.

Patellar reflex Reflex occur when patellar ligament is tapped, characterized by contraction of quadriceps and extrusion of leg.

Visceral reflex Organic reflex.

Refractometer (*re-frak-tom'e-ter*) An instrument to measure the degree of refraction in translucent substances especially the media of the eye.

Refractory (*re-frak'to-ri*) Pertaining to a disorder that is resistant to the treatment; intractable.

Regimen (*rej'i-men*) A regulation of the mode of living, diet, exercise, etc. for health or therapy.

Regional enteritis A chronic inflammatory disease of the intestines, especially in the colon and ileum associated with ulcers and fistulae.

Regorafenib A kinase inhibitor used to treat patients with metastatic colorectal cancer, unresectable, locally advanced, or metastatic gastrointestinal stromal tumors, and hepatocellular carcinoma.

Regurgitant (*re-garji-tant*) Backward flow.

Regurgitant murmur A cardiac murmur caused by a defective valve allowing blood flow backward as in pansystolic murmur of mitral incompetence and early diastolic murmur of aortic incompetence.

Regurgitation (*re-ger'ji-ta'shun*) A backward flow as in return of swallowed food or drink from the stomach back into the mouth or the backflow of blood through an incompetent valve.

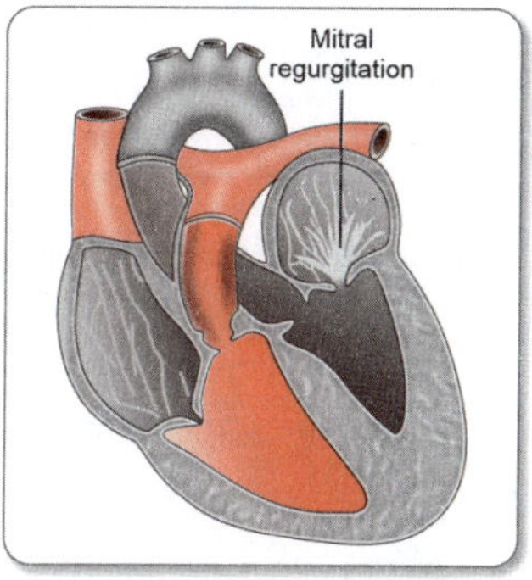

Mitral valve regurgitation

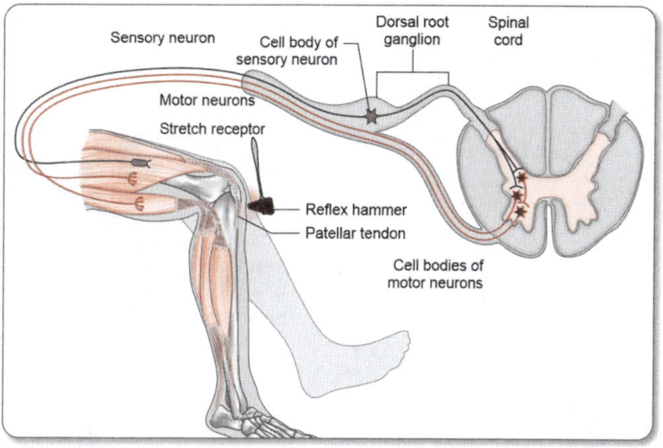

Patellar reflex

Rehabilitation (*re-ha-bil'i-ta'shun*) Restoration of ability to function.

Reid index Hypertrophy of mucus glands in chronic bronchitis can be quantified. It is based on ratio of the thickness of the submucous glands to that of the bronchial wall (from the basement membrane of epithelium to cartilage). Normally it is <0.4. It reaches 0.7-0.8.

Reiter's syndrome (*ri'terz*) Occurrence of urethritis, conjunctivitis and arthritis. It usually follows a case of nongonococcal urethritis, named after Hans Reiter, German hygienist.

Rejection (*re-jek'shun*) Refuse to accept; incompatibility in a transplanted organ; an immune reaction evoked by allografted organs.

Acute rejection Occurrence during the first six months of transplantation mediated by T cell-dependent immune response.

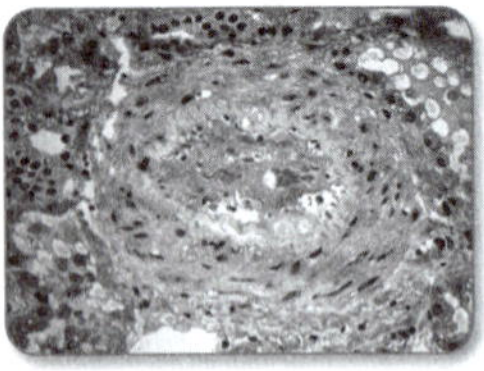

Acute rejection— renal histology

Chronic allograft rejection Occurrence after first six months, most common cause of graft failure and nonimmune factors may contribute to pathogenesis.

Hyperacute rejection Immediate graft destruction due to ABO or pre-formed anti-HLA antibodies.

Relapse (*re'laps*) Recurrence or recrudescence.

Relapsing fevers A group of diseases due to infection by spirochetes of the genus Borrelia transmitted by body lice or soft ticks; vagabond fever.

Relative analgesia Inhalational sedation technique (nitrous oxide and oxygen is used).

Relative bradycardia Normally for each half degree centigrade rise of temperature the pulse rate quickens by 10 beats. The pulse-temperature relationship is not maintained in typhoid, meningitis, cerebral abscess, dengue fever, hepatitis and burns where the pulse rate is relatively slow when compared to the temperature.

Relative tachycardia The pulse rate quickens out of proportion to the temperature in cases of rheumatic fever, diphtheria, clostridial infections, tuberculosis and thyrotoxicosis.

Relaxant Relaxing; Lessening or reducing tension; an agent that lessens the tension.

Muscle relaxant A class of drug that effectively decreases skeletal muscle function which in turn produces a tranquilizing effect.

Relaxation (*re'lak-sa'shun*) Loosening, lengthening or dilatation; any conversion of a system to a state requiring less energy.

Relaxation therapy A therapy that helps reduce muscle tension and stress, lowers blood pressure and controls pain.

Relaxin An insulin-like polypeptide produced by the corpus luteum that relaxes ligaments at symphysis pubis and sacroiliac joints.

Reline Process of resurfacing the tissue side of a removable prosthesis with new base material.

Rem Acronym for roentgen equivalent man; the dosage in rads that will cause the same amount of biological injury as one rad of X-rays or gamma rays.

REM Rapid eye movement.

REM sleep Rapid eye movement sleep. A segment of normal sleep cycle where eye muscles contract rapidly and dreaming occurs in which the usual high amplitude slow brain waves seen by EEG are replaced by rapid eye movement, rapid, low voltage irregular EEG activity, a pattern similar to that seen in an awake person.

Remission (*re-mish'un*) Partial or complete disappearance of symptoms or lesions.

Renal Relating to kidney

Renal anuria Cessation of urine production due to diseases of the kidney.

Renal arteriography Injection of contrast material into the aorta to investigate suspected renal artery stenosis or hemorrhage.

Renal artery stenosis Atheromatous narrowing of the renal artery leading to secondary hypertension.

Renal biopsy Study of renal tissue to establish the nature and extent of renal disease.

Renal calculus Renal stone, may be of calcium oxalate, phosphate, uric acid and urates, cystine or rarely xanthine indigo matrix stone, may be asymptomatic or present with dull aching pain.

Renal calyx The first part in the system of ducts in the kidney carrying urine from the renal pyramid of the cortex to the renal pelvis for excretion through the ureters.

Renal capsule A connective tissue capsule surrounding the kidney.

Renal colic A gripping pain which comes in waves with freedom from pain between the attacks. It starts in loin and then radiates downward obliquely across abdomen toward groin and the patient is found rolling in bed.

Renal dialysis Treatment method used for the management of acute or chronic renal failure where the excretory function of the kidney are partially replaced by dialysis wherein the blood is diffused across a semipermeable membrane.

Renal failure Failure of excretory function of the kidneys, leading to retention of nitrogen waste products of metabolism.

Acute renal failure (ARC) Is a sudden and usually reversible loss of renal function, which develops over a period of days or weeks.

Chronic renal failure (CRF) Is an irreversible deterioration in renal function which develops over a period of years.

Renal function Kidney regulates the volume and composition of body fluids. It is the main source of erythropoietin. Kidney is essential for the metabolism of vitamin D and it secretes renin.

Renal glycosuria An autosomal recessive condition in which there is glycosuria without hyperglycemia. The patients are asymptomatic and have a normal glucose tolerance test.

Renal hypertension Hypertension resulting from kidney disease.

Renal osteodystrophy A metabolic bone disease accompanying CRF. It consists of a mixture of osteomalacia, osteitis fibrosa, osteoporosis and osteosclerosis.

Renal papillary necrosis An analgesic nephropathy developing from long continued ingestion of analgesic drugs.

Renal papilloma A premalignant growth arising in the renal pelvis that presents as painless, profuse and paroxysmal hematuria.

Renal pelvis A funnel-shaped dilatation that drains urine from the kidney to ureter.

Renal pyramid One of the conical masses of tissue that form the kidney medulla that consist of the loops of the Henle and the collecting tubules of nephrons.

Renal rickets A condition characterized by rachitic changes in the skeleton due to chronic nephritis.

Renal sclerosis Atherosclerosis of the arterioles of the kidney.

Renal transplantation Kidney graft to restore normal kidney function and to correct the metabolic abnormalities of CRF.

Renal tuberculosis Occurs secondarily to the presence of primary lesion elsewhere, presents with increased frequency of micturition both during day and night and urine is sterile on ordinary culture.

Renal tubular acidosis A condition caused by functional defects in the distal renal tubules with loss of ability to form ammonia and to exchange hydrogen ions. The glomerular filtration rate is normal, but there is persistent metabolic acidosis and hyperchloremia and markedly decreased urinary excretion of acid.

Renal tubule The part of nephron that leads from the glomerulus to the collecting tubules.

Renal ultrasound A quick, noninvasive method of renal, it shows renal size and dilatation of the collecting duct and cysts.

Renal cell carcinoma Malignant cells are formed in the tubules of the kidney.

Renin (*re'nin*) Proteolytic enzyme produced in the juxtaglomerular apparatus that converts angiotensinogen to angiotensin. It occurs in response to a reduction in renal perfusion pressure.

Rennin (*ren'in*) Chymosin, a milk-curdling enzyme found in the gastric juices of infants.

Renography (*re'nog'ra-fi*) Radiography of the kidney.

Reovirus (*re-o-vi'rus*) A double stranded RNA virus family which includes orthoreovirus, orbivirus and rotavirus, which may produce gastroenteritis, or rhinopharyngitis.

Replication (*rep'li-ka'shun*) The process of copying, reproducing or duplicating; the process of synthesizing a daughter DNA molecule from a parent DNA 'template'.

Repolarization (*re'po-lar-i-za'shun*) The process by which the membrane cell or fiber gets repolarized.

Repositor (*re-poz'i-tar*) Programmed for acting over a prolonged period.

Repression (*re-presh'un*) Removal of ideas, impulses or affects from consciousness. *psy* Unconscious psychological mechanism in which painful or unacceptable ideas, memories or feelings are removed from conscious awareness or recall.

Reproductive system The male and female organs and connecting tubes and glands necessary for sexual intercourse and production of offspring.

Female Reproductive system Consists of the ovaries, fallopian tubes, uterus, vagina, clitoris and vulva.

Male reproductive system Consists of the testes, epididymis, vas deferens, seminal vesicles, ejaculatory duct, prostate and penis.

RES Reticuloendothelial system.

Resection (*re-sek'shun*) Surgical removal; excision.

Resectoscope (*re-sek'to-skop*) An endoscope for transurethral removal of lesions in the urethra, prostate or bladder.

Reserpine (*re-ser'pin*) An alkaloid isolated from *Rauwolfia serpentina* used as an antihypertensive.

Residual/Reserve volume The amount of air that remains in the lungs and passage ways after a maximal expiration.

Resistance (*re-zis'tans*) Ability to remain unaffected.

Resistance ratio (RR) A ratio of the minimal inhibitory concentration of a test strain to that of the control strain.

Resolution Regression; the minimum distance or degree of separation between two points that can be identified as distinct.

Resorcinol (*ra-sor'si-nol*) A 1,3-isomer (or meta-isomer) of benzenediol with the formula $C_6H_4(OH)_2$, used in the manufacturing of resins, plastics, dyes, medicine, and numerous other organic chemical compounds.

Resorption (*ri-sorp'shun*) Act of removal by absorption.

Respiration (*res-pi-ra'shun*) The act of breathing with the lungs, consisting of inhalation of the oxygen and exhalation of carbon dioxide.

Cheyne-Stokes respiration A specific form of periodic breathing (waxing and waning amplitude of flow or tidal volume) characterized by a crescendo-decrescendo pattern of respiration between central apneas or central hypopneas.

Respiration rate The number of inspirations per minute.

Respirator Ventilator.

Respirator brain Global necrotic softening of the cerebral cortex. It is noted in 'brain dead' persons who are kept alive by ventilatory support.

Respiratory distress syndrome, acute (ARDS) A severe, life-threatening catastrophe occurring suddenly in patients without any evidence of previous lung diseases. The condition is characterized by marked dyspnea, progressive hypoxemia, reduced pulmonary compliance, marked impairment in oxygen transportation despite ventilatory assistance and roentgenographic evidence of bilateral pulmonary infiltrates. It needs ventilatory support and PEEP.

Respiratory quotient (RQ) (RQ) Ratio of the volume of CO_2 produced to the volume of O_2 consumed per unit of time at steady state conditions.

Respiratory syncytial virus (RSV) Most frequent cause of lower respiratory tract disease of infants and children.

Respiratory Pertaining to respiratory system.

Respiratory acidosis An acid base disturbance developing from an increase in $PaCO_2$. In a sustained elevation in $PaCO_2$, there is a rise in the level of plasma bicarbonate.

Respiratory alkalosis An acid base disturbance where CO_2 in the arterial blood is below normal range. There is hyperventilation causing an increased elimination of CO_2. There is reduction in H^+ ions and pH is raised.

Respiratory failure An inability of the respiratory system to keep the arterial blood gases at normal level while breathing ambient air at rest at sea level and the individual exhibits the partial pressure of oxygen below 60 mm Hg with or without an elevation of carbon dioxide tension above 49 mm Hg in the arterial blood. It may be acute with threat to life within minutes to hours or days or chronic developing over a prolonged period due to smouldering disease in the lung.

Respiratory quotient (RQ) Ratio of the volume of CO_2 produced to the volume of O_2 consumed per unit of time at steady state conditions.

Respiratory syndrome An immune response to high dose rifampicin therapy characterized by a flu-like complex, dyspnea, wheezing, leukopenia and thrombocytopenia.

Respiratory system Organs responsible for exchange of gases between inspired air and blood in the alveolar capillaries. They provide a surface for transfer of gases through which blood gets rid of carbon dioxide and absorbs oxygen. It maintains the arterial oxygen and carbon dioxide tensions at constant levels of 100 mm and 40 mm respectively with variations in a very narrow range and maintenance of normal acid-base balance of the body.

Response (*re-spons'*) Reaction to any stimulus.

Restiform body A cord like bundle of nerve fibers lying on each side of the medulla oblongata and connecting it with the cerebellum.

Restoration (*res-to-ra'shun*) Replacement of the lost structure.

Restriction enzyme (restriction endonuclease) An enzyme that cuts DNA at specific sites.

Retainer (*re-ta'nar*) *dent* An orthodontic appliance that is worn to stabiles teeth in a new position.

Retardation (*re-tar-dashun*) A slowness of development.

Retching Dry vomiting.

Rete (*re'te*) Net, network.

Reteplase Thrombolytic medication, works by dissolving the harmful blood clots in the blood vessels. This restores the blood flow to the affected tissue, thereby preventing tissue death and improving outcomes.

Retention (*re-ten'shun*) A holding back; retaining.

Urinary retention The inability to completely or partially empty the bladder.

Reticular activating system Is a network of neurons located in the brain stem that project anteriorly to the hypothalamus to mediate behavior, as well as both posteriorly to the thalamus and directly to the cortex for activation of awake (desynchronized cortical EEG patterns).

Reticular fibers Type of fibers in connective tissue composed of type III collagen secreted by reticular cells.

Reticular formation A small, thick cluster of neurones within the brain stem controlling breathing, heart beat, blood pressure and consciousness.

Reticulin (*re-tik'u-lin*) A scleroprotein present in the connective tissue framework.

Reticulocyte (*re-tik'u-lo-sit*) A young red blood cell containing residual ribosomal RNA.

Reticulocyte count Enumeration of reticulocytes to evaluate red cell production in the bone marrow.

Reticulocytopenia (*re-tik'u-lo-si-to-pen-ia*) A decrease in the number of circulating reticulocytes.

Reticulocytosis (*retik'u-lo-si-to'sis*) An increase in the number of circulating reticulocytes.

Reticuloendothelial system (RES) A system involved in defense against infection and disposal of the products of breakdown of cells.

Reticuloendotheliosis (histoocytotis X) (*re-tik'u-lo-en'do-the-li-o-sis*) Proliferation of reticuloendothelial system.

Reticulosis (*re-tik'u-lo-sis*) Proliferation of reticuloendothelial cells such as histiocytes, or monocytes.

Reticulum (*re-tik-u-lum*) A fine network of connective tissue fibers between cells.

Retina (*ret-i-na*) The light-sensitive membrane which lines the inside of the back of the eye, on which light are focused. It is 10-layered and continuous with the optic nerve, and transmits the visual impulses through the optic nerve to the brain.

Retinaculum (*ret-i-nak'u-lum*) A strong fibrous band.

Retinal (retinene) (*ret'i-nal*) Related to retina; aldehyde of retinol, derived from the absorbed dietary carotenoids.

Retinal-renal syndrome Nephronophthisis associated with retinal degeneration.

Retinitis (*ret-i-nitis*) Inflammation of the retina.

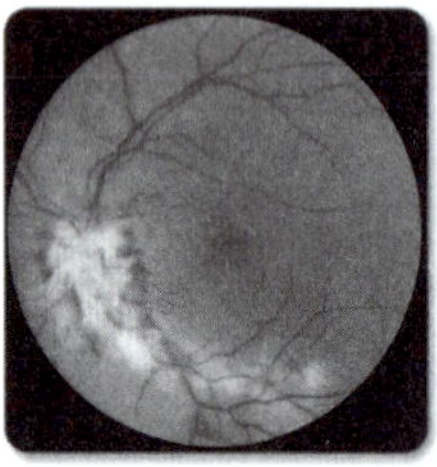

Cytomegalovirus retinitis with papillary involvement

Retinitis pigmentosa Retinal degeneration characterized by night blindness and progressive centripetal loss of visual fields progressing to blindness.

Retinitis proliferans Serous products leaking from new vessels formed in diabetic retinopathy stimulate a connective tissue reaction.

Retinoblastoma (*ret-i-no-blas-to'ma*) A malignant tumor of the retina that affects infants and children.

Endophytic retinoblastoma Retinoblastoma begins from inner layer.

Exophytic retinoblastoma Retinoblastoma begins from outer layer.

Retinol (*ret'i-nol*) A form of vitamin A, Fat soluble vitamin. Used as active ingredients in various skincare products.

Retinopathy (*ret-i-nop'a-thi*) A degenerative disorder of the retina.

Diabetic retinopathy A diabetes complication that affects eyes. It is caused by damage to the blood vessels of the light-sensitive tissue at the back of the eye (retina). There is widespread capillary nonperfusion. Retinal photocoagulation is indicated at an early stage of development.

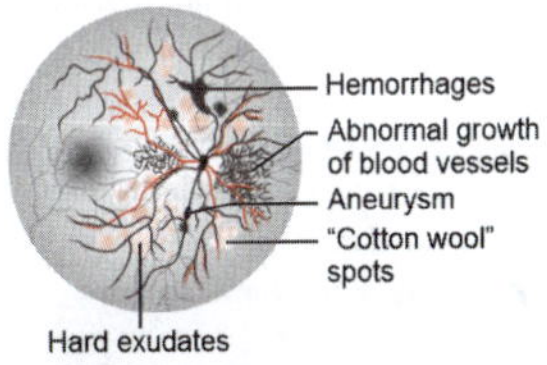

Fundal image of proliferative type of diabetic retinopathy

Hypertensive retinopathy A condition developing in individuals having prolonged hypertension. It consists of arteriolar narrowing due to vasoconstriction and intimal hyalinization (Grade I); extensive vascular thickening imparting a copper (column of blood still visible) or silver (no longer visible) 'wire' appearance with 'nicking' of the veins where they are crossed by arteries (Grade II); hemorrhages within the nerve fiber layer, exudates and marked nicking (Grade III); and edema of optic disk (Grade IV).

Stellate retinopathy Retinopathy not associated with hypertension but exhibit same symptoms as hypertensive retinopathy.

Retinoschisis (*ret'i-nos'ki-sis*) Splitting of sensory layers of the retina resulting in a fixed, smooth, convex, transparent elevation.

Retinoscope (*reti-no-skop*) An optical device used in retinoscopy.

Retraction (*re-trak'shun*) Drawing back; posterior movement.

Retraction ring Refer Bandl's ring.

Retractor (*re-trak'tor*) An instrument to draw aside the structures.

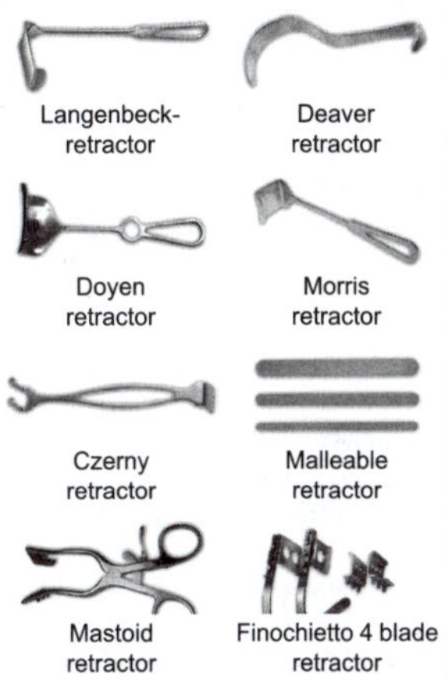

Retractors used in surgery

Retrobulbar neuritis (optic neuritis) Neuropathy affecting the optic nerve.

Retroflexion (*re-tro-flek'shun*) Backward bending.

Retrograde (*re-tro-grad*) Moving backward; degenerative.

Retrograde amnesia Loss of memory regarding the events preceding the accident.

Retrograde ejaculation An ejaculation of semen in a reverse direction into the urinary bladder.

Retrograde flow Regurgitation.

Retrograde infection An infection that spreads along a tube or duct against the flow of secretions or excretions.

Retrograde pyelography A radiologic technique to examine the structures of the collecting system of the kidneys, wherein a radiopaque contrast medium is injected through a urinary catheter into the ureters and calyces of the pelvis of the kidney. It is useful in locating a urinary tract obstruction.

Retroperitoneal fibrosis (RPF) A chronic inflammatory process of unknown etiology in which fibrous tissue surrounds the large blood vessels in the lower lumbar region.

Retropulsion (*retro-pul'shun*) An involuntary backward walking.

Retroversion (*re-tro-ver'zhun*) Turning backward.

Retrovirus (*re-tro-vi-rus*) An RNA virus possessing reverse transcriptase. It can insert and efficiently express its own genetic-information in a host cell's genome by transcribing its own RNA to DNA that is integrated with a host cells genome.

Retrusion (*re-troo'zhan*) The act of moving a tooth backward.

Rett's syndrome A rare genetic neurological disorder that occurs almost exclusively in girls, rarely in boys; caused by X-chromosome mutation. Hallmark is near constant repetitive hand movements.

Reverse transcriptase *mol* An RNA dependent DNA polymerase that is capable of copying genomic RNA into DNA, catalyzing the synthesis of DNA using retroviral RNA as a template.

Reverse transcriptase inhibitors Agents preventing the spread of infectious virus to uninfected cells but do not affect replication of the HIV genome once integrated into the host cell.

Reye's syndrome Occurrence of brain and liver damage following a viral infection and it may be related to taking aspirin for treatment of infection. There is vomiting, hepatic dysfunction, and minimal neurologic impairment often preceded by viral upper respiratory tract infection. It affects children under 15, is named after Ralph Reye, Australian pathologist.

Rh Rhesus

Rh blood group A blood group classified by the presence or absence of a Rh factor on the surface of red blood cells.

Rh factor An antigenic substance present in the erythrocytes. The person having the factor is Rh^+ (Rh positive), a person lacking the factor is Rh^- (Rh negative).

Rh immune globulin An Rh immune globulin concentrate used to prevent the maternal immunization against the infant's Rh group D antigen.

Rh incompatibility Lack of compatibility between two groups of blood cells that are antigenically different due to the presence of the Rh factor in one group and absence of the Rh factor in another.

Rhabdomyoma (*rab'do-mi-o'ma*) A benign tumor of skeletal muscle. Rhabdomyomas are the most common type of cardiac tumors seen in infants and children. Cardiac rhabdomyomas usually grow in the muscles of the left and right ventricles (the lower chambers of the heart).

Rhabdomyosarcoma (*rab'do-mi-o-sar-ko'ma*) A rare type of cancer that forms in soft tissue—specifically skeletal muscle tissue or sometimes hollow organs such as the bladder or uterus. It can occur at any age, but it most often affects children.

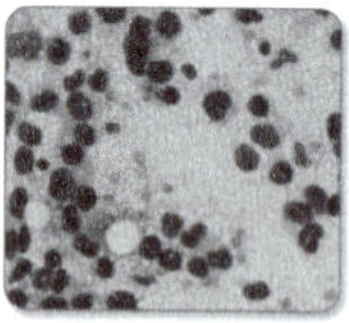

Rhabdomyosarcoma showing characteristic —round, spindled and plumper rhabdoid cells

Rhagades (*raga-des*) Cracks or fissures at mucocutaneous junctions.

R factor An episome in bacteria that is responsible for drug resistance.

Rheumatic (*ru-mati'k*) Relating to rheumatism.

Rheumatic fever A condition affecting children or young adults that is triggered by infection with group A streptococci which possess antigens that cross-react with human connective tissue particularly heart valve glycoprotein. It is a systemic illness presenting with fever, anorexia, lethargy and joint pains. The diagnosis is based on Jones Criteria (*see* Jones Criteria).

Rheumatic heart disease Damage to heart valves and heart muscle resulting from rheumatic fever.

Rheumatism (*ru'ma-tizm*) A painful condition arising from articular or other elements of musculoskeletal system.

Muscular rheumatism Fibrositis.

Palindromic rheumatism Repeated attacks of arthritis and periarthritis without pyrexia and do not causes irriversible joint changes.

Rheumatoid Resembling rheumatism.

Rheumatoid arthritis An autoimmune inflammatory arthropathy presenting with morning stiffness in and around joints lasting at least one hour before maximum improvement, soft tissue swelling of three or more joint, swelling of the proximal interphalangeal, metacarpophalangeal or wrist joints, symmetric arthritis.

Rheumatoid factors (RF) Polyclonal IgM antibodies produced by synovial neutrophils in a majority of patients with rheumatoid arthritis, which may be demonstrated by erythrocyte agglutination (Rose-Waalar test) or latex agglutination test.

Rheumatoid nodule A mass consisting of central necrosis surrounded by successive rims of fibrinoid degeneration, fibrosis and palisaded serous membranes and lung parenchyma in some patients with rheumatoid arthritis.

Rheumatoid pneumonitis Diffuse interstitial fibrosis encountered infrequently in rheumatoid arthritis.

Rheumatology (*roo"me-tol'o-je*) The branch of medicine that deals with painful, typically inflammatory or infectious conditions of the joints and other parts of the musculoskeletal system.

Rhexis (*rek'sis*) Rupture of a vessel or organ.

Rhin-(rhino-) Referring to nose.

Rhinencephalon (*ri-nen-sef'a-lon*) The part of the cerebral hemisphere containing structures of the sense of the smell.

Rhinitis (*ri-ni'tis*) Inflammation of nasal mucosa, which causes sneezing, nasal discharge and facial discomfort.

Allergic rhinitis Occurs as an immediate hypersensitivity reaction to allergens in the nasal mucosa.

Atrophic rhinitis A chronic condition characterized by symptoms of crusting, purulent discharge, nasal obstruction, and halitosis.

Fibrinous rhinitis Membranous.

Membranous rhinitis Chronic rhinitis with false membrane formation.

Nonseasonal allergic rhinitis Rhinitis occurring through out the year.

Tuberculous rhinitis Rhinitis due to tuberculous.

Vasomotor rhinitis Rhinitis caused by physical or chemical irritants.

Rhinolith (*rino-lith*) Nasal calculus.

Rhinology (*rino'lo-ji*) Medical science concerned with the nose and its diseases.

Rhinomycosis (*ri'no-mi-kosis*) Fungal infection of the nasal mucous membrane.

Rhinophyma (*ri'no-fi-ma*) Bulbous deformity and redness of the nose. It occurs as a severe complication of rosacea, occurring primarily in elderly men.

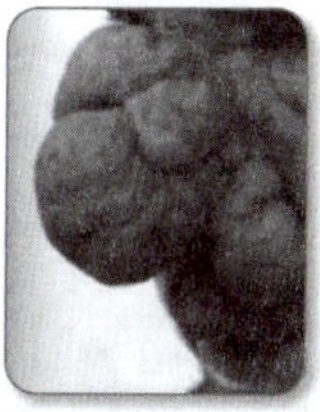

Rhinophyma

Rhinoplasty (*rino-plas-ti*) A surgical procedure to change the structure of the nose either for cosmetic purpose or to correct an injury or deformity.

Rhinorrhea (*ri-no-re'ah*) A discharge from the nasal mucosa.

Cerebrospinal fluid rhinorrhea Discharge of CSF though nose.

Rhinoscleroma (*ri-no-skle-ro'ma*) A chronic granulomatous condition affecting the nose, upper lip, oral cavity and upper air way.

Rhinoscopy (*ri'no-skopi*) Visualization of the nasal cavity.

Anterior rhinoscopy Examination of anterior part of the nasal cavity by nasal speculum under good illumination.

Posterior rhinoscopy Visualization of posterior nares by placing a mirror behind the uvula and soft palate.

Rhinosporidiosis (*rino-spo-rid-i-o'sis*) Chronic granulomatous condition of nasal mucosa due to *Rhinosporidium seeberi*, an yeast-like organism.

Rhinovirus (*ri'no-virus*) Virus associated with common cold.

Rhipicephalus (*ri"pi-sefa-bs*) Belongs to genus of ixodid ticks that are parasitic on many mammals and some birds and include vectors of serious diseases.

Rhizotomy (*ri-zot'o-mi*) Section of the nerve roots.

Rhodnius (*rod'ne-as*) A genus of South American insects of Family Reduviidae, a major vector of Chagas disease, an illness caused by *Trypanosoma cruzi*.

Rhodopsin (*ro-dop'sin*) Visual purple.

Rhombencephalon (*rom"ben-sefa-lon*) Also known as hindbrain, a developmental categorization of portions of the central nervous system in vertebrates.

Rhomboid (*rom'boyd*) Oblique with unequal sides.

Rhonchus (*rong'kus*) Wheezy continuous, dry adventitious respiratory sound having a musical pitch. pl. **ronchi**.

Sibilant rhonchus Obstruction of smaller bronchi result in high-pitched rhonchi as whistling or squeaking sounds.

Sonorous rhonchus Obstruction of larger bronchi producing low pitched, snoring quality sounds.

Rhythm method A contraceptive method where unprotected intercourse is allowed shortly after a menstrual period or before the onset of the next period.

Rib Costa, one of the 12 pairs of elastic bony structure forming thoracic cage.

Rib cage The bony framework of bones attached to the spine and the sternum that supports the chest wall and protects the heart, lungs and other organs in the chest.

Ribonuclease (*ri-bo-nu'kle-as*) RNase, an enzyme that catalysis the hydrolysis of ribonucleic acid.

Ribonucleic acid (*ribo-nu-kle'ik*) RNA, a ribonucleoside present in all cells in the nuclei and cytoplasm that helps to decode the genetic instructions carried in the DNA of cell.

Ribose (*ri'bos*) Pentose present in RNA.

Ribosome (*ri-bo-som*) A particle of ribonucleoprotein found inside cell which plays an important role in the protein synthesis.

Rib-tip syndrome Sharp episodic pain at the costal margin caused by hypermotility of the anterior end of tenth rib, often due to trauma.

Rice water stools Clear and watery diarrhea with flecks of mucus giving an appearance of water boiled rice, an appearance seen in cholera.

Richter's syndrome (*rik'terz*) A large cell lymphomatous transformation as a terminal event in chronic lymphocytic leukemia described by August Richter, US pathologist.

Richter's hernia A hernia wherein a portion of the circumference of the bowel is strangulated. It is common in femoral hernia. The diagnosis is delayed as the patient is able to pass flatus and feces, named after August Richter, German surgeon.

Ricin A highly toxic protein obtained from the pressed seeds of the castor oil plant from the waste left when castor beans are made into castor oil.

Rickets (*rik'ets*) A vitamin D deficiency seen primarily in infancy and childhood associated with excess production and deficient calcification of osteoid tissue resulting in bony deformities, like bow legs and knock knee. It responds to vitamin D and calcium supplementation.

Adult rickets Osteomalacia.

Familial rickets A genetic condition causing rickets.

Fetal rickets Achondroplasia.

Renal rickets Rickets resulting from chronic renal insufficiency.

Vitamin D dependent rickets Characterized by early-onset rickets due to the inability to maintain adequate concentrations of active forms of vitamin D or a failure to respond fully to activated vitamin D.

Vitamin D resistant rickets A group of rare disease characterized by lack of reaction to vitamin D administered in doses sufficient to manage patients with rickets caused by vitamin D deficiency.

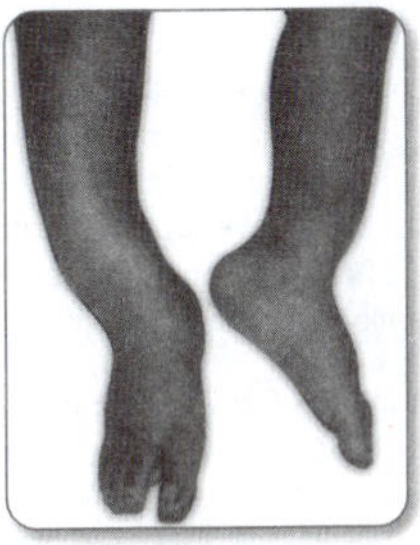

Vitamin D deficiency rickets

X-linked hypophosphatemic rickets A rare genetic disorder related to low levels of phosphate in the blood, termed hypophosphatemia.

Rickettsialpox A mite-borne infectious skin disease caused by Rickettsia akari.

Ridge *(rij)* A projection or projecting structure; crest; a long, narrow, raised part of a surface, especially a high edge of a hill or mountain.

Dental ridge Linear elevation on the crown of teeth.

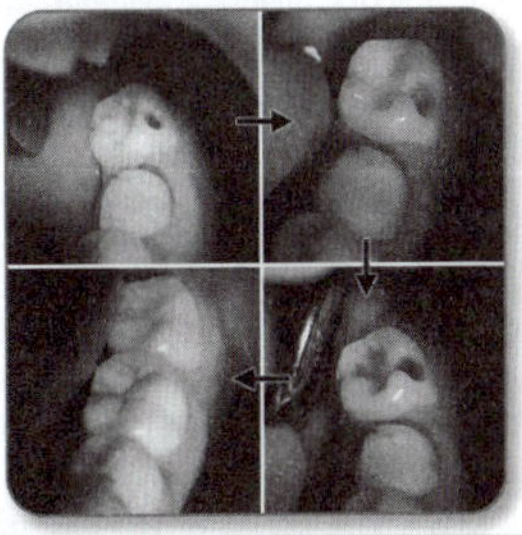

Dental ridge care

Mammary ridge Primordium specific for development of mammary gland.

Rete ridge Epithelial extensions that project into underlying connective tissue in both skin and mucous membrane.

Urogenital ridge Structure give rise to gonads, adrenal cortex, kidney and reproductive tract.

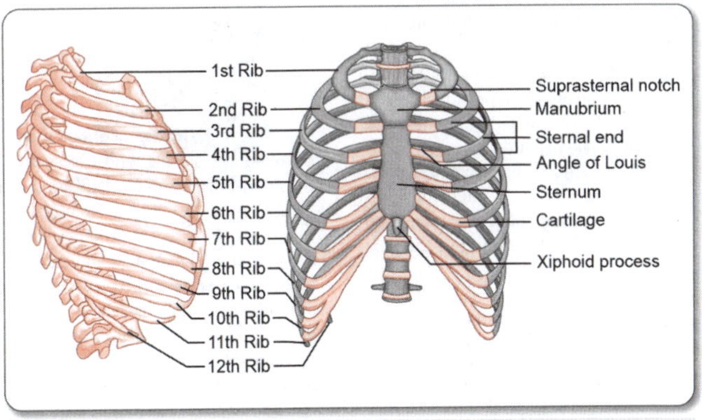

Rib cage

Rifabutin A broad spectrum antibiotic used to treat Mycobacterium avium complex disease in patients with HIV.

Rifampin (*rif-am'pin*) A semisynthetic derivative of rifamycin, with the antibacterial actions and uses of the rifamycin group; administered orally or intravenously.

Rifamycin (*rif'a-mi'sin*) A group of antibiotics whose activity depends on its high affinity for prokaryotic RNA polymerase inhibiting bacterial DNA-dependent RNA synthesis, used to treat traveler's diarrhea.

Rift valley fever Viral, zoonotic disease which causes disease in humans, ranging from mild flue-like illness to severe hemorrhagic fever that can be fatal.

Rigidity (*ri-jid-i-ti*) Stiffness; assumption of a rigid posture, against all efforts to be moved.

Cogwheel rigidity Resistance less uniform and diminishing in jerky steps when the rigidity and tremors coexist.

Decerebrate rigidity Also known as extensor posturing, it is the involuntary extensor positioning of the arms, flexion of the hands, with knee extension and plantar flexion when stimulated as a result of a midbrain lesion.

Decorticate rigidity A condition characterized by abnormal posturing of the limbs that is associated with injury to the brainstem.

Hysterical rigidity Resistance to passive movements is proportional to the amount of force applied.

Lead pipe rigidity Resistance felt to the same degree throughout passive movement.

Paratonic rigidity An uniform resistance during all phases of passive movements as in catatonic states and dementia.

Rigor (*rig'er*) Stiff; violent attack of shivering.

Rigor mortis Stiffening of muscles that occurs after death. There is rigid contraction of skeletal muscles that is first seen in the jaw 2–4 hours after death, later appearing on the trunk and extremities, reaching its peak at 48 hours, disappearing in the same order of its development; cadaveric rigidity.

Rima A narrow elongated opening between two symmetric margins.

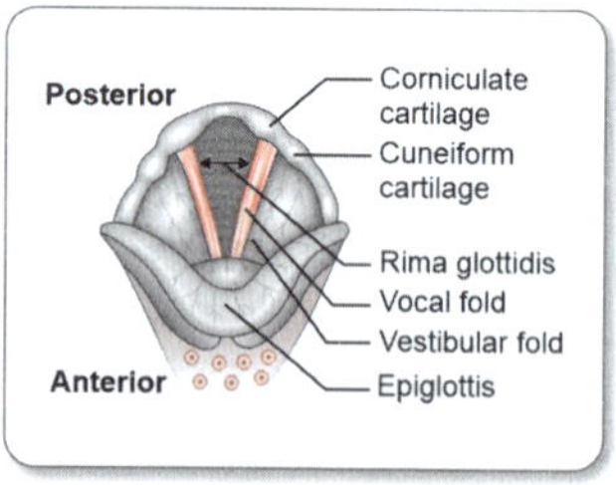

Anatomy of larynx showing Rima glottidis - Glottis (open)

Ring A circular band or structure.

Contraceptive ring A type of birth control method, worn inside the vagina.

Cytoplasmic ring Ring formed to assist the import of materials from cytoplasm into nucleus.

Hernial ring A well defined defect in transverse aponeurosis.

Kayser-Fleischer ring Golden brown deposit at the level of Descemet's membrane of cornea, seen in Wilson's disease.

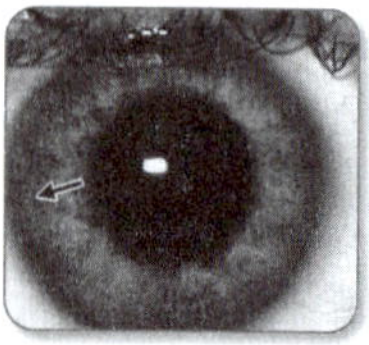

Kayser-Fleischer ring

Ring abscess Histological appearance of an abscess seen in infective endocarditis which consists of a central focus of neutrophils, necrosis and bacteria surrounded by fibroblasts and fibrosis.

Ring enhancement CT finding in the brain consisting of a radiolucent zone surrounded by a faint radio dense rim, which in turn is surrounded by a second radiolucent zone outside of the rim. These rings correspond to regional edema, hyper vascularity, and hypercellularity.

Ring shadows Annular thickening of the bronchial walls seen by a plain roentgenogram in bronchiectasis.

Ringer's solution (Ringer's mixture) A physiological saline solution that typically contains sodium chloride and salts of potassium and calcium.

Ringworm (tinea) Dermatophyte, tinea capable of invading the keratinized tissue of skin, nail or hair. The lesions begin as a scaly plaque spreading centrifugally with central clearing.

Rinne's test Normally the sound is conducted, better through the air than bone. A vibrating tuning fork is placed on the mastoid process on one side while the other ear is closed. When the patient stops hearing the sound, the tines of the fork are brought near the ear and noted whether the patient still hears the sound. In diseases of middle ear the bone conduction is better than air conduction. In nerve deafness both are lost, named after Heinrich Rinne, German otologist.

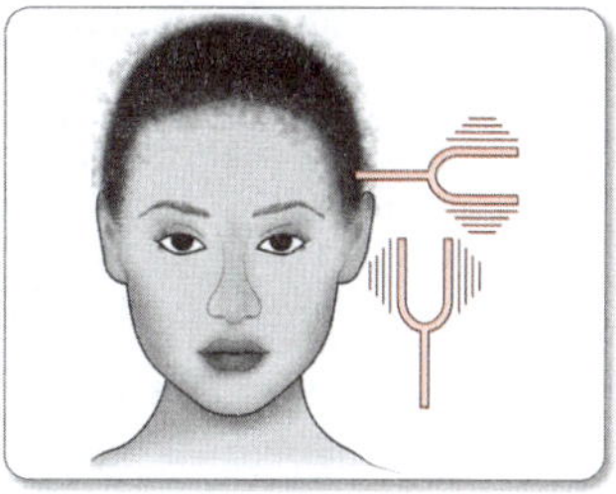

Rinne's test

Risk The probability of suffering from a particular disease.

Risk assessment The process by which new chemical substances are evaluated for their potential impact on human health.

Risk management Activities involved in reducing the risks of injury to the patients.

Risk ratio (RR) The probability of the occurrence of a disease in a group that has been exposed to some environmental, medicinal, microbial, or toxic influence, relative to its probability in a randomly selected population.

Risperidone A benzisoxazole preparation for psychosis.

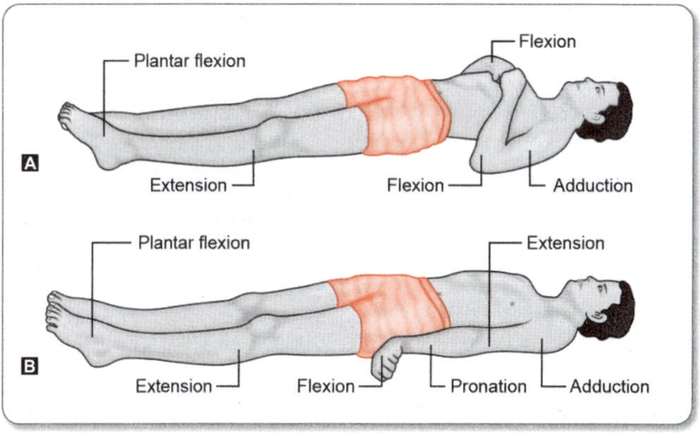

A. *Decorticate rigidity;* ***B.*** *Decerebrate rigidity*

Risus sardonicus Grinning facial expression seen in tetanus.

Rituximab (*ri-tuk'si-mab*) A monoclonal antibody which is anti CD20 chimeric antibody presents with human IgG1 immunoglobulin constant regions and variable regions from an anti CD20 murine antibody, used to treat certain autoimmune diseases and types of cancer.

River blindness Infection with filarial worm, Onchocerca, causing blindness due to punctate keratitis, corneal fibrosis, iridocyclitis, glaucoma and optic atrophy; it is named river blindness because the blackfly that transmits the infection lives and breeds near fast-flowing streams and rivers, mostly near remote rural villages. The infection can result in visual impairment and sometimes blindness.

RNA (ribonucleic acid) Ribonucleic acid.

Negative sense RNA Group of RNA with genetic content being antisense complementary to mRNA.

Positive sense RNA Having positive sense single stranded RNA.

Ribosomal RNA Forms protein synthesizing organelles known as ribosome.

RNA interference The inhibition of gene expression by noncoding RNA molecules.

RNA polymerase Enzyme that copy strands of RNA from DNA template.

Transfer RNA RNA helps in decoding a messenger RNA sequence into protein.

Rocky mountain spotted fever (spotted fever, tick fever) An infectious disease caused by *R. rickettsii* transmitted by ticks and characterized by small pink spots on the wrists and ankle, enlargement of regional lymph nodes. It responds to tetracycline or chloramphenicol.

Rod A straight slender cylinder; photosensitive cell of the retina, that contains rhodopsin which adapts the eye to detect low intensity light.

Olfactory rods Rods help in smell.

Retinal rods Rods present in retina and help in vision.

Rodent ulcer A deeply invasive basal cell carcinoma.

Roentgen (*ront'gen*) The international unit of dose exposure to X- or gamma-radiation, named after the discoverer of X-rays, Wilhelm Conrad Roentgen, German physicist.

Roentgenology (*rent'gen-olo-ji*) Radiology concerned with study of the diagnostic and therapeutic uses of X-rays.

Romana's sign Unilateral firm reddish swelling of the lids in Chaga's disease, described by Cecilio Romana, Argentine physician.

Romanowsky effect Romanowsky staining (A mixture of methylene blue, azure and eosin) produces wide range of color shades, allowing cellular components to be easily differentiated. The phenomenon is called Romanowsky effect or metachromasia.

Romberg sign A special test to demonstrate incoordination in the lower limbs, especially sensory ataxia. The patient loses balance when standing erect, feet together and eyes closed, named after Moritz' Romberg, German physician.

Rongeur (*ron-zhur*) Forceps useful to nip the bone.

Root *(root)* The embedded part of an organ or structure such as hair, tooth or nerve.

Root canal A pulp filled channel in a root of a tooth; a treatment in which diseased tissue from this part of tooth is removed and cavity is filled with an inert material.

Root file A small metal hand instrument used for cleaning and shaping a root canal

Root filling A material placed in the root canal of a tooth to seal the space previously occupied by the dental pulp.

Rorschach test (*ror'shak*) *psy* A psychological projective assessment test in which a person is asked to respond to a series of ink blots by saying what image or emotion each one evokes; ink blot test named after Hermann Rorschach, Swiss psychiatrist.

Rosacea (*ro-za'she-a*) A chronic inflammatory facial eruption consisting of erythema often accompanied by papules.

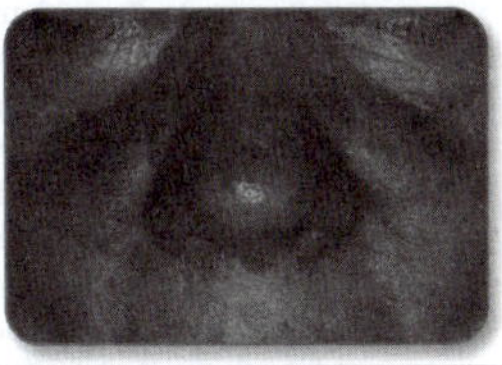

Rosacea

Roseola (*ro-ze'o-la*) Rose-red colored small eruptions.

Roseola infantum An infectious disease that primarily affects young children and is characterized by irritability, fever and rash.

Rose-Waaler test An anti-immunoglobulin test with sheep erythrocytes sensitized with rabbit anti-sheep erythrocyte IgE. If the test serum contains 'rheumatoid factor it combines with the membrane-bound IgE and causes agglutination.

Rostellum (*ros-tel'um*) The anterior part of the scolex of a tapeworm with a row of hooks.

Rostrum (*ros'trum*) Beak-like structure.

Rotator A muscle that helps a part to turn circularly.

Rotator cuff The musculotendinous covering of the shoulder joint, bounded inferiorly by the subscapularis muscles, superiorly by the supraspinatus muscle and posteriorly by the infraspinatus and teres muscles.

Rothera's test A method of testing urine for the presence of acetone or autoacetic acid—a sign of diabetes mellitus.

Roth's spots Round or oval white spots seen in the retina in subacute bacterial endocarditis, named after Moritz Roth, Swiss physician.

Roughage (*ruf'ij*) Indigestible food material.

Rouleaux (*roo-lo'*) Stacking of red blood cells occurring in presence of increased plasma fibrinogen and globulins.

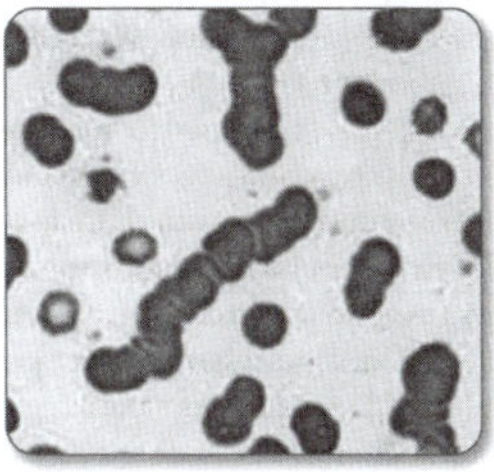

Rouleaux formation of human RBCs

Round window A round opening in the medial wall of the middle ear leading into the cochlea.

Roundworm A nematode belonging to the phylum Nemathelminths.

Rovsing's sign (*rov'singz*) Application of pressure on the left iliac fossa causes pain in the right iliac fossa in acute appendicitis, named after Nils Rovsing, Danish surgeon.

RSV Respiratory syncytial virus.

Rubber dam A thin sheet of latex rubber for isolating one or more teeth during a dental procedure.

Rubefacient (*ru-be-fa'shent*) Agent causing a reddening of the skin; a counter irritant producing redness on application to the skin surface.

Rubella embryopathy Any congenital abnormality in infant caused by maternal rubella in early stages of pregnancy.

Rubeola (*ru-be'o-la*) Also known as measles, a highly contagious, an airborne disease which spreads easily from one person to the next through the coughs and sneezes of infected people. It is vaccine-preventable infectious disease caused by measles virus.

Rubidium (*Rb*) A silver-white, metallic, active element resembling potassium, used in photoelectric cells and radio vacuum tubes.

Rubor Redness of the skin generally around the site of wound.

Rubrospinal tract A descending pathway that starts as axons of the neurons present in the red nucleus and terminates by synapsing with the interneurons in the spinal cord. It is part of the extrapyramidal system and is important for regulating the activity of the motor neurons.

Ruffini's corpuscles *(roo-fe'nez)* Certain nerve endings concerned in the perception of pressure and warmth, named after Angelo Ruffini, Italian anatomist.

Ruga A fold; a wrinkle, pl. **rugae**.

Rule *(rul)* Criterion or standard.

Rule of forceps A rule giving a hint about the handle of the forceps to be used on which side of the mother to be: left blade, left handle and left side of mother; right blade, right handle and right side of mother.

Rule of nine A quick method to assess the extent of burns on the skin surface. The head, upper extremities on either side, anterior or posterior surface of lower extremities on either side, represent 9% of skin surface, the anterior and posterior trunk represent 18% each and the inguinal area 1%.

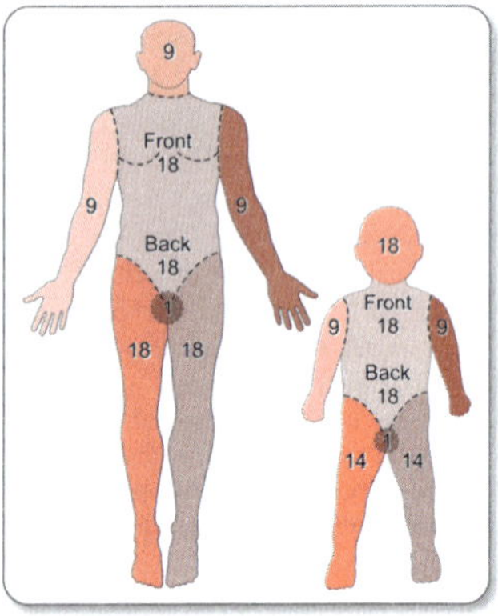

Rule of nine

Rumination syndrome Regurgitation of food 10–15 minutes following deglutition, which may be brought out or chewed and swallowed may be noted in those with emotional and intellectual defects or in children with marasmus.

Rupture *(rup'chur)* A break or a tear in continuity of an organ or body tissue.

Rusty lungs Brown induration of the lungs due to accumulation of hemosiderin laden macrophages.

Rusty sputum Sputum composed of bacteria, hemorrhage, mucus and sloughed tissue seen in pneumonia produced by *Streptococcus pneumonia.*

Rutherford *(ruth'ar-ford)* A unit of activity equal to the quantity of a radioactive nuclide required to produce one million disintegrations per second.

Ruxolitinib A kinase inhibitor used to treat various types of myelofibrosis, polycythemia vera in patients who have not responded to or cannot tolerate hydroxyurea, and to treat graft-versus-host disease in cases that are refractory to steroid treatment.

Rx Recipe, prescription.

Ryle's tube A thin, flexible rubber tube of 75 cm length, having markings at 30.5 cm, 40 cm and 57 cm indicating the position of the tip of the tube in the cardiac end of the stomach, in the stomach and duodenum respectively when each mark is opposite the teeth. The tube has a blind bulbous end containing a lead shot and is perforated by several small holes at the sides 2 cm from the tip, named after Jhon Ryle, professor of Social Medicine at Oxford.

S

Sabin vaccine A live oral vaccine to prevent poliomyelitis prepared by Albert Sabin, Russian-born US virologist.

Sac (*sak*) A pouch; a bag-like organ or structure.

Abdominal sac The part of the embryonic celom that develops into the abdominal cavity.

Air sac Alveolar sac.

Allantoic sac Expanded portion of the allantois that becomes part of the placenta in many mammals.

Alveolar sac Air sacs from which alveoli arise. Alveoli are the terminal, blind-ending structures. They are connected with the respiratory bronchiole through alveolar ducts. Alveoli have a continuous layer of epithelial cells. The elastic reticular framework, small arterioles and a meshwork of capillaries surround the alveoli. Gas exchange occurs mostly in blind-ended alveolar ductal system and alveoli

Amniotic sac Amnion.

Chorionic sac Chorion that encloses developing embryo.

Conjunctival sac The potential space lined by conjunctiva between the eyelids and the anterior surface of the eyeball.

Dental sac The mesenchymal tissue surrounding a developing tooth.

Endolymphatic sac The blind expanded distal end of the endolymphatic duct.

Heart sac Pericardium.

Hernial sac A sac-like protrusion of peritoneum containing a herniated structure.

Lacrimal sac Dilated upper end of the nasolacrimal duct situated in the groove of the lacrimal bone.

Lesser peritoneal sac Omental bursa.

Yolk sac The extra embryonic membrane that connects with the midgut.

Sacchar- (saccharo-) (*sak'a-ras*) An enzyme that catalyzes the breakdown of disaccharides to monosaccharides such as sucrose to dextrose.

Saccharide (*sak'a-rid*) One of a series of carbohydrates such as monosaccharides, disaccharides, oligosaccharides and polysaccharides.

Saccharin (*sak'a-rin*) A white synthetic crystalline compound that is sweeter

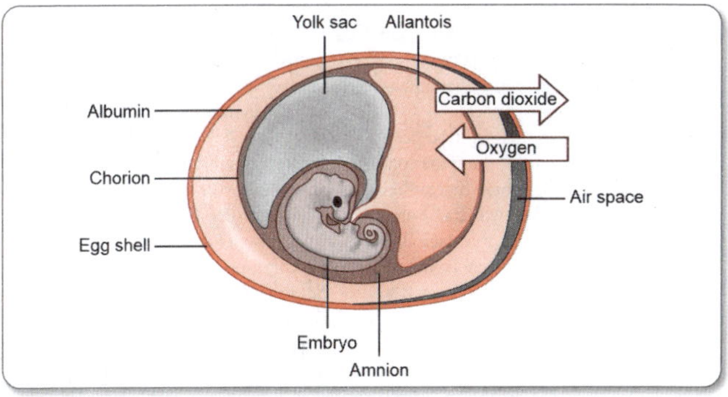

Yolk sac

than sugar, and used as a non-nutritive sweetener.

Saccharin clearance time Test to measure rate of ciliary movement of mucus by putting a saccharin tablet on inferior turbinate and appreciating sweet taste in the pharynx.

Saccharomyces (*sak'a-ro-mi'sez*) A genus of yeasts.

Saccharomyces boulardii This species is used as a probiotic in treatment of diarrhea.

Saccharomyces carlsbergensis A species used in microbiological assay in measuring vitamin B6 in the urine, and in the brewing of beer; also seen in some cases of mycosis of stomach.

Saccharomyces cerevisiae Brewers' yeast or bakers' yeast, a species with oval or spherical cells, used for alcoholic fermentation and leavening in bread; sometimes causes lung disease.

Saccharomyces fragilis A species that is sometimes part of the normal flora of the human throat and gastrointestinal tract but can also cause opportunistic infection.

Sacculus (saccule) (*sak'u-lus*) Pl. **sacculi**. Saccule.

Saccus (*sak'us*) Pl. **sacci**. A sac.

Sacralization (*sa'kral-i-za'shun*) Fusion of the fifth lumbar vertebra with the sacrum.

Sacral vertebrae One of the fused vertebrae forming the sacrum.

Sacroiliitis (*sak'ro-il'e-i'tis*) Inflammation of the sacroiliac joints, usually caused by ankylosing spondylitis, that causes aching pain in the lower back.

Sacrum (*sa'krum*) The large, triangular bone in the lower part of the spine consisting five united vertebrae that sit like a wedge between the two iliac bones and articulations form the sacroiliac joints, name borrowed from Egyptians who considered the bone was sacred to Osiris, their God of resurrection.

Scimitar Sacrum A deformed sacrum resembling a short curved sword accompanied by anorectal or neural anomalies.

Saddle joint A joint at the base of the thumb that has two inter-locking saddle-shaped surfaces.

Sadism (*sad'izm*) Sexual gratification by inflicting mental or physical pain on others, named after Marquis de Sade, French author.

Anal Sadism With regard to psychoanalytic theory, the displaying of demanding urges in the anal stage of psychosexual development, concerning the deterioration of an item and its ownership and management. It is developed in adults as anal-aggressive personality.

Oral Sadism Characterized by the advent of aggressiveness, by ambivalence, and by the anxiety associated with the destruction of the loved object and the fear of being devoured in turn by that object.

Phallic Sadism In classical psychoanalytic theory, aggression that is associated with the child's phallic stage of psychosexual development. The child interprets sexual intercourse as a violent, aggressive activity on the part of the man and particularly on the part of the penis.

Sexual Sadism The condition of experiencing sexual arousal in response to the extreme pain, suffering or humiliation of others.

Safe period An interval of the menstrual cycle when fertilization is considered to be least likely.

Safe sex The practice of protecting oneself and one's partner from sexually transmitted diseases by using condoms.

Safranin (safranine) Stain used in histology and cytology.

Sagittal (*saj'i-t'l*) Arrow-like; situated in the direction of the sagittal suture; in an anteroposterior direction.

Sagittal outlet Diameter of pelvic brim from lower end of sacrum to lower edge of symphysis.

Sagittal plane A vertical plane through the longitudinal axis of the trunk dividing the body into two parts.

Sagittal sulcus A groove in the inner surface of the parietal bones, forming a channel for the superior sagittal sinus.

Sagittal suture Interparietal suture, line of union between two parietal bones.

Sagittal suture Interparietal suture, line of union between two parietal bones.

Sahli's method (*sah'lez*) Conversion of hemoglobin into acid hematin by adding HCI and comparing the color with a standard color scale to estimate hemoglobin, named after Hermann Sahli, Bern physician.

Saint's triad Hiatus hernia, gall stones and diverticulosis, named after J. Saint, South African surgeon.

St Anthony's fire Inflammation of the skin associated with ergot poisoning.

Salbutamol (*sal-bu-ta'mol*) A beta-2 adrenergic agent that combines with beta-2 receptors on bronchial smooth muscle to increase production of cyclic AMP and reverse airway obstruction used as a bronchodilator.

Salicylamide (*sali-sil-am'id*) An amide salt of salicylic acid used as an analgesic and antipyretic.

Salicylic acid (*sal'i-sil'ik*) A whity crystalline acid derived from phenol. Its salt as sodium salicylate acts as an analgesic. Topically it is a keratolytic agent.

Salicylism (*sal'i-sil'ism*) A toxic condition caused by an overdose of salicylic acid or its salts presenting with tinnitus, nausea and vomiting. There is a severe metabolic acidosis and a large anion gap.

Saline (normal saline) (*sa'lin*) Salty; containing salt or a salt solution.

Hypertonic saline An aqueous solution of sodium chloride of greater than 0.85%.

Hypotonic saline An aqueous solution of sodium chloride of less than 0.85%.

Isotonic saline A 0.9% solution of sodium chloride with an osmolality similar to that of blood serum.

Physiological saline An isotonic aqueous solution of sodium chloride.

Saline cathartic A salt capable of evacuation of the bowel.

Saline enema Enema containing sodium chloride solution to induce peristalsis and evacuation.

Saliva (*sa-li'va*) A secretion of salivary glands and oral mucous glands. It consists of inorganic substances and enzymes and daily secretion is about 1.5 liter. It initiates digestion of starches, moistens the oral mucosa, and lubricates food for tasting, chewing and swallowing.

Saliva ejector A device used during dental work to remove saliva.

Salivary gland Three pairs of glands - parotid, submandibular and sublingual glands - that secrete saliva to initiate digestion. The saliva travels from the glands through ducts into the mouth.

Salivation (*sal'i-va'shun*) The act of secretion of saliva.

Salk vaccine (*sawk*) An injectable, formalin-inactivated vaccine of poliomyelitis virus, used to induce immunity against the disease, prepared by Jonas Salk, US microbiologist.

Salmonella (*sal'mo-nel'a*) A genus of gram-negative, motile bacteria belonging to the family Enterobacteriaceae. The pathogenic species causes food poisoning and enteric fever. The organisms are named after Daniel Salmon, US veterinarian. S. cholerae suis is a species occurring in pigs which may cause gastroenteritis in humans. S. paratyphi is a group of organisms of Salmonella types A, B, and C, causing paratyphoid fever. S. typhimurium is a species responsible for acute gastroenteritis.

Salmonellosis (*sal'mo-ne-lo'sis*) Infection with organisms of the genus Salmonella. Salmonella species other than S. typhi are very common causes of food poisoning.

Salping- (salpingo-) (*sal'pin-je-on*) A point at the inferior surface of the apex of the petrous portion of a temporal bone.

Salpingectomy (*sal'pin-jek'to-me*) Surgical removal of one or both fallopian tubes; tubectomy.

Salpingitis (*sal'pin-ji'tis*) Inflammation or infection of fallopian tube or the eustachian tube.

Chronic intestinal Salpingitis Inflammation of the fallopian tubes, caused by bacterial infection, usually follows an acute attack. The infection is milder, longer lasting and may not produce many noticeable symptoms.

Hemorrhagic Salpingitis Salpingitis associated with bleeding.

Pseudofollicular Salpingitis Inflammation of the uterine tube characterized by agglutination of its walls, causing a formation of saccules.

Acute Salpingitis The fallopian tubes become red and swollen, and secrete extra fluid so that the inner walls of the tubes often stick together.

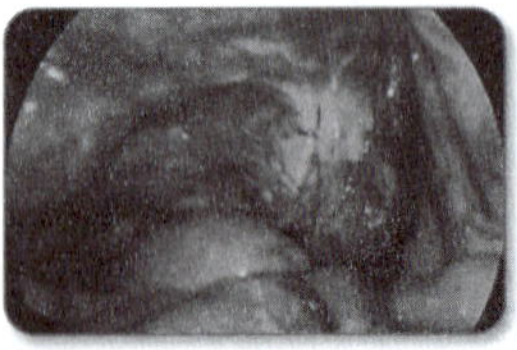

Acute salpingitis with dense adhesions that obscure the ovary. Dye has been instilled into the swollen uterine tube on the right (blue)

Salpingography (*sal'ping-gog'ra-fe*) Radiographic examination of fallopian tubes after injection of a radiopaque contrast medium. It is performed to test the patency of the tubes.

Salpingo-oophoritis (*sal-ping'go-o'of'o-ri'tis*) Inflammation of a fallopian tube and ovary.

Salpingostomy (*sal-pingo-os'to-me*) A surgical procedure to make an opening in a blocked fallopian tube.

Salt wasting disease A condition of excessive loss of sodium from the body seen in patients with renal cystic disease, obstructive uropathy, tubulointestinal disease, adrenocortical insufficiency or gastrointestinal disease. These patients require a high sodium and water intake to prevent fluid depletion and worsening of renal function; Salt losing syndrome.

Sanatorium (*san'a-to're-um*) An institution for treatment of sick persons with chronic diseases such as tuberculosis or mental disorders, and for recuperation of health under medical supervision.

Sandfly Any of various two-winged flies belonging to the genus Phlebotomus that transmit leishmaniasis, and sandfly fever.

Sandfly fever A mild viral illness resembling influenza without respiratory manifestations, transmitted by sandfly Phlebotomus papatasi.

Sandfly fever (pappataci fever) A mild viral illness resembling influenza without respiratory manifestations, transmitted by sandfly Phlebotomus papatasi.

Sandpaper skin Coarse, bumpy, cool, pale hypotrichous skin in hypothyroidism.

Sanguineous (*sang-gwin'e-us*) Pertaining to blood; abundance of blood.

Sanies (*sa'ne-ez*) A fetid discharge containing serum, pus and blood.

Saphena (*sa-fe'na*) A saphenous vein.

Saphena varix Single varix formed at origin of great saphenous vein.

Saphenous vein (saphena) Blood vessels in the legs that help send blood from the legs and feet back up to the heart.

Sapremia A toxic state in the blood that results from the presence of toxic products of putrefactive bacteria.

Saprophyte (*sap'ro-fit*) Any organism living on decaying or dead organic matter such as higher fungi; adj. **saprophytic**.

Sarc- (sarco-) Combining word for flesh.

Sarcocele (*sar'ko-sel*) Fleshy tumor of the testis.

Sarcocystis (*sar'ko-sis'tis*) A genus of parasitic protozoa living in the host's muscles.

Sarcoid 1 Stage 1 of sarcoidosis, characterized by a condition where inflammed cells join together to make tiny lumps called granuloma.

Sarcoidosis (*sar'koi-do'sis*) A chronic progressive multisystem granulomatous disorder of unknown etiology; characterized by enhanced cell-mediated immune processes at the site of involvement. There is widespread non-caseating granulomas and the histologic pattern is uniformly the same in all affected organs. It affects especially the lungs, lymph, nodes, liver, skin and eyes. Intrathoracic involvement is noted in 90% of all patients of sarcoidosis. Cough and progressively increasing breathlessness are most common respiratory symptoms. Erythema nodosum, fever, polyarthralgia and hilar adenopathy are characteristics during the early stages of disease.

Sarcolemma (*sar'ko-lem'a*) The plasma membrane of a striated muscle fiber.

Sarcoma (*sar-ko'ma*) A tumor or cancer arising from any tissue including muscle, fat, bone or blood vessels other than skin and mucous membranes.

Ewing sarcoma A highly malignant, metastatic, primary tumor of bone, closely related to a primitive neuroectodermal tumor; it is usually found in the diaphysis of long bones, ribs, or flat bones of children or adolescents. Characteristics include saucerization of the cortex, patchy, permeative destruction, and often a large soft tissue mass; the most common symptoms include pain, swelling, leukocytosis, and fever.

Fascial sarcoma A sarcoma arising in the fasciae about the joints, especially in the lower limbs.

Fibroblastic sarcoma The fibroblastic form of osteosarcoma.

Fowl sarcoma A transmissible sarcoma of the chicken.

Giant cell sarcoma A form of giant cell tumor of bone (q.v.) that arises malignant de novo, rather than transforming to malignancy; sarcoma characterized by large anaplastic (giant) cells.

Granulocytic sarcoma Chloroma.

Hemangioendothelial sarcoma Hemangiosarcoma.

Hodgkin sarcoma Hodgkin disease, lymphocyte depletion type.

Kaposi sarcoma A multicentric, malignant neoplastic vascular proliferation characterized by bluish-red cutaneous nodules, usually on the lower limbs, that slowly increase in size and number and spread to more proximal sites. The tumors have endothelium-lined channels and vascular spaces mixed with aggregates of spindle-shaped cells; they may remain confined to skin and subcutaneous tissue, but widespread visceral involvement may occur. The condition is endemic in certain parts of Central Africa and Central and Eastern Europe, and a virulent and disseminated form occurs in immunocompromised patients. It is caused by human herpesvirus 8.

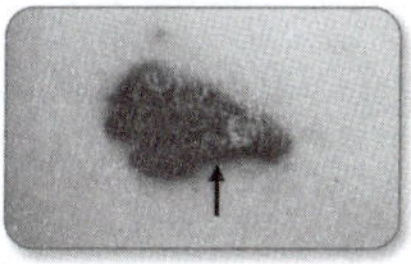

Kaposi sarcoma

Kupffer cell sarcoma Hepatic angiosarcoma.

Lymphatic sarcoma Diffuse lymphoma.

Melanotic sarcoma Malignant melanoma.

Mixed cell sarcoma Malignant mesenchymoma.

Multiple idiopathic hemorrhagic sarcoma Kaposi sarcoma

Sarcomatosis (*sar'ko-ma-to'sis*) A condition characerized by the presence and spread of sarcomas.

Sarcomere (*sar'ko-mer*) The contractile unit of a myofibril. It consists of myosin and actin filaments arranged between two Z discs.

Sarcoplasm (myoplasm) (*sar'ko-plazm*) The cytoplasm of striated muscle.

Sarcoplasmic reticulum A complex network of specialized smooth endoplasmic reticulum important in transmitting the electrical impulse as well as in storage of calcium ions.

Sarcoptes (*sar-kop'tez*) A genus of Acarina that includes the mites that infest humans and animals. Sarcoptes scabiei causes scabies in humans.

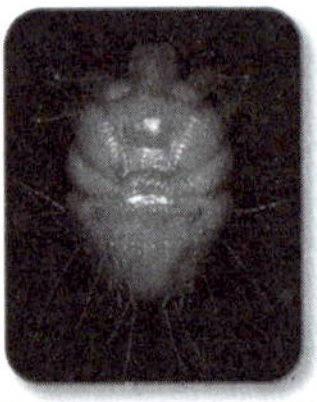

Sarcoptes scabiei

Sartorius (*sar-to're-us*) The longest muscle in the body, *see* Table of muscles.

Satyriasis (*sat'i-ri'-a-sis*) An excessive and often uncontrollable sexual desire in the male.

Saucerization (*saw-ser-i-za'shun*) The creation of a shallow depression to facilitate drainage; a disciform defect that parallels the shaft of long bones on a plain film in fibrosarcoma with bony involvement.

Sayre's jacket (*sarz*) A jacket of plaster of Paris worn to support the spine, named after Lewis Sayre, US surgeon.

Scab (*skab*) Crust of a wound, ulcer.

Scabicide (*ska'bi-sid*) An agent that kills mites such as causative agents of scabies.

Scabies (*ska'bez*) A condition caused by itch mite, Sarcoptes scabiei hominis. It is transmitted by direct contact and causes an intensely pruritic linear eruption corresponding to the tracks of the burrowing mite, commonly affects children and pruritus result in excoriation and secondary pyoderma.

Scala (*ska'la*) Any one of the three spiral passages of the cochlea of the inner ear.

Scala media The cochlear duct lying between the scala tympani and scala vestibuli. Its floor contains the spiral organ of Corti.

Scala tympani The cochlear duct filled with perilymph lying below the spiral lamina.

Scala vestibuli The cochlear duct forming the upper portion of the bony canal. It extends from the oval window to the tip of the cochlea.

Scald (*skawld*) A burn to the skin and underlying tissues caused by moist heat and steam.

Scale (*skal*) A small, dry, thin exfoliation occurring from the upper layers of the skin; a film of tarter encrusting the teeth; an instrument for weighting; a graduated measure.

Scalenus A group of 3 pairs of muscles in the lateral neck–scalenus anterior, scalenus medius and scalenus posterior.

Scalenus syndrome (thoracic outlet syndrome) The compression occurs in a scalenus triangle, which bordered anteriorly by anterior scalenus muscle posteriorly by scalenus medius and the first rib inferiorly.

Scaler (*ska'ler*) An instrument used for removal of stains and adherent deposits on the teeth.

Chisel scaler Periodontal chisel.

Sickle scaler A scaler that removes tenacious supragingival or subgingival deposits; it has a sickle-like blade with flattened sides and a trapezoidal cross section.

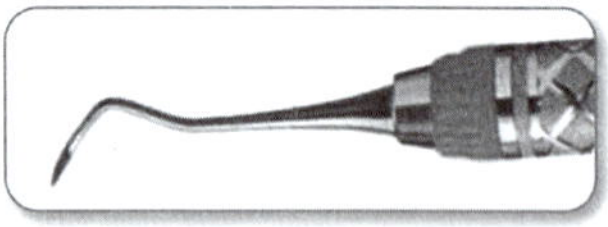

Sickle scaler

Scalpel (*skal'pel*) A small, straight surgical knife.

Scan An image obtained from computed tomography, ultrasound or magnetic resonance imaging.

Scanning speech A slurring speech with tendency to separate syllables in cerebellar diseases.

Scaphocephaly (*skaf'o-sef'a-le*) A deformed head projectin[illegible] kneel of a boat. Sagittal fusion results in long narrow skull with sagittal ridge.

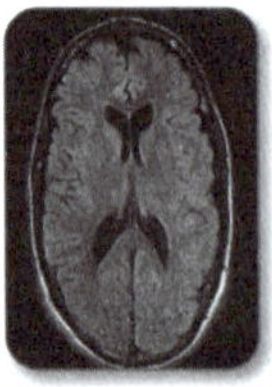

Scaphocephaly in brain— CT scan

Scaphoid (*skaf'oyd*) Depression.

Scaphoid abdomen Sunken abdomen where the anterior abdominal wall is hollowed in and presents a concavity to the horizontal plane when looked at from the sides.

Scaphoid fracture The most common carpal fracture produced by fall on outstretched hand.

Scaphoid bone One of the carpal bones on the thumb side of the wrist, just above the radius.

Scapula (scapula-) (*skap'u-la*) Pl. **scapulae.** The large, triangular bone that forms the posterior part of the shoulder. It articulates with clavicle and the humerus.

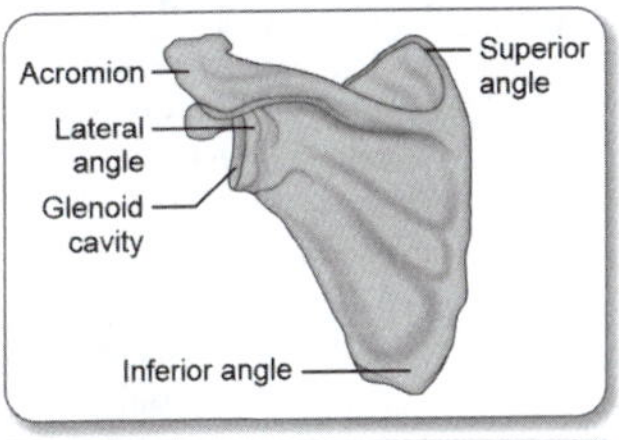

Scapula

Winged scapula Prominent medial border of the scapula, may be due to paralysis of serrates anterior or trapezius muscles.

Scapula (*skap'u-lar*) Pertaining to the shoulder blade.

Scar (*skar*) Cicatrix; fibrous trace of destructive lesion of tissue.

Scar cancer Lung cancer developing in preexisting scars.

Scarification (*skar'ifi-ka'shun*) Making multiple small skin incisions with a sharp point.

Scarlatina (*skar'la-te'na*) Scarlet fever due to hemolytic streptococcus.

Scarlet fever Erythrogenic toxin produced by Streptococcus pyogenes causing pharyngitis, strawberry tongue, generalized blanching erythema of face with circumoral pallor and linear petechiae.

Scarpa's triangle Femoral triangle named after Antony Scarpa, Italian surgeon.

Schick test Intradermal injection of diphtheria toxin to determine immunity status. Lack of antibody is indicated erythema, named after Bela Schick, Hungaria, US pediatrician.

Schilling test A test using radioactive vitamin B_{12} to assess the gastrointestinal absorption of vitamin B_{12} to diagnose primary pernicious anemia, named after Robert Schilling, US hematologist.

Schindylesis (*skin'di-le'sis*) An articulation in which one bone is received into a cleft of another.

Schistoglossia A congenital fissure or cleft of the tongue.

Schistosoma (Bilharzia) (*shis'to-so'ma*) A genus of blood flukes that cause infection in man on entry through the skin. It includes *S. haematobium*, *S. japonicum* and *S. mansoni*. They belong to phylum Platyhelminthes, class Trematoda.

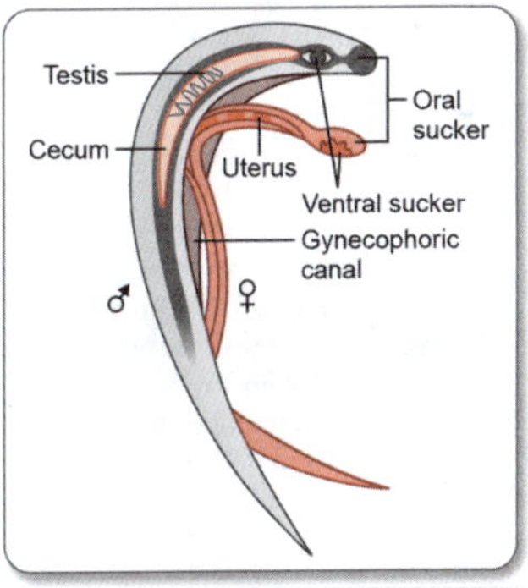

Schistosoma haematobium—male and female

Schistosomiasis (bilharziasis) (*shis'to-so-mi-a-sis*) Three species of the genus Schistosoma (*S. haematobium*, *S. mansoni* and *S. japonicum*) are the causative agents of schistosomiasis. The ovum passed in the urine or feces of infected persons gains entry into freshwater. A ciliated miracidium is liberated and it enters an intermediate host, a freshwater snail where it multiplies. A large number of cercariae are liberated which penetrate the skin or mucosa of definite host, human where they pass through the lung and reach liver and mature. The manifestations are painless terminal hematuria, frequency of micturition, pain, pyelonephritis, hydronephrosis, and uremia (*S. hematobium*), abdominal pain, frequent stools with blood-stained mucus, hepatomegaly, portal hypertension, hematemesis and ascites (*S. mansoni*) features resembling infection with *S. mansoni* with added neurologic features (*S. japonicum*).

Schizogony (*ski'zog'o-ne*) The asexual reproduction of a sporozoon parasite by multiple fission of the nucleus and later segmentation of cytoplasm to produce merozoites.

Schizoid personality Introspective, solitary, shy behavior.

Schizont (*skiz'ont*) Multinucleated stage during schizogony.

Schizonticide An agent selectively destructive of the schizont of a sporozoin parasite.

Schizophrenia (*skiz'o-fre'ne-a*) A disorder of thinking and perception, and inappropriate or blunted mood.

Catatonic schizophrenia Marked psychomotor disturbance which alternates between hyperkinesis and stupor.

Chronic schizophrenia Schizophrenia exhibiting thought disorder and negative symptoms of underactivity, lack of drive, social withdrawal and emotional emptiness.

Hebephrenic schizophrenia Schizophrenia characterized by a markedly shallow and inappropriate mood.

Negative schizophrenia Schizophrenia having a slow and insidious onset, apathy, social withdrawal, lack of motivation and underlying abnormalities of brain structure.

Paranoid schizophrenia Schizophrenia with insidious onset, with delusions of persecutory nature with hallucinatory voices.

Positive schizophrenia Schizophrenia is characterized with prominent delusions and hallucinations and normal structure of the brain.

Simple schizophrenia Schizophrenia exhibiting insidious deterioration of the personality.

Schizotypal (*skit'so-ti'pal*) One of a group of conditions informally called "eccentric" personality disorders. People who have these disorders often seem odd or peculiar to others. They also may show unusual thinking patterns and behaviors.

Schlemm's canal A circular canal found within the posterior part of the corneoscleral junction.

Schonlein-Henoch purpura An autoimmune disorder causing inflammation and bleeding in the small blood vessels.

Schuffner's dots Stippling of red blood cells infected with malarial parasite *Plasmodium vivax*, named after Wilful Schuffner, German parasitologist.

Schwann cell (*shwan*) One of the cells of the peripheral nervous system producing myelin sheath and neurilemma of peripheral nerve fibers, named after Theodor Schwann, German anatomist.

Schwannoma (*shwa-no'ma*) A tumor of Schwann cells; neurilemmomas are benign schwannoma and true or malignant schwannoma are Schwannomas, occurring as malignant peripheral nerve sheath tumors.

Sciatica (*si'at'i-ka*) Pain in the distribution of sciatic nerve due to lateral disc protrusion on L4 and/or L5 spinal nerve roots.

Sciatic nerve The nerve that travels from the buttocks and down each leg.

Scintigram (*sin'ti-gram*) Scintiscan.

Scintillascope An instrument for detecting and measuring the intensity of high energy radiation.

Scintillator Substances that emit fluorescence when exposed to radiations such as X-rays and γ-rays.

Scintiscan (*sin'ti-skan*) The record obtained by scanning, that gives a photographic display of the distribution of internally administered radiopharmaceutical.

Scirrhous (*skir'us*) Hard; indurated.

Scissura (Scissure) A cleft or elongated opening in a body or surface created by as if by cutting.

Sclera (sclerotic coat) (*skler'a*) White of the eye; a fibrous tunic forming the outer envelope of the eye.

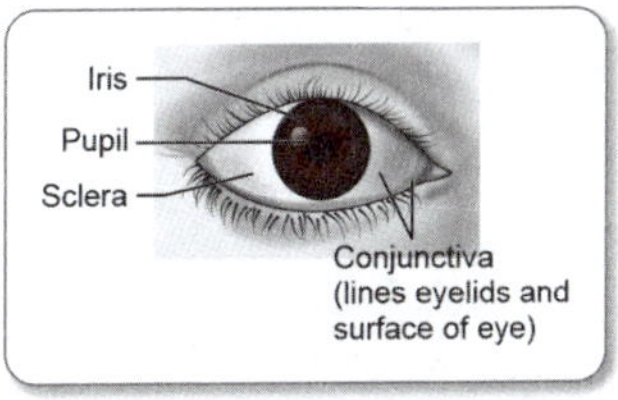

Sclera

Sclerectomy (*skle-rek'to-me*) Excision of a portion of the sclera.

Scleritis (*skle-ritis*) Inflammation of the sclera.

Anterior scleritis Inflammation affecting the sclera adjoining the limbus of the cornea.

Posterior scleritis Inflammation of the sclera underlying retina and choroid.

Necrotizing scleritis Associated with rheumatoid arthritis.

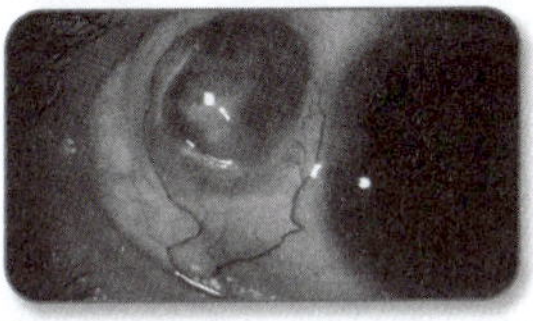

Necrotizing scleritis

Scleroderma (*skler'o-der'ma*) Widespread thickening and fibrosis of the skin due to accumulation of excess collagen and polyglycans, a manifestation of systemic sclerosis.

Systemic scleroderma A rare chronic disease of unknown cause characterized by diffuse fibrosis and vascular abnormalities in the skin, joints, and internal organs (especially the esophagus, lower gastrointestinal tract, lungs, heart, and kidneys). Common symptoms include Raynaud syndrome, polyarthralgia, dysphagia, heartburn, and swelling and eventually skin tightening and contractures of the fingers. Lung, heart, and kidney involvement accounts for most deaths. Diagnosis is clinical, but laboratory tests support the diagnosis and aid in prognostication. Specific treatment is difficult, and emphasis is often on treatment of complications.

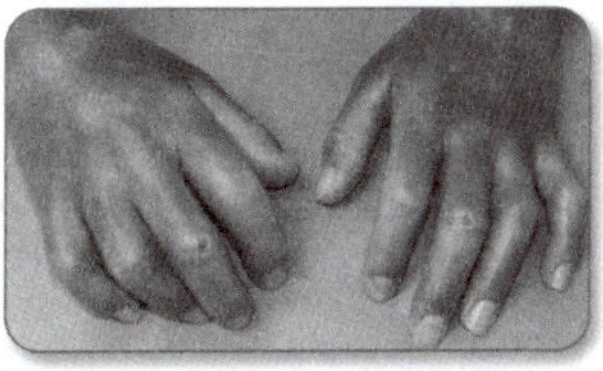

Systemic scleroderma with characteristic shiny skin and fixed claw-like position of the fingers caused by acro-osteolysis and flexion contractures

Scleroma (*skle-ro'ma*) A circumscribed indurated focus of granulation tissue in the skin or mucous membrane.

Scleromalacia (*skler'o-ma-la'shea*) Degeneration and softening of the sclera.

Scleronychia Thickening, hardening and yellowing of the nail plate, possibly combined with onycholysis. The nail plate is increasingly.

Sclerosis (*skle-ro'sis*) An induration of tissue due to excess fibrosis; induration of nervous structures; thickening and hardening of the layers in the wall of an artery.

Amyotrophic lateral sclerosis A variant of motor neuron disease causing degeneration of motor tracts of the lateral columns, distal and proximal muscle wasting and weakness, fasciculations, spasticity, exaggerated reflexes and extensor plantars.

Arterial sclerosis Arteriosclerosis; hardening of the arteries.

Lateral sclerosis Sclerosis of the lateral column of the spinal cord.

Multiple sclerosis Occurrence of plaque of inflammatory demyelination in more than one anatomical site at more than one time such as periventricular regions of the brain, the optic nerves and subpial regions of the spinal cord. It presents a relapsing and remitting clinical course with optic neuritis, relapsing and remitting sensory symptoms, and acute brain non-compressive paraparesis.

Systemic sclerosis A generalized disorder of connective tissue characterized by widespread thickening and fibrosis of the skin and obliterative lesions of the arterioles and capillaries. It presents with Raynaud's phenomenon, sclerodactyly, tightness, telangiectasias, arthralgia, dysphagia, interstitial pulmonary fibrosis.

Tuberous sclerosis An abnormal development of mesodermal tissue occurring as a genetic defect involving skin and the nervous system manifesting with features of epilepsy, mental retardation and adenoma sebaceum at an early age.

Sclerotherapy (*skler'o-ther'a-pe*) Injection of sclerosing agents in the treatment of piles or varicose veins.

Sclerotic (*skle-rot'ik*) Relating to or characterized by sclerosis; scleral.

Sclerotome (*skler'o-tom*) Knife used in sclerotomy; a group of mesenchymal cells migrating from mesodermal somite toward notochord.

Sclerotomy (*skle-rot'o-me*) Incision of the sclera.

Scotch tape test Retrieval of eggs of Enterobius vermicular from the perianal region in children by application of an adhesive tape.

Scolex (*sko'leks*) Pl. **scoleces**. Head of tapeworm, attached by suckers and frequently, by rostellar hooks to the wall of intestine.

Scoliosis (*sko'le-o'sis*) Lateral curvature of the vertebral column. adj. **scoliotic**.

Functional scoliosis A non-structural reversible lateral curvature of the spine.

Structural scoliosis An irreversible lateral curvature of the spine with fixed rotation of the vertebrae.

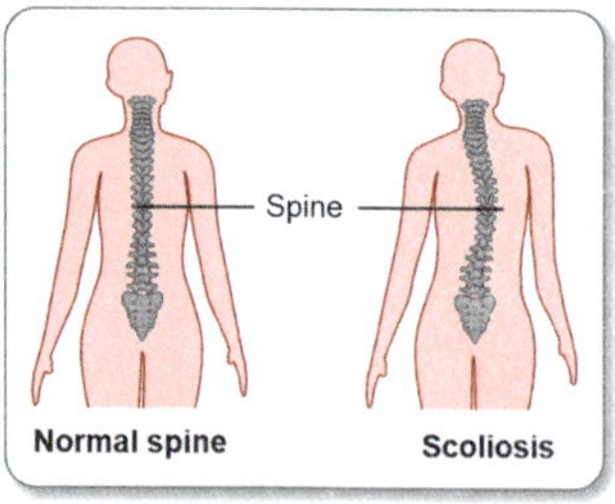

Scoliosis

Scopolamine (hyoscine) A medication used to manage and treat postoperative nausea and vomiting and motion sickness. It is an anticholinergic drug.

Scorbutic (*skor-bu'tik*) Pertaining to or affected by scurvy.

Scotoma (*sko-to'ma*) Pl. **scotomata**; Localized loss of vision within otherwise normal lung fields.

Scotometer A device used to measure size, shape and intensity of scatoma.

Scotopic Vision with full dark adaptation.

Screening (*skren'ing*) A process in which a large population group is evaluated for the possible presence of a morbid condition by measuring clinical parameters; initial patient evaluation; a fluoroscopic examination.

Scrotum (*skro'tum*) A musculocutaneous sac containing testes. It is formed of skin, a network of nonstriated muscle fibers (dartos), cremasteric muscle and fascia and serous coverings of the testes and epididymis. adj. **scrotal**.

Lymph scrotum Elephantiasis of the scrotum.

Scrotal tongue Grooved or fissured tongue, which allows food particles to stick and later colonized by bacteria.

Watering-can scrotum Presence of multiple sinuses on the under surface of the scrotum and the perineum discharging urine.

Scrub typhus (tsutsugamushi disease) Rickettsial infection caused by *R. tsutsugamushi* transmitted by mites.

Scruple Moral principles or beliefs that make one unwilling to do something that seems wrong.

Scurf Thin dry scales detached from the epidermis especially in an abnormal skin condition; dandruff.

Scurvy (*sker've*) Vitamin C deficiency manifesting in children with features of irritability, enlargement of ends of long bones, beading of costochondral junctions, subcutaneous echymosis, swollen gums and hemorrhage.

Scybalum (*sib'a-lum*) Hard mass of fecal material in the intestine.

Seasickness (*se'sik-nes*) A result of a conflict in the inner ear, where the human balance mechanism resides, and is caused by a vessel's erratic motion on the water.

Sebaceous (*se-ba'shus*) Pertaining to or secreting sebum.

Sebaceous cyst (steatoma) A benign encapsulated, subepidermal nodule field with keratin material.

Sebaceous gland Microscopic glands found in hair follicles that secrete sebum.

Seborrhea (*seb'o-re'a*) Excessive secretion of sebum. adj. **seborrhoeic**.

Seborrhea sicca An accumulation on the skin, especially the scalp, of dry scales; dandruff.

Sebum (*se'bum*) Oily secretion of the sebaceous glands, composed of fat and epithelial debris.

Secondary Arising from some earlier event or condition; later in time; metastasis of a tumor.

Secondary amenorrhea Cessation of menstruation after being once established.

Secondary hemorrhage Bleeding from infection of wound with damage to vessels.

Secondary hydrocephalus Increase in volume of cerebrospinal fluid due to shrinkage of brain.

Secondary optic atrophy Optic atrophy due to loss of retinal ganglion cells.

Second messenger Chemical that sends genetic instructions after those received from messenger RNA, which enables turning genes on or off.

Second opinion An advice from a second health professional as to the correctness of the diagnosis and appropriateness of suggested line of treatment.

Secondary care Health care provided by a specialist in a community hospital to a patient who has been referred by a primary care physician.

Secondary sexual characteristics These appear during puberty. In humans, secondary sexual characteristics include enlarged breasts and widened hips of females, facial hair and Adam's apples in males and pubic hair on both.

Secretagogue (*se-kret'a-gog*) Stimulating secretion; an agent that stimulates secretion; an agent that increases gastrointestinal secretion of electrolyte and fluid by increasing adenylate cyclase activity or by increasing calcium in the cytosol.

Secretin (*se-kre'tin*) A helical peptide produced by S cells in the upper small intestine, released by acid, bile or fat into the intestinal lumen, stimulating the release of water and bicarbonate from pancreas, neutralizing gastric acid, stimulating intestinal motility and release of bile and gastric acid and inhibiting gastrin.

Secretion (*se-kre-shun*) Material produced by and separated from gland or cell; the process involved in it.

Section (*sek'shun*) An act of cutting; a cut surface; a segment or subdivision of an organ.

Abdominal section Laparotomy.

Cesarean section Incision through the abdominal wall and uterus for extraction of the fetus.

Cross section A section perpendicular to the long axis of an organ.

Frozen section A thin section of tissue cut from a frozen specimen, used for rapid histologic diagnosis.

Perineal section Section through the perineum.

Serial section One of a number of consecutive sections.

Sedation (*se-da'shun*) Making calm, allaying irritability or excitation by drugs.

Sedative (*sed'a-tiv*) Calming; quieting; an agent causing such an effect.

Sedimentation (*sed'i-men-ta'shun*) The settling out of sediment.

Sedimentation rate The distance red blood cells travel in one hour in a sample of blood as they settle at the bottom of a test tube.

Segment (*segment*) Adj. **segmental**. A part or section of an organ or body; one of the serial divisions of an animal.

Bronchopulmonary segment A wedge-shaped lung supplied by segmental bronchus.

Hepatic segment Segment of the liver made up of smaller units (lobules) comprising of a central vein, radiating sinusoids separated from each other by hepatocytes and peripheral portal tracts.

Internodal segment The portion of a myelinated nerve between two successive nodes.

Mesodermal segment A somite.

Uterine segment The lower end of the uterus joining with the cervical canal, which during pregnancy expands to become lower part of the uterine cavity and the upper part of the gravid uterus becomes thicker whose contractions provide the expulsory force in labor.

Seizure (*se-zhur*) The sudden attack or recurrence of a disease; an episode caused by an electrical discharge from the brain.

Absence seizure Petit mal. The attacks are brief and more frequent, and are caused by a general discharge which does not spread out of the hemisphere and there is no loss of posture.

Partial motor seizure Rhythmical jerking or sustained spasm of contralateral face, arm, trunk and leg as the electrical activity arises in precentral gyrus.

Partial sensory seizure Seizures arising in the sensory cortex exhibit unpleasant tingling or electric sensations in the contralateral face and limbs.

Tonic clonic seizure An aura followed by rigidity, unconsciousness, which a few moments later is periodically relaxed causing clonic jerks.

Sella turcica Pituitary fossa, also known as Turk's saddle; midline part of superior surface of the body of the sphenoid bone, consisting of tuberculum sellae, hypophyseal fossa and dorsum sellae.

Selegiline (*se-lej'i-len*) A selective monoamine oxidase type B inhibitor enhancing action of dopamine used in the symptomatic treatment of Parkinsonism.

Semeiology The study of signs.

Semen (seminal fluid) (*se'men*) Material of male ejaculation containing secretions from seminal vesicle and prostate.

Semi Combining word for half.

Semicircular canals Three tiny fluid filled tubes in the inner ear that helps to keep body's sense of balance.

Semilunar cartilage (*se'mi-lu'nar*) Half moon; crescent.

Semilunar valve The heart valve at the base of the aorta and the pulmonary artery, consisting of cusps or flaps that prevent the backflow of the blood during systole.

Seminal vesicle Small glands that produce the majority of the fluid that makes up semen, although they do not have a role in producing sperm.

Seminiferous tubule (*se'mi-nifer-us*) Carrying or conducting the semen, referring to the tubules of the testis.

Seminoma (*se'mi-noma*) Testicular tumor presenting in the fourth decade of life as chronic painless enlargement of testicle. Testis is uniformly enlarged, and smooth. There is loss of testicular sensation.

Anaplastic seminoma Tumors with overall morphologic features of seminoma but with more than three mitotic figures per high-powered field (HPF), cellular irregularity, no fibrovascular septae, few lymphocytes, focal necrosis, and pleomorphic cells with non-clear cytoplasm.

Classical seminoma A malignant germ cell tumor that involves most commonly the testicle or less frequently the mediastinum, the retroperitoneum, or other extra-gonadal sites.

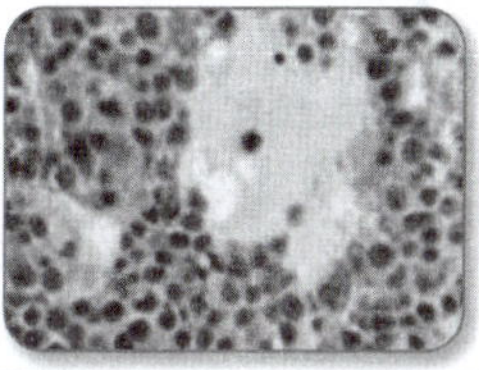

Classical seminoma with large nuclei and clear cytoplasm

Ovarian seminoma Seminoma of ovary.

Spermatocytic seminoma A polymorphous triphasic germ cell neoplasm recapitulating spermatogonia development and unrelated to germ cell neoplasia in situ (GCNIS).

Semipermeable membrane (*seme-per'me-a-b'l*) Allowing passage only of certain molecules.

Semiprone A position in which patient in lying on side between a lateral and prone position with the upper knee drawn up toward the chest and the lower arm drawn behind parallel to the back.

Senescence (*se'nes'ens*) The process of growing old; the phenomenon by which normal diploid cells lose the ability to divide.

Replication senescence Human diploid fibroblasts at the end of their proliferative lifespan, remain alive in a rested state and it occurs after about 60 cell divisions.

Senile Pertaining to an old age.

Senile dementia Progressive neurodegenerative disease which may be primary (Alzheimer's disease) or secondary to vascular degeneration from atherosclerosis.

Senile miosis Pupil becoming small and irregular in old age.

Senile plaque Neuritic plaque composed of a core of extracellular amyloid surrounded by a spherical mass of axons and dendrites in the grey matter.

Senile purpura Easy bruising and bleeding into the skin due to atrophy of the vascular supporting tissue.

Senna (*sen'ah*) Extract of leaves or pods of Cassia angustifolia, used as purgative.

Sensation (*sen-sa'shun*) Appreciation of sensation obtained from sources outside and inside the body.

Sense (*sens*) Feeling; a faculty by which objects are perceived.

Color sense The ability to distinguish differences in color.

Joint sense Sense of passive movement.

Kinesthetic sense Muscular sense.

Light sense Ability to distinguish the degree of intensity of light.

Muscular sense A consciousness of the muscular movement needed in a given act.

Pain sense Ability to appreciate prick of a pin.

Position sense Ability to place a limb in a particular position.

Pressure sense Ability to feel different degrees of pressure on the body surface.

Special sense One of the five senses related to the organs of sight, hearing, smell, taste and touch.

Static sense The sense that makes it possible to maintain equilibrium.

Temperature sense The ability to detect temperature.

Time sense Ability to detect differences in time intervals.

Touch sense A primary sensation to recognize touch when different dermatomes are touched.

Vibration sense Appreciation of vibrations.

Visceral sense The perception of existence of the internal organs.

Sense organ The specialized organs composed of sensory neurons, which help us to perceive and respond to our surroundings such as eyes, ears, nose, tongue and skin.

Sensibility (*sen'si-bil'i-te*) The capability of perceiving sensory stimuli.

Sensitive (*sen'si-tiv*) Capable of perceiving sensations; responding to a stimulus; a person rendered susceptible by previous exposure.

Sensitivity (*sen'si-tiv'i-te*) *stat* The degree to which a test or clinical assay is capable of confirming or supporting the diagnosis of a disease.

Anaphylactic sensitivity Sensitivity to allergens, it is a severe reaction that happens when an over-release of chemicals puts the person into shock.

Antibiotic sensitivity Refers to how responsive antimicrobials are to bacteria.

Insulin sensitivity Refers to how responsive your cells are to insulin.

Sensitization (*sen'si-ti-za'shun*) Immunization; exposure to allergen that results in the development of hypersensitivity; a condition of being made sensitive to a specific antigen such as a protein or pollen; the process of making an individual susceptible to a substance by repeated injections.

Central sensitization Corresponds to an enhancement in the functional status of neurons and circuits in nociceptive pathways throughout the neuraxis caused by increase in membrane excitability, synaptic efficacy, or a reduced inhibition.

Rh sensitization Can occur when a person with Rh-negative blood is exposed to Rh-positive blood.

Spinal sensitization Sensitization in spinal cord.

Sensory (*sen'sor-e*) Pertaining to sensation.

Sensory ataxia Ataxia due to posterior column lesions increased with eyes closed.

Sensory deafness Sensorineural deafness.

Sensory dysphasia Receptive dysphasia.

Sensory discrimination Ability to discriminate between the stimulus of two blunt points of a divider or two pins when applied simultaneously over the skin while the eyes are closed.

Sensory extinction Failure to perceive the stimulus such as touch or pinprick applied simultaneously, occurs in parietal lobe lesions.

Sensory cortex All of the areas in the brain that lets humans process sensory input.

Sensory nerve The nerve which carries signals to brain to help feel, touch, taste, smell and see.

Separation anxiety Mental health condition that causes excessive fear or anxiety when separated from a loved one or anticipating separation.

Sepsis (*sep'sis*) Presence of pathogens or their toxins in the blood or tissues.

Sepsis syndrome A systemic inflammatory response to infection exhibiting hypothermia or hyperthermia, tachycardia, tachypnea, a focus of infection, positive blood cultures, one or more end organ dysfunction, hypoxemia, and oliguria, initiating a systemic inflammatory response that adversely affects the blood flow to the vital organs.

Septal defect An opening in the septum (interatrial or interventricular) between the left and right sides of the heart.

Septic (*sep'tik*) Pertaining to sepsis.

Septic arthritis Inflammation of joint by infection.

Septic shock A septic shock syndrome with hypotension.

Septicemia (*sep'ti-se'me-a*) Disease produced by multiplication of pathogenic organisms in the circulating blood.

Cryptogenic septic Systemic infection of the blood by pathogenic microorganisms, especially bacteria, that originate from a localized source.

Plague septic A systemic disease involving infection of the blood and is most commonly spread by bites from infected fleas.

Septra A synthetic combination of Trimethoprim and sulfamethoxazole, which is antibacterial in action.

Septum (*sep'tum*) Pl. **septa**. A thin wall dividing two cavities or masses of soft tissue.

Septum primum defect A hole low in the interatrial septum, often involving AV valves.

Septum secundum defect A hole in the middle of the interatrial septum.

Interventricular septum of heart, septum. interventriculare cordis [TA] The partition that separates the left ventricle from the right ventricle, consisting of a muscular and a membranous part; called also ventricular.

Sequel (*se'k wel*) Sequela.

Sequence (*se'kwens*) Order of succession; a series of things following in a certain order.

Raw sequence Individual unassembled sequence reads, produced by sequencing of clones containing DNA inserts.

Pierre Robin sequence (PRS) A triad of micrognathia, glossoptosis, and airway obstruction. Infants frequently present at birth with a hypoplastic mandible and difficulty breathing. The smaller mandible displaces the tongue posteriorly, resulting in obstruction of the airway.

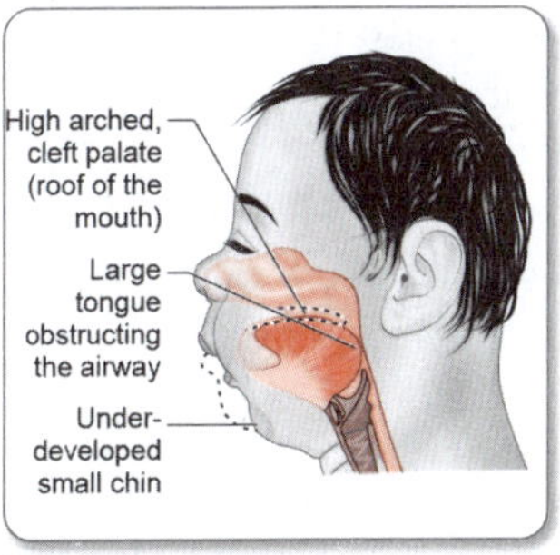

Pierre Robin sequence showing triad of symptoms

Sequestration (*se'kwes-tra'shun*) A part separated from the surrounding healthy tissue; loss of blood or its fluid not participating in the circulation.

Bronchopulmonary sequestration An area of non-functioning abnormal segment of lung parenchyma receiving its blood supply from a systemic artery and has no connection with tracheobronchial tree.

Sequestrectomy (*se-kwes-trek'to-me*) Surgical removal of a sequestrum.

Sequestrum (*se-kwes'trum*) Pl. **sequestra**. A piece of necrosed tissue, usually bone separated from the surrounding healthy tissue.

Serine (*ser'en*) A nonessential amino acid found in many proteins.

Serine proteases A family of proteolytic enzymes that includes coagulation cascade enzymes, trypsin and chymotrypsin.

Seroconversion (*ser'o-con-ver'zhun*) The change of an immune status from that of non-production of a particular antibody to a state of detectable production.

Serofibrinous (*ser'o-fi'bri-nus*) Composed of serum and fibrin, as in serofibrinous exudate.

Serology (*ser-ol'o-je*) Study of serum in immunological aspects; results of immunological tests on the serum. adj. **serologic**.

Seropus (*ser'o-pus*) Serum mixed with pus.

Serosa (*se-ro'sa*) Any flattened cell layer lining serous membranes; the chorion. adj. **serosal**.

Serositis (*ser'o-si'tis*) Pl. **serositides**. Inflammation of a serous membrane.

Serotherapy (*sero-ther'a-pe*) Treatment of an infection by injection of immune serum or antitoxin.

Serotonin (*sero'to'nin*) 5-Hydroxytryptamine, a molecule secreted by activated platelets. It is a potent vasoconstrictor and a neurotransmitter in CNS.

Serotonin syndrome A clinical triad of mental status changes, autonomic hyperactivity and neuromuscular abnormalities, often encountered following overdose of proserotonergic agents.

Serotype (*ser'o-tip*) The type of a microorganism determined by its constituent antigens.

Serous (*ser'us*) Pertaining to or resembling serum; producing or containing serum; serosal; secreting watery fluid as parotid gland.

Serous cystadenoma Ovarian cyst with watery contents and papillary ingrowth into the cavity.

Serous membrane (serosa) A membrane that lines a body cavity, such as pleural, pericardial and peritoneal cavities that do not open to the exterior.

Serpiginous (*ser-pig'i-nus*) Creeping, having a wavy or serrated margin.

Serpiginous tract A twisted vermiform radiolucency surrounded by a sclerotic rim in long bones in pyogenic osteomyelitis.

Serpiginous ulcer Ulcer of irregular shape which shows healing in one area while spreading in another.

Serratus Any of the several muscles taking origin from ribs or vertebrae by separate slips.

Sertoli cells Supporting cells of testicular germinal layers, named after Enrice Sertoli, Italian physician.

Sertraline (*ser'tra-len*) A selective inhibitor of the reuptake of serotonin.

Serum (blood serum) (*ser'um*) Pl. **sera**. The fluid component of blood from which the coagulation factors have been removed.

Serum protein Any protein in the blood serum.

Convalescent serum Convalescent serum is blood serum obtained from one who has recovered from an infectious disease. It is considered to be rich in antibodies which is effective against the infectious agent of the said disease.

Inactivated serum The heating of the serum, mitigates or eliminates a broad range of generally disturbing effects of the serum.

Blood serum The fluid and solute component of blood which does not play a role in clotting.

Serum hepatitis Type B viral hepatitis.

Serum sickness An immune response noted after reexposure to an antigen to which a person has been previously sensitized. The presence of soluble circulating immune complexes to cause urticaria, fever, adenopathy and occasionally arthritis.

Sesamoid bone (*ses'a-moid*) A type of bone that develops in some tendons where they cross the ends of long bones.

Sessile (*ses'il*) Attached to a structure by a broad base.

Seton A thin thread inserted beneath the skin to provide drainage or to guide subsequent passage of a tube.

Sexarche When a person first engages in sexual intercourse.

Sex chromatin A small dense mass of chromatin attached to the inner nuclear membrane of the nuclei in female somatic cells of all mammalian species.

Sex chromosome The 23rd pair of chromosomes, designated X and Y, which determine the genetic sex of an individual.

Sex hormone Steroid hormones primarily produced by the gonads, such as ovary in females and testes in males. Two major classes of sex hormones are estrogen and androgens. Females have high circulating levels of estrogens and males have higher circulating levels of androgens.

Sex-limited (*seks'-lim'i-ted*) Occurring in one sex only.

Sex-linked (*seks'linkd*) Transmitted by a gene located on the X-chromosome, hence, carried by the mother and expressed by the son.

Sexology (*sek-sol'o-je*) The scientific study of sex and sexuality.

Sex ratio The ratio of females to males, expressed as X women for every 1000 men.

Sexual abuse Sexual assault, rape or sexual molestation.

SGPT Serum glutamic pyruvic transaminase, named as serum alanine transaminase.

Shaking palsy Parkinson's syndrome; a degenerative disorder of the central nervous system characterized by tremor and impaired muscular coordination.

Shaping (*shap'ing*) A technique of behavior therapy to produce new behavior.

Sheath (*sheth*) A tubular covering, shell or protective layer.

Caudal sheath Constituting or relating to a tail.

Dermal sheath Sheath that surrounds the outside of the hair follicle containing progenitor cells that maintain and regenerate the dermal papilla, a key component for hair growth.

Myelin sheath An extended and modified plasma membrane that is wrapped around the nerve axon in a spiral fashion.

Neumann sheath The thin layer of dentine immediately surrounding each dentinal tubule.

Tendon sheath A membrane that wraps around a tendon, which allows the tendon to stretch and prevents it from adhering to the overlying fascia.

Sheehan's syndrome Hypopituitarism due to an infarct of the pituitary following postpartum hemorrhage, manifesting in partial or total loss of thyroid, adrenocortical and gonadal functions, named after Harold Sheehan, British pathologist.

Shigella (*shi-gel'ah*) Genus of gram-negative non-motile bacilli, cause bacillary dysentery; *Shigella boydii* agent causing dysentery; *Shigella dysenteriae* shiga bacillus responsible for most severe dysentery; *Shigella flexneri Flexnor bacillus*; *Shigella shiga*, *Shigella dysenteriae Shigella sonnei* agents causing mild dysentery.

Shigellosis (*shi'gel-lo'sis*) Infection with shigella organisms; bacillary dysentery.

Shingles (*shing'g'lz*) Herpes roster; band-like involvement of neurocutaneous tissues.

Shock (*shok*) A profound hemodynamic disturbance characterized by the failure of the circulatory system to maintain adequate perfusion of vital organs; a sudden disturbance of mental equilibrium.

Anaphylactic shock An immediate hypersensitivity reaction following exposure to a specific antigen by a sensitized individual.

Cardiogenic shock Shock resulting from failure to maintain circulation or mechanical obstruction of the heart.

Electric shock Shock resulting from passage of electric current through any part of the body.

Hemorrhagic shock Condition due to insufficient amount of blood in the circulatory system.

Insulin shock Condition resulting from overdose of insulin causing reduction of blood sugar below normal level.

Mental shock Shock due to emotional stress.

Neurogenic shock Shock due to decreased peripheral vascular resistance from damage to brain or the spinal cord.

Shock lung ARDS.

Septic shock Shock associated with overwhelming infection.

Spinal shock Flaccid paralysis and loss of all sensations and reflex activity below the level of injury to spinal cord.

Traumatic shock Shock due to injury or surgery.

Shoulder girdle (pectoral girdle) (*shol'der*) The junction of clavicle and scapula where the arm joins the trunk.

Frozen shoulder A common cause of shoulder stiffness; adhesive capsulitis.

Shoulder blade Scapula.

Shoulder-hand syndrome Swollen and painful hand and shoulder pain, with limitation of movements.

Shoulder pad sign Enlargement of glenohumeral joint due to periarticular accumulation of amyloid.

Shunt Diversion of blood from existing or normal channel to another.

Arteriovenous shunt The passage of blood directly from arteries to veins without passing through the capillary network.

Left-to-right shunt Acyanotic shunt wherein the right and left sides of heart communicate by an atrial or ventricular septal defect and patent ductus arteriosus. It leads to pulmonary congestion and later pulmonary hypertension.

Mesocaval shunt Anastomosis of the side of superior mesenteric vein to the inferior vena cava to control portal hypertension.

Portacaval shunt Surgical anastomosis between the portal vein and inferior vena cava.

SIADH Syndrome of inappropriate antidiuretic hormone secretion. It is characterized by excess secretion of vasopressin, low plasma osmolarity, water retention and dilutional hyponatremia noted as an ectopic hormone production in carcinoma, ACTH, deficiency, untreated Addison's disease, pneumonia, tuberculosis, use of PEEP and chromophobe adenoma.

Sial- (slalo-) Combining word for saliva; salivary glands.

Sialadenitis (*si-al-ad'en-it'is*) Inflammation of a salivary gland.

Sialagogue (*si-al'a-gog*) An agent which stimulates the salivary secretion. adj. **sialogogic**.

Sialic acid A group of reducing amino acids which are 9-carbon monosaccharides, and are found especially as components of blood glycoproteins and mucoproteins. Sialic acid play important roles in cell-cell interactions communications, signaling and immune reactions.

Sialögrahy (ptyalography) Radiographic examination of the salivary glands.

Sialolith (*si-al'o-lith*) A calculus in the salivary ducts or glands.

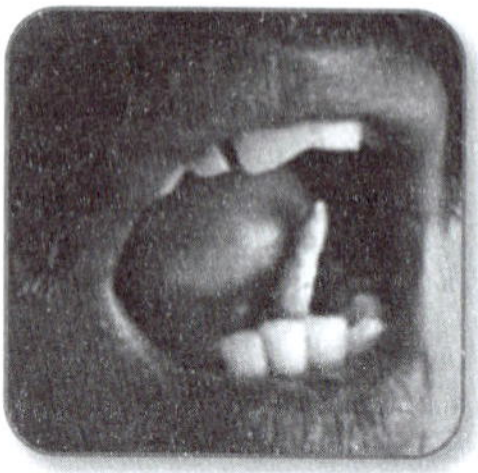

Sialolith

Sialorrhea (*si-al'o-re'a*) Increased flow of saliva.

Siamese twins Conjoined gestational products due to a failure in division of the yolk sac or due to a delay in monovular separation, mostly they are joined in the chest. Chang and Eng Bunker were most famous twins born in Siam (now Thailand).

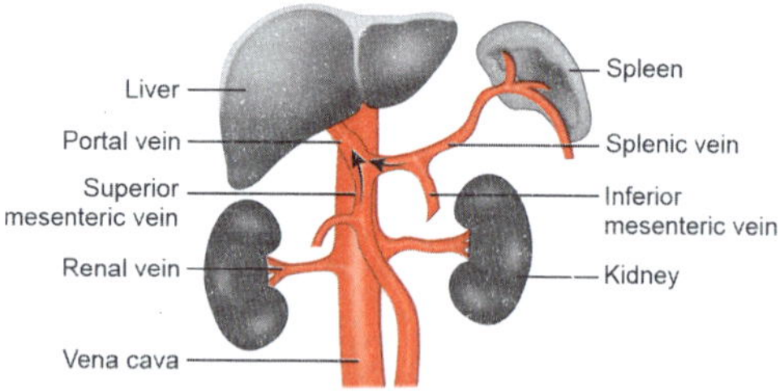

Portacaval shunt

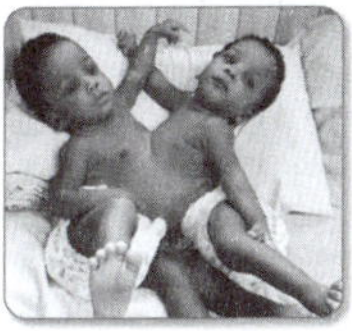

Siamese twins

Sib Person related especially by blood.

Sibilant (*sib'i-lant*) Whistling; hissing.

Sibilant rhonchi High-pitched rhonchi as whistling or squeaking sounds arise from obstruction of smaller bronchi.

Sibling (sib) (*sib-ling*) Offspring of same two parents.

Sickle cell The distorted sickle-shaped red blood cells, that result when the hemoglobin (has an altered amino acid structure of polypeptide) is deoxygenated, molecules of hemoglobin polymerize to form pseudocrystalline structures (tactoids) which distort red cell membrane and the process gets reversed when reoxygenated. The distortion of red cell membrane may become permanent to make the red cells to assume sickle shape constantly. Such cells increase blood viscosity, traverse capillaries poorly and obstruct the blood flow.

Sickle cell disease A congenital hemoglobinopathy caused by a point mutation on the gene that encodes hemoglobin resulting in a defective functioning of hemoglobin causing the red blood cells to 'sickle' when deoxygenated, that includes sickle cell anemia.

Sideroblast (*sid'er-o-blast*) Red cell precursor with hemosiderin granules in the cytoplasm.

Siderocyte (*sid'er-o-sit*) Red blood cell with iron containing granules.

Sideropenia (*sid'er-o-pe'ne-a*) Iron deficiency in the body or blood. adj. **sideropenic**.

Siderosis (*sid'er-o'sis*) Iron overload; pneumoconiosis from inhalation of dust or fumes containing iron particles.

Siemens (*se'menz*) (*S*) A unit referring to the conductance of one ampere per volt in a body with an ohm resistance.

Sievert (SV) The unit of radiation absorption in the international system of units.

Sigmoid- (*sig'moid*) Shaped like the letter C or S; the sigmoid colon.

Sigmoid colon (sigmoid flexure) The S-shaped portion of large intestine that begins at the level of the left iliac crest, projects inward to the midline, and terminates at the rectum.

Sigmoidectomy (*sig'moi-dek'to-me*) Surgical removal of a part or whole of the sigmoid colon.

Sigmoidoscope Rigid tubular speculum introduced through anus to visualize sigmoid colon.

Sigmoidoscopy (*sig'moi-dos'ko-pe*) Examination of the interior of sigmoid colon by a sigmoidoscope.

Sign (*sin*) Finding elicited by making a general and systemic examination and it represents the objective evidence of disease; a conventional or arbitrary mark, figure or symbol used technically as an arbitrary or conventional symbol.

Aaron sign A feeling of distress and pain in the epigastric, umbilical and precordial regions, on steady pressure over McBurney point.

Allis sign Also known as Galeazzi test, used to assess for hip dislocation, primarily in order to test for developmental dysplasia of the hip.

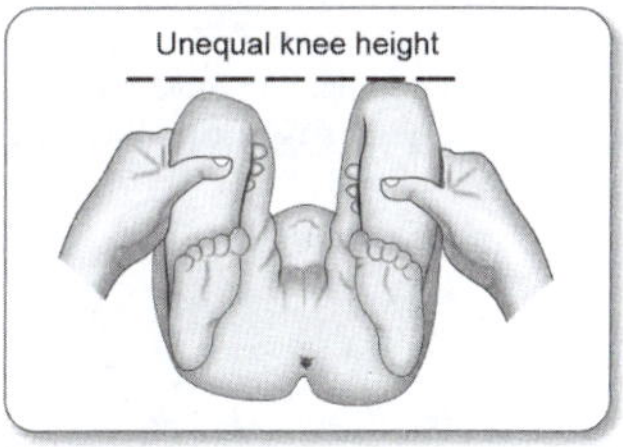

Allis sign

Babinski sign A cutaneous reflex in which the big toe moves upward on stimulation of the sole of the foot.

Battle sign Bruising over the mastoid process. It is retroauricular or mastoid ecchymosis that is typically the result of head trauma.

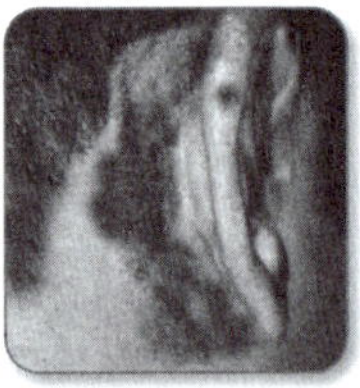

Battle sign

Bergman sign A radiographic finding in which (1) the ureter is dilated distal to a ureteral obstruction and (2) a catheter, passed retrograde, coils in the dilated ureter.

Brown sign Pulsation of the glomus tumor in the middle ear when positive pressure is applied to the external auditory canal during otoscopy.

Chadwick sign A nonspecific, early sign of pregnancy that is typically characterized by a bluish discoloration of the cervix, vagina, and vulva.

Cheyne-Stokes sign A type of breathing disorder characterized by cyclical episodes of apnea and hyperventilation.

Codman sign A periosteal reaction that occurs when bone lesions grow so aggressively that they lift the periosteum off the bone and do not allow the periosteum to lay down new bone.

Crowe sign The presence of axillary (armpit) freckling in people with neurofibromatosis type I (von Recklinghausen's disease).

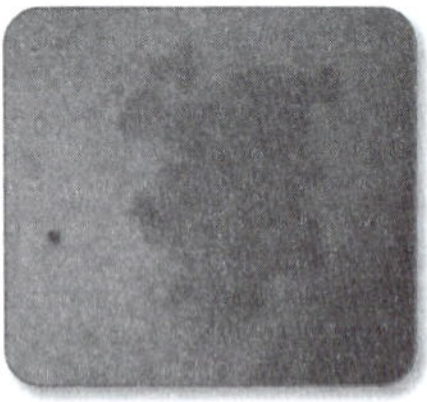

Crowe sign

Double bubble sign A feature of pediatric imaging seen on radiographs or prenatal ultrasound in which two air filled bubbles are seen in the abdomen, representing two discontinuous loops of bowel in a proximal, or 'high,' small bowel obstruction.

Gorlin sign The ability to touch the tip of the nose with the tongue.

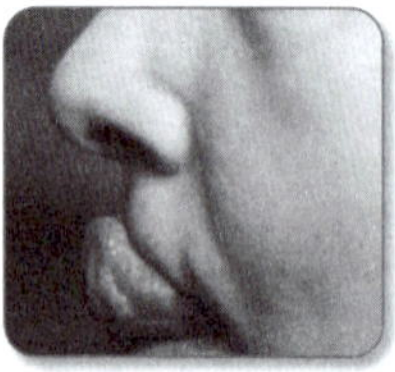

Gorlin sign

Glasgow sign A systolic murmur heard over the brachial artery in aortic aneurysm.

Hamman sign A "mediastinal crunch" heard upon auscultation in the setting of mediastinal emphysema (air in the mediastinum).

Hoffmann sign An involuntary flexion movement of the thumb and or index finger when the examiner flicks the fingernail of the middle finger down. It is suggestive of corticospinal tract dysfunction localized to the cervical segments of the spinal cord.

Murphy sign Elicited in patients with acute cholecystitis by asking the patient to take in and hold a deep breath while palpating the right subcostal area.

Nikolsky sign A skin finding in which the top layers of the skin slip away from the lower layers when rubbed. Nikolsky sign is a condition caused by a staphylococcal infection in which the superficial layers of skin slip free from the lower layers with a slight rubbing pressure.

Plummer sign A clinical sign in which there is onycholysis, or separation of the nail from the nail bed, particularly affecting the ring and little fingers.

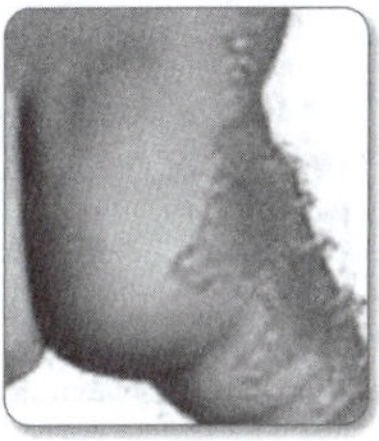

Nikolsky sign

Setting sun sign An ophthalmologic sign in young children resulting from upward-gaze paresis. In this condition, the eyes appear driven downward, the sclera may be seen between the upper eyelid and the iris, and part of the lower pupil may be covered by the lower eyelid.

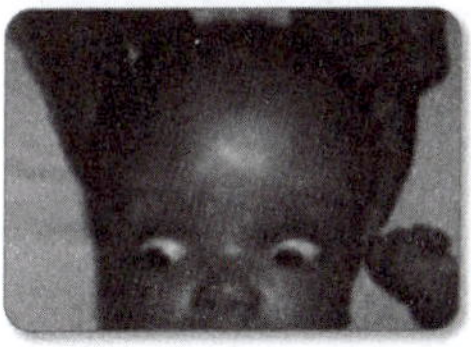

Setting sun sign

String sign A radiographic finding on an upper GI series, in which the patient is given a radio-opaque material, such as barium, to drink. Used in diagnosing Hypertrophic Pyloric Stenosis (HPS).

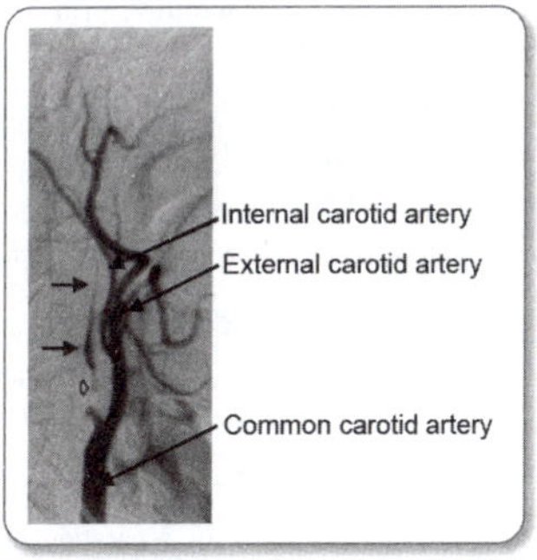

String sign in angiography

Table: Signs and symbols

+	death
♂	male
♀	female
+	excess of acid reaction, positive reaction
—	deficiency of alkaline reaction, negative reaction
ac	before meals, ante cibum
Ag	silver, argentums
Al	aluminum
aq	water, aqua
aq dist.	distilled water
As	arsenic
Au	gold, aurum
Ba	barium
Bi	bismuth
bid	twice a day, bis in die
Br	bromine
C	carbon
c	with, cum
Ca	calcium
Cap	capsule
Cd	cadmium
cib	food or meals, cibum
Cl	chlorine
Cm	curium
c/o	complains of
coch	spoonful, cochleare
Cr	chromium
Cu	copper, cuprum
d	day

Contd...

D & C	dilatation and curettage
D/s	dextrose in saline
D/w	dextrose in water
Dx	diagnosis
et al	and others, et alit; elsewhere et alibi
ex aq	with water
F	fluorine
Fe	iron, ferrum
Ga	gallium,
gt	drops, guttae
H	hydrogen
He	helium
Hg	mercury, hydrargyrum
hs	at bed time, just before going to sleep, hora somni
Hx	history
I	iodine
K	potassium, kalium
Li	lithium
Mg	magnesium
mst	mixture, mistura
Mn	manganese
N	nitrogen
Na	sodium, natrium
Nd	neodymium
Ni	nickel
NR	do not repeat, non repetatur
O	oxygen
OD	right eye, ocular dexter
Od	once daily
Oh	every hour, omni hora
On	every night, omni nocte
OS	left eye, oculus sinister
Ou	in each eye, oculo ultra
P	phosphorus
Pb	lead, plumbum
pc	after food, post cibum
Po	by mouth, per os
PR	through the rectum, per rectum
Prn	as occasion arises, given when necessary, pro re nata
Pulv	powder, pulvis
PV	through the vagina, per vagina
Px	past history
Q2h	every second hour, quaque secunda hora
Q3h	every third hour, quaque quarta hora
Q4h	every four hour, quaque quarta hora
Qd	every day, quaque die
Qh	every hour, quaque hora
Qn	every night, quaque nocte
Qs	as much as will suffice, quan-tum sufficit
Rx	take though, sign of Jupiter, used to propitiate the God in writing a prescription
Rh^{-}	Rhesus (factor) negative
Rh^{+}	Rhesus (factor) positive
R/O	rule out
S	signa, signetur label indicating directions to be written on a package or label for the use of the patient

Contd...

S & s	signs and symptoms
S1	first heart sound
S2	second heart sound
S3	third heart sound
S4	fourth heart sound
Si op sit	if it is necessary, si opus sit
Sol	solution, solutio
Ss	one half, semis
SD	Standard deviation stat SD, an interval consisting of the 95 percent of observed values
Stat	immediately, statim
Syr	syrup, syrupus
tid	three times a day, ter in die
Tin	tincture, tincutra
Ung	ointment, unguentum
Ut	dict, as directed, ut dictum
W/v	weight in volume
W/w	weight in weight
X	sex chromosome, female will have two X chromosomes
XX	chromosome pair resulting in offspring with female characteristics
XY	chromosome pair resulting in offspring with male characteristics
Y	sex chromosome, male will have one X and one Y chromosome

Silicosis (*sil'i-ko'sis*) A chronic fibrosis of the lungs caused by prolonged exposure to free silica. Radiologically it shows finely nodular, rounded opacities predominantly in the upper lung lobes. The condition may progress to massive fibrosis.

Accelerated silicosis Upper zone fibrosis progressing at an intermediate rate.

Acute silicosis Silicoproteinosis developing in individuals in overwhelming exposure of pure silica particles.

Chronic silicosis Progressive, nodular interstitial fibrosis from inhalation of low concentrations of silica.

Conglomerate silicosis Presence of both small nodules of simple silicosis and confluent nodules.

Silver sulfadiazone (*sil'ver*) A sulfa-derived antibiotic medication used to prevent and treat wound infection in patients with 2nd and 3rd degree burns.

Silver impregnation Silver complexes applied to demonstrate reticulin.

Silver nitrate An antiseptic and astringent.

Simmonds' disease A condition of atrophy of pituitary causing loss of function of thyroid, adrenals and gonads, cachexia and premature senility, named after Morris Simmonds, German Physician.

Simulium (*si-mu'le-am*) A genus of black flies, which may transmit diseases such as onchocerciasis (*river blindness*). It is a large genus with several hundred species, and 41 subgenera.

Sinew (*sin'u*) A tendon of a muscle.

Weeping sinew An encysted ganglion containing synovial fluid.

Singultus (*sing-gul'tus*) Hiccup.

Sinoatrial node (SA node) Modified muscle cells with spontaneous rhythm acting as cardiac pacemaker, located in the right atrium beneath the opening of superior vena cava.

Sinus (*si'nus*) A hollow in a bone, as paranasal sinus; a channel for blood as vascular sinus; any cavity having a narrow opening.

Accessory nasal sinus One of the paranasal sinuses: frontal, maxillary, ethmoidal and sphenoidal.

Anal sinus The grooves between the anal columns.

Aortic sinus The space between each semilunar valve and the wall of the aorta.

Carotid sinus Dilatation of the common carotid artery at its bifurcation, that contains baroreceptors.

Cavernous sinus A paired dural sinus on either side of sella turcica and communicating across the midline, containing internal carotid artery and abducent nerve.

Coronary sinus A short venous trunk receiving the veins of the heart, that runs in the posterior part of coronary sulcus and empties into the right atrium.

Ducal sinuses Endothelium lined venous channels in the dura mater.

Ethmoidal sinuses Paranasal sinuses in the ethmoidal bone.

Frontal sinus One of the paired paranasal sinuses in the frontal bone each communicating with the middle meatus of the ipsilateral nasal cavity.

Intercavernous sinuses The anterior and posterior anastomoses between the cavernous sinuses.

Lactiferous sinus A circumscribed spindle shaped dilatation of the lactiferous duct prior to its entry into the nipple.

Lymphatic sinus Irregular tortuous spaces within the lymph nodes through which lymph passes.

Mastoid sinuses Numerous small intercommunicating cavities in the mastoid process of temporal bone.

Maxillary sinus The air cavity in the body of its maxilla communicating with the middle meatus of the nose.

Occipital sinus A venous sinus in the attached margin of falx cerebelli extending to the foramen magnum.

Paranasal sinuses Accessory nasal sinuses.

Pilonidal sinus A pit in the sacral region.

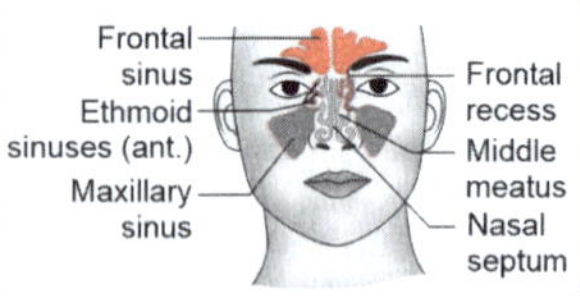

Paranasal sinuses

Pleural sinus Pleural cavity.

Prostatic sinus Groove on either side of the urethral crest in the prostatic part of the urethra.

Rectus sinus A venous sinus at the junction of the falx cerebri and the cerebellar tentorium.

Renal sinus The cavity of the kidney containing calyces and pelvis.

Sagittal sinus An unpaired dural sinus in the lower margin of the falx cerebri (inferior) and in the sagittal groove (superior).

Sigmoid sinus S-shaped dural sinus lying on the mastoid process of the occipital bone.

Sinus of valsalva Aortic sinus.

Sinus of venae cavae The portion of the cavity of right atrium of the heart receiving the blood from venae cavae.

Sinus venosus A cavity at the caudal end of embryonic cardiac tube.

Sphenoidal sinus One of a pair of cavities in the sphenoid bone communicating with the nasal cavity.

Sphenoparietal sinus Either of two sinuses of dura mater draining into the cavernous sinus.

Splenic sinus A dilated venous sinus in the substance of spleen.

Straight sinus Rectus sinus.

Tarsal sinus A canal formed by the groove of the talus and the groove of calcaneum.

Transverse sinus A sinus that unites the two inferior petrosal sinuses of the cranium; venous network in the dura over the basilar process of occipital bone; passage in the pericardium between the origins of great vessels and atria.

Tympanic sinus A deep recess in the posterior part of the tympanic cavity.

Urogenital sinus The ventral part of the cloaca that gives rise to lower part of the bladder in both sexes, the prostatic portion of male urethra, and to urethra and vestibule in the female.

Uterine sinus A small vascular channel in the endometrium.

Venous sinus A sinus carrying venous blood.

Sinus arrhythmia Commonly encountered variation of normal sinus rhythm. More often in children and young adults. Respirations lead to vagal stimuli resulting in R-R interval variations.

Sinusitis (*si'nu-si'tis*) Inflammation of the mucous membrane of a paranasal sinus.

Sinusoid (*si'nu-soyd*) A microscopic space or passage for blood in organs like liver or spleen.

Sinus venosus A cavity at the caudal end of embryonic cardiac tube.

Siphonage (*si-fun-ij*) The use of the siphon as in gastric lavage.

Sirenomelia (*si"ren-o-me'le-a*) Also called mermaid syndrome, a rare congenital deformity in which the legs are fused together. Apodal symmelia.

Sitosterol A type of chemical called a plant sterol. It is similar to cholesterol and is found in fruits, vegetables, nuts, and seeds. Beta-sitosterol might help reduce cholesterol levels by limiting the amount of cholesterol that is able to enter the body.

Sitz bath A warm bath in which just the buttocks and genital areas are soaked in water.

Sjogren's syndrome An autoimmune disorder characterized by lymphocytic infiltration of salivary and lacrimal glands leading to xerostomia and keratoconjunctivitis sicca, named after Henrick Sjogren, Swedish ophthalmologist.

Skatole (methyl indole) (*skat'ol*) Methyl indole produced by decomposition of proteins, especially tryptophan, in the intestine.

Skeletal muscle A highly organized tissue composed of bundles of muscle fibers (myofibers) which certain several myofibrils. They are part of voluntary muscular system and are typically attached by tendons to bones of a skeleton.

Skeleton (*skel'e-ton*) The bony framework of the body in vertebrates (endoskeleton) or hard outer envelope of insects (exoskeleton); all dry parts of the body after removal of soft parts; all bones of the body taken together.

Appendicular skeleton The bones of the limbs including the pectoral and pelvic girdles.

Axial skeleton The bones of the head and trunk excluding the pectoral and pelvic girdles.

Skew (*skyu*) *stat* Deviating from a straight line.

Skia Pertaining to shade of darkness.

Skiagram (*ski'a-gram*) A picture or photograph made up of shadows or outlines; a roentgenogram.

Skin The largest organ in the body consisting of epidermis and dermis. The epidermis is continuously renewing, stratified squamous epithelium that keratinizes. Innermost layer of epidermis is stratum germinativum in which keratinocytes are formed. Above it stratum spinosum is present in which progressive stages of keratinization occurs. Stratum granulosum overlies this layer where the cells become flat and contain keratohyalin granules. Stratum lucidum and stratum corneum are the most superficial layers.

Skin traction Extension of fracture by pulling on the adhesive plaster applied to the skin.

Skin graft Skin used to cover the skin surfaces with third degree burns.

Skull (*skul*) The cranium; the bony framework of the head composed of cranial and facial bones.

Sleep (*slep*) To take rest by relaxation of consciousness; to slumber. It is a nonhomogeneous phenomenon having two distinct forms: rapid eye movement (REM) sleep and non-rapid eye movement (NREM) sleep, REM sleep shows bursts of rapid eye movements. The skeletal muscle tone is decreased. NREM sleep exhibits four stages demonstrating a progression in a cyclic fashion throughout the night in a normal adult and are governed by the 100 minute ultradian rhythm.

Sleep apnea Absence of airflow at the nose and mouth for at least 10 seconds during sleep. The apneic episodes are repetitive and result in sleep arousal and they occur at a rate greater than 20 episodes per hour of sleep.

Sleepwalking Somnambulism, walking in sleep.

Sleeping sickness African trypanosomiasis.

Slipped disc Herniation of nucleus pulposus of the intervertebral disc through its capsule, and press on ligaments, nerve roots or occasionally spinal arteries.

Slit lamp A low power microscope with a specialized illuminating system for examining the anterior segment of the eye.

Slough (*sluf*) Necrotic tissue that is getting cast off from viable part of the body.

Small cell carcinoma Tumor of the lung arising from the bronchial epithelium that grows rapidly and metastatize to hilar lymph nodes and mediastinum. The cells are loosely arranged and contain oval, round or fusiform nuclei with finely stippled chromatin. The cytoplasm is scanty. They contain neurosecretory granules and often produce the endocrine paraneoplastic manifestations; SSC.

Small cuff syndrome Occurrence of gross error in auscultatory systolic and diastolic values when a small cuff is used to determine arterial pressures; non-hypertension.

Smallpox (*small'poks*) Variola, a disease eradicated from the globe. An acute eruptive contagious disease caused by pox virus marked by fever, chills, headache followed by papules which become umbilicated vesicles and later pustules. They get dried and form scab and fall leaving a permanent mark on the skin.

Smear (*smer*) A specimen for microscopic examination prepared by spreading the material across the glass slide.

Smegma (*smeg'ma*) Sebum and keratinous debris collected under foreskin.

Smooth muscle (involuntary muscle) An organ specialized for contraction, composed of smooth muscle fibers, located in the walls of hollow internal structures.

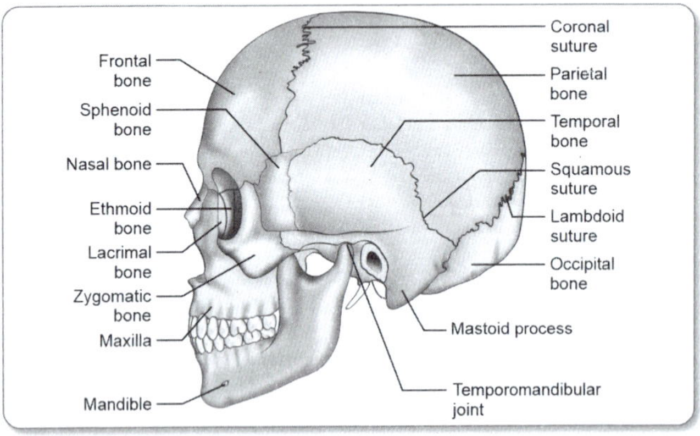

Skull lateral view

Sneeze (*S*) An involuntary sudden, violent and audible expulsion of air through the mouth and nose.

Snellen's chart To test visual acuity by asking the patient to read letters on the chart at a distance of six meters. The construction of the letters is such that the test letter is visible to the normal eye at 60 meters and the seventh (penultimate) line can be read at a distance of six meters. The individual who can read all letters, has a visual acuity of 6/6 named after Herman Snellen, Dutch ophthalmologist.

Snore (*snor*) A harsh buzzing noise in a sleeping person from vibration of redundant soft palate.

Snow blindness Ultraviolet keratitis and severe blepharospasm.

Snuffles (*snuf'alz*) To snuff or sniff usually audibly and repeatedly; to breathe through an obstructed nose with a sniffing sound; to speak through or as if through the nose; whine.

Social medicine Branch of medicine concerned with identification and modification of features of social organization that promotes illness.

Socket (*sok'it*) A hollow or depression into which a corresponding part fits.

Tooth socket The cavities in upper and lower jaw in which teeth are embedded.

Sodium Alkaline metal, atomic no. 11, symbol Na.

Sodium flumide A white crystalline powder used as a dental prophylactic of caries.

Sodium nitrate Antidote for cyanide poisoning.

Sodium nitroprusside An antihypertensive and a powerful vasodilator.

Sodium pump ATPase-based enzyme active transport system of cell membrane that actively moves sodium ions out of the cell and potassium ions into the cell at the expense of cellular ATP. It enables to keep the ionic concentrations at physiological levels.

Sodium sulphate A saline cathartic.

Sodium thiosulphate Antidote for cyanide poisoning.

Sodium aminosalicylate Antibiotic primarily used to treat tuberculosis.

Sodium bicarbonate $NaHCO_3$, baking soda used as a gastric and systemic antacid, to alkalize urine.

Sodium fusidate An antibiotic used to treat skin infections and eye infections.

Sodium hydroxide (caustic soda) Caustic soda NaOH, a caustic.

Sodium salicylate Analgesic and antipyretic.

Sodium valproate Used to treat epilepsy and bipolar disorder.

Sodoku (*so'do-koo*) Japanese name for the spirillary form of rat-bite fever.

Sodomy (*so'do-me*) Anal intercourse, copulation of man and animal.

Soft sore (chancroid) a notifiable infections disease. It is a sexually transmitted disease that causes ulcers on the genitals.

Soleus A calf muscle that is one of the two muscles making up the calf called the triceps surae. It is attached to the tibia fibulae and to a tissue connection between the two bones.

Soma (*so'ma*) The body as distinguished from mind; the body tissue; the cell body.

Somat Combining word for body; viscera.

Somatic (*so-mat'ik*) Pertaining to body or body wall.

Somatic cell Any cell in an organism which is not a germ cell.

Somatic cell division In which the parent cell duplicates itself to produce two daughter cells.

Somatic cell genetic disorder Defects in DNA in specific somatic cells (cancer).

Somatic cell hybrid A hybrid formed from fusion together of different cells from different species. Human and rodent hybrids are used for human gene mapping.

Somatic mutation A mutation which occurs in any cell that will not become a germ cell.

Somatic mutation A deleterious genetic variation occurring in any cell of the body except sperm and egg cells.

Somatic nervous system The portion of peripheral nervous system consisting of somatic efferent fibers that run between the CNS and the skeletal muscles and skin.

Somatization (*so'ma-tiza'shun*) Expression of mental disorder as apparent physical disease.

Somatization disorder Briquet syndrome.

Somatomedin (*so'ma-to-me'din*) A group of proteins produced predominantly by the liver when growth hormones act on target tissue. Somatomedins inhibit the release of growth hormones by acting directly on anterior pituitary and by stimulating the secretion of somatostatin from the hypothalamus.

Somatopleure (*so-mat'o-plur*) The embryonic body wall made of ectoderm and somatic mesoderm.

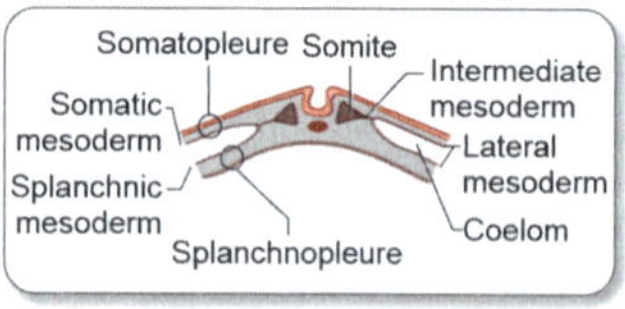

Somatopleure and splanchnopleure on transverse section through embryonic disc of a 21-day-embryo

Somatostatin (growth-hormone-release inhibiting factor) (*so'ma-to-stat'in*) A hormone that inhibits the release of somatotropin, and secretion of insulin and gastrin. It is produced by the hypothalamus and delta cells of pancreas.

Somatotrophin (*so-mat'o-tro'fin*) Pituitary growth hormone.

Somatotype (*so-mat'o-tip*) Body configuration. It may be ectomorph, endomorph or mesomorph.

Somite (*so'mit*) Block of mesodermal cells in a developing embryo that forms skeletal muscles (myotome), a connective tissue (dermatome) and a vertebrae (sclerotome).

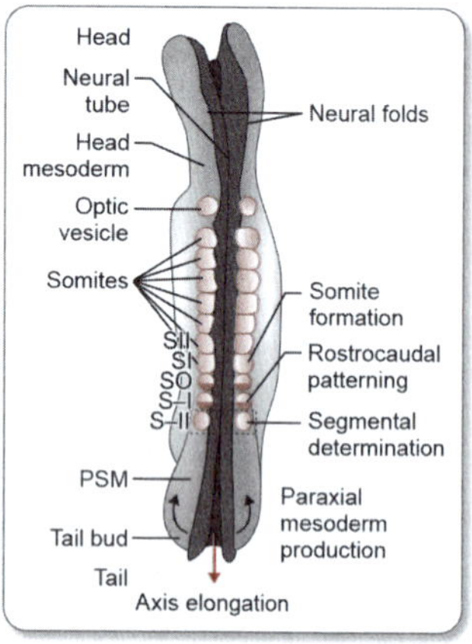

Somites in a 22-day-embryo

Somnambulism (noctambulation) (*som-nam'bu-lizm*) Sleep walking.

Somnolence A hypnotic trance; sleepiness

Sonoplacentography Ultrasonography if the pregnant uterus in order to determine the position of the placenta during pregnancy.

Soporific (*sop'o-rif'ik*) Producing deep sleep; an agent that produces deep sleep.

Sorbitol (*sor'bi-tol*) Hexahydroxyhexane, a sugar substitute for diabetics.

Sorbitol cataract Due to excess sorbitol in the lens its hyperglycemic state.

Sordes (*sor'dez*) A dark brown crust-like collection on the lips, teeth and gums of a person with dehydration in chronic debilitating disease.

Sore (*sor*) A lesion of the skin or mucous membrane; a wound, ulcer; painful.

Sore throat Inflammation of the pharynx, larynx and tonsils often caused by hemolytic streptococcus or adenovirus.

Sotalol Beta-blocker used in hypertension.

Souffle (*soo'fl*) A soft, blowing, auscultatory sound; called also bruit de soufflet.

Cardiac souffle Any cardiac or vascular murmur of a blowing quality.

Funic souffle (Funicular souffle) A hissing souffle synchronous with the fetal heart sounds, and supposed to be produced in the umbilical cord.

Mammary souffle A functional cardiac murmur with a blowing sound, heard over the breasts in late pregnancy and during lactation; it may be either restricted to systole or continuous.

Placental souffle A souffle supposed to be produced by the blood current in the placenta.

Uterine souffle A sound made by the blood within the arteries of the gravid uterus.

Sound Noise; vibrations produced by a sounding body transmitted by the air and perceived by the internal ear; an elongated, cylindrical, usually curved instrument is used for exploring the bladder or other cavities of the body, dilating strictures of the urethra or esophagus, or detecting the presence of a foreign body in a body cavity; healthy.

Amphoric breath sound A variant of bronchial breathing where a number of high-pitched sounds overlap the fundamental low-pitched sounds.

Bowel sound Sound gurgling and bubbling sounds (borborygmi) due to the peristaltic action of the intestinal wall on the contents (fluid and air) within.

Breath sound Sounds due to the penetration of the air into the normal lung tissue and its expulsion.

Bronchial sound An abnormal breath sound with a pause between inspiration and expiration and expiratory phase being longer and harsher than inspiratory phase.

Bronchovesicular breath sound An intermediate type of breathing having features of vesicular and bronchial breathing.

Cavernous breath sound A low-pitched bronchial breath sound.

Cracked pot sound A tympanitic percussion note in internal hydrocephalus in children with separation of sutures from raised intracranial tension.

Ejection sound A high-pitched clicking sound heard just after the first heart sound.

Fetal heart sound Sound produced by contraction of the fetal heart.

First sound Sound due to the closure of atrioventricular valves and it heralds the beginning of the ventricular systole.

Fourth heart sound Sound occurs from the vibrations generated from vigorous contraction of the atria and is heard in late diastole.

Friction sound Friction rub produced by inflamed opposing pleural surfaces.

Heart sounds One of the sounds heard on auscultation over the heart.

Korotkoff's sound Sounds heard over an artery when blood pressure is measured by the auscultatory method.

Pistol shot sound Sound coinciding first heart sound audible over brachial and femoral artery in hyperkinetic circulatory state and aortic incompetence.

Second heart sound Sound due to the closure of the aortic and pulmonary valves and it occurs at the end of the systole.

Succussion sound A splashing sound elicited in a patient with hydro- or pyopneumothorax.

Tambours sound A heart sound from aortic or pulmonary valve closure giving a booming and ringing quality like that of a drum.

Third heart sound Sound produced by the ventricular wall during transition in from rapid early diastolic flow to the slow rate of passive distension of the ventricle and it occurs early in the diastole.

Tracheal breath sound Loud, low-pitched breath sounds audible over trachea.

Tubular breath sound A high-pitched bronchial breath sound.

Urethral sound A device to explore urethra.

Uterine sound Used to gauge the depth and position of the uterine cavity.

Vesicular breath sound Normal breath sound.

White sound A sound made up of all audible frequencies.

Soutter's tube Cylinder of spiral wire introduced into the esophagus to preserve its lumen in inoperable carcinoma, named after H. Soutter, UK surgeon.

Space maintainer *dent* An orthodontic appliance that is worn to prevent adjacent teeth from moving into the space left by an unerupted or prematurely lost teeth.

Sparganosis An infection by the plerocercoid larva or sparganum developing in humans, usually subcutaneously.

Sparganum (*spahr'ga-nam*) A ribbon-shaped motile worm that migrates to skeletal muscles or subcutaneous tissue where it produces growing nodules.

Spasm (*spazm*) An involuntary contraction of the muscles occurring in an exaggerated form as in tetanus, hydrophobia, strychnine poisoning.

Clonic spasm Spasm interrupted by relaxations.

Tonic spasm Continuous contractions of the muscles.

Spasmodic (*spaz-mod'ik*) Of the nature of a spasm.

Spasmodic dysmenorrhea Dysfunction of menstruation accompanied by painful contractions of the uterus.

Spasmodic dysphonia A chronic phonatory disorder with jerky, effortful strained sounds with laryngeal discomfort.

Spasmodic torticollis Intermittent turning of head to one side with muscle contractions.

Spasmolytic A drug or treatment able to relieve spasm of smooth muscles.

Spasmus nutans A disorder affecting infants and young children. It involves rapid, uncontrolled eye movements, head bobbling and sometimes, holding the neck in an abnormal position.

Spastic colon Irritable bowel syndrome.

Spasticity (*spas-tis'i-te*) Increased muscle tone due to lesions of pyramidal tract.

Clasp-knife spasticity Resistance being felt at the beginning of passive flexion in spasticity and it gives way suddenly on continued pressure. The muscles feel firm.

Spastic paralysis Paralysis with tonic spasm of the affected muscles and with increased tendon reflexes.

Spatula (*spach'u-la*) A flat, blunt instrument for spreading plasters and for mixing ointments.

Species (*spe'shez*) A taxonomic category subordinate to a genus and superior to subspecies.

Species specific Characteristic of a particular species.

Specific gravity The density of an object divided by the density of water.

Specificity (*spes'i-fis'i-te*) The degree of an enzyme's selectivity for a substrate; the avidity of an antibody for an antigen; the condition of being specific, of having a fixed relation to a single cause or to a definite result; the proportion of individuals with negative test results for the disease that the test is intended to reveal.

SPECT Single photon emission computerized tomography, a method for reconstructing cross-sectional images of radiotracer distribution in an organ, used to evaluate acute ischemic episodes of the brain, vascular dementia, and myocardial perfusion.

Spectinomycin (*spek'ti-no-mi'sin*) An aminocyclitol antibiotic used in penicillin-resistant gonorrhea.

Spectrograph A instrument used to separate and measure the wavelengths present in electromagnetic radiations and to measure the relative amount of radiation at each wavelength.

Spectrometer Measures the reflection or transmission of light by an object, usually in wavelength range from 360 nanometers to 760 nanometers.

Spectrophotometer (*spek'tro-fo-tom'e-ter*) Measures the full color spectrum and produces spectral color data that is typically not detected by the human eye.

Spectroscope (*spek'tro-skop*) An instrument for forming and examining spectra of luminous bodies.

Specular reflection The mirror-like reflection of light or other waves that occurs when light hits a smooth surface and reflects at the same angle.

Speculum (*spek'u-lum*) Pl. **specula**. An instrument for exposing the interior of a passage or cavity of the body.

Graves speculum A type of two-valved vaginal speculum.

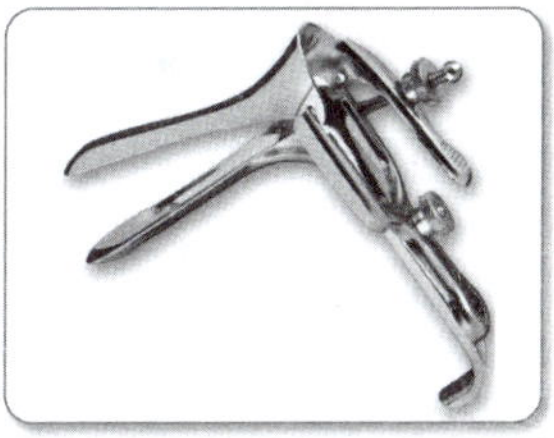

Graves speculum

Lid speculum An appliance for keeping the eyelids apart. Also called eye or eyelids blepharostat.

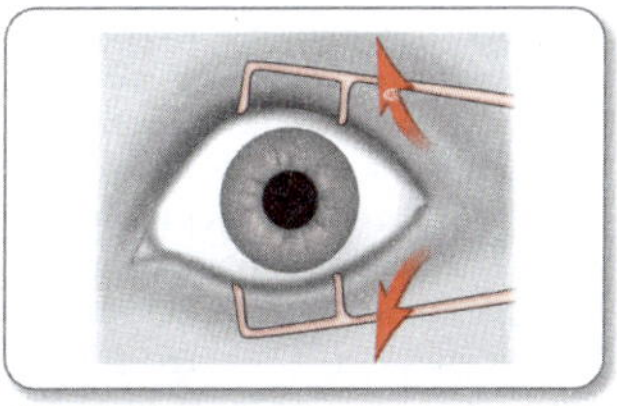

Lid speculum

Nasal speculum A medical tool used by the ENT physicians to examine the anterior part of the nose.

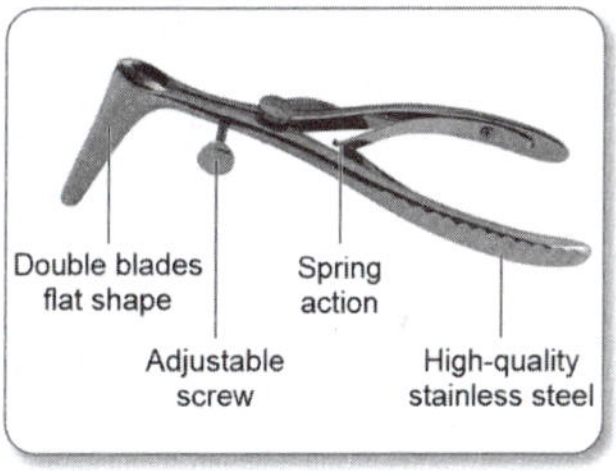

Nasal speculum

Speech therapy (*spech*) That which is spoken; the power of speaking.

Speech audiometry Determination of percentage of words recognized at varying levels of loudness.

Speech center Formation of speech is a cortical function and the centers are situated in the left hemisphere in the right handed individuals as the dominant hemisphere. The center is situated in the form of a quadrilateral consisting of visual area (calcarine salcus of the occipital lobe), auditory area (superior temporal gyrus), Broca's area (3rd frontal convolution), writing center (2nd frontal convolution) and their associated fibers in between.

Sperm Spermatozoon; semen.

Sperm antibody An antibody directed against the sperm heads or tails.

Spermatic artery (*sper-mat'ik*) Pertaining to the semen; seminal.

Spermatic cord A supporting structure extending from a testis to the deep inguinal ring, that includes vas deferens, arteries, veins, lymphatics, nerves, cremaster muscle and connective tissue.

Spermatid (*sper'ma-tid*) Spermatoblast; a cell derived from spermatocyte, and develops into spermatozoon.

Spermatocele An abnormal sac (cyst) that develops in the epididymis. The fluid is usually clear or milky white and may contain sperms.

Spermatocyte (*sper-mat'o-sit*) A cell developing from a spermatogonium that gives rise to spermatozoa.

Spermatogenesis (*sper'ma-to-jen'e-sis*) The formation and development of spermatozoa in the seminiferous tubules of the testes.

Spermatogonium (*sper'ma-to-go'ne-um*) An undifferentiated germ cell of a male that takes its origin in a seminal tubule. pl. **spermatogonia**.

Spermatorrhea Excessive emission of semen without orgasm or erection.

Spermatozoon (sperm) (*sper'ma-to-zo'on)* A mature sperm cell, *see* Sperm.

Spermaturia (*sper'ma-tu're-a*) A discharge of semen with urine.

Sperm count A measure of the number of spermatozoa per ejaculation or per measured amount of semen; used as an indication of a man's fertility.

Spermicide (*sper'-mi-sid*) An agent that kills spermatozoa. Also called spermatocide.

Spermiogenesis (*sper'me-o-jen'e-sis*) The maturation of spermatids into spermatozoa.

Spherocyte (*sfer'o-sit*) A small globular, completely hemoglobinated erythrocyte without central pallor seen in hereditary spherocytosis.

Spherocytosis (*sfer'o-si-to'sis*) A defect in erythrocyte membrane causing an increase in osmotic fragility and autohemolysis.

Hereditary spherocytosis An autosomal dominant condition exhibiting anemia, intermittent jaundice, splenomegaly, gallstones and leg ulcers.

Spheroid (*sfe'roid*) A local axonal dilatation filled with degenerated organelles.

Sphincter (*sfingk'ter*) A circular muscle constricting an orifice.

Bladder sphincter The smooth muscle about the opening of bladder into the urethra.

Cardiac sphincter The smooth muscle at the esophagogastric junction.

Pyloric sphincter The smooth muscle around the opening of the stomach into the duodenum.

Sphincter ani The sphincter that closes the anus. It consists of sphincter ani externus of striated muscle and sphincter ani internus of smooth muscle.

Sphincter of oddi A circular muscle at the opening of the common bile duct and main pancreatic ducts in the duodenum.

Sphincterectomy (*sfingk'ter-ek'to-me*) Surgical removal of a sphincter.

Sphincterotomy (*sfingk'ter-oto-me*) Incision of a sphincter.

Sphingomyelin (*sfing'go-mie'e-lin*) Cera-midephosphocholine compound.

Sphingosine (*sfing'go-sen*) A long chain, monounsaturated aliphatic amino alcohol found in sphingomyelin.

Sphygmocardiograph An instrument for measuring blood pressure, especially arterial blood pressure.

Sphygmograph (*sfig'mo-graf*) An instrument to record the movement, form and force of the arterial pulse.

Sphygmomanometer (*sfig'mo-ma-nom'e-ter*) An instrument for measuring the arterial blood pressure.

Sphygmophone A device by which a pulse may be heard.

Sphygmoscope (*sfig'mo-skop*) An instrument making the pulse beat visible.

Spica (*spi'ka*) Figure of eight bandage or plaster especially as applied to bigger joints.

Spicule (*spik'ul*) A sharp, needle-like body.

Spina bifida (rachischisis) Failure of closure of the spinal canal due to defective fusion of the vertebral arch in the lumbosacral region and is associated with depression, pigmentation or presence of hair.

Spinal accessory nerve XI cranial nerve, essential for neck and shoulder movement, the intrinsic musculature of the larynx and the sensitive afferences of the trapezius and sternocleidomastoid musculature.

Spinal anesthesia A neuraxial technique where local anesthetic is placed directly in the intrathecal place.

Spinal column The central axis of weight bearing column which supports the head as well as transforms the weight of the trunk and abdomen to the legs; provides structure and flexibility to the body.

Spinal (*spi'n'l*) pertaining to a spine or to the vertebral column.

Spinal cord An elongated mass of nerve tissue located in the vertebral canal from which 31 pains of spinal nerves originate.

Spinal shock A flaccid paralysis below the site of spinal injury.

Spinal tap Withdrawal of cerebrospinal fluid from the subarachnoid space in the lumbar region.

Spindle (*spin'd'l*) Any fusiform cell or structure; a structure consists of microtubules that help in the alignment and movement of chromosomes during cell division.

Muscle spindle Small, spindle-shaped sensory receptors located in skeletal muscle tissue, and they run parallel to the main muscle fibers (extrafusal fibers).

Spine (*spin*) Spina; the spinal column.

Kissing spine A term referring to close approximation of adjacent spinous processes due to degenerative changes of the spine.

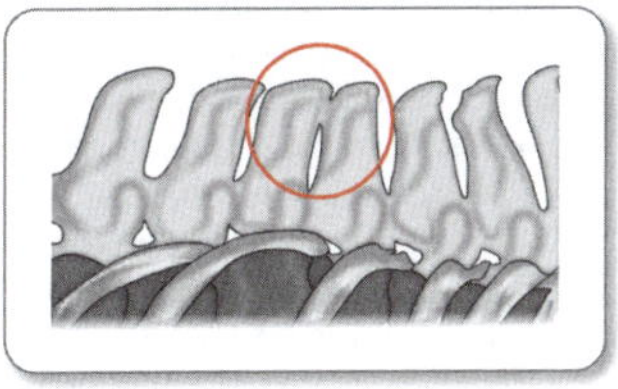

Kissing spine

Spinocerebellar degeneration (*spi'no-ser'e-bel'ar*) An inherited (autosomal dominant) progressive, neurogenerative and heterogenous disease that mainly affects the cerebellum.

Spiral (*spi'ral*) winding about a center like coil.

Curschmann's spiral Coiled mucous fibrils sometimes found in sputum of patients with bronchial asthma.

Spiral computed tomography Helical CT medical imaging method in which a large image volume is obtained by continuous rotation of the detector and scanning images at a speed of 10 mm/sec in a single breath.

Spiral organ The organ of hearing consists of supporting cells and hair cells that rest on the basilar membrane and extend into the endolymph.

Spirillum (*spi-ril'um*) A spiral-shaped bacterium; an organism of the genus. pl. **spirilla**.

Spirochaetes (*spi'ro-ke'tez*) A member of the phylum Spirochaetota, which contains distinctive diderm gram-negative bacteria, most of which have long, helically coiled cells. Spirochaetes are chemoheterotrophic in nature, with lengths between 3 and 500 μm and diameters around 0.09 to at least 3 μm. Also known as spirochete.

Spirograph (*spi'ro-graf*) A device for representing graphically the lung volumes and its subdivisions.

Spirometer (*spi'rom'e-ter*) A device that measures the volume of air inhaled or

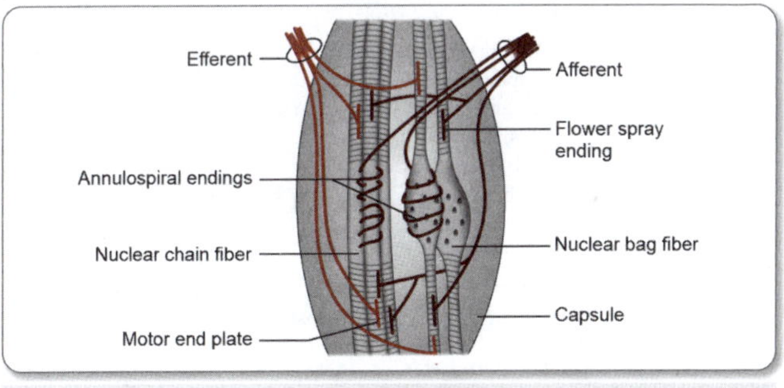

Cross-section of a muscle spindle showing the intrafusal fibers and afferent and efferent endings (Diagrammatic)

exhaled out of the lungs and records the time over which the volume changes. Vital capacity and its subdivisions are obtained. The spirometers may be of closed system—wet type (Bell spirometer with a water-seal) or dry type (bellows, piston, wedge spirometer) or open system (using a pneumotachograph with a differential pressure transducer or turbine or vane type volume transducer).

Spironolactone (*spir'o-no-lak'ton*) A diuretic that blocks the action of aldosterone on the distal convoluted tubules and collecting tubules of the kidney.

Spitz-Holter valve A one way valve used to drain cerebrospinal fluid in order to control hydrocephalus.

Splanch- (splanchno-) Combining word for viscera, viscus, splanchnic nerve.

Splanchnic (*splangk'nik*) Pertaining to the viscera.

Splanchnic nerves (*splangk'nik*) Paired ganglionic autonomic nerves running along either side of the vertebral column.

Splanchnocranium The portion of the skull that arises from the first 3 branchial arches and forms the supporting structure of the jaws.

Splanchnopleure The double layer formed by the association of the lower layer of the lateral plate of mesoderm with the underlying entoderm, which develops into the embryonic viscera.

Spleen (*splen*) A large mass of lymphatic tissue between the fundus of the stomach and the diaphragm that functions in phagocytosis, production of lymphocytes, and blood storage. It has an outer capsule of dense connective tissue and smooth muscle fibers, from which trabeculae extend into the pulp consisting of lymphocytes and a network of venous sinuses.

Floating spleen Also known as wandering spleen, refers to a spleen that does not have normal fixed ligamentous attachments (gastrosplenic and splenorenal ligaments).

Sago spleen A morbid condition of the spleen, produced by amyloid degeneration of the organ, in which a cross-section shows scattered gray translucent bodies looking like grains of sago.

Waxy spleen A condition of amyloid degeneration of the spleen, affecting chiefly the extrasinusoidal tissue spaces of the pulp.

Splenectomy (*sple-nek'to-me*) Excision of the spleen.

Splenitis (*sple-ni'tis*) Inflammation of the spleen.

Splenium (*sple'ne-um*) A band-like structure; a bandage or compress.

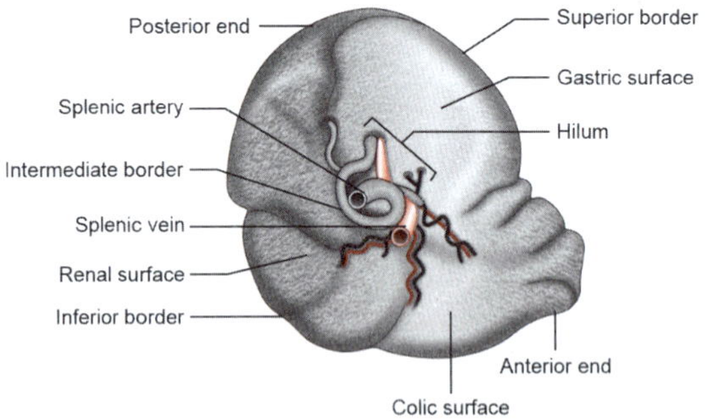

Visceral surface of spleen

Splenomegaly (*sple'no-mega-le*) Enlargement of the spleen. Spleen is enlarged in infections (enteric fever, septicemia infective hepatitis, brucellosis, malaria, kalaazar, subacute infective endocarditis), congestion (portal hypertension, noncirrhotic portal fibrosis, tropical splenomegaly), anemias, leukemias, myelofibrosis, amyloidosis, lipid storage disorders, Felty's syndrome and Still's disease.

Congestive splenomegaly A disorder in which, the spleen becomes engorged with blood because of impaired flow through the splenic vein, which empties into the portal vein.

Hemolytic splenomegaly Splenomegaly seen in hemolytic anemia.

Siderotic splenomegaly Also known as Gamna-Gandy bodies, it is the most commonly encountered in portal hypertension. The pathophysiological process is the result of microhemorrhage resulting in hemosiderin and calcium deposition followed by fibroblastic reaction.

Splenorenal anastomosis An anastomosis between the splenic vein and renal vein of the left kidney, made especially for the relief of the portal hypertension.

Splint A rigid device for holding broken bones in place or easing pain.

Air splint Use to immobilize the distal joints and to restore motion and control at the proximal joints.

Angle splint A brace across two pieces that meet at an angle.

Banjo splint A thin piece of wood or other rigid material used to immobilize a fractured or dislocated bone, or to maintain any part of the body in a fixed position.

Anderson splint A skeletal traction splint with pins inserted into proximal and distal ends of a fracture; reduction is obtained by an external plate attached to the pins.

Anchor splint An apparatus used to support and immobilize a fractured jaw; wire loops are fitted around the teeth and an external rod is used to hold the device in place.

Essig type splint A stainless steel wire passed labially and lingually around a segment of the dental arch and held in position by individual ligature wires around the contact areas of the teeth; it is used to stabilize fractured or repositioned teeth and the involved alveolar bone.

Fracture splint A supportive device used to keep in place any suspected fracture in one's arm or leg.

Keller-blake splint A hinged half ring modification of the Thomas splint for fracture of the femur.

Occlusal splint Intra-oral devices mostly indicated to modify the occlusal relationship between maxillar and mandibular dental arches.

Ulnar deviation splint Also known as ulnar drift, is a hand deformity in which the swelling of the metacarpophalangeal joints (the big knuckles at the base of the fingers) causes the fingers to become displaced, tending toward the little finger.

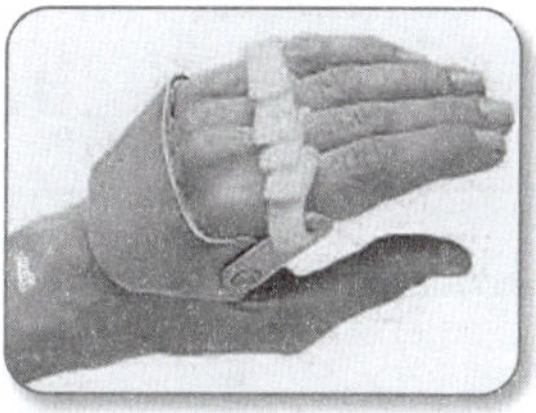

Ulnar deviation splint

Wrist splint A brace that looks like a fingerless glove. It stabilizes your wrist in a straight and sometimes slightly bent-back position.

Splitting (*split'ing*) The division of a single object into two or more parts; the cleavage of a covalent bond, fragmenting the molecule involved; division of a well-defined morbid condition into smaller subtypes; *psy* a psychological defense mechanism in which the individual deals with emotional conflict by compartmentalizing positive and negative qualities into separate parts.

Fixed splitting The splitting is wide and fixed exhibiting no expiratory variations in ASD.

Narrow splitting Splitting becomes narrowed with increased resistance in the pulmonary vascular bed, as in Eisenmenger's complex.

Paradoxical splitting Delayed closure of the aortic component may cause splitting to become narrow and pulmonary closure sound precedes the aortic closure sound.

Splitting of first heart sound Noted as 'l-lub' over the lower end of the sternum on its left side in right bundle branch block due to delay in the onset of the right ventricular systole.

Splitting of second heart sound The pulmonary valve closes later than the aortic valve and is recognized in the form of split second heart sound in the pulmonary area.

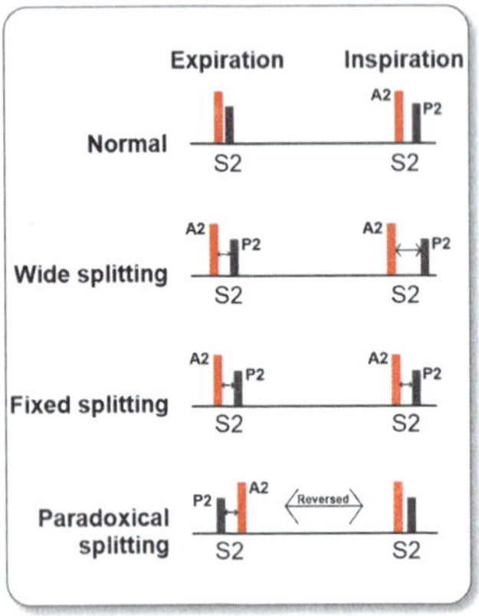

Splitting of second sound

Wide splitting Wide splitting when there is delay in the closure of the pulmonary valve, as in RBBB and pulmonary stenosis.

Spondylitis (*spon'di-li'tis*) Inflammation of vertebra.

Ankylosing spondylitis A chronic inflammatory arthritis with a predilection for the sacroiliac joints and spine. It manifests by progressive stiffening and fusion of the axial skeleton.

Spondylitis deformans Arthritis and osteitis deformans affecting the spinal column. There is ossification of ligaments and bony ankylosis of the intervertebral articulations to result in kyphosis and rigidity.

Tuberculous spondylitis Pott's disease. Tuberculous infection of the spine with a gibbus of spine.

Spondylolisthesis (*spon'di-lo-lis'the-sis*) forward displacement of a vertebra over the one below. It is associated with low back pain aggravated by standing and walking. There can be nerve root compression.

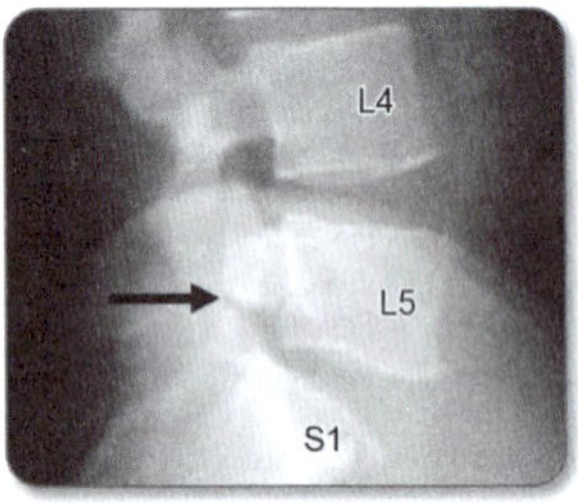

Spondylolisthesis - Straight lateral radiograph of L4-S1 level of spine - arrow showing lucency at the pars area.

Spondylosis (*spon'di-lo'sis*) Ankylosis of a vertebral joint; any degenerative lesion of the spine.

Cervical spondylosis Disc degeneration with associated osteophyte formation and osteoarthritis of the joints of cervical spine. It is associated with cervical radiculopathy.

Lumbar spondylosis Degenerative changes in the disks and lumbar spine, associated with low back pain and features of nerve root compression.

Spondylosyndesis (*spon'di-lo-sin-de'sis*) Spinal fusion.

Spongioblast (*spun'je-o-blast*) A neuroepithelial filiform ependyma cell.

Spongioblastoma (*spun'je-o-blas-to'ma*) A malignant tumor derived from spongioblasts.

Spontaneous Involuntary; produced of itself.

Spontaneous bacterial peritonitis Increased susceptibility of patients with cirrhosis to infection of ascitic fluid characterized by sudden onset of abdominal pain, rebound tenderness, absence bowel sounds and fever.

Spontaneous subcortical hematoma A form of cerebral hemorrhage without hypertension.

Sporadic (*spo-rad'ic*) Occurring singly and is neither epidemic nor endemic.

Spot A circumscribed area; a macula.

Bitot's spot Small foamy gray triangular deposits of keratinized epithelium in the conjunctiva associated with vitamin A deficiency.

Blind spot The optic disc, the site of entrance of the optic nerve and it is not sensitive to light.

Brushfield spot Small, white or greyish/brown spots on the periphery of the iris in the human eye due to aggregation of connective tissue, a normal constituent of the iris stroma. The spots are named after the physician Thomas Brushfield, who first described them in his 1924 M.D. thesis.

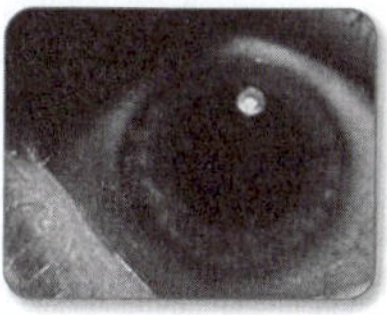

Brushfield spot

Sporicide (*spor'i-sid*) An agent which kills the spores, adj. **sporicidal**.

Sporocyst (*spor'o-sist*) Any cyst containing reproductive cells like spores; a stage in the life cycle of a trematode in the first intermediate host where the germinal sac contains germ cells; a stage in the life cycle of certain protozoa contained within a oocyst.

Sporogony (*spo-rog'o-ne*) Formation of sporozoites in sporozoan protozoa. It is an asexual division within the sporocyte.

Sporotrichosis (*spor'o-tri-ko'sis*) Infection with *Sporotrichum schenckii* through the wounds presenting with granulomatous lesion, ulcer, and lymphatic spread.

Sporozoa (*spor'o-zo'an*) Sporozoon, an individual organism of sporozoa; relating to the sporozoa.

Sporozoite (*spor'o-zo'it*) Spore forms of protozoa.

Spotted fever Group of rickettsial infections; meningococcal meningitis or septicemia with petechial rash.

Sprain (*spran*) Partial tear of joint ligament.

Sprengel deformity A complex anomaly associated with malposition and dysplasia of the scapula; may also involve atropy, which causes disfigurement and limitation of shoulder movement.

Sprue (psilosis) (*sproo*) A chronic malabsorption syndrome with steatorrhea; in dentistry, the hole made of wax or metal through which molten metal is allowed to flow into a mold.

Collagenous sprue Extensive deposition of collagen in the lamina propria of the colon that does not respond to withdrawal of dietary gluten.

Nontropical sprue Celiac disease where patients are intolerant to the proteins found in wheat (gluten and gliadin).

Tropical sprue Chronic progressive malabsorption in a patient in or from tropics with partial villous atrophy presenting with diarrhea, abdominal distension, anorexia, fatigue and weight loss. It responds to tetracyclines.

Spud Spade shaped small surgical instrument used to remove a foreign object from the eye.

Spur A small projection from any structure.

Sputum (*spu'tum*) Spit; expectoration. The material expelled by coughing contains cellular debris, mucus, blood, pus and micro-organisms.

Bloody sputum Hemoptysis.

Nummular sputum Sputum in discoid masses resembling a coin.

Rusty sputum A reddish brown expectoration in lobar pneumonia.

Squalene A triterpene that carries oxygen independent of the hemoglobin. It can carry oxygen directly to the cell membranes throughout the body and reach the regions having low oxygen supply.

Squama (*skwah'ma*) Pl. **squamae**. A thin plate of bone; an epidermic scale.

Squamous bone Upper anterior portion of temporal bone.

Squamous epithelium The flat form of epithelial cells.

Squint (*skwint*) Strabismus; an abnormality in which the right and left visual axes fail to meet toward an objective point simultaneously.

Concomitant squint; non-paralytic squint An imbalance in the action of opposing muscles and squint is present at rest in all directions of gaze and it is not associated with diplopia.

Paralytic squint Due to weakness of one or more extraocular muscles; the squint is noticeable when the patient attempts to move the eye in the direction of action of paralyzed muscle and diplopia occurs in such positions of the eyes which depend upon the contractions of the paralyzed muscles.

Stadium (*sta'de-um*) A stage or period in the progress of the disease.

Stadium decrementi The period of decrease in severity of a disease.

Stadium fluorescentiae The stage of eruption in an exanthematous disease.

Stadium incrementi The period of increase in the intensity of a disease.

Stadium sudoris The sweating stage of malaria.

Stage (*staj*) A period in the course of a disease; distribution and extent of spread of a malignancy; the part of microscope on which the slide is placed for examination.

Algid stage Period marked by collapse in cholera.

Amphibolic stage The stage of an infectious disease between the acme and decline at a time when outcome is not certain.

Anal stage The second stage of psychosexual development in a child when its activities and interests are on the anal zone.

Cold stage The period of chills or rigor in malaria.

Defervescent stage The period of decline in fever.

Eruptive stage The period of appearance of exanthema; tooth eruption.

Exoerythrocytic stage Developmental stage of malarial parasite outside of red blood cells, in the liver parenchymal cells.

Expulsive stage of labor The stage of dilatation of uterine cervix during which child is expelled from uterus; second stage of labor.

First stage of labor Period when the fetal head is molded and cervix dilated.

Fourth stage of labor The post partum period following expulsion of the placenta.

Hot stage Period of pyrexia malaria.

Imperfect stage The asexual life cycle, phase of a fungus.

Intuitive stage A stage of development in child when a child's thought processes are determined by the most prominent aspects of the stimuli.

Latent stage Incubation period.

Oral stage The earliest stage of psychosexual development when the infant's needs and expressions are centered on the oral zone to be followed by anal stage.

Phallic stage The third stage of psychosexual development during which period of sexual interest of the child is centered on the penis in boys and clitoris in girls. It is preceded by anal stage.

Preeruptive stage A stage in infectious disease before appearance of eruption.

Prodromal stage Incubation period.

Second stage of labor Expulsive stage of labor.

Stage of labor The placental stage of labor.

Sweating stage Occurrence of sweating as a terminal stage of malaria third.

Staghorn calculus A renal stone of magnesium ammonium phosphate with broad arborescence filling the renal pelvicalyceal system.

Stagnant loop syndrome (Blind loop syndrome) occurs when food does not move normally through a section of intestine during digestion.

Stain (*stan*) Dye used in histologic and bacteriologic examinations; a procedure in which the dye and reagents are used to color the constituents of cells and tissues.

Acid fast stain Stain containing carbol fuchsin which is retained by mycobacteria.

Acid stain A stain in which the anion is the colored component of the dye molecule. Eosin is commonly used to stain the cytoplasm.

Basic stain A stain in which the cation is the colored component of the dye molecule. Methylene blue is employed to stain nuclear elements of the cells.

Contrast stain Differential stain that facilitates differentiation of various elements in a specimen.

Counter stain A contrast stain used after staining of specific elements of a tissue.

Dental stain Discoloration accumulating on the surface of teeth or dentures.

Differential stain A stain that helps to differentiate among different types of bacteria.

Double stain A mixture of acid and basic stains.

Giemsa stain A stain contains azure II-eosin and azure II used for staining Negri bodies, differential staining of blood smears and chromosomes.

Gram's stain A method of differential staining of bacteria which are stained with crystal violet, washed and then flooded with iodine solution. It stains bacteria either dark or purple. Then, acetone is added. It decolorizes the gram-negative bacteria without affecting gram-positive ones. Then it is counter-stained with safranine or neutral red. Gram-positive organisms appear violet and gram-negative organisms appear red against pink background.

Haematoxylin-eosin stain A mixture of a haematoxylin in distilled water and aqueous eosin solution to stain tissues. Nuclei are stained a deep blue-black with haematoxylin and cytoplasm is stained pink after counter staining with eosin.

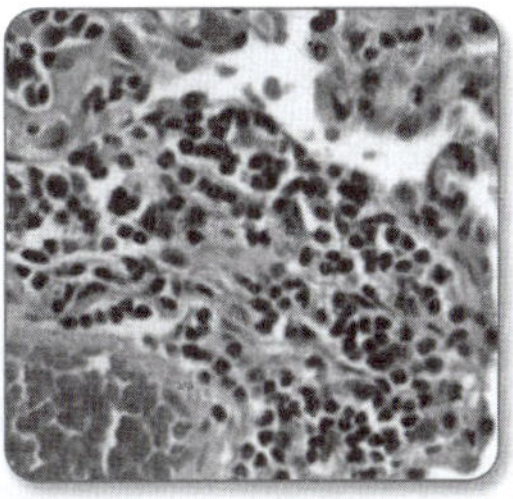

Haematoxylin-eosin staining

Immunofluorescent stain Staining resulting from a combination of fluorescent antibody with antigen specific for the antibody.

Intravital stain A stain which is taken up by living cells after parenteral administration.

Iodine stain Stain for amebae, amyloid, cellulose and starch.

Metachromatic stain A stain having an ability to produce different colors on staining cells and tissues.

Papanicolaou stain *see* Papanicolaou stain.

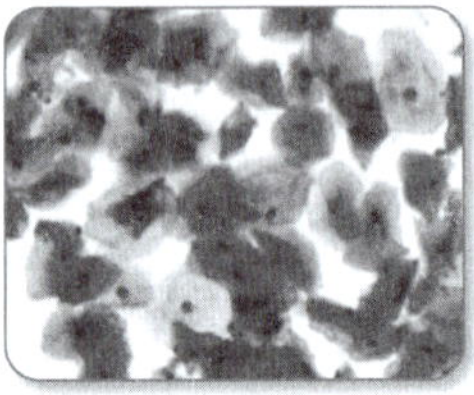

Papanicolaou stain - histological

Port-wine stain A birthmark in which swollen blood vessels create a reddish-purplish discoloration of the skin.

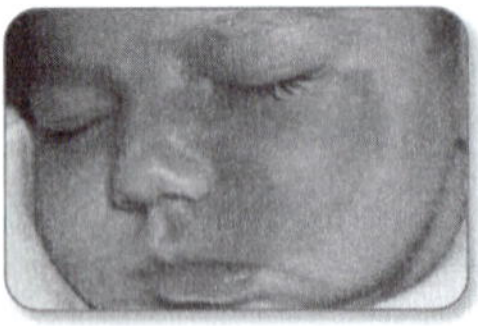

Port-wine stain

Supravital stain Stain that colors living cells or tissues that have been removed from the body.

Vital stain Intravital stain.

Wright's stain A polychrome stain contains eosin and methylene blue used for demonstration of cells and malarial parasites.

Stamey procedure Involves passing a single-holed ligature carrier (Stamey needle) through two small suprapubic incisions either side of the midline, through the retropubic space to ipsilateral transvaginal incisions either side of the bladder neck.

Stammering (stuttering) (*stam'er-ing*) A speed disorder with hesitation and repetition of sounds.

Stanolone (*stan'o-lon*) An androgen and anabolic steroid (AAS) medication derived from dihydrotestosterone (DHT).

Stanozolol (*stan'o-zo-lol*) Anabolic steroid.

Stanya (*S*) Breast milk.

Stapedectomy (*sta'pe-dek'to-me*) Excision of stapes.

Stapes (*sta'pes*) A small stirrup-shaped bone in the middle ear

Staphylectomy Surgical excision of the uvula.

Staphylococcus (*staf'a-lo-kok'as*) A genus of gram-positive bacteria in the family Staphylococcaceae from the order Bacillales. Under the microscope, they appear spherical, and form in grapelike clusters. Staphylococcus species are facultative anaerobic organisms. pl. **staphylococci**.

Staphylococcus aureus An agent responsible for wide variety of suppurative conditions.

Staphylococcus epidermidis Commonly found on normal skin.

Staphylococcus saprophyticus An agent that may cause urinary tract infections.

Staphyloma (*staf'i-lo-ma*) Herniation of sclera or cornea with uvea included.

Anterior staphyloma A localized defect in the anterior eye wall with protrusion of uveal tissue due to alterations in scleral thickness and structure.

Posterior staphyloma An outpouching of the wall of the eye that has a radius of curvature that is less than the surrounding curvature of the wall of the eye.

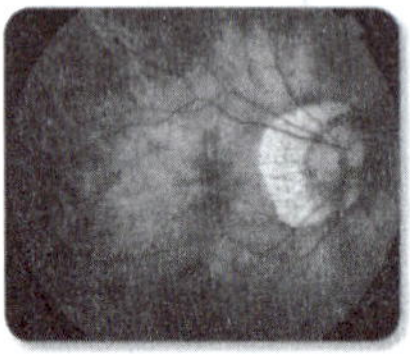

Posterior staphyloma

Staphylorrhaphy (palatorrhaphy, uraniscorrhaphy) (*staf'i-lora'a-fe*) Suture of a cleft palate.

Starch Polymers of glucose linked by 1–4 glycoside linkages. Nutrient found in cereals, roots and legumes, providing largest proportion of calories. They are digested promptly by amylase, or slowly digested or escape digestion.

Starling law Energy of contraction of heart muscle varies directly with the length of muscle fibers at the end of diastole, named after Ernest Starling a British physiologist.

Starvation A condition of being without food for a long period of time resulting in undernutrition and loss of weight.

Stasis (*sta'sis*) Stoppage of flow, growth or activity.

Status asthmaticus Acute severe asthma.

Status epilepticus A major attack of epilepsy succeeding another without the patient regaining awareness between attacks.

Status lymphaticus A constitutional hereditary anomaly characterized by hypoplasia of the cardiovascular apparatus, hyperplasia of the thymus gland and of the lymphoid tissues in other localities and by congenital structural defects in different parts of viscera.

Steapsin Other name for the enzyme lipase.

Stearic acid (*ste-ar'ik*) Straight-chain saturated 18-carbon fatty acid, used in ointments, suppositories and soaps.

Steal-(steato-) (*stel*) Diversion of blood via alternate routes or reversed flow. A partial blockage of a large artery causing a temporary ischemia in one segment of its territory by diverting the blood to cater to the excessive demands in another.

Steatoma (*ste'a-to'ma*) Lipoma; a fatty mass within a sebaceous cyst. pl **steotomata.**

Steatopygia (*ste'a-to-pij'e-a*) Excessive fatness of the buttocks.

Steatorrhoea (*ste'a-to-re'a*) Excess amount of fat in the feces.

Steatosis (*ste'a-to'sis*) Fatty degeneration of the liver.

Macrovascular steatosis A single fat globule fills the liver cell and pushes the nucleus to the periphery, found in alcoholism, obesity, diabetes mellitus, starvation and malabsorption.

Microvascular steatosis Small fat vacuoles giving the liver cells foamy appearance found in fatty liver of pregnancy, Reye's syndrome, certain inherited metabolic disorders and drugs.

Stellate fracture A fracture with many fissures that radiate from central point of injury.

Stellate ganglia Fused lower cervical and first thoracic ganglia of the sympathetic chain.

Stellwag's sign Infrequent blinking in thyrotoxicosis, named after Carl Stellwag, an Austrian ophthalmologist.

Stem cell Any stalk-like structure. **Stem cell** an undifferentiated cell that can differentiate in more than one direction.

Stem cell factor Growth factor influencing proliferation and differentiation of stem cells.

Stenopeic (*sten'o-pe'ik*) Having a narrow opening; slit.

Stenosis (*ste-no'sis*) A stricture or narrowing of any canal, especially of the cardiac valves.

Aortic stenosis Narrowing of the aortic valve orifice or of the aorta near the valve.

Cicatricial stenosis Stenosis from any contracted cicatrix.

Hypertrophic pyloric stenosis Congenital pyloric stenosis due to hypertrophy of the pyloric sphincter presenting with projectile vomiting in second or third week of life.

Idiopathic hypertrophic subaortic stenosis Left ventricular outflow obstruction due to hypertrophy of the ventricular septum.

Lumbar stenosis Narrowing of lumbar canal from overgrowth of laminae of vertebrae.

Mitral stenosis Narrowing of the mitral valve.

Pulmonary stenosis Narrowing of the opening between pulmonary artery and the right ventricle.

Pyloric stenosis Hypertrophy of the walls of pyloric orifice causing obstruction.

Tricuspid stenosis Narrowing of the orifice of the tricuspid valve.

Stenostomia (stenostomy) Abnormal narrowing of an opening such as the opening of the bile duct.

Stensen's duct Parotid duct, named after Niels Stensen, a Danish anatomist.

Sterc(o) Combining word for feces.

Stercobilin (*ster'ko-bi'lin*) Brown-orange-red pigment, an oxidized product of stercobilinogen, excreted in the stool.

Stercolith (*ster'ko-lith*) Fecalith.

Stercoraceous (*ster'ka-ra'shas*) Fecal.

Stereognosis (*ster'e-og-no'sis*) Recognition of the commonly used object by feeling its size, shape, weight and form when kept in hand while the eyes are closed and it is dependent on the sense of touch, position and movement.

Stereoscopic vision Binocular vision having perception of the shape, depth and distance of an object.

Stereotaxy (*sti'ri-o'ta-ksi*) Three-dimensional target localization.

Stereotypy (*ster'e-o-ti'pe*) Repetition of meaningless, often bizarre action.

Sterile (*ster'il*) Aseptic, free from living microorganisms; barren; not fertile.

Sterility (*sta-rili-te*) Physiological inability to effect sexual reproduction in a living thing; freedom from the presence of viable microorganisms.

Sterilization (*ster'i-li-za'shun*) A process that destroys pathogens by autoclaving pressurized moist heat or by dry heat; any procedure like vasectomy or tubectomy making an individual incapable of reproduction.

Sternebra (*ster'ne-bra*) Any of the segments of the sternum in early life that fuse to form the body of the sternum.

Sternocleidomastoid muscle (*ster'no-kli'do-mas'toid*) Pertaining to the sternum, clavicle and mastoid process.

Sternohyoid (*ster'no-hi'oid*) Pertaining to the sternum and hyoid bone.

Sternomastoid muscle (*ster'no-mas'toid*) Pertaining to the sternum and mastoid process.

Sternomastoid tumor Fibromatosis colli of infancy, is a rare benign mass in the muscle on the side of the neck; appears in a newborn usually between the 2nd and 4th weeks of life.

Sternotomy (*ster-not'o-me*) Operative cutting through the sternum.

Sternum (*ster'num*) Breastbone.

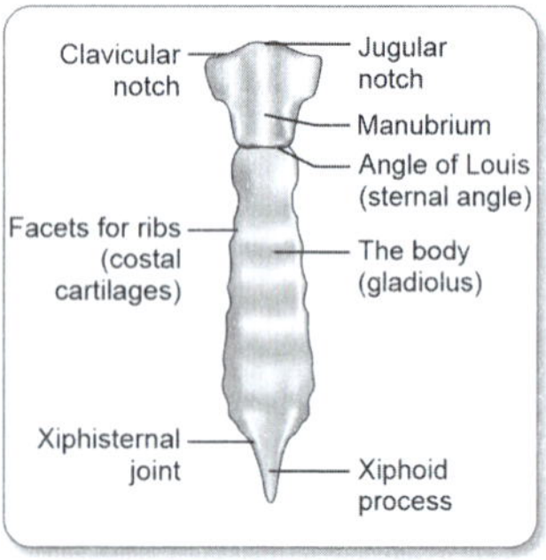

Sternum - Anterior view

Sternutator (*ster-nu'ta-tor'e*) Causing sneezing.

Steroid (*ster'oid*) Any of a group of polycyclic compounds containing in its chemical nucleus cyclopentanoperhydrophenanthrene ring.

Sterol (*ster'ol*) A steroid of 27 or more carbon atoms with one OH group.

Stertor (*ster'tor*) The act of snoring.

Steth- (stetho-) Combining word for chest.

Stethalgia (*ste-thal'je-a*) Pain in the chests.

Stethogoniometer (*steth'o-go'ne-om'e-ter*) An apparatus for the measurement of curvature of the chest.

Stethometer (*steth-om'e-ter*) An instrument to measure circular dimension or expansion of the chest.

Stethoscope (*steth'o-skop*) An instrument consisting of ear piece, metal frame, rubber or plastic tube and chest piece (bell and diaphragm) used to transmit sounds produced in the body to the examiner's ears.

Sthenia (*sthe'ne-a*) A condition of activity.

Stibophen Antihelminthic drug used by intramuscular injection.

Stigma (*stig'ma*) Visible evidence of a disease; any spot or blemish on the skin; mark of disgrace.

Stilbestrol Synthetic estrogen used in cancer of prostate and breast.

Stilet (*sti'let*) A slender probe.

Stillbirth (*stil'berth*) Delivery of a dead fetus.

Stillbirth ratio The number of still births per thousand still and live births in the same period.

Still's disease Juvenile rheumatoid arthritis, named after Sir George Still, British physician.

Stimulant (*stim'u-lant*) Stimulating; an agent that increases activity.

Stimulus (*stim'u-lus*) Stimulant; that which can elicit response in an excitable tissue. pl. **stimuli**.

Stippling (*stip'ling*) Punctate appearance; red white granularity in a radiolucent background.

Stirrup (*stir'up*) stapes.

Stitch (*stich*) Suture; a momentary sharp pain.

Stokes-Adams syndrome (Adams-stokes syndrome) A syndrome characterized by slow or absent pulse, vertigo, syncope, convulsions and sometimes, Cheyne-stokes respiration.

Stoma (*sto'ma*) The mouth; a minute opening; an artificial opening between two cavities or canals.

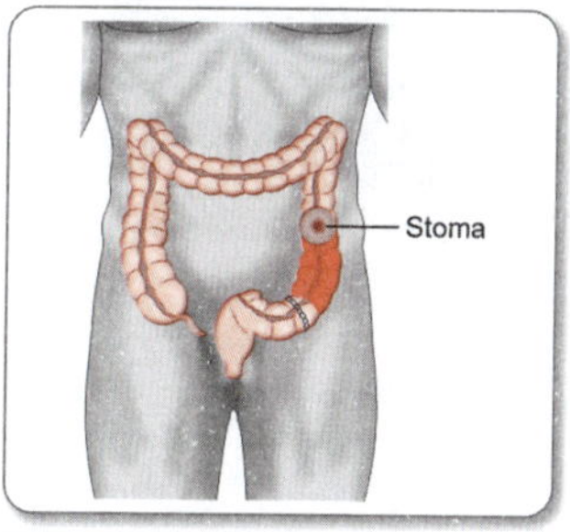

Stoma - colorectal

Stomach (*stom'ak*) The J-shaped musculo-membranous enlargement of the alimentary canal directly under the diaphragm in the epigastric, umbilical and left hypochondriac regions of the abdomen, between the esophagus and small intestine. It consists of a cardiac part, a fundus, a body and a pyloric part. Its glands secrete gastric juice which when mixed with food forms chyme making it suitable for further digestion.

Cascade stomach A form of hourglass stomach in which there is constriction between the cardiac and pyloric portions.

Hourglass stomach Division of stomach into two parts by scar in chronic duodenal ulcer resembling an hourglass in shape.

Leather bottle stomach A type of stomach with hypertrophy of its walls by infiltration with malignant tissue.

Watermelon stomach Gastric antral vascular ectasia where linear angioid streaks converge at the pylorus in the pattern reminiscent of watermelon, which presents with acute gastric bleeding or chronic iron deficiency anemia.

Stomachic (*sto-mak'ik*) Gastric; a medicine that promotes the functional activity of the stomach.

Stomal ulcer Ulcer at the site of gastrojejunostomy.

Stomat- (stomato-) Combining word for mouth.

Stomatitis (*sto'ma-ti-tis*) Inflammation of the mucous membrane of the mouth.

Nicotine stomatitis A reaction seen on the roof of the mouth caused by extreme heat in the mouth, most commonly from smoking. It is also known as including nicotinic stomatitis, stomatitis nicotina and smoker's keratosis.

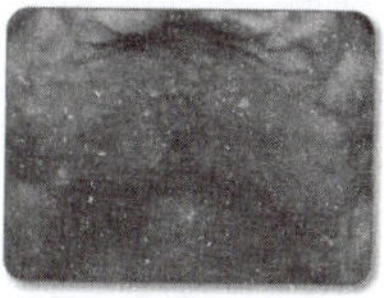

Nicotine stomatitis

Stomatology (*sto'ma-tol'o-je*) Branch of medicine concerned with the mouth and its diseases.

Stomodeum (*sto'ma-de'um*) An ectodermal depression at the cranial end of an embryo that forms front part of the mouth.

-stomy (-ostomy) Combining word for creation of an opening into or a communication between.

Stone (*ston*) A calculus.

Bile duct stone Common bile duct stone may develop from biliary sludge due to dysfunction of sphincter of Oddi many years after cholecystectomy or may migrate from the gallbladder.

Dental stone A hemihydrate of gypsum used in the preparation of dental models.

Gallbladder stone Gall stones which may be cholesterol or pigment stones.

Salivary stone A calcified stone present in the ducts of salivary glands.

Urinary tract stone Aggregates of crystals and small amount of protein and glycoprotein found as sand anywhere in the urinary tract or as a round stone in the bladder.

Stool (*stul*) Feces; evacuation of the bowel.

Bloody stool Blood in the stools as in dysentery.

Fatty stool Stools containing fat as in malabsorption syndrome and pancreatic disease.

Lienteric stool Stool that contains undigested material.

Mucous stool Stools containing large amount of mucus.

Pea soup stool Liquid stools of enteric fever.

Pipe stem stool Stools resembling a pipe stem in stricture of rectum.

Rice water stool Watery stools in cholera.

Tarry stool Stools appearing like a tar as in upper GI bleed.

Strabismus (heterotropia) (*stra-biz'mus*) Failure of eyes to fix at the same point; squint.

Strain (*stran*) To exert to the utmost; subline of species; a hereditary tendency; to filter.

Strangulated (*strang'gu-la-ted*) Constricted so as to prevent passage of sufficient amount of air, as through the trachea or to cut off venous return as in a hernia.

Strangulation (*strang'gu-la'shun*) Asphyxiation by neck compression; passage of a motile tissue through an orifice, as in hernia, tight enough to stop blood flow.

Strangury (*strang'gu-re*) Frequent painful passage of urine.

Stratum (*stra'tum*) A layer; pl. **strata**.

Stratum basalis The outer layer of the endometrium next to the myometrium that is maintained during menstruation and gestation.

Stratum functionalis The inner layer of endometrium; the layer next to the uterine cavity that is shed during menstruation and that forms the maternal part of the placenta during gestation.

Stratum germinativum Multiplying layer of the epidermis.

Streak (*strek*) A line or stria.

Angioid streak Bilateral, narrow, irregular lines deep to the retina configured in a radiating fashion emanating from the optic disc, which result from breaks in a weakened Bruch's membrane.

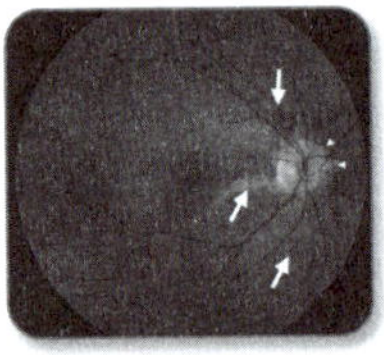

Angioid streak

Streptobacillus (*strep'to-ba-sil'lus*) A genus of gram-negative bacteria that are highly pleomorphic; S. moniliformis is a causative agent of rat bite fever.

Streptococcus (*strep'to-kok'us*) A genus of gram-positive cocci dividing in one direction only forming chains. Some of the species are highly pathogenic.

Alpha hemolytic streptococcus Streptococci causing partial hemolysis of blood on blood agar plates.

Beta hemolytic streptococcus Streptococci causing complete hemolysis of the blood in blood agar plates.

Streptococcus agalactiae A group of beta hemolytic species found in raw milk responsible for sepsis in newborn and endometritis in post-partum women.

Streptococcus faecalis An enterococcus found in the alimentary tract that may cause urinary tract infections.

Streptococcus pneumoniae An oval or spherical, gram-positive cocci possessing a capsule with more than 80 serological strains and is responsible for lobar pneumonia and other infections in different parts of the body.

Streptococcus pyogenes Any of the group of beta hemolytic streptococci causing suppuration.

Streptococcus viridans A group of alpha hemolytic streptococci found in upper respiratory tract and a common agent causing subacute infective endocarditis.

Streptodornase (*strep'to-dor'nas*) DNA-splitting enzyme produced by group A streptococci.

Streptokinase (*strep'to-ki'nas*) A streptococcus produced plasminogen activator that increases plasmin levels to dissolve recently formed clots.

Streptolysin (*strop-tol'i-sin*) Hemolysin of hemolytic streptococci.

Streptomyces (*strep'to-mi'sez*) A group of soil bacteria order Actinomycetales that are a source of various antibiotics.

Streptomycin (*strep'to-mi'sin*) An aminoglycoside antibiotic obtained from Streptomyces griseus effective against mycobacteria, and a variety of aerobic gram-negative bacilli and some gram positive bacteria.

Stretch receptor Mechanoreceptors responsive to distention of various organs and muscles, neurologically linked to medulla *via* afferent nerve fibers.

Stretch reflex (myotatic reflex) A lower motor neuron reaction in which stretching of the muscle makes it contract.

Stria A streak-like, linear atrophic, pink, purple or white line on the skin due to changes in the connective tissue. pl **striae.**

Stria gravidarum Curved pink streaks on lower abdomen following pregnancy due to stretch damage to elastic tissue in the skin.

Striae distensae A form of scarring on the skin with an off-color hue.

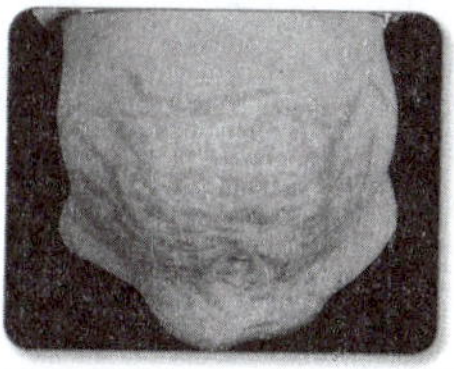

Striae distensae in a man with Cushing syndrome

Striated muscle (*stri'at-ed*) Muscles having stripes or striaes; These are voluntary muscles e.g., cardiac muscles and skeletal muscles.

Stricture (*strik'chur*) An abnormal narrowing of a duct or passage.

Stricturoplasty A surgical procedure performed to alleviate bowel narrowing due to scar tissue that has built up in the intestinal wall from an inflammatory condition like Crohn disease.

Stridor (*stri'dor*) A loud, musical sound of constant pitch heard in laryngeal or intratracheal obstruction. The crowing sounds are accompanied by supraclavicular inspiratory retraction.

String of pearls sign An abdominal radiograph showing small bowel obstruction that has resulted in markedly dilated small bowel revealing a line of gas bubbles trapped between the valvulae conniventes.

Strobila Segments of a tapeworm.

Stroke (apoplexy) (*strok*) Rapidly developing clinical symptoms and/or signs of focal (at times global) disturbance of cerebral function, with symptoms lasting for more than 24 hours or leading to death with no apparent cause other than that of vascular origin.

Heat stroke *see* Heat stroke.

Ischemic stroke Sudden onset of stroke due to diminished blood supply to the brain.

Paralytic stroke Sudden onset of paralysis from an injury to the brain or spinal cord.

Stroke in evolution Cerebral ischemia progressing to hemiplegia over several hours.

Stroke volume Amount of blood pumped by either ventricle per beat and it is dependent upon end-diastolic pressure and peripheral vascular resistance (after load).

Stroke work External work performed by the ventricle with each beat. It maintains perfusion and oxygen delivery to all organs.

Stroma (*stro'ma*) Supporting connective tissue of epithelial organ. pl. **Stromata**.

Strongyloides (*stron'ji-loi-dez*) A very small nematode (2 mm × 0.4 mm) parasites commonly found in the small intestine. The eggs hatch in the intestine and larvae are passed in the stool. They moult in moist soil and become infective filariform larvae and penetrate human skin and undergo a developmental cycle.

Strongyloides stercoralis Human pathogenic parasitic roundworm causing the disease strongyloidiasis.

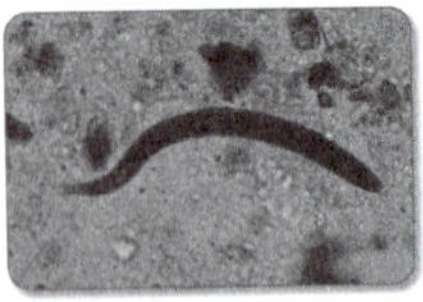

Strongyloides stercoralis

Strongyloidiasis (strongyloidosis) (*stron'ji-loi-di'a-sis*) Infestation with the namatode Strongyloides stercoralis presenting with itchy rash, abdominal pain, steatorrhea, and weight loss; also called **strongyloidosis**.

Systemic strongyloidiasis Stronglyloides hyperinfestation syndrome occurring in association with immune suppression presenting with diarrhea, pneumonia and meningoencephalopathies.

Struma (*stru'ma*) (*Ger*) Goiter, name from a Bulgarian river Struma showing high incidence of the condition.

Strychnine (*strik'nin*) A poisonous alkaloid from Strychnos nux-vomica. It causes excitation of all parts of central nervous system by blocking neural impulses and is used in experimental pharmacology.

Stunning (*stun'ing*) Loss of function.

Stupor (*stu'per*) A state wherein the patient shows response on vigorous stimuli but sinks back to the original state as soon as the painful stimulus is withdrawn.

Sturge-Weber syndrome Encephalo-trigeminal angiomatosis presenting as cutaneous vascular port-wine naevus on the face, contralateral hemiparesis and hemiatrophy, glaucoma and seizures, named after William Sturge and Frederick Weber, British physicians.

Stuttering (*Stut'er-ing*) A defective speech pattern wherein there is staccato repetition of the first phoneme of a spoken phrase; intermittent progression of disease.

Stye (*Sti*) Also called hordeolum; a painful red bump on the edge of your eyelid.

Stylet (stilet, stylus) (*sti'lit*) A wire running through a catheter or cannula to make it stiff or to clear its passage; a slender probe.

Styloglossus Paired extrinsic muscle of the tongue.

Stylohyoid (*sti'lo-hi'oid*) Pertaining to the styloid process and hyoid hone.

Styloid process (*sti'loid*) A conical prolongation of the lateral surface of the distal extremity of the radius that gives attachment to several tendons and ligaments.

Stylus (*sti'lus*) Stylet; a probe or slender wire or needle for stiffening or clearing a canal; a pointed medicinal preparation in the form of a stick.

Styptic (*stip'tik*) Astringent; hemostatic.

Sub- Combining word for under; near; almost.

Subacute (*sub-a-kut*) A condition between acute and chronic.

Subacute combined degeneration of cord A combined system disease and funicular myelitis characterized by progressive spastic and ataxic paraparesis and distal neuropathy due to vitamin B12 deficiency. There is symmetric demyelination in posterior and lateral columns.

Subacute infective endocarditis A microbial infection of a heart valve, the lining of a cardiac chamber or blood vessel or a congenital abnormality like septal defect presenting with fever, tiredness, night sweats, weight loss, new signs of valve dysfunction or heart failure. There may be features of embolic stroke or peripheral arterial embolism. Other features are purpura, petechial hemorrhages, splinter hemorrhage, Osler's nodes, digital clubbing, splenomegaly and microscopic hematuria.

Subacute necrotic myelitis A progressive ascending motor, sensory and autonomic paralysis due to necrosis and distension of the spinal cord.

Subacute sclerosing panencephalitis (SSPE) A slow form of measles encephalitis affecting children and adolescents, has an insidious onset manifesting with poor performance in studies, incoordination, ataxia, pyramidal and extrapyramidal manifestations, aphasia and optic atrophy.

Subacute combined degeneration of the cord A combined system disease and funicular myelitis characterized by progressive spastic and ataxic paraparesis and distal neuropathy due to vitamin B12 deficiency. There is symmetric demyelination in posterior and lateral columns.

Subarachnoid hemorrhage Bleeding into the subarachnoid space. It results in blood spilling over into the cerebrospinal flow resulting in bloody CSF. It presents with sudden severe headache, which frequently spreads to the cervical region, nausea, vomiting with loss of consciousness. There is neck stiffness, focal neurologic deficit and/or cranial nerve palsy.

Subarachnoid space Space between the arachnoid and pia mater filled with cerebrospinal fluid.

Subclavian artery Located under the clavicle, this artery moves oxygen rich blood from heart to upper body.

Subclinical (*sub-kl'in'i-k'l*) Without obvious clinical manifestations.

Subconscious (*sub-kon'shus*) Partially conscious; occurrence of mental processes without the individual being aware of their occurrence.

Subcutaneous (*sub'ku-ta'ne-us*) Beneath the skin.

Subdural (*sub-dur'al*) Between the dura mater and arachnoid.

Subdural hematoma Venous blood after trauma.

Subependymoma (*sub'ep-en'di-mo'ma*) Benign tumors in the ventricles that grow from the ventricular wall into the spinal fluid spaces within the brain. These lesions may obstruct spinal fluid flow and/or put pressure on surrounding structures, causing symptoms including headaches and confusion.

Subinvolution (*sub'in-vo-lu'shun*) Incomplete involution.

Sublimation (*sub'li-ma'shun*) The conversion of a solid directly into a gas; diversion of primitive impulse into acceptable activity.

Subliminal (*sub-lim'i-n'l*) Below the threshold of consciousness.

Sublingual (*sub-ling'gwal*) Beneath the tongue.

Subluxation (*sub-luk-sa'shun*) Incomplete dislocation, especially when joint surfaces remain in contact but displaced from normal position.

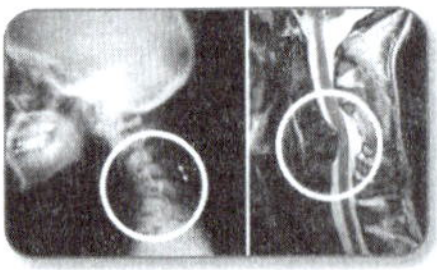

Severe subluxation of cervical vertebra

Submandibular gland Submaxillary gland; below the mandible.

Submentovertical (SMV) Longest effective diameter of the fetal head as in brow presentation.

Submucosa (*sub'mu-ko'sa*) Beneath a mucous membrane.

Submucous fibrosis of mouth Severe fibrosis of structures of oral cavity affecting mobility.

Subphrenic abscess Abscess between the liver and diaphragm.

Substitution (*sub'sti-tu'shun*) Replacement of an atom or group in a compound by another; *psy* an unconscious defense mechanism by which an unacceptable thing is replaced by one that is acceptable.

Substitution therapy Replacement of substances normally produced by body especially hormones.

Substrate (*sub'strat*) Specific substance acted on by enzyme.

Subsultus Twitch.

Subtertian fever Occurring more often than every second day.

Subthalamic nucleus (*sub"tha-lam'ik*) Inferior to the thalamus; pertaining to the subthalamus.

Succinylcholine (*suk'si-nil-ko'len*) A short-acting neuromuscular relaxant.

Succus (*suk'us*) Juice; any fluid obtained from a living tissue as secretion especially the digestive juices.

Succus entericus Intestinal juice.

Succussion (*su-kush'un*) A shaking.

Succussion splash A splashing sound audible over the chest in hydro- or pyo-pneumothorax while the chest is jerked to-and-fro. It is also heard in conditions of severe distension of the stomach, herniation of stomach or of intestine into the thorax and over a large cavity containing fluid and air in the lung.

Sucking wound Wound of chest wall communicating with pleura.

Sucralfate A basic aluminum salt of sucrose octasulfate. It has no effect on acid secretion but binds to fibroblast growth factor and to ulcer base reducing the excess of pepsin and acid in peptic ulcer.

Sucrose (*su'kros*) Saccharum, a disaccharide made up of glucose and fructose.

Suction (*suk'shun*) The act of drawing, as fluids by exhausting the air.

Nasogastric suction The suction of fluid, solid or gaseous material from the gastrointestinal tract by use of tube introduced into the stomach or intestine through the nares.

Post-tussive suction A sucking noise audible immediately after coughing over a cavity in the lung.

Suction abortion The removal of products of conception from the uterus by a device that sucks the tissues away from the lining of the uterus.

Suction biopsy A method to obtain tissues by a device that applies suction.

Sudamen (*su-da'men*) Minute epidermal vesicles produced by excessive sweating over a prolonged period.

Sudden infant death syndrome Sudden death of a baby less than 1 year of age; and unexplained cause ever after investigation, autopsy and a review of clinical history.

Sudeck atrophy Complex regional pain syndrome, developing after injury, surgery, stroke or heart attack.

Sudor (*soo'dor*) Sweat, perspiration.

Sudorific (*su'do-rif'ik*) Causing sweat.

Suffocation (*suf'o-ka'shun*) Asphyxiation.

Suffusion (*su-fu'zhun*) Extravasation; reddening of the surface; condition of being wet with a fluid; the act of pouring fluid over the body.

Sugar (*shug'ar*) A carbohydrate, that is the chief source of energy.

Extrinsic sugar Extracted, refined or concentrated sugar such as sucrose.

Intrinsic sugar Naturally incorporated sugars in the cellular structure of fruits or milk.

Sugar coating Gray-pink plaque like elevations of cerebellar folia seen with medulloblastoma.

Sugar intolerance Diarrhea due to osmotic effect on unabsorbed sugar.

Sugar substitutes A group of carbohydrates such as fructose, sorbitol and xylitol used as replacements of usual dietary sugars in diabetics.

Sugar tumor A benign lung tumor with increased vascularity and polygonal glycogen filled clear cells.

Suggestion (*sug-jes'chun*) Implanting of an idea in the mind of another by some word or act; incitement.

Post hypnotic suggestion The act of exercising control over a hypnotized person by communicating some belief or words.

Suicide (*su'i-sid*) The act of taking one's own life.

Attempted suicide An attempt that does not inevitably involve fatal intent.

Sulcus (*sul'kus*) A groove, furrow, fissure especially of the brain or slight depression.

Alveololingual sulcus The space in the floor of the mouth between the base of the tongue and the alveolar ridge.

Calcarine sulcus A fissure on the medial surface of the occipital lobe of the brain, separating the cuneus from lingual gyrus.

Central sulcus A fissure on the lateral surface of each cerebral hemisphere at the border between the frontal and parietal lobes.

Cingulate sulcus A fissure on the medial surface of the cerebral hemisphere binding the gypus cinguli and paracentral lobule.

Collateral sulcus A deep sagittal fissure on the undersurface of the temporal lobe between the fusiform and hippocampal gyri.

Coronary sulcus Atrioventricular groove on the outer surface of the heart.

Frontal sulcus Fissure on outer surface of each frontal lobe of cerebrum.

Gingival sulcus The space between the surface of the tooth and free gingiva.

Hippocampal sulcus A shallow groove on the medial side of hippocampal gyrus.

Intraparietal sulcus A groove that separates parietal lobe into a superior and inferior parietal lobule.

Olfactory sulcus Groove on the inferior surface of each frontal lobe of cerebrum.

Precentral sulcus A fissure demarcating the anterior border of precentral gyrus.

Scleral sulcus A slight groove at the line of union of sclera and cornea.

Sulcus cuits The ridges on the skin of the palmar surface of the fingers and toes.

Sulcus gluteus Furrow between the buttock and thigh.

Sulcus matricis unguis The cutaneous furrow in which the lateral border of nail is situated.

Sulfacetamide (*sul'fati-set'amid*) Soluble sulfonamide used in the treatment of ophthalmic infections.

Sulfadoxine A long acting sulfonamide used for the treatment or prevention of malaria.

Sulfa drug Sulfonamides drugs.

Sulfaphenazole A long lasting sulphonamide antibiotic used in the treatment of leprosy.

Sulfamethizole *(sul'fa-meth'i-zol)* Rapidly excreted sulfonamide used in urinary tract infection.

Sulfamethoxazole (*sul'fa-meth-ok'sa-zol*) A sulfonamide preparation used in combination with trimethoprim.

Sulfaphenazole Antibacterial, sulphonamide drug.

Sulfasalazine (*sul'fa-sal'a-zen*) Sulfonamide possessing no antibacterial activity used in ulcerative colitis. It is a 5-amino salicylic acid bound by an azo bond to sulfapyridine. The colonic bacteria break the azo bond to release aminosalicylate which has an anti-inflammatory effect on colonic mucosa.

Sulfinpyrazone (*sul'fin-pi'ra-zon*) An uricosuric agent used in gout.

Sulfisoxazole (*sul'fi-sok'sa-zol*) A short-acting sulfonamide preparation.

Sulfobromophthalein (*sul'fo-bro'mo-thal'e-in*) A sulfur and bromine containing compound used in testing hepatic function.

Sulfonamide (sulfa drug) (*sul-fon'a-mid*) Para-amino benzene sulfonamide group of antibacterial agents. They have a synergistic action with trimethoprim, dapsone and pyrimethamine.

Sulfone (*sul'fon*) An oxidation product of sulfur compound in which two hydrocarbon radicals are attached to –SO_2- group. Dapsone is a preparation of sulfone.

Sulfonylurea (*sul'fo-nil-u-re'a*) Hypoglycemic agent whose action is mediated through stimulation of the release of insulin from the pancreatic beta cells, and may also reduce the hepatic release of glucose and diminish insulin resistance. They are used in the treatment of non-obese patients with type 2 diabetes who fail to respond to dietary measures alone.

First generation sulfonylurea Chlorpropamide, tolbutamide and tolazamide.

Second generation sulfonylurea Glipizide, glicazide and glybenclamide.

Sulfur (*sul'fur*) A pale yellow crystalline element, atomic no. 6.

Sulfur granules Yellow aggregates of filamentous branching actinomycotic bacteria.

Sulfur test A pinch of flowers of sulfur when sprinkled on urine sample placed in a beaker, sulfur sinks in presence of bile salts due to lowering of surface tension of urine.

Sulfuric acid (*sul-fur'ik*) H_2SO_4, a colorless, corrosive liquid.

Sulindac A nonsteroidal anti-inflammatory drug of the aryl alkanoic acid class, used primarily to treat conditions characterized by acute or chronic inflammation.

Sunburn (*sun'bern*) Erythema caused by exposure to critical amounts of ultraviolet light.

Sunstroke (*sun-strok*) Heat stroke; the most severe form of hyperthermia, or heat-related illness.

Superego *psy* The ethical component of the personality which provides the moral standards by which the ego operates. The superego's criticisms, prohibitions, and inhibitions form a person's conscience, and its positive aspirations and ideals represent one's idealized self-image, or "ego ideal".

Superfecundation (*su'per-fe'kun-da'shun*) Fertilization of a second ovum by a second sperm after one has already been fertilized.

Superfetation (*su'per-fe-ta'shun*) Fertilization and subsequent development of a second ovum after the first has already been implanted in the uterus.

Superficial (*su'per-fish'al*) Situated near the surface of the body; cursory.

Superinfection (*su'per-in-fek'shun*) An infection that occurs when the native flora of the body have been markedly reduced, often by antibiotic therapy, allowing invasion by opportunistic organisms.

Superior (*su-per'e-or*) Situated above; directed upward; situated near the vertex of the head.

Superior mesenteric artery syndrome Condition due to compression of superior mesenteric artery presenting with postprandial epigastric pain, distension, nausea and weight loss.

Superior vena cava obstruction Obstruction of superior vena cava presenting with bilateral engorgement of the jugular veins, and edema affecting the face, neck and arms.

Supernumerary (*su'per-nu'mer-ar'e*) Exceeding the normal number.

Supernumerary marker chromosome A small chromosome containing a centromere occasionally seen in tissue culture, often in a mosaic state.

Supination (*su'pi-na'shun*) Rotation of the forearm and hand so that the palm faces forward or upward. Also: a corresponding movement of the foot and leg in which the foot rolls outward with an elevated arch.

Supine (*su'pin*) Lying on the back with the face upward.

Suppository (*su-poz'i-tor'e*) A solid cone-shaped medicated pellet made up of inert substance, that is inserted into the rectum or vagina where it melts and releases the drug.

Suppression (*su-presh'un*) Arrest of secretion of a fluid; deliberately excluding from conscious thought; stopping an abnormal flow or discharge; masking of a phenotypic expression of a mutation.

Bone marrow suppression When fewer blood cells are made in the bone marrow. It is a common side effect of some strong medicines, such as chemotherapy.

Immune suppression A state of temporary or permanent dysfunction of the immune response resulting from problem with the immune system, leading to increased susceptibility to disease.

Overdrive suppression The suppression of intrinsic cellular automaticity by a rapid outside stimulus; In cardiology, this refers to the inhibitory effect of a faster pacemaker on a slower pacemaker.

Suppuration (*sup'u-ra'shun*) The formation of pus.

Supra- Combining word for above; over.

Supraorbital (*su'pra-or'bi-tal*) Superior to the orbit.

Supraorbital (*su'pra-or'bi-tal*) Superior to the orbit.

Supravital staining Staining of living cells after removal from organism (in vitro) usually applied to the slide preparation of detached cells.

Suramin Agent used in the treatment of trypanosomiasis and onchocerciasis.

Surfactant (*sur-fak'tant*) A chemically heterogeneous material consisting of phospholipids and proteins that are present in the alveolar epithelium as a surface active lining complex. It provides a film at the interface between the air and liquid and reduces the surface tension in the lungs. It is necessary for the normal expansion of fetal lung when the infant is transferred from fluid to gaseous environment.

Surgeon (*ser'jun*) A medical practitioner specialized in surgery and treats disease, injury and deformity by operation or manipulation.

Surgery (*ser'jer-e*) That branch of medicine which treats diseases, injuries and deformities by operation or manipulation; a place in a hospital where surgery is performed; performance or procedures of an operation.

Ablative surgery Operation in which a part is removed.

Ambulatory surgery Undertaking operation on patients who are admitted to and discharged from the hospital on the same day.

Aseptic surgery Operation carried out under aseptic conditions.

Conservative surgery Surgery in which as much as possible a part or structure is retained.

Cosmetic surgery Surgery to improve the appearance.

Cytoreductive surgery Debulking operation; a procedure that aims to completely remove all macroscopic disease; a common treatment for ovarian cancer and it aims to remove the tumor and any nearby tissues.

Dental surgery Oral and maxillofacial surgery.

Exploratory surgery An operation undertaken to establish diagnosis.

General surgery That which deals with surgical problems of all kinds.

Major surgery Involving increased risk to the life.

Manipulative surgery Use of manipulation in surgery or bone setting.

Maxillofacial surgery The branch of dentistry concerned with diagnosis and surgical and adjunctive treatment of injuries and deformities of the oral and maxillofacial region.

Minor surgery A simple operative procedure not causing risk to life.

Open heart surgery Concerned with correction of intracardiac disease under direct vision.

Orthopedic surgery Surgical correction of musculoskeletal diseases, injuries and deformities.

Plastic surgery Concerned with the restoration, reconstruction and improvement of shape and appearance of body structures.

Radical surgery Designed to remove a large area of damaged or neoplastic tissue or adjoining areas of lymphatic drainage.

Reconstructive surgery Plastic surgery.

Second look surgery Undertaken at a later date after original operation to detect recurrence of the disease.

Stereotaxic surgery Operation to produce sharply circumscribed lesions in specific regions of the brain after locating the structure by three-dimensional coordinates.

Subtotal surgery An operation in which only a portion of the organ is removed.

Surgical Pertaining to surgery.

Surgical diathermy Application of a high frequency alternating current through the body tissue and the concentration of current to produce an area of high current density liberating heat.

Surgical drain An appliance inserted into a body cavity or wound to allow drainage of fluid, pus or air.

Surgical emphysema Presence of gas in the subcutaneous tissue which gives a peculiar crackling sensation to the examining fingers and it is like palpating a horse hair mattress. It may be due to trauma leading to fractured ribs or nasal bone, or infections such as gas gangrene or following administration of saline by subcutaneous route or intercostal tubal drainage subcutaneous emphysema.

Surgical jaundice Obstructive jaundice.

Surgical spares Material used to close surgical incisions.

Surgical ventricular restoration Surgical procedure to remodel a ventricle damaged by a heart attack or heart failure.

Surrogate pregnancy Bearing child with an intention of handing over to another whatever source of ova or sperm.

Susac's syndrome Retinocochleocerebral vasculopathy affecting brain, hearing in adults, named after John Susac of US who described the condition in 1979.

Susceptibility (*su-sep"ti-bili-te*) The state of being readily affected or acted upon; diminished immunity to a disease, especially an infection.

Suspensory ligament A ligament that supports a body part, especially an organ.

Suture (*su'chur*) Surgical stitch used to close an incision of a wound; the surgical material so used; sutura.

Absorbable suture A surgical suture material that can be digested by body tissues.

Apposition suture A suture of the skin only.

Approximation suture A suture that pulls together the deep tissues.

Atraumatic suture A suture affixed to the end of an eyeless needle.

Blanket suture A continuous lock-stick to approximate the skin of a wound.

Continuous suture An uninterrupted series of stitches using one suture fastened at each end by a knot.

Cranial suture The suture between the bones of the skull.

Interrupted suture Suture created by passing a needle through both sides of a wound and knotting the ends of the suture material together to one side.

Swab (*swob*) A wad of cotton or gauze attached to one end of a slender stick used for applying medication, removing a substance from a surface or obtaining a piece of tissue or secretion for bacteriological examination.

Swallowing (deglutition) (*swal'o-ing*) A complicated process initiated voluntarily, then completed reflexly enabling the movement of food from mouth through the pharynx and oesophagus to the stomach.

Sweat (*swet*) Secretion of sweat glands of the skin, a colorless fluid containing sodium chloride, urea and fatty substances. It cools the body by evaporation and also eliminates waste material.

Sweat gland A simple coiled tubular gland found on the body. The coiled secreting part lies in the subcutaneous tissue and the duct passes through dermis and epidermis to its opening, sweat pore. The sweat glands are more numerous in the palms and soles.

Symbiosis (*sim'bi-o'sis*) Living together of two organisms of different species; *psy* mutually interdependence of two persons.

Symblepharon (*sim-blef'a-ron*) Adhesion of one or both eyelids to the eyeball.

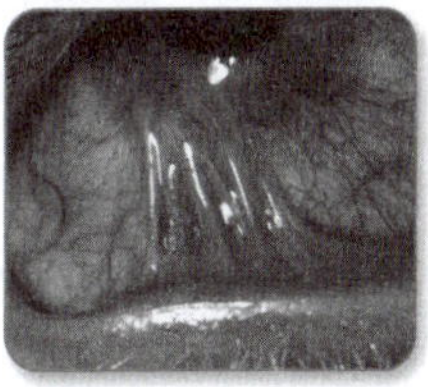

Symblepharon

Symbolism (*sim'bo-lizm*) An abnormal mental state in which everything that happens is considered by the individual as symbolic of his thoughts; a process involved in the disguised representation in consciousness of unconscious events.

Symmelia (*si-me'le-a*) A developmental anomaly characterized by an apparent fusion of the lower limbs; also known as mermaid malformation.

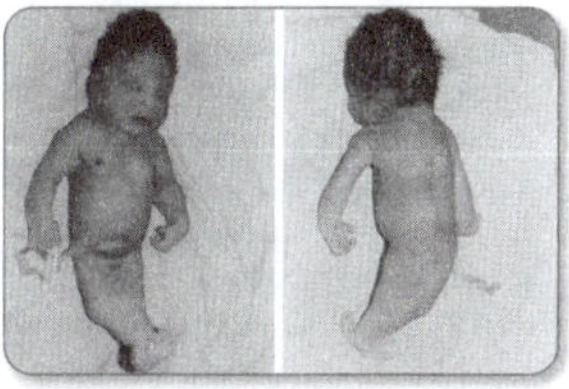

Symmelia

Symmetry (*sim'e-tre*) Equality; correspondence in the shape, size and relative position of parts on opposite sides of the body.

Icosahedral symmetry A mathematical property of objects indicating that an object has the same symmetries as a regular icosahedron.

Helical symmetry In 3D geometry and higher, a screw axis (or rotary translation) is a combination of a rotation and a translation along the rotation axis.

Radial symmetry A symmetry in which the sides exhibit correspondence or regularity of parts around a central axis.

Sympathectomy (*sim'pa-thek'to-me*) Excision of a segment of a sympathetic nerve or of one or more sympathetic ganglia.

Sympathetic nervous system One of the two sub-divisions of the autonomic nervous system, having cell bodies of preganglionic neurons in the lateral gray columns of the thoracic segment and first two or three lumbar segments of spinal cord (thoracolumbar).

Sympathetic chain ganglion A cluster of cell bodies of postganglionic sympathetic neurons lateral to the vertebral column, close to the body of a vertebra. These ganglia extend downward through the neck, thorax and abdomen to the coccyx on both sides of the vertebral column and are connected to one another to form a chain on either side of the vertebral column.

Sympathetic meningitis Mild aseptic meningitis produced by an infective lesion close to meninges.

Sympathetic ophthalmia Autoimmune uveitis in one eye induced by injury to other.

Sympathin A substance norepinephrine, secreted by sympathetic nerve endings which acts as chemical mediator.

Sympathoblast (*sim-path'o-blast*) A primitive cell from the neural crest glia which forms the adrenal medulla.

Sympatholytic (*sim'pa-tho-litik*) Antagonism to or inhibition of transmission of impulses from the postganglionic fibers to effector organs, inhibiting the smooth muscle contraction and glandular activity.

Sympathomimetic (*sim'pa-tho-mi'met'ik*) Producing effects that mimic those caused by the sympathetic nervous system; an agent that produces such an effect.

Sympathy (*sim'pa-the*) The mutual correlation between two organs, systems or parts of the body; an emotional concern for and sharing of mental and emotional state of another person.

Symphysiotomy (*sim-fiz'e-ot'o-me*) Division of symphysis pubis to facilitate labor, very rarely performed.

Symphysis (*sim'fi-sis*) A line of union; a form of cartilaginous joint without cavity.

Mental symphysis The fibrocartilaginous union of the two halves of the mandible that gets ossified during the first year.

Pubic symphysis The firm fibrocartilaginous joint between the two pubic bones.

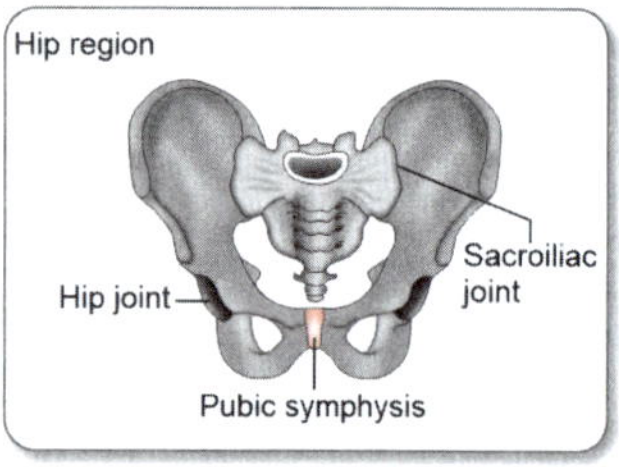

Pubic symphysis

Sympodia (sirenomelia) (*sim'po'de-a*) Fusion of lower extremities.

Symptomatology (semeiology) (*simp'to-ma-tol'o-je*) The branch of medicine dealing with symptoms of various diseases; all the manifestations of a given disease.

Synalgia Reffered pain.

Synapse (*sin'aps*) The functional junction between the neurons or between a neuron and an effector such as a muscle or gland. The transmission of impulse occurs by a chemical transmitter or by a direct propagation of the bioelectric potential.

Axodendritic synapse A type of synapse, formed by one between the axon of the neuron and the dendrites of another.

Axosomatic synapse One between the axow of one neuron and the body of another.

Axoaxonic synapse Type of synapse formed by one between the axon of one neuron and the axon of another neuron.

Synarthrosis (*sin-ar-thro'sis*) An immobile joint; joint without synovial cavity.

Synchilia (syncheilia) (*sin-ki'le-a*) Congenital adhesion of lips.

Synchondrosis (*sin'kon-dro'sis*) A cartilaginous joint in which the connecting material is a hyaline cartilage or fibrocartilage.

Syncope (fainting) A transient loss of consciousness accompanied by loss of postural tone and followed by spontaneous recovery.

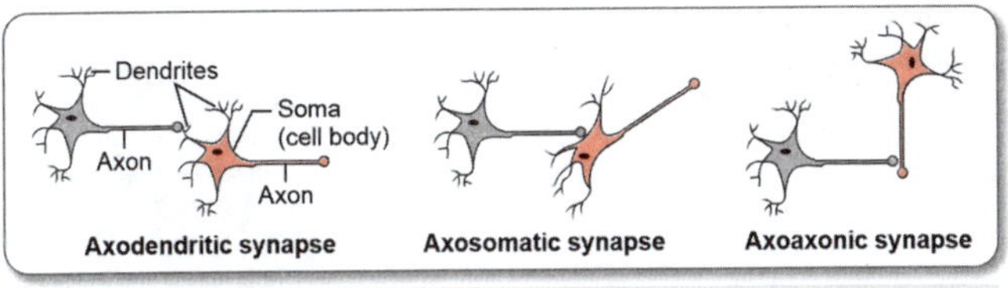

Three different types of synapses

Cardiac syncope Syncope of cardiac origin due to severe obstruction to cardiac output or disturbances of cardiac rhythm.

Carotid syncope Compression of carotid sinus leading to syncope that may be cardioinhibitory manifesting in bradycardia, sinus standstill and AV block that can be prevented by atropine, or vasodepressor manifesting with hypotension prevented by atropine or adrenaline.

Cough syncope Markedly raised intrathoracic pressure during paroxysms of prolonged bouts of cough producing syncopal attack.

Defecation syncope Sudden rectal emptying producing syncope.

Micturition syncope Syncope during or immediately after passing urine.

Multifactorial syncope Precipitation of syncope in elderly by vascular instability from diseases or physical stresses.

Neurologic syncope Syncope due to obstruction of vertebrobasilar artery and is associated with neurologic signs.

Orthostatic syncope Occurrence of syncope when a person assumes upright posture and it is due to uncompensated gravitational stress on circulation.

Syncytiotrophoblast (plasmoditrophoblast) (*sin-sit'e-o-trof'o-blast*) The outer syncytial layer of the trophoblast.

Syncytium (*sin-sish'e-am*) A multinucleate mass of protoplasm produced by the merging of cells.

Syndactyly (*sin-dak'ti-le*) Fusion of fingers which may be cutaneous due to bridging of soft tissues or osseous due to bony fusion.

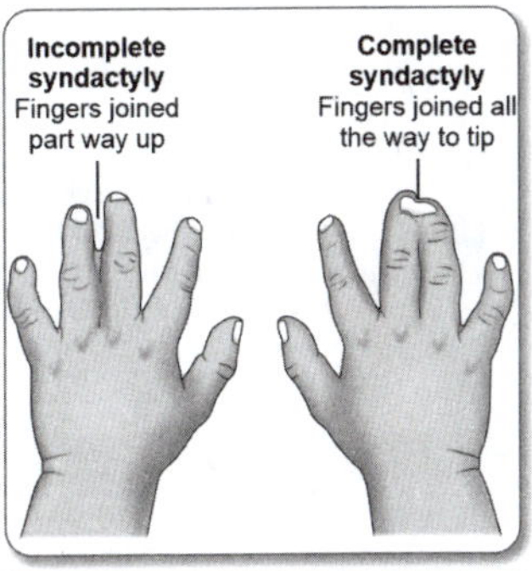

Syndactyly of the hand in Apert syndrome

Syndesm- (syndesmo-) Combining word for connective tissue; ligament.

Syndesmography (*sin"dez-mog'ra-fe*) Description of the ligaments.

Syndesmology (*sin-dez'-mol'o-je*) Study of the ligaments and joints.

Syndesmophyte Bony out growths from the spinal ligaments as they attach to adjacent vertebral bodies.

Syndesmoplasty (*sin-dez'mo-plas'te*) Plastic surgery of a ligament.

Syndesmosis (*sin'dez-mo'sis*) A joint in which the bones are united by interosseous membrane or ligament.

Syndrome (*sin'drom*) A group of signs and symptoms of disease occurring together.

Apert syndrome Also known as acrocephalosyndactyly, it is a genetic disorder that causes fusion of the skull, hands, and feet bones. It is characterized by deformities of the skull, face, teeth, and limbs.

Carpal tunnel syndrome An entrapment neuropathy characterized by pain and burning or tingling paresthesia in the fingers and hand, sometimes extending to the elbow. Symptoms result from compression of the median nerve in the carpal tunnel.

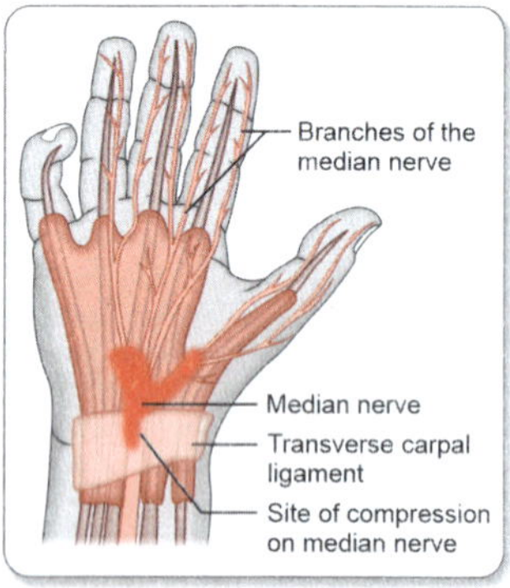

Carpal tunnel syndrome

Cushing syndrome A complex of symptoms caused by hyperadrenocorticism due to either a neoplasm of the adrenal cortex or adenohypophysis, or to excessive intake of glucocorticoids. Symptoms may include adiposity of the face, neck, and trunk; kyphosis from osteoporosis of the spine; hypertension; diabetes mellitus; amenorrhea and hypertrichosis in females; impotence in males; dusky complexion with purple striae; polycythemia; and muscular wasting and weakness. When secondary to excessive pituitary secretion of corticotropin, it is known as Cushing disease.

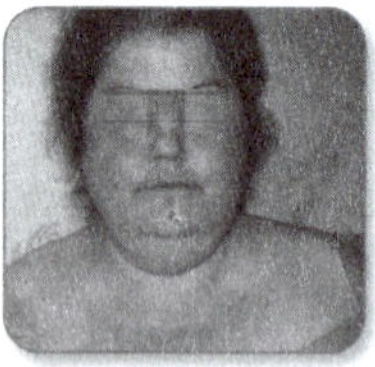

Cushing syndrome

De Lange syndrome A congenital syndrome in which severe mental retardation is associated with many abnormalities, including short stature (Amsterdam dwarf), brachycephaly, low-set ears, webbed neck, Cupid's-bow mouth, depressed bridge of the nose with the end tilted up and forward-directed nostrils, arched heavy eyebrows meeting at the midline, unruly coarse hair growing low on the forehead and neck, and flat spadelike hands with short tapering fingers. Called also Brachmann-de Lange or Cornelia de Lange syndrome.

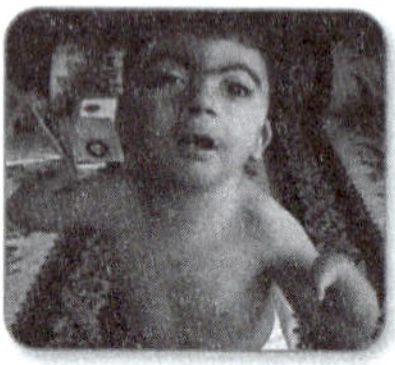

De Lange syndrome

Down syndrome A genetic disorder caused by the presence of all or a portion of a third chromosome 21. It is usually associated with developmental delays, mild to moderate intellectual disability, and characteristic physical features.

Ehlers-Danlos syndrome A group of hereditary connective tissue disorders that manifest clinically with skin hyperelasticity, hypermobility of joints, atrophic scarring, and fragility of blood vessels.

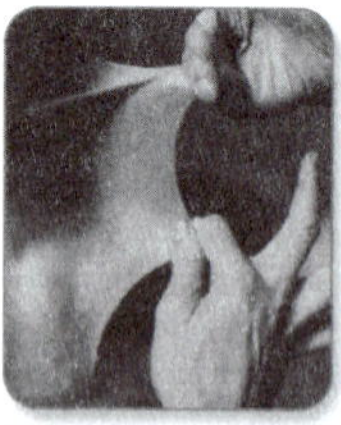

Ehlers-Danlos syndrome

Fetal alcohol syndrome A group of conditions that can occur in a person who is exposed to alcohol as a result of their mother drinking during pregnancy. Symptoms can include an abnormal appearance, short height, low body weight, small head size, poor coordination, behavioral problems, learning difficulties, and problems with hearing and sight.

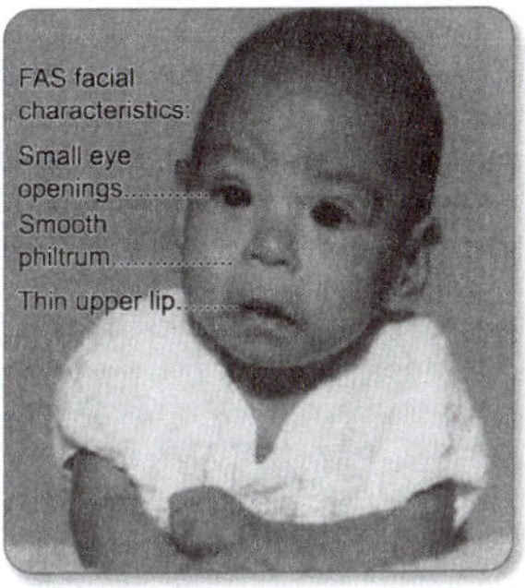

Fetal alcohol syndrome-FAS

Marfan syndrome A genetic condition that affects connective tissue, which provides support for the body and organs. Marfan syndrome can damage the blood vessels, heart, eyes, skin, lungs, and the bones of the hips, spine, feet, and rib cage. The most serious complications involve the heart and aorta, with an increased risk of mitral valve prolapse and aortic aneurysm.

Polycystic ovary syndrome The most common endocrine disorder in women of reproductive age, characterized by many cysts in the ovaries. Symptoms include irregular menstrual periods, heavy periods, excess hair, acne, pelvic pain, difficulty getting pregnant, and patches of thick, darker, velvety skin. The primary characteristics of this syndrome include hyperandrogenism, anovulation, insulin resistance, and neuroendocrine disruption.

Prune belly syndrome A rare congenitally acquired disorder primarily characterized by the clinical triad of deficient abdominal musculature, cryptorchidism, and urinary tract abnormalities.

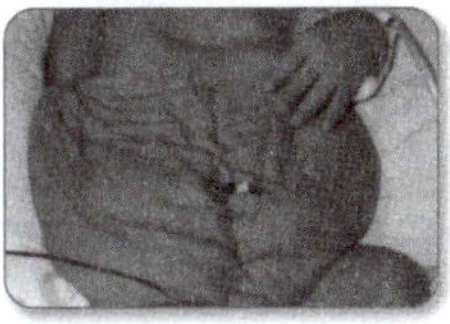

Prune belly syndrome

Syndrome X Insulin resistance with central truncal obesity, impaired glucose tolerance, hypertriglyceridemia, hypertension and accelerated atherosclerosis.

Synechia (*si-nek'e-a*) Adhesion especially of iris, cornea and conjunctiva. pl. **Synechiae**.

Annular synechia An adhesion of iris to the lens throughout its entire pupillary margin.

Anterior synechia An adhesion of the iris to the cornea.

Posterior synechia An adhesion of the iris to the lens.

Synechia vulvae A congenital fusion of the labia minora.

Total synechia An adhesion of the entire surface of the iris to the lens.

Syneresis (*si-ner'i-sis*) Release of part of fluid content of gel.

Synergist (*si-ner'i-jist*) A structure or a drug that aids the action of another.

Syngeneic (*sin'je-ne'ik*) Same species; genetically identical; immunologically compatible, accepting grafts from each other.

Synoptophore An instrument used in orthoptics to test binocular vision.

Synostosis (*sin-os-to'sis*) A joint in which the dense fibrous connective tissue uniting the adjacent bones at a suture has been replaced by bone, resulting in a complete fusion across the suture line.

Synovectomy (*sin'o-vek'to-me*) Resection of overgrown synovium in rheumatoid arthritis to prevent destruction of joint cartilage.

Synovia (synovial fluid) (*si-no've-a*) Synovial fluid in the joint cavity, which is highly viscous due to presence of hyaluronic acid synthesized by type B cells. It also contains electrolytes, albumin, glucose and water that have their origin from filtration from subsynovial capillaries. The fluid maintains the nutrition of the avascular articular cartilage and lubricates the joint.

Synovial (*si-nove-al*) Pertaining to synovium; pertaining to or secreting synovia.

Synovial membrane (synovium) A smooth joint cavity with one or two cells. A thin barrier that lines the inside of some of the joints. The cells are of connective of origin and are of two types: type A (a phagocytic cell) and type B (fibroblast with well developed endoplasmic reticulum).

Synovioma (*si-nove-o'ma*) A highly malignant synovial sarcoma occurring in the knee, ankle, foot or other joints.

Synovitis (*sin'o-vi'tis*) Inflammation of a synovial membrane.

Pigmented villonodular synovitis Synovial proliferation forming brown nodular masses, probably caused by hemangiomas of synovial membrane that become traumatized, resulting in synovial hyperplasia and inflammation; it is characterized by episodic monoarticular pain and swelling, with joint locking and hemorrhagic effusions.

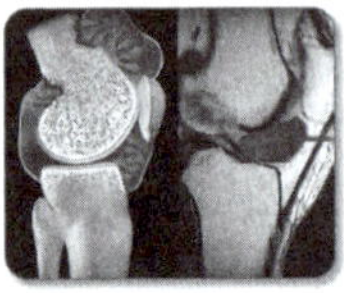

Pigmented villonodular synovitis.

Synovium (*si-novi-am*) Synovial membrane.

Syphilid (syphilide) (*sif'i-lid*) Any of the skin lesions of secondary syphilis.

Syphilis (*sif'i-lis*) A sexually transmitted disease due to infection with Treponema pallidum.

Acquired syphilis Condition begins as a painless ulcer at the site of infection usually on the genitals a urged regional lymph nodes are enlarged (primary syphilis). 6–8 weeks later there is macular or papular rash, mucosal ulcers and lymphadenopathy (secondary syphilis). Later, there is development of gumma (syphilitic granuloma) affecting skin, mucosa and bones (tertiary syphilis). Cardiovascular syphilis and neurosyphilis develop at a quaternary stage.

Congenital syphilis Fetus developing syphilis by contacting it from the mother. The child may be born dead, or present with vesicles, bullae and mucosal ulcers, hepatosplenomegaly and CNS involvement.

Latent syphilis Syphilis characterized by seroreactivity without other evidence of primary, secondary, or tertiary disease.

Primary syphilis A solitary, small firm red painless papule on the genital area quickly becomes a painless ulcer with a well-defined margin and an indurated base. Characterized by chancre(s) at the point of entry of the *T. pallidum spirochete. T. pallidum* uses its spiral shape to twist into the skin.

Secondary syphilis A systemic disease, with the patient often presenting with a variety of symptoms, such as malaise, sore throat, headache, weight loss, low-grade fever, pruritus, and muscle aches, in addition to the dermatologic manifestations.

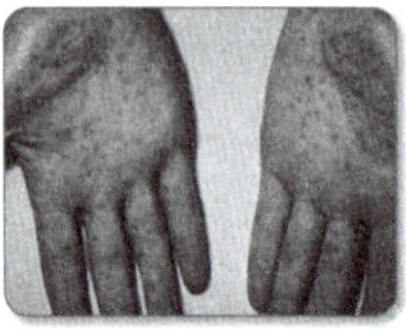

Palmar rash in secondary syphilis

Tertiary syphilis Refers to gummas, cardiovascular syphilis, psychiatric manifestations (e.g., memory loss or personality changes), or late neurosyphilis.

Syringe (*sir'inj*) An instrument used for injecting or withdrawing fluids.

Air syringe A small, fine nozzled syringe through which air is forced to blow debris from or to dry a cavity in preparing teeth for restoration.

Chip syringe Air syringe.

Dental syringe A small syringe containing an anesthetic solution used in operative dentistry.

Hypodermic syringe A small syringe, with a calibrated barrel, used to administer drugs into the subcutaneous tissue.

Luer-Lok syringe A glass syringe with a metal tip and locking device to secure needle, used for intravenous or hypodermic use.

Syringobulbia (*si-ring'go-bul'be-a*) Development of fluid filled cavity in the medulla presenting with dysarthria, palatal palsy, Horner's syndrome, nystagmus and sensory loss on the face.

Syringocystadenoma (syringoma) (*si-ring'go-sis'ted-e-no'ma*) Papilloma of sweat gland ducts.

Syringomyelia (*si-ring'go-mi-e'le-a*) Development of a fluid filled cavity near the center of the spinal cord and the expanding cavity disrupts the spinothalamic tract, damage anterior horn cells and compress long fiber tracts. It is characterized by dissociated sensory loss (loss of pain and temperature sensation with preservation of posterior column modalities), trophic lesions, wasting of small muscles of hand, and upper motor neuron lesion signs in the lower limb.

System (*sis'tim*) The association of organs that have common functions.

Alimentary system Digestive system.

Autonomic nervous system That part of the nervous system which represents motor innervation to smooth muscle of internal organs, cardiac muscle and glands. It consists of two distinct mutually antagonistic divisions as sympathetic and parasympathetic systems, the name has been derived as it was thought to be self-governing or spontaneous.

Cardiovascular system The heart and blood vessels by which blood is pumped and circulated through the body.

CD system Cluster designation, a system for classifying cell surface markers expressed by lymphocytes.

Centimeter-gram-seconds system (CGS) Metric system expressing fundamental physical units of length, mass and time and those units derived from them, in centimeters, grams and seconds.

Central nervous system (CNS) That portion of nervous system consisting of the brain and spinal cord.

Centroencephalic system The neurons in the brainstem.

Chromaffin system Chromaffin cells of the body staining readily with chromium salts, found along sympathetic nerves, in adrenal medulla, and in various other organs.

Circulatory system A system concerned with circulation of nutrient fluids that includes cardiovascular and lymphatic systems.

Conducting system of the heart A system of specialized muscle fibers that generate and transmit electrical discharges and coordinate contractions, comprising the sinus node, atrioventricular node, Bundle of His and bundle branches and their terminal ramifications into Purkinje system.

Digestive system Alimentary system from the mouth to anus with associated organs and glands concerned with ingestion, digestion and absorption of food stuffs and nutrients, and elimination of undigested material.

Endocrine system Ductless glands secreting hormones into the blood which include pituitary, pineal body, thyroid, parathyroid, pancreas and adrenal glands, paraganglia and gonads.

Extrapyramidal motor system Basal ganglia (corpus striatum), its associated structures (substantia nigra, subthalamic nucleus) and its descending connections with the midbrain, concerned with maintenance of equilibrium and muscle tone.

Genitourinary system Urogenital system.

Haversian system Basic unit of compact bone consisting of a haversian canal and its concentrically arranged lamellae.

Hexaxial reference system A series of lines used in electrocardiography to describe the potentials of the heart in the frontal plane by diagramming vectors that represent the standard bipolar limb leads and the augmented unipolar limb leads.

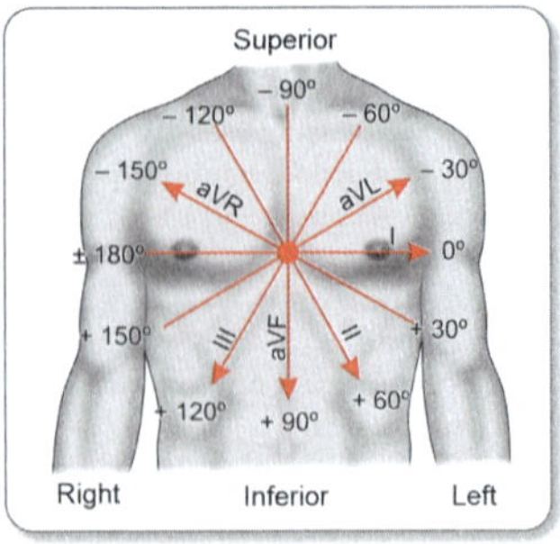

Hexaxial reference system

Hematopoietic system The tissues concerned with the production of blood including the bone marrow and lymph nodes.

Hypothalamohypophyseal portal system A system of veins from median eminence of the hypothalamus passes downward along the stalk and pars tuberalis of the hypophysis and reaches anterior lobe of the pituitary where they arborize into a second capillary bed and convey releasing factors to the anterior lobe.

Limbic system A heterogeneous group of brain structures at or near the edge (limbus) of the medial wall of the cerebral hemisphere (hippocampus, amygdala and gyrus funiculatus).

Lymphatic system The lymphatic vessels, lymph nodes and lymphoid tissue.

Lymphoreticular system The tissues of the lymphoid and reticuloendothelial systems.

Masticatory system The bony and soft structures of the face and mouth involved in mastication; jaws, teeth, temporomandibular articulations, masticatory muscles, tongue, lips, cheeks and oral mucosa.

Muscular system Voluntary or skeletal muscles of the body.

Nervous system Spinal cord, ganglia and nerves.

Neuromuscular system The muscles of the body collectively and the nerves supplying them.

Parasympathetic nervous system One of the two subdivisions of the autonomic nervous system having cell bodies of preganglionic neurons in, the nuclei of the brain stem and in the lateral gray matter of the sacral portion of the spinal cord.

Peripheral nervous system That part of the nervous system, other than the CNS.

Portal system An arrangement of vessels in which blood after passing through one capillary bed enters a second capillary network.

Properdin system An alternate pathway for complement consisting of many distinct proteins that react in a serial manner and activate C3.

Renal system Urinary system.

Reproductive system Male or female gonads, associated ducts and external genitalia.

Respiratory system The system concerned with the supply of oxygen to and elimination of carbon dioxide from the cells of the body and maintenance of normal acid base balance. It consists of gas conducting airways and lungs (alveoli, terminal and respiratory bronchioles and blood vessels surrounding the alveoli).

Reticular activating system (RAS) That part of brain stem reticular formation (an extensive branched nerve cells) that receives collaterals from the ascending sensory pathways and project to the higher centers. When it is activated, a generalized alert or arousal behavior results.

Reticuloendothelial system The network of cells of different organs concerned with phagocytosis found in connective tissue and lymphatic structures, Kupffer cells, histiocytes, alveolar macrophages, and microglia.

Skeletal system The bony framework of the body.

Stomatognathic system All structures involved in speech and in reception, mastication and deglutition of food.

Sympathetic nervous system One of the two divisions of autonomic nervous system having cell bodies in the preganglionic neurons in the lateral gray columns of the thoracic segments and first two or three lumbar segments of the spinal cord.

Urinary system The kidneys, ureters, bladder and urethra.

Urogenital system Genitourinary system, consisting of organs involved in the formation and excretion of urine and in reproduction.

Vascular system Circulatory system consisting of cardiovascular and lymphatics.

Vegetative nervous system Autonomic nervous system.

Systemic (*sis-tem'ik*) Affecting the whole body: generalized; relating to a system.

Systemic inflammatory response (SIR) A part of metabolic response to injury that may be sepsis, trauma, or burns. It is associated with encephalopathy, spiking fever, marked tachycardia, hyperventilation, signs of increased sympathetic tone, bleeding and leukocytosis.

Systemic lupus erythematosus (SLE) An autoimmune disorder of undetermined etiology with a variety of clinical manifestations. There is non-organ specific autoimmunity with the presence of a group of autoantibodies directed against components of the cell nucleus, such as antinuclear antibody, circulating immune complexes and widespread immunologically determined tissue damage. It is characterized by arthritis, arthralgia, fever, photosensitive erythematous, butterfly rash across the face, livedo reticularis, Raynaud's phenomenon, pericarditis, myocarditis, endocarditis, pleurisy, fibrosing alveolitis, acute lupus pneumonitis, nephrotic syndrome and renal failure.

Systemic mycosis Systemic infection by fungi acquired by inhalation.

Systemic vasculitis Generalized inflammation of blood vessels that may be a primary disorder or may be part of or secondary to another disease process such as SLE. There is infiltration of one or more layers of the blood vessels with polymorphonuclear cells in acute stage and with lymphocytes in the chronic stage. There may be giant cells, granuloma and fibrinoid necrosis. The vasculitis may affect large vessels (Giant cell arteritis, Takayasu's arteritis) medium sized vessels (Polyarteritis nodosa, Kawasaki's disease) or small vessels (Wegener's granulomatosis, Churg-Strauss syndrome, Henoch-Schonlein purpura).

Systemic inflammatory response syndrome A systemic inflammatory response to the invasion of microorganisms and their breakdown products; SIRS.

Systole (*sis'to-le*) The phase of contraction of the heart muscle especially of the ventricles in the cardiac cycle.

Systolic Pertaining to systole.

Systolic bladder Excessively contracted bladder following tuberculous fibrosis.

Systolic blood pressure The force exerted by blood on arterial walls during ventricular contraction.

Systolic hypertension Marked rise in systolic blood pressure without rise of diastolic blood pressure.

T

Tabes (*ta'bez*) Any chronic condition leading to wasting of the body.

Tabes dorsalis Syphilis of the spinal cord and its appendages. There is degeneration of sensory neurons and wasting of dorsal columns and optic atrophy characterized by lightning pains, ataxia, and visual failure.

Tablet (*tab'let*) A small piece of solid dosage form of a medication.

Compressed tablet A tablet made by forcibly compressing the powdered substances.

Enteric-coated tablet Tablet having an outer layer resisting dissolution by gastric juice.

Sublingual tablet Small, flat, oval tablet kept beneath the tongue to permit direct absorption.

Taboparesis (*ta'bo-par-e'sis*) A combined form of tabes dorsalis and general paralysis of insane.

TAB vaccine A combined vaccine used to produce immunity against diseases typhoid, paratyphoid A and B.

Tachy A combining word for, meaning rapid.

Tachycardia (*tak-e-kar'de-a*) Increased heart rate. It occurs during and immediately after exercise, in febrile conditions, thyrotoxicosis, anemia, anxiety, nervousness, congestive heart failure, after hemorrhage, paroxysmal tachycardia, atrial fibrillation and atrial flutter. Tachycardia acts to increase the amount of oxygen delivered to the cells of the body by increasing the heart rate.

Atrial tachycardia Rapid heart rate arising from an atrial focus with less than 200 beats per minute.

Bidirectional ventricular tachycardia A rare form of ventricular tachycardia with right bundle branch block and alternating polarity of QRS in the frontal axis.

Nodal tachycardia Tachycardia occurring because of an increase in rhythmicity of the AV node over the SA node.

Paroxysmal atrial tachycardia (PAT) Episodes of atrial tachycardia beginning and ending suddenly.

Paroxysmal supraventricular tachycardia Rapid ectopic atrial beats originating proximal to bifurcation of bundle or in an accessory pathway. It is sudden in origin and transient in nature.

Sinus tachycardia Tachycardia originating in the sinus node. It is normal during exercise or anxiety and occurs abnormally associated with shock, hypotension, hypoxia, congestive heart failure, fever, and various high output states.

Supraventricular tachycardia (SVT) A regular tachycardia with a rate of between 140 and 220 due to reentry within the AV node.

Ventricular tachycardia A rapid succession of beats arising from a ventricular focus at a rate greater than 100 beats per minute.

Tachyphrasia A communication disorder involving rapid, unintelligible speech.

Tachyphrenia The sensation that thoughts are moving too quickly.

Tachyphylaxis (*tak'e-fi-lak'sis*) Rapid immunization against the effects of toxic doses of a substance; repeated administration of some drugs results in a marked decrease in effectiveness.

Tachypnea (*tak'ip-ne'a*) Increased respiratory rate. Normal rate of respiration is 16–20 per minute at rest in a normal adult. The rate is increased in pneumonia, pleurisy, hypoxic conditions, cardiac failure, during excitement, exertion and fever.

Tacrolimus (*tak'ro-li'mas*) An immunosuppressive drug. After allogenic organ transplant, the risk of organ rejection is moderate. To lower the risk of organ rejection, tacrolimus is given.

Tactile (*tak'til*) Pertaining to the sense of touch.

Tactile agnosia An impairment of tactile object recognition caused by unilateral damage to parietotemporal cortices.

Tactile anesthesia Lack of sense of touch in the fingers.

Tactile corpuscles Minute elongated bodies enclosing the afferent fibers and serving as receptor for touch or slight pressure. They are located in dermal papillae just beneath the epidermis and are found in large numbers on fingertips, toes, soles, palms, lips, nipples and tip of tongue.

Tactile discrimination Ability to localize two points of pressure on the surface of the skin.

Tactile disk Tiny expanded end of a secondary nerve fiber in the epidermis and in hair roots.

Tactile hyperesthesia An abnormal increase in the sense of touch.

Tactile image A mental concept of an object perceived through the sense of touch.

Tactile localization Ability to accurately identify the site of tactile stimulation.

Tactile sensation The sensation of touch.

Tactile system Part of the nervous system concerned with sense of touch.

Tactile vocal fremitus (TVF) Detection of vibrations transmitted to the palpating hand from the larynx through the bronchi, lungs and chest wall. It is increased in solidified lung or superficial cavity, and diminished in airways obstruction, collapse, fibrosis, pleural effusion, pneumothorax and pleural thickening.

Taenia (*te'ne-a*) A genus of large tapeworms of the family Taeniidae; a flat band or strip of tissue.

Taenia coli One of three large bands of the large intestine into which muscular fibers are collected.

Taenia echinococcus Dog is the definitive host of the tiny tapeworm *E. granulosus*. Man acquires the disease by handling a dog or drinking contaminated water with eggs. The embryo through blood reaches liver or lung or brain and gives rise to multiple cysts referred as hydatid cysts.

Taenia saginata Beef tapeworm. It has a scolex of the size of a pinhead and four suckers. The adult worm produces little or no intestinal upset. The segments appear in the stool. Praziquantel is drug of choice.

Taenia solium Pork tapeworm. The scolex has in addition to sucker, two circular rows of hooklets. Adult gets the disease by eating undercooked pork containing cysticerci. The larvae liberated from eggs in the stomach, get distributed to different parts of the body where they develop and cysticercosis in the brain causes epilepsy, personality changes, and staggering gait.

Taeniacide (taenicide) (*ta'ne-a-sid*) An agent that destroys tapeworms; also teniacide.

Taeniafuge (*ta'ne-a-fuj'*) An agent that expels tapeworms from the body of their host also teniafuge.

Taeniasis (*tenia-sis*) Infestation with tapeworms of the genus *Taenia*; also teniasis.

Tagamet A histamine receptor antagonist used to treat and prevent certain types of ulcer and to inhibit stomach acid production.

Takayasu's disease Pulseless disease or aortic arch syndrome, named after Japanese ophthalmologist, Michishige Takayasu. It is a chronic inflammatory granulomatous panarteritis of elastic arteries such as aorta and its major branches; common in women and is associated with loss of pulse.

Talalgia (*tal-al'je-a*) Pain in the heel or ankle.

Talipes (*tali-pez*) Clubfoot, a congenital deformity wherein the foot is twisted out of shape and position.

Talipes arcuatus High plantar arch.

Talipes calcaneovalgus Dorsiflexed and abducted (evertion) foot and its dorsum lies almost in contact with the skin. There is tightness of the dorsolateral soft tissue, responds to repeated manual stretching and should be begun immediately after birth.

Talipes calcaneus Fixed dorsiflexion and walking on heel.

Talipes equinovarus Clubfoot; the foot is adducted and inverted and is held equinus (plantar flexion) at the ankle. It requires operative correction in early infancy.

Talipes planus Flatfoot.

Talipes valgus Outward turning of foot.

Talipes varus Inward turning of foot.

Talus (astragalus) (*ta'lus*) Articulation between the upper tarsal bone and the lower ends of tibia and fibula to form ankle joint.

Tambour (*tam-boor*) A shallow, drum-shaped appliance.

Tamoxifen (*ta-moks'i-fen*) Selective estrogen receptor modulator without androgen activity, used to treat early estrogen receptor-positive breast cancer.

Tampon (*tam'pon*) A pack of cotton wool or gauze useful to stop hemorrhage, or absorb secretions.

Tamponade (*tam'pon-ad*) Pathologic compression of a part; insertion of tampon to stop bleeding.

Balloon tamponade Producing pressure against some object by a catheter surrounded by an elongated balloon, often to arrest oesophageal bleeding from varices.

Cardiac tamponade Pathologic condition resulting from accumulation of excess fluid in the pericardium.

Tantalum (*tan'ta-lum*) A noncorrosive and malleable metal used to make prosthetic appliances or plates, atomic no. 73.

Tapetum (*ta-pe'tum*) A membranous layer.

Tapotement (percussion) (*ta-pot'men't*) Percussion with hand of tissue while massaging.

Tapping (*tap'ing*) Withdrawal of fluid from a body cavity. Example includes paracentesis.

Target cell Helmet cell, an abnormal erythrocyte with a rounded deeply staining area surrounded by lightly staining area which in turn is surrounded by dense cytoplasm at the periphery of the cell.

Target organ An organ intended to receive a therapeutic dose of irradiation; an organ most affected by a specific hormone.

Tarsal (*tar'sal*) Referring to the edge of an eyelid; instep; any of the bones of the tarsus (back part of the foot).

Tarsal bone Any one of seven bones making up the tarsus of foot consisting of the talus, calcaneus, cobotil, navicular and three cuneiforms.

Tarsal coalition A painful rigid flat foot deformity due to a congenital fusion or failure of segmentation between two or more tarsal bones and peroneal muscle spasm but without true spasticity.

Tarsal tunnel syndrome Compression of posterior tibial nerve following long standing or walking, presents with pain, paresthesis and cyanosis of foot.

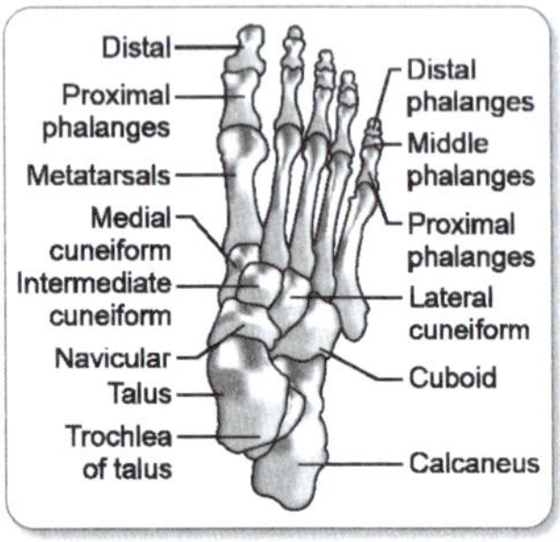

Tarsal and metatarsal bones

Tarsalgia (*tar-salje-a*) Pain in the ankle or foot.

Tarsal gland One of numerous modified sebaceous glands on the inner surfaces of eyelids.

Tarsectomy (*tar-sek'to-me*) Operative procedure to remove tarsus of the foot; excision of all or part of the tarsus of an eyelid.

Tarsitis (*tar-si'tis*) Inflammation of the tarsus or margin of an eyelid.

Tarsoplasty (*tar'so-plast'e*) Blepharoplasty.

Tarsorrhapy (*tar-sor'a-fe*) Suturing of the eyelids to protect the cornea when the person cannot close the eyelids.

Tarsus (*tar'sus*) Articulation between the foot and the leg where talus articulates with tibia and fibula, the cuboid and cuneiform bones with the metatarsals; connective tissue framework that provides internal support for the eyelid.

Tartar (*tar'tar*) Potassium bitartrate; a hard crust-like deposit on teeth.

Tartrate (*tar'trat*) Any salt of tartaric acid.

Taste A chemical sense-dependent upon sense organs on the surface of the tongue. The nerve impulses are carried to the brain by the lingual and glossopharyngeal nerves from the anterior two-thirds and posterior-third of the tongue, respectively.

Aftertaste The persistence of a taste sensation after removal of original stimulus.

Taste area Area in the cerebral cortex.

Taste cells Neuroepithelial cells within a taste bud that act as receptors for the taste sense.

Taste buds Oval sensory end organs located on the surface of tongue also found on soft palate, epiglottis and portions of the pharynx. Each bud contains sensory and gustatory cells and supporting cells. When stimulated by chemical stimuli, they produce one or a combination of the four fundamental taste sensations—sweet, bitter, sour and salty.

Taurine (*taw'rin*) A product of taurocholic acid which is present in bile.

Taurocholic acid A bile acid taurine conjugate of cholic acid involved in the emulsification of fats.

TAVR Transcatheter aortic valve replacement.

Taxis (*tak'sis*) A movement of an organism toward or away from the stimulus; application of force in the manual replacement of a displaced or injured part.

Tay-Sachs disease (amaurotic familial idiocy) (*ta'saks*) An autosomal recessive disorder presenting with mental and physical retardation, blindness, cherryred spots on the macula, spasticity, enlarged head and convulsions. It is due to an absence of an enzyme, hexosaminidase—a necessary in the metabolism of sphingolipid, described by Warren Tay, British physician and Bernard Sachs, US neurologist.

TCR T-cell receptor is a protein complex found on the surface of T cells and recognizes antigens in an immune reaction.

Tear gas Sulfur dioxide; used to disperse rioters.

Technetium-99 (*tek-ne'she-um*) A radioactive element obtained in the fission of uranium atomic weight 99 widely used radioisotope studies.

Tectospinal tract Nerve tract that coordinates head and eye movements.

Tectum (*tek'tum*) Any roof-like structure.

Teeth (*teth*) Hard bony projections in the jaws.

Anterior teeth Teeth located close to the midline of the dental arch on either side of the jaw.

Deciduous teeth 20 teeth making up the first dentition, which are shed and replaced by the permanent teeth.

Hutchinson's teeth Upper central permanent incisors are peg-shaped and notched in congenital syphilis, named after Sir Jonathan Hutchinson, English surgeon.

Milk teeth Deciduous teeth.

Moon teeth The dome-shaped first permanent molars, named after Henry Moon, English surgeon.

Permanent teeth The teeth that develop as second dentition replacing the deciduous teeth. They are 32 in number, 16 in each jaw. They include incisors (central and lateral), canines (cuspids), premolars (bicuspids) and molars.

Tegmen (*teg-men*) A covering.

Tegmentum (*teg-men'tum*) A covering or roof; the dorsal portion of cruri cerebri of the midbrain.

Teichopsia (*ti'kop'sea*) A temporary visual impairment associated with migraine.

Tela (*te'la*) A thin web-like structure or tissue.

Telangiectasis (*tel-an'je-ek-to-sis*) The site on the skin containing dilated small blood vessels.

Telangiitis (*tel-an-je-itis*) Inflammation of the capillaries; an obsolute term for capillaritis.

Teleceptor (*tel'e-sep'tor*) An organ, such as the eye, that can receive sense stimuli from a distance; such nerve endings exist in the eyes, ears, and nose.

Telegony A theory of heredity saying that offspring can inherit the characteristics of a previous mate of the female parent.

Telencephalon (*tel-en-sefa-lon*) Most highly developed anterior part of the forebrain consisting chiefly of cerebral hemispheres.

Telepaque (*tela-pak*) Trademark for a preparation of iopanoic acid.

Telepathology (*tel'e-pa-thol'o-je*) Transmission of digitized images of pathology specimens over telecommunication network for study at a far-off place.

Teleratidography The transmission of radiological patient images from tests such as X-rays, CT and MRI, from one location to another for getting further opinions or studies.

Teleradiography (*tel'e-ra"de-og'rafe*) Process whereby images are transferred to distant locations for the purpose of interpretation and diagnosis.

Teletherapy (*tel-e-ther'-a-pe*) Treatment wherein the source of the therapeutic agent (radiation) is away from the body; teleradiotherapy.

Telocentric (*tel'o-sen'trik*) Having the centromere terminally placed so that there is only one chromosomal arm.

Telodendron (*tel'o-den'dron*) The terminal arborization of a nerve fiber used originally of dendrites but now especially of the main arborization of an axon.

Telophase (*tel'o-faz*) The final stage of mitosis wherein the nucleus is formed from each group of chromosomes produced by anaphase or meiosis following the migration of chromosomes to the poles of the cell.

Temazepam (*ta-maz'e-pam*) A benzodiazepine sedative hypnotic used to treat insomnia symptoms, such as trouble falling or staying asleep.

Temple (*tem'pl*) The flattened lateral side of the head above the zygomatic arch.

Temporal (*tem'por-al*) Relating to the temple; pertaining to time.

Temporal arteritis Inflammation of arteries of head referred as giant cell arteritis in elderly persons. It is associated with severe headaches and scalp tenderness. The temporal arteries are thickened and tender. Corticosteroids are useful.

Temporal bone A bone on either side of skull at its base. It is composed of squamous, mastoid and petrous portions, the latter enclosing the receptors for hearing and equilibrium.

Temporalis (*tem'po-ralis*) Pertaining to the temple.

Temporal lobe One of the two lower side lobes of the cerebral hemisphere that perceives sounds and smell, and controls balance. The dominant temporal lobe is involved in verbal comprehension. Music processing occurs in both temporal lobes, rhythm being processed on the dominant side and melody/pitch more on the nondominant side.

Temporal lobe epilepsy A form of epilepsy in which abnormal electrical discharges are confined to one of the temporal lobes. It presents with hallucinations and abnormal sensations of taste and smell.

Temporomandibular joint syndrome Incordinated function of the jaw joints and their supporting muscles and ligaments. It is characterized by headache, facial pain and restriction of jaw movement.

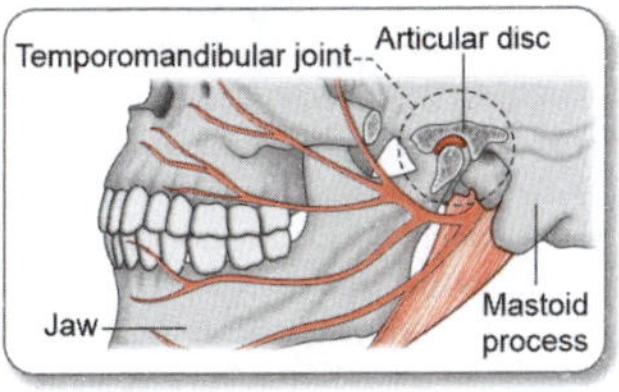

Temporomandibular joint

Tenaculum (*te-nak'u-lum*) A small, sharp pointed hook set in a handle to seize and hold the tissues in operations.

Tendinitis (*ten'di-ni'tis*) Painful inflammation of a tendon caused by injury, overuse or prolonged pressure rotator; tendonitis; tenonitis.

Cuff tendinitis Shoulder pain from pressure on the tendons of shoulder especially that of supraspinatus. It follows injury or overuse during activities involving repeated elevation of the arm as in cricket.

Tendon (*ten'don*) A dense, inelastic fibrous cord of connective tissue by which muscle gets attached to a bone or other structure.

Tendon reflex A reflex act in which a muscle contracts when its tendon is percussed.

Tendon transfer A surgical procedure in which a tendon is repositioned to make a muscle perform a new function.

Tendon organ (Golgi tendon organ) A tree like sensory ending enclosed in a spindle-like connective tissue capsule, that lies near the junction of a tendon with a muscle.

Tenesmus Painful straining to pass stools and less commonly urine.

Tenia A flat ribbon like structure in the body.

Tennis elbow Damage by repeated small injuries and overuse at the attachment of forearm extensors to the lateral epicondyle of humerus and presenting with pain. There is tenderness on the lateral epicondyle and in the outer part of the antecubital fossa. Pronation of the forearm accentuates the pain.

Tenon's capsule (*te'nonz*) Fascial sheath of eyeball in which it rotates, named after French surgeon, Jacques Tenon.

Tenoplasty (*ten'o-plaste*) The surgical repair of a defect in a tendon.

Tenorrhaphy (*ten-or'a-fe*) Suture of a divided tendon.

Tenosynovitis (peritendinitis) (*ten'o'sin'o-vi'tis*) Inflammation of the synovial lining of a tendon sheath. It is caused by mechanical irritation or by bacterial infection.

Tenotomy (*te-not'o-me*) Surgical division of a tendon.

Tenovaginitis (*ten'o-vaj'in-i'tis*) A mild chronic inflammation or thickening of the fibrous wall of the sheath that surrounds a tendon. The cause is unknown.

TENS Transcutaneous electrical/electronic nerve stimulation.

Tensor (*ten'sor*) A muscle that stretches or tightens some part of the body.

Tensor fascia lata Mucocutaneous flap.

Tensor tympani Small muscle lying in a bony canal above eustachian tube whose tendon is inserted on malleolus. It helps to dampen excessive vibrations.

Tent Covering over bed to maintain a controlled atmosphere.

Tentorium (*ten-to're-um*) A tent or a membranous covering.

Tentorium cerebelli The process of dura mater between the cerebrum and cerebellum supporting the occipital lobes.

Teratogenesis (*ter'a-toje-ne-sis*) The production of physical defects in the embryo or fetus; production of a monstrous growth.

Teratology (*ter-a-tol'o-je*) Study of fetal malformations.

Teratoma (*ter-a-to'ma*) A neoplasm representing all the germinal layers of embryo usually found in an ovary, testis and mediastinum.

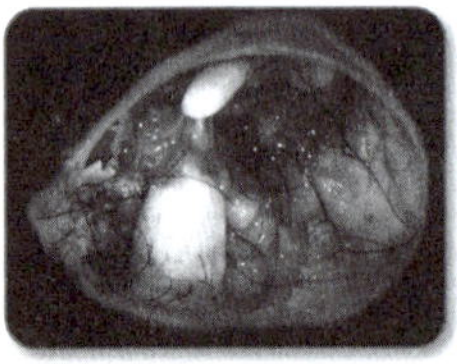

Ovarian teratoma

Terbutaline A sympathomimetic bronchodilator.

Terconazole An antifungal drug that is mainly used to treat vaginal yeast infections.

Teres (*te'rez*) Long and round.

Terfenadine H_1 receptor blocking antihistamine.

Terpene (*tur'pen*) Any of a class of hydrocarbons occurring widely in plants and animals and empirically regarded as built up from isoprene, a hydrocarbon consisting of five carbon atoms attached to eight hydrogen atoms (C_5H_8).

Terramycin Oxytetracycline is proprietary term of terramycin. It is a broad spectrum antibiotic which acts by inhibiting production of bacterial protein.

Tertian fever Fever characterized by febrile paroxysms occurring every third day as in malaria that may be benign (*Plasmodium vivax*) or malignant (*P. falciparum*).

Tertiary health care Health care offered at super-speciality institutions.

Tesla A unit of measure of magnetic strength, named after Nikola Tesla, US physicist.

Testicle (*tes'ti-k'l*) The testis; male sex organs suspended in the scrotum.

Testis (*tes'tis*) The male gonad situated on either side in the scrotum, produces sperms and testosterone. Each testis contains hundreds of compartments containing tiny tubes called seminiferous tubules in which sperms are produced. Sperms mature in the epididymis at the back of the testis before passing into the vas deferens. pl. **testes**.

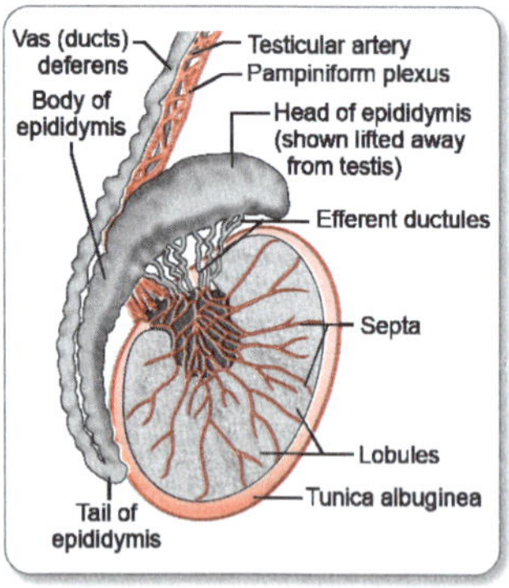

Testis

Testis determining factor A protein encoded by a gene on the short arm of Y chromosome which is responsible for development of primary male organs.

Test meal A meal of small quantity and composition given to aid chemical analysis of the stomach contents or radiological examination of the stomach.

Testosterone (*tes-tos'ter-on*) A sex hormone that stimulates bone and muscle growth and the development of male characteristics. It is produced by the testes and in small amounts by the ovaries.

Test tube baby A full-term gestational product resulting from in vitro fertilization of an egg that was implanted in a uterus and carried to term.

Tetanolysin (*tet'a-nol'i-sin*) The hemolytic fraction of the exotoxin formed by *Clostridium tetani*.

Tetanospasmin (*tet'a-no-spas'min*) A neurotoxin of *Clostridium tetani*, that is most toxic substance known to man, causing profound muscle spasms due to tetanospasmin, blockage of the release of glycine.

Tetanus (lockjaw) (*tet'a-nus*) An infectious often fatal disease characterized by violent tonic muscle spasms and rigidity caused by toxin of *Clostridium tetani*. It presents initially with trismus, tonic rigidity involving muscles of the face, neck and trunk. The back is slightly arched and there is board-like abdominal wall. Contraction of the frontalis and the muscles of the angles of the mouth gives rise to the risus sardonicus. Violent spasms lasting for a few seconds to 3–4 minutes occur. Death may occur from exhaustion, asphyxia or aspiration pneumonia. Active immunization prevents the development of tetanus. Tetanus toxoid is commonly given in combination with the diphtheria toxoid and pertussis vaccine in childhood. Tetanus toxoid booster has to be given every 10 years.

Tetanus antitoxin An antibody that develops in the humans or other animals (horses) as a result of infection by tetanus organism or inoculation with tetanus toxoid.

Tetanus immunoglobulin Immunoglobulin from human blood for use in persons not previously immunized against tetanus.

Tetanus neonatorum Umbilical infection due to dressing with mud, dung, etc.

Tetanus toxoid A highly effective vaccine for *C. tetani* that selectively elicits helper immune response.

Tetany (*tet'a-ne*) Severe tonic muscle spasm often due to a deficiency of ionized calcium from low blood calcium or respiratory alkalosis.

Tetracycline (*tet'ra-si'klen*) A broad-spectrum antibiotic active against most pathogenic bacteria, rickettsias, chlamydias and mycoplasma.

Tetrad (*tet'rad*) A group of four similar or related entities.

Tetradactyly (*tet'ra-dak'ti-le*) Four digits on the hand or foot.

Tetrahydrocannabinol (THC) (*tet'ra-hi'dro-ka-nab'i-nol*) The major psychoactive component and one of the 113 cannabinoids recognized in cannabis, used to manage chemotherapy-induced nausea and vomiting and for appetite stimulation in HIV/AIDS anorexia.

Tetrahydrozoline (*tet'ra-hi-droz'o-len*) An alpha-adrenergic agonist used in the temporary symptomatic relief of discomfort and redness of the eyes due to minor irritations, as well as alleviate nasal congestion.

Tetralogy of fallot A congenital heart disease characterized by ventricular septal defect, pulmonary stenosis, overriding of aorta and hypertrophy of right ventricle present with cyanosis, hypoxic spells, squatting after exertion, clubbing, needs shunt surgery, named after Etienne Fallot, French physician.

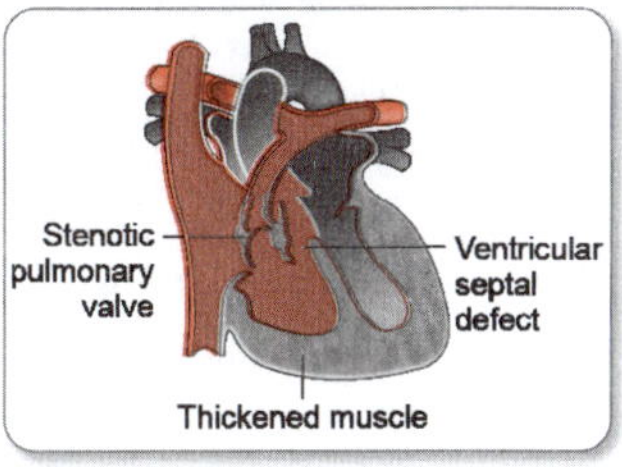

Tetralogy of Fallot

Tetraplegia (*tet'ra-pleje-a*) Paralysis of all four limbs.

T fracture A type of intercondylar fracture of the distal femur that occurs in falls from a height with the feet extended resulting in a violent impact of femur on the tibial plateau.

TGF Transforming growth factor; group of distinct polypeptides that have been isolated from virus-transformed rodent cells, capable of altering cell phenotype.

Thalamic syndrome Infarction of sensory tracts in or below thalamus presenting with hemianesthesia and severe pain on minimal stimulus.

Thalamotomy (*thal'a-mot'o-me*) A neurosurgical procedure which aims at creating local lesions with the help of thermal energy in the thalamic region of the brain.

Thalamus (*thal-a-mus*) An ovoid gray nuclear mass deep within the brain in the lateral wall of lateral ventricle through which sensory impulses pass to reach the cerebral cortex. It may also play a part in long-term memory.

Thalassemia (Cooley's anemia) (*thal-a-se'me-a*) A hereditary hemolytic anemia having decreased synthesis of hemoglobin polypeptide chains.

α-thalassemia Defective formation of α-chains.

Thalassemia major Homozygous β-chain defect with a reduction of Hb-A and an increase of Hb-F.

Thalassemia minor Heterozygous chain defect with mild hypochromic anemia without iron deficiency.

Thalidomide (*tha-lid'o-mid*) Hypnotic and antiemetic, teratogenic. Its use was abandoned as it caused severe fetal malformations, if taken in early pregnancy. Now has found new indications as an immunosuppressive agent.

Thallium (*thal'e-um*) A heavy, soft malleable metallic, radioactive element, atomic no. 81.

Thallium scanning A radionuclide scanning to assess the heart function by determining how well different area of heart muscle absorb thallium after it has been injected into the blood.

Theca (*the'ka*) Sheath enclosing an organ or structure.

Theca cell tumor A benign, yellow, solid ovarian tumor.

Thenar (*the'nar*) The palm of the hand or sole of the foot; fleshy part on the outside of the palm of the hand.

Thenar eminence A prominence at the base of the thumb.

Thenar fascia A thin membrane covering the short muscles of the thumb.

Thenar muscle The abductor or flexor muscle of the thumb.

Theobromine Principal alkaloid of the cacao bean.

Theophylline (*the'o-fil'in*) Xanthine compound inhibiting breakdown of cyclic AMP; an alkaloid found with caffeine in tea leaves.

Therapeutic index The ratio of drug's toxic level to therapeutic level.

Therapeutic window The range of a drug's concentration in which the desired effect occurs, below which there is little desired effect and above which toxic effects appear; the gap between the dose needed to provide desired effect and that needed for undesired effect.

Therapeutics (*the'r-a-pyu'tiks*) Branch of medicine concerned with the details of treatment of disease.

Therm (*thurm*) Any of a several units of heat; a unit for quantity of heat that equals 100,000 British thermal units.

Thermalgesia (*ther'mal-je'ze-a*) Pain caused by heat.

Thermanesthesia (*ther'm-an'es-the' ze-a*) Loss of ability to feel cold or heat.

Thermoanalgesia (*ther'mo-an'al-je-si-a*) A condition in which the application of heat produces pain.

Thermocautery (*ther'mo-kaw'ter-e*) Cautery (destruction of tissue) by heat.

Thermocoagulation (*ther'mo-ko-ag-u-la'shun*) Coagulation of tissue by the action of high frequency currents.

Thermography (*ther-mog'ra-fe*) Technique of obtaining an image of the heat distribution over the surface of an object.

Thermolysis (*ther-mol'i-sis*) The breakdown of molecules by the action of heat.

Thermometer (*ther-mom'e-ter*) An instrument for measuring temperature.

Thermophore (*ther'mo-for*) An instrument or apparatus to retain heat; used in therapeutic local application.

Thermoreceptor (*ther-mo-re-sep'tor*) A sensory receptor stimulated by a rise in body temperature.

Thermotaxis (*ther"mo-tak'sis*) The regular normal adjustment of body temperature.

Thermotherapy (*ther'mo-ther'a-pe*) Treatment of disease by means of heat.

Thiabendazole Broad-spectrum antihelmintic, effective against most types of roundworms in the gut.

Thiamine The first component of B complex; aneurin; vitamin B_1. It is essential for energy production, and nerve and muscle function.

Thiersch graft (split-skin graft) A skin graft that consists of thin strips of epithelium with the tops of dermal papillae, split off with a sharp knife.

Thimble bladder Grossly contracted and fibrosed bladder.

Thioguanine (*thi'o-gwa'nen*) An anti-neoplastic anti-metabolite used in the treatment of several forms of leukemia including acute nonlymphocytic leukemia.

Thiopental (*thi'o-pen'tal*) An ultra-short-acting depressant of the central nervous system which induces hypnosis and anesthesia, but not analgesia.

Thiophilic Having an attraction to sulfur.

Thiopropazate Antipsychotic of the phenothiazine class. It is a prodrug to perphenazine.

Thioridazine (*thi'o-rid'a-zen*) A phenothiazine antipsychotic used to treat schizophrenia and generalized anxiety disorder.

Thiotepa Alkylating cytotoxic agent.

Thiothixene (*thi'o-thik'sen*) An antipsychotic medicine that is used to treat schizophrenia.

Thiouracil Antithyroid drug.

Thoracectomy (*thor'a-sek'to-me*) Surgical resection of a portion of a rib.

Thoracentesis (*tho'ra-sen-te'sis*) Aspiration of fluid from the pleural space.

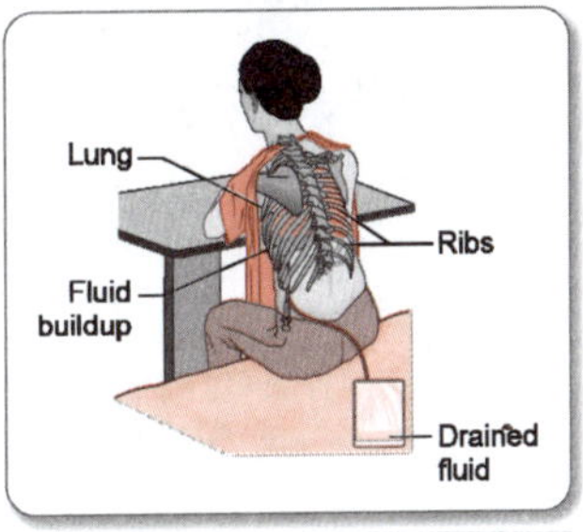

Thoracentesis

Thoracic cavity A space inside the chest containing heart, lungs and other organs and tissues.

Thoracic duct The main trunk of lymphatic system opening into venous system. The duct enters the thoracic cavity posteriorly to the esophagus and to the right of the aorta. In the superior mediastinum, the duct arches to the left crossing the midline at approximately the level of T_4 to T_6 vertebrae and merges with the left internal jugular vein.

Thoracic inlet injury Traumatic injury to the base of the neck involving superior mediastinal vessels.

Thoracic outlet syndrome Scalenus syndrome. A condition caused by compression of brachial plexus and subclavian artery between a cervical rib and the scalenus anticus muscle.

Thoracocentesis Procedure done to remove fluid from the thoracic cavity.

Thoracoplasty (*tho'ra-ko-plas'te*) Surgical removal of the ribs facilitating the chest wall to move in and cause compression of a diseased lung.

Thoracoscope (*tho'ra-ko-skop*) An endoscope facilitating the examination of the pleural cavity.

Thoracostenosis (*thor'a-ko-s'te-no'sis*) Abnormal contraction of the thorax.

Thoracotomy (*tho'ra-kot'o-me*) A surgical procedure in which chest is opened for operation on a diseased lung, heart or other organ lying in the thoracic cavity.

Thorax (*tho'raks*) Region of the trunk between the neck and abdomen; the chest. By drawing certain imaginary vertical lines, the thorax is divided into various regions such as supraclavicular, suprasternal, clavicular, infraclavicular, mammary between third and sixth costal cartilages, inframammary between the sixth rib and costal arch, sternal, axillary, infra-axillary, suprascapular, scapular (supraspinous and infraspinous), interscapular and infrascapular regions.

Thorium (*thor'e-um*) A chemical element with atomic number 90 and is represented by the symbol 'Th' in the periodic table.

Threadworm *Enterobius vermicularis*; pinworm.

Threonine (Thr, T) (*threo-nen*) A precursor to the amino acids glycine and serine.

Threshold (*thresh'old*) Limit of perception; point above which the substance is eliminated.

Threshold dose The minimum dose that will produce an effect on the patient.

Threshold limit value The concentration of an airborne chemical or potentially toxic or radioactive substance below which persons may work over an eight-hour period without known adverse effect.

Thrombasthenia (*throm'bas-the-ne-a*) Defective clot retraction due to a platelet abnormality causing bleeding.

Thrombectomy (*throm-bek'to-me*) Removal of a thrombus from a blood vessel, to restore blood flow.

Thrombin (*throm'bin*) The enzyme which converts fibrinogen into fibrin.

Thromboangiitis (*throm'bo-an'je-i'tis*) Inflammation of inner wall of a blood vessel with thrombosis.

Thrombocyte (*throm'bo-sit*) A blood platelet which aids coagulation of the blood.

Thrombocythemia (*throm'bo-si-the' me-a*) An increase in the number of circulating blood platelets.

Thrombocytopenia (*throm'bo-sito-pe'nea*) The decrease in the number of circulating blood platelets.

Thrombocytopenic purpura A bleeding disorder that results from a deficiency of platelets in the blood. It is characterized by purple or reddish brown discolored areas on the skin.

Thrombocytosis (*throm'bo-si-to'sis*) Increased number of platelets in the peripheral blood.

Thromboembolism (*throm'bo-em'bo-lizm*) Obstruction of a blood vessel by a fragment that has broken off from a thrombus elsewhere in the circulation.

Thromboendarterectomy (*throm'bo-end'ar-ter-ek'to-me*) Removal of an obstructing thrombus together with the inner lining of an obstructed artery.

Thromboendarteritis (*throm'bo-end-ar'ter-i'tis*) Inflammation of the inner lining of an artery with formation of thrombus.

Thrombogenesis (*throm'bo-jen'e-sis*) The formation of blood clots.

Thrombokinase (*throm'bo-ki-naze*) A clotting factor that is activated by tissue injury.

Thrombolysis (*throm-bol'i-sis*) Dissolution of a thrombus.

Thrombolytic (*throm'bo-lit'ik*) An agent used in breaking up a thrombus.

Thrombophlebitis (*throm'bo-fle-bi'tis*) Inflammation of a vein often with the formation of a thrombus in part of a vein present near the surface of the body.

Thrombophlebitis migrans Thrombosis developing and receding in different parts of the body, often associated with carcinoma of pancreas.

Thromboplastin (thrombokinase) (*throm'bo-plas'tin*) A substance necessary in the coagulation, which facilitates conversion of prothrombin to thrombin in presence of calcium ions.

Thrombopoiesis (*throm'bo-poy-e'sis*) Formation of thrombus.

Thrombosis (*throm'bo'sis*) The formation of a fibrinous clot in any part of the circulatory system.

Coronary thrombosis Thrombosis of a coronary artery, a common cause of myocardial infarction.

Deep vein thrombosis (DVT) Thrombosis of veins in the legs or pelvis. It is encouraged by low cardiac output, sluggish flow, increased coagulability of blood, endothelial damage, postoperative and postpartum states and in carcinoma.

Thrombotic thrombocytopenic purpura (TTP) A rare condition of thrombocytopenia, and normal coagulation factors presenting with splenomegaly, varying neurologic signs, disseminated intravascular coagulation and fever.

Thrombus (*throm'bus*) A fibrinous clot consisting of platelets, fibrin and cellular elements which obstructs a blood vessel or is formed in one of the chambers of the heart.

Thrush White creamy patches on the oral mucosa caused by a fungus, *Candida albicans*; candidiasis.

THV Transcatheter heart valve.

Thymectomy (*thi-mek'to-me*) Surgical removal of the thymus gland.

Thymic aplasia Congenital absence of the thymus. It is caused by genetic mutations.

Thymidine (*thi'mi-den*) A nucleoside present in deoxyribonucleic acid.

Thymine (*thi'min*) A pyrimidine base present in DNA where it is paired with adenine.

Thymitis (*thi-mi'tis*) Inflammation of the thymus.

Thymocyte (*thi'mo-sit*) A cell formed in the thymus as the precursor of T (thymus derived) lymphocyte.

Thymoma (*thi-mo'ma*) A tumor of thymus.

Thymus (*thi'mus*) A lymphoid gland situated in the anterior mediastinum playing an important role in the development of immunologic competence. It weighs 10–35 g at birth, increasing to 20–50 g by puberty, involuting to 5 g or less in elderly. It consists of two flat symmetric lobes and contain cortex and medulla. The cortex is a dense lymphoid tissue containing thymocytes in large number. Medulla contains less number of thymocytes and thymic (Hassall's) corpuscles.

Thyrocalcitonin (calcitonin) (*thi'ro-kal'si-to'nin*) A polypeptide hormone elaborated by thyroid gland.

Thyrocele A swelling of the thyroid gland.

Thyroglobulin (*thi'ro-glob'u-lin*) An iodine- containing protein.

Thyrohyoid (*thi'ro-hi'oyd*) Pertaining to the thyroid gland or cartilage and the hyoid bone.

Thyroid cartilage Largest cartilage of the larynx which projects in men as 'Adam's apple'.

Thyroidectomy (*thi'roid-ek'to-me*) Surgical removal of all or a part of thyroid gland, in situations of hyperthyroidism, goiter or thyroid tumors.

Thyroid gland An endocrine gland in the base of the neck on either side of the lower part of larynx and upper part of the trachea. It consists of two lateral lobes connected by an isthmus. It contains a large number of follicles that contain a homogeneous substance (colloid). It contains thyroglobulin with active substances like thyroxine and triiodothyronine.

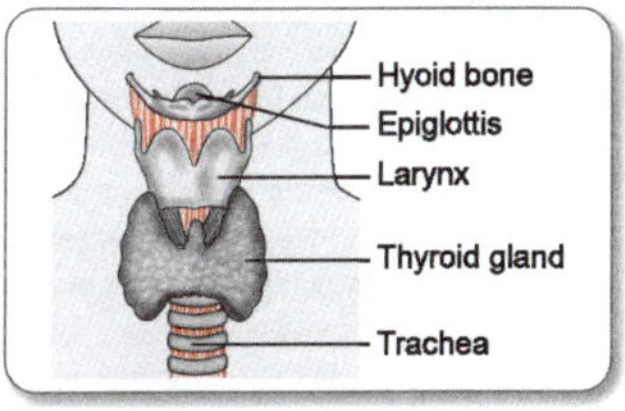

Thyroid gland

Thyroid hormone Hormones secreted by the thyroid gland.

Thyroiditis (*thi-roid-i'tis*) Inflammation of the thyroid gland.

Hashimoto's thyroiditis A condition of goitrous hypothyroidism presenting with a small or moderately sized diffuse goiter which is firm or rubbery in consistency. Thyroxine therapy is indicated, named after Hakaru Hashimoto, Japanese surgeon.

Postpartum thyroiditis Unmasking of previously unrecognized subclinical autoimmune thyroid disease, within 6 months of delivery.

Riedel's thyroiditis A rare condition in which there is extensive infiltration of the thyroid and surrounding structures with fibrous tissue. It presents with a slow-growing goiter which is irregular and hard, named after Bernhard Riedel, German surgeon.

Subacute thyroiditis A virus (Coxsackie, mumps or adenovirus) induced inflammation of thyroid gland which results in release of colloid and its constituents into the circulation. There is hyperthyroidism characterized by pain in the region of thyroid gland, raised levels of thyroid hormones and systemic abnormalities.

Thyroid stimulating hormone A hormone secreted by the pituitary gland that stimulates the thyroid gland to increase its secretion of hormones.

Thyroxine (*thi'roks'in*) A thyroid hormone of the thyroid gland. It helps to control the rate of energy production in the body.

Tibia (*tib'e-a*) The inner, thick bone of the leg extending from the knee to the ankle articulating with the femur above and talus below; the shin-bone.

Saber tibia A deformed tibia that is curved outward due to gummatous periostitis of syphilis.

Tibia valga A bulging of legs in which the convexity is inward.

Tibia vara A bowing of the legs in which the convexity is outward.

Tibialis (*tib'e-a'lis*) Either of two muscles of the calf of the leg.

Tic (*tik*) Twitching; a sudden, repetitive involuntary muscular contraction including eye blinking, facial gestures and shoulder shrugging.

Tic douloureux Trigeminal neuralgia, paroxysmal severe pain over the face.

Tick (*tik*) A small, eight-legged blood-sucking creature, some of which spread infectious diseases such as Lyme disease, Kyasanur forest disease and Rocky Mountain spotted fever.

Tick typhus *Rickettsia* infection transmitted by ticks.

Tietze's syndrome (costochondritis) Costochondritis; a painful condition resulting from inflammation of the cartilages that attach the ribs to the sternum, named after Alexander Tietze, German surgeon.

Timolol Beta-blocker used in hypertension, myocardial ischemia and glaucoma.

Tincture (*tink'chur*) An alcoholic solution, containing medicinal substances.

Tincture of iodine An alcoholic solution of iodine.

Tinea (*tin'e-a*) Superficial fungal infection affecting the skin, hair or nails; ringworm.

Tinea barbae Fungal involvement of hairs of beard region presenting as localized boggy swellings.

Tinea capitis Fungal infection primarily involving scalp hair, occurs mainly in children.

Tinea corporis Tinea infection of the surface of the skin of the trunk, face and extremities and presents as markedly itchy circular or irregular lesions.

Tinea cruris Tinea lesions in the groin seen in adult males.

Tinea interdigitale Fungal infection of interdigital spaces between adjoining toes or finger.

Tinea manuum Fungal infection of the palms and it is markedly itchy.

Tinea pedis Fungal infection of the soles that appear as circumscribed areas of scaling and fissures in adults.

Tinea unguium Fungal infection of nails.

Tinea versicolor Fungal infection by *Malassezia furfur* forming discrete hypo- or hyperpigmented macules with overlying fine scaling over the trunk, proximal extremities and face.

Tinel's sign (*ti'nelz*) Nerve regeneration indicated by occurrence of tingling sensation on percussion over the site of nerve injury, named after Jules Tinel, French neurosurgeon.

Tinnitus (*tin-i'tus*) A persistent ringing sound heard in the ear.

Tinzaparin (*tin-zap'a-rin*) A low- molecular-weight heparin used for the treatment of acute symptomatic deep vein thrombosis with or without pulmonary embolism when administered in conjunction with warfarin.

Tirofiban (*tiro-fiban*) A reversible antagonist of fibrinogen binding to the GP IIb/IIIa receptor, the major platelet surface receptor involved in platelet aggregation.

Tissue (*tish'u*) An aggregation of similar cells united to perform a particular function.

Tissue typing A series of tests of a donor and recipient before transplant surgery.

Tissue culture Growth of tissue *in vitro* on artificial media.

Tissue type plasminogen activator (tPA) A thrombolytic protease that converts plasminogen into plasmin, activating fibrinolysis, without affecting the circulating plasminogen or fibrinogen.

Titer (*ti'ter*) The quantity of a substance required to produce a reaction with a given volume of another substance.

Antibody titer A measure of the amount of antibody against a particular antigen present in the blood.

Titubation (*tit'u-ba'shun*) Shaking of the trunk and head; staggering.

T lymphocyte A type of thymic lymphoid cell that fights infections and cancer cells directly.

TNM classification Tumor, nodes, metastases; an international system for staging cancer by giving numerical values to each of these.

Tobacco (*to-bak'o*) Dried leaves of *Nicotiana tabacum*. It contains nicotine. It is widely used in the form of cigarettes, *beedis*, cigars, snuff and chewing tobacco.

Tobramycin An aminoglycoside antibiotic.

Tocography (*to'ko-gra'fi*) An obstetric procedure to record uterine muscle contractions during childbirth.

Tocopherol (*to-kof'er-ol*) Vitamin E.

Todd's palsy Prolonged episodes of partial seizures may leave paresis of the involved limb lasting for several hours after the seizure ceases, named after Robert Todd, British physician.

Todd's paralysis (Todd's palsy) Prolonged episodes of partial seizures may leave paresis of the involved limb lasting for several hours after the seizure ceases, named after Robert Todd, British physician.

Tofranil Imipiramine is sold under the brand name tofranil. It is a tricyclic antidepressant, used in treatment of depression, anxiety and panic disorders.

Tolazamide (*tol-az'a-mid*) A sulfonylurea used in the treatment of noninsulin-dependent diabetes mellitus.

Tolazoline (*tol-az'o-len*) An alpha-adrenergic blocking agent used to produce peripheral vasodilation.

Tolbutamide An oral hypoglycemic agent of sulfonylurea group.

Tolerance (*tol'er-ans*) The ability to endure without ill effect; endurance; need to take increasingly higher doses of a drug to obtain the same effect.

Tolnaftate (*tol-naf-tate*) Topically used antifungal agent for ringworm.

Toluidine blue A basic thiazine dye, used as a biological stain.

Tomography (*to'mog'ra-fe*) Body section roentgenography; laminography. A diagnostic imaging technique that produces a cross-sectional image of an organ or part of the body.

Computed tomography CT; tomography in which transverse planes of tissue are swept by radiographic beam and a computerized analysis of variance in absorption produces a precise reconstructed image of that area.

Computerized axial tomography (CAT) Computed tomography in which cross-sectional scans are made of a bodily structure.

Single-photon emission computed tomography (SPECT) An imaging method for reconstructing cross-sectional images of radiotracer distributions.

Tongue (*tung*) The movable muscular organ on the floor of mouth functioning in tasting, eating and speaking. It consists of a body and root and is attached by muscles to the hyoid bone below, mandible in front, styloid process behind and the palate above and by the mucous membrane to the floor of the month, the lateral walls of pharynx and the epiglottis. The surface of the tongue has numerous papillae (filiform, fungiform and vallate). Taste buds are present on the papillae especially the vallate papillae. The mucous and serous glands open on the surface.

Black hairy tongue Fungal infection associated with a brown fur due to elongated growth of the filiform papillae without desquamation.

Geographic tongue Appearance of a map on the tongue due to localized irregular red areas of desquamation of filiform papillae surrounded by a whitish border.

Magenta tongue A magenta-colored tongue in riboflavin deficiency.

Scrotal tongue A furrowed and fissured tongue resembling the skin of the scrotum.

Smooth tongue Smooth surface tongue due to atrophy of papillae as in anemia.

Strawberry tongue Red tongue in scarlet fever due to hypertrophy of fungiform papillae.

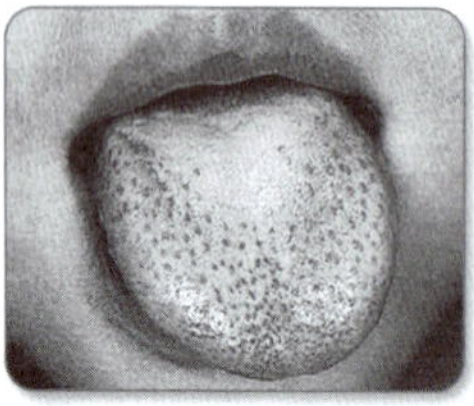

Strawberry tongue

Tongue-tie A midline mucosal fold on the undersurface of the tongue, binding it to the floor of the mouth impeding its movements.

Tonic (*ton'ik*) Continuous tension; a substance that invigorates or strengthens.

Tonic atrophy Wasting of muscles with active reflexes.

Tonic clonic fits Grand mal seizures.

Tonic phase Early rigid stage of contraction of all muscles as in major fits.

Tonic pupil Delayed reaction to light and accommodation.

Tonic reflex Maintenance of muscle tone.

Tonicity (*to'nis'i-te*) Tone; property of possessing tone; a physiological process dependent upon the selectively permeable characteristics of a membrane.

Tonofibril (*ton'o-fibril*) A thin fibril made up of tonofilaments.

Tonography (*to-nog'ra-fe*) The measurement and recording of intraocular pressure while the eyeball is subjected to pressure over a period of several minutes.

Tonometer (ophthalmotonometer) (*ton-om'e-ter*) An instrument to measure tension of a gas in a liquid or pressure usually intraocular pressure; an instrument to measure frequencies of tones as a tuning fork.

Tonsil (*ton'sil*) A small oval mass of lymphoid tissue on each side of the fauces; rounded projection toward the midline of the posterior end of lower surface of each cerebral hemisphere.

Lingual tonsil Mass of lymphoid tissue in the root of the tongue.

Nasal tonsil Lymphoid tissue on the nasal septum.

Palatine tonsil A mass of lymphoid tissue lying in the tonsillar fossa on each side of the oral pharynx between the glossopalatine and pharyngopalatine arches; faucial tonsil.

Pharyngeal tonsil Lymphoid tissue on the roof of the posterior wall of the nasopharynx.

Tonsillectomy (*ton-sil-ek'to-me*) The operative removal of a tonsil or the tonsils. It is performed in those with recurrent severe tonsillitis.

Tonsillitis (*ton-sil-i'tis*) Inflammation of the tonsils, especially faucial tonsil. It has a sudden onset with fever, chills, headache, pain in tonsils while swallowing. The tonsils appear enlarged and red.

Tonsillotomy (*ton'si-lot'o-me*) Incision of a tonsil.

Tonus (tone) (*to'nus*) The slight, continuous tension in muscle.

Tooth (*toth*) One of a set of small hard bodies attached in a row to each jaw, pl. **teeth**. They cut, grind and process food in the mouth for ingestion. Each tooth consists of a crown which projects above the gum, two to four roots embedded in the alveolus and a neck between the crown and the root. Each tooth contains a cavity filled with pulp, and it is richly supplied with blood vessels and nerves. The solid portion of the tooth consists of dentin; and the enamel covers the exposed portion of the crown. Two sets of teeth appear at different periods of life; the 20 deciduous teeth appear during infancy and 32 permanent teeth during childhood and early adulthood.

Impacted tooth A tooth that is unable to erupt due to adjacent teeth or malposition of the tooth.

Tooth surface The external aspect of tooth that has labial, lingual, menial, distal and occlusal surfaces.

Topagnosis A symptom of a disease or damage to the brain in which a person cannot identify a part of body that has been touched.

Topectomy (*to-pek'to-me*) Excision of part of the cerebral cortex for the relief of unmanageable pain or especially as a treatment for certain mental disorders.

Tophus (*to'fus*) A chalky deposit of urates in the soft tissue about joint and in the pinna of the ear. pl. **tophi**.

Topical A particular part of the body; pertaining to matters of current interest.

Topiramate (*to-pira-mat*) An anticonvulsant prescribed for preventing epileptic seizures and migraine headaches.

Topography (*to-pog'ra-fe*) The physical features of a surface.

Topotecan (*to'po-te'kan*) An antineoplastic agent used to treat ovarian cancer, small cell lung cancer, or cervical cancer.

Tormina Severe pain in the stomach.

Torpor Lack of response to normal stimulus; apathy; inactivity.

Torsemide (*tor'se-mid*) A diuretic related to sulfonylurea, used in treatment of edema and hypertension, administered orally or intravenously.

Torsion (*tor'shun*) The act of twisting.

Torsion dystonia A disorder of basal ganglia exhibiting a prolonged muscular contraction and the part of the body thrown into spasm.

Torsion of testicle Twisting of the cord that is attached to a testicle. It interrupts its blood supply and may destroy it.

Torticollis (wryneck) (*tor'ti-kol'is*) Wry neck, a contracted state of the cervical muscles causing twisting of the neck and inclination of the head to one side.

Toruloma A tumor like lesion in the lungs resulting from cryptococcosis.

Torulosis (*tor-u-lo'sis*) Cryptococcosis.

Tourette's syndrome (TS) A disorder characterized by recurrent twitching, snorting and sniffing noises and involuntary shouting of obscenities. *see* Gilles de la Tourette's syndrome.

Tourniquet (*toor'ni-ket*) An appliance to compress a blood vessel to reduce blood flow.

Tourniquet test Capillary fragility test. Appearance of 10 or more petechiae within a circle of 2.5 cm in diameter on the forearm when the sphygmomano meter cuff is left inflated for 15 minutes on the arm at a pressure midway between the systolic and diastolic pressures. It may occur in thrombocytopenia, nonthrombocytopenic purpura and scurvy.

Towne's projection An angled anteroposterior radiograph of the skull.

Toxemia (*toks-e'me-a*) A general intoxication due to a presence of toxins in the bloodstream.

Toxemia of pregnancy Preeclampsia or eclampsia.

Toxic (*toks'ik*) Pertaining to a poison.

Toxic epidermal necrolysis (TEN) A severe mucocutaneous reaction pattern characterized by fever, systemic toxicity, tenderness, erythema and widespread exfoliation.

Toxic megacolon An acute colitis with partial or complete colonic dilatation occurring as a life-threatening complication of ulcerative colitis and Crohn's disease.

Toxic state A condition typically seen in third week of typhoid at which the patient is markedly sick, disoriented and having greatest risk for intestinal perforation and hemorrhage.

Toxic vacuolization Rounded 'empty' cytoplasmic spaces within neutrophils seen in gram-negative bacteremia and endotoxemia.

Toxicity (*toks-isi-te*) The quality of being poisonous.

Toxicology (*toks'i-kol'o-je*) Scientific study of poisons, its effects, manifestations and treatment.

Toxicosis (*toks'i-ko'sis*) Any disorder produced by the action of a poison.

Toxic shock syndrome (TSS) A life-threatening condition caused by staphylococci associated most often with the use of some highly absorbable tampons.

Toxin (*toks'in*) Any of a group of poisonous substances produced by microorganisms, or plants or of animal origin.

Toxocara A nematode worm, *Toxocara canis* or *T. cati*.

Toxocariasis (visceral larva migrans) Infestation with the larvae of roundworms of the genus *Toxocara* that normally live in the intestines of dogs.

Toxoid (*toks'oyd*) A modified bacterial exotoxin which has lost its toxicity but retains the property of stimulating the formation of antibodies.

Toxoplasma (*toks'o-plas'ma*) An intracellular protozoan parasite of genus Sporozoa.

Toxoplasmosis A protozoan parasitic disease caused by *Toxoplasma gondii*.

Acquired toxoplasmosis Toxoplasma organism invades lymph nodes and spleen. It may be asymptomatic or present with features of pneumonia, or enlarged lymph nodes.

Congenital toxoplasmosis Occurs from transmission from mother infected during pregnancy to fetus. The manifestations are cerebral with hydrocephalus or microcephaly associated with convulsion, tremors or paralysis.

Trabecular bone Also called cancellous bone is porous bone composed of trabeculated bone tissue.

Trabeculectomy A type of glaucoma surgery performed on the eye that creates a new pathway for fluid inside the eye to be drained.

Tracer Readily recognizable element, usually radioactive or radical introduced into a metabolite.

Trachea (*tra'ke-a*) Windpipe; the cartilaginous tube from the larynx to its bifurcation into the right and left main bronchi; trachea is 12 cm long and consists of a framework of 16–20 C-shaped cartilaginous plates with a dense connective tissue.

Tracheal tug Downward pull with each pulsation of the heart seen in aortic aneurysm.

Tracheitis (*tra'ke-i'tis*) Inflammation of the trachea usually caused by infection.

Trachelitis (*tra'ke-li'tis*) Inflammation of the trachea.

Tracheostomy (tracheotomy) (*tra'ke-os'to-me*) The surgical creation of an opening into the trachea through the neck. It provides an airway during tracheal obstruction.

Tracheotomy (*tra'ke-ot'o-me*) Incision of the trachea through the skin and muscles of the neck in which a tube is inserted into the trachea to keep the airway open.

Trachoma (*tra-ko'ma*) A chronic infection of the conjunctiva and cornea caused by *Chlamydia trachomatis*. Transmission occurs by direct contact and the condition responds to tetracycline, or erythromycin.

Tract (*trakt*) Bundle of nerve fibers having common origin and termination and subserving similar function; a number of organs arranged in series subserving a common function.

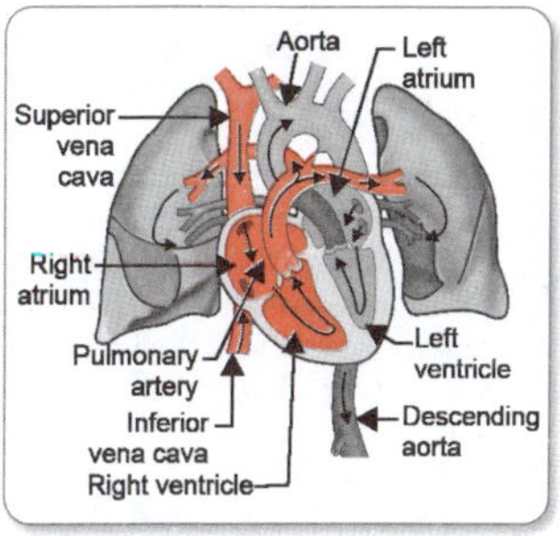

Flow tract of heart

Traction (*trak'shun*) A procedure of exerting a pulling force, along the long axis of a structure. To align two adjoining structures or to hold them in place. A traction technique is used to align some types of fracture of the femur.

Tractotomy (*trak-tot'o-me*) The surgical severing of nerve tracts especially in the medulla of the brain, typically to relieve intractable pain or mental illness, or in research.

Tragus (*tra'gus*) Cartilaginous projection anterior to the external opening of the ear.

Trailing phenomenon Perceptual abnormality associated with hallucinogenic drugs where moving objects appear as a series of discrete and discontinuous images.

Tramadol (*tram'a-dol"*) A centrally-acting opioid agonist and SNRI (serotonin/norepinephrine reuptake inhibitor) used for the management of moderate to severe pain in adults.

Trance (*trans*) A profound degree of sleep from which the person cannot be aroused easily.

Transcervical balloon tuboplasty A procedure attempting to re-establish the patency of fallopian tubes.

Tranquilizer (*tran'kwi-liz'er*) An agent which has calming effect without inducing sleep.

Trans- Prefix meaning through; across.

Transaminase (*trans-am'in-as*) An enzyme that catalyzes the reversible transfer of an amino group.

Transamination (*trans'am-i-na'shan*) Means the transfer of an amine group from α-amino acid to α-keto acid (amino acid without an amine group), thus creating a new α-amino acid and α-keto acid. This pathway is responsible for the deamination of most amino acids.

Transcription (*tran-skrip'shun*) Synthesis of a single-stranded RNA molecule from a double-standard DNA template in the nucleus, during protein production.

Transcription activator A protein that binds to DNA, activating its transcription machinery.

Transcription factors DNA-binding proteins necessary for gene activity.

Transcription unit A DNA sequence that is transcribed into a coherent peptide.

Transduction (*trans-duk'shun*) Transfer of genetic material from one cell to another by viral infection.

Transection (*tran-sek'shun*) A cross section cut transversely.

Transfection(*trans-fek'shun*) Acquisition of new genetic markers by incorporation of added DNA into eukaryotic cells.?

Transferase (*trans-fer-as*) Any of the enzymes that catalyzes the transfer of an organic group from one compound to another.

Transference *psy* The process that develops during psychoanalysis in which the patient redirects feelings about early life figures toward analyst.

Transferrin (siderophilin) (*trans-fer'rin*) Serum beta- globulin that binds and transports iron, throughout the body in the bloodstream.

Transfer RNA A molecule of RNA that picks up a specific amino acid in a cell and joins it with other amino acid in a correct sequence to make a particular protein.

Transfusion (*trans-fu'shun*) Administration of blood or blood components directly into the bloodstream.

Transfusion medicine A subspecialty involved in patient management through administration of blood cells and blood products.

Transfusion reaction Any untoward response to nonself blood products which elicit febrile reactions that are either minor from nonspecific leukocyte derived pyrogens or major due to a true immune reaction.

Transient ischemic attack (TIA) A brief interruption in the blood supply to the brain that results in temporary impaired sensation, movement, vision or speech. The disability is less than 24 hours duration. TlAs often precede cerebral infarctions or strokes.

Transillumination (*trans'il-lu'mi-na' shun*) The passage of light through body tissues for purpose of diagnosis.

Translation (*trans'la'shun*) The conversion of genetically coded instructions into a sequence of amino acids to make an essential protein inside a cell.

Translocation (*tra'ns-lo'ka'shun*) A chromosomal segment that has been broken off and reinserted in a different place in the genome; rearrangement of genetic information on a chromosome.

Transmethylation (*trans'meth-a-la'shan*) The transfer of a methyl group from one compound to another.

Transplantation (*trans'plan-ta'shun*) The grafting of tissues or organ taken from the same body or from another to replace a malfunctioning part.

Transplantation rejection Host immune responses evoked when an allograft tissue is transplanted into a recipient.

Transposition (*trnas'po-zishun*) Displacement of a viscus to opposite side.

Transposition of the great vessels A serious, rare heart problem in which two main arteries leaving the heart are reversed.

Transrectal ultrasound An imaging test in which a probe inserted into the rectum gives off sound waves to create a picture of the prostate on a screen: TRUS.

Transsexualism A gender identity disorder characterized by a persistent belief on the part of the affected individuals that they belong to the opposite sex.

Female transsexualism Present masculine appearance and behavior.

Male transsexualism Behaves that he will grow up to be a woman and lose his genitals.

Transudation (*trans-u-da'shun*) The passage of fluid through a membrane or tissue surface.

Transurethral (*trans-u-re'thral*) Performed through the urethra.

Transurethral needle ablation Destruction by heat energy that directs radio waves through needles that are inserted into the prostate gland; TUNA.

Transurethral prostatectomy Removal of prostate with a resectoscope which is passed up through the urethra.

Transurethral resection of the prostate (TURP) An operation that involves removing a part of the prostate gland that surrounds the urethra.

Transverse process The bony projection on either side of the vertebrae.

Transvestism (*trans-vest'izm*) A sexual deviation having an excessive desire to wear the dress of the opposite sex.

Tranylcypromine (*tran'il-sipro-men*) A monoamine oxidase inhibitor (MAOI) used the treatment of major depressive episode without melancholia.

Trapezium (*tra-pe'ze-um*) A quadrilateral plane figure of which no two sides are parallel; the first bone on the radial side of the distal row of the bones of the wrist.

Os trapezium It articulates with the base of metacarpal bone of the thumb.

Trapezius (*tra-pe'ze-us*) A broad flat muscle on either side of upper and back the neck, shoulders and thorax.

Trapezoid (*trap'e-zoyd*) Having the shape of a four-sided place with two sides parallel and two diverging.

Trapped lung A portion of infected lobe of the lung and visceral pleura fixing the affected lung in a partially collapsed state, seen in empyema.

Trauma (*traw'ma*) A wound or physical injury, a severe emotional shock.

Trauma center A hospital providing care for critically injured patients.

Trauma score Numerical grading system that combines the Glasgow Coma scale and measurement of cardiopulmonary function as a gauge of severity of injury and to predict the outcome.

Traumatic (*traw-mat'ik*) Produced by a trauma.

Traumatology (*traw-ma-tol'oje*) The branch of surgery dealing with wounds or injuries.

Trazodone A serotonin uptake inhibitor used to treat major depressive disorder.

Trematode (*trem'a-tod*) Any parasitic platyhelminth or flatworm of the class Trematoda, having one or more external suckers; fluke.

Tremor (*trem'or*) Regular rhythmic oscilatory movements around a fixed axis due to alternating contraction and relaxation of the muscles.

Essential tremor Coarse postural termor noted in upper extremity, head and neck. Noted with muscle contraction, exaggerated by emotional and physical stress.

Flapping tremor Movements simulating the beating of wings with rapid flexion and extensions at the wrist and metacarpophalangeal joints seen in hepatic precoma, respiratory and renal failure.

Hysterical tremor Variable tremors with a bizarre picture involving a limb or whole body.

Intention tremor Appearance of tremors in a limb with a goal-directed action due to loss of modulating effect of cerebellum on voluntary movement, seen in brain stem or cerebellar disease.

Kinetic tremor Intention tremor; tremor due to affection of cerebellum and its outflow pathways.

Pill-rolling tremor Tremors as rotary movements between index finger and the thumb.

Postural tremor Fine tremors at a fast rate in a limb held in an antigravity posture noted in situations of catecholamine excess such as thyrotoxicosis, anxiety state, hypoglycemia and in alcoholism.

Static tremor Rapid tremors which are rhythmically alternating in flexor and extensor muscles that are marked at rest as in Parkinsonism.

Toxic tremor Postural tremors seen in excess smoking and ingestion of drugs such as caffeine, theophylline, amphetamine, beta-2 agonists and tricyclic antidepressants.

Trench foot (immersion foot) Cold trauma due to prolonged exposure to cold.

Trendelenburg position Marked head down tilt of whole body especially for pelvic operations.

Trephine (*tre-fin'*) A saw for removal of a circular disk of bone; an instrument for removal of a circular area of cornea.

Treponema (*trep"o-ne'ma*) A spirochete bacterium that is parasitic or pathogenic in humans and warm-blooded animals, including the causal agents of syphilis and yaws; a genus of spiral shaped bacteria. *T. carateum* causative agent of pinta, *T. pallidum* causative agent of syphilis, *T. pertenue* causative agent of yaws.

Treponematosis (*trep'o-ne-ma-to'sis*) A disease or infection caused by a *Treponema.*

Tretinoin (*tret'i-noin"*) A form of retinoic acid, applied to the skin to treat acne and other disorders.

Triad (*tri'ad*) A group of three entities; an association of three clinical or pathologic findings, characteristic of a disease.

Triamcinolone (*tri'am-sin'a-lon*) A glucocorticoid drug used chiefly in the form of its acetal or acetate derivatives especially in treating skin disorders, asthma, and allergic rhinitis.

Triamterene (*tri-am'ter-en*) A potassium-sparing diuretic that is used in the management of hypertension.

Triangle (*tri'ang-g'l*) A three-cornered area.

Codman triangle A wedge-shaped periosteal elevation of bone seen on a plain film of the long bones characteristic of Ewing's sarcoma.

Triangle test A method to investigate the neighborhood of the shoulder joint for bony injury. The triangle is formed by three bony points, namely the tip of acromion, the tip of the coracoid process and the most prominent part of the great tuberosity of the humerus.

Triangular bandage A square bandage folded diagonally.

Triatoma (*tri-at'o-ma*) Any member of the genus *Triatoma* of assassin bugs.

Triaziquone A drug, member of aziridines alkylating agents, is used in chemotherapy. It can react with DNA to form intrastrand crosslinks.

Triazolam (*tri-a'zo-lam*) A form of benzodiazepine prescribed for sleeping pill.

Triceps (*tri'seps*) A muscle that arises from three heads.

Triceps muscle A muscle at the back of the upper part of the arm that straightens the elbow joint.

Triceps skinfold thickness Estimation of corporal fat by measuring on the right arm halfway between the olecranon process of the elbow and the acromial process of scapula.

Trichiasis (*trik-i'a-sis*) A condition of ingrowing eyelashes that causes them to rub against eyeball.

Trichinella (*trik'i-nel'a*) A nematode, *Trichinella spiralis*, that causes trichinosis, the adults of which live in the intestine and produce larvae that encyst in the muscle tissue, especially in pigs, rats, and humans.

Trichinosis (trichiniasis) (*trik'in-o'sis*) Disease due to *Trichinella spiralis* which spreads by eating undercooked meat. Symptoms occur from secondary invasion of tissues mainly striated muscle in which larvae encyst. Initially the condition presents with diarrhea, later by fever, edema of face, eyelids and conjunctiva, stiffness, pain and tenderness of muscle. There is eosinophilia and albendazole is useful. Also called trichinellosis.

Trichlormethiazide (*tri-klor'me-thi'a-zid*) A diuretic with properties similar to those of hydrochlorothiazide.

Trichoadenoma (*trik'o-ad'e-no'ma*) Benign follicular tumors that usually present as slow-growing dermal masses.

Trichobezoar (*trik'o-be'zor*) A hair ball formed in the stomach or intestine.

Trichoblastoma (*trik'o-blas-to'ma*) A rare, slow-growing, benign cutaneous tumor derived from follicular germinative cells.

Trichoglossia (*trik'o-glos'e-a*) Hairy tongue due to thickening of papillae.

Trichology (*trik'o-logi*) The sturdy of the hair and scalp in healthy and disease condition.

Trichomonas (*trik'o-mo'nas*) A parasitic flagellate protozoan called *Trichomonas vaginalis* that is sexually transmitted.

Trichomoniasis (*trik'o-mo-ni-a-sis*) Infection with *T. vaginalis*, common in women, presents with burning, redness and itching of vulvar tissue and profuse vaginal discharge; it may be malodorous. Metronidazole is useful.

Trichomycosis (*trik'o-mi-ko'sis*) A mild infection of the hair under the armpit caused by *Corynebacterium tenuis* bacterium.

Trichophyton (*tri-kof'it-on*) A genus of imperfect fungi.

Trichophyton rubrum Causes dermatophytic infection where this fungus remains confined to stratum corneum only.

Trichorrhexis (*trik'o-rek'sis*) Brittleness of the hair.

Trichosis (*tri-ko'sis*) Hairiness.

Trichosporon (*tri-kos'po-ron*) A genus of anamorphic fungi in the family Trichosporonaceae.

Trichotillomania (*trik'o-till'o-man-ia*) Compulsive hair pulling.

Trichromatic (*tri'kro-mat'ik*) Having or using three colors.

Trichuriasis (*trik'-u-ri'a-sis*) Infection caused by nematode, *Trichuris*. Intense infections in children present with persistent diarrhea or rectal prolapse and stunting. Treatment is with mebendazole.

Trichuris (*tri-ku'ris*) An intestinal nematode, whipworm. *T. trichiura* a species of *Trichuris* that infects humans when the ova are ingested. The larvae develop into adults which inhabit the large intestine, cecum, lower ileum and anal canal.

Tricuspid valve The valve that guards the opening between the right atrium and right ventricle, and it has largest circumference.

Tridactyl Having three fingers or toes.

Trifluoperazine A phenothiazine used to treat depression, anxiety, and agitation.

Trifocal lenses Lenses that have three regions which corrects far distance, intermediate and near vision.

Trigeminal nerve Fifth cranial nerve.

Trigeminal neuralgia (tic douloureux) Also called as tic dolourex is a type of chronic pain disorder that involves sudden attacks of severe facial pain.

Trigeminy *ECG* A form of arrhythmia in which every third QRS wave is a ventricular premature beat.

Trigger finger Thickening and constriction of the mouth of a fibrous digital sheath interfering with the free gliding of the contracted flexor tendons. It may affect the fingers in middle aged and the thumb in infants. In adults, there is tenderness at the base of affected finger and locking of the finger in full flexion. Infants are unable to straighten the thumb which is locked in flexion. The treatment consists of incising the mouth of the fibrous flexor sheath longitudinally.

Triglyceride Glycerol with all three hydroxyls linked to fatty acids.

Trigone (*tri'gon*) A triangular area.

Trigone of bladder A triangular area at the base of the bladder between the two openings of the ureter and urethra.

Trigonitis (*trig'o-ni'tis*) A condition of inflammation of the trigone region of the bladder.

Trigonocephaly (*trig'o-no-sefa-le*) Premature fusion of the metopic suture leading to deformation of anterior calvarium causing keel shaped deformity of forehead.

Trihexyphenidyl (*tri-hek"si-fen'i-dil*) An antispasmodic drug used as an adjunct drug in the management of parkinsonism and as a treatment for extrapyramidal symptoms caused by drugs affecting the central nervous system.

Triiodothyronine Also known as T_3, is a thyroid hormone, which regulates several developmental, metabolic, and neural activities throughout the body.

Trimeprazine (*tri-mep'ra-zen*) An antihistamine agent used to prevent and relieve allergic conditions which cause pruritus and other allergic skin conditions, including urticaria.

Trimester (*tri-mes'ter*) One of the three periods of approximately 3 months each into which pregnancy is divided.

Trimethadione (*tri'meth-a-di'on*) An anticonvulsant agent indicated for the control of treatment-refractory petit mal seizures.

Trimethobenzamide (*tri-meth'o-ben'za-mid*) An antiemetic used to treat postoperative nausea and vomiting and nausea associated with gastroenteritis.

Trimethoprim TMP, folic acid antagonist.

Trimethoprim-sulfamethoxazole SMX, a combination of antibacterial agent formulated as a 1:20 ratio of TMP to SMX, effective against genitourinary, gastrointestinal and respiratory tract infections and to treat *Pneumocystis carinii* pneumonia.

Trimipramine (*tri-mip'ra-men*) A tricyclic antidepressant that is used to treat symptoms of depression.

Trinitrophenol (*tri'ni'tro-fe'nol*) A toxic sparingly soluble crystalline yellow acid used as a dye, antiseptic, and explosive.

Triose (*tri'os*) A monosaccharide, or simple sugar, containing three carbon atoms.

Triploid (*trip'loid*) Containing three homologous sets of chromosomes.

Triquetral bone The third carpal bone in the proximal row, enumerated from the radial side; any Wormian bone.

Trismus (*tris'mus*) Spasm of muscles of mastication with difficulty to open the mouth and in mastication; lock jaw.

Trisomy (*tri'so-me*) Condition of having three identical chromosomes instead of the normal two in a cell.

Trisomy 13 Mental defect, microphthalmia, polydactyly and congenital heart disease; Patau's syndrome.

Trisomy 18 Mental defect, micrognathia, deformed hands and feet, congenital heart disease; Edward's syndrome.

Trisomy 21 Down's syndrome; mongolism.

Tritanope (*tri'ta-nop*) A condition where a person cannot distinguish between blue and yellow colors.

Trocar (*tro'kar*) a sharp-pointed obturator contained in a cannula to pierce the wall of a cavity.

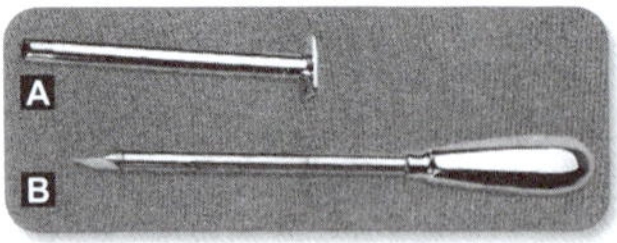

***A.** Trocar with handle; **B.** Cannula*

Trochanter (*tro-kan'ter*) Either of the two processes below the neck of the femur.

Greater trochanter A thick process at the upper end of femur projecting upward externally to the union of the neck and shaft.

Lesser trochanter A conical tuberosity on the inner and posterior surface of the upper end of the femur at the junction of shaft and neck.

Third trochanter An unusually prominent gluteal ridge of the femur.

Troche (*tro'ke*) Lozenge. It releases drug as it dissolves in the mouth.

Trochlea (*trok'le-a*) A pulley-shaped structure.

Trochoid (*tro'koid*) The curve described by a fixed point on the radius or extended radius of a circle as the circle rolls along a straight line.

Trombicula (*trom-bik'u-la*) The chigger mite.

Tromethamine A proton acceptor used for the prevention and correction of metabolic acidosis associated with various clinical conditions, such as cardiac bypass surgery.

Trophoblast (*trof'o-blast*) A layer of extraembryonic ectodermal tissue on the outside of blastocyst. It develops into placenta and amniotic sac.

Trophozoite (*trof'o-zo'it*) The active, motile feeding stage of a protozoan.

-trophy Referring to nutrition or growth.

-tropic Of direction. Movement in response to a stimulus; aim of a specific object; hormones stimulating specific object.

Tropical ulcer (Naga sore) Ulceration of legs and feet seen in malnourished, bare-footed laborers with multiple infections in tropics.

Tropocollagen (*tro'po-kola-jen*) The structural unit of a collagen fiber.

Truncus (*trung'kus*) A stem; trunk.

Truncus arteriosus The arterial trunk from the embryonic heart.

Trunk That portion of the body exclusive of the head and limbs; the main stem of a nerve, lymphatic or blood vessel.

Celiac trunk The trunk arising from abdominal aorta that supplies blood to the stomach, duodenum, liver, gallbladder, pancreas and spleen.

Pulmonary trunk The great vessel arising from the right ventricle of the heart that gives the right and left pulmonary arteries to the lungs.

Sympathetic trunk The two long chains of ganglia connected by sympathetic nerve fibers that extend along the vertebral column.

Truss (*trus*) An elastic appliance to retain a reduced hernia within the abdominal cavity.

Trypanocide (*tri-pan'o-sid*) A drug or substance that kills trypanosomes.

Trypanosoma (*tri'pan-o-so'ma*) A protozoan parasite with a whiplike flagella. ***T. cruzi*** causative agent of American trypanosomiasis. ***T. gambiense*** causative agent of African sleeping sickness. ***T. rhodesiense*** causative agent of sleeping sickness in East Aftrica.

Trypanosomiasis (*tri-pan'o-so-mi'a-sis*) Infection with protozoa of the genus *Trypanosoma.*

Trypsin (*trip'sin*) A proteolytic enzyme formed in the intestine from the action of enterokinase of intestinal juice on trypsinogen secreted by pancreas. It catalyzes the hydrolysis of peptide bonds in partly digested proteins.

Trypsinogen (*trip-sin'o-gen*) A proenzyme found in pancreatic juice.

Tryptophan (*trip'to-fan*) An essential amino acid. It is found in high concentration in animal and fish protein. It is a precursor of serotonin.

Tsetse (*she'she*) Blood-sucking diptera confined to Africa. It is an important transmitter of trypanosomes, the causative agents of African sleeping sickness.

TSH Thyroid-stimulating hormone.

Tsutsugamushi disease (*t-sut-sug-a-mu' shi*) An acute infectious disease of man; scrub typhus.

Tubal Pertaining to a tube, especially fallopian tube.

Tubal ligation A female sterilization procedure in which the fallopian tubes are surgically tied off and cut.

Tubal reanastomosis A surgical reconstruction procedure when the cut ends of a fallopian tube are joined together.

Tubal pregnancy Implantation of a fertilized egg in a fallopian tube. It is associated with severe abdominal pain and light vaginal bleeding.

Tube (*tub*) A long hollow cylindrical structure.

Stomach tube A rubber tube to introduce food or to perform a wash.

Tube feeding Providing fluid and food into the stomach through a nasogastric tube.

Test tube A glass tube closed at one end.

Uterine tube Fallopian tube.

Tuber (*tu'ber*) A swelling, protuberance.

Tuber cinereum A part of the base of hypothalamus that is connected by infundibulum with the posterior pituitary.

Tubercle (*tu'ber-kl*) Small, rounded nodule produced by infection with *Mycobacterium tuberculosis*; a small rounded elevation on a bone; a small nodule.

Tubercular (*tu-ber'ku-lar*) Resembling tubercles.

Tubercular chancre Extremely rare form of primary cutaneous tuberculosis with painless nodules which breakdown in a week to form an ulcer with enlargement of regional lymph nodes.

Tuberculid (*tu-ber'ku-lid*) A popular eruption probably due to allergy to tuberculosis.

Tuberculin (*tu-ber'ku-lin*) A sterile liquid containing the growth products of or specific substances extracted from the tubercle bacillus.

Tuberculin test A test to determine the presence of tuberculosis infection based on positive reaction to tuberculin. It is useful in epidemiological survey to get a picture of prevalence of tuberculosis in a community and to select a group requiring BCG vaccination. The test is performed by either old tuberculin or tuberculin-purified protein derivative. Mantoux test, Heaf's test or tine test are useful.

Tuberculoma (*tu-ber'ku-lo'ma*) A tumor-like mass from an enlarged caseous tubercle.

Tuberculosis (*tu-ber'ku-lo'sis*) An infectious disease caused by *Mycobacterium tuberculosis*. Lungs form the common site of the disease. Other sites are gastrointestinal and genitourinary systems, CNS, bones, joints, lymph nodes and skin.

Avian tuberculosis Tuberculosis of birds caused by *Mycobacterium avium*.

Bovine tuberculosis Tuberculosis of cattle caused by *Mycobacterium bovis*.

Endogenous tuberculosis Tuberculosis originating from a primary lesion.

Exogenous tuberculosis Tuberculosis acquired from an exogenous source.

Miliary tuberculosis Presence of widespread lesions of tuberculosis occurring after a hematogenous dissemination of tubercle bacilli. It occurs in individuals who have inadequate cell-mediated immunity.

Multidrug-resistant tuberculosis (MDR-TB) *Mycobacterium tuberculosis* that is resistant to therapy with a variety of antituberculosis agents that had been effective in treatment.

Open tuberculosis Tuberculosis in which the tubercle bacilli are present in the sputum.

Postprimary tuberculosis The pathological changes are as a result of interaction between tubercle bacilli and the host immunological responses. Tubercle is the primary lesion of tuberculosis, which undergoes caseous necrosis and forms a cavity. It can undergo fibrosis or get disseminated. Clinically it presents with fever, cough, loss of weight and hemoptysis. The condition is diagnosed by chest radiograph and sputum examination for presence of acid-fast bacteria. It is treated with short-course chemotherapy using rifampicin, isoniazid (INH), pyrazinamide, ethambutol and/or streptomycin.

Primary tuberculosis Lesion due to an infection with *M. tuberculosis* in individuals who have never had previous experience with tubercle bacilli. The spread of the disease is by inhalation of airborne droplet nuclei containing tubercle bacilli. It is characterized by formation of tubercles and caseation, fibrosis and calcification.

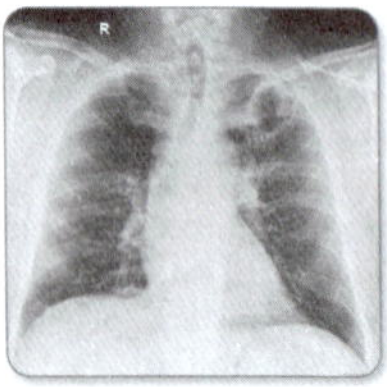

X-ray of primary tuberculosis

Tuberosity (*tu-ber-osi-te*) An elevation or protuberance.

Tuberous (tuberos) (*too'bar-us*) A rare genetic condition that causes mainly noncancerous (benign) tumors to develop in different parts of the body.

Tuberous sclerosis (epiloia) An autosomal dominant condition with hamartomas affecting many systems. Classically it is characterized by mental retardation, epilepsy and skin lesions like small white oval (ash leaf) macules or pink or yellowish papules on the center of the face (adenoma sabaceum).

Tubo- Relating to, or affecting a fallopian tube and ovary.

Tuboabdominal (*too'bo-ab-dom'i-nal*) Pertaining to fallopian tube and abdomen.

Tubo-ovarian (*tu'bo-o-va're-an*) Pertaining to a uterine tube and ovary.

Tubotympanum (*too'bo-tim'pa-num*) Consists of Eustachian (auditory) tube and tympanomastoid cavities form an anatomic and functional whole that cannot easily be divided.

Tubule (*tu'bul*) A small tube.

Renal tubule The part of a nephron through which renal filtrate from the renal corpuscle flows and is changed to urine by absorption and secretion.

Tularemia (rabbit fever) (*tu-lar-e'me-a*) A bacterial infection by *Francisella tularensis*. It is transmitted by ticks or acquired while skinning infected wild rabbits. It presents as a skin ulcer and painful regional lymphadenopathy. Streptomycin, gentamicin and tetracyclines are useful. It is named after Tulare in California where disease was first discovered.

Tulle gras A close-meshed net cut into squares and impregnated with soft paraffin, Peruvian balsam and vegetable oil to treat raw surfaces.

Tumefaction (*tu'me-fak'shun*) A swelling.

Tumescence (*tu-mes'ens*) Swollen.

Tumid Swollen.

Tumor (*tu'mor*) Swelling, one of the cardinal signs of inflammation; a neoplastic growth with an uncontrolled, multiplication of cells.

Tumor-associated antigens Molecules such as CA 19-9, CA 125 and CA 195 that may be associated with specific tumors.

Tumor necrosis factor TNF, a molecule that mediates shock and tumor-related cachexia divided into TNF-α and TNF-β.

Tumor promoter Cocarcinogen. A substance that has no intrinsic carcinogenic potential, but which when applied repeatedly, is capable of amplifying the cancer-inducing effects of other substances.

Tumor seeding The spillage of tumor cells and then subsequent growth into tumor colonies. The spillage can occur from an operative field and along needle biopsy tracts.

Tumor-specific antigen A substance secreted by some tumors and in some conditions.

Tumor suppressor gene A growth regulatory gene that encodes a protein capable of suppressing malignant transformation.

Tumor marker Nonspecific substances, which under certain circumstances can be used to detect recurrence. The tumor markers include carcinoembryonic antigen—CEA, oncofetal antigens (α-fetoprotein), and tumor associated antigens (CA 125, CA 19-9).

Tunica (*tu'ni-ka*) A covering or coat.

Tunica albuginea White fibrous capsule of testis.

Tunica vaginalis Serous cavity surrounding testis and epididymis.

Turbinate bone 3 pairs of long thin bones covered with a layer of tissue that can expand, which are present inside walls of the nose.

Turbinectomy (*tur'bi-nek'to-me*) Surgical excision of a nasal concha.

Turbinotomy (*tur'bi-not'o-me*) The surgical cutting of a nasal concha (turbinate bone).

Turcot's disease (*tur'kotz*) Autosomal recessive condition described by Jacques Turcot, Canadian physician. Characterized by colonic adenomatous polyps and glioblastomas of the central nervous system.

Turgescence (*tur-jes'ens*) Swelling of a part.

Turgor Normal consistency of living tissue; distension.

Turner's syndrome A genetic disorder affecting females who have only one X chromosome, described by Henry Turner, US physician. There is failure of the ovaries to respond to pituitary hormone stimulation. It is characterized by amenorrhea, failure of sexual maturation, short stature, webbing of neck and cubital valgus.

Turricephaly (*tur'i-sefa-le*) A disorder in which the top of the skull is pointed or conical owing to premature closure of the coronal and lambdoid sutures.

Tussis A voluntary or involuntary act that clears the throat and breathing passage of foreign particles, microbes, irritants, fluids, and mucus.

Twilight state Disturbed consciousness with hallucinations.

Twilight sleep A dream-like state of conscious sedation.

Twin One of two offsprings born at one birth.

Fraternal twin Twin comes from two separate fertilized ova and the two individuals growing from them are like ordinary siblings except that they are born together.

Identical twin Twin coming from the same fertilized ova which instead of growing into one individual, becomes split into two. The nuclei of the two cells contain exactly the same hereditary determinants. Such twins resemble each other, in almost complete detail.

Tylosis (*ti-lo'sis*) Formation of a callus; palmoplantar hyperkeratosis.

Tympanic (*tim-pan'ik*) Pertaining to the tympanum.

Tympanic membrane Eardrum.

Tympanic resonance A sound produced by percussion over an air fitted cavity or gas-filled cavity.

Tympanites (meteorism) (*tim-pan-i'tez*) Distension of the abdomen due to presence of gas or air in the intestine or in the peritoneal cavity.

Tympanoplasty (*tim'pan-o-plas'te*) Surgical procedure to repair the hearing mechanism of the middle ear. It consists of repair of the eardrum and/or repositioning of the tiny bones of the middle ear to treat hearing loss.

Tympanotomy (*tim'pa-not'o-me*) Incision into the tympanum.

Tympanum (*tim'pan-um*) The cavity of middle ear.

Typhilitis Inflammation of the cecum.

Typhoid fever Caused by *S. typhi* which is transmitted by the fecal-oral route. The bacilli localize mainly in the lymphoid tissue of the small intestine in the Peyer's patches where they ulcerate. It presents with fever, headache, myalgia, bradycardia, constipation, splenomegaly, abdominal distension, diarrhoea and delirium. It may be associated with complications such as haemorrhage, perforation and septicemia. Ciprofloxacin, amoxycillin, cotrimoxazole and chloramphenicol are effective. Injectable or oral vaccines are available for prevention.

Typhus (spotted fever) (*ti'fus*) Arthropod-borne infectious disease caused by *Rickettsia*. Rickettsiae multiply in vascular endothelial cells and produce lesions in different parts of the body. The common clinical features are fever, severe prostration, mental disturbance and often rash.

Endemic typhus fever Flea-borne typhus caused by *R. mooseri*; the clinical features resemble those of a mild louse-borne typhus.

Epidemic typhus fever Louse-borne typhus caused by *R. prowazekii*. It has sudden onset with malaise, headache, fever, pain in the back and limbs and rash. There is splenomegaly, dry tongue, condition responds to tetracycline or chloramphenicol.

Tyramine (*ti'ra-men*) A decarboxylation product of tyrosine and it is a sympathomimetic amine.

Tyrosinosis (*ti'ro-sin-o'sis*) A rare disorder of tyrosine metabolism, wherein there is an increased urinary excretion of tyrosyl metabolites following ingestion of tyrosine.

U

Ubiquinone (*u-bik'-wi-non*) Coenzyme Q, a protein that acts as a hydrogen carrier which is linked to intramitochondrial electron transport cascade.

Ulcer (*ul'ser*) A circumscribed depressed lesion on the skin or mucous membrane of any internal organ following sloughing of necrotic inflammation.

Buruli ulcer Necrotizing ulcer of skin and subcutaneous tissue of the extremities from My. ulcerans, named after Buruli in Uganda.

Corneal ulcer Ulcer in the cornea.

Curling's ulcer An ulcer of the duodenum following severe burns.

Decubitus ulcer An ulceration caused by prolonged pressure in a patient who is bedridden for a prolonged period of time, pressure sore.

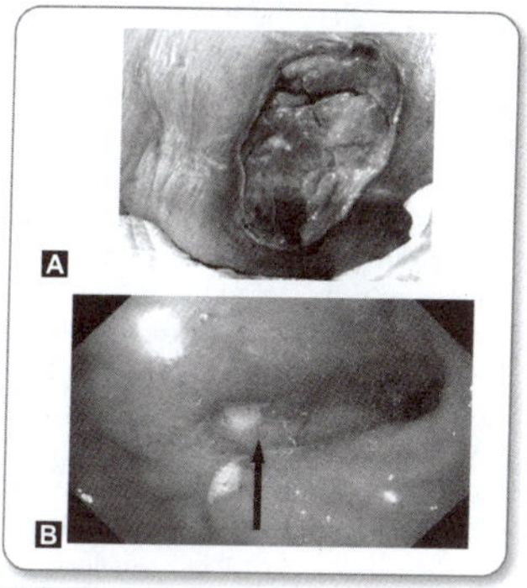

Endoscopic appearance of ulcer:
***A.** Decubitus ulcer; **B.** Gastric ulcer*

Flask ulcer Flask-shaped ulcer in the intestine in amoebic dysentery.

Girdle ulcer A tuberculous ulcer spreading along the wall of the intestine in an encircling manner.

Gwalior ulcer Cutaneous leishmaniasis.

Hunner's ulcer Chronic interstitial cystitis with ulcers involving all layers of the bladder.

Kissing ulcer Ulcers developing on directly opposing surfaces of the stomach in lesser curvature.

Peptic ulcer A group of ulcerating lesions affecting the upper gastrointestinal tract.

Phagedenic ulcer Ulcer that spreads rapidly causing disintegration of tissues with slough and discharge.

Preauricular ulcer Ulcer at the root of helix with a preauricular sinus.

Prosthetic ulcer Ulcer over the gums due to an ill-fitting denture.

Serpiginous ulcer A creeping ulcer that heals in one part and extends to another.

Stress ulcer Peptic ulcer developing front stress such as burns, surgery, prolonged corticosteroid therapy, acute infections or cerebral trauma.

Traumatic ulcer An ulcer due to a local injury.

Trophic ulcer An ulcer due to imperfect nutrition of the part.

Varicose ulcer Ulcer in the leg associated with varicose veins.

Venous ulcer Ulcer on ankle due to venous insufficiency.

Ulceration (*ul'ser-a'shun*) The formation of an ulcer.

Ulcerative colitis A nonspecific inflammation of large bowel especially rectum characterized by diarrhea with blood and mucus. It occurs in young and middle aged adults of either sex. It runs a chronic course with remissions and relapses. Corticosteroids and sulphasalazine are used in treatment.

Ulcerogangrenous (*ul'ser-o-gang'gre-nus*) An ulcer that contains gangrenous tissue.

Ulcerous (*ul'ser-us*) Affected with ulceration.

Ulegyria (*u'le-giy're-a*) A defect of the cerebral cortex showing narrow and distorted gyri.

Uletic (*u-let'ik*) Pertaining to the gums.

Ullmann's line (*ul'manz*) A line from the anterior edge of the first sacral vertebra when extended upward at a right angle to the superior surface of the sacrum will pass through the last lumbar vertebra in spondylolisthesis, named after Emerich Ullmann, Hungarian surgeon.

Ulna (*ul'na*) The larger of the two bones of the forearm lying parallel with the radius. It extends from the elbow to the wrist on the side of the little finger. It articulates with the humerus and with the head of the radius above and bones of the carpus below. pl. **ulnae.**

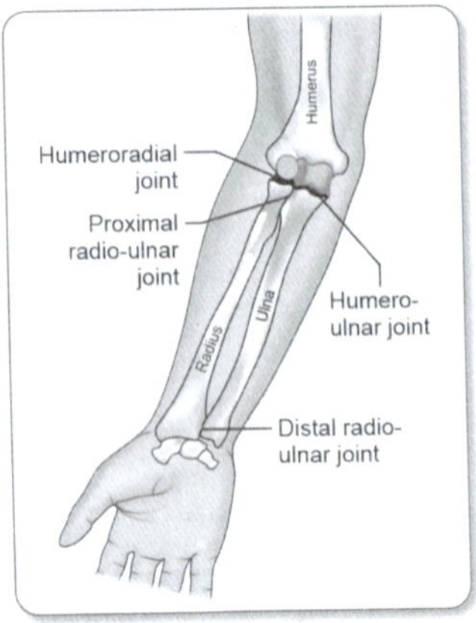

Bones of forearm showing ulna and radius with joints

Ulnar artery One of the terminal branches of the brachial artery. Originating in cubital fossa, supplies muscles of forearm and palm, contributes in anastomosis around elbow joint and terminates in palm by joining superficial palmar arch.

Ulnar nerve One of the 5 terminal branches of the brachial plexus, arising from the medial cord.

Ulocarcinoma (*u'lo-kar'sino'ma*) Carcinoma of the gums.

Ulorrhagia (*u'lo-ra'jea*) Bleeding from gums.

Ultimobranchial body (*ul'ti-mo-brang' ke-al*) Embryonic pharyngeal pouches getting separated from the pharynx and incorporated into substance of thyroid gland, and secrete calcitonin.

Ultracentrifuge (*ul'trah-sen'-tri-fuj*) A high speed centrifuge for subjecting solutions to forces many times that of gravity and producing concentration differences depending on the weight of the molecule.

Ultrafiltration (*ul'tra-fil-tra'shun*) Filtration through an ultrafilter capable of removing very minute particles.

Ultramicroscope (*ul'tra-mi'kro-skop*) An instrument using scattering phenomenon to detect the position of objects too small to be seen by an ordinary microscope. adj. **ultramicroscopic**.

Ultrasonics (*ul'tra-son'iks*) The branch of science that deals with ultrasonic phenomenon.

Ultrasonography (*ul'tra-sono-gra-fe*) A process of imaging deep structures of the body based on the differences in the acoustic impedance of different tissues, electricity applied 10 a piezoelectric crystal in the transducer causes a high frequency mechanical vibration. The transducer generates the ultra-sound beam and detect the returning echo.

Doppler ultrasonography Measurement of velocities of moving fluid such as blood based on principles of the Doppler effect, there is shift in frequency between emitted ultrasonic waves and their echoes.

Duplex ultrasonography An ultrasonographic modality combining B mode display with pulsed Doppler signals and it reflects motions within a tissue such as blood flow.

Endoscopic ultrasonography A procedure in which endoscopy is combined with ultrasound to obtain images of the internal organs in the chest, abdomen, colon and its adjacent structures.

Gray-scale ultrasonography Refers to a two-dimensional image in which the desired organs and tissues are depicted as points of variable brightness.

Intravascular ultrasonography An imaging test that creates images of the heart and blood vessels from the inside of the body.

Pulsed wave doppler ultrasonography Uses the Doppler principle that moving objects change the characteristic of sound waves.

Transcranial ultrasonography A painless test that uses sound waves to detect pathology that affect blood flow in your brain.

Transrectal ultrasonography Procedure that uses sound waves to create a video image of the prostate gland.

Ultrasound (ultrasonic waves) (*ultra sownd*) Sound waves having frequency higher than the range audible to the human ear (over 20000 vibrations per second).

Real time ultrasound A sonographic procedure providing rapid, multiple images of an anatomical structure in the form of motion.

Ultrasound scanning A diagnostic imaging procedure wherein high frequency sound waves are passed into the body and reflected back, on which a computer builds up an image of internal structures.

Ultrasound therapy Ultrasonic waves when projected as a beam from a transducer penetrate and strike the tissues and the energy is converted into heat which is used for relief of pain.

Ultrastructure (*ul'tra-struk'tur*) The fine structure of tissues such as membranes microtubules and microfilaments visible on electro microscopic study.

Ultraviolet rays (*ul'tra-vi'o-let*) Beyond the visible violet portion of the spectrum.

Ultraviolet radiation The segment of the electromagnetic spectrum lying between 200 and 400 nm.

Ultraviolet therapy Treatment with ultraviolet radiation.

Umbilical cord (*umbil'ikal*) Pertaining to umbilicus or umbilical cord.

Umbilical adenoma A pedunculated, raspberry-like mass in the umbilicus.

Umbilical carcinoma A secondary carcinomatous nodule at the umbilicus, The cord structure connect the umbilicus of the fetus with the placenta in the gravid uterus, and carry two umbilical arteries and a vein.

Umbilical fissure The part of hepatic longitudinal fissure in which the umbilical vein is located.

Umbilical fistula A fistulous tract in the umbilicus may discharge urine (urachal fistula), feces (patent omphalomesenteric duct) or mucus.

Umbilical hernia A hernia of the umbilicus. It may be congenital seen in infants or acquired where a scar gives way.

Umbilical sepsis Infection of umbilicus by careless handling or cutting of the cord without antiseptic measures.

Umbilical vesicle The part of the embryonic yolk sac leading from the umbilicus.

Umbilicus (omphalus) (*um-bil'i-kus*) The depressed area of scar in the middle of the abdominal wall where the umbilical cord was attached to the fetus; navel.

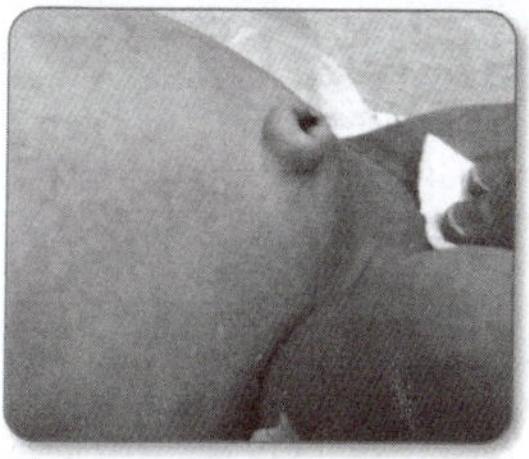

Umbilicus (navel)

Umbo (*um'bo*) A rounded elevation; the slight projection at the center of the inner surface of the tympanic membrane.

Unciform bone Hamate bone on ulnar side of distal row of the carpus.

Uncinaria (*un'sin-a-ri'a*) Nematodes having a hook-like structure.

Uncinate seizure Conditions characterized by recurrent paroxysmal neuronal discharges which arise from a focal region of the brain.

Unconscious (*un-kon'shus*) Inability to respond to any sensory stimuli or being unaware of the surroundings; insensible.

Unconsciousness (*un-kon'shus-nes*) A state of loss of awareness from which a person cannot be aroused.

Uncus (*unk'us*) Hook-shaped structure; hooked anterior portion of hippocampal gyrus, one of the convolutions on the inferior surface of the temporal lobe.

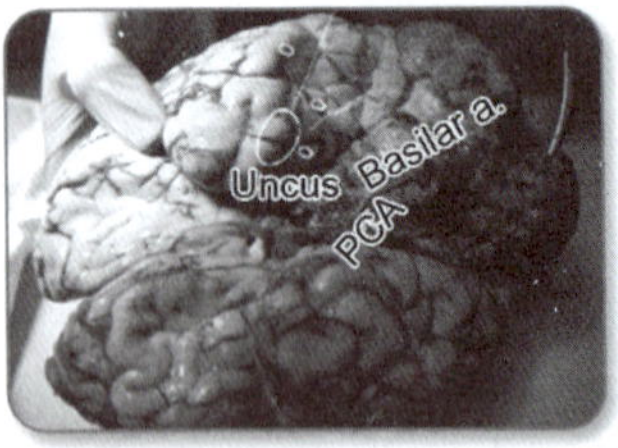

Uncus

Undulant fever brucellosis.

Ungual (*ung'gwal*) Pertaining to the nails.

Ungual phalanx Terminal phalanx of each finger and toe

Ungual tuberosity Spatula-shaped extremity of terminal phalanx that gives support to the nails.

Unguis (*ung'gwis*) A finger nail or toe nail; the lacrimal bone; white prominence on floor of the posterior horn of the lateral ventricle. pl. **ungues.**

UNICEF United Nations International Children's Emergency Fund.

Unicellular (*u'ni-sel'u-lar*) Having one cell such as protozoa or bacteria.

Unifascicular (*u'ni-fa-sik'u-lar*) A single bundle, or fasciculus.

Unigravida (*u'ni-grav'i-da*) Primigravida; woman pregnant for the first time.

Unilateral (*uni-lat'er-al*) Affecting only one side.

Unilateral hyperlucent lung syndrome A small unilateral transradiant lung or a lobe with poor ventilation and perfusion, named after MacLeod, and Swyer and James.

Unipolar disorder A mood disorder with recurrent depression.

Uniovular (*u'ni-ov'u-lar*) Arising from one ovum.

Unipara (*u-nip'a-ra*) A woman having one pregnancy over 20 weeks.

United Nations International Children's Emergency Fund UNICEF, one of the specialized agencies of the United Nation with activities covering programs of assistance in child survival, protection and development and undertaken a campaign for a "child health revolution".

United States Pharmacopeia (USP) A pharmacopeia for the United States published annually by the United States Pharmacopeial Convention, a nonprofit organization that owns the trademark and also owns the copyright on the pharmacopeia itself. It is an independent, scientific nonprofit organization focused on building trust in the supply of safe, quality medicines. It includes also assays and tests for the determination of strength, quality, and purity.

Univalent (*uni-va'lent*) Monovalent.

University of Wisconsin preservation solution 1 liter of solution at 4°C is perfused through the donor portal vein and 2–3 liters through the aorta to perfuse the liver and kidneys. This enables extension of organ storage such as liver after retrieval.

Unoprostone (*uno-pros'ton*) An antiglaucoma agent that increases the outflow of aqueous humor and reduces the elevated intraocular pressure; used in the treatment of open angle glaucoma and ocular hypertension, applied topically.

Upper airway obstruction Obstruction in upper airway may occur from inhalation of foreign bodies, acute edema or infections. The condition may also develop slowly from tumors, tracheal stenosis and laryngeal abnormalities enabling examination of the esophagus, stomach and duodenum.

Upper GI Term for radiocontrast studies of the upper gastrointestinal tract.

Upper motor neuron (UMN) A descending fiber (corticospinal or pyramidal) system with cells of origin in the precentral gyrus of cerebral cortex, that descends and after decussation to the opposite side innervates cranial nerve nuclei and the anterior horn cells.

Upper respiratory tract URT consists of nose, nasopharynx and larynx lined by vascular mucous membranes with ciliated epithelium. It participates in air conditioning, swallowing.

Urachus (*u'ra-kus*) Remnant of allantois, a canal present in the fetus between the umbilicus and the apex of the bladder, which changes as a fibrous cord after. adj. **urachal**.

Uracil (*ur'-ah-sil*) A pyrimidine base.

Uraniscoplasty (*u'ran-is'ko-plas'te*) Repair of cleft palate.

Uraniscorrhaphy (*u'ran-is-kor'ra-fe*) Suturing of cleft palate.

Uraniscus (*u'rah-nis'kus*) The palate.

Uranorrhaphy (*u-ran-or-ra-fe*) Suturing of a cleft palate.

Uratemia (*u'ra-te'me-a*) Presence of urates in the blood.

Uraturia (*u'rah-tu're-a*) Urates in the urine.

Urbach-Oppenheim disease (*ur'bak-ope' en-him*) Necrobiosis lipoidius diabeticorum, described by Erich Urbach and Maurice Oppenheim, US dermatologists.

Urbanization Migration of people to cities because of employment opportunities, attraction of better living conditions and availability of social services.

Urceiform (*ur-se'i-form*) Pitcher-shaped.

Urea (*u-re'a*) The chief nitrogenous end product of protein metabolism.

Urea breath test Test to determine the amount of urease in *Helicobacter pylori* infection.

Urea clearance Measurement of renal function, which is dependent on glomerular filtration rate and tubular reabsorption.

Urea frost Minute white flaky deposits of urea on the skin of the face in patients with advanced uremia.

Urease (*u're-as*) An enzyme that promotes the breakdown of urea into ammonia and carbon dioxide, first enzyme to be prepared in the crystalline state.

Urecchysis (*u'rek'i-sis*) The extravasation of urine into the tissue.

Uremia (*u-re'me-a*) Accumulation of excess amount of nitrogenous end products of protein metabolism due to renal insufficiency. adj. **uremic**.

Postrenal uremia Conditions preventing urine already formed from being excreted out of the body from obstructions in the urinary tract.

Prerenal uremia Poor renal blood flow resulting in renal failure.

Renal uremia Disorders of kidney with deranged or destroyed parenchyma.

Uremia serositis A syndrome of pericarditis, pleural effusion and sometimes ascites

Uremia syndrome Condition noted when BUN exceeds 100 mg/dL.

Ureter (*u-re'ter*) One of a pair of long slender muscular tubes that convey urine from the pelvis of the kidney to the base of the bladder.

Bifid ureter A congenital renal tract abnormality due to some error or disturbance during development.

Ectopic ureter A congenital renal anomaly seen as a result of abnormal caudal migration of the ureteral bud during its insertion to the urinary bladder.

Lower pole ureter The ureter draining the lower pole of a duplex kidney.

Pipestem ureter A thickened, firm and fixed, aperistaltic ureter that extends from the kidney to bladder in advanced tuberculosis of the urinary tract.

Retroiliac ureter A rare condition where the ureter passes behind the iliac vessels.

Ureteral stenting Threading of thin catheter into segments of the ureter.

Ureterectomy (*u-re'ter-ek'to-me*) Surgical removal of a ureter or a segment of it.

Ureteritis (*u-re'ter-i'tis*) An inflammation of a ureter.

Ureterocele (*u-re'ter-o-sel*) A ballooning at the end of the ureter inside the bladder. It appears as a thin-walled balloon inside the bladder.

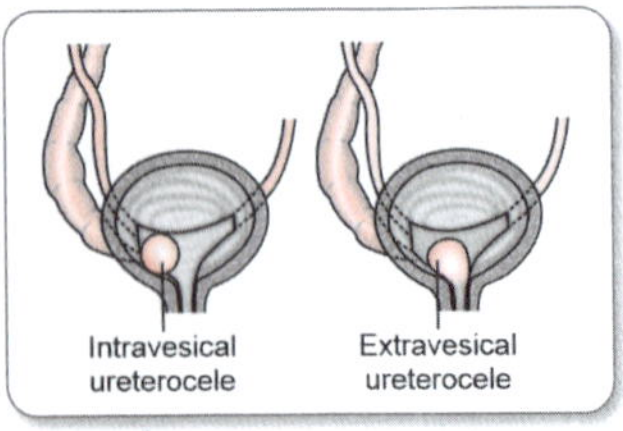

Ureterocele

Extravesical or Ectopic ureterocele Ureterocele that extends into bladder neck or urethra.

Prolapsed ureterocele Represents a dilated intravesicular component of the ureter inserting ectopically just above the bladder neck, commonly seen in girls, presented as bladder outlet obstruction.

Ureterocolostomy (*u-re'ter-o-ko-los'to-me*) Surgical anastomosis of a ureter to the colon.

Ureterohydronephrosis (*u-re'ter-o-hi' dro-ne-fro'sis*) Dilatation of ureter and pelvis of the kidney. This may occur from a mechanical or inflammatory obstruction in the urinary tract.

Ureteroenterostomy (*u-re'ter-o'en'ter-os-to-me*) The surgically created anastomosis between a ureter and the intestine.

Ureterolith (*u-re'ter-o-lith*) A stone in the ureter.

Ureterolithotomy (*u-re'ter'o-li-th-ot'o-me*) Surgical removal of a stone from a ureter.

Ureterolysis (*u-re'ter-ol'i-sis*) Rupture of the ureter; surgical procedure of separating the ureter from adhesions; paralysis of the ureter.

Ureteroneocystostomy (*u-re'ter-o-ne'o-sis-tos'to-me*) Transplantation of a ureter to a different site in the bladder.

Ureteronephrectomy (*u-re'ter-o-nef-rek'to-me*) Excision of a kidney and its ureter.

Ureteroplasty (*u-re'ter-o-plas'te*) Surgical reconstruction of the ureter.

Ureteropyelenephritis A complication of an ascending urinary tract infection that spreads from the bladder to the kidneys.

Ureteroscope (*u-re'ter-o-skop*) Fiberoptic endoscope to visualize the ureter.

Ureteroscopy (*u-reter-o-sko'pe*) Examination of the ureter by ureteroscope.

Ureterosigmoidostomy (*u-re'ter-o-sig-moyd-os-to-me*) Anastomosis of a ureter to the sigmoid colon.

Ureterostomy (*u-re'ter-os'to-me*) Attachment of the divided distal end of a ureter to the skin of the lower abdomen.

Ureterotomy (*u-re'ter-ot'o-me*) Incision of a ureter.

Urethra (*u-re'thra*) A membranous canal for the external discharge of urine from the bladder.

Bulbous urethra The portion of corpus spongiosum that lies between the split corpora cavernosa in the superficial perineal space.

Female urethra Relatively simple tubular structure that has the sole purpose of conducting urine from the bladder to the outside of the body.

Male urethra A dynamic fibromuscular tube which serves as the terminal region of both the male urinary and reproductive systems.

Penile urethra Largest and terminal part of the urethra.

Prostatic urethra The part of the urethra that passes through the prostate. It is about 3–4 cm long.

Spinning top urethra Nonobstructive posterior urethral dilatation seen on voiding cystourethrography, most commonly found in female.

Spongiose urethra The longest part of the male urethra, and present in the corpus spongiosum of the penis.

Urethritis (*u're-thri'tis*) Inflammation of the urethra.

Gonococcal urethritis Infection of urethra by *Neisseria gonorrhoeae* causing dysuria and purulent discharge.

Nongonococcal urethritis NGU, urethritis of nongonococcal origin, milder than gonococcal urethritis.

Urethrocele (*u-re'thro-sel*) Prolapse of the female urethra into the vagina caused by a weakness in the muscles of the front wall of the vagina.

Urethrocystogram (*u-re'thro-sis'to-gram*) A roentgenogram of the urethra and bladder.

Urethrography (*u-re-throg'ra-fe*) The roentgenographic study of the urethra.

Retrograde urethrography A routine radiologic procedure (most typically in males) used to image the integrity of the urethra.

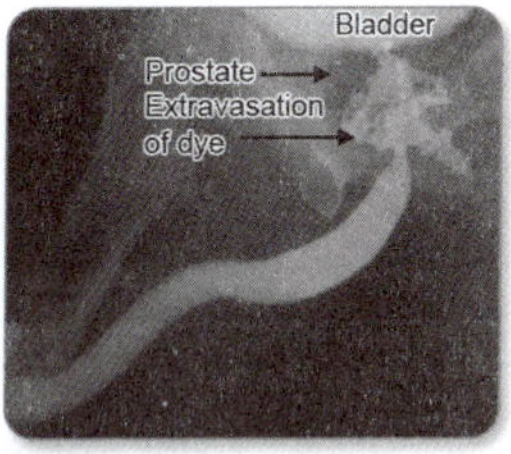

Retrourethrography

Urethropenile (*u-re'thro-pe'nil*) Pertaining to the urethra and the penis.

Urethroplasty (*u-re'thro-plas'te*) Surgical repair of a wound or a defect of the urethra.

Urethrorrhaphy (*ure-thro-r'a-fe*) Suture of the urethra.

Urethrorrhea (*u-re'thro-rea*) An abnormal discharge from the urethra.

Urethroscope (*u-re'thro-skop*) A lighted instrument to examine the interior of the urethra.

Urethrostaxis (*u-re'thro-stak'sis*) Discharge or oozing of blood from the urethra.

Urethrostenosis (*u-re'thro-ste-no'sis*) Stricture of the urethra.

Urethrostomy (*u're-thros'to-me*) Surgical formation of an opening of urethra at the perineal surface.

Urethrotomy (*u-re'throt'o-me*) Incision of a urethral stricture.

Urethrotrigonitis (*u-re"thro-tri"go-ni-tis*) Inflammation of the urethra and trigone of the bladder.

Uric acid (*u'rik*) An acid occurring as an end product of purine metabolism.

Uricosuric drug Drugs that promote the excretion of uric acid; used in patients having gout.

Uridine (*u'ri-den*) A nucleoside from nucleic acid, which on hydrolysis yields uracil and ribose.

Uridrosis The presence of excessive amounts of urea in sweat.

Urinalysis (*u-ri-nal'i-sis*) Physical, chemical and microscopic examination of urine for diagnostic purpose.

Urinary bladder Receptacle for urine excreted by the kidneys.

Urinary tract The structures involved in the formation, storage and excretion of urine-kidneys, ureters, bladder and urethra.

Urination (micturition) (*u'ri-na'shun*) The act of passing urine, micturition.

Urine (*u'rin*) The fluid formed by the kidneys, transported by the ureters, stored in the bladder and eliminated through urethra during micturition. adj. **urinary**.

Chylous urine Milky urine from presence of chyle or fat.

Cloudy urine Urine with cloudy appearance which may be due to presence of phosphates, urates or pus.

Febrile urine Passage of high colored, concentrated urine.

Midstream urine A specimen of urine collected while voiding urine. It eliminates organisms in urethra to a great extent as many of them come out at the beginning or at the end of urinary stream.

Residual urine Urine remaining in the bladder after urination.

Uriniferous tubule Nephrons or kidney tubules.

Urinogenital System consisting of urinary system and genital system.

Urinometer (*u'ri-nome'ter*) An instrument to determine the specific gravity of urine or other fluids; hydrometer. It has calibrations from 1.000 to 1.060 for a temperature of 15°C.

Urobilinogen (*u'ro-bi-lin'o-jen*) Product obtained following reduction of bilirubin. A red color appears when Ehrlich's aldehyde reagent is added to urine.

Urocele (*u'ro-sel*) Distension of the scrotum with extravasated urine.

Urochezia (*u"ro-ke'zhea*) Presence of urine in the feces.

Urodynamics (*u'ro-di-nam'iks*) The dynamics of the propulsion and flow of urine in the urinary tract. adj. **urodynamic**.

Uroflowmeter (*u'ro-flo-me-ter*) Calculates the amount of urine passed, the flow rate in milliliters per second, and the length of time it takes to empty the bladder.

Urofollitropin (*u'ro-fol'i-tro'pin*) A preparation of gonadotropins from the urine of postmenopausal women, it administered by subcutaneous injection.

Urogenital sinus Outpouching of hindgut from which bladder and urethra develop.

Urography (*u-ro-g'ra-fe*) Roentgenography of any portion of the urinary tract.

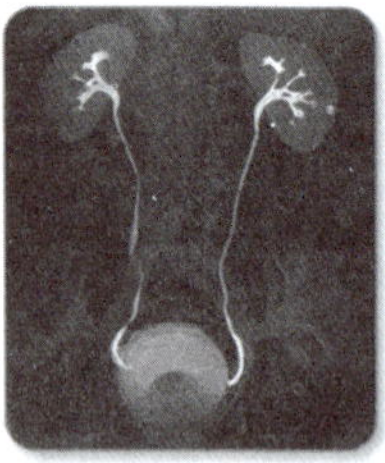

MR urography

Intravenous urography Urography after intravenous injection of an opaque medium which is rapidly excreted in the urine.

Retrograde urography Urography after injection of a contrast medium into the bladder through urethra.

Urogynecology (*u'ro-gi'ne-kol'o-je*) Urogynecology is a surgical subspecialty of urology and gynecology that deals with pelvic floor disorders, originally applied only to the lower female urinary tract but now including a wide range of disorders, such as fecal or urinary incontinence or prolapse of the bladder or uterus.

Urokinase (*u-ro-ki'nas*) A proteolytic enzyme activating the fibrinolytic system by converting the plasminogen to plasmin. It is used as a thrombolytic agent.

Urolith (*u'ro-lith*) A stone in the urinary tract.

Urolithiasis (*u'ro-li-thi'a-sis*) The formation of urinary stone and the resultant disorder.

Urology (*u-rol'o-je*) The branch of medicine concerned with the study of disorders of the urinary tract and of the reproductive system of the male.

Uroporphyrin (*u'ro-por'fi-rin*) Degradation product formed, which is excreted in the urine along coproporphyrin and urine may turn reddish-brown on standing.

Urticaria (hives, nettle rash) (*ur-ti-ka're-a*) Sudden eruption of transitory, itchy wheals of variable size and shape due to a particular food or food additive, a drug and rarely an underlying systemic disease; hives; adj. **urticarial**.

Uterine (*u'ter-in*) Related to the uterus.

Uterine apoplexy A uterus in which myometrial vessels have been stripped of a protective endometrium and are actively bleeding.

Uterine bleeding Bleeding from uterus either physiologically (menstruation) or pathologically (menorrhagia, polymenorrhea). It can occur as a non-menstrual bleeding (metrorrhagia), withdrawal bleeding (following estrogen therapy) or breakthrough bleeding from progestational agents).

Uterine inertia Inability of the uterus to produce sufficiently strong contractions during labor to move the fetus through the birth canal.

Uterine prolapse Descent of the uterus from its normal position.

Uterine souffle A vascular sound audible in a pregnant uterus.

Uterine subinvolution Failure of the uterus to return to normal size after childbirth.

Uterine tube One of the two small fallopian tubes attached to either side of the uterus.

Utero-ovarian (*u'ter-o-o-va're-an*) Pertaining to uterus and ovary.

Uterosalpingography (hysterosalpingography) (*u'ter-o-sal-ping-og'ra-fe*) Radiography of the uterus and fallopian tubes after the introduction of a contrast medium.

Uterus (womb) (*u'ter-us*) A hollow pear-shaped muscular organ of female reproductive system situated in the pelvis which allows the fertilized ovum to implant and provide nourishment to the developing fetus. It consists of a main part (corpus) with an elongated lower part (cervix) with an opening at the end (os). The upper rounded part of the uterus is the fundus at each end of which is the cornua where the uterine tubes join it.

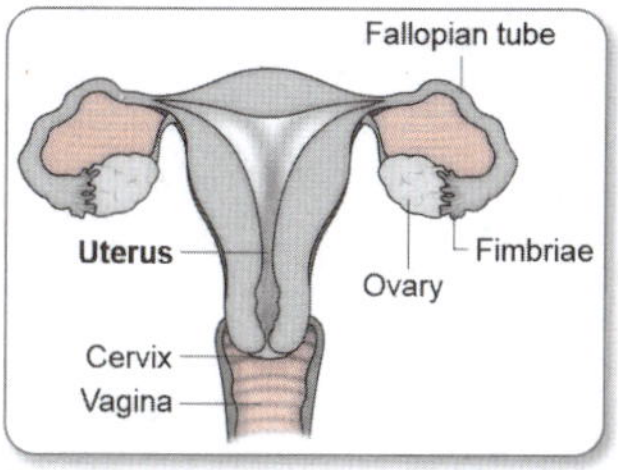

Uterus

Bicornuate uterus Uterus having two lateral horns.

Double uterus Uterus bicorpus.

Gravid uterus The pregnant uterus.

Inversion uterus A turning inside out of the uterus.

Involution uterus Uterus diminishing in its size following delivery.

Parturient uterus Uterine contractions of labor.

Prolapse uterus Downward displacement of uterus which may be of first degree with cervix being within the vaginal orifice; second degree-with-cervix outside the vaginal orifice or third degree-with whole uterus remaining outside the vaginal orifice.

Rudimentary uterus Hypoplastic uterus measuring 1–3 cm in length.

Septate uterus Uterus divided into two cavities by a septum.

Unicornuate uterus A one-horned uterus where one half is developed and the other undeveloped or absent.

Uterus rupture May be spontaneous due to weakening of the uterine wall of previous cesarean section scar or trauma during pregnancy.

Utricle A small bag like structure in the body, especially in the inner ear that helps to control balance.

Uvea (uveal tract) (*uve-a*) Tunica vasculosa bulbi. The pigmented vascular layer of the eye consisting of the choroid, ciliary body and the iris.

Uveal tract Consists of the iris, the ciliary body and the choroid. All of these form a continuous layer within the eye.

Uveitis (*u-ve-i'tis*) Inflammation of the uvea.

Uveoparotitis (Uveoparotid fever) (*u've-o-par-o-ti'tis*) Inflammation of the uvea and the parotid gland.

Uvula (*u'vu-la*) The conical fleshy mass of tissue projecting down from the posterior border of the soft palate.

Bifid uvula Split uvula, part of inferior vermis of cerebellum belonging to Paleocerebellum.

Palatine uvula A soft conic projection from the back edge of the middle of the soft palate, consists of connective tissue, racemose glands and some muscular fibers.

Uvula of bladder A rounded elevation at the bladder neck in males, formed by convergence of muscle fibers terminating in the urethra.

Uvula of cerebellum Cerebellar uvula forms a considerable portion of the inferior vermis; it is separated on either side from the tonsil by the sulcus vallecula indented on its surface by shallow farrows.

Uvula vesicae Elevation on the trigone immediately posterior to the urethral orifice produced by the median lobe of prostate.

Uvulectomy (*u'vu-lek'to-me*) Surgical removal of the uvula.

Uvulitis (*u'vu-li'tis*) Inflammation of the uvula.

Uvulopalatopharyngoplasty (*u"vu-lo-pal"a-to"fe-ring'go-plas"te*) Extensive surgical resection of the soft palate in the oropharynx. The procedure is to increase the size of the airway by removal of the uvula, part of the soft palate and other redundant pharyngeal tissue.

Uvuloptosis (*u'vu-lop-to'sis*) Elongation or relaxation of the palate.

Uvulotome (*u'vu-lo-tom*) An instrument for cutting the uvula.

V

Vaccination (*vak'si-na'shun*) The inoculation of vaccine to produce immunity; immunization.

Vaccine (*vak'sen*) A suspension of live, live-attenuated, killed, complete or incomplete microorganisms or products obtained therefrom which contains antigens, administered to induce active immunity against a specific infectious disease.

Acellular pertussis vaccine A vaccine that protects against whooping cough (pertussis), contain inactivated pertussis toxin (PT) and may contain one or more other bacterial components.

Anthrax vaccine A vaccine that can help prevent anthrax, a serious infection caused by the bacterium *Bacillus anthracis*.

Autogenous vaccine A killed vaccine prepared from antigens (Virus or Bacteria) that is caused of an outbreak and return to use for control and prevention in those farms.

Bacterial vaccine Contains killed or attenuated bacteria that activate the immune system.

BCG vaccine Bacille Calmette-Guérin, protects against tuberculosis, which is also known as TB. Given intradermally into left upper arm (at the insertion of deltoid).

Conjugate vaccine A type of subunit vaccine where antigens are linked to polysaccharides (from the outer coat of microbes) to stimulate immunity.

Diphtheria vaccine A toxoid vaccine against diphtheria, an illness caused by *Corynebacterium diphtheriae* given intramuscularly.

DTap vaccine The booster shot should be given at ages 11–12, and to older teens and adults who have not yet had a booster with pertussis coverage.

Haemophilus B vaccine Conjugate vaccine used to prevent Haemophilus influenzae type b (Hib) infection. Available in combination with the diphtheria/tetanus/pertussis vaccine, and in combination with the hepatitis B vaccine.

Hepatitis B vaccine A vaccine that prevents hepatitis B. The first dose is recommended within 24 hours of birth with either two or three more doses given after that. Given Intramuscularly.

Inactivated vaccine Killed vaccine. Organisms killed by heat or chemicals when injected into the body stimulate active immunity (pertussis, cholera, typhoid, rabies, Salk vaccine).

Live vaccine Vaccines prepared from live-attenuated organisms (BCG, oral polio, measles).

MMR vaccine A vaccine against measles, mumps, and rubella (German measles), abbreviated as MMR. The first dose is generally given to children around 9 months to 15 months of age, with a second dose at 15 months to 6 years of age, with at least four weeks between the doses. Given intramuscularly.

Polio vaccine Vaccines used to prevent poliomyelitis (polio). Two types are used— An inactivated poliovirus given by injection (IPV) and a weakened poliovirus given by mouth (OPV), Given orally.

Rabies vaccine A vaccine used to prevent rabies. Given IM.

Sabin vaccine Live polio vaccine.

Salk vaccine Killed polio vaccine administered parenterally.

Vaccine lymph Material obtained from cowpox.

Vaccinia (*vak-sin'e-a*) Cowpox.

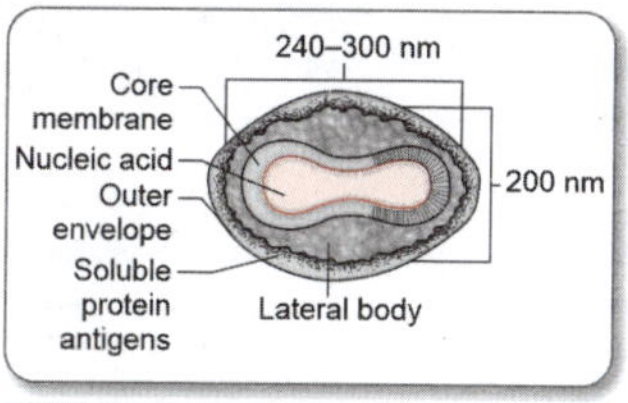

Vaccinia virus

Fetal vaccinia A known, but extremely rare, complication that can occur after smallpox vaccine is given in pregnancy.

Generalized vaccinia A rare, self-limiting complication of the smallpox vaccination that is caused by the systemic spread of the virus from the inoculation site.

Progressive vaccinia A rare cutaneous condition caused by the vaccinia virus, characterized by painless but progressive necrosis and ulceration.

Vacuole (*vak'u-ol*) Small cavity formed within the protoplasm of a cell.

Contractile vacuole A subcellular structure (organelle) involved in osmoregulation. It is found predominantly in protists and in unicellular algae. It was previously known as pulsatile or pulsating vacuole.

Food vacuole Also known as digestive vacuole a membrane-enclosed sac, which has a digestive function, presented in unicellular protozoans such as amoeba, plasmodium, etc.

Vacuum (*vak'u-um*) A space devoid of air.

Vacuum aspiration A method of removal of fetus and placenta using a suction device and can be carried out in early pregnancy up to 14th week.

Vacuum sign A normal radiologic finding noted when traction is applied to a joint causing coalescence of gas within a joint. It disappears in effusion.

VAD A ventricular assist device (VAD) is an electromechanical device for assisting cardiac circulation, pumps blood from ventricles to other parts of body.

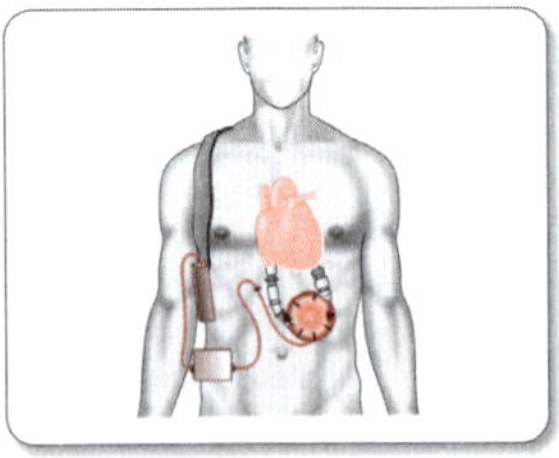

Ventricular assist device

Vagina (*va-ji'na*) A muscular canal, in the female extending from the vulva to the uterine cervix; a sheath.

Vagina bulbi Sheath of eyeball—connective tissue that forms the capsule enclosing the posterior part of the eyeball, extending anteriorly to the conjunctival fornix, and continuous with the muscular fascia of the eye.

Vaginismus (*vaj'in-iz'mus*) An involuntary spasm and tightening of the opening of the vagina and perineal muscles preventing intercourse.

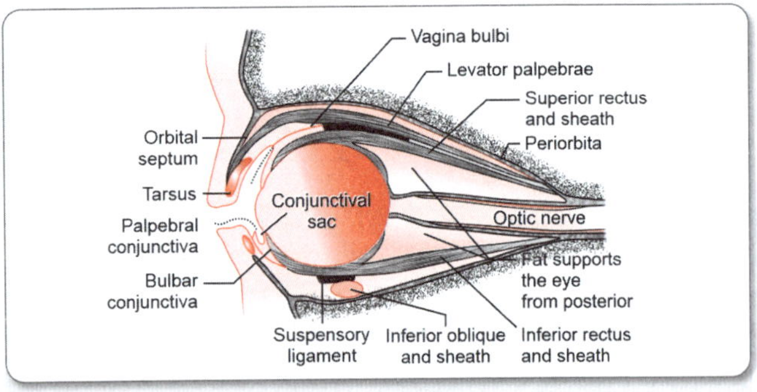

Sagittal section through the eyeball showing vagina bulbi

Vaginitis (*vaj-in-i'tis*) Inflammation of the vagina and it can be caused by infection, allergic reaction or estrogen deficiency.

Vaginodynia (*vaj'i-no-din'e-a*) Pain in Vagina.

Vaginoplasty (colpoplasty) (*vaj'i-no-plas'te*) Plastic surgery of the vagina; called also colpoplasty.

Vaginoperineorrhaphy (*vaj'i-no-per'i-ne-or'ah-fe*) Suture repair of the vagina and perineum.

Vaginopexy (*vaj'i-no-pek'se*) Colpopexy.

Vaginoscope (*vaj'in-o-skop*) A vaginal speculum.

Vaginotomy (*vaj'i-not'o-me*) Colpotomy.

Vagotomy (*va-got'o-me*) Interruption of the impulses transmitted by vagus nerve by its surgical division.

Vagovagal Controls contraction of the gastrointestinal muscle layers in response to distension of the tract by food.

Vagus nerve Either of the tenth crania nerves that regulate various functions such as swallowing, talking, heart rate and digestion. This mixed cranial nerve takes its origin in an elongated nucleus in the floor of the fourth ventricle and emerges along the internal aspect of the medulla and leave the skull through the jugular foramen along with 9th and 11th cranial nerves. It carries sensation from the pharynx, larynx, esophagus, heart, respiratory passages, and abdominal viscera. The motor fibers innervate the muscles of the soft palate, pharynx, and larynx.

Valgus (*val'gus*) Bent outward.

Validity (*va-lid'i-te*) *stat* Extent to which figure derived from the test actually measures intended object in statistics.

Valine (*val'en*) An essential amino acid.

Vallum (*val'um*) A wall.

Vallecula (*val-lek'u-la*) A depression or furrow on any surface.

Valsalva's maneuver (*val-salvaz*)Increase of intrathoracic pressure by forcible exhalation effort against closed glottis, named after Italian anatomist, Antonio Valsalva.

Valsartan (*val-sahr'tan*) Angiotensin II receptor antagonist having similar effects to ACE inhibitors. It does not influence bradykinin metabolism and does not cause cough.

Valve (*valv*) A membranous fold in a canal or passage to allow flow in one direction and to retard or to prevent regurgitation of the contents passing through it.

Valvotomy (valvulotomy) (*val-vot'o-me*) A surgical procedure of opening or slitting of a narrowed heart valve.

Valvula (*val'vu-la*) A small valve.

Valvula venosa Venous valve; any of the small cusps or folds found in the tunica intima of many veins, serving to prevent backflow of blood.

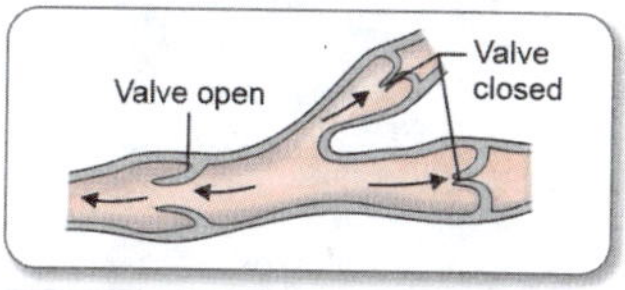

Venous valves

Valvulitis Inflammation of a valve especially of the heart.

Vancomycin Glycopeptide bactericidal antibiotic and is indicated in serious infections such as endocarditis or septicemia.

Van den Bergh reaction Test to distinguish unconjugated from conjugated bilirubin, named after Dutch physician, Van den Bergh.

Vaquez-osler disease Polycythemia rubra vera named after Louis Vaquez, French physician.

Varicella (*var'i-sel'a*) Chickenpox.

Varices (*var'i-sez*) Plural of varix.

Varicocele (*var'i-ko-sel'*) Abnormal dilation and enlargement of the scrotal venous pampiniform plexus which drains blood from each testicle and is accompanied by a constant pulling, dragging, or dull pain in the scrotum. Since the presence of excess blood in the scrotum increases temperature, the condition is thought to be linked to male factor infertility.

Varicocelectomy (*var'i-ko-se-lek'to-me*) Ligation and excision of the enlarged veins of a varicocele. Varicose condition of the veins of the spermatic cord surrounding a testicle in the scrotum giving a sensation like a bag of worms.

Varicography (*var'i-kog'ra-fe*) Roentgennologic visualization of varicose veins following injection of a radiopaque medium.

Varicose veins Enlarged and twisted veins just below the skin, usually in the legs.

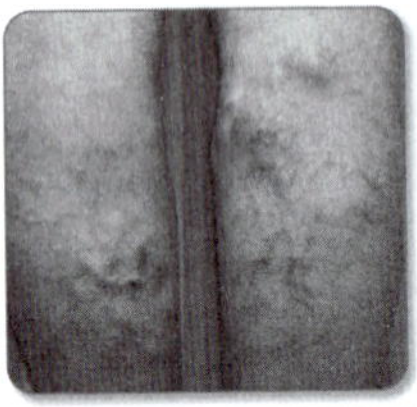

Varicose veins

Varicotomy (*var'i-kot'o-me*) Incision into a varix or a varicose vein.

Variola (*va-ri'o-la*) Smallpox.

Variola caprina Goatpox.

Variola hemorrha'gica Hemorrhagic smallpox.

Variola major The classic severe form of smallpox.

Variola minor A mild form of smallpox that was found only in certain parts of South America and Africa.

Variola ovina Sheep-pox.

Varioloid (*va-ri'o-loid'*) Resembling smallpox; called also varioliform.

Varix (*va'riks*) An enlarged and tortuous vein, artery or lymphatic vessel.

Varus (*va'rus*) Bent inward; bending with outward convexity.

Vas (*vas*) Any canal to carry a fluid. pl. **vasa.**

Vasa vasorum The small nutrient arteries and the veins in the walls of the larger blood vessels.

Vascular (*vas'ku-lar*) Relating to blood vessels.

Vascular headache A headache caused by spasm of blood vessels in the brain and scalp.

Vascular sling A congenital malformation in which the left pulmonary artery arises from the right pulmonary artery, crossing to the left between the trachea and esophagus forming a sling around the trachea. It is associated with tracheal stenosis with stridor, wheeze and choking.

Vascularization (*vas'ku-lar-i-za'shun*) Formation of new blood vessels.

Vascular system Circulatory system that includes vessels that carry blood and lymph through the body.

Vasculitis (*vas'ku-li'tis*) Inflammation of blood vessels, leading to end-organ or tissue damage.

Large vessel vasculitis Temporal arteritis, pulseless disease.

Medium size vasculitis Polyarteritis nodosa, Kawasaki disease.

Small vessel vasculitis Microscopic polyangiitis, Wegener's granulomatosis, Churg-Strauss syndrome, Leukocytoclastic vasculitis, Henoch-Schonlein purpura and essential mixed cryoglobulinemia.

Vas deferens One of a pair of narrow elongated tubes of 47 cm length that store and carry sperms from the testicles to ejaculatory duct which empties into the prostatic urethra.

Vasectomy (*vas-ek'to-me*) Surgical interruption of the vas deferens by excision of a portion of it to prevent sperm reaching the urethra; a male sterilizing procedure following which the man is capable of ejaculation normally but semen is devoid of sperms.

Vaso- Relation to a vessel or to a duct.

Vasoactive (*vas'o-ak'tiv*) Exerting influence upon the caliber of blood vessels.

Vasoactive intestinal polypeptide (VIP) A neuropeptide present in the nerve fibers of smooth muscle, blood vessels and in the glands of the upper respiratory tract. It stimulates adenylate cyclase causing potent vasodilation, pancreatic and intestinal secretion, inhibition of gastric acid secretion, increased cardiac output, glycogenolysis, bronchodilation and inhibition of macromolecule release from mucous glands.

Vasoactive substances A group of circulating substances that regulate vascular tone causing either vasodilation (atrial natriuretic peptide, kinins and VIP) or vasoconstriction (angiotensin II, adrenaline and noradrenaline and vasopressin).

Vasoconstriction (*vaso-kon-strik'shun*) The diminution of the caliber of blood vessels.

Vasoconstrictor (*vas'o-kon-strik'tor*) An agent causing constriction of the blood vessels.

Vasodilation (*vas'o-di-la'shun*) An increase in diameter of blood vessels especially arteries.

Vasodilator (*vas'o-di-la'tor*) An agent causing dilatation or relaxation of the blood vessels.

Vasoepididymostomy (*vas'o-ep'i-did-i-mos'to-me*) Surgical procedures designed to bypass an obstruction in the male genital tract or by which vasectomies are reversed.

Vasoligation (*vas'o-li-ga'shun*) Ligation of the ductus (vas) deferens.

Vasomotor (*vas'o-mo'tor*) An agent regulating the diameter of the blood vessels.

Vasomotor rhinitis Rhinorrhea, and sneezing without any evidence of infection or allergy.

Vasomotor center A portion of the medulla oblongata. Together with the cardiovascular center and respiratory center, it regulates blood pressure.

Vasomotor nerve The nerve of the autonomic nervous system that controls the diameter of blood vessels.

Vasopressin (antidiuretic hormone, ADH) (*vas'o-pres'in*) Also known as antidiuretic hormone (ADH) or arginine vasopressin (AVP) a hormone synthesized from the AVP gene as a peptide prohormone in neurons in the hypothalamus, and is converted to AVP. It acts to promote the retention of water by kidney and increases blood pressure.

Vasopressor (*vas'o-pres'or*) An agent causing contraction of the muscular tissue of the capillaries and arteries and raising the blood pressure.

Vasospasm (*vas'o-spazm*) Spasm of the blood vessels causing a decrease in their caliber.

Vasotomy (*va-sot'o-me*) Incision into or cutting of the ductus deferens (vas deferens); also known as vasopuncture and vasostomy.

Vasovagal (*vas'o-va'gal*) Relating to the action of vagus nerve on the blood vessels.

Vasovagal attacks A sudden slowing of the heart causing temporary loss of consciousness; fainting.

Vasovasostomy (*vas'o-va-sos'to-me*) Surgical reanastomosis of vasa deferentia in a vasectomized person.

Vasovesiculitis Inflammation of seminal vesicles and vas deferens.

Vastus (*vas'tus*) Vast, great, extensive.

VATS Video-assisted thoracic surgery.

VBAC Vaginal birth after cesarean.

VC Vital capacity.

VCG Vector cardiogram.

VD Venereal disease.

VDH Valvular disease of the heart.

VDRL Venereal disease research laboratories.

Vector (*vek'tor*) An invertebrate animal acting as a carrier transmitting an infective agent from one host to another; *mol* a cloning vehicle such as plasmid, phage, cosmid, yeast, artificial chromosome into which DNA to be cloned can be inserted.

Vector competence The ability to acquire, maintain and transmit an infectious agent.

Vectorcardiography (*vek'tor-kar'de-o-gra-fe*) A method to determine the direction and magnitude of electromotive forces of the heart as represented by vector loops.

Vegetation (*vej-e-ta'shun*) A morbid growth; variably sized excrescences found on the heart valves.

Bacterial vegetation Friable necrotic lesions on the valves.

Lupus erythematous vegetation Lesions consisting mucoid substance, fibrinoid degeneration and collagenous fibrosis on tricuspid and mitral valve.

Nonbacterial thrombotic vegetation Small foci of organizing thrombi along the line of the valve leaflet's closure or on either side of the ventricle.

Verrucous vegetation Small irregular fibrinous excrescences usually occurring along the line of closure of the cardiac valve cusps, sometimes extending into the mural endocardium or chordae tendineae, and rarely also present on the left ventricular papillary muscles.

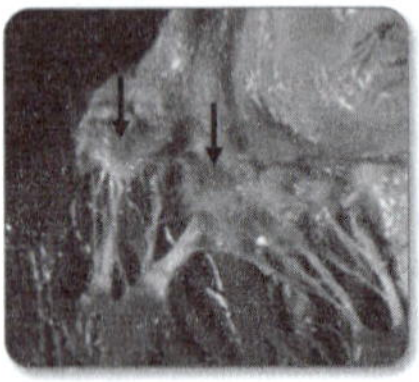

Verrucous vegetations (arrows) along the line of closure of the mitral valve leaflet in acute rheumatic mitral valvulitis superimposed on chronic rheumatic heart disease

Vegetative (*veje-ta'tiv*) To exist in an inactive and passive way devoid of mental activities.

Vehicle (*ve'hi-kel*) A substance having no therapeutic action used as a medium for active remedies *mol* a self-replicating DNA molecule such as virus, plasmid or phage that serves as a vector for insertion of a segment of DNA into a host.

Vein (*van*) One of the systems of branching vessels carrying deoxygenated blood from various parts of the body to the heart (*see* **Table**).

Velamen (velamentum) (*ve-la'man*) A membrane, velum, meninx, or tegument.

Vellus (*vel'us*) Fine body hair which appears after fall of the lanugo hair and present before puberty.

Velum (*ve'lum*) A covering.

Vena (*ve'na*) A vein. pl. **venae.**

Vena cava Either of two large veins that drain deoxygenated blood from the body into the right atrium of the heart.

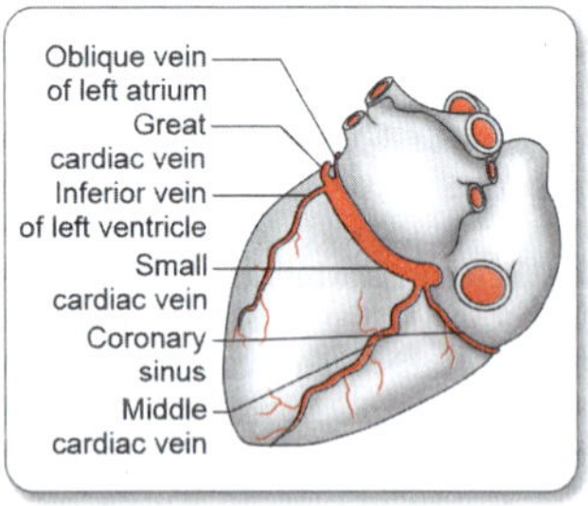

Middle and great cardiac veins in a posterior view

Venacavogram (*ve-na-kavo-gram*) The film obtained by venacavography.

Veneer (*ve-ner*) A thin surface laid over a base of common material; *dent* a layer of tooth-colored material such as porcelain or composite resin attached to and covering the surface of a natural tooth or a metal crown.

Venereal disease (VD) Any sexually transmitted disease which includes syphilis, gonorrhea, AIDS, nonspecific urethritis, chlamydiosis and chancroid.

Venereology (*ve-nerè-olò-je*) The branch of medicine dealing with the study and treatment of venereal disease.

Venesection (*venè-sek'shun*) Phlebotomy.

Venipuncture (venipuncture) (*ven'i-punk'chur*) Puncture of a vein with a needle to withdraw blood or to inject fluid or drugs.

Venisuture (*ven'-su'chur*) Phleborrhaphy.

Veno- Pertaining to or of veins.

Venoclysis (*ve'nok'li-sis*) Intravenous infusion.

Venogram (*ve'no-gram*) Phlebogram.

Venography (phlebography) (*ve-nog'ra-fe*) A diagnostic imaging procedure to examine veins following injection of a contrast medium.

Table: Veins

Axillary vein	Present in axilla accompanying axillary artery. Continues as subclavian vein at the outer border of the 1st rib.
Azygos vein	On the right side in front of vertebra, begins as lumbar azygos vein ends into superior vena cava.
Basilic vein	Begins on the ulnar side on the dorsum of hand, ascends, joins cubital veins, becomes deep in the upper arm, and continues as axillary vein.
Basivertebral vein	Emerges from foramina on posterior surface of vertebral bodies, communicates with external vertebral plexus, opens into anterior internal vertebral plexus.
Brachiocephalic vein	Two large trunks at the root of the neck formed by union of internal jugular and subclavian vein. They unite to form superior vena cava.
Cardiac vein (great)	Begins at the apex of the heart, lies in anterior interventricular groove, enters the beginning of coronary sinus.
Cardiac vein (middle)	Begins at the apex of the heart, lies in posterior interventricular groove and ends in the coronary sinus near its termination.
Cardiac vein (small)	Runs in the coronary sulcus posteriorly, opens into the end of coronary sinus, drains back of right atrium and ventricle.
Cephalic veins	Begins from the dorsal venous network on radial side of hands, ascends on the forearm, gives median cubital vein, ends in the axillary vein just below the clavicle.
Cerebellar vein (inferior)	Placed on the inferior surface of cerebellum, includes median and lateral vessels, drains into straight sinus, sigmoid sinus, or petrosal sinuses.
Cerebral vein (anterior)	Small vein accompanying anterior cerebral artery. Joins to form basal vein which ends into great cerebral vein.
Cerebral vein (great)	Formed by union of internal cerebral veins, opens into straight sinus.
Cerebral vein (inferior)	Drains inferior surface of cerebral hemispheres. Communicate with superior sagittal, cavernous, superior petrosal and transverse sinus through superior, basal, and middle cerebral veins.
Cerebral vein (internal)	Right and left vein, drains internal deep parts at cerebral hemispheres unite to form great cerebral vein.
Cerebral vein (middle, deep)	Runs in the floor of lateral cerebral sulcus, drain insula and neighboring gyri, joins basal vein.
Cerebral vein (middle, superficial)	Begins on the lateral surface of hemisphere, ends in the cavernous sinus.

Contd...

Cerebral vein (superior)	8–12 in number, drains superolateral and medial surfaces of hemisphere, open into superior sagittal sinus against the current of blood in it.
Cubital vein (median)	Present in front of elbow region. Communicates with cephalic vein and deep veins. Joins basilic vein.
Cystic vein	Runs between gallbladder and liver, vary considerably, drains gallbladder and cystic duct, joins hepatic veins.
Diploic vein	Occupy diploe of the cranial bones, develops after 2 years of age. They are devoid of valves and communicate with meningeal veins and sinuses of dura mater frontal, temporal, parietal, and occipital bones.
Dorsal vein of penis (deep)	Drains glans penis and corpora cavernosa, enters prostatic plexus, communicates with internal pudendal veins.
Dorsal vein of penis (superficial)	Drains prepuce and skin of the penis, ends in external pudendal vein .
Emissary vein	Passes through openings in skull bones. Communicates scalp veins with cranial venous sinuses, e.g., mastoid, parietal and condylar.
Facial vein	Formed by union of supraorbital and supratrochlear vein, ends in internal jugular vein. It has no valves and communicates with cavernous sinus through ophthalmic and pterygoid venous plexus.
Femoral vein	Begins as continuation of popliteal vein, receives many tributaries, communicates with great saphenous vein, becomes external iliac vein at the margin of inguinal ligament.
Hemiazygos vein	Starts on the left in front of vertebral column, ends in azygos vein, communicates with left renal vein drains lower intercostal spaces.
Hemiazygos vein accessory	Ascends in front of thoracic vertebra on the left, drains 4–6 intercostal spaces, joins azygos vein.
Hepatic vein	Commence in the liver as intralobular veins, opens into sublobular veins, which unite to form hepatic veins, ends into inferior vena cava.
Iliac vein (common)	Result from the union of external and internal iliac veins lies in front of sacroiliac joint. Veins of two sides unite to form inferior vena cava.
Iliac vein (external)	Upward continuation of femoral vein, begins behind inguinal ligament, joins internal iliac vein to form common iliac vein.
Iliac vein (internal)	Formed by confluence of the veins, draining pelvis corresponding to the branches of the internal iliac artery. Joins external iliac vein to form common iliac vein.

Contd...

Intercostal vein (posterior)	Eleven on each side run with branches of posterior intercostal arteries, first intercostal ends in brachiocephalic vein. Other veins open into azygos vein.
Intervertebral vein	Drains veins from spinal cord, communicates with vertebral venous plexus, ends in vertebral, intercostal, lumbar, and sacral veins.
Jugular vein (anterior)	Starts at the level of hyoid bone, communicates with internal jugular vein, ends into external jugular vein.
Jugular vein (external)	Drains mostly scalp and face, formed by union of retro-mandibular vein and posterior auricular vein, ends into subclavian vein.
Jugular vein (internal)	Collects blood from brain, face, and neck. Begins at the jugular foramen as continuation of sigmoid sinus. It joins subclavian vein to form brachiocephalic vein.
Meningeal vein (middle)	Communicates with superior sagittal sinus, diploic veins and middle cerebral veins, drains meninges, ends in cavernous sinus or pterygoid venous plexus.
Paraumbilical vein	Establishes anastomosis between the veins of anterior abdominal wall and portal vein, runs along *ligamentum teres*, ends in left branch of portal vein.
Popliteal vein	Formed by union of tibial veins, runs in popliteal fossa, becomes femoral vein.
Portal vein	Formed by union of superior mesenteric and splenic vein at the level of second lumbar vertebra, enters *porta hepatis*, divides into right and left branch to enter substance of liver.
Pulmonary vein	Commences in the capillary network in the walls of alveoli of lungs, joining together, ultimately two veins emerge from each lung, opens separately in the upper posterior part of the left atrium.
Rectal vein (inferior)	Formed by external rectal venous plexus in the lower part, drains into internal pudendal vein.
Rectal vein (middle)	Begins in the rectal venous plexus, receives tributaries from bladder, prostate, seminal vesicle, ends in internal iliac vein.
Rectal vein (superior)	Starts from the rectal venous plexus, continues as inferior mesenteric vein.
Retromandibular vein	Descends in the parotid glands, divides into anterior and posterior branches. Anterior branch joins posterior auricular to form external jugular vein.
Saphenous vein (great)	Longest in the body, begins on the medial margin of foot, ends in femoral vein, has 10–15 valves, and communicates with deep veins of the leg.

Contd...

Saphenous vein small	Begins as continuation of lateral marginal vein of foot ends in popliteal vein, has 10–12 valves and communicates with deep veins of leg and great saphenous vein.
Splenic vein	Starts from union of splenic tributaries, ends behind the neck of the pancreas by uniting with superior mesenteric vein to form portal vein .
Subclavian vein	Continuation of axillary vein, unites with the internal jugular to form the brachiocephalic vein.
Testicular vein	Formed by tributaries of veins of epididymis, emerge at the back of testis, ascends as pampiniform plexus, coalesce into two veins, becomes single vein which opens into inferior vena cava (right) and left renal vein (left).
Thyroid vein (middle)	Drains lower part of thyroid gland, larynx and trachea joins internal jugular vein.
Thyroid vein (superior)	Formed by superficial tributaries, drains thyroid gland, ends by joining internal jugular or facial vein.
Vena cava (inferior)	Formed by junction of two common iliac veins, in front of lumbar 5th vertebra, ascends, perforates the diaphragm, passing through pericardium, opens in the lower part of right atrium.
Vena cava (superior)	Collects blood from upper half of body, formed by junction of right and left brachiocephalic veins, opens in the upper part of right atrium.

Venom (*ven'om*) A poison which certain snakes or insects secrete and introduce into the victims by biting or stinging.

Venoscan Study for deep vein thrombosis by injection of technetium-labelled fibrinogen.

Venosclerosis (*ve-no-skle-ro'sis*) Phlebosclerosis.?

Ventilation (*ven'ti-la'shun*) Process of exchange of gas between the lungs and ambient air; replacement of vitiated air by a supply of fresh outdoor air, and control of the quality of incoming air with regard to its temperature, provide an environment that is comfortable and free from risk of infection.

Alveolar ventilation Ventilation of alveoli where gas exchange takes place.

Controlled mandatory ventilation CMV, it is done by intermittent positive pressure ventilation through an endotracheal tube.

Dead space ventilation Ventilation occurring in alveoli which are not perfused with blood and ventilation becomes ineffective.

Intermittent mandatory ventilation IMV, used for weaning the patients from controlled ventilation. It maintains respiratory muscle function and prevents asynchronous breathing.

Intermittent positive-pressure ventilation IPPV, it assists in delivery of bronchodilator aerosols and humidification of the bronchial passages.

Mechanical ventilation Artificial ventilation from exhaust, fans and air conditioning; the partial or complete replacement of a patient's own respiratory muscle function by external mechanical support to improve gas exchange and reduce the work of breathing.

Natural ventilation Simple system of ventilating small houses, school and offices.

Noninvasive intermittent positive pressure ventilation NIPPV, provides pressure support of 25 cm H_2O at the onset of inspiration which ceases at the onset of expiration. It may be applied *via* a face or nasal mask.

Noninvasive negative pressure ventilation NINPV, it operates by producing negative pressures within an internal tank or iron lung that increases all or part of the thorax. It has been replaced by NIPPV.

Pressure support ventilation PSV, breaths initiated by the patient are assisted by a preset positive pressure supplement. It may help weaning from CMV or SIMV.

Synchronized intermittent mandatory ventilation SIMV, the ventilator is programmed to deliver a predetermined number of mechanical breaths of specified tidal volume after a suitable pause in the patient's spontaneous ventilatory efforts. It may help weaning from CMV.

Ventilation scan An image produced by radionuclide scanning of the lungs following inhalation of a radioactive gas.

Ventilation-perfusion imaging Useful in the detection of pulmonary thromboemboli, which appear as 'filling defect'. ^{131}Xe gas is inhaled in ventilation scan and 99 m Tc-labelled macroaggregates of albumin microspheres are injected intravenously, the particles becoming transiently trapped in pulmonary micro vessels providing the 'perfusion' scan.

Ventilation-perfusion ratio Measure of efficiency of gas transfer in the lung. Perfusion defect is indicated by a ratio above 1; and a ratio below 1 indicates ventilation defect.

Ventilator A machine that takes over the breathing of a person who is unable to breath on his or her own.

Ventouse A cup shaped device used to help in delivery by putting it over the baby's head and using suction to pull the baby out of the mother's body.

Ventral (*ven'tral*) Toward the belly surface.

Ventral hernia A hernia through the abdominal wall especially in the epigastrium.

Ventricle (*ven'trik-l*) A small cavity referring to either of the two lower thick-walled chambers on each side of the heart or one of a series of intercommunicating cavities of the brain filled with cerebrospinal fluid.

Ventriculo-caval shunt Communication through a tube from lateral ventricle *via* jugular vein to superior vena cava in hydrocephalus.

Ventricular folds False vocal cord is one of mucous membrane, each enclosing a narrow bond of fibrous tissue the vestibular ligament, which is attached to the angle of the thyoid cartilage immediately below the attachment of epiglottis.

Ventriculitis (*ven-trik-u-li'tis*) Inflammation of a ventricle.

Ventriculoatriostomy Surgical estabishment of a shunt to drain CSF from the ventricle of the brain to the right atrium.

Ventriculogram (*ven-trik'u-lo-gram*) A roentgenogram of the cerebral ventricle following injection of air or gas as a contrast medium.

Ventriculography (*ven-trik'u-lo'gra-fe*) Roentgenography of the cerebral ventricle or ventricle of the heart following injection of a contrast medium.

Ventriculoscopy (*ven-trik"u-los'ko-pe*) A minimal invasive procedure for examination of the cerebral ventricles by means of an endoscope or cystoscope.

Ventriculostomy (*ven-trik'u-los'to-me*) The formation of a drain for cerebrospinal fluid from the ventricles of the brain.

Ventriculotomy (*ven-trik'u-lot'o-me*) Incision of a ventricle of the brain or heart.

Vermiform (*ver'mi-form*) Resembling a worm in shape.

Vertex (*ver'teks*) A summit or top; the highest point; the crown of the head.

Vesicoureteric reflux Backward flow during the process of micturition, of urine from urinary bladder to ureter which results in recurrent ascending urinary infection.

Vestibulo-ocular (*ves-tib'u-lo-ok'u-lar*) Belonging to the vestibular and oculomotor nerves; to the maintenance of visual stability during head movements.

Videoendoscopy (*vid'e-o-en'do-skop'e*) A flexible endoscope whose tip is equipped with a video camera that transmits a signal that is converted to an image on a color monitor.

Videofluoroscopy (*vid'e-o-floo'r"os'ko-pe*) A radiographic technique in which an image displayed on an intensifying screen is scanned by a television camera and displayed on a television monitor.

Vinblastine (*vin-blas'ten*) A chemotherapeutic alkaloid that interferes with the microtubules of the mitotic spindle causing the lysis of rapidly dividing cells. Used in the treatment of Hodgkin's disease, leukemia and other lymphoproliferative disorders.

Vincristine (*vin-kris'ten*) A chemotherapeutic alkaloid that interrupts the mitotic spindles causing lysis of proliferating cells. Used to treat leukemia and other malignancies.

Vinculum (*ving'ku-lum*) A term used in anatomy to denote a band or bandlike structure.

Vindesine A plant alkaloid that inhibits cell division by binding to tubulin and disrupting the mitotic spindle.

Viomycin (*vi-o-mi'sin*) Aminoglycoside antibiotic having relatively weak antituberculosis activity. Poorly absorbed from gastrointestinal tract; administered intramuscularly. It is ototoxic and nephrotoxic.

VIP (vasoactive intestinal peptide) Vasoactive intestinal polypeptide, found throughout the gut. It inhibits gastric secretion but increases pancreatic and intestinal secretions, increases cardiac output, glycogenolysis and bronchodilation.

Vipoma An endocrine tumor in the gut or pancreas producing vasoactive intestinal polypeptide.

Viral pneumonia Acute infection of the lung caused by any one of a number of viruses such as entero viruses, influenza A and B.

Virchow's sign Enlargement of left supraclavicular lymph nodes in gastric carcinoma.

Viremia (*vi-re'me-a*) The presence of viruses in the blood.

Virilism (*vir'il-izm*) Development or possession of male secondary sex characters in a female or prepubertal male; a female disorder in which there is development of secondary male sexual characteristics.

Virilization (*vir'i-li-za'shun*) The development of male secondary sex characters in female due to overproduction of androgens. The features include hirsutism, temporal balding, deepened voice, acne, enlarged clitoris.

Virology (*vi-rol'o-je*) A branch of microbiology concerned with viruses and viral diseases.

Virulence (*vir'u-lens*) The relative ability of a microorganism to cause disease by overcoming body defenses; being extremely poisonous.

Virus (*vi'rus*) Any of a group of ultramicroscopic infectious agents that reproduce only in living cells. They contain either RNA or DNA, but not both. The virus genome is enclosed in a protein shell and in some cases by a lipid envelope. They are intracellular diverting host cell's metabolites to its own reproduction. Glycoproteins on the virus surface recognize specific cellular receptors which determine the cells that virus infects and hence the type of disease produced; a program designed to damage a computer system.

Visceral arch Also known as pharyngeal arch; these are pieces of cartilages or bones that support the pharyngeal region of vertebrates and also help attach the jaws with the skull.

Visceral cleft Any of a series of paired openings leading from the pharynx to the ectoderm on each side of the neck area in a chordata embryo.

Visceral pouch Structure seen in the embryonic development of vertebrates between pharyngeal arches.

Viscero Organs of body especially larger organs within serous cavities of the trunk.

Viscus (*vis'kas*) An internal organ of the body especially—one (such as the heart, liver, or intestine) located in the great cavity of the trunk proper.

Visual acuity Sharpness of vision.

Visual field Field of vision.

Visual purple A red or purple pigment in the retina of various vertebrates including human beings that is sensitive to dim light and functions in right vision.

Visuoauditory (*vizh'oo-o-aw'di-tor'e*) Relating to simultaneous stimulation of, the senses of both hearing and sight.

Vital capacity Maximum volume of air that can be exhaled or inhaled following a maximum expiratory or inspiratory effort respectively.

Vital center Any of collections of nerve cells in the brain that acts as governing centre for different vital body functions.

Vitallium (*vi-tal'e-um*) An alloy of 65% cobalt, 30% chromium, 5% molybdenum, and other substances; used in dentistry and artificial joints, because of its resistance to corrosion. Also used for components of turbochargers because of its thermal resistance.

Vital staining (intravital staining) Staining of living cells or tissues by injecting a stain.

Vital statistics Statistics concerned to human life or the conditions affecting human life and maintenance of population.

Vitamin (*vi'ta-minz*) A group of organic substances present in foods essential in small quantities for normal functioning of the body (*see* **Tables**).

Vitellus (*vi-tel'us*) Yolk.

Vitiligo (leukoderma) (*vit-il-i'go*) Depigmented macule of variable size and shape in the skin or any part of the body including the mucous membranes of the lips and genitalia. There is no other change in the skin and it is due to lack of melanin formation by the melanocytes.

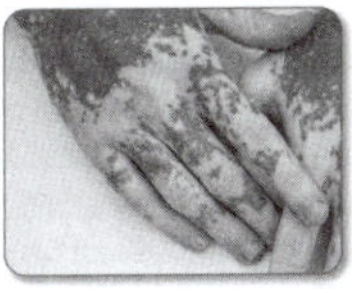

Vitiligo

Vitrectomy (*vi-trek'to-me*) Removal of vitreous.

Vitreous humor (vitreous body) The transparent, gelatinous substance filling the posterior chamber of the eye.

Viviparous (*viv-ip'ar-us*) Bearing living young.

Vivisection (*viv'i-sek'shun*) The performance of surgical procedures upon living animals for the experimental purpose.

VLDL Very low-density lipoprotein. It transports triglycerides to tissues to be used as energy or stored as fat. High level in the blood is associated with ischemic heart disease.

Vocal cord dysfunction syndrome VCDS Throat tightness and loss of voice from incomplete adduction of the vocal cord. The attacks are rapid to develop and to dissolve.

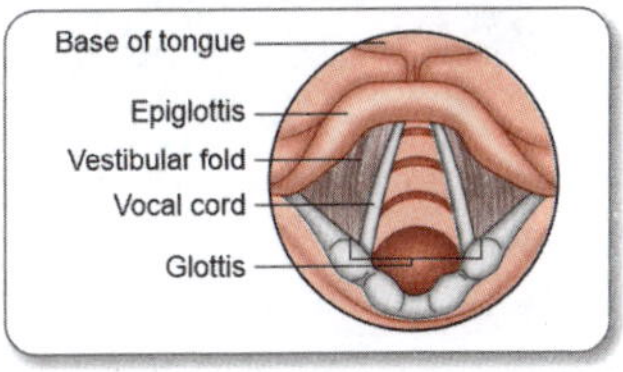

Vocal cord

VOD Veno-occlusive disease.

Vocal fremitus A vibration transmitted through the body.

Vocal resonance An assessment of the density of lung tissues performed by auscultating the chest and asking the patient to speak.

Von Hippel-Lindau disease (*hip'el-lin'dow*) Hemangioblastoma of the cerebellum associated with angioma of the retina and cysts of the pancreas and kidneys. There may be polycythemia, named after Eugen von Hippel, German ophthalmologist and Arvid Lindau, Swedish pathologist.

Von Willebrand disease A congenital bleeding disorder due to the deficiency of factor VIII presenting with bleeding tendency at an early age usually as epistaxis and easy bruising. There is prolonged bleeding time, named after Erik von Willebrand, Finnish physician.

Volar (*vo'lar*) Pertaining to flexor surface.

Volsella (*vol-sel'ah*) Vulsella.

Volt SI unit of electric potential

Voluntary admission Admission with the consent of the person diagnosed with signs of mental illness into a health facility or mental health.

Voluntary hospital A private nonprofit hospital that is operated under individual.

Voluntary muscle A muscle that you choose to move, such as in the arms and legs.

Volvulus (*vol'vu-lus*) Twisting or knotting.

Volvulus of intestine Twisting of a loop intestine that causes intestinal obstruction.

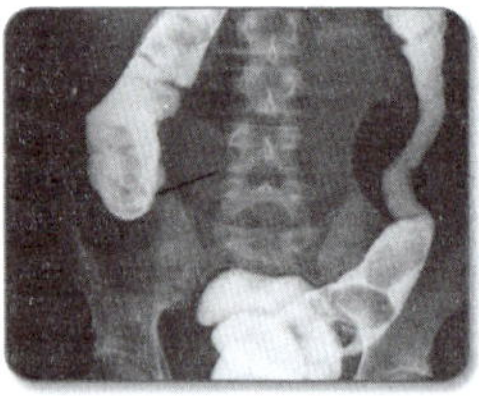

Transverse colon volvulus

Vomer (*vo'mer*) The unpaired flat bone of the nasal septum.

Vomit (*vom'it*) To eject contents of the stomach through the mouth.

Bilious vomit Has a green or bright yellow color, indicating larger amounts of bile in the stomach.

Black vomit Dark-colored vomit due to oxidation.

Coffee-ground vomit Like coffee grounds, occur due to the presence of coagulated blood in the vomit.

Vomiting (*vom'it-ing*) Expulsion of the contents of the stomach through the mouth.

Anticipatory vomiting Conditioned, learned, or psychological nausea and vomiting.

Bilious vomiting Dark green color vomiting due to obstruction at the level of or distal to the ampulla of Vater in the descending duodenum.

Delayed vomiting Occurs 24 hours after chemotherapy and may last up to 5 days.

Fecal vomiting An unusual symptom associated with gastrocolic fistulas, coprophagy and violent reverse peristalsis.

Functional vomiting Frequent episodes of recurrent vomiting that is not self-induced nor medication induced, and occurs in the absence of eating disorders, major psychiatric diseases, abnormalities in the gut or central nervous system, or metabolic diseases that can explain the symptom.

Obstructive vomiting Vomiting due to intestinal vomiting.

Pernicious vomiting A complication of pregnancy that affects various areas of the woman's health, including homeostasis, electrolytes, and kidney function, and may also have adverse fetal consequences.

Psychological vomiting Refers to persistent or recurrent vomiting in the absence of any obvious organic cause and resulting from a psychological mechanism.

Table: Vitamins and their actions, daily requirement and effects

Name	Alternative name	Action	Daily requirement	Effects of deficiency	Effects from excess intake
Fat soluble					
Vitamin A	Retinol	Night vision, epithelial function, antioxidant	1 mg	Night blindness, xerophthalmia, perifollicular hyperkeratosis	Raised intracranial pressure, liver damage, skin changes
Vitamin D	Vitamin D_2 Vitamin D_3	Calcium. Metabolism	3 mcg	Rickets, osteomalacia	hypercalcemia
Vitamin E	Tocopherols	Red cell function, antioxidant	10 mg	Mild hemolytic neuropathy in children	
Vitamin K		Synthesis of clotting factors (II, VII, IX, X)	100 mcg	Bleeding	
Water soluble					
Thiamine	Vitamin B_1	Carbohydrate metabolism	1 mg	Beri-beri, peripheral neuropathy, Wernicke-Korsakoff syndrome	
Riboflavin	Vitamin B_2	Cellular oxidation	1.5 mg	Angular stomatitis, cheilosis	
Niacin	Nicotinic acid, nicotinamide	Cellular oxidation	15–20 mg	Pellagra	Flushing
Vitamin B_6	Pyridoxine	Transamination decarboxylation	3 mg	Peripheral neuropathy	

Contd...

Name	Alternative name	Action	Daily requirement	Effects of deficiency	Effects from excess intake
Folate	Folic acid	Hemopoiesis	200 mcg	Megaloblastic anemia	
Vitamin B_{12}	Cobalamin	Hemopoiesis	3 mcg	Megaloblastic anemia, subacute combined degeneration of the spinal cord	
Vitamin C	Ascorbic acid	Collagen synthesis; antioxidant	30–60 mg	Scurvy, impaired healing, bleeding into tissues and joints	Raised urinary oxalate and urate

Table: Sources of different vitamins

Fat soluble vitamins	Sources	Water soluble vitamins	Sources
A	Animal foods—liver, fish, egg yolk, milk, ghee, cheese, butter and as carotene in dark green leafy vegetables, carrot, pumpkin, papaya, mangoes, red palm oil	Thiamine	Cereals, sprouting green leafy vegetables, liver, pork, legumes
		Riboflavin	Liver, meat, eggs, kidney, milk and other dairy products, green leafy vegetables, sprouted cereals and pulses
D	Exposure to ultraviolet radiation of sun light, milk, butter, cheese, egg yolk, fish liver oils	Niacin	Liver, pulses, whole cereals, fish, meat, milk, eggs, groundnut, coffee
E	All vegetable oils, wheatgerm, egg yolk, butter, peas	Pyridoxine	Yeast, liver, meat, whole grain cereals, groundnuts, banana, legumes
K	Green leafy vegetables, liver, pulses, also synthesized by colonic bacteria	Folic acid	Yeast, liver, nuts, green vegetables, chocolate
		Vitamin B_{12}	Meat, liver, egg, dairy products, yeast
		Vitamin C	Fresh fruits, green leafy vegetables, germinating pulses

Von Hippel-Lindau disease (*hipel-lindow*) Hemangioblastoma of the cerebellum associated with angioma of the retina and cysts of the pancreas and kidneys. There may be polycythemia, named after Eugen von Hippel, German ophthalmologist and Arvid Lindau, Swedish pathologist.

Von Recklinghausen's disease (*rek'ling-how'zenz*) Generalized neurofibromatosis, a hereditary disorder characterized by multiple nodules all over the body and it may be associated with 'café au lait' spots; primary hyperparathyroidism exhibiting osteitis fibrosa cystica, named after Friedrich von Recklinghausen, German pathologist.

Voyeurism (*voi'yer-izm*) Sexual gratification derived from looking at sexual objects or acts.

Vulsella (volsella) (*vul-sel'a*) A forceps with claw-like hooks at the end of each blade.

Vulva (*vul'va*) External visible part of female genitalia consisting of the clitoris and the labia, vestibule of the vagina and the opening of the urethra and of the vagina; pudendum.

Vulvectomy (*val-vek'to-me*) Excision of the vulva.

Vulvitis (*vul-vi'tis*) Inflammation of the vulva, caused by infection, allergic reaction and ageing.

Atrophic vulvitis An inflammatory condition associated with low estrogen levels.

Diabetic vulvitis Vulvitis due to diabetes.

Erosive vulvitis The presence of erosive changes in the vulva, vagina, or both areas constitutes a major diagnostic and therapeutic challenge for clinicians.

Leukoplakic vulvitis Characterized by a pink-red vulva with overlying gray-white keratin and involved labium majus, nympholabial furrow, preputium clitoridis, and commissura labiorum posterior.

Ulcerative vulvitis Ulcerative inflammatory condition of vulva.

Vulvovaginitis *(vul'vo-vaji-ni'tis)* Inflammation of the vulva and vagina by an infection.

W

W Chemical symbol for the element tungsten; a unit of hardness of X-rays.

Waardenburg's syndrome (*vah-denbergz*) A genetic disorder characterized by wide-bridge of nose, frontal white blaze of hair, growing together of the two eyebrows, white eyelashes, lateral displacement of the inner canthi, cutaneous hypopigmentation and deafness, described by Petrus Waardenburg, Dutch ophthalmologist.

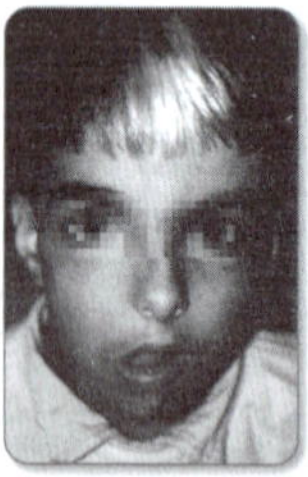

Waardenburg's syndrome

Waldeyer's ring Lymphoid tissue formed by the lingual, pharyngeal and faucial tonsils arranged in the form of a ring at the level of the nasopharynx and oropharynx.

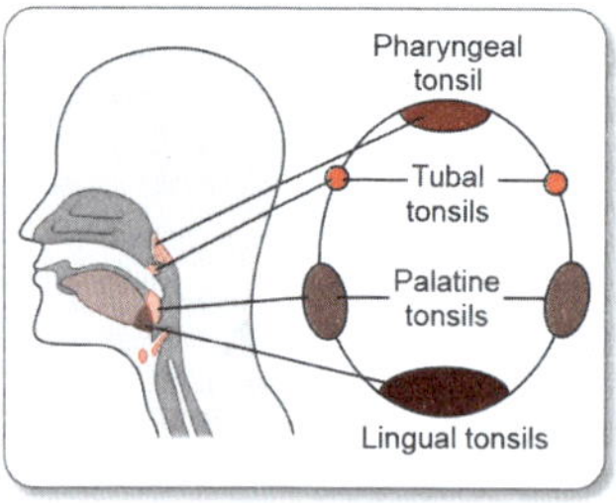

Waldeyer's ring of lymphoid tissues

Warfarin An oral anticoagulant commonly used to treat and prevent clots.

WAGR syndrome Acronym for Wilms tumor, aniridia, genitourinary anomalies and mental retardation syndrome.

Walter Reed staging A system for clinical staging of AIDS.

Wandering (*wahn'der-ing*) Moving about; not fined.

Wandering abscess Abscess appearing on a site distant from its origin.

Wandering pacemaker Dual rhythm wherein both SA and AV nodes discharge spontaneously with variable asynchronicity.

Wart (*wort*) A circumscribed cutaneous elevation due to hypertrophy of the papillae and hyperplasia of all layers of the epidermis.

Genital wart A wart of the genitalia caused by human papilloma virus (HPV).

Periungual warts Dry looking bumps around fingers or toe nails resembling cauliflower.

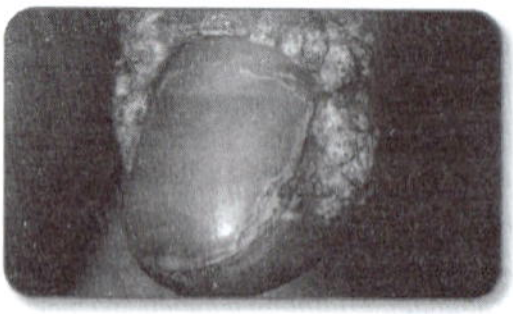

Periungual wart

Plane wart Smooth, round, polygonal, flat or slightly raised lesion noted on the face and dorsum of the hands.

Plantar wart Small shiny rounded flat painful lesion beneath pressure points.

Seborrheic wart Benign epidermal tumor showing raised and stuck-on appearance, unrelated to sebaceous glands.

Water wart Molluscum contagiosa, shiny white, hemispherical lesions with an umbilicated look.

Warren incision An incision following the thoracomammary fold, permitting access to any part of the breast.

Warren shunt Anastomosis of the splenic end of the divided splenic vein to the left renal vein.

Warthin's tumor Adenolymphoma of parotid gland that contains both epithelial and lymphoid tissues which produce a slowly growing painless swelling in the lower part of parotid gland.

Wasserman reaction (*wos'er-man*) A complement fixation test to diagnose syphilis, named after August Wasserman, a German bacteriologist. It is used to detect the presence of the bacterium Treponema pallidum.

Water bed A rubber mattress partially filled with warm water.

Water brash The mixing of saliva and gastric acids that have risen to the throat; heartburn.

Waters' projection Occipitomental or parietocanthial projection is an angled PA radiograph of the skull with the patient gazing slightly upwards.

Watt (*wot*) A unit of electric power, being the work done at the rate of 1 joule per second, named after James Watt, a Scottish engineer.

Waterhouse-Friderichsen syndrome (*wah'ter-hous frid'er-iksen*) Fatal vasomotor collapse and shock in meningococcal infection due to hemorrhage into the adrenal gland, named after Rupert Waterhouse, an English physician and Carl Friderichsen, a Danish physician.

Water-lily sign Rupture of hydatid cyst giving a radiological shadow of an air and water-filled cavity with a floating membrane.

Weal Mark on the skin made by a blow of stick or whip.

Weber-Christian disease Relapsing febrile non-suppurative nodules in subcutaneous tissue with central depression, noted in a generalized disorder of fat metabolism, named after Frederick Weber, English physician and Henry Christian, American physician.

Weber's syndrome Ipsilateral oculomotor paralysis and contralateral paralysis of the face, arm and leg due to a damage to pyramidal tract in the brainstem.

Weber's test Test performed by placing the stem of vibrating tuning fork on the head in the midline and asking the patient whether the tune is heard in both the ears or better in one ear than in the other. In unilateral conduction deafness, the tune is appreciated in the affected ear and in unilateral nerve deafness the tune is appreciated in unaffected ear, named after Friedrich Weber, a German otologist.

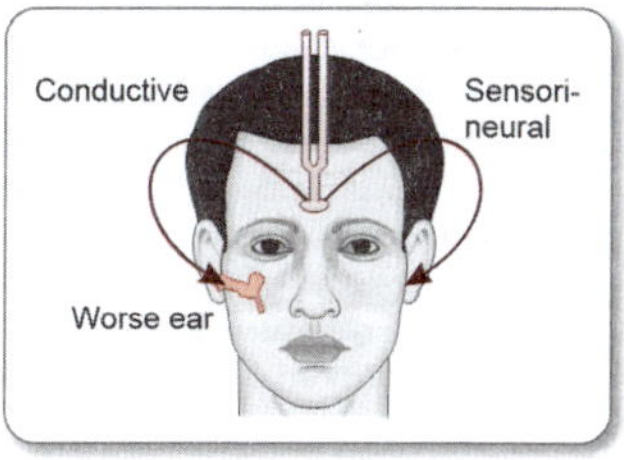

Weber's test

Wechsler scales Most widely used intelligence scales, applied to assess intellectual abilities, and cognitive understanding.

Wegener's granulomatosis (*veg'nerz*) A triad of necrotizing angiitis and aseptic necrosis of the upper respiratory tract and paranasal sinuses, granulomatous pulmonary vasculitis, and a nonspecific segmental necrotizing glomerulonephritis, named after Friedrich Wegener, a German pathologist. The level of antineutrophil cytoplasmic autoantibodies reflects the activity of the disease and is treated with immunosuppressive agents.

Weil-felix reaction Serological test to diagnose rickettsial disease.

Weil's disease Leptospirosis caused by leptospira interrogans with heptocellular involvement.

Welch's bacillus (*welsh'ez*) *Clostridium perfringens*, the causative organism of gas gangrene, named after William Welch, American pathologist.

Wen Sebaceous cyst of the scalp; epidermal cyst.

Wernicke's disease (*ver'ni-kez*) Hemorrhagic polioencephalitis.

Wernicke's encephalopathy Cerebral form of thiamine deficiency often presenting acutely, usually in an alcoholic where the patient is confused and shows ophthalmoplegia.

Wertheim's hysterectomy A radial operation done for cervical cancer in which uterus, the upper vagina, broad ligaments and parametrium are removed along with regional lymph nodes.

Wharton'a jelly Substance of the umbilical cord consisting of a special form of embryonic connective tissue consisting of small stellate cells with long processes, which anastomose with each other, the meshes of which are filled with a gelatinous material.

Wheal (weal) Urticarial lesion presenting on the skin as a smooth, slightly elevated area which is redder or paler than the surrounding skin accompanied by itching. Example: Multiple wheal.

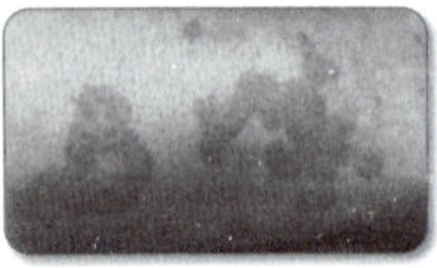

Multiple wheals

Wheal and flare reaction A rapid response to a skin allergy characterized by the development of a red itchy spot in the area where the allergen is injected.

Wheeze (*hwez*) A continuous high pitched whistling sound heard in patients with generalized airways obstruction; rhonchi.

WHIM syndrome An autosomal dominant disorder characterized by warts, hypogammaglobulinemia, infections and myelokanthexis.

Whiplash injury (*hwip'lash*) An injury to the spine at the junction of the fourth and fifth cervical vertebrae occurring from a rapid acceleration or deceleration of the body where upper four cervical vertebrae act as the lash a lower three-act as the handle of the whip. Such injuries are common in rear-end auto collisions, and sometimes in football players.

Whipple's disease (*hwip'elz*) Intestinal lipodystrophy, named after George Whipple, American pathologist. It presents with malabsorption, weight, loss, enlarged lymph nodes, fever, pigmentation, anemia and joint pains.

Whipple's procedure Radical pancreatoduodenectomy, named after Allen Whipple, an American surgeon.

Whipple's operation An operation to treat tumors and other conditions in the pancreas, small intestine and bile ducts.

Whipworm (*hwip'wurm*) A roundworm *Trichuris trichiura* often parasitic in human intestines. The adult worms are found in the large intestine with their anterior ends deeply embedded in the mucosa and measure 30–50 mm in length. Female worm produces 5000 eggs each day. The eggs appear like grenades.

White blood cell Leukocytes; white cells.

White leg Phlegmasia alba dolens occurs during puerperium from deep vein thrombosis.

White matter Nervous system composed of white medullated nerve fibers.

Whitlow (felon) (*wit'lo*) An inflammation of deeper tissues of a finger or toe especially of the terminal phalanx usually terminating in suppuration.

Herpetic whitlow Cutaneous herpes simplex on the terminal segment of a finger, forms deep coalescing vesicles with tissue destruction, also known as herpetic paronychia.

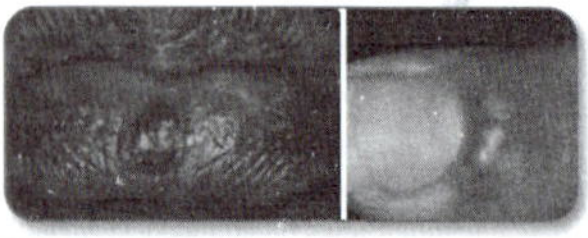

Herpetic whitlow

Melanotic whitlow Subungual melanoma.

Thecal whitlow Suppurative tenosynovitis of the terminal phalanx of a finger.

Whoop (*hoop*) The sonorous and compulsive inspiration of whooping cough.

Whooping cough (*hoop'ing kawf*) Infection from *Bordetella pertussis* characterized by catarrh of respiratory tract and paroxysms of cough ending with a whooping inspiration.

Wilms tumor (*vilmz*) Nephroblastoma, named after Marx Wilms, the German surgeon, it occurs in children of ages 1–7 years of age, arises from the entrapped embryonic nephrogenic tissue and presents with enlargement of kidney. There can be pain, fever and hypertension. Kidney is of enormous size, soft in consistency and the shape is lost.

Windpipe (*wind'pip*) Trachea.

Wisdom tooth (*wiz'dom*) Last molar tooth on either side of jaw usually erupting between 18 and 25 years.

Wiskott-Aldrich syndrome (*wis'kot-awl'drich*) A sex-linked recessive disorder with a defect in both T and B cell function. It is characterized by eczema, thrombocytopenia with bleeding tendency, and infections.

Witch milk Galactorrhea in newborn.

Witzel's operation (*vit'selz*) Gastrostomy, named after Friedrich Witzel, a German surgeon.

Withdrawal Stopping of administration of a drug especially a narcotic or an alcohol to which the individual has become addict either physiologically or pathologically.

Withdrawal behavior The physical or psychological removal of oneself from a stressor.

Withdrawal bleeding Occurrence of vaginal bleeding following discontinuation of hormonal medication, noted at the end of each cycle of oral contraceptive pill.

Withdrawal method A contraceptive technique where male withdraws his penis before occurrence of ejaculation.

Withdrawal syndrome Physical and psychological disturbances expressed by a narcotic addict when deprived of the required drug dosage.

Wolffian body (*wool'fean*) Mesonephros, described by Kaspar Wolff, a German anatomist.

Wolffian duct Mesonephric duct in the embryo extending from the mesonephros to the cloaca.

Wolman's disease An inherited metabolic disorder in which infants show hepatosplenomegaly, adrenal calcification and foam cells in the bone marrow, named after Moshe Wolman, an Israeli physician.

Womb (*woom*) Uterus which protects and nourishes the fetus.

Womb-leasing Surrogate motherhood.

Womb stone Calcified hydatidiform mole or fibroid.

Wood's light (*woodz*) Long wavelength ultraviolet light used in the diagnosis of fungal infections of the scalp, named after Robert Wood, an American physicist.

Woodworker's lung Extrinsic allergic alveolitis developing from inhalation of oak, cedar and mahogany wood dust.

Word blindness Infarction in the distribution of posterior cerebral artery, tumor or hemorrhage resulting in an inability to comprehend written words; visual aphasia; alexia.

Wormian bone (*wur'me-an*) Small, irregular bones in the course of the cranial sutures, described by Olaus Worm, a Danish anatomist.

Wound (*wund*) Injury caused by physical means wherein there is disruption of the normal continuity of structures.

Lacerated wound A torn wound with ragged edges.

Nonpenetrating wound Wound in which surface of the skin remains intact.

Open wound Contusion in which skin is broken.

Penetrating wound Wound in which the causative weapon or bullet entered the body and emerged.

Puncture wound Wound by a sharp pointed instrument.

Wound irrigation The rinsing of a wound by a medicated solution, water or antibiotic liquid preparation.

Wound repair Restoration of the normal structure following an injury.

W-plasty Plastic surgery to repair straight scars requiring the redistribution of tension.

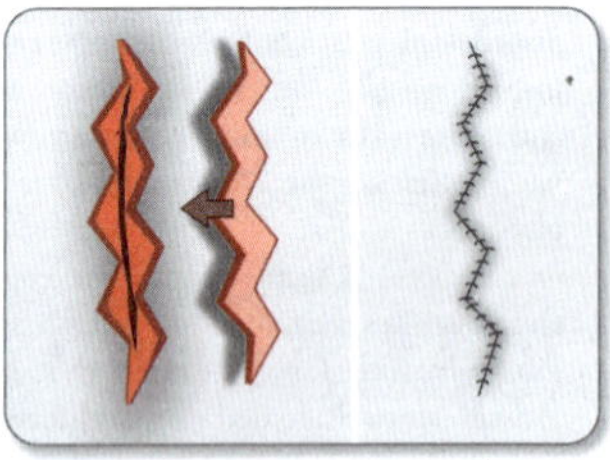

W-plasty

Wrist (*rist*) region of the articulation between the forearm and hands; carpus.

Wrist band An identifying label attached to a patient's wrist at the time of admission to a hospital.

Wrist drop (rist'drop) Paralysis of the extensors of the hand and fingers from radial nerve lesions due to injury, compression or lead palsy; drop hand.

Wry neck (ri'*neck*) Torticollis; a contracted state of one or more muscles of the neck resulting in a characteristic attitude of the head. There is lateral inclination of the head toward the shoulder on the affected side.

Wuchereria *(vu'ker-e're-a)* Filarial nematodes, named after Otto Wocherer, a German physician.

Wuchereria bancrofti White thread-like nematode which causes lymphangitic filariasis.

Wuchereria malayi Brugia malayi.

X

Xanthelasma (*zan-thah-laz'ma*) Subcutaneous cholesterol deposits at the inner margins of the eyelids, that are most common in normocholesterolemic elderly or hypercholesterolemia younger subjects.

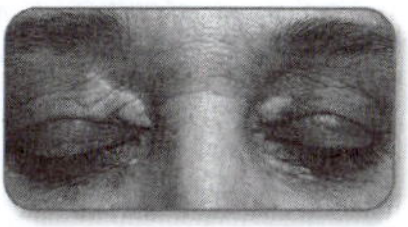

Xanthelasma showing cutaneous cholesterol deposits

Xanthemia (*zan-the'mi-a*) Presence of yellow coloring matter in the blood; carotenemia.

Xanthine (*zan'thin*) Sympathomimetic agent affecting cyclic 3', 5' AMP system of the bronchial smooth muscle and cause bronchodilatation; a purine base found in body tissues and fluids; oxidation product of guanine and hypoxanthine.

Xanthine oxidase An enzyme facilitating breakdown of purines.

Xanthinuria (*zan'thin-ur'i-a*) Excretion of large amounts of xanthine in the urine; a hereditary disorder of purine metabolism due to a deficiency of the enzyme, xanthine oxidase, causing excess elimination of xanthine in urine, and may be associated with xanthine stones in the urinary tract; xanthuria.

Xanthochromia (*zan'tho-kro'mi-a*) An yellowish discoloration, as of the skin or cerebrospinal fluid.

Xanthoma (*zan-tho'-ma*) Xanthomata, raised yellow papule, nodule or plaque-like lesions in the skin on tendons from deposition of lipid-laden histiocytes found in hypercholesterolemia, hypertriglyceridemia, lipoprotein lipase deficiency or b lipoproteinemia.

Eruptive xanthoma Wax yellow lesions especially over extensors of the elbows and knees, and on the back and buttocks, in patients exhibiting severe hyperlipidemia.

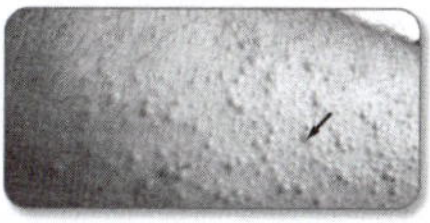

Eruptive xanthoma

Xanthoma disseminatum Presence of xanthoma throughout the body especially on the face, in the tendon sheaths and mucous membranes.

Xanthoma palpebrarum Small yellow-gray plaques around the eyes.

Xanthoma planum Yellowish macules or plaques.

Xanthoma tendinosum Subcutaneous nodules on the dorsal aspect of fingers and the Achilles tendon.

Xanthoma tuberosum Nodules over the elbows and knees.

Xanthomatosis (*zan'tho-ma-to'sis*) An accumulation of an excess of lipids in the internal organs due to an altered metabolism of lipids with hypercholesterolemia; X-disseminatum or multiplex.

Cerebrotendinous xanthomatosis A lipid storage disease characterized by infantile-onset diarrhea, childhood-onset cataract, adolescent to young adult-onset tendon xanthomas, and adult-onset progressive neurologic dysfunction (dementia, psychiatric disturbances, pyramidal and/or cerebellar signs, dystonia, atypical parkinsonism, peripheral neuropathy, and seizures).

Hypercholesterolemic xanthomatosis A condition in which hypercholesterolemia and xanthomas occur in the setting of hepatic cholestasis.

Primary familial xanthomatosis An autosomal dominant disorder that causes severe elevations in total cholesterol and low-density lipoprotein cholesterol.

Wolman xanthomatosis A lethal rare autosomal recessive disorder defined by the deficiency of acid lipase enzyme.

Xanthomatosis bulbi A metabolic disorder characterized by excessive accumulation of lipids in the body and a resulting spread of xanthomas.

Xanthophyll (*zan'tho-fil*) A yellow pigment derived from carotene.

Xanthopsia (*zan-thop'si-a*) Abnormal vision in which all objects appear yellow.

Xanthuria (*zan-thu're-a*) Excretion of excess of xanthine in the urine; xanthinuria.

X-chromosome A chromosome that determines female sex characteristics. In the normal female, there are two X chromosomes, and in the male one X chromosome and one Y chromosome.

X-disease Aflatoxicosis occurring after consumption of groundnuts contaminated by *Aspergillus flavus* that produce aflatoxin.

XDR-TB Extensively drug-resistant tuberculosis; MDR-TB that is also resistant to any fluoroquinolone, and to at least one of three injectable second-line antituberculosis drugs (capreomycin, kanamycin, amikacin).

Xenodiagnosis (*zen'o-dia'g-no'-sis*) A biologic diagnosis of some diseases caused by insects, ticks or vectors by feeding uninfected vectors on patient and later examining them for infection.

Xenogeneic (*zen'o-jen-e'ik*) Xenogenic; tissues from individuals of different species utilized in transplantation.

Xenograft (*zen'o-graft*) A graft of tissue transplanted between animals of different species, that are closely (concordant) or distantly (discordant) related; heterograft.

Xenophobia (*zen'o-fo'bi-a*) An irrational fear of strangers, and strange customs.

Xenopsylla (*zen'op-sil'a*) A genus of fleas, common example being *Xenopsylla cheopis* the rat flea, which carries plague bacillus from rodents to man.

Xeroderma (*zer'o-der'ma*) Dry, rough discolored skin.

Xeroderma pigmentosum An autosomal recessive disorder presenting with photodermatosis. There is defective repair of the damaged DNA induced by sunlight due to an enzymatic deficiency.

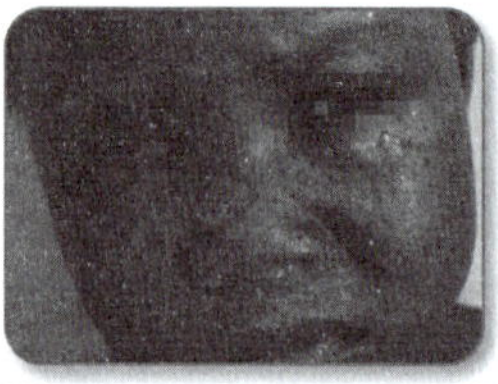

Xeroderma pigmentosum

Xerogram (*zir'o-gram*) Image produced by xerography.

Xerography (*zerog'ra-fe*) A method of radiography to obtain image on paper; xeroradiography.

Xerophthalmia (*zer'of-thal'me-a*) Abnormal dryness of conjunctiva and cornea due to keratinization from vitamin A deficiency and it may also occur in Sjogren's syndrome; xeroma.

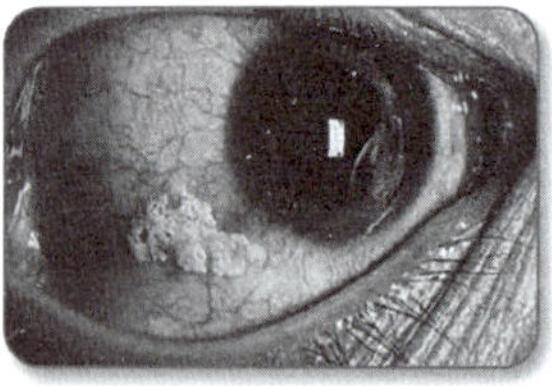

Bitot's spot in xerophthalmia

Xerosis (*ze-ro'sis*) Dryness of the conjunctiva, cornea, skin or mucous membranes.

Xerosis conjunctivae A dry, thickened and pigmented bulbar conjunctiva.

Xerosis corneae A dull, hazy and lusterless cornea.

Xerosis cutis Refers to dry skin, and is a common condition which results in skin roughness, tightness, flaking, and scaling.

Xerosis superficialis Dry skin of superficial skin.

Xerostomia (*zer'o-sto'me-a*) Dryness of oropharyngeal mucosa due to decreased or arrested salivary secretion, and is characteristic of Sjogren's syndrome and it may also occur in HIV-1 and *Candida* infection, malignancy and systemic sclerosis.

X-knife system A high-tech radiation treatment for brain tumors and the knife performs a method of zapping brain tumors with highly focused, high-dose beams of radiation generated by a linear accelerator.

Xiphisternum (*zif'i-ster'num*) Xiphoid process, lowest part of the three segments of the sternum. adj. **xiphisternal**.

Xiphoid process (Xiphoid cartilage) The lowest portion of the sternum; a sword-shaped cartilaginous process to which no ribs are attached.

X-linkage Sex linkage; disorders determined by mutant genes carried on the X chromosomes.

X-rays (*eks' rae*) Roentgen ray named after discoverer, Wilhelm Rontgen German physicist; electromagnetic radiation similar to light but of shorter wavelength and capable of penetrating solids; a radiogram made by X-rays.

X-ray film A radiograph made by projecting X-rays through organs or structures of the body onto a photographic film.

X-ray fluoroscopy Real-time imaging using an X-ray source that projects through the patient onto a fluorescent screen or image intensifier.

X-ray pelvimetry A radiographic examination used to determine the dimensions of the bony pelvis of a pregnant woman.

Xylene (dimethy lbenzene) (*zi'len*) Dimethylbenzene. Useful as a solvent in microscopy; aromatic hydrocarbon, which is depressant of central nervous system.

Xylometazoline (*zi'lo-met'a-zo'len*) An adrenergic agent used topically as a vasoconstrictor to reduce swelling and congestion of the nasal mucosa.

Xylose (*zi'los*) An aldopentose, wood sugar, used to test intestinal absorptive capacity.

48, XXXX syndrome Rare disorder of sex chromosomes characterized by menstrual irregularity, infertility and mental retardation.

47, XXY syndrome Klinefelter's syndrome.

48, XXXY syndrome Sex chromosome abnormality characterized by multiple X chromosomes accompanied by one Y chromosome, with mental and growth retardation and testicular atrophy.

Y

Y cartilage Most elastic cartilage consisting of elastic fibers in a flexible fibrous matrix. It is yellow and found in the external ear, auditory tube, epiglottis and the larynx.

Yawning (*yawn'ing*) Taking deep inspiration with mouth wide open.

Yaws (pian, frambesia) (*yawz*) A chronic, epidemic, nonvenereal infectious and tropical disease caused by *Treponema pertenue* which spreads by direct contact usually in children (Usually under 15 years), and is characterized by an initial granulomatous lesion usually in the lower limb which converts into painless papule and then grows into papilloma (Mother Yaw) which ultimately gets crusted leaving behind a scar.

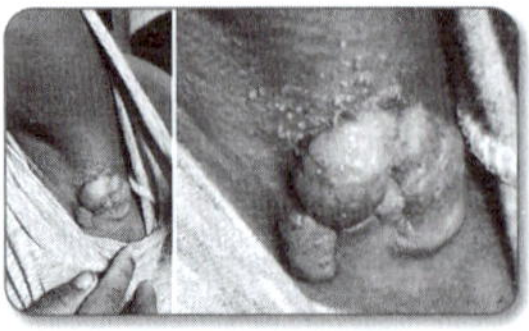

Secondary lesions of yaws in a child

Crab yaws Yaws characterized by hyperkeratosis with fissuring and ulceration of the soles.

Forest yaws Pian bois.

Y chromosome A sex chromosome carrying genes which produce male characteristics in human.

Yeast (*yest*) Single celled rounded fungus of the family Saccharomycetaceae, that multiplies by budding and it can transform to a mycelial stage or remain single celled; frothy yellow fungus capable of fermenting carbohydrates.

Yellow fever An acute, often fatal infection seen in Africa and South America between latitudes of 15° North and 15° South of the equator, transmitted by mosquito, *Aedes aegypti* and characterized by high fever, vomiting, jaundice and bleeding.

Y fracture A Y-shaped intercondylar fracture.

Yellow spot Y.S. A small circular yellow area on the retina opposite the pupil which is the point of clearest vision; yellow nodule on anterior end of vocal cords.

Yellow vision Xanthopsia, a color vision deficiency in which objects appear yellow in color due to yellowing of optical media of eye.

Yersinia (*yer-sin'i-a*) A genus of non-motile, nonencapsulated ovoid or rod-shaped, bi-polar staining gram-negative bacteria belonging to the family Enterobacteriaceae.

Yersinia enterocolitica Causes febrile enterocolitis or yersiniosis.

Yersinia pestis Causes plague in humans and rodents.

Yersinia pseudotuberculosis A bacterial illness causing acute mesenteric lymphadenitis.

Yolk (deutoplasm) (*yok*) Yellow of the egg; stored nutrient in the ovum entering into the formation of the embryo.

Yolk stalk The umbilical duct connecting yolk sac with the embryo

Yolk sac carcinoma A nonseminomatous germ cell lesion.

Yolk sac (vitelline sac) Membranous sac surrounding yolk in the embryo.

Young's operation (*Yungz*) Partial prostatectomy, described by Baltimore urologist, Hugh Young.

Yuzpe regimen A form of emergency contraception in which two oral contraceptive pills, which contain estrogen and progestin hormones with each dose containing 100 micrograms of ethinyl estradiol and 1.0 mg of norgestril giving a total amount of active progestin of 0.5 mg per dose, are taken to prevent unwanted pregnancy.

Yttrium-90 A radioactive trivalent metallic element used in the treatment of pituitary tumors.

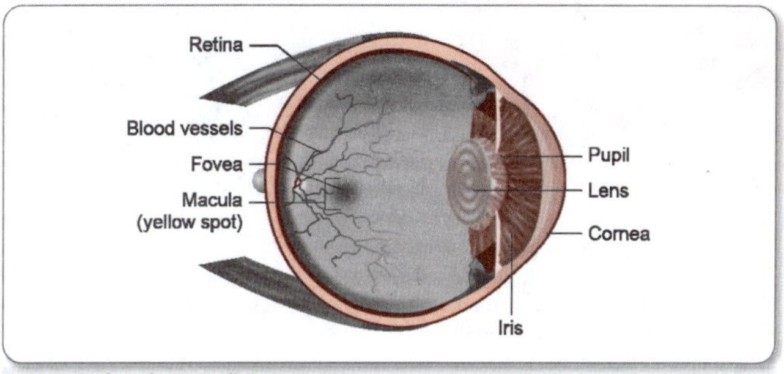

Anatomy of eye showing yellow spot

Z

Zahn infarct A subcapsular, wedge-shaped lesion in the liver characterized by sinusoidal dilatation from obstructed intrahepatic portal veins, named after Friedrich Zahn, a German-born Swiss Pathologist.

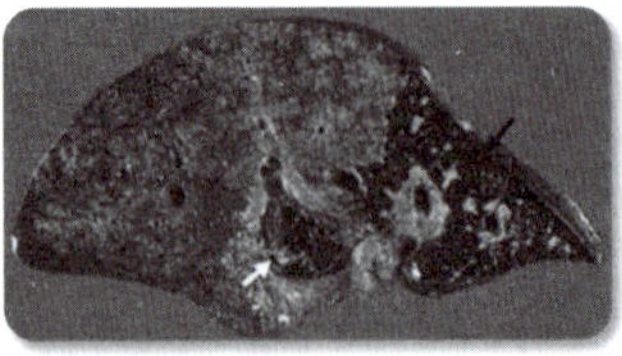

Zahn infarct

Z-band A thin, dark band passing through transversely across the striated muscle fiber.

Zebra body myopathy A congenital, non-progressive myopathy with presence of striped and rod-shaped bodies in muscle fibers, visible on electron microscopy.

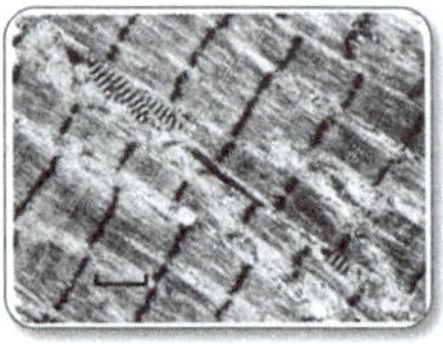

Zebra body myopathy

Zein (*ze'in*) Corn protein.

Zeis's glands (*ze'is*) Sebaceous glands in the lid margin, described by a German ophthalmologist, Eduard Zeis.

Zellweger syndrome Cerebrohepatorenal syndrome, described by Hans Zellweger, US pediatrician.

Zenker's degeneration (*zeng'kerz*) Degeneration of skeletal muscles especially in typhoid, described by Freidrich Zenker, German pathologist; zenkerism.

Zidovudin (*zi-do-vu-den*) A thymidine analogue which inhibits the human immunodeficiency virus reverse transcriptase thereby impairing viral replication; ZDV.

Ziehen's test (*ze'henz*) Test for mental functions requiring description of difference between contrasting objects, such as cat and dog, described by a German neurologist, Gerog Ziehen.

Zinc oxide White odorless, water insoluble powder used as antiseptic and astringent

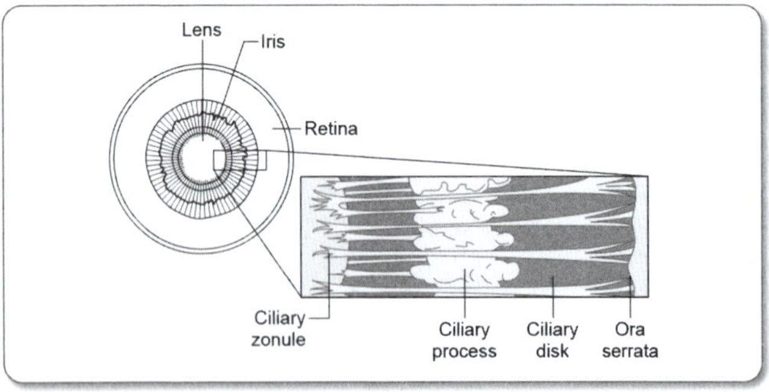

Zonule ciliaris

in the treatment of some skin disorders and also acts as a reflector of sunlight.

Zinc sulphate Colorless crystalline powder used as an astringent and as an emetic.

Zollinger-ellison syndrome (*zol'lin-ger-el'li-son*) Gastrin syndrome; tumors or hyperplasia of the D cells of the islets of the pancreas secreting large amounts of gastrin, stimulate the parietal cells of the stomach to secrete maximal amount of gastric acid resulting in severe peptic ulceration, diarrhea, occasionally with malabsorption.

Zona pellucida A thick transparent non-cellular membranous envelope of the ovum comprises of uniform thickness.

Zonula (*zo'nu-la*) Little zone or area, pl. **zonulae**.

Zonula ciliaris Suspensory ligament of the lens.

Zonula ocludens Intracellular tight junctions that regulate the intestinal epithelial barrier, and its permeability.

Zonule (zonula) (*zo'nu-l*) Tiny thread-like fibers that hold the eye's lens firmly in place; work with the ciliary muscles to help the lens accommodate.

Zonulolysis (*zo-nu-lol'i'sis*) Disintegration of the ciliary zonule by enzymes instilled into the anterior chamber.

Zoo blot A method to detect conservation of DNA sequence during evolution among different species.

Zoonosis (*zo-o-no'sis*) Any infectious or parasitic disease transmissible to man from animals, pl. **zoonoses**; adj. **zoonotic**.

Zoophilism Attraction or love for animals; emotional attachment to animals.

Zoophobia (*zo'o-fo'be-a*) Abnormal fear of animals.

Zoopsia (*zo-op'se-ah*) A hallucination in which the patient thinks he sees animals.

Z-plasty (*ze'plas-te*) A plastic operation for relaxation of scar contractures by Z-shaped incision, and transposition of two triangular flaps in such a way so that their apices cross the line of contracture.

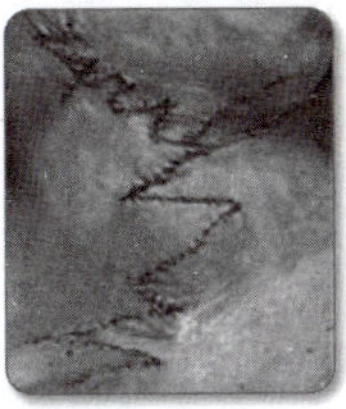

Z-plasty technique

Zoospermia (*zo'o-sper'me-a*) The presence of live spermatozoa in the ejaculated semen.

Zwitterion (*zvit'er-ion*) (*Ger*) An ion having both positive and negative regions of charge; dipolar ion.

Zygoma (*zi-go'ma*) The zygomatic process of the temporal bone fused with zygomatic bone, forming an arch.

Zygomatic arch (zygoma) The bony arch below the orbit of the skull formed by the union of the processes of temporal and zygomatic bone; forming the prominence of the cheek and part of the orbit.

Zygomatic bone (zygoma, molar bone) The bone that forms the prominent part of the cheek and the outer side of the eye socket.

Zygote (*zi'got*) The cell produced by zygosis; adj. **zygotic**.

Zygotene (*zi'go-ten*) Second stage during prophase in meiosis I of cell division during which homologous chromosomes begin to pair.

Zymogen (*zi-mo-jen*) Any substance that may change into an enzyme due to some internal alteration; proenzyme.

Zymolysis (*zi-mo-lie'sis*) Digestive and fermentative action of enzymes.

Zymosis (*zi-mo'sis*) Fermentation; an infectious disease.

Zymotic disease (*zi-mot'ik*) An infectious disease caused by germs introduced into the body from outside which act in a manner similar to fermentation.

ZZ Homozygous phenotype as in a_1- antitrypsin deficiency.

Notes

Notes

Notes

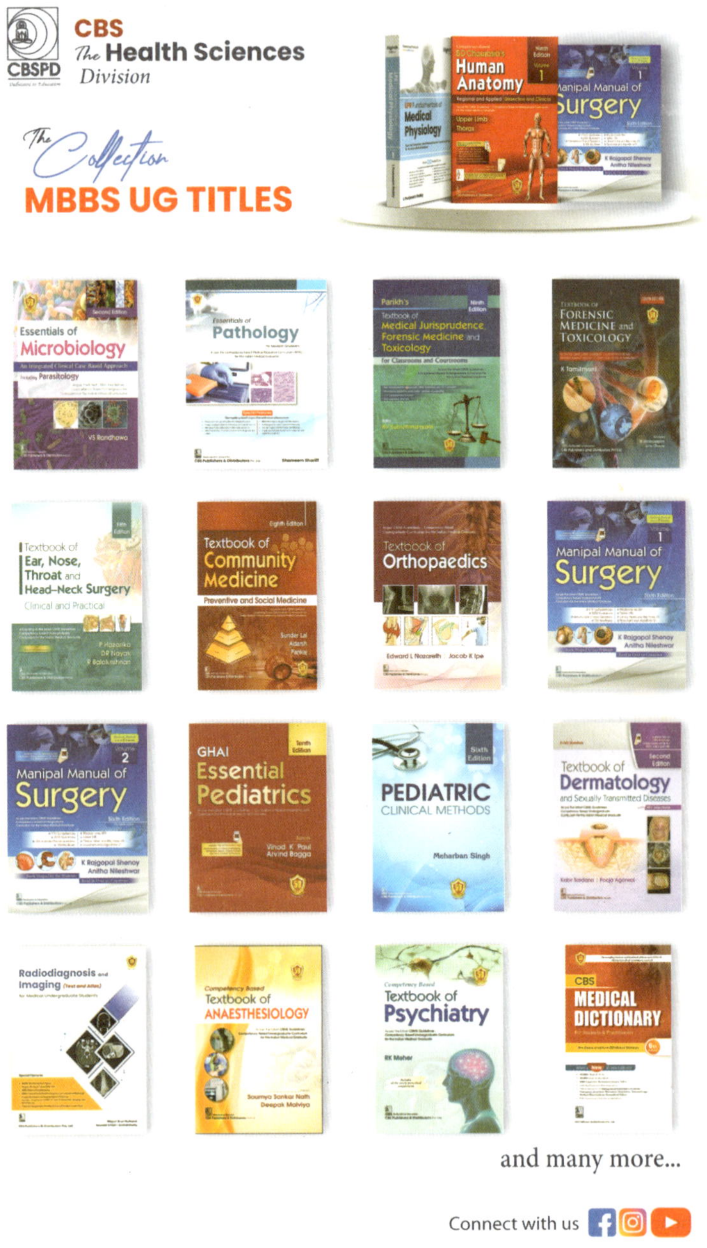
CBS
The Health Sciences
Division
CBSPD
The Collection
MBBS UG TITLES
Human Anatomy
Medical Physiology
Manipal Manual of Surgery
Essentials of Microbiology
Essentials of Pathology
Parikh's Textbook of Medical Jurisprudence, Forensic Medicine and Toxicology
Textbook of Forensic Medicine and Toxicology
Textbook of Ear, Nose, Throat and Head–Neck Surgery
Clinical and Practical
Textbook of Community Medicine
Preventive and Social Medicine
Textbook of Orthopaedics
Manipal Manual of Surgery
GHAI Essential Pediatrics
PEDIATRIC CLINICAL METHODS
Textbook of Dermatology and Sexually Transmitted Diseases
Radiodiagnosis and Imaging
Competency Based Textbook of ANAESTHESIOLOGY
Textbook of Psychiatry
CBS MEDICAL DICTIONARY
and many more...
Connect with us

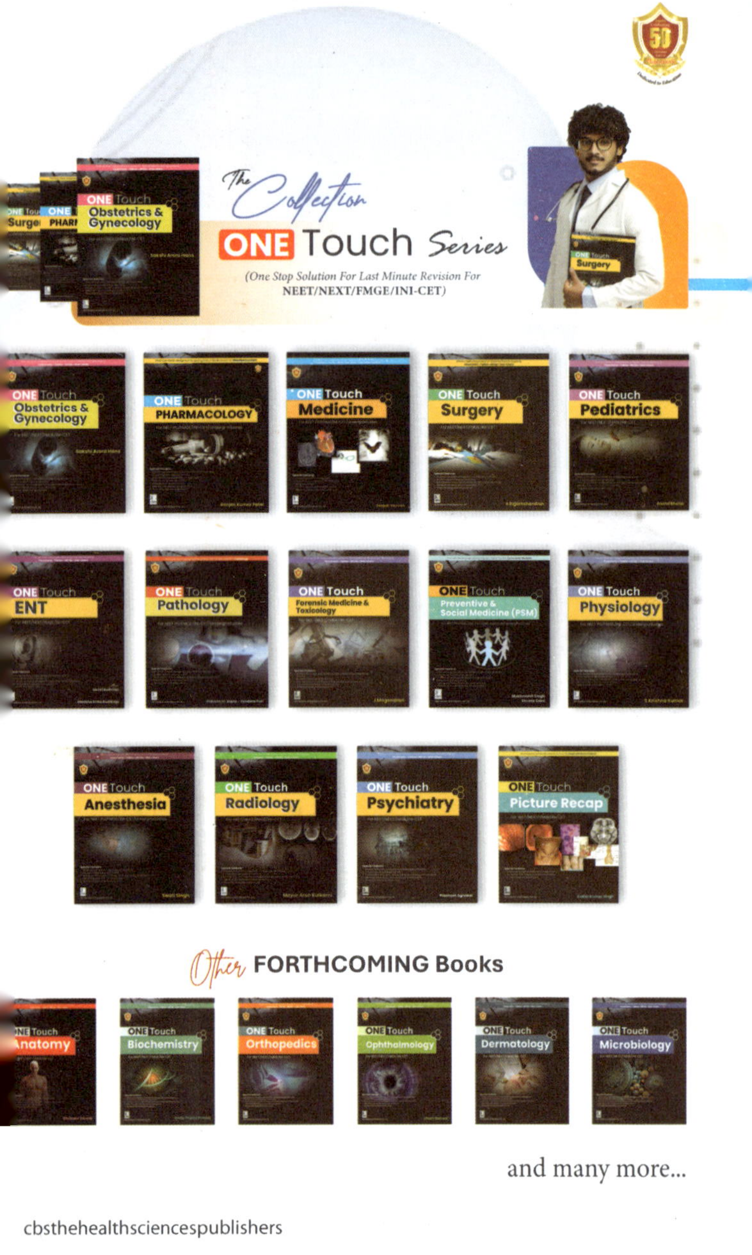
The Collection
ONE Touch Series
(One Stop Solution For Last Minute Revision For
NEET/NEXT/FMGE/INI-CET)
ONE Touch Obstetrics & Gynecology
ONE Touch PHARMACOLOGY
ONE Touch Medicine
ONE Touch Surgery
ONE Touch Pediatrics
ONE Touch ENT
ONE Touch Pathology
ONE Touch Forensic Medicine & Toxicology
ONE Touch Preventive & Social Medicine (PSM)
ONE Touch Physiology
ONE Touch Anesthesia
ONE Touch Radiology
ONE Touch Psychiatry
ONE Touch Picture Recap
Other FORTHCOMING Books
ONE Touch Anatomy
ONE Touch Biochemistry
ONE Touch Orthopedics
ONE Touch Ophthalmology
ONE Touch Dermatology
ONE Touch Microbiology
and many more...
cbsthehealthsciencespublishers